AF358144

XIII° CONGRÈS INTERNATIONAL DE MÉDECINE. PARIS 1900

SECTION DE MÉDECINE DE L'ENFANCE

SECTION DE CHIRURGIE DE L'ENFANCE

Les Comptes rendus des Travaux des Sections du XIIIe Congrès international de Médecine sont publiés en 17 volumes ainsi répartis :

1. Anatomie descriptive et comparée. — Histologie et Embryologie. — Physiologie. Physique et Chimie biologiques.
2. Pathologie générale. Pathologie expérimentale.
3. Anatomie pathologique. — Bactériologie. Parasitologie.
4. Pathologie interne.
5. Médecine de l'enfance. — Chirurgie de l'enfance.
6. Thérapeutique. Pharmacologie. Matière médicale.
7. Neurologie.
8. Psychiatrie.
9. Dermatologie et Syphiligraphie.
10. Chirurgie générale.
11. Chirurgie urinaire.
12. Ophtalmologie.
13. Laryngologie. Rhinologie. — Otologie.
14. Stomatologie.
15. Obstétrique. — Gynécologie.
16. Médecine légale.
17. Médecine et chirurgie militaires : Sous-sections de Chirurgie, d'Épidémiologie et Hygiène, de Médecine navale, de Médecine coloniale.

Chaque volume est vendu séparément 5 fr. — On peut souscrire pour l'ensemble des 17 volumes au prix de 50 fr.

*Chaque congressiste reçoit gratuitement **le volume de la section à laquelle il a été inscrit. Il peut se procurer les volumes des autres sections au prix de 4 fr. et souscrire à l'ensemble au prix de 45 fr.***

14157. — Imprimerie Lahure, 9, rue de Fleurus, à Paris.

XIIIᵉ CONGRÈS INTERNATIONAL DE MÉDECINE. PARIS 1900

COMPTES RENDUS

Publiés sous la direction de **A. CHAUFFARD**. Secrétaire général

SECTION

DE

Médecine de l'Enfance

COMPTES RENDUS PUBLIÉS PAR

M. MARFAN

Secrétaire de la Section

SECTION

DE

Chirurgie de l'Enfance

COMPTES RENDUS PUBLIÉS PAR

MM. VILLEMIN et BROCA

Secrétaires de la Section

PARIS

MASSON ET Cⁱᵉ, ÉDITEURS

LIBRAIRES DE L'ACADÉMIE DE MÉDECINE

120, BOULEVARD SAINT-GERMAIN

SECTION DE MÉDECINE DE L'ENFANCE

COMPTES RENDUS

publiés par M. MARFAN

Secrétaire de la Section.

MÉDECINE DE L'ENFANCE

COMITÉ D'ORGANISATION DE LA SECTION

Président d'honneur : M. BERGERON.

Président : M. GRANCHER.

Vice-Présidents : MM. SEVESTRE et HUTINEL.

Secrétaire : M. MARFAN.

Secrétaire adjoint : M. L. GUINON.

Membres : MM. D'HEILLY, HUTINEL, MOIZARD, COMBY, JOSIAS, NETTER, VARIOT, RICHARDIÈRE (Paris); BAUMEL (Montpellier); MOUSSOUS (Bordeaux); WEILL (Lyon); BÉZY (Toulouse); HAUSHALTER (Nancy); AUSSET (Lille).

La section de Médecine de l'Enfance a commencé ses travaux le vendredi 2 août, à 9 heures du matin. Après une allocution de M. le professeur GRANCHER, président, elle a procédé à la nomination des présidents d'honneur et des vice-présidents.

Ont été nommés :

Présidents d'honneur : ALVAREZ (Madrid), BAGINSKY (Berlin), BOKAY (Buda-Pest), COMBE (Lausanne), CONCETTI (Rome), DELL' ARCA (Buenos-Ayres), D'ESPINE (Genève), ESCHERICH (Gratz), FILATOW (Moscou), HEUBNER (Berlin), JACOBI (New York), JABLOKOFF (Saint-Pétersbourg), JOHANNESSEN (Christiania), MAC MILLAN (Édimbourg), Martinez VARGAS (Barcelone), MONTI (Vienne), SEITZ (Munich), THOMESCO (Bucarest), VIOLI (Constantinople).

Vice-Présidents : AUSSET (Lille), BAUMEL (Montpellier), BÉZY (Toulouse), DELMAS (Bordeaux), HAUSHALTER (Nancy), MOUSSOUS (Bordeaux), SAINT-PHILIPPE (Bordeaux), WEILL (Lyon).

La section de Médecine de l'Enfance a tenu dix séances, à la Sorbonne (amphithéâtre Turgot).

Quatre questions avaient été choisies par le Comité pour être l'objet de rapports : 1° *De l'allaitement artificiel et en particulier de l'emploi du lait stérilisé.* Rapporteurs : MM. JACOBI (New-York), HEUBNER (Berlin), JOHANNESSEN (Christiania), MONTI (Vienne), VARIOT (Paris). — 2° *Infections et intoxications gastro-intestinales chez l'enfant du premier âge.* Rapporteurs : MM. BAGINSKY (Berlin), ESCHERICH (Gratz), F. FEDE (Naples), Martinez VARGAS (Barcelone), MARFAN (Paris). — 3° *Tuberculose infantile.* Rapporteurs : M. D'ESPINE (Genève), HUTINEL (Paris), RICHARDIÈRE (Paris), MOUSSOUS (Bordeaux). — 4° *Méningites aiguës non tuberculeuses.* Rapporteurs : MM. MYA (Florence), CONCETTI (Rome), NETTER (Paris).

En outre, le Comité avait spécialement attiré l'attention sur les questions suivantes : *Sérumthérapie antidiphtérique; Rhumatisme infantile et*

*ses rapports avec les affections du cœur et la chorée; Alcoolisme des enfants;
Constipation; Maladies du thymus.*

Enfin de nombreuses communications ont été faites sur des sujets
divers.

Dans le compte rendu de ces travaux, nous n'avons pas suivi l'ordre
dans lequel les rapports et communications ont été faits dans les séances:
il nous a paru préférable de grouper ensemble toutes celles qui se rapportent au même sujet.

Les comptes rendus des discussions ont été faits par MM. les Dʳˢ Saint-
Céne, Léon Bernard, Guillemot, Thiercelin, Critzmann et Froin.

La séance de clôture a eu lieu dans la matinée du jeudi 9 août. Elle
s'est terminée par une allocution de M. le professeur Grancher, président. Nous la reproduisons à la fin de ces comptes rendus.

I

ALLAITEMENT: ALIMENTATION ET HYGIÈNE
DES ENFANTS

I. — Rapports sur l'allaitement artificiel
et en particulier sur l'emploi du lait stérilisé.

ARTIFICIAL ALIMENTATION

RAPPORT

By prof A. JACOBI. MD. LLD.,

of New-York

When, 25 years ago I wrote on Infant Hygiene in the first volume
of *Gerhardt's Handbuch der Kinderkrankheiten*, I quoted 500 books
and essays published on that subject. To-day there are probably
5000. The majority of them are journal articles or small pamphlets
containing the results of individual researches on the chemical composition of woman's and of cow's milk, or of one or more of its constituents. They are generally accompanied by more or less dictatorial
precepts referring to artificial feeding of the infant: these precepts do not, in their majority, claim to be founded on experience,
but only that they are scientific, and that for that reason the
healthy baby is bound to thrive, and the sick baby to recover, on them,

and to kindly overlook the fact that chemistry is after all not physiology, and a living infant's stomach no test tube.

Other books or pamphlets are written to order, in the service and in the interest of manufacturers of proprietary foods. It is to be regretted that honest laboratory workers and clinicians should be found willing to spend their time and efforts on these products, and that medical journals pay them earnest attention.

Some of these prescriptions are followed by a desert of priority claims, replies and counterreplies, so that those of us who work in the nursery and hospital and sickchamber are not always fire-proof against suspecting that class of soi-disant scientific productions which exhibit a caviling spirit characteristic of ambitious mediocrity. There is no Malthus yet to strangle literary progeny when in its embryonal stage. That is a pity. I share the regret I believe I saw expressed lately that there is the same possibility of harm done by indiscriminate literary production that may be attended by universal suffrage, and the further regret that hygiene and medicine appear to be relegated by some of us to the dead walls of a laboratory only.

As far as I am concerned, I shall at once declare my point of view. Science of man is not tied down to chemical and mathematical formulae, or to a microscopical observation and a stained bacterium, with all their accurate or inaccurate results: it lives also in exact observations of facts connected with the living organism, particularly when they are repeated a hundred and a thousand fold.

To give a report of everything that has been done for infant hygiene, and for the subject of sterilization as a part of it during the last dozen years or more I considered absolutely superfluous after studying the most modern literature, and particularly three books, those of Monti, of Marfan, and the new edition of Biedert which are both compendious and comprehensive. What I shall say therefore, is either critical, or the result of my experience, based upon careful observation and honest sympathy with the living and dying infant. If in the main some of it agrees with what after a practical experience of twenty years I wrote twenty five years ago, the accumulated evidence should encourage and direct further observations. My plea may not always agree with accepted theories or some of the existing analyses; it frequently happens that theories had to be modified after the facts were established.

Substitutes of mother's milk were made in accordance with the results of chemical analyses of woman's and of cow's milk. What is mother's milk? Is that known, or is the milk of one mother, or of many mothers, identical? How is it that a baby will thrive on the milk of one woman and not on that of the other? The mildest way in which Monti puts the results of what we know is this : that the constituents of woman's milk are « *more or less* constant », and it is « *only some* that vary ». But the facts are worse. The analyses of woman's milk are contradictory, not two are alike. The percentages of albumin vary least, those of sugar and fat considerably. A woman's milk will change during every minute's nursing, from morning to night, is changed by food, state of health, menstruation, lactation, and *still the baby thrives.*

Thus there is no sameness in human milk and no possibility of arranging a perfect and uniform substitute for every kind of it.

The differences between the casein of woman's and of cow's milk have been studied extensively, since Hammarsten, 50 years ago, but to this moment it is not clear, whether the albuminoid which is found (more in the woman than in the cow) besides casein, is coordinate to it, or a derivatum.

According to E. Pfeiffer casein is the only albuminoid in milk. Whatever else is found, is a product of disintegration; there are no other nitrogenous materials (« extractive substances »), but it is admitted that nitrogen varies considerably in amount.

On the other hand in Immanuel Munk's opinion (*Virch. Arch.*, Vol. 154) nitrogen plays a different role altogether. In his researches referring to the question how much nitrogen there is in albumin and how much in extractive substances, he comes to the following conclusions : Total nitrogenous substances in cow's milk 15,7 p. c., in woman's milk 15,76. Of this total sum there is in extractive materials in cow's milk 6(4,8-8,6) p. c., in woman's 8,7 p. c. In his calculations the albuminoids in woman's milk amount to 1,19-1,57 p. c., while it is only calcium and phosphorus that is found in twice the quantity in the latter. There is more syntonin in cow's milk casein, and more lime (6.6 p. c. compared with 5.2 p. c. in woman's milk, Leymann) more phosphorus in woman's (0,84) than in cow's milk (0,68), less sulphur in woman's milk (0.74) than in cow's milk (1.11). In « Lab » ferment the casein of cow's milk coagulates in coarser lumps than woman's milk : *they are modified by the introduction of milk-sugar, of fat, of chloride of sodium, and of dextrinized or other flours*[1].

---

1. Beside the chemical, there are probably many physical differences; for according to Michael Cohn (*Berl. Med. Gesellschaft*, of May 16th 1900) not even the elements of woman's milk are of a uniform construction. On its corpuscles there are spherical bodies (first noticed by Heidenhayn) in which there are con-

The casein of woman's milk is not so easily thrown out by acids or salts as that of cow's milk, and is more readily dissolved in an excess of acid. Wroblewski demonstrated that woman's casein retains, during pepsin digestion, its nuclein in solution. *This* proteid with its ample supply of phosphorus is fully digested: artificial gastric juice, however, does not fully digest the nuclein of *cow's* casein, of which a « paranuclein » is deposited undigested and undissolved. Besides, these are those according to whom woman's casein contains an additional albuminoid which is not identical with either the known casein or albumin (Koplik, *N. Y. Med Jour.*, April 15th 1895).

According to Schlossmann, of the albuminoids in woman's milk 65 per cent. are casein, 57 per cent. lacto-albumin, the latter of which is absorbed directly. There is moreover, according to Wroblewski, in the human milk another proteid rich in sulphur, poor in carbonhydrate: and according to some, albumoses and peptones, that also would be directly absorbable.

Of nucleon (V. Wittmaack and M. Siegfried, *Zeitsch. f. phys. Chem.*, XXII) there is contained in cow's milk 0.057, in goat's milk 0,110, and in woman's 0,124 per c. In cow's milk the phosphorus of the nucleon amounts to 6 p. c. of the total amount of phosphorus contained in the milk; in woman's milk 41,5 p. c. That means that in cow's milk not one half of its phosphorus is in the organic combinations of casein and nucleon; in woman's milk almost all of it. In cow's milk the phosphorus not utilized for organic combinations is contained in the inferior phosphates. That explains why good cow's milk with its anorganic phosphates may give a baby rachitis, while *good* breast milk does not at all (*Kassowitz's statement (see below) notwithstanding*[1].)

There are some modern observations which seem to prove conclusively that the caseins of different milks cannot be equal, any more than the blood corpuscles of different animals. Bordet discovered the fact that the fluids of cells, and tissues, and the blood sera of animals become influenced by the substances with which the latter are treated. Subsequently Wassermann, aided by A. Schülze (*Proceedings of the Society for internal medicine of Berlin*, meeting of July 2 nd. 1900) injected 10 cmc. of sterilized milk under the skin of rabbits daily a fortnight in succession. After that time their blood

---

tained fat globules and sometimes an epithelial nucleus. They are always present, and many a milk exhibits a great many of them, but its digestibility does not suffer from that fact.

1. We should not forget that improper food is not the only, probably not even the most important cause of rickets.

serum acquired the property of coagulating cow's milk. that is its proteid. Similarly other animals were treated with goat's and others with woman's milk, with the result that their blood sera would eliminate the albuminate either of goat's milk or of human milk, respectively. In every case this specific coagulating effect was observed in that kind of milk only with which the animal was previously treated.

It has often struck me as an incongruity when I observed how eagerly. almost fanatically. for important purposes it is true. the slightest differences were studied in the organic composition — with little result only — and no attention was paid to the mineral constituents of milks. It is particularly phosphorus. potassium. sodium, iron and calcium that should be looked after. Cow's milk contains twice as much phosphorus as woman's milk, *but* in anorganic combinations. Iron is held in both milks in about equal amounts, much less however than in cereals. and still much less than in fruit, vegetables, meat and the yellow of egg. Potassium is represented in a somewhat larger quantity in the milk of herbivores. In 1000 parts of desiccated woman's milk potassium is found to be 5-6, sodium 1-2. in desiccated cow's milk. potassium 9-17. sodium 1-10 p. c. Thus it appears that when cow's milk is substituted for woman's milk, some chloride of sodium should be added (when cereals are added, the percentage of the sodium salt should be much higher). the more so as solid coagulation by rennet is prevented by the sodium chlorid. This is the rule I have always obeyed and taught. It gratifies me to notice that in the person of Tweifel. in his new book on Rachitis, 1900, a well known authority rises in favor of full amounts of chloride of sodium. He contends that rachitis is due, besides an insufficient amount of soluble and absorbable lime salts, to the *low percentage of chlorid of sodium*, which F. Pfeiffer found to be less than one tenth of one (0,1) p. c. in the milk of women whose children were rachitical. Tweifel tells us that one half of the working women of Saxony nurse their children, but that the bread they can buy, is not salted. In regard to the quantity of the tablesalt to be added to the food of infants he is not over particular. He adds a thimble full (5 grams) to 500 cubic centimetres of food which consists of equal parts of milk and a 6 1 2 p. c. solution of milksugar.

Calcium is represented in 1000 parts of (desiccated) woman's milk with 0.245. in cow's milk. 1.51 p. c. The latter figure is certainly high. Bunge from whom I quote these figures adds that as organic substances act as sources of organic force by decomposition, or transmutation, and as salts are either saturated with oxygen or are chlorids and need no more oxygen. there is surely a disproportion between cow's milk and the organic want of the nursling. Now do I believe that therefore cow's milk should be taken in hand and strained and decomposed and modified to get the surplus calcium out? By no means. If we have to rely on cow's milk. and cannot have breastmilk under our imperfect social and sanitary conditions, why! let us be grateful that nature is not so cruel as she is believed to be and permits of a good deal of generous latitude in the feeding of babies. a great deal more than our laboratory tyrants.

Is it true that iron-clad rules as to the composition of a substitute are to the point or justified? Everybody knows that all these questions are not answered, but fifty substitutes are based upon fifty contradictory and uncertain chemical analyses.

In my opinion only one great progress has been made in infant feeding these dozens of years, viz : the more or less universal introduction of heating cow's milk and all other substances employed in infant feeding.

Sterilization, pasteurization, and tyndallisation are different methods of heating cow's milk to preserve it or to prepare it for its use as infant food. As long as sterile milk cannot be had with the usual dairy habits, as long as it takes a long time to get the milk from the producer to the consumer, as long as tuberculosis may be transmitted, at least now and then, by the milk of a tuberculous cow, or. what is more frequent, as long as scarlet fever and diphteria are met with in the houses and about the clothing and on the hands of dairy men and women, and as long as typhoid germs are contained in the water used for washing utensils, or for adulterating the original article. some such method cannot be dispensed with.

A very few figures will demonstrate the dangers. E. Cantley (26th *Ann. Rep. of the Local Gov.* Board Suppl., p. 245), when discussing the thriving of typhoid bacilli in milk, reports he found in 1 cmc. in January 142 800, in July 8 119 200. Of indiscriminate bacteria Bunge found in 1 cmc. of fresh milk 9000. after 1 hour 51750. after 9 hours 120 000. after 24 hours 5 600 000, and remarks that a brief sterilization did not destroy all of them. P. Ignard (Thèse de Paris, 1899) reports that in unsterilized milk living cholera bacilli were found after 6 days. typhoid after 35, and tubercle bacilli after 10 days. in butter respectively 52. 21 and 50 days.

How unexpectedly great the dangers may be from what is generally called fresh milk, is shown by Leslie Eastes (*Ann. de Méd. et de Chir. Inf.*, 1900, p. 126). He examined 186 specimens of milks furnished by healthboards and farmers from all parts of England. He found tubercle bacilli in 11, pus in 47, muco-pus in 77, blood in 24, streptococci in 106, and colostrum corpuscles in 16, surely a bad showing.

If that were the rule the suggestion that only summer, milk, and milk consumed in large cities should be pasteurized and sterilized, and that this process was superfluous in the country, and in winter, would not be in accordance with the dangers thus exhibited. But such conditions are exceptional, and in most cases local. Fresh and good milk is not expected to hold more than 10000 bacteria, which must not be pathogenous. Still, Rabinowitsch and Kempner (*Z. f. Hyg. u. Inf. Krkh.*, XXXI. p. 157), collating the results obtained by various observers, found tubercle bacilli in from 44 to 61 p. c. of all the specimens of market milk, though tuberculosis of the cows was incipient only and the udders not diseased; and Max Beck (*Viertely. f. öff. Ges.*, XXXII. 1900, p. 445) reports the occurrence of pathogenous bacteria in 80 p. c. of all the specimens of milk sold in Berlin, streptococci in 62, and tubercle bacilli in 50 p. c.

What is the object of heating to 100° or less or more, and its effect? Besides expelling air, it destroys the germ of typhoid fever, Asiatic cholera, diphteria and tuberculosis, and staphylo and streptococcus, also the bacillus aërogenes and the numerous other germs which transform milk sugar into lactic acid, and those which increase the virulence of the intestinal saprophytes mostly belonging to the proteus and coli order. By so doing it prevents numerous cases of gastro-enteritis, nephritis and degeneration of the liver and pancreas, of pneumonia and otitis, all of which we see in connection with intestinal disorders, mostly or perhaps always without the intervention of the blood current, in which bacilli are rarely found.

There are exceptions to this universal efficacy. Heins found cholera bacilli in sterilized milk after 4 weeks, typhoid after 4 months, and according to D' Lydia Rabinowitsch (*D. Med. Woch.*, 1900, p. 490, No 50) experiments made in the Institute for Infectious Diseases in Berlin appear to prove that occasionally tubercle bacilli are not killed by less than 100°. Organisms surrounded by fat seem to require more than the average heat to be destroyed; in accordance with the finding of Ignard whom I just quoted, which appear to prove that butter unsterilized would preserve cholera and tubercle bacilli much longer than unsterilized milk. If that be beyond doubt, butter and rich milk would retain their infesting qualities longer then average milk with a moderate percentage of fat.

Still, while all this is true in exceptional cases, the main object of destroying microbes by heat is accomplished as a rule.

This wonderful effect is generally obtained even below the boiling point. Tubercle bacilli (Hueppe) and the other germs named died at 80° C. in 10 minutes, at 68° in 30 minutes, with occasional exceptions. For the purposes of infant feeding it is of the greatest import that the lactic acid fermentation should be prevented or interrupted. This can be accomplished when from 2 to 5 hours only in summer, and from 6 to 8 hours in winter are consumed between milking and heating. More time should not elapse, for Russel and Farrington found that milk containing as little as 1/5 100 of 1 per cent of lactic acid was too sour for efficient pasteurization. I imagine therefore that when Koplik protested against gastro-enteritis, and insisted upon sterilization as a general rule he was carried to that extreme opinion by the fact that his milk cannot possibly reach him in New York City within 2 or 3 hours after milking. There is, however, no complete effect obtained by mere pasteurization because in it the lactic acid germs are not all destroyed. It is good, however, that should be so, for their presence is a restraint to the unchecked growth of more dangerous bacilli.

The taste of milk begins to change at 75° C. (Duclaux), the milk albumin is altered at about 65-70°, according to some at 60°. Dairymen ascertained that fact from their experience in cheesemaking. Jemma found that pepsin hydrochloric acid digests milk sterilized at 100° C. more slowly than it does raw milk. During sterilization lime salts are thrown out, phosphorus combinations are disintegrated, nitrogenous substances are liable to be decomposed into tyrosin, peptotoxin and ammonium, lecithin is destroyed, fat changed both chemically and physically. During a long continued sterilization casein and nucleon are likely to undergo marked changes, and the sugar is found at the bottom as a brown deposit. That is mainly so when excessively high temperatures are employed, for instance 110° (by wholesale sterilizers), " surchauffage ", which causes the production of peptone by the action of chlorine or casein, or 100-105° in steam-heat. Even these high temperatures do not accomplish actual and complete sterilization in all cases. Chemical toxins are not changed by them even by greater heat, and spores are very obstinate ; such as those of bacterium subtile for instance, and tyrothrix ; which resist the usual methods.

Tyndallisation is called the process of daily boiling. The first day the microbes are killed; when spores grow out, they are killed the next day. Three such daily boilings sterilized in Soxhlet's observation absolutely. Dahl exposed milk five times to a temperature of 100° 1/2 hour. That is similar to what I have practiced and advised the people both rich and poor, these nearly forty years. In my Intestinal Diseases of Infancy and Childhood, 1887, p. 18, I have the following : " After boiling, milk destined for the use of a baby during the day should be kept in clean bottles containing from 5 to 6 ounces (90.0-180.0), filled up to the cork, and the bottles then turned upside down in a cold place ; such will keep longer than milk preserved in the usual way. Before being used it should be heated in a water-bath ; and by repeating this heating of the whole amount of the day's milk several times during the twenty four hours, fermentation will be retarded and digestibility improved. " The same teaching is found in my contributions to *Gerhardt's Handb. d. Kinderk.*, Vol. I, 1876, second ed. 1882, and to *Bruck's Hygiene.* Such advice, taught by me these forty years, had its local effect, I am certain. It took however the initiative of Soxhlet whose immortal merit it is to have systematized and popularized the necessity of boiling and thereby sterilizing milk in single portions for use of infants.

Should milk be pasteurized or sterilized at home, or should it be procured from a manufacturer who keeps a stock on hand? These latter wares can never be guaranteed, and when they are dangerous, no taste or odor need betray them. Obstinate spores that were not destroyed during sterilization, will grow out, and most easily when, as is always the case in such preparations, the milder and undangerous bacteria have all perished. Thus occasional dangers and deaths will occur, and the lesson to be derived from these occurrences is that domestic daily sterilization for 10 minutes, or pasteurization twice that time, of fresh pure milk, obtained as soon as possible after milking, is far preferable to the wholesale manufacturing of a marketable stock, which now and then is kept and sold, not to betray its secrets, in intransparent bottles.

It is just such milk as has been kept for sale, in which the cream will permanently separate from the milk. This process begins during the first week, and in later cases (Ann. d. Gaz. XVI.) found 45.5 p. c. of all the cream in that condition.

According to A. Weber (*Arb. ausd. Kaiserl. Ges Amt.*, XVII. 1900, p. 108) the present wholesale procedures of sterilizing milk cannot furnish milk that is absolutely free from germs. The nearer the milk he investigated approached absolute sterilization, the more readily could the gross changes occasioned by sterilizing be noticed.

He found Flügge's " poisonous peptonizing bacteria " three times in one hundred and fifty specimens of commercial sterilized milk.

They were " hay bacilli " which cause a strong decomposition of albumin and copious development of sulphide of hydrogen. It is particularly this rapid putrefaction which proves dangerous to the nursling.

While in sterilized milk the anaerobicmicrobes are not numerous nor important, according to the same author, the aërobic kinds are able to peptonize milk in from one to two days (some species in from five to seven), and to cause putrefaction and produce sulphid of hydrogen. Raw milk is indeed protected by its milk sugar, which by being transformed into lactic acid destroys the effect of peptonizing bacteria: in sterilized milk the latter are apt to predominate.

Consequently, domestic daily sterilization (or pasteurization) is to be preferred to wholesale production. That is why even Henri de Rothschild's advice is not unobjectionable. He attributes all the failures of sterizilation to its erroneous methods only; he advises not to use the wholesale product when it is more than 8 to 10 days old, and only in flasks of from 50 to 150 cmc., and prefers daily home sterilization of 45 minutes each. Even in this, as we shall see, there are mistakes.

The destruction of microbes by heat forms such a progress over all previous methods of employing milk, that its disadvantages are too apt to be overlooked. In some cases heat is insufficient in its effects, obstinate bacteria not being destroyed, in other instances its excessive effect proves dangerous by destroying milk elements. While appreciating the latter danger which is due to prolonged heating mostly, we should never forget however, that the advantages of heating derived from the destruction of microbes, either directly pathogenous, or indirectly so by increasing the virulence of saprophytes, are incalculable. But with every degree beyond pasteurization the disintegration of the milk becomes more marked: therefore it appears that from 65 to 68 degrees should be employed, though it may be found wiser to extend the process over a longer time.

The lower the degree of heat which may be expected to destroy lactic acid or pathogenous microbes, the more easily the integrity of milk in preserved. Now, Theobald Smith found (*Jour. Exper. Med.*, 1899, vol. IV, n° 2) that in distilled water, in physiological solutions of sodium chloride, in beefbroth, or in milk, *when heated to 60° C. (140° F.)*, tubercle bacilli die mostly in from 5 to 10, all of them in

from 15 to 20 minutes. The membrane however which is formed o
milk even at 60° C., keeps tubercle bacilli alive even after 60 minutes;
that is why its formation should be prevented by stirring, or it should
be removed[1].

This low temperature preserves also the taste of milk and is a very
borderline only of the temperature that coagulates lactalbumin. The
confirmation of these observations made by one of the most reliable
experimenters will not be wanting; then nothing will be required
except a cheap and handy apparatus to prevent milk from getting
warmed beyond 60°, thus preserving the freshness of milk and reduc-
ing or removing its dangers.

One of the latter is scurvy which is a frequent occurrence after
feeding with sterilized milk. In an address delivered in one of the
general Assemblies of the Eleventh International Congress in 1894
(" Non nocere ", *Transac. of 11th. Intern. Cong.* and *N. Y. Med.
Record*. May 19. 1894) I could make the statement that some of my
cases of infantile scurvy were those in which the patients had been
on an *exclusive* diet of sterilized milk. I have seen many of the same
kind since. They were not the first however that had been observed, and since that time their number has increased. In n° 8 of the
Semaine Médicale of 1899. Netter publishes a similar one and gives a
rich literature. Of the 379 cases of scurvy collected by the American
Pediatric Society. 107 occurred in infants brought up on sterilized
milk without or with some addition. Of 67 cases collected by Von
Starck (*Deutsche Med. Woch.* octobre 15th, 1898) 14 were brought
up according to Soxhlet. 2 Gaertner. 2 Biedert. Of 48 German cases
collected by Von Stare. 15 were attributed to sterilized milk. As
early as 1895 (*Medecine Med. Woch.*, n° 42. 1895). he complained of
the occurrence of Barlow's disease since in Holstein milk sterilized
by manufactories had been introduced. It would be a mistake however to believe that it is such sterilized milk only as has been kept for
some time, that causes scurvy. Every one of my cases was of domestic daily make. Indeed I do not know that manufacturer's sterilized
milk, the " Dauermilch " of the Germans is used at all in my part of
the world. To imply however that I believe sterilized milk to be
the, the only cause, of scurvy would be a mistake. Referring to a

1. W. Hesse (*Z. f. Hyg. u. Inf. Krkh.*. XXXIV. 1900, p. 546) states 60° C. suffice
to destroy the microbes of typhoid fever. Asiatic cholera. diphteria. plague. bac.
coli communis, staph. erysipelatos. pyog. aureus and albus. bac. cholerae
suum. bac. rhusiopathiæ suum. b. septicaemiæ haemorrhagica. and b. muri-
septicaemiæ.

case of Fruitnight's which occurred in a baby fed at the mother's breast. Marfan (*L'Allaitement*, p. 512), denies the connection between scurvy and sterilized milk and adds that whenever it apparently existed, it was overfeeding which caused the disease. But it is a fact that scurvy is frequent now, and was quite rare many years ago, before and after the first cases of Moeller's. If I were to count all the cases of "acute rickets" and "acute purpura" observed by me during the first 25 years of my active life and call them scurvy, they would not reach the number of genuine cases I meet now within a single year. There *always was* overfeeding, but little scurvy.

Though there be a reason to consider *sterilized* milk to be *the* cause of scurvy, it is *one* of the causes. In the American Pediatric Society's 379 cases 20 were fed on *pasteurized*, and 14 on peptonized milk; 129 on proprietary foods; 10 cases were developed at the breast, 5 on raw milk, and 2 on a mixture of breast milk and artificial food. Some of my cases were fed on pasteurized milk. Three such were communicated to me by Dr. L. Emmet Holt; he makes the statement that daily pasteurization lasted 20 minutes in one case, 45 minutes in each of the others. This close observer declares himself to be opposed to pasteurization as a routine practice. The *long duration* of either sterilization or pasteurization appears to have a good deal of bad influence. The worst of my cases were those in which the parents proudly stated the routine time of sterilization to have been 40 minutes or one hour.

While being so positive in my convictions, it is but just to say that many of my cases were not in connection with sterilized milk as exclusive food. In some cases it was mixed with water, in one case with oatmealwater (2 : 1), in many the feeding was wavering and unsystematical. A child of 2 months had been at the breast ½ month, on condensed milk and water 5 weeks, on sterilized milk and barley water 4 weeks, on barley water and egg albumin 2 weeks, on malted milk 2 months, on sterilized milk and barley water since; one had been fed on sterilized milk and oatmealwater, on unstrained thick gruel and a daily dose of meat juice. One bad case, a year old, had been fed on carefully pasteurized milk, prepared daily by a beneficent layman for nine months, and three more months on a mixture of the same milk with barley water, prepared in the same institution. Denekamp's case, quoted by Netter, in which a scurvy child, that had been fed on buttermilk, was cured by raw milk, belongs to that class and may well be quoted to support A. Caillé's opinion, that scurvy is a ptomaine poisoning, caused by every improper food employed too long. Again however the question arises in our minds, why it is, that formerly. though babies were overfed[1] and improperly and badly fed all the time. scurvy was rare amongst the very poor and the very rich. and that it has become frequent in those classes, which can afford to spend much time on destructive sterilization of milk and much money on proprietary foods.

One of the most systematic attempts at finding a substitute for mother's milk partly by means of sterilization has been made by Prof. T. M. Rotch of Harvard University. He calls his process "modification of milk". the preparation "modified milk". The milk to be prepared must come from a large dairy, in as much as most infections come from small ones: that is a demand experience, taught me also these forty years. The usual precautions are ordered in securing transporting and cooling it. In the laboratory it is "separated " by a centrifuge. having 6800 revolutions every minute, more than 110 every second. The cream thus obtained is mixed with the proteïd, with milksugar. with water. a little lime water, everything in fixed proportion and sterilized in separate bottles. each containing the amount destined for a meal. The newly born is given much less than one. less than $\frac{1}{2}$ p. c. of proteïd. and the intention is to increase or to diminish now this. now the other ingredient, until the exact mixture is found, which suits the baby. In opposition to his former views, which then were very categoric. he frequently selects at present decoctions of barley or oatmeal in place of water as part of the mixture. Here are his axioms :

"Try until you find the exact proportion." The principal object is to be able to write "500 different prescriptions". In his enthusiasm for exactness he went so far as to say. that not so much on especial food was wanted as the principle of prescribing exactly. By prescribing once or more times he feels certain. he finds a substitute for mother's milk. Which mother's milk? we ask. Let me select *only one*. Johannessen and Wang (*Zeitschr. f. Phys. Chem..* Vol. XXIV) found in breastmilk the following differences : albumin 0,9-1.5 p. c.,

---

1 Overfeeding. like hasty feeding. is mainly seen during artificial alimentation: the latter is not frequent at the breast. for to fill himself with the contents of a mamma. takes time and labor and generally fatigues the little gourmand. Bad results of overfeeding are frequent. not so many acute deaths, as chronic disorders. Adiposity. pallor. lymphatism. eczema. tetany. furunculosis, polyuria. large defecations. large bellies. constipation or diarrhoea. vomiting and tympanites. These are frequent occurrences : though I am not prepared to follow Schlossmann (*Jahrb. f. Kinderh. N. F.* vol. 48) who tells us that tympanites. constipation and bloated and pallid face are seen only in babies whose amylaceous meals are undigested and fermented. and in none others. particularly not in those that suffer from the putrefaction of albuminoids.

fat 2,7-4,6 p. c., sugar 5,9-7,55 p. c. They also found the amount of sugar to be less, but that of albumin and of fat larger towards the end of nursing, and they found the fat to reach its minimum in the course of the night. Now, if the principle of prescribing exactly is uppermost, can we expect to follow mother's milk in all its alterations, caused by individual differences, by morning or evening, hunger and overfeeding, menstruation and illness, and feed it to the infant in all its wavering conditions. That is impossible, the baby is given his uniform compound a long time. If you and I should eat the same things exactly and in the same quantities during all the conditions of one wavering health, how should even we fare, adult and robust? I ask, should we do it? We should protest and refuse. But the baby must, until there is an apparent reason for a change. This change Rotch tries to meet. He gives his preparations in health and disease: "modified milk" is always the proper thing. Summer complaint, which contraindicates milk, is said to do well with "modified" milk; I hope, I know, it is so "modified" in these cases, that very little of any milk is left in the preparation. The question, whether all babies thrive on this "modified" milk, has often been answered. Many have replied in the negative; my positive experience is, that very many thrive on it a certain time — for the mixture is sterilized in single feeding bottles holding prescribed quantities —, and that very many become rachitical. Mild forms of craniotabes, which require the addition of animal food and of phosphorus and antirachitical treatment generally, I have seen in many instances. There is no food in the world, on which every baby would thrive and thrive always, not even breastmilk. If any there be, it is not modified milk.

Rotch himself says: "The digestive capabilities of infants differ just as do those of adults, and nature therefore provides a variety of good breastmilks adapted to the individual idiosyncrasy of the special infant." With this fact impressed upon us, we can well see, that in artificial feeding no routine mixture will in all cases prove successful.

This " modified milk " feeding has become frequent in our large cities, Boston originally, New York, Philadelphia, Chicago. It is expected that a baby has a prescription given by the doctor, and that the daily portions are prepared in and sent from the laboratory. But the most frequent procedure is that people will apply at the laboratory, and the barmaid in charge will prescribe according to the printed schedules of proportions which are said to correspond with certain ages, a very unscientific application of a method which was meant to be the very essence of scientific accuracy adapted to the individual case. One reason why D' Rotch insists upon the laboratory furnishing the separate meals, is that he does not trust mothers in regard to accuracy and to cleanliness (*Festschrift in honor of doctor Jacobi*. New York 1900. p. 518). I must admit. I am of a different opinion. I know of flies and of cockroaches in the " modified milk " bottles sent from the laboratory. That they were also sterilized, does not help the case. indeed the larger the number of strangers and paid employees who are to do your work, the greater is the danger of neglect.

The method is very expensive. The annual income of many a working man would have to be spent on the baby's feeding. The objections raised to this, and the urgent necessity of finding substitutes for the population at large, rich and poor alike, make Rotch say (*Boston Med. Surg. Journal*. Sept. 1895, p. 293) that " the advance in infant feeding was very much impeded by the cry in New York a few years ago for cheap food for the poor ".

There can be no doubt that the end aimed at by D' Rotch is partly obtained by securing a reliable and approximately fresh milk and by sterilizing it in small portions. That however the 6800 revolutions a minute should leave the milk intact. that after the mixture of its " disjecta membra " we should again have milk is not very probable. Lunin (*Dis. Dorpat*, 1880) fed mice on milk and they lived, but they died when the constituent parts of milk were recompounded.

The " fat milk " (Fettmilch) of Gartner is also obtained by centrifuging and sterilizing. According to Escherich's analysis of woman's and of cow's milk this preparation is to contain casein 1,76, fat 3, and sugar 2.4 per cent. It is preserved in tin cans which are favorable to occasional decomposition. Bad odor, discoloration, and fat swimming on top are frequent occurrences. It is expected to be given indefinitely and no consideration is paid to the fact that woman's milk (not to speak of colostrum) contains more albumin and salts and less fat in the first few months. but less albumin and salts and more fat later[1]. It is advertised. in boastful and sometimes unintelligible terms. according to the methods of low commercialism. at least in America. and is distrusted for that very reason, by the very best part of the profession.

---

1. According to Emil Pfeiffer the percentages of albumin decrease until the end of the 5th month. those of sugar decrease. those of fat and of salts differ very much. particularly the former. On the other hand Heubner (*B. Kl. Woch.*. 1894. n° 57) accepts the analysis of Franz Hoffman according to which from the third week to the termination of lactation there is albumin in mother's milk. 1.05. fat 4.07 sugar 7.05 and salts 0.21 p. c.

The identity of milksugar in woman's and in cow's milk is very doubtful, and the milksugar of the market is quite often impure. That alone makes it desirable in many instances to substitute cane sugar if this afford the same advantage. For four dozen years I made that very substitution and have continued to do so. Part of any kind of sugar, like dextrin, peptone and salt solutions also, is absorbed in the stomach, part of the milksugar of the milk is changed into lactic acid by the bacterium lactis aerogenes and bacterium coli, bacillus acidi paralactici (*not identical with Hueppe's bac. acidi lactici*: Y. Kozai, *Z. Hyg.*, 51, p. 557) and perhaps twenty more different germs. Possibly however, there is an additional source of lactic acid which appears in digestion from 1 2 to 1 hour after a meal, for it seems that this short time is not sufficient to give rise to such formidable masses of microbes as are required for the purpose of transformation. Probably therefore, there are several kinds of lactic acid, which differ not only in proportion to the temperatures in which coagulation takes place and to the composition of the nutrient soil of the bacteria. All of this appears to be sub judice, however. Absorption of milksugar need not always be direct however. Some of the milksugar which was not absorbed as such, is perhaps (Dastre) decomposed by microbic action or by hydrochloric acid, or some unknown ferment into gelactose and glucose, and then absorbed (Portier *in Soc. biol.*, April 2nd. 1898).

When 8 tenths of one per cent of the milksugar contained in the whole milk in the stomach are changed into lactic acid, no more lactic acid is produced. Ordinarily this limit is reached when about one fourth of the milksugar has been changed into lactic acid. If at that period, however, lactic acid be neutralized by an alcali, then more milksugar is changed into lactic acid. In this way the amount of lactic acid present in the digestive tract and of its various derivata depends on accidents only, that is mainly on the presence or absence of an alcali, and it appears that in every preparation of cow's milk selected for the use of an infant there is milksugar enough to supply the needs of the digestive process. Moreover, a goodly part of the milksugar introduced even in woman's milk is eliminated unchanged, for Blauberg (*Studien über Säuglingsfäces*, p. 55) found the desiccated nursling's feces to contain from 0.22 to 0.59 per cent of milksugar. Escherich found besides, that peptones which form in milk when kept are destroyed by acid fermentation, and concludes that another carbohydrate should rather take the place of milksugar. It appears after all this that it *is easier to give too much milksugar than too little*, and that the careful weighing and measuring of copious quantities of milksugar is of doubtful value. It appears also that my method of adding to the cow's milkmixtures destined for infants and children, not milksugar, but canesugar, in quantities estimated rather than anxiously weighed, was correct and is justified by modern research[1].

That fat calories should be replaced by milksugar as has been proposed, appears as an outrage except to those who mistake the infant for a retort. At last :

The anti-fermentative action of milksugar or rather of lactic acid displayed during the putrefaction of albuminoids, is shared by other sugars and by starch.

And Miura proved that the small intestine of the fetus and the newly born (and later on?) have an inverting ferment which makes cane sugar absorbable.

Marfan gives cane sugar because there are traders who give no pure milksugar and declares he finds no inconvenience in so doing. Evidently he has come to the same conclusions that I have arrived at by a clinical experience of nearly half a century.

According to what I said above, a milk mixture in which 25 per cent of milk are contained, holds milksugar enough for the purposes of lactic acid production and of digestion.

I may here also be permitted to remind my hearers of my old recommendation to increase the amount of (cane) sugar in the food of infants when constipated, as a further proof of the identical effect of the different varieties of sugar.

Generally modern modification of cow's milk is not considered

[1]. The amount of organic heat that is produced by the combustion of carbohydrates is expressed in calories. Now it is easy enough to calculate then theoretically, by combining their carbon and hydrogen with the accessible oxygen, but practically this calculation is rendered futile by the condition of the digestive organs of the child, of his respiration, of the surrounding temperature, of the purity of the air, all of which modify metabolism. Nothing can be thought of that is more deceptive than this calculation of calories. Rubner, for instance, declares 245 parts of milk sugar isodynamic with 190 of fat, and Soxhlet — great and meritorious man — pronounces equal parts of cow's milk and of a twelve per cent of sugar of milk solution to be isodynamic with mother's milk. That is why the substitutions of one carbohydrate for the other has been advised. I admit that is all right for chemistry, and atomistic composition, but ask the baby for its opinion, which will be as follows : " first I am constipated with sterilized milk, then I am purged with milksugar. " As to me, its reminds me of Moliere, when one consultant says to the other : You let me bleed him, and I shall let you purge him. The baby will also say : " Yesterday the temperature of the air was dry and 15° C., I was out all day, and felt splendid, and had some use for all the calories I got, to-day the air is humid and 50° C., I am at home and feel sick, and shall be sicker if I have to take all your calories. "

appropriate unless some cream is added to it. Voit taught us indeed that fat in the food prevents loss both of the fat and of the albumin of the tissues; but other carbohydrates do the same. Its percentage in cow's milk is very varying; when high it is considered dangerous by Monti and others. Still Schlossmann pronounces the belief in the injuriousness of fat to be " antiquated ", the excessive elimination of ammonium in the urine, indicating as increase of acid intoxication, nothwithstanding[1]. Fat is added by Biedert and many others for two reasons, viz : 1st to increase the nutritiousness of a food, and 2nd, to increase the digestibility of casein. I, on the contrary, have from year to year been more convinced that the fat of cow's milk should rather be reduced than otherwise. If that is, as Shakespeare said " madness ", there is " method in the madness ".

The normal feces of the nursling were long known, since Wegscheider to consist to the amount of 9 per cent, or much more, of digested cream. Lately W. Knöpfelmacher (*W. Med. Woch.* N°. 30, 1897) found that the fat of the feces of the adult and advanced child while they were fed on milk, consisted of from 12 to 20 per cent olein; of which the larger portion came from the digestive juices, the smaller from the unabsorbed fat of the milk. The fecal fat of the nursling however, contained from 28,8, 57,8 olein, only 5 per cent of which was due to the digestive juices; all the rest belonged to the unabsorbed milk fat. Thus we may conclude that the latter is less utilized by the nursling than by the adult.

According to Heubner (*Berl. klin. Woch.*, I, 1899) in the breastfed infant 5,9 p. c., in the cow milk fed baby, 5.5 p. c., in the infant with " weak intestines " 15 p. c. of the fat introduced into the stomach is expelled undigested.

Now if so much is expelled unchanged, and it seems useless, and superfluous — I refuse to enter into teleological discussions on the benign intentions of providence — the addition of cow's cream to cow's milk should not appear a sine qua non in the preparation of infant's food, the reason or alleged reason for that addition being that the amount of fat in cow's milk is so much inferior to that of woman's milk. Still, Heubner's investigations just quoted, prove that the feces of the nursling excrete nearly the same percentage of fat whether fed on breast or on cow's milk.

It is to this day inconceivable to me that in that connection other analyses (also modern) should be persistently overlooked. There is

1. G. T. PALMER feeds infants on raw milk containing 4-6 p. c. of fat (*N. Y. med. Journ.*, sept. 8th 1900, and obtaines good results.

Söldner with 3,26 p. c. of fat in woman's milk, there is Marfan (p. 10) who draws the average from Gautier, Féry, Gautrelet, Guiraud, Pfeiffer and Michel, which is 3,7 p. c. of fat for cow's, and 3,8 p. c. for woman's milk. And in the face of these data cow's milk fat is added to infant food, equally in winter and in summer, while Esquimaux have told us long ago that it is they that require fat, and ancient Hebrews that it should be prohibited in broiling climates, or seasons. Nor has the frequency of (Biedert's) fat diarrhoea, which has been noticed even in infants nursed by their own mothers, been a warning.

Moreover the fat of cow's milk differs from that of woman's milk. The latter has more oleic acid, less volatile acid than cow's milk; woman's milk contains its fat in a finer emulsion, contains from two to four times as many fat globules as are contained in equally fat cow's milk (Schlossmann). This condition makes it more digestible; it is assumed, and reasonably so, that the fine fat globules may be absorbed directly through the epithelia of the intestinal villi. Moreover, cow's milk fat before it is used undergoes changes. When taken after slow rising it is apt to acidulate, when sterilized and centrifuged it is changed chemically and physically, when frozen it separates from the milk and does not mix again.

All of these facts and considerations and the low percentage in fat of asses milk, which was known to agree best with nurslings and to be inferior to woman's milk only (according to Vernois and Becquerel's analyses made 59 years ago) have led me to reduce rather than to increase the fat of the cow's milk used for infant feeding. I meet with no fat diarrhoea and no excessive acidity when babies are fed according to that rule.

R. v. Ranke's recent favorable experiences with asses milk (*Festschrift in honor of A. Jacobi*, New York, 1900) administered to young infants, one of which did not thrive at all previously; Klemm's report (Dresden, 1898) on asses milk employed for the first two or three months, Marfan's corrobarative opinion (*Allaitement*, p. 299), and the earlier result of Parrot and West, leave no doubt as to the favorable effect of asses milk, with its low percentage of fat, at all events in the first few months of infant life[1]. Asses milk is digestible and wholesome

1. According to Bunge (*Phys. Chemie*, 4th Edition, 1899), There is in the milk of.

	Woman	Cow	Asses
Albuminoid	1.7	3.5	2.5
Fat	3.8	3.7	1.6
Salts	0.2	0.7	0.5

not in spite but because of its low percentage of fat, and in spite of
its albuminoid being contained in larger quantities in asses than in
woman's milk.

What is proven for babies in the first months, I also claim for older
infants. For them some fat may be added to asses' milk, perhaps,
while the stools are being watched for undigested cream, but I know
they do better with less fat than under the influence of laboratory
analyses, not two of which are alike, is generally considered their due.
I insist that a series of clinical observations made prudently and cri-
tically and extensively, must and will be esteemed as equivalent to
the results of measures and scales and microscopes: I say equivalent,
neither superior, nor inferior, for there is no more virtue in the limi-
ted and boastful experimenter, than in the onesided and narrow prac-
titioner. That is why to me it has been a source of great satisfaction
to notice that in the writings of the last few years clinical experience
is frequently appealed to and called in as evidence; and from that
point of view I again appeal to the medical profession from this plat-
form than which I know of none more public, and more authoritative,
to revise theories and practices that I firmly believe to be wrong and
dangerous.

The question of the dilution of cow's milk to make it acceptable
and digestible is not easily answered, because there are some, even
many, babies that appear to be almost inaccessible to injury. They
seem to thrive on almost anything. Still everybody appears to agree
on this that in case of sickness at least undiluted cow's milk is not
tolerated. In France particularly the gospel of undiluted cow's milk
has been preached extensively.

Parrot resorts to sterilized milk when mother's milk is not tolerated.
H. Rothschild details the cases of 6 newly born babies that were suc-
cessfully fed on sterilized milk, Mauchamp believes that it comple-
tely replaces maternal milk. What he however (p. 494) calls its
" curative " effect cannot refer to anything but the destruction of dangerous germs by heat. And Chaternikoff reports (Thèse de Paris, 1899)
on 4 creches, in which pure sterilized milk as administered with
" practically ", (?) she says " no mortality at all. "

My experience is, however, that there is not a more frequent cause
of dyspepsia except excessive summer heat and senseless amylaceous
foods, than undiluted cow's milk in the well and the sick.

In atrophic conditions dilution as well as diminution of nutriment
is a necessity; in bad cases of fat diarrhoea in which even dextrinized
flour and skimmed milk and mother's milk pass unchanged, even Bie-

dert dilutes his cream mixture with three or four or probably more times its quantity of water: such is the result of his experience. What is found by experience to be indicated in disease is applicable to the normal condition, also as the result of experience. I have ever been convinced that the dilutions usually prescribed are insufficient. Now if there were such a thing as *condensed woman's* milk, we should readily agree upon the method of dilution. But in artifical feeding we deal with cow's milk which is not only dense but also chemically different. The dilution for the newly born should be from four or six to one, and for a baby of six months one to one. So much for the regard to be paid to digestion. There are more reasons however for a high degree of dilution: such as I have published and preached without much avail, for one voice cannot carry far. It should be easily admitted however, by this time, that our babies are not given enough water. Breast and bottle contain food, not water. When babies are hungry they cry, when they are thirsty they speak the same language. In either case they are given food, and no drink. That is why babies should frequently be offered water, in some shape or other and it is easiest to add it to their food. The objection made to this plan is that it leads to dilatation of the stomach. I firmly believe that objection has been constructed at the desk. I have not yet seen such a case, and the rapid muscular action of the almost vertical stomach endowed with good circular fibres, and the rapid absorption of fluids containing salts or sugar from it and from the long intestine with its well developed lymph apparatus and very vascular villi renders gastric dilatation very improbable, probably impossible. Water does not act like bulky indigestible food: in the condition in which it is in the infants stomach, viz. with salts and sugar, it is readily absorbed. I have moreover seen diabetics drink five and ten litres of water and more daily, for years, and no dilatation of the stomach from that cause: and three or five hundred more cmc. of water given to a baby in the course of twenty four hours are no danger. But they are a blessing in more than one way. The frequency of uric acid infarction in the newly born, leading in many instances to the formation of renal calculus which is quite frequent, or to nephritis which is *very very* frequent, is best corrected by flushing the kidneys from an early time. These many years that I and my pupils have insisted upon copious dilution of the food of the newly born and young infant, I have seen many less colics from nephro-lithiasis and less cases of nephritis than formerly. Still nephritis is unfortunately very frequent; but then it has so many causes that one single measure cannot obviate all of them.

The selection of the diluent need not be discussed just now. But simple dilution of cow's milk with unmodified water is without avail in obviating the tendency of the milk to form tough and more and less indigestible curds. That is what I have been teaching these forty years, and which I find is acknowledged by chemists such as Chittenden and by clinical observers.

The observation made by Raudnitz (*Arch. Anat. u. Phys.*, Suppl., p. 267) that milk mixed with water leaves the stomach sooner than undiluted milk, if confirmed, need not prove the greater digestibility of the mixture.

Again I wish to emphasize the necessity of considerable proper dilution of the food of the newly born, if artificial, and the frequent administration of water if natural. Colostrum contains much more nitrogenous substance (5-5 pour 100) than the milk of the 10 th day and afterwards, and demands even more dilution than the mammary secretion when regularly established. It is very probable that loss of weight in the newly born will be observed less frequently when plenty of water is administered.

If water is not the proper diluent of cow's milk, what is it? Cereal decoctions have always been preferred by me, partly because, partly inspite of their containing amylum.

Amylum shares some of the properties of all carbohydrates. As early as 1881 Voit (*Handb. d. Physiol. by Hermann*, vol. VI, I, 159) proved their equivalence with milksugar and grapesugar in regard to their effect on the decomposition of albuminoids. While feeding carbohydrates, the consumption of the latter (albuminoids) is diminished and becomes in part unnecessary. Increase of muscle goes to a certain extent hand in hand with the diminution, in the food, of albumin and with the increase of carbohydrates. That agrees perfectly with the experience Gregor had lately (*Arch. f. Kinderh.*, 1900) when he found that his infants when nourished on milk containing sufficient quantities of amylum were more active, and less rachitical than the average, and with Kassowitz's experience according to which 50 pour 100 of his rachitic infants were indeed breastfed, not to speak of my own observations, now extending over much more than forty years and made on tens of thousands of infants in whom *not exactly large* amounts of amylum but cereals containing a *small percentage* of amylum, were proven to add to health and strength in preference to anything else when combined with milk, and with sugar and salts in the average cases, and in cases of incipient rachitis with animal food.

It is understood, and Biedert and Escherich (*Ges. f. Kind.* Wiesbaden, 1887) emphasized the fact, that milksugar cannot be tolerated
in sufficient quantities to have all the effect claimed for carbohydrates.
Nor is dextrinized flour-malt even in Arthur Keller's opinion the best
or only carbohydrate to be employed.   Though using it in preference
he admits that safety lies mainly in the admixture of wheatflour to
his maltsugar, the latter when not so mixed giving rise to diarrhoea.
He states distinctly that the beneficient effect in doubtful cases must
be due to the amylum of the wheat, in as much as all the other constituents of the wheat are contained in the malt also.   Thus he too
attributes the principal effect to the amylum.

This leads us to the consideration of amylum from another point
of view.   Not only does it save feeding with albumin, the excess of
which leads so easily to intestinal putrefaction, not only is it (together
with other carbohydrates) the principal source of muscular force in
general and of the heart in particular. mainly in acute diseases (and
probably better than alcohol). but it acts as a direct intestinal anti-
septic.   I need not prove that, as it is a generally accepted fact.

Now then, what should be the material to be used for dilution of
cow's milk?   My objections to the use of pure or sterilized water are
given above.   Old men in the profession may remember that I always
recommended cereals. mainly oatmeal or barley, the raw, and not the
dextrinized material. in such a proportion, that about a tablespoonful
of the powder was boiled in a litre of water. 1/2 hour or more or less
down to half a litre. this decoction to be used in certain proportions,
as indicated above. with the sugared and salted cow's milk; the
whole to be boiled. or sterilized, before using.   I selected these
cereals for the reason that they contained plenty of iron and other
salts. and vegetable albumin. and as *little* amylum as any cereals or
farinacea are known to contain.

Now an additional word on the admissibility of amylum, in small
or moderate quantities. in the food of the infant.

Heubner (*Berl. klin. Woch.*, 1895. n° 10) was converted to believe
in the good there is in flour feeding by the observation that infants
sick with gastro-intestinal disorders bear and require flour, and that
nurslings before the fourth month of life dextrinize and absorb it.
He prefers simple flours. mainly oats and rice. to any compound.
To him and to Carstens (*Verh. Ges. Kind..* Lubeck, 1895) a good deal
of change in the public medical opinion in regard to the estimation in
which flours are held. is due.   For indeed, my labors of 1876 and
long before (*Infant Diet.* 1872 and 1875. rules and regulations of the

New York Board of Health, and papers on the same subject covering the last forty years) have long been forgotten and seldom enjoy the honor of being quoted in our fast living time.

Now it appears to be considered fair to accept that milk becomes more digestible by the addition of flour decoctions, and that starch is not only changed in the upper but also in the lower intestine, even of moribund infants an occurrence which need not even depend on the presence of microbes (Miura, *Zeitsch. f. Biol.* N. F., XIV, p. 266).

I suggest that whatever is possible in the sick and in the moribund, is not difficult in the well.

Is amylum digested by the very young?

Schiffer (*Ub. d. saccharificirenden Eigenschaften des Kindl. Speichels, Dubois u. Reichert's Arch.*, IV, 1872, p. 469, and *Berl. kl. Woch.*, 1872, n° 29) proved the transformation of starch within from 5 to 10 minutes into sugar in the mouths of babies, of whom one was 2 hours, one 16 days, and one 2 months old. Zweifel (*Unters. üb. d. Verdauungsapparat der Neugebornen.* Berlin. 1874) demonstrated the diastatic effect of the parotid of an infant of 7 days within 4 minutes; even in the case of one that died on the 18th day of its life of gastro-enteritis, there was some little diastatic action in the parotid infusion. Korowin, in his last paper on the subject (*Arch. Kinderheilk.*, 1875, p. 581), says verbally : There is a distinct diastatic influence of the oral secretion from the first minute. It increases with every month. Infusions of the parotid prepared at different periods after death, will transform starch. Infusions of the pancreas of infants that died in the first three weeks had no diastatic action; it begins with the fourth week, but remains feeble to the end of the first year.

These and other facts I have carefully stated in my contribution to *Gerhardt's Handbuch*, vol. I, 1876, and in the second edition 1882, pp. 99-105, and in many other publications, and taught them dozens of years. They have been just as carefully neglected, and, if ever some of them were quoted, they were mostly quoted erroneously. Even Marfan makes a mistake (*L'allaitement*, p. 116) when he says, referring to Korowin and others : " En somme ce ferment est absent ou en très petite quantité dans les premiers temps de la vie; à la vérité, le jeune enfant n'en a pas besoin, puisque le lait ne renferme point d'amidon. Mais on comprend les dangers qu'il y a à alimenter les nouveau-nés et les nourrissons avec des féculents avant la fin de première année. " I do not share any teleological points of view ; nature does not mind them, she kills and cures, prevents or destroys with sublime indifference. A similar mistake has been made with unusual pertinacity by a late writer, Gregor (*Ub. d. Verwendung d. Mehles. in d. Säuglingsernährung. Arch. f. Kinderheilk.* 1900, vol. XXIX), who for that reason comes to wrong conclusions. His case becomes no better by his adding to his mistakes when (to mention only one example), he cites me amongst the thorough going adversaries of farinaceous admixtures to infant foods, and adds that there is " no sufficient clinical experience " on the subject, before his own. Unfortunately, most " clinical experiences " were made with excessive quantities of starch, for instance those referred to by Henoch and von Dusch[1].

Whenever flours are mentioned, the question is always not of a rational administration, but of an excessive, or exclusive supply, and the terrors of the latter are attributed to the former. That is not a very conclusive method of reasoning and not exactly " scientific ".

Let me say a final word on the feces of babies fed on my mixtures. There is very little if any fat in them, the large masses of casein (and fat) which are frequently found after exclusive cow's milk feeding in the constipated or diarrhoeic stools are not found, and there is very little amylum noticed in them, and sometimes none at all. If there is, it is not enough to do harm; it is indifferent.

Do I say that my method is infaillible? By no means. What I claim is that I have been more successful with it than with any other, and I have the advantage of having began and continued it upon the foundation of clinical experience now of nearly half a century, and find my position fortified through the researches and the failures of others.

Without cow's milk no substitute infant food, mine included can be thought of. That is why the one great desideratum will always remain, viz. good milk. Individualism and competition have seemed always to work in the direction of deterioration of that article, for commerce knows no pity. It is in some instances however that I know of, that honorable dealing and financial success went hand in hand. There are gentlemen in every profession or trade.

Municipal strict superintendence may do a good deal for the protection of infant life, and has accomplished some. Efficient aid may come from the future changes in the structure of human society; at present the exertions of states lie still too much in the direction of

---

1. Alle so genannten Kindermehle mit Einschluss der Liebig'schen Suppe sind wegen ihres *hohen Gehaltes on Särkemehl* für die Ernährung der Säuglinge in den ersten Lebensmonaten ungeeignet (*Deutsche Med. Woch.*, 1883, p. 591).

mutual destruction as that of Emperors in that of giving no quarter;
and still, fair beginnings have been made everywhere leaning
towards the acknowledgement of mutual responsibilities. Call it
what you please, socialism or otherwise, I believe the time will come
when even babies will be considered entitled to live, and to live in
the enjoyment of health.

RÉSUMÉ DU RAPPORT

Les analyses du lait humain ont donné des résultats différents ou
contradictoires. Les unes y indiquent des modifications pour les différentes périodes de la lactation, les autres n'en indiquent pas : de
même, on a admis ou approximativement apprécié les changements
apportés par la menstruation, par l'alimentation, par la maladie ; on
les a rarement mesurés. On n'a pas suffisamment élucidé la nature
simple ou composée de la substance protéique. Si ce lait possède en
outre une qualité essentielle et vitale, la chimie ne l'a pas encore
reconnue. C'est pourquoi, devant cette incertitude, on a indiqué tant
de moyens différents pour remplacer le lait humain, et que des chimistes ou même de célèbres cliniciens ont expérimenté tant de produits commerciaux. Si le lait de femme était un corps toujours identique, on serait en droit de rechercher une substance exactement
équivalente. Mais la nature est plus libérale que les chimistes et diver-
sifie davantage ses produits. Le lait est quelquefois amélioré, quelquefois détérioré par la chaleur. Exposés dix ou quinze minutes à la
température de 68 degrés à 70 degrés, le B. coli et le B. lactis aerogenes sont détruits ; exposés plus longtemps à la chaleur, les germes
pathogènes sont tués ; à 80 degrés, l'albumine se coagule, l'odeur et
la saveur du lait sont modifiées ; même à 70 degrés, la caséine est
modifiée, de sorte que sa valeur marchande est diminuée. L'ébullition
fait déposer une partie de l'albumine, détruit la lécithine, altère chimiquement et physiquement les substances grasses. L'ébullition prolongée exagère encore les transformations de la caséine et des
nucléines. Pour détruire les spores résistantes, il faut maintenir une
température élevée pendant quelques heures ; d'ailleurs, leur nocivité
n'est pas complètement démontrée.

Bouilli, stérilisé ou pasteurisé, le lait de vache ne reproduit jamais
le lait humain : sans être un agent curatif, il présente le grand avantage
de ne contenir ni ferment, ni germe pathogène : c'est pourquoi il

devient indispensable dans les grandes villes et pendant certaines épidémies, enfin chaque fois qu'il est impossible de se procurer du lait frais et pur. Lorsqu'il constitue exclusivement l'alimentation d'un enfant, le lait de vache, coupé ou non d'eau, est susceptible de déterminer la constipation, la diarrhée, le rachitisme ou le scorbut. Pour réaliser l'action antibactérienne, la chaleur doit être suivie d'un refroidissement rapide, mais non de la congélation. Dans l'allaitement artificiel, surtout pour le nouveau-né, la composition hétérogène du lait de vache rend nécessaire la dilution de ce lait. Et même les enfants nourris au sein, lorsque le lait maternel n'est pas suffisant, doivent recevoir de l'eau, pour prévenir la perte de poids, la néphrite et la lithiase rénale, ces deux affections étant fréquentes, surtout la néphrite. L'ingestion de grandes quantités de liquide ne diminue pas la motilité de l'estomac, et ne provoque pas la dilatation de l'organe, d'abord parce que l'enfant normal n'est pas glouton, et aussi parce que l'absorption suit immédiatement l'ingestion. La digestion de la caséine du lait de femme est aussi facile ou moins facile, selon les observateurs, que celle de la caséine du lait de vache. Quand le lait de vache est dilué avec une décoction de céréales, la caséine se précipite en flocons finement divisés ; mais certains auteurs soutiennent que les céréales n'ont pas plus d'effet que l'eau. Et cependant ces mêmes auteurs pensent que la dilution hydrique du lait de vache est nécessaire. Cette contradiction est écartée pour ceux qui recommandent l'usage des farines dextrinées pour le coupage du lait de vache. La quantité de substances amylacées, que contiennent les céréales, a été par erreur considérée comme non digestible, malgré les nombreuses expériences qui ont prouvé le contraire. Les décoctions de céréales conviennent pour diluer l'excès de caséine du lait de vache. Le lactose est partiellement absorbé dans l'estomac, partiellement dans l'intestin, partiellement transformé en acide lactique : il est nécessaire à la digestion, et est antiseptique. Mais il est impossible d'en donner une quantité équivalente dans ses effets à ceux que produisent les farineux. En outre, les peptones du lait se détruisent par la fermentation acide. C'est pourquoi le sucre de lait ne doit pas être donné en grande quantité, mais les autres hydrates de carbone peuvent le remplacer. On doit se servir du sucre de canne, car le lait de vache, qui constitue l'allaitement artificiel, contient assez de lactose pour la digestion. En outre, il existe dans l'intestin de l'enfant un ferment qui transforme le sucre de canne et le rend absorbable ; et enfin tous les hydrates de carbone ont le même pouvoir de préserver l'albumine de la putréfaction.

La graisse est ajoutée au lait de vache dans le but d'augmenter ses propriétés nutritives (en empêchant la perte de la graisse et de l'albumine dans les tissus) et de diviser la caséine en particules minimes.

Il faut se souvenir cependant que même le lait de femme contient souvent assez de graisse pour causer de la diarrhée, que les selles normales de l'enfant contiennent de la graisse pure en quantité considérable. Les globules de graisse du lait de vache sont plus grands, moins abondants et moins absorbables que ceux du lait de femme : ces deux variétés de graisse ne sont pas chimiquement semblables. Enfin, quand l'enfant est nourri au lait de vache, les urines contiennent souvent de l'ammoniaque, et l'intestin des substances toxiques.

Les substances minérales sont différentes dans le lait de vache et dans le lait de femme. L'addition de chlorure de sodium au lait de vache est requise par des raisons physiologiques et chimiques.

Il est préférable de préparer soi-même le lait, dans l'allaitement artificiel, plutôt que de l'acheter dans le commerce. En effet, la séparation et la reconstitution des parties constituantes du lait de vache par des moyens mécaniques est un procédé d'une valeur douteuse. L'expérience du médecin et du public valent en général au moins autant que les théories émanées des laboratoires ou développées dans la littérature médicale, qui ne reposent que sur des faits sans jugement.

UEBER KÜNSTLICHE ERNÄHRUNG DES SÄUGLINGS

RAPPORT

von O. HEUBNER,

in Berlin.

Die Lehre von der Ernährung der Erwachsenen hat viel an Klarheit und Sicherheit gewonnen, seitdem man deren Vorgänge unter das grosse Grundgesetz von der Erhaltung der Energie einzuordnen gelernt hat. Der Fortschritt unserer Einsicht in die natürliche und künstliche Ernährung des Säuglings steht nicht minder unter dem Zeichen dieses Gesetzes. Die Bilanz des Kräftestromes, der durch den Säugling hindurchgeht, wird die zukünftige Forschung der Gesetze der künstlichen Ernährung nie aus den Augen verlieren dürfen. Alle Einnahmen und alle Ausgaben ebenso wie das Wachsthum des jugendlichen Organismus lassen sich gemeinsam an diesem Maasstabe messen, dessen Einheit wir als Kalorie bezeichnen. — Kalorisch gewerthet müssen in Zukunft die verschiedenen Nahrungen werden, die wir bei der künstlichen Ernährung verwenden: eine Forderung, der ohne grosse Schwierigkeit entsprochen werden kann, die aber freilich erst in ihren ersten Anfängen befriedigt zu werden beginnt, da noch sehr wenig Unterlagen hierfür vorhanden sind. Vor Allem ist es nöthig, die Nahrungsformen direkt kalorimetrisch zu bestimmen durch experimentelle Erforschung ihrer Verbrennungswärme, denn die Berechnung derselben aus der chemischen Zusammensetzung leidet schon an dem Mangel, dass diese letztere für die meisten in Frage kommenden Nahrungen, also hauptsächlich die Milch und ihre Präparate, noch nicht genügend genau bekannt ist. Die ersten Schritte auf dem eben bezeichneten Wege hat *Rubner* gethan, indem er die Verbrennungswärme oder mit anderen Worten den Energievorrath der Muttermilch, sowie der Kuhmilch, durch den Verbrennungsversuch feststellte.

Noch in einer zweiten Beziehung aber sind die Unterlagen für eine wissenschaftliche Betrachtung der künstlichen Ernährung höchst mangelhaft, — insofern in der Litteratur bisher nur sehr spärliche fortlaufende Beobachtungen künstlicher Ernährung von gesunden Kindern mit genauer täglicher Abmessung der Nahrungszufuhr sowie regelmässigen Gewichtsbestimmungen durch das ganze erste Lebensjahr, oder auch nur einen etwas grösseren Theil desselben hindurch, vorhanden sind. Wo aber genaue Protokolle über Körpergewichte, über Qualität und Quantität einer Nahrung vorliegen, da lassen sich vermittelst der kalorischen Rechnung die Beziehungen zwischen Nahrung und deren Werth für den Säugling viel besser erkennen, als wenn man blos etwa das Volumen oder die chemische Zusammensetzung der Nahrung in Betracht zieht.

Es ist mir gelungen wenigstens eine kleine Reihe solcher Beobachtungen aus der Litteratur und durch die Güte einiger Kollegen zu sammeln. Ich berechnete nun den Nahrungswerth in der Weise, dass ich zunächst in bekannter Weise für jede einzelne Woche das mittlere Kindesgewicht feststellte und sodann den Tageswerth der Nahrung in der nämlichen Woche kalorisch berechnete. Für die Kuhmilch setzte ich bei diesen Berechnungen den von *Rubner* gefundenen Werth von 690 Kalorieen pro Liter Kuhmilch, für die Frauenmilch das Mittel zwischen 2 Bestimmungen *Rubner's* mit rund 650 Kalorieen pro 1000 Gramm ein.

Waren complicirtere Nahrungsweisen angewendet (Biedert's Rahmgemisch, Loeflund's peptonisirte Milch), so berechnete ich Eiweiss und Kohlenhydrate mit rund 4, um deren Kalorieenwerth zu erhalten, Fett mit rund 9 kalorieen das Gram. — Nun wurde die so erhaltene Kalorieenzahl durch die Zahl des mittleren Gewichtes der betreffenden Woche dividirt und so die Energiezufuhr pro Kilo Kind für eine mehr oder weniger grosse Periode des Säuglingsalters. soweit eben die genauen Angaben der Autoren reichten, Woche für Woche festgestellt. — Auf diese Weise habe ich eine Reihe von Kurven gewonnen. aus denen die Beziehungen zwischen Energiezufuhr und Körpergewichtszunahme in recht klarer Weise hervorgehen.

Da es sich in diesen Kurven um *gesunde* Kinder oder wenigstens um solche Kinder handelt. deren Verdauung nicht gestört war. so darf angenommen werden, dass die Resorption und Verwerthung der zugeführten Nahrung in physiologischer Weise vor sich ging.

Ich zeige Ihnen zuerst die Kurve eines Brustkindes. Sie stammt von dem bekannten lehrreichen Fall Dr. Feer's. wo die Stillungsperiode genau berichtet ist. Sie bemerken auf dem unteren Theil jeder Tafel die getrunkenen Tagesmengen schwarz schraffirt und in diese die Energiezufuhr pro Kilo Körpersubstanz in Kalorieeneinheiten roth eingetragen. Darüber ist die Gewichtszunahme der gleichnamigen Lebensperiode in einer ansteigenden Linie aufgetragen.

Sie bemerken nun sehr deutlich, wie die Gewichtskurve des Feer'schen Kindes vom 1. bis in den 5. Monat hinein am steilsten ansteigt, während einer Zeit, wo die Energiezufuhr pro Kilo Kind erheblich über 100 Kalorieen beträgt, ja fast einen Monat lang bis auf 125 Kalorieen und selbst darüber ansteigt. Eine zweite Periode, die sich übrigens noch weiter gliedern liesse, erstreckt sich von der 11. bis zur 24. Woche. während deren der Anstieg weniger steil ist. Ziehen Sie durch Anfangs- und Endpunkt jeder der beiden Perioden eine Gerade, so bemerken Sie sogleich. wie der Winkel, den die Linie II mit der Abscisse bildet, kleiner ist als derjenige der Linie I. Während nun in der ersten Hälfte dieser zweiten Periode die von der Mutterbrust gelieferte Energiezufuhr (bis zur 16. Woche) noch 100 Kalorieen und etwas darüber betrug, sinkt sie in der zweiten Hälfte auf 85-90 Kalorieen. Die schlechteste Zunahme erfolgt in der dritten Periode, durch Linie III gekennzeichnet, von der 25. bis zur 50. Woche. Hier sinkt die Energiezufuhr auf 75. Ja, wenn man in Rücksicht zieht, dass die Milch der Mutter um diese Zeit wahrscheinlich kalorieenärmer ist. als ich aus den beiden Zahlen *Rubner's* durchschnittlich der Rechnung zu Grunde gelegt habe, so dürften wir hier wahrscheinlich den kalorieenärmsten Abschnitt der ganzen Stillungszeit vor uns haben.

Erst in der letzten Periode unserer Kurve, der Linie IV entsprechend, wird das Ansteigen des Gewichtes wieder etwas steiler. Jetzt tritt an Stelle der versiegenden Muttermilch die Energiezufuhr durch Kuhmilch. Die tägliche Energiezufuhr beträgt 75 Kalorieen pro Kilo.

Misst man die Winkel, welche die 4 Linien mit der Abscissenaxe bilden, aus, so ergiebt sich für

1) ein Winkel von $59^{0}45'$, d. h. Wachsthum, = Tang. $59^{0}45' = 0,8502$.
2) » » » $22^{0}45'$, » » = » $22^{0}45' = 0,4061$.
3) » » » $7^{0}10'$, » » = » $7^{0}15' = 0,1246$.
4) » » » $14^{0}0'$, » » = » $14^{0}0' = 0,2495$.

Lassen wir die 4. Periode, wo die künstliche Ernährung Platz greift, ausser Betracht, so ergiebt sich für die ersten zwei Drittel des Säuglingsjahres eine ganz deutliche Proportion zwischen Wachsthumsintensität und Energiezufuhr. Man kann sagen, dass in diesem Falle bei normaler, natürlicher Säuglingsernährung die tägliche Kalorieenzufuhr pro Kilo während des ersten Drittels des Jahres nicht unter 100 und während der ersten Hälfte nicht unter 90 sinkt. Ich will aber auf diese absolute Zahl nicht etwa das entscheidende Gewicht legen, denn ich gebe gern zu, dass weitere genaue Bestimmungen der Verbrennungswärme der Muttermilch in deren verschiedenen Absonderungsperioden und Ausmessungen der gelieferten Gewichtsmengen diese Zahl ändern werden. Deutlich ist aber unter allen Umständen, dass auch unter ganz regelrechter Ernährung das langsamere Tempo der Zunahme in der späteren Säuglingszeit in direkter Beziehung zu der geringeren Energiezufuhr pro Kilo Körper steht.

Auf die Volumina der Nahrung kommt es dabei, wie Sie sehen, gar nicht an; diese waren während der Periode der stärksten Zunahme kleiner als später.

Vergleichen wir nun hiermit die zweite Kurve, die von einem künstlich genährten Säugling stammt. Sie ist von meinem früheren Assistenten, Herrn Privatdocent Dr. *Finkelstein*, in der Privatpraxis beobachtet; alle Maassnahmen, die zur Berechnung gedient haben, sind von ihm genau controllirt.

Die Kurve beginnt allerdings erst mit der 7. Woche; die ersten 6 Wochen vergingen mit dem Versuch der Ernährung an der Ammenbrust, der aber wegen Unfähigkeit der Ammen aufgegeben wurde. Die künstliche Ernährung wurde hier in der Weise durchgeführt, dass mit zunehmendem Körpergewicht die Concentration der Nahrung, mit anderen Worten, ihr Energiegehalt in gleichem Verhältniss ge-

steigert wurde. Hier sehen wir nun keine Abnahme der Wachsthumsgeschwindigkeit in der zweiten Hälfte des Säuglingsjahres, sondern
eine Zunahme. Wir können drei Perioden unterscheiden, die erste
von der 7. bis zur 22. Woche (Linie I), die zweite von der 25. bis zur
52. Woche (Linie II), die dritte von der 55. bis zur 56. Woche (Linie III).
Die Winkel, die diese Linien mit der Abscissenachse bilden, und
welche die Wachsthumsgeschwindigkeit ausdrücken, betragen

$$\text{für Linie} \quad \text{I} = 22°30', \text{ d. h. Wachsthum.} = 0.4142.$$
$$\text{» } \quad \text{» } \quad \text{II} \quad 26°50', \quad \text{»} \qquad \text{»} \qquad 0.4986.$$
$$\text{» } \quad \text{» } \quad \text{III} \quad 45°50', \quad \text{»} \qquad \text{»} \qquad = 1.0180.$$

Das Kind wächst also hier im 5. Vierteljahr rapider als je vorher.
Betrachten wir nun die täglich pro Kilo zugeführte Energie, so sehen
wir sie während der ganzen Zeit nie unter 100 sinken und fast immer
um 125 sich halten.

Es ist nun sehr interessant zu sehen, wie die gleiche Energiezufuhr
bei dem künstlich genährten Kinde im 2. und 5. Lebensmonat weniger
Erfolg für die Wachsthumsgeschwindigkeit hat als beim Brustkinde.
Während das letztere bei einer Zufuhr von 120-125 Kalorieen eine
Wachsthumsgeschwindigkeit von 0,8502 zeigt, ist sie beim Flaschenkinde im selben Alter nur 0.4142. Da haben wir den Ausdruck der
Ueberlegenheit der natürlichen Nahrung über die künstliche. Die
gleiche Wachsthumsgeschwindigkeit wie das Flaschenkind bei Zufuhr
von 125 Kalorieen zeigt das Brustkind schon bei einer Zufuhr von
90 bis 100 (nämlich in der zweiten Periode).

Später aber gleicht sich das Verhältniss aus, ja im 5. Vierteljahr
übertrifft die Wachsthumsgeschwindigkeit des Flaschenkindes sogar
die des Brustkindes bei gleicher Energiezufuhr.

Es geht also aus dieser Betrachtung hervor, dass der Energiegehalt
der täglichen Zufuhr nicht unter ein gewisses Maass sinken darf, das
vorläufig beim künstlich genährten Kinde mit 100 Kalorieen pro Kilo
angenommen werden mag, ohne das normale Gedeihen des Kindes
zu gefährden.

Aber, meine Herren, es darf auch nach oben hin dieses Maass nicht
überschritten werden. Das lehrt uns das Beispiel der 11. Woche in
unserer zweiten Kurve. Als hier versucht wurde, dem grösser gewordenen Flaschenkinde durch concentrirtere Nahrung die gleiche
Energiemenge pro Kilo zuzuführen wie fünf Wochen vorher, da nahm
es zwar eine Woche lang stärker zu als vorher, aber dann bekam es
eine Verdauungsstörung, die erst wieder ausgeglichen werden musste,
bis die eigentliche Ernährung wieder begonnen werden konnte. Die

Verdauungsorgane waren nicht im Stande, die grössere Energiemenge in der zugeführten Form längere Zeit zu verarbeiten. Hier haben Sie ein klassisches Beispiel der sogenannten Ueberernährung. Als aber nachher, in der 15. Woche, fast die gleiche Energie, aber in einer anderen Form, einer anderen Mischung der einzelnen Nährstoffe, zugeführt wird, gelingt es den Verdauungsorganen, die Nahrung zu bewältigen, und das Wachsthum vollzieht sich weiterhin in befriedigender Weise.

Ganz in der nämlichen Weise nun habe ich die Verhältnisse in den übrigen Fällen, die ich mir in der gleichen Weise darzustellen vermochte, immer wieder gefunden. Das Wachsthum und Gedeihen geht mit dem *Energiequotienten* in gleichlaufendem Verhältniss, d. h. mit der *Energiemenge*, die dem Körper *pro Kilo Körpergewicht* zugeführt wird.

In Kurve III sehen Sie die Ernährung einer sehr schwachen Frühgeburt dargestellt. Es war das Kind eines Chemikers, der den Gehalt der Nahrung an Nährstoffen bis zum Jahresende genau berechnet hat. Die Zahlen verdanke ich Herrn *Camerer* in Urach.

Die täglich zugeführte Energie steigt hier im Allgemeinen noch höher als bei dem ersten Flaschenkinde, und es hat den Anschein, als ob dieser Fall einen noch höheren Durchschnittsbetrag an Zufuhr nöthig gehabt hätte als das Brustkind, denn obwohl diese im letzten Vierteljahr fast immer noch erheblich mehr als 100 Kalorieen pro Kilo beträgt, steht die Gewichtszunahme von der 40. bis zur 52. Woche fast still. — Das Kind ist aber später gut in die Höhe gekommen, ist jetzt 8 Jahre alt, gesund, aber noch immer etwas dünn, wie *Camerer* schreibt.

Die noch übrigen vier Kurven stellen nur Fragmente der gesammten Säuglingsperiode dar. An dieser Kurve IV hier sehen Sie die ersten fünf Wochen eines ebenfalls zu früh geborenen Kindes dargestellt (Anfangsgewicht 1855 Gramm), das vom ersten Lebenstage an künstlich genährt worden ist; auch hier bemerken Sie, wie die Zunahme erst beginnt, nachdem die Energiezufuhr auf 105 bis 110 Kalorieen pro Kilo gesteigert worden ist.

Von besonderem Interesse sind aber die drei letzten Kurven, die ich Ihnen zeige. Sie stammen aus einer schon vor 20 Jahren von *Biedert* veröffentlichten Studie über die Nahrungsminima bei der Säuglingsernährung. *Biedert* hat dort sehr genaue Angaben über die jeweilig gewählte Zusammensetzung der Nahrung gemacht, sodass auch hier eine Berechnung in dem von mir angegebenen Sinne möglich ist. Da stellt sich denn heraus, dass auch bei seiner sogenannten Minimalnahrung die Kinder fast ausnahmlos nur dann ordentlich zunahmen, wenn der Kalorieenwerth der Zufuhr pro Kilo auf 100, ja sehr vielfach auf weit über 100, sogar nahe an 150 stieg!

An dieser ersten Kurve sehen Sie ein Beispiel, wo *Biedert* die Ernährung an der Ammenbrust — wegen Diarrhoeen des Kindes. — Aber sie nehmen ja auch Anfangs ab und dann langsam zu, um erst nach etwa 6 Tagen das Anfangsgewicht wieder zu erreichen.

Für diese Zeit nun bis zum 10. Lebenstage hat vor Kurzem Cramer[1] Beobachtungen veröffentlicht, die zu allen bisherigen Erfahrungen in schroffem Widerspruch stehen. So hat er z. B. bei einem Neugeborenen nach der Abnahme der ersten Tage vom 4. bis zum 10. Lebenstage eine Zunahme von durchschnittlich 46.6 Gramm pro die erzielt bei einer Ernährung, die, nach der hier erörterten Methode berechnet, pro Kilo Körpergewicht täglich 10 bis 50 Kalorieen an Energie zuführte — also in den ersten Tagen der Zunahme erheblich weniger, als der ruhende Erwachsene nöthig hat! Dahingegen begann in meinen beiden Fällen von Frühgeburt bei künstlicher Ernährung die Zunahme nicht eher, als bis die Zufuhr 100 Kalorieen pro Kilo erreicht hatte.

Auch alle sonstigen Erfahrungen, z. B. die von *A. Schmidt*, von *Finkelstein* aus meiner Klinik, aus der Klinik von *Budin* (vergl. *Finkelstein, Ueber Pflege kleiner Frühgeburten, Therapie der Gegenwart*, März 1900), lehren, dass wenigstens schwache und zarte Kinder nur bei bedeutend höherer Zufuhr zunehmen.

Ich vermag den Widerspruch vor der Hand nicht zu lösen.

Geringer als später scheint vielleicht das Energiebedürfniss des Kindes in der 1. Woche zu sein. Aber unter allen Umständen wäre es sehr erwünscht, bei Wiederholung der Ernährungsversuche in den ersten Lebenstagen auch möglichst genaue kalorische Messungen der zugeführten Nahrung vorzunehmen.

Meine Herren, das thatsächliche Material, was Ich Ihnen zur Begründung meiner Anschauung vorlege, ist, wie ich gar nicht verkenne, noch ein recht spärliches. Die Ursache liegt eben darin, dass über die künstliche Ernährung gesunder Kinder in der Litteratur noch äusserst wenig fortlaufende Beobachtungen mit so sorgfältigen Angaben vorliegen, um genügende Unterlagen für die vorgeführten Berechnungen zu gewähren. Von darmkranken oder von Darmkrankheiten reconvalescenten Kindern hätte ich viel grösseres Material sammeln können.

---

1. *Deutsche med. Wochenschrift*, No. 2, 1900; *Klinische Vorträge*, Neue Folge, No. 265, 1900.

Hier kam aber sofort noch eine unbekannte Grösse für die Rechnung ins Spiel, nämlich der Grad der mehr oder weniger gestörten Ausnützung der zugeführten Energie. Für gesunde Säuglinge darf diese absichtlich so einschränkte, dass das Kind nicht ganz 100 Kaloriëen bekam. Während dieser ganzen Zeit Stillstand des Körpergewichts. Als aber dann der Nährwerth der Nahrung auf 125 Kaloriëen stieg, da stieg auch das Körpergewicht, obwohl die Diarrhoeen zunächst fortdauerten.

An der zweiten Kurve sehen wir bei 85 bis 90 Kaloriëen pro Kilo Zufuhr allerdings eine Zunahme eintreten und zwar unter einem Winkel von 21°15′, aber nachdem der Nährwerth auf nahezu 140 Kaloriëen pro Kilo gesteigert ist, erreicht das Wachsthum einen Winkel von 58°15′.

Bei der letzten Kurve endlich zeigt sich auch eine ziemlich **genaue** Congruenz zwischen Wachsthum intensität und Kaloriëenwerth der Nahrung. Der letztere ist, solange Gewichtszunahme eintritt, immer höher als 100 Kaloriëen. — Erwähnenswerth ist in diesem Falle der Umstand, dass die Zufuhr sehr grosser Nahrungs*volumina* den Nutzen der Nahrung wenigstens nicht erheblich beeinträchtigt zu haben scheint, so lange als der Gehalt dieser Mengen an Nährwerth nicht zu niedrig wurde. Dem hier dargestellten Kinde wurden im Alter von 6 bis 8 Monaten täglich über 1 1/2 Liter Flüssigkeit eingeführt.

Trotz der grösseren Arbeit, die damit dem Körper aufgebürdet wurde, erfolgte doch in den betreffenden Monaten ein **Wachsthum**, dessen Raschheit durch einen Winkel von 52°40′ (in obigem Sinne) ausgedrückt wird. Freilich erhielt das Kind dabei eine tägliche Energiezufuhr von meist 125, ja mehrfach selbst über 150 Kaloriëen pro Kilo.

Der Parallelismus zwischen dem Energiewerth der zugeführten Nahrung scheint nun, soweit sich aus den bisher von mir studirten Fällen schliessen lässt, während des ganzen Säuglingsalters in Geltung zu sein. Auch gegen das Ende des ersten Lebensjahres hin sehen wir eine noch erheblichere Zunahme des Körpers eintreten, wo der Nährwerth der Zufuhr immer von Neuem auf 100 Kaloriëen pro Kilo erhöht wird, während die Zunahme um so geringer wird, je mehr die Zahl unter 100 sinkt. Für die ersten Wochen des Lebens, besonders für die erste Woche mit ihrer sogenannten physiologischen Abnahme, bieten meine Kurven noch ein zu spärliches Material, um hier mit Sicherheit sich zu äussern. Aus der Mutterbrust erhalten die Kinder für gewöhnlich während dieser Lebensperiode keine 100 Kaloriëen pro Kilo, auch gegenüber künstlicher Nahrung auf Grund der vorhandenen

Stoffwechselversuche als eine recht gute angenommen werden.

Nun aber stimmen alle Kurven, Zunahme, Stillstand oder Abnahme des Körpergewichtes, so genau mit der grösseren oder geringeren Zufuhr von Energie in der Nahrung überein, und ist fast überall die Zahl von 100 Kalorieen pro Kilo der Pegel, der nicht unterschritten werden darf, wenn eine gute Zunahme erfolgen soll, dass es wohl erlaubt ist, bis auf Weiteres hier ein Gesetz oder eine Regel zu erblicken, von der Ausnahmen vor der Hand noch nicht vorliegen. Da aber die gute Zunahme eines Säuglings der sicherste Maassstab für den Werth einer Ernährungsmethode ist, so könnte man diese Regel auch etwa so formuliren : die wichtigste Eigenschaft für jede Art künstlicher Ernährung des Säuglings ist ihr Gehalt an potentieller Energie.

Es kommt also in erster Linie auf die *chemische* Zusammensetzung der Nahrung *nicht* an. — In der That sind die Kurven, die ich Ihnen vorgelegt habe, mit chemisch ganz verschiedenen Nahrungsmitteln erzielt. Wir finden, abgesehen von der Muttermilch, darunter meine Mischungen von 1/5 und 2/5 Kuhmilch, dieselbe Mischung mit Zusatz von Kindermehl, peptonisirte Kindermilch (nach *Loeflund*), gemischte Ernährung mit Brust- und Kuhmilch, *Biedert'sches* Rahmgemisch : überall war — wenn die Nahrung überhaupt vertragen wurde, und das war eben durchweg der Fall — die Zunahme lediglich vom Energiewerth der täglichen Zufuhr abhängig.

Meine Herren, es wird Ihnen nicht entgehen, dass mit dieser Erkenntniss, wenn sie sich weiterhin bestätigen sollte, der Lehre von der Säuglingsernährung eine neue Wendung gegeben wird, eine Wendung, die ich schon 1897 in meiner Schrift *Ueber Säuglingsernährung und Säuglingsspitäler*[1] anzubahnen versuchte, für die mir aber damals noch die jetzt ausgeführten rechnerischen Grundlagen fehlten. Sehr gestützt wird diese veränderte Auffassung durch die trefflichen Ausführungen *Camerer's* im *Jahrbuch für Kinderheilkunde*.[2] Gestützt ist sie aber auch, was die von mir aufgestellte Zahl an Energiezufuhr anlangt, bereits durch das Experiment. In unserem ersten Stoffwechselversuch[3] hatten *Rubner* und *ich* bewiesen, dass eine Energiezufuhr von 70 Kalorieen pro Kilo Kind nicht ganz ausreichte, um den Bestand des Säuglingskörpers zu erhalten (2-monatliches Kind), also unter dem normalen Bedürfniss lag. Die Zufuhr war in diesem Falle zu 91.6 % ausgenützt worden, der wirkliche Ver-

---

1. Berlin, 1897, Hirschwald.
2. Band LI, Seite 26 bis 54, *Die Verdauungsarbeit*, u. s. w.
3. *Die natürliche Ernährung eines Säuglings. Zeitschrift für Biologie.* Band 36.

brauch 64.12 Kalorieen pro Tag und Kilo. Dahingegen betrug in
unserem zweiten Stoffwechselversuch an einem 7 1/2-monatlichen
Kinde[1], das bei einer Ernährung mit reiner Kuhmilch ziemlich gut
zunahm, die Bruttozufuhr der mit der Nahrung incorporirten Energie
menge 96.27 Kalorieen, eine Zahl, die sich also wieder fast genau der
aus unseren Kurven gewonnenen Zahl 100 anschliesst. Von der obigen
Bruttoeinnahme an Energie wurden in unserem Falle 12,2 % zum
Körperwachsthum verbraucht. Die dem Körper wirklich zu Gute
kommende Energie belief sich auf 89.8 Kalorieen pro Kilo, die physiologische Ausnützung der zugeführten Energie auf 95,9 %. Man darf
aus diesen experimentellen Erfahrungen wohl den Schluss ziehen,
dass beim gesunden Säugling mindestens 90 % der zugeführten
Energie wirklich durch den Körper hindurchgeht und zu einem Achtel
oder Neuntel im Körper aufgespeichert wird. Ja, es ist sogar wahrscheinlich, dass diese Zahlen unter ganz normalen Verhältnissen noch
höher sind als in unseren Versuchen.

Wir verlassen mit der so gewonnenen Anschauung, wenn ich mich
so ausdrücken darf, den *chemisch-physiologischen* Standpunkt bei
der Betrachtung der Säuglingsernährung und begeben uns auf den
physiologisch-physikalischen. Und, meine Herren, ich spreche es hier
als meine Ueberzeugung aus, dass wir mit dieser Art der Betrachtung
ungleich besser vorwärts kommen werden als mit der bisherigen.

Es muss doch zugestanden werden, dass die zahlreichen Bemühungen der Chemiker uns noch keineswegs zu klareren Begriffen
und besonders nicht zu einem zielbewussten Vorgehen in der künstlichen Ernährung geführt haben. Das gleiche Präparat, das dem einen
sehr gute Dienste leistete, versagte bei dem andereu und umgekehrt.
Das Universalrecept für die künstliche Säuglingsernährung, das geben
Sie wohl Alle zu, ist noch nicht gefunden, — und ich füge hinzu : *wird
nie gefunden werden.* Denn wir haben es in jedem einzelnen Falle mit
einem neuen Individuum zu thun, auf das die übliche Regel mög-
licher Weise nicht ohne Weiteres passen wird. Aber der Werth an
Energiezufuhr, den das Kind braucht, der nicht unter, aber auch
nicht zu weit überschritten werden darf, das ist wahrscheinlich eine
feste Norm, nach der wir uns in jedem einzelnen Falle richten müssen,
und mit der wir klar rechnen können.

Nun würde ich aber missverstanden werden, wenn man annehmen
würde, dass ich mit der Voranstellung dieses Begriffes in der Säuglingsernährung etwa die chemische Zusammensetzung der Säuglings-

<hr>

1. *Zeitschrift für Biologie.* Band XXXVIII. Seite 544 u. 545.

nahrung für etwas Gleichgiltiges erachten würde. Dieser kommt vielmehr bei der Ernährung schwacher und darmkranker Kinder auch nach meiner Meinung die grösste Bedeutung zu. Bei der künstlichen Ernährung normaler und gesunder Säuglinge können die Vorschriften über die Zusammensetzung der Nahrung verhältnissmässig einfach gestaltet werden : Man kommt bei guter Ueberwachung im Allgemeinen mit den von mir angegebenen 1/2 oder 2.5 Milchmischungen oder mit der Vorschrift, wie sie *Marfan* in seinem Werke über die Säuglingsernährung anräth, ganz gut aus. Ich möchte nur anführen, dass es sich nach den in unserer Klinik und auch früher schon von einzelnen Aerzten gesammelten Erfahrungen empfiehlt, die Milch statt mit reinem Milchzuckerwasser, mit einer dünnen (vierprocentigen) *Mehl*suppe zu mischen. Zur Zubereitung dieser Mehlsuppe aber sind die präparirten Kindermehle (im Allgemeinen aus Zwieback oder Biscuit hergestellt) den einfachen Mehlen, wie Hafer- und Gerstenmehl, vorzuziehen. Mit derartig hergestellter Milch kann man, unter steter Berücksichtigung der nöthigen Energiezufuhr, gesunde Kinder bis zum Ende ihrer Säuglingsperiode ohne Schwierigkeit in die Höhe bringen.

Es darf nur eins nicht fehlen : die möglichste bakterielle Reinheit. Diese aber haben die Bemühungen der Aerzte im letzten Vierteljahrhundert dank der Anregung *Soxhlet's* in durchaus befriedigender Weise erreicht, so dass über diesen Punkt nichts mehr zu sagen ist und nur rühmend hervorgehoben werden darf, dass wir in dieser Errungenschaft wohl den grössten Fortschritt in der Säuglingsernährung zu betrachten haben, den uns das 19. Jahrhundert gebracht hat.

Wenn es aber gilt, schwache und kranke Kinder zu ernähren, da kommen wir sehr häufig mit obigen einfachen Vorschriften nicht aus, und da haben wir nun in den Schätzen uns umzuschen, die uns erfinderische Gelehrte, wie *Biedert*, *Backhaus*, *Gärtner*, *Keller*, *de Jager* u. A., und unter ihrem Einfluss wieder die unermüdliche Industrie an die Hand geben.

Die Sache ist nur die, dass man nicht von vornherein bestimmen kann, welches der nach den verschiedenen theoretischen Ueberlegungen ihrer Erfinder hergestellten Ersatzmittel der Muttermilch für das einzelne Kind, das man gerade vor sich hat, das richtige und passendste ist. Nach den auf meiner Klinik gemachten Erfahrungen gehört z. B. die nach *Keller* modificirte alte *Liebig'sche* Suppe zu denjenigen Nährmitteln, die von recht vielen darmschwachen Säuglingen viele Wochen lang mit sehr gutem Nutzen genossen wird. Sie

versagt nur ziemlich oft bei sehr jungen und bei frühgeborenen
Kindern, auch wenn man sie noch verdünnt. Andererseits haben wir
aber auch recht schwache Frühgeburten mit dieser Nahrung in die
Höhe kommen sehen. Häufiger als diese fettarme und kohlenhydrat-
reiche Nahrung sehen wir gerade bei frühgeborenen Kindern die
entgegengesetzte Nahrung gute Zunahme bewirken, die fettreiche
und zuckerärmere Fettmilch in Gestalt des *Biedert'schen* Rahm-
gemisches und besonders auch der von *Backhaus* erdachten peptoni-
sirten Fettmilch.

Doch kamen andererseits wieder Frühgeburten vor, bei denen diese
Fettmilch nach kurzem Gebrauche sehr schlecht verdaut wurde und
zu Störungen führte, die sich schwer und langsam oder auch gar
nicht wieder ausglichen.

Bei einzelnen Kindern erwies sich die *trockne peptonisirte* Kuhmilch,
wie sie von der englischen Firma Allen and Hanbury unter dem Namen
Allenbury in den Handel gebracht wird, als besonders gut ausnütz-
bare, bekömmliche und gutes Wachsthum befördernde Nahrung;
andere Male war wieder Nichts damit zu erreichen.

Die früheren Assistenten meiner Klinik, Docent Dr. *Finkelstein* und
Dr. *Bendix*, werden über diese Erfahrungen in einer Reihe von Mittheilungen eingehenden Bericht erstatten.

Man könnte meinen und hat gemeint, dass die gute Wirkung der
Liebig'schen Suppe zu einem erheblichen Theile auf ihre alkalische
Beschaffenheit zurückzuführen ist.

Wir haben aber in den letzten Monaten Versuche mit einem saueren
Nahrungsmittel von ziemlich hohem Eiweissgehalt, aber geringem
Fettgehalt angestellt — mit der Buttermilch in der von *de Jager*
empfohlenen Zubereitung, — das in einigen recht schlimmen Fällen,
besonders in einem geradezu verzweifelten Fall schwerster Atrophie
mit multiplen Phlegmonen, überraschende Erfolge erzielt hat.

So sehen wir bei scheinbar gleichartigen Erkrankungen die gleiche
Nahrung das eine Mal gut, das andere Mal schlecht bekommen, und
umgekehrt ganz verschieden zusammengesetzte Nährmittel ganz
ähnliche Erfolge erzielen. Es gilt auch hier der Satz : der Säugling
selbst mit schwachem Darm vermag mit sehr verschieden zusammen-
gesetzter Nahrung sein Energiebedürfniss zu befriedigen, vorausgesetzt, dass sie ihm rein zugeführt wird und genügende Energie
enthält.

Der Umstand, dass mit zwei chemisch so entgegengesetzten
Nahrungen, wie es die Buttermilch und die *Liebig'sche* Suppe sind,
ähnliche Erfolge erzielbar sind — wir gaben diese Nahrungen einem

sehr elenden Kinde sogar abwechselnd am selben Tage, zu verschiedenen Mahlzeiten, — veranlasste mich den Verbrennungswerth dieser beiden Suppen ermitteln zu lassen. Mein Kollege Professor *Rubner* hatte die Güte diese Bestimmungen selbst auszuführen, die besonders bei der Liebig'schen Suppe grosse Schwierigkeiten bereiteten. Es ergab sich das bemerkenswerthe Resultat, dass beide Nahrungsmittel einen hohen Energiegehalt haben, die Buttermilch 700 Kalorieen im Liter, die Liebig'sche Suppe sogar 800, also fast um 100 Kalorieen mehr als die gehaltreichste Frauenmilch. Um den nöthigen Energiewerth zuzuführen braucht man also von diesen beiden Suppen verhältnissmässig kleine Volumina. Stoffwechselversuche haben ergeben, dass auch ihre Ausnützung in schwachen Därmen eine verhältnissmässig sehr gute ist.

So führt uns dieser letzte Aufschluss wieder an den Anfang unserer Betrachtung, auf die Wichtigkeit der Werthung der Säuglingsnahrung nach ihrem Energiegehalt zurück.

Meine Herren, der Fortschritt in dieser Richtung ist nur möglich unter Erfüllung zweier Anforderungen :

1. Es muss in möglichst grossem Umfange der Verbrennungswerth der hauptsächlichen Nährmittel des Säuglings durch das direkte Experiment festgestellt werden.

2. Es müssen möglichst zahlreiche fortlaufende Beobachtungen von Einzelfällen über die Qualität der täglichen Zufuhr bei künstlicher Ernährung gut gedeihender Säuglinge angestellt werden. Den Ablauf des gesunden Verhaltens müssen wir noch viel genauer kennen lernen als dieses bisher der Fall.

Ich würde mich glücklich schätzen, wenn meine kleine Mittheilung den Erfolg hätte, recht zahlreiche Kollegen zur Anstellung solcher Beobachtungen anzuregen.

Wir gehen damit einen neuen Weg, sagen wir einen Seitenweg. der uns aber, mit reicher Frucht beladen, auf die Hauptstrasse zurückführen wird !

RÉSUMÉ DU RAPPORT

On ne peut établir scientifiquement un procédé d'alimentation artificielle des nourrissons que par l'étude du nourrisson sain et né à terme, et non par celle du nourrisson malade. De même que l'on ne pourrait se baser sur la diète d'un malade pour régler le régime d'un ouvrier sain, de même on ne peut conclure d'échecs ou de succès obtenus sur des enfants dyspeptiques, à la meilleure manière d'alimenter le nourrisson normal. C'est cependant ce que font encore fréquemment les médecins, sans doute parce qu'ils ont le plus souvent affaire à des enfants malades. C'est pourquoi nous ne possédons pas une somme relativement importante de documents, qui puissent scientifiquement servir à établir la méthode la plus rationnelle d'alimentation artificielle. Chaque année des centaines de mille d'enfants sont nourris artificiellement avec succès pendant leur première année; et pourtant les observations poursuivies longtemps, de manière à nous renseigner sur le mode qualificatif et quantitatif de l'alimentation artificielle quotidienne d'enfants dont la croissance s'est bien effectuée, ne sont pas aussi exactes que celles qui concernent l'allaitement maternel. Voilà pourquoi nous trouvons sur cette question plus d'idées théoriques que de faits probants.

Mais, de tout temps, le bon sens des nourrices a compris que rien ne pouvait mieux remplacer le lait de femme que le lait animal, ce que confirme l'analyse chimique. Celle-ci montre, en effet, que le lait de nos animaux domestiques, surtout de la vache et de la chèvre (du moins, en ce qui concerne les principes nutritifs), ne diffèrent pas plus du lait de femme que les diverses sortes de viande ne diffèrent entre elles : ainsi en est-il des viandes de porc et de bœuf, que l'enfant comme l'adulte mange cependant alternativement ou successivement. Leur valeur nutritive générale, leur énergie potentielle sont dans les deux cas à peu près les mêmes (650 à 700 calories par litre).

L'intestin du nourrisson sain est capable de digérer le lait de vache tout aussi bien que le lait de femme. Seulement, le travail digestif est plus grand dans le premier cas que dans le deuxième, car les grosses molécules protéiques exigent un effort digestif plus considérable que les petites molécules hydrocarbonées ; or, la composition du lait de vache est surtout riche en molécules protéiques, celle du lait de femme en molécules hydrocarbonées. Il en résulte qu'une plus grande quantité de résidus reste dans les intestins après la digestion du lait animal qu'après celle du lait de femme. Mais toutes les recherches faites jusqu'ici sur les échanges organiques du nourrisson démontrent que celui-ci est parfaitement capable de trouver la ration d'entretien nécessaire dans le lait de vache, pourvu qu'il en absorbe la quantité équivalente à celle que lui livrerait le sein maternel au temps correspondant du développement. Naturellement, cette quantité varie entre certaines limites physiologiques.

L'allaitement artificiel doit ne pas dépasser cette juste mesure du dosage quotidien exact du lait animal. coupé ou non, mêlé ou non avec tel ou tel ingrédient.

C'est d'abord la détermination de règles exactes qui présente les plus grandes difficultés de l'alimentation artificielle.

D'autres difficultés de l'alimentation artificielle proviennent des dangers d'infection et de décomposition, auxquels le lait animal se trouve exposé avant son ingestion même: le lait maternel est prémuni contre ces dangers. On n'a appris à les éviter dans l'allaitement artificiel. que depuis que l'on a compris l'insuffisance de la propreté macroscopique et la nécessité de l'asepsie. En cette matière. la fabrication du lait stérilisé constitue le plus grand progrès du siècle. Pour réaliser cette condition d'une manière satisfaisante on n'a pas besoin de chauffer le lait une demi-heure à 100 degrés: il suffit de le faire bouillir pendant cinq minutes, dix au plus. Et même un lait chauffé pendant vingt-cinq minutes à 62 degrés paraît subir une stérilisation parfaite sans présenter les modifications fâcheuses de sa saveur et de sa valeur nutritive (Forster).

Si nous avons à nourrir artificiellement un nourrisson dyspeptique. c'est une tout autre affaire. Ici. le pouvoir digestif de l'intestin est troublé, ainsi que les modifications régulières des substances nutritives. C'est pourquoi l'énergie. acquise par l'élaboration des mêmes ingesta, est plus faible qu'à l'état normal. D'après des recherches de ces dernières années. ce n'est pas la protéine qui semble présenter les plus grandes difficultés, comme on le croyait il y a peu de temps, mais la graisse du lait. Au reste. ce fait est conforme à ce qu'ont montré les travaux analogues poursuivis chez l'adulte. Mais la trop grande proportion de matières azotées dans le lait peut également devenir dangereuse: et même le sucre. s'il n'est pas parfaitement brûlé. peut porter obstacle aux bons effets de l'alimentation.

Maintenant. le régime doit chercher à atteindre le but par une voie indirecte. On doit diminuer la quantité de graisse et de substance protéique du lait en le diminuant au tiers avec de l'eau bouillie: et. pour compenser la diminution énergétique ainsi réalisée. augmenter la quantité de sucre jusqu'à ce qu'elle corresponde à celle du lait maternel (7 pour 100). Outre cela. on peut encore enrichir le lait moins concentré que le lait naturel par un autre hydrate de carbone. Dans ce but, la soupe à la farine de biscotte est bien préférable à la simple farine (d'orge ou de froment. ou d'avoine. ou de riz).

De plus. on peut essayer de faciliter la digestion des substances azotées par une digestion artificielle préalable (lait peptonisé. lait de Voltmer. de Backhaus et autres en Allemagne).

D'autres médecins préfèrent diminuer seulement la quantité de substances protéiques du lait, tandis qu'ils cherchent à conserver la quantité originelle de graisse, en centrifugeant le lait dilué, de manière à obtenir 1 pour 100 de caséine, et 5 pour 100 de graisse (Gœrtner's Fettmilch) ou, en ajoutant des quantités exactement mesurées de crème au lait dilué (mélanges de Biedert) ou au petit lait (Monti).

Enfin, on a aussi remplacé avec succès le sucre de lait par un autre sucre plus parfaitement brûlé par les tissus de l'organisme, la maltose (Liebig's Suppe, Keller's Malzsuppe).

Voilà les principes les plus importants, qu'on a le plus souvent appliqués jusqu'ici pour la préparation des laits artificiels pour nourrissons débilités et malades.

On réussit avec l'une ou l'autre des méthodes indiquées, mais en tâtonnant : nous n'avons pas encore dépassé ce stade d'action thérapeutique. Si toutes donnent des échecs, c'est toujours au lait maternel qu'on revient : il est encore supérieur à tous les procédés d'alimentation artificielle, lorsqu'il s'agit d'une maladie grave.

LES PRINCIPES SCIENTIFIQUES POUR LA PRODUCTION D'UNE NOURRITURE PRESQUE ÉQUIVALENTE AU LAIT DE FEMME

RAPPORT

par M. le professeur MONTI,

de Vienne.

Dans les dernières dizaines d'années, les confrères de toutes les nations se sont efforcés d'approfondir la question de l'alimentation artificielle des nourrissons et ont inventé de nombreuses méthodes.

Dans toutes ces méthodes, on a tâché de compenser les différences entre le lait de femme et celui de vache d'une façon trop exclusive : les unes tâchent de balancer la trop haute teneur en caséine par la dilution, les autres corrigent le défaut de sucre et de graisse par l'addition de sucre, de lait et de graisse. Mais jamais la qualité totale de la nourriture ne fut prise en considération, de sorte que d'après l'une des méthodes on donne trop peu d'albumine, d'après l'autre trop de graisse.

Sans doute, il y a des nourrissons qui se développent bien, même quand ils sont nourris d'après ces divers procédés, malgré les défauts qu'ils ont, mais on n'a pas encore trouvé un procédé d'alimentation équivalent à l'alimentation par le lait de femme.

Récemment M. *Heubner* a proposé une méthode d'alimentation basée sur la valeur en calories. Mais comme le fait très bien remarquer Baginsky, les chiffres de calories donnent peut-être des points d'appui généraux pour l'alimentation, mais jamais cette base théorique ne pourra nous aider à remplacer en pratique l'albumine par la graisse ou la graisse par les hydrates de carbone.

L'organisme infantile ne peut prospérer que lorsqu'il reçoit une nourriture, qui contient les substances chimiques nécessaires pour le développement de son corps. A cet égard, je suis d'accord avec Baginsky, qui dit que l'organisme infantile supporte mieux une nourriture qualitativement incorrecte qu'une mixture dont la composition quantitative correspond exactement aux exigences théoriques de la loi des calories. Nous savons très bien que, lorsque l'organisme a besoin de graisse, on n'obtient pas la même chose quand on remplace la graisse par le sucre, quoique celui-ci ait la même valeur en calories que celle-là. Enfin la caséine n'est pas équivalente à l'albumine soluble pour la digestion des enfants.

Le même auteur qui, il y a 15 ans, avait combattu chaleureusement la dilution du lait, alors en usage (dilution diminuant avec le progrès de l'âge de l'enfant), et qui affirmait hautement que la dilution du lait de vache avec des parties égales d'eau suffit complètement pour toute la période de l'allaitement, est aujourd'hui d'avis que la dilution du lait avec de l'eau n'a d'autre but que de mouiller les langes et que le nourrisson sain peut digérer les éléments nutritifs du lait de vache aussi bien que ceux du lait de femme. M. Heubner admet bien que le travail de digestion est plus grand pour le lait de vache que pour celui de femme, parce qu'une plus grande quantité d'albumine et une plus petite quantité d'hydrates de carbone participent à la production d'énergie et parce que la grosse molécule d'albumine est plus difficilement dissociée que la petite molécule de sucre. Heubner admet également qu'après la digestion du lait de vache le résidu fécal est beaucoup plus grand qu'après la digestion du lait de femme. L'opinion qu'un nouveau-né, nourri au lait de vache pur peut se développer aussi bien qu'un enfant nourri au sein, ne saurait être généralisée. Pour prouver cette affirmation, il ne suffit pas de faire un petit nombre de recherches, il faut continuer les recherches plusieurs mois sur le même individu. On observe alors que l'enfant supporte bien le lait pur quelques semaines, mais que le résidu fécal est 4 à 5 fois plus grand que celui d'un enfant nourri au sein et que son poids reste bien au-dessous de celui des enfants nourris au lait de femme, les fermentations ou la pourriture des matières fécales produisent de temps à autre des troubles de la fonction intestinale, qui entravent le développement de l'enfant, troubles qui, à leur tour, donnent lieu à un arrêt de développement.

Nous savons que le lait de femme ne peut être remplacé que par un lait d'animal dont la composition se rapproche le plus de celui-là. Mais il nous manque une base pour accommoder ce lait aux exigences du nourrisson. Les opinions des différents auteurs sur cette question sont si divergentes que leur discussion ne correspondrait pas au but de cette assemblée. Si l'on veut faire quelque chose de durable dans cette matière, il faut d'abord s'entendre sur les principes d'après lesquels on peut rapprocher le lait d'animal de celui de la femme.

Il est vrai que c'est difficile, mais possible, car l'affirmation de Heubner, qui dit que le lait de vache se distingue à peine au point de vue des matières nutritives principales du lait de femme, est erronée, comme nous le verrons plus tard.

Il s'ensuit qu'un rapport sur la valeur des méthodes connues de l'alimentation artificielle des nourrissons ne serait pas fructueux dans cette assemblée, parce que les confrères ne sont pas encore d'accord sur les principes fondamentaux de cette question.

Je ne ferai donc pas une critique des diverses méthodes d'alimentation artificielle, mais je me permettrai de soumettre à l'appréciation de cette haute assemblée quelques propositions qui nous permettront peut-être de poser des principes généraux, d'après lesquels l'alimentation artificielle des nourrissons pourrait devenir presque équivalente à l'alimentation naturelle par le lait de femme et être ainsi accommodée aux facultés digestives et aux exigences des nourrissons.

Il va sans dire que la qualité et la composition du lait de femme doivent former les éléments fondamentaux de ces principes, et que la question de l'alimentation artificielle des nourrissons ne sera résolue que lorsque nous réussirons à imiter aussi complètement que possible la composition du lait de femme.

Je fais abstraction de l'emploi du lait de différentes espèces animales, telles que l'ânesse, la chèvre, etc., etc et des divers succédanés artificiels du lait et je me borne seulement au lait de vache, qui est presque partout employé pour l'alimentation artificielle des enfants.

I

Acidité.

Je veux d'abord discuter la qualité du lait de vache qui diffère le plus de celle du lait de femme, et contribue le plus à l'échec de l'alimentation artificielle; c'est l'acidité. Nous nous servons pour le dosage de l'acidité du lait d'une solution normale de soude (à 1 10), que nous employons pour le titrage de 5 centimètres cubes de lait.

D'après les recherches de mes assistants, MM. Wolf et Friedjung, le lait de femme récent a une acidité de 0, 1, tandis que le lait de vache non bouilli présente une acidité qui, selon la saison et la durée de la conservation, arrive à 1, 1 et même au delà.

Cette différence des deux sortes de lait a de graves conséquences. Tandis que le lait de femme coagule lentement en fins flocons quand on ajoute de la présure, la coagulation du lait de vache se fait rapidement et en grands flocons et oppose à l'action des sucs digestifs une résistance beaucoup plus grande que le lait de femme.

Cet inconvénient fut reconnu par tous les auteurs et en effet on a cherché par divers moyens à abaisser le degré de l'acidité du lait de vache. D'après les recherches faites par mes assistants Wolf et Friedjung, sous ma direction, on peut abaisser l'acidité du lait de vache par la cuisson jusqu'à 0,9 : par la stérilisation à la suite de la précipitation des sels calcaires seulement jusqu'à 1, 0.

L'abaissement de l'acidité peut être atteint le mieux par la dilution avec de l'eau ou d'autres liquides. Plus la dilution est grande, plus l'acidité diminue. C'est ainsi qu'on arrive par un coupage avec une quantité égale d'eau à une acidité de 0, 55. Mais on n'arrive jamais à réduire l'acidité du lait de vache à celle du lait de femme par le coupage à l'eau. De là la nécessité d'ajouter un alcali.

Toutes les sortes de lait destinées à l'alimentation artificielle ont un trop haut degré d'acidité. C'est ainsi que le lait de Gaertner et celui de Backhaus ont une acidité de 0,5 à 0,6. Le mélange de lait et de petit-lait (que je désigne par le nom « lait de nourrisson ») a une acidité de 0,7 à 0,8 qui doit être réduite.

Pour rapprocher la coagulabilité du lait de vache destiné à l'alimentation artificielle du lait de femme, il faut lui ajouter une certaine quantité d'alcali.

Cette proposition n'est pas nouvelle. Déjà Alfred Vogel a observé que, lorsqu'on ajoute du carbonate de soude au lait de vache dilué avec de l'eau, celui-ci se comporte de même que celui de femme quand on le traite avec la présure et l'acide chlorhydrique.

D'après les recherches mentionnées de mes assistants, une quantité de 5 grammes de carbonate de soude par litre suffit pour abaisser l'acidité du lait de vache à celle du lait de femme. Si l'on dilue le lait de vache avec des parties égales d'eau, il suffit d'ajouter 2 grammes et demi de carbonate de soude; à une dilution de une partie de lait et deux parties d'eau, il ne faut ajouter que un gramme et 70 centigrammes de carbonate de soude. Lorsqu'on dilue le lait avec du petit-lait dans une proportion de 1 : 1, on peut donner au mélange l'acidité du lait de femme par l'addition de 4 grammes de carbonate par litre du mélange. L'addition de bicarbonate de soude d'après la proposition de Ashby ne peut pas produire un pareil degré d'acidité.

Je crois donc que, quelle que soit la manière de coupage du lait, l'acidité de la nourriture artificielle administrée au nourrisson doit être la même que celle du lait de femme. Le but peut être atteint par le carbonate de soude.

II

Coagulation par la présure.

La manière dont se comportent les différents mélanges vis-à-vis de la présure est importante pour l'appréciation de la valeur des méthodes d'alimentation artificielle au lait de vache.

D'après les recherches faites dans mon laboratoire par mes assistants, 5 centimètres cubes de lait de vache non cuit coagulent lorsqu'on ajoute 0,5 centimètre cube de présure française, dans un délai de 5 minutes, et forment un caillot dur; pour le lait cuit cette coagulation a lieu en 12 et pour le lait stérilisé en 15 minutes. Le lait dilué avec de l'eau se comporte d'une façon variable selon le degré de dilution : un mélange d'une partie de lait et de deux parties d'eau coagule sous l'action de la présure en 17 minutes, le mélange de parties égales de lait et d'eau coagule en 14 minutes et le mélange de deux parties de lait et d'une partie d'eau en 10 minutes.

Le lait de Backhaus ne coagule qu'après trois quarts d'heure N° I en fins flocons, N° II en flocons moyens et N° III en caillot dur. Le lait de Gaertner coagule également en trois quarts d'heure en fins flocons. Le lait de nourrisson introduit par moi dans la pratique coagule dans la proportion d'une partie de lait sur deux parties de petit-lait au bout de 15 minutes en flocons très fins.

Le lait de femme ne coagule pas sous l'action de la présure seule.

Les choses se passent autrement quand l'acidité du lait de vache est abaissée jusqu'à celle du lait de femme par l'addition d'un alcali. D'après les recherches de mes assistants, la coagulation est retardée par l'alcali et le caillot est moins dur, mais il reste toujours une différence entre le lait de vache et celui de femme. Seulement, le mélange de lait et de petit-lait montre une coagulation analogue à celle du lait de femme.

Au point de vue de la coagulation, aucune des méthodes usuelles ne correspond aux exigences mentionnées. Seulement, l'abaissement de l'acidité du lait de vache donne lieu à une coagulation analogue à celle du lait de femme sous l'action de la présure.

III

Matières albuminoïdes.

L'accommodation des matières albuminoïdes du lait de vache à celles du lait de femme présente des difficultés sérieuses. La quantité de caséine du lait de femme est inférieure, celle de l'albumine soluble (lactalbumine et lactoglobine) est plus forte que dans le lait de vache. La proportion varie selon l'âge du lait de femme, c'est-à-dire selon l'intervalle qui s'est écoulé depuis l'accouchement.

Quoiqu'il n'y ait pas d'analyses exactes du lait de femme dans les différentes périodes de la lactation en nombre suffisant pour permettre des conclusions sûres et malgré les différences individuelles, nos connaissances actuelles suffisent pour établir les chiffres moyens suivants concernant la teneur du lait de femme en albumine dans les différentes périodes de la lactation.

Ordinairement on distingue le premier lait, qui suffit aux besoins de l'enfant dans les premières quatre à six semaines de la vie; le jeune lait qui suffit pour les facultés digestives du nourrisson du 2ᵉ au 4ᵉ mois; le lait mûr, qui satisfait l'enfant jusqu'à l'âge de 7 mois et le lait vieux qui montre déjà une diminution des substances nécessaires pour le développement du corps et nous force de compléter la nourriture par des aliments étrangers.

	caséine	d'albumine soluble.
100 parties premier lait contiennent approximativement	1.55	1.62
— du jeune lait	0.85	1.19
— du lait mûr	0.99	1.0
— du lait vieux	0.76	0.84

Il s'ensuit que la quantité d'albumine diminue dans le cours de la lactation, mais que la quantité d'albumine soluble dépasse toujours celle de la caséine.

On emploie généralement pour l'alimentation artificielle du lait de vache, provenant de plusieurs animaux, un mélange, qui contient des quantités variables de caséine et d'albumine soluble. Assurément le lait n'est pas le même dans les différentes villes, je ne parle que du lait de Vienne. Celui-ci contient 2.41 pour 100 de caséine et 0,80 — 1 pour 100 d'albumine soluble.

Si nous voulons employer un lait pareil pour l'alimentation artificielle, il faut diminuer la quantité de caséine comme dans le lait de femme dans les différentes périodes de la lactation et rapprocher la quantité d'albumine soluble autant que possible de celle du lait de femme.

Les méthodes connues ont tâché de réduire la quantité de caséine du lait de vache par l'addition d'un liquide exempt d'albumine, mais le coupage diminue également la quantité déjà trop petite d'albumine soluble.

Si l'on coupe le lait de vache avec deux parties d'eau pour en former une nourriture pour le nouveau-né, ce mélange contient 0,81 pour 100 de caséine et 0,24 à 0,55 d'albumine soluble, tandis que le lait de femme à cette période contient 1,55 pour 100 de caséine et 1,62 pour 100 d'albumine soluble. Ce mélange ne correspond pas au premier lait, il est insuffisant pour un nouveau-né, parce qu'il contient trop peu d'albumine soluble et même de caséine. Si l'on voulait employer ce mélange comme nourriture au delà du premier mois, comme succédané du lait de femme, qui contient 0,85 pour 100 de caséine et 1,19 pour 100 d'albumine soluble, la quantité de caséine serait à peu près suffisante, mais celle de l'albumine soluble serait beaucoup inférieure aux exigences. En outre, la caséine du lait de vache étant moins digestible que celle du lait de femme, il y aurait des troubles digestifs.

Quand on dilue le lait de vache avec des parties égales d'eau, la teneur du mélange en caséine s'élève à 1,21 pour 100 et celle de l'albumine soluble à 0,40 — 0,50 pour 100, mais ce mélange ne remplace pas le lait de femme mûr, qui contient 0,99 pour 100 de caséine et 1 pour 100 d'albumine soluble. Ledit mélange contient la caséine en abondance, mais presque la moitié de la quantité nécessaire d'albumine soluble.

Ces faits prouvent que la dilution du lait de vache avec des parties égales d'eau ne suffit pas pour l'alimentation des nourrissons depuis la naissance jusqu'à l'âge de neuf mois, et qu'elle ne correspond pas aux conditions du lait de femme.

Le mélange de deux parties de lait de vache et une partie d'eau.

proposé par beaucoup d'auteurs comme succédané du lait vieux ne satisfait non plus à toutes les exigences, parce qu'il contient 1,65 pour 100 de caséine et 0,55 à 0,66 pour 100 d'albumine soluble.

Il s'ensuit qu'aucune manière de dilution du lait de vache avec de l'eau ne peut pas accommoder les albumines de ce lait à celles du lait de femme, et que ces mélanges sont très pauvres en albumine soluble. Mais nous savons que le nourrisson ne peut pas résorber une nourriture composée principalement de caséine de la même manière que celle qui contient un surplus d'albumine soluble, car celle-ci est résorbée directement, tandis que la caséine subit sous l'influence du suc gastrique une série de transformations avant d'être absorbée comme peptone. Une nourriture composée principalement de caséine produit chez le nouveau-né des troubles digestifs, parce que le suc gastrique ne peut pas transformer toute la caséine en peptone. C'est pourquoi le lait de femme contient dans les premières semaines et mois beaucoup plus d'albumine soluble, qui peut être absorbée, même par le suc gastrique des enfants du premier âge. Plus l'enfant se développe, plus la quantité de lactalbumine diminue dans le lait, parce que la faculté digestive de l'estomac augmente et l'enfant peut digérer une nourriture qui contient relativement beaucoup de caséine.

C'est pourquoi toutes les méthodes d'alimentation artificielle qui ne tiennent pas compte de cette relation entre l'albumine soluble et la caséine donnent des résultats défavorables dans les premiers trois mois, malgré l'observation stricte de toutes les règles concernant la quantité de la nourriture et les intervalles parmi les repas.

Pour accommoder les matières albuminoïdes du lait de vache à celles du lait de femme, il faut donc réduire la quantité de caséine et augmenter celle de l'albumine soluble. Ce but ne peut être atteint que par le coupage du lait de vache par un liquide, qui contient de l'albumine soluble. D'après mon expérience, ce but ne peut être atteint qu'avec le petit-lait.

On prépare le petit-lait de la manière suivante : On chauffe 900 grammes de lait à 40 degrés, et on ajoute deux cuillères à café d'essence de présure. Après la coagulation, on agite le mélange et on le filtre par un linge fin. Pour éliminer toute trace de présure, on chauffe le petit-lait avant de l'employer à 60 degrés. Le petit-lait préparé du lait frais présente une réaction alcaline et contient 0,80 à 1 gramme d'albumine soluble et un reste, environ 0,05 de caséine.

Si l'on mêle une partie de lait avec deux parties de petit-lait pour remplacer le premier lait, qui contient 1,55 pour 100 de caséine et 1,62 pour 100 d'albumine soluble, le mélange contient 0,82 de caséine et 0.80 à 1 gramme d'albumine soluble. Le défaut de caséine n'est pas nuisible, parce que, comme nous verrons plus tard, la caséine de lait de vache, à cause de sa composition différente, est plus difficilement digérée par l'estomac du nouveau-né. Il est vrai que dans cette méthode la quantité d'albumine soluble est inférieure à celle du premier lait de femme, mais elle est toutefois trois fois plus grande que dans le mélange analogue à l'eau. Le nouveau-né, qui recevra cette nourriture, n'augmentera pas de volume dans la même mesure qu'avec le lait de femme, mais il n'aura pas les troubles digestifs si désagréables.

Le jeune lait de femme contient 0,85, le lait mûr 0,99, et le lait vieux 0,76 pour 100 de caséine et 1,19, 1,0 et 0,84 pour 100 d'albumine soluble. Si nous mélons le lait de vache et le petit-lait en quantités égales pour remplacer le lait de femme dans les trois périodes de lactation, le mélange contiendra 1,22 pour 100 de caséine et 0,80 — 1,0 d'albumine soluble, soit un peu plus de caséine que dans le lait de femme. Mais cette différence a trait à une époque où l'enfant augmente le plus de poids, elle n'est donc pas nuisible. En tout cas la proportion est beaucoup plus favorable que dans le coupage à l'eau. A l'époque où l'enfant devrait recevoir du lait jeune, la teneur du mélange en albumine soluble est un peu moindre, plus tard elle est égale à celle du lait de femme, et c'est pourquoi les enfants digèrent mieux cette nourriture.

Bien que le coupage du lait de vache avec du petit-lait ne fournisse pas la même teneur en caséine et en albumine soluble pour toutes les périodes de lactation que dans le lait de femme, on obtient avec ce mélange des résultats beaucoup plus favorables qu'avec la dilution à l'eau. Je vous assure que j'ai obtenu avec ce mélange les meilleurs résultats, quoiqu'il ne puisse remplacer le lait de femme dans tous les cas.

Une autre difficulté dans l'accommodation du lait de vache aux conditions du lait de femme est la différence des deux sortes de caséine.

La caséine du lait de femme est précipitée difficilement par des sels et des acides, le précipité se dissout dans un excès d'acide, et la diges ion de ce précipité avec la pepsine ne donne pas de pseudo-nucléine.

La caséine du lait de vache est facilement précipitée par des sels et des acides, le précipité se dissout dans un excès d'acide et appartient au groupe des nucléo-albumines. Ces différences sont en accord avec la différence dans la composition chimique :

	C	H	N	P	S	O
Caséine du lait de femme	52.24	7.52	14.90	0,68	11,17	25,66
— de vache	55.00	7.00	25.70	0.85	0,80	22,65

Cette différence ne peut pas être conservée, mais la quantité suffisante d'albumine soluble contenue dans le petit-lait permet une meilleure utilisation des albumines que lorsqu'on emploie le lait coupé d'eau.

Cela est prouvé par une série d'expériences faites sous ma direction par mes assistants Wolf et Friedjung avec toutes les méthodes d'alimentation artificielle. Les différents mélanges des diverses méthodes furent traités de la façon suivante :

Cinq centimètres cubes du mélange furent mêlés avec 0,5 centimètre cube de présure. Au bout d'un quart d'heure on a ajouté 1 gramme de pepsine, 20 gouttes d'acide chlorhydrique et 100 grammes d'eau distillée. La digestion fut continuée pendant trois heures. **Pendant ce temps** le mélange fut agité toutes les dix minutes pour imiter les conditions de la digestion stomacale, puis on a filtré et pesé le résidu. Le poids moyen de ce résidu était :

de 2.8 grammes en employant du lait non écrémé.

    1.8   —   —   — non écrémé stérilisé.

    0.9   un mélange de 1 partie lait :
                                        2 parties d'eau.

1,1   grammes en employant un mélange de 1 partie de lait et 1 d'eau.

1,5   —   —   2   1

1,1   —   le lait de Gaertner.

0,4   —   le lait de Backhaus. . . . . N° I

1,7   —   —   — . . . . . N° II

2,0   —   —   — . . . . . N° III

0,7   —   le lait des nourrisons. . . . 1:2

1,2   —   — 1:1

Traces   —   le lait de femme.

On voit donc qu'au point de vue de la digestion de la caséine aucune méthode d'alimentation artificielle n'équivaut au lait de femme : toutefois le mélange de lait et de petit-lait donne des résultats très favorables. De plus, en approchant le degré d'acidité à celui du lait de femme par un alcali, les résultats de l'essai de digestion avec celui dit « lait de nourrissons » s'approchent de ceux du lait de femme.

Quoique le mélange de lait et de petit-lait ne soit pas un succédané complet du lait de femme, les échecs de cette méthode sont beaucoup moins fréquents que ceux des autres méthodes d'alimentation artificielle

IV

Graisses.

Une autre difficulté consiste dans l'accommodation de la graisse du lait de vache à celle du lait de femme.

La graisse du lait de femme est relativement pauvre en acides volatils et les graisses non volatiles contiennent pour la moitié de l'acide oléinique: parmi les graisses solides, les acides miristique et palmitique prédominent sur l'acide stéarique.

Le lait de vache contient environ 70 pour 100 d'acides graisseux volatils, et les acides non volatils sont formés seulement de 0,5 — 0,1 pour 100 d'oléine, le reste sont les acides palmitique et stéarique. En outre on trouve dans la graisse du lait de vache les acides caprylique, laurique et arachique, lécithine et cholestérine.

Outre ces différences, la relation entre la graisse et les albumines est bien différente dans les deux sortes de lait. Selon Goroup-Besanez, il y a dans le lait de femme sur 100 parties d'albumine 68, dans celui de vache 79 parties de graisse. Cette différence serait encore plus grande après d'autres auteurs.

Par la dilution du lait de vache avec de l'eau, la quantité de graisse devient trop basse, et la relation entre la graisse et les albumines est trop déplacée. Pour obvier à cet inconvénient, on a ajouté une certaine quantité de graisse de lait de vache. Mais cette graisse est difficilement émulsionnée dans l'organisme infantile par la bile et le suc pancréatique et passe pour la plupart par le canal digestif sans être résorbée. Un séjour prolongé de cette graisse dans l'intestin des enfants peut donner lieu à l'auto-intoxication aux acides gras.

L'addition de graisse du lait de vache est nuisible d'après mes expériences et les méthodes qui l'emploient sont à regretter.

Si l'on dilue le lait avec du petit-lait au lieu d'eau, la teneur de la nourriture en graisse est beaucoup plus favorable, parce que le petit-lait préparé de la façon décrite contient 1 pour 100 de graisse. Lorsqu'on agite le petit-lait fortement avant la filtration, la quantité de graisse peut monter, selon Ashby, jusqu'à 2 pour 100, de sorte que le mélange de lait de vache et de petit-lait contienne presque la même quantité de graisse que le lait de femme. Lorsque le petit-lait ne contient que 1 pour 100 de graisse :

le mélange de lait de vache et petit-lait 1:2 contient 1,88 0/0 de graisse.
            —   1:1   2,33 0/0

D'après mes recherches sur le lait de femme, une teneur de 2 pour 100 de graisse suffit complètement pour l'alimentation, quoiqu'il supporte aussi 3 pour 100. Un lait qui contient un peu moins de 2 pour 100 n'est pas très désavantageux pour le nourrisson, parce que la graisse de lait de vache est sans cela mal utilisée par ces organes digestifs. Par la dilution 1 : 1, dans les mois ultérieurs, la quantité de graisse devient égale à celle du lait de femme. C'est pourquoi l'addition de graisse est inutile dans cette méthode.

Dans le lait de femme, la graisse se trouve dans une fine émulsion et contribue par sa fine suspension à la coagulation du lait et à la précipitation de la caséine en fins flocons.

Dans le lait de vache, la graisse se trouve en gouttelettes grosses. L'addition de graisse obtenue par l'appareil centrifugeur provoque des conditions défavorables pour la digestion du nourrisson et devient nuisible. Lorsqu'on soumet le lait à l'action de la centrifugation, d'après la proposition de Gaertner, la structure de la graisse devient défavorable et sa résorption difficile.

Ce n'est donc que par la dilution au petit-lait que le lait de vache se rapproche au point de vue de la graisse le plus du lait de femme. Toutefois la relation entre l'albumine et la graisse n'est pas idéale, mais elle est encore meilleure que lorsqu'on ajoute de la graisse.

Le lait de vache contient moins de sucre que celui de femme. Cette proportion devient encore plus défavorable par la dilution à l'eau. Pour obvier à cet inconvénient, on a proposé d'ajouter du sucre de lait; on a voulu même remplacer le défaut de graisses par un excès de lactose. C'est ainsi que la méthode de Soxhlet, Heubner-Hoffmann diluent le lait avec des solutions qui contiennent jusqu'à 1.2 pour 100 de sucre, et celle de Marfan avec une solution à 10 pour 100 de sucre.

L'expérience pratique montre cependant que ces quantités de sucre calculées d'après des vues théoriques, ne sont pas bien utilisées par le nourrisson. Dans ces méthodes d'alimentation, le sucre devient la *proie* des bactéries de l'intestin grêle et donne lieu à la fermentation d'acide lactique qui, selon son intensité, donne lieu à des dyspepsies ou à des catarrhes de l'intestin grêle. Ces méthodes sont donc plutôt nuisibles; en tout cas elles ne peuvent pas rapprocher le lait de vache de celui de femme.

Lorsqu'on dilue le lait de vache avec du petit-lait au lieu de solutions sucrées, la teneur naturelle du lait en sucre (4,5 à 5 pour 100) ne se change pas, parce que le petit-lait contient toute la quantité primitive du sucre, tandis que dans

```
le mélange à l'eau 1:2 la quantité du sucre tombe à   1.5    16
       —               1:2                        —    2.25  2.50
                       2:1                        —    5.0   5.50
```

L'avantage du coupage au petit-lait au point de vue de la teneur en sucre est donc évident, d'autant plus que la solution naturelle de sucre du lait est meilleure que les solutions artificielles de sucre.

Une autre cause d'échec de l'alimentation artificielle doit être cherchée dans les sels minéraux, dont la quantité contenue dans le lait de vache dépasse celle du lait de femme. C'est ainsi que le lait de vache contient six fois plus de Ca O et quatre fois plus de P_2O_5 et en somme 0.70 pour 100 de sels, tandis que le lait de femme n'en a que 0,15 à 0.55 pour 100. La dilution à l'eau fait en partie disparaître cette disproportion, tandis que celle au petit-lait la conserve, parce que le petit-lait contient toutes les substances minérales du lait. Malgré cela les résultats de l'alimentation avec le mélange de lait et petit-lait ne sont pas défavorables, en tout cas plus favorables qu'avec le lait dilué d'eau.

Le lait de femme est presque toujours stérile et ne peut infecter par des bactéries que lorsqu'il provient de personnes malades.

Le lait de vache contient toutes les bactéries du lait et parfois même des microbes pathogènes, comme celui de la dipthérie, de la tuberculose, des fièvres typhoïdes, etc. Le lait de vache ne doit donc pas être administré à l'état cru, il faut d'abord éloigner le *danger* des microbes. On a proposé dans ce but plusieurs procédés.

Nous faisons abstraction des moyens chimiques et mécaniques (force centrifuge, froid, etc.), les uns altèrent trop le lait, les autres sont insuffisants.

Par la simple cuisson du lait, la plupart des bactéries pathogènes est tuée, mais le lait n'est pas durable, parce que les bactéries du lait peuvent se développer encore et *tourner* le lait.

L'échauffement du lait à 60 degrés pendant dix minutes suffit pour tuer les microbes pathogènes sans altérer le lait, mais les ferments de la caséine, le bacillus subtilis, le bacillus thyrothrix tenuis, le bacillus mesentericus vulgatus résistent à ces températures, et même après la cuisson à 100 degrés, il reste des spores de ces bacilles qui peuvent encore se développer.

Mais l'action des hautes températures altère le goût du lait et la composition chimique de ses éléments: par l'altération de la lactose, le lait a un goût de caramel, la lactalbumine coagule, d'après Hammarsten, déjà à 72 - 84 degrés, la caséine coagule dans un pareil lait en flocons gros et durs: la fine émulsion des globules lactés est détruite, les acides graisseux sont mis en liberté et donnent au lait un goût désagréable, même les sels sont transformés dans une forme insoluble et sont précipités. De cette manière on crée des conditions défavorables à la digestion et l'utilisation de la nourriture devient difficile.

Il faut donc employer une méthode de stérilisation, qui soit dépourvue de ces inconvénients. Soxhlet a le grand mérite d'avoir créé une pareille méthode.

Du lait tiré proprement est chauffé en petites portions en flacons fermés à la température de l'eau bouillante pendant 35 à 40 minutes. Comme les flacons restent fermés, ils sont protégés contre toute infection ultérieure.

Mais par la cuisson prolongée, le lait subit les altérations mentionnées, et pourtant d'après les recherches de Flügge, les saprophytes ne sont pas complètement tués, mais ils sont seulement réduits à un minimum, et il reste encore une quantité de spores qui peuvent se développer.

D'après ma longue expérience clinique, je dois dire que le lait stérilisé selon le procédé de Soxhlet n'est pas si bien utilisé que le lait simplement cuit. La quantité des excréments est plus grande et les dyspepsies, les catarrhes intestinaux, sont aussi fréquents qu'avec le lait non stérilisé, parce que les bactéries intestinales agissent sur les restes non digérés du lait stérilisé, qui subissent la fermentation d'acide lactique ou la putréfaction. Cela a eu lieu même quand on observe les mesures les plus rigoureuses de *propreté*, et les prescriptions exactes au point de vue de la quantité des portions. C'est ainsi qu'on voit des nourrissons nourris au lait stérilisé augmentant parfois de poids, mais que ce poids reste enfin au-dessous de celui des enfants nourris au sein. Les enfants nourris par le lait stérilisé deviennent aussi anémiques et rachitiques.

Je ne peux donc pas me rallier à l'opinion de ceux qui croient que les enfants nourris d'après le procédé de Soxhlet se développent aussi bien que ceux nourris au sein. C'est là *une exagération*. D'autres auteurs sont du même avis.

Je devais donc recourir à la stérilisation d'après Soxhlet, de même qu'à la stérilisation fractionnée, d'autant plus que dans le lait mêlé au petit-lait l'albumine soluble est coagulée par ces procédés.

Je fais donc chauffer le lait à 60—70 degrés pendant dix minutes, puis je le laisse refroidir jusqu'à 6 degrés, et je le conserve à cette température jusqu'au moment de l'emploi. Ce procédé est actuellement le meilleur, et je suis convaincu que la plupart des confrères partageront mon avis.

Il va sans dire que les détails du procédé de Soxhlet : cuisson par portions, empêchement d'une infection nouvelle, etc., doivent être appliqués également dans la méthode que je viens de proposer, et qu'à cet égard les mérites de Soxhlet restent sans restriction.

Il est vrai que cette méthode ne saurait non plus atteindre le lait de femme. Il serait à désirer qu'on puisse stériliser le lait sans le cuire. Mais les procédés proposés jusqu'à ce jour ne suffisent pas, les filtres laissent passer une partie des microbes et les filtres, comme ceux de Chamberland, qui retiennent les microbes ne laissent pas passer le lait.

Marmier et Abraham ont obtenu des succès brillants avec la stérilisation de l'eau par l'ozone. Peut-être ce procédé sera-t-il utile aussi pour le lait.

Il nous reste encore à aborder la question de savoir si, avec l'accommodation si complète que possible du lait de vache au lait de femme, on réussit à administrer au nourrisson la même quantité quotidienne des principaux éléments : caséine, albumine soluble, graisse, sucre et sels, qu'avec la nourriture naturelle. La grandeur des repas étant différente selon la capacité de l'estomac du nourrisson, ces conditions sont dans toutes les méthodes connues différentes de celles de l'alimentation naturelle.

Pour mieux faire ressortir ces conditions, j'ai réuni dans un tableau les quantités quotidiennes des matières mentionnées, que le nourrisson reçoit aux différents âges d'après les diverses méthodes d'alimentation.

Dans la première semaine, 240 grammes de nourriture suffisent pour un enfant d'un poids au-dessous de 5 kilogrammes. Quand il est nourri avec du lait de femme, il reçoit 5,24 grammes de caséine et 5,89 grammes d'albumine soluble : avec le mélange de lait et d'eau 1 : 2, il reçoit 1,94 de caséine et 0,65 — 0,79 d'albumine soluble, soit une quantité absolument insuffisante : avec le mélange de lait et petit-lait 1 : 2, il reçoit 1,97 caséine et 1,92 à 2,40 d'albumine soluble. La quantité trop basse de caséine n'est pas nuisible, celle de l'albumine soluble satisfait parfaitement aux besoins d'un pareil enfant.

Dans les deuxième et troisième semaines il reçoit une nourriture quotidienne de 515 grammes, ce qui fait avec le lait de femme, 4,25 grammes de caséine et 5,20 grammes d'albumine soluble : avec le mélange de lait et d'eau 1 : 2, il reçoit 2,55 grammes de caséine et 0,85 — 1,04 grammes d'albumine soluble; avec le mélange de lait et petit-lait 1 : 2, il reçoit 2,58 grammes de caséine et 2,52 grammes d'albumine soluble. Dans le coupage avec l'eau, la quantité d'albumine soluble est trop basse, tandis que dans le mélange de lait et petit-lait, elle correspond toutefois aux exigences de l'enfant.

Dans la quatrième semaine, l'enfant reçoit avec une quantité de 420 grammes par jour avec le lait de femme 5,67 grammes de caséine et 6,80 grammes d'albumine soluble : avec le mélange de lait et d'eau

1 : 2, il reçoit 5,40 grammes de caséine et 1,15 — 1.59 d'albumine soluble, soit trop peu ; avec le mélange de lait et de petit-lait 1 : 2, il reçoit 5.44 grammes de caséine et 5.56 — 4.20 grammes d'albumine soluble.

Des conditions analogues se trouvent dans les semaines ultérieures.

La quantité quotidienne de graisse qu'un enfant reçoit avec le lait dilué d'eau est beaucoup inférieure à celle qu'il reçoit avec le lait de femme. Dans le mélange de lait et de petit-lait, cette quantité est également inférieure, mais toutefois elle suffit aux besoins du nourrisson.

La quantité du sucre est aussi inférieure dans le lait coupé d'eau à celui du lait de femme, tandis que dans le lait coupé de petit-lait, la teneur en sucre suffit aux besoins du nourrisson.

La quantité des sels dépasse dans toutes les méthodes d'alimentation artificielle celle du lait de femme.

De tout ce que nous venons d'exposer, il s'ensuit qu'aucune méthode d'alimentation artificielle ne fournit au nourrisson la même quantité quotidienne de caséine, d'albumine soluble, de graisse, de sucre et de sels que le lait de femme. C'est pourquoi l'alimentation artificielle ne peut pas mener au même développement de l'enfant que l'alimentation par le lait de femme.

De tous les procédés d'alimentation artificielle, celui du lait coupé de petit-lait se rapproche le plus des conditions naturelles.

STÉRILISATION DU LAIT ET MODE D'EMPLOI DU LAIT STÉRILISÉ

RAPPORT

par M. le docteur Axel JOHANNESSEN,

Professeur de l'Université de Kristiania

La section de Pédiatrie du Congrès international de Paris, 1900, m'a prié de fournir un rapport sur *Les procédés de stérilisation et résultats de l'emploi du lait stérilisé*. Je remercie la section de l'honneur qu'elle m'a ainsi fait et je lui suis reconnaissant de m'avoir donné l'occasion, à moi, représentant d'un petit pays isolé, d'apporter au milieu d'un auditoire si distingué ma modeste part contributive à l'étude de cette délicate et complexe question : *L'alimentation de l'enfant*.

Le peu de temps qui m'est accordé pour ce discours ne me permet pas d'entrer dans tous les détails du sujet.

Et d'abord, que comprend-on par lait stérilisé ?

On peut appeler lait stérilisé, dans la vraie signification du mot, tout lait dans lequel non seulement les bactéries, mais encore leurs spores sont détruites de manière qu'aucune culture nouvelle ne puisse se développer.

Pour obtenir cette complète stérilisation, on peut procéder de différentes façons.

Premièrement en faisant bouillir le lait très longtemps : 6 à 7 heures à une température de 100 degrés centigrades ; ou bien, en élevant la température et en diminuant proportionnellement la durée du chauffage. A 102, 105 degrés, on fait bouillir 3 heures 1/2 à 4 heures ; à 105 degrés, 1 heure ; à 107, 108 degrés, une demi-heure ; à 110 degrés, un quart d'heure.

Mais, par ce procédé, le lait subit de grandes modifications, il acquiert une teinte brun foncé et un goût désagréable de caoutchouc et ne peut, par conséquent, servir à l'alimentation.

On a essayé d'autres méthodes qui consistent à chauffer le lait à la vapeur d'eau sous pression, ce qui permet d'obtenir une plus haute élévation de température.

On a aussi employé le chauffage discontinu, ou tyndallisation, qui consiste à porter trois fois le lait à une température voisine de 100 degrés, une fois tous les jours pendant trois jours.

On parvient ainsi à avoir un lait stérilisé qui n'a pas perdu plus de son goût et de sa couleur que le lait bouilli.

Mais il a fallu renoncer à faire disparaître tout germe de bactéries et se contenter d'une stérilisation qui surtout détruit les organismes pathogènes vivants et autres bactéries qui ne résistent pas à une température supérieure à 100 degrés : cependant les spores de certaines bactéries, qui ont une plus grande vitalité, ne sont pas anéanties à cette température et peuvent encore se développer dans le lait.

Le point d'ébullition du lait est à 100 ou 101 degrés, mais avec le chauffage ordinaire on n'arrive guère qu'à 96 ou 98 degrés ; pour détruire, à ce degré thermique, les différentes bactéries, il est alors nécessaire que l'ébullition se prolonge pendant un certain temps. Cette durée peut être de 5 minutes ou trois quarts d'heure peu importe, l'essentiel est que le lait, immédiatement après la cuisson, soit placé dans un endroit d'une température au-dessous de 18 degrés. Un récipient quelconque, fermé ou ouvert, est suffisant pour cette cuisson.

On doit procéder avec une propreté rigoureuse, car, si les bouteilles destinées à contenir le lait n'étaient pas stériles, on courrait le danger d'une nouvelle infection.

La cuisson se fait également dans les bouteilles mêmes, au bain-marie. Cette méthode peut être employée dans les grandes industries ou dans les familles, lorsqu'on veut obtenir un lait stérilisé en partie.

On s'est demandé s'il était vraiment désirable de soumettre le lait à une température d'environ 100 degrés, laquelle lui fait acquérir un goût fade de bouilli, alors qu'une stérilisation complète ne peut être obtenue. De plus, ainsi que nous le verrons plus tard, le lait subit par ce procédé des altérations qui ne sont pas sans importance dans le rôle qu'il doit jouer comme succédané du lait de femme.

On a alors essayé d'appliquer au lait les mêmes principes que Pasteur, dès 1869, avait employés pour la conservation du vin, de la bière et autres liquides, méthode que l'on a appelée *pasteurisation*. La température peut varier entre 56 et 80 degrés.

Un lait est dit pasteurisé lorsqu'il a été chauffé durant 15 minutes à 75 degrés ou durant 50 minutes à 68 degrés.

Il est démontré que la température critique pour les bactéries pathogènes est entre 58 et 60 degrés ; pour les bacilles de la tuberculose, elle est un peu plus élevée, probablement vers 75 degrés et après 10 minutes de cuisson.

Toutefois, il résulte des recherches de Bitter qu'un chauffage porté à une moindre température, mais d'une plus longue durée, peut donner les mêmes résultats.

Avec la pasteurisation, comme avec la stérilisation partielle, il est indispensable, immédiatement après l'opération, de conserver le lait dans un endroit frais. La température préférable est de 12 à 14 degrés.

La stérilisation du lait a pris pour point de départ la loi établie par Pasteur, que les tissus et les humeurs d'un individu sain ne contiennent pas de germes, à moins qu'ils ne soient venus du monde extérieur. Il est cependant certain que le lait d'une femme en bonne santé n'est pas exempt de bactéries, mais, évidemment, ces bactéries sont venues du dehors et ont pénétré dans les canaux galactophores : toutefois, il est démontré que les premières portions du liquide recueilli sont seules contaminées, ensuite le lait est stérile.

Les bactéries qui se montrent dans le lait de vache appartiennent à deux groupes : celles du premier groupe peuvent provenir de la malpropreté, soit pendant, soit après la traite ; celles du deuxième groupe de la vache elle-même et, dans ce cas, elles sont susceptibles de transmettre la maladie dont la bête est atteinte.

Parmi les bactéries du premier groupe, on a étudié principalement les bacilles de l'acide lactique et les bacilles qui décomposent la caséine.

L'action de ces dernières bactéries, dont quelques espèces ont une influence nocive sur le canal intestinal et donnent de la diarrhée aux lapins et aux jeunes chiens, a été en partie attribuée à la peptonisation et en partie aux toxines (Flügge et Lübbert).

Quant aux bactéries anaérobies, comme le bacillus butyricus (Botkin et autres), l'opinion paraît mieux s'accorder sur leur importance et, quoique l'on reconnaisse leur nocuité, leur rôle est fort restreint parce qu'ils altèrent le lait à un tel point qu'il ne peut être consommé.

Indépendamment de ces bactéries, on en a observé d'autres, appartenant au même groupe, qui produisent parfois des phénomènes d'intoxication et donnent au lait une coloration rouge, jaune, bleue.

Mossler, Zundel et Demme ont fait des descriptions de l'état pathologique d'enfants qui avaient absorbé de ce lait et, dernièrement, un rapport a paru relatant la mort d'un enfant qui avait bu du lait infecté par des bacilles lactiques érythrogènes (Hueppe).

D'un autre côté, Baron essaya de démontrer que ces bactéries, de même que les bactéries du lait visqueux filant, n'étaient pas dangereuses.

Il est peut-être intéressant de savoir qu'en Norvège on consomme très bien ce lait visqueux. La coagulation est produite par des feuilles de *Pinguicula palustris* dans lesquelles on trouve en symbiose un microbe qui rend le lait visqueux. (*Streptrococcus hollandicus*, Weigmann.)

Le deuxième groupe des bactéries se compose d'organismes pathogènes. Elles peuvent provenir en partie de la malpropreté et en partie de la vache malade. Basch et Weleminsky supposent que ce sont seulement les bactéries qui peuvent arriver dans le lait qui sont capables de causer des hémorragies et autres accidents dans les glandes mammaires. Probablement qu'une lésion préexistante peut amener les mêmes désordres. Cette hypothèse est très douteuse pourtant en ce qui concerne les bacilles de la tuberculose même, quoiqu'on ait trouvé assez souvent qu'une femme tuberculeuse peut produire un lait stérile (Bang).

Au Congrès de la tuberculose tenu à Berlin en 1899, Bollinger a fait ressortir que le lait des animaux tuberculeux a des propriétés infectieuses non seulement par une mamelle tuberculeuse et par la tuberculose générale, mais aussi par la tuberculose locale.

Pour la plupart des autres maladies infectieuses on n'est pas d'accord à l'égard de leur transmission par le lait. Quelques-uns ont supposé que plusieurs maladies infectieuses de l'espèce humaine pouvaient paraître chez la vache et directement arriver au lait par un pis malade ou sain ; d'autres, que l'existence de pareilles bactéries spécifiques provenaient, accidentellement, de la contamination d'un individu malade.

Il est clair maintenant que la destruction de ces bactéries est désirable et nécessaire.

Cette méthode, produisant une bonne alimentation artificielle pour l'enfant nouveau-né qui a à lutter contre les bactéries, il est parfaitement explicable qu'elle ait pris une grande extension et rallié de nombreux et enthousiastes partisans ; en outre, elle s'accorde complètement avec les idées qu'on a maintenant sur l'étiologie des maladies.

Considérables sont aussi les rapports sur les bons résultats qu'on a obtenus avec un lait ainsi traité.

Il deviendra cependant bientôt évident que cette méthode n'est que le premier maillon dans la chaîne des conditions requises pour obtenir un bon succédané du lait de la mère.

Il sera d'abord nécessaire de savoir si le lait a déjà subi des modifications bacillaires avant le commencement du chauffage — modifications causées, soit par la négligence, soit par la malpropreté — et ensuite jusqu'à quel point un long transport, durant de fortes chaleurs, est favorable au développement des bactéries.

Ainsi, il faut faire ressortir, et le public doit comprendre, que la cuisson ne peut pas neutraliser l'influence nocive qu'une falsification ou qu'un défaut dans la nourriture des vaches peuvent avoir sur la qualité nutritive du lait, pas plus qu'elle ne peut tuer les spores de certaines bactéries, même si l'on porte le liquide à une ébullition prolongée à 100 degrés ; il faudrait pour cela arriver à 120 degrés.

Et ces spores peuvent encore se développer et donner naissance à de nouvelles bactéries qui, comme Soxhlet l'a déjà démontré dès 1891, sont capables de changer complètement le goût et l'aspect du lait par la fermentation de l'acide butyrique. Ces bactéries peptonisent la caséine au début, sans toutefois modifier le goût du lait ; plus tard, elles donnent au liquide de l'amertume.

La cuisson est loin d'avoir une action mortelle sur ces bactéries, bien au contraire, elles semblent se développer plus richement dans le lait bouilli que dans le lait cru et cela parce que la cuisson détruit les bacilles lactiques qui ont le pouvoir, en raison de leur grande quantité, d'empêcher d'autres bactéries de se développer (Soxhlet et Flügge).

Cependant, même si les bactéries sont tuées par l'ébullition, il peut encore se produire des toxines nuisibles qui ne sont pas détruites, comme le tyrotoxicon de Vaughan, les bactéries de Flügge (nᵒˢ 1, 5 et 7), le bacille nᵒ 1 de Lubbert, dans laquelle le corps du bacille vivant est montré empoisonné et, enfin, la toxine que Pasquale de Michele a trouvée formée dans le lait contenant des bacilles de la tuberculose, même après la destruction de ceux-ci.

Les empoisonnements causés par ces toxines revêtent un caractère aigu, mais je désire indiquer qu'ils peuvent aussi devenir chroniques. Je crois que la maladie appelée scorbut infantile (maladie de Barlow) doit venir de pareils empoisonnements chimiques.

Il faut se rappeler que plusieurs de ces toxines ne sont pas influencées par une courte cuisson et que, par conséquent, elles peuvent aussi développer leur action dans le lait dit stérilisé.

Cette manière de voir est également partagée par M. le professeur Torup à la suite d'analyses faites, à ce point de vue, sur le scorbut arctique à propos de l'expédition polaire de Nansen. Il paraît que partout où le scorbut s'est déclaré on a pu constater que les aliments avaient subi une plus ou moins grande décomposition, alors que le manque de végétaux qu'on avait supposé devoir jouer un grand rôle dans le développement de ces états a fait voir qu'il était sans importance (Nansen et Johansen sont restés 9 mois sans manger de végétaux : ils se sont nourris seulement de viande et de lard gelés).

Torup a, en outre, été capable, en faisant ingérer à des chiens une nourriture décomposée de la sorte, de produire chez eux un état pathologique ressemblant complètement aux graves formes du scorbut.

Harley a récemment, à la suite d'expériences faites sur des singes, entièrement confirmé ces résultats.

J'ai fait voir précédemment que la soi-disant stérilisation ordinaire ne neutralise pas toujours (jamais peut-être) les dangers que le lait, suivant son origine et son traitement, implique sous le rapport hygiénique.

J'arrive maintenant à montrer que la stérilisation elle-même fait subir au lait des modifications qui ne sont pas sans valeur dans la nourriture lactée.

Il est clair que par la cuisson à air libre le lait perd de son contenu d'eau — circonstance qui ne joue aucun rôle, excepté lorsqu'il est donné sans coupage.

La pasteurisation du lait peut, suivant les analyses de Woll, changer son poids spécifique ; 12 échantillons ont montré une baisse de 1,03303 à 1/0528.

La viscosité peut aussi, d'après les mêmes analyses, diminuer par la pasteurisation non seulement pour le lait mais encore pour la crème. Par la stérilisation, sous pression de vapeur d'eau, la viscosité diminue pour la crème, mais très peu pour le lait.

Par le chauffage le goût du lait s'altère. Des essais faits, pour la première fois en 1889, par M. Fjord, professeur à l'Institut agronomique de Copenhague, ont montré que le changement qui s'opère dans le goût du lait commence à 80 degrés ou, suivant Duclaux, à 75 degrés.

Thörner a pensé que la cause de cette modification peut être attribuée à la perte de CO_2. Cet auteur suppose encore qu'on peut empêcher cette altération par l'introduction de ce même gaz.

Je serais disposé à croire que le goût de bouilli provient de la décomposition des acides non saturés.

La faculté de caséifier le lait par l'action du lab-ferment est ordinairement perdue par la cuisson. Quelques-uns, comme Schaeffer, ont cru que la cause était due au départ de CO_2, quelques-uns encore, comme Enhlin, ont pensé que la quantité d'acide était diminuée, d'autres enfin, comme Ad. Meyer, que le défaut de caséification dépend de la haute température elle-même. Söldder a cependant montré que la raison de ce changement est à chercher dans les sels du lait, parce que les sels de calcium, par la cuisson, se transforment en partie en phosphate de calcium insoluble (principalement $Ca_3(PO_4)_2$. D'un autre côté, Hammarsten et, dernièrement, Arthus ont montré les grandes et décisives influences que les sels de chaux solubles exercent sur la caséification du lait. Cette caséification peut de nouveau avoir lieu lorsqu'on fait dissoudre les phosphates de calcium insolubles, soit en ajoutant avec précaution de l'acide phosphatique (Engling), soit par une introduction d'acide carbonique (Schaeffer et Söldner).

D'après de récentes recherches, les matières protéiques du lait se divisent en : *caséine*, *lactalbumine*, *lactoglobuline*. La caséine ne se coagule pas avant 150 degrés dans un vase fermé, mais il se forme, par l'ébullition, une pellicule à la surface du lait.

Soxhlet et Stohmann expliquent l'établissement de cette pellicule comme un dessèchement relatif de la surface du lait.

La lactalbumine et la lactoglobuline se coagulent de la même manière que les albumines et les globulines ordinaires.

Soxhlet et Rubner profitent, conséquemment, de l'absence de l'albu-

mine coagulable, après la précipitation de la caséine par l'acide,
pour constater si le lait a été cuit.

Mais, ainsi qu'il arrive toujours quand les substances albuminoïdes
se coagulent par la chaleur, il restera dans la solution, en même temps
que se fait la modification insoluble et coagulée, une partie d'albumine, soit comme un produit de la décomposition, soit comme un
reste inattaqué à cause des changements dans le liquide par la cuisson.

On voit, quand on a précipité toute la caséine du lait bouilli par un
moyen absolu de précipitation (Kalialun, p. ex.), qu'on peut toujours
avoir dans le liquide filtré avec le tanin assez de résidu provenant
d'une matière protéique.

M. Sebelien a bien voulu faire une série de recherches qui ont
montré qu'environ la moitié de l'azote contenue comme albumine
se dérobe à la coagulation par la stérilisation.

M. Sebelien a aussi observé à propos du degré de température où
se produit la coagulation que cette dernière, pour la **lactoglobuline**,
arrive vers 750 degrés dans une solution de 5,10 p. 100 de Nacl ; pour la
lactalbumine, elle varie suivant la quantité de Nacl de **72 à 84 degrés**.

Récemment Siegfried a trouvé dans le lait une substance qui,
selon lui, appartiendrait au groupe des **mucléo-protéides** et qu'il a
nommée acide *phospho-carnique* ou *nucleon*. On a attribué à la présence supposée de cette substance, de même qu'à ses rapports au lait
stérilisé, une certaine importance pour la nourriture de l'enfant.
Cependant, il convient d'attendre de nouvelles recherches sur les propriétés et sur la composition chimique de cette substance avant de
commencer à s'occuper de son rôle à cet égard.

Les résultats avec la méthode de Siegfried peuvent être facilement
compromis par différentes matières qui se trouvent dans le lait.

En outre de cette combinaison de phosphore, Stoklasa a montré
que le phosphore se trouve aussi dans la lécithine qui s'altère par la
cuisson. Suivant les recherches de Siegfried et de Stoklasa, le phosphore serait contenu dans le lait de femme 7 fois autant que dans le
lait de vache lié aux matières organiques.

Pour Keller et Knaeppelmacher le phosphore contenu dans le lait
de femme paraît être beaucoup mieux utilisé que le phosphore du lait
de vache.

Il est évident que les matières protéiques contenant du phosphore
surtout comme la lécithine qui, d'après Chabrie, a une grande importance pour le développement de l'organisme et pour la formation du
squelette, se trouvent non seulement en différentes quantités, mais

aussi dans des combinaisons chimiques toutes différentes dans les deux espèces de lait. La cuisson peut encore rendre le lait de vache plus pauvre en combinaisons organiques phosphoriques.

On peut donc conclure que ces faits ne sont pas sans importance pour la nutrition de l'enfant.

Quant à la graisse, on sait qu'une stérilisation à une température plus haute que 100 degrés ou qu'une plus longue cuisson à cette même température la modifient. Elle ne peut rester plus longtemps à l'état de fine émulsion, elle monte à la surface en une couche solidifiée.

Il est facile de s'imaginer qu'une stérilisation intensive, sous une haute pression, peut saponifier la graisse neutre et volatiliser les acides gras.

Autant que je sache, il n'existe pas de recherches à ce sujet.

Il est évident que les modifications de la graisse dans les rapports physiologiques ne sont pas sans valeur.

L'enfant au sein absorbe beaucoup plus de graisse comparativement qu'un adulte (la relation est de 4,27, 0,75 en 24 heures par kilo de son poids).

On peut considérer comme certain, en tout cas, que la plus grande partie de la graisse du lait est résorbée sans décomposition, elle est seulement transformée au contact du ferment que Henriot a découvert dans le sérum du sang.

La graisse doit être pour cette raison finement émulsionnée et les recherches montrent aussi que la graisse du lait de femme est constituée en globules plus nombreux et plus fins que celle du lait de vache.

D'après Woll, une pasteurisation n'a aucune influence sur le volume ou sur la quantité des globules gras.

Tant qu'au sucre de lait, il est susceptible d'être modifié par de plus hautes températures ; à 110 degrés, il subit une décomposition qui va en s'aggravant avec l'élévation de la température.

Le lait qui a été stérilisé 10 minutes à 120 degrés acquiert une couleur jaune brun très prononcée causée par une formation de caramel. Peut-être se forme-t-il en même temps quelque acide (acide lactique Wroblewsky). De plus, le pouvoir de la réduction du liquide de Fehling est attiré.

Ainsi que nous l'avons vu, les sels de lait peuvent aussi, par la cuisson, subir des changements. Je mentionnerai les recherches faites par Henkel, Scheibe et Vaudin, sur le grand rôle que joue l'acide citrique dans le lait de vache et dans la solubilité des phosphates de calcium. Par la stérilisation, il se produit une modification dans l'état du lait.

amenée par la précipitation du citrate de chaux et du phosphate tricalcique.

Évidemment la retentissante conclusion de Bunge que les substances minérales se trouvent dans le lait en même proportion que dans l'organisme ne peut plus se soutenir depuis les dernières recherches faites par Camerer et Söldner.

Suivant Koeppe, il semble résulter que les sels jouent un grand rôle sous le rapport de la résorption de la nourriture. Il constate aussi une concordance, passée jusqu'ici inaperçue, entre le lait de femme et celui de vache quant à la dépression du point de congélation et à la pression osmotique dans les deux liquides — concordance qui, bien que la quantité d'albumine et de sucre soit si différente dans les deux espèces de lait, est amenée par les sels.

Il est donc permis d'admettre qu'une variation dans les quantités relatives des différentes matières n'est pas sans importance pour le rôle du lait dans l'alimentation.

Indépendamment des substances déjà nommées qui, par l'ébullition, subissent des modifications plus ou moins grandes, le lait possède certainement d'autres propriétés qui ne sont pas encore complètement mises en lumière, mais dont on peut néanmoins avoir idée, grâce aux recherches déjà faites.

Je rappellerai ainsi l'enzyme diastatique que Moro a signalé dans le lait de femme et l'enzyme protéolytique décelé par Babcock et Russel en 1897. Ces enzymes sont détruits par le chauffage.

Il existe encore d'autres recherches qui laissent soupçonner qu'il se trouve dans le lait frais plusieurs autres matières inconnues et dont la présence se révèle par certaines réactions, mais qui perdent cette faculté à la cuisson. Quelques-unes paraissent encore montrer que le lait frais possède certaines propriétés qui peuvent avoir une influence sur diverses espèces de bactéries.

Fokker a attribué au lait frais des propriétés antiseptiques sur les bactéries de l'acide lactique parce que le lait stérilisé, où sont ensemencées ces bactéries, se coagule plus vite que le lait frais. D'autres auteurs, comme Hesse et Baseman, ont fait des recherches sur les relations du lait frais avec les bactéries du choléra.

Quelques antitoxines peuvent même se transmettre dans le lait; c'est d'ailleurs ce qui résulte des recherches de Ehrlich, Brieger, Cohn et Wassermann, faites avec du lait de chèvres immunisées contre le tétanos et la diphtérie.

Félix Klemperer a pu transporter, à l'aide d'irrigations par l'anus, du lait d'une chèvre immunisée contre la fièvre typhoïde à une nouvelle accouchée et il a trouvé que le lait de cette femme avait une influence immunisante sur des souris infectées avec des bacilles typhiques.

Il semble certain que les célèbres recherches de changement de nourrice qu'a faites Ehrlich ont démontré que le lait des bêtes immunisées avec des antitoxines de l'abrine, de la ricine et du tétanos, avait un pouvoir immunisant sur les petits qui tétaient ces animaux ; mais, d'après Vaillard, ce résultat n'aurait lieu, en général, qu'avec les bêtes employées à l'essai, c'est-à-dire avec des souris.

Vidal et Sicard ont obtenu le même résultat avec la substance agglutinante typhique. Ils ne réussirent à communiquer la réaction agglutinante qu'au lait de ces mêmes bêtes. Cette expérience est cependant en contradiction avec les observations de : Achard, Bensaude, Thiercelin, Lenoble, Castaigne, Landouzy et Griffon, qui tous ont trouvé que le lait des mères atteintes de la fièvre typhoïde et que le sang des enfants qu'elles allaitaient possédaient cette même réaction.

Schmid et Pflanz ont prouvé que le lait de femme a des propriétés antitoxiques sur la toxine diphtérique, mais que, pour paralyser une certaine quantité de cette matière, il faudrait quinze fois autant de lait que de sérum sanguin.

Un cas intéressant est rapporté de Norvège par M. Bang. Un enfant qui souffrait d'un goitre fut guéri en tétant sa mère qui, elle aussi, ayant la même affection, était traitée avec l'iodothyrine.

Quant aux maladies contagieuses, le lait ne semble pas avoir une propriété immunisante contre la rougeole ; pour la coqueluche, on ne sait encore rien de positif (Neumann).

Il est évident que toutes les recherches précitées — recherches fort loin d'ailleurs d'être terminées — nous posent la question de savoir si la cuisson du lait est d'une grande importance pour l'enfant. Sauf les bactéries pathogènes, les qualités du lait *après* la cuisson dépendent des qualités qu'il avait *avant*. Le but de tout travail futur sera donc d'arriver à obtenir un lait dès le début exempt, autant que possible, de bactéries — résultat auquel on peut parvenir par un examen minutieux des animaux et par une hygiène absolue de l'étable. Ensuite les bactéries pathogènes qui peuvent se trouver dans le lait devront être détruites, sans que ses bonnes qualités soient altérées.

Pour le moment, cela se fait de la meilleure manière en pasteurisant le lait et en le refroidissant ensuite.

Il est encore un point sur lequel je me permets d'attirer votre attention.

Comme l'alimentation artificielle se fait d'après la méthode de Soxhlet, l'enfant aura pour chaque repas une composition de lait tout à fait homogène. Des recherches que j'ai faites à cet égard, il résulte que l'albumine, la graisse et le sucre, ont un pourcentage peu variable dans les différents repas journaliers; tandis qu'une série d'observations sur l'alimentation naturelle montrent, pour les mêmes substances, des variations très considérables, — variations qui, en ce qui concerne les sels, sont établies par Koeppe. Il arrive aussi que le lait des deux mamelles diffère beaucoup. Il existe également des recherches qui semblent prouver qu'il se produit des changements dans la composition du lait suivant que s'avance la période de la lactation; il n'est pas douteux que ces modifications répondent au développement et au besoin de nourriture de l'enfant.

EMPLOI MÉTHODIQUE DU LAIT STÉRILISÉ INDUSTRIELLEMENT POUR L'ALLAITEMENT ARTIFICIEL DANS LES GRANDES VILLES

RAPPORT

par M. le docteur G. VARIOT.

Médecin de l'Hôpital des Enfants-Malades.

La destruction des germes pathogènes aussi bien que des saprophytes étant obtenue par la stérilisation du lait, tous les médecins sont à peu près d'accord pour accepter la nécessité de la stérilisation, et pour en reconnaître les avantages dans l'allaitement artificiel.

Mais les appareils du type Soxhlet, qui peuvent être si utiles à la campagne et dans les endroits où il est aisé de se procurer de bon lait frais et pur, dont on connaît exactement la provenance, ne sont pas toujours applicables dans les grandes cités et surtout à Paris; car les laits peuvent être fermentés, mouillés, adultérés, sophistiqués de bien des manières avant d'arriver au consommateur. Ce n'est pas l'ébullition prolongée dans les appareils stérilisateurs qui rendra au lait les qualités qu'il aura perdues durant le transport ou par des manipulations frauduleuses.

A Paris, les laits vendus à bas prix, à la portée de la classe populaire, subissent toute espèce d'altérations et même de fraudes, qu'il est impossible de réprimer par la surveillance la plus stricte. Les mesures de police sont impuissantes à entraver la fraude, au témoignage de M. Girard, directeur du laboratoire municipal.

C'est pour parer à des inconvénients si graves, quand il s'agit de l'allaitement artificiel, que bon nombre de médecins ont pensé à recourir au lait stérilisé industriellement à 115 degrés environ, au lieu de production. dans les pays d'herbages. embouteillés dans des flacons de capacité réduite (1/2 ou 1/4 de litre). hermétiquement fermés avec des bouchons de liège paraffinés.

A Paris, en ce moment. les médecins qui s'occupent de faire progresser l'art de l'allaitement se divisent en deux groupes.

Dans le premier groupe, dont M. Budin est incontestablement le chef, se rangent ceux qui conservent leurs préférences au lait préparé dans les appareils de Soxhlet: la majorité des accoucheurs partage les opinions de M. Budin.

L'autre groupe se compose surtout des médecins d'enfants qui. ayant bien reconnu les défauts de la stérilisation tardive, considèrent l'emploi du lait stérilisé industriellement comme une nécessité devant laquelle il faut savoir se plier dans les grandes cités. Mes collègues des hôpitaux. MM. Comby et Marfan en particulier se sont prononcés dans ce sens. Parmi les accoucheurs. je citerai M. Bonnaire qui est venu s'adjoindre à nous.

J'ai repris moi-même sur une grande échelle l'expérience faite par mes collègues, et en quatre années j'ai fait distribuer, à prix réduit, 160 000 litres de lait stérilisé industriellement à plus de huit cents nourrissons que j'ai inspectés chaque semaine et dont j'ai surveillé la croissance et le développement par des pesées régulières.

Voici les avantages pratiques que nous avons reconnus au maniement du lait stérilisé industriellement, après ces essais multiples et prolongés :

1º Il se conserve intact, à l'abri de toute fermentation, aussi bien l'été que l'hiver. non seulement pendant la durée du transport mais encore pendant un délai assez long.

2º Le mouillage, l'écrémage, les sophistications et les fraudes diverses si communes pour le lait ordinaire transporté à Paris. sont à peu près impossibles avec des flacons de capacité *réduite* fermés hermétiquement avec des bouchons de liège paraffinés. La fraude s'exercerait sans profit sur de si faibles quantités de lait, et c'est peut-être la garantie la plus assurée que l'on puisse avoir de la pureté du lait.

3º La conservation prolongée de ce lait en rend l'emploi et le maniement bien plus faciles que pour le lait frais qui s'altère si rapidement.

Nous avons pu. au dispensaire de Belleville. sans grand embarras, distribuer chaque jour 150 litres de lait. soit 500 bouteilles: le samedi on distribue jusqu'à 500 litres, 600 bouteilles pour deux journées. Il faudrait de grandes ressources, un outillage compliqué, un personnel spécial, pour faire de semblables distributions avec les appareils de Soxhlet. A l'instigation de M. Budin, on a installé, depuis plusieurs années rue du Chemin-Vert des appareils stérilisateurs pour fournir du lait à 50 ou 40 nourrissons. Il suffit de comparer la distribution de lait de la rue du Chemin-Vert à celle du dispensaire de Belleville pour se rendre compte que dans ce dernier établissement nous obtenons des résultats bien plus importants par des moyens plus simples et à moins de frais.

Les membres du Congrès qui s'intéressent au fonctionnement de ces distributions de lait pourront aller vérifier, *de visu*, ce que nous avançons : nous nous mettons bien volontiers à leur disposition pour les guider dans cette inspection.

Le lait stérilisé industriellement que nous avons manié en grand à Belleville est le même que celui adopté dans nos hôpitaux de Paris il y a déjà une dizaine d'années. Il vient de la vallée de Bray et est fourni par des vaches de race normande : ces vaches vivent la plus grande partie de l'année nuit et jour dans l'herbage et ne sont soumises à la stabulation que pendant les grands froids.

Avant d'être accepté à l'usine, le lait est dégusté par des employés spéciaux et fréquemment analysé.

La composition moyenne de ce lait est la suivante pour un litre :

Extrait	150 grammes.
Beurre	59 gr. 2.
Lactose hydraté.	46 gr. 4.
Caséine	57 gr.
Cendres. . . :	7 gr. 9.

Phosphate tricalcique 4 gr. 91 (compris dans les cendres totales).

Ce lait est donc un lait moyen riche en phosphates.

C'est par des chauffages à des températures atteignant 115°, alternant avec des refroidissements rapides, que les bouteilles de lait, bouchées à l'avance, sont stérilisées dans d'immenses étuves à vapeur.

Après la stérilisation, qui n'altère en rien sa couleur, ce lait a un goût de cuit assez prononcé, mais dont les enfants s'accommodent bien.

Mode d'administration du lait. — Graduation des tétées suivant l'âge et le poids des enfants. — Lait coupé et lait pur. — D'après l'expérience générale, un des plus grands écueils de l'allaitement artificiel, surtout dans les deux ou trois premiers mois de la vie, consiste dans la suralimentation, soit que les mères n'espacent pas suffisamment les tétées, soit qu'elles chargent trop les biberons. La stérilisation du lait ne met pas à l'abri des accidents d'intolérance gastrique et des autres troubles dyspeptiques qui suivent la suralimentation. Il importe donc au plus haut point de bien régler le nourrisson en appliquant les principes connus pour espacer les tétées et pour proportionner, à chaque tétée, la quantité de lait à l'âge et au poids de l'enfant, c'est-à-dire à la capacité physiologique variable de l'estomac et du tube digestif.

Bien qu'il y ait à cet égard des écarts individuels dont il faudra tenir compte dans la pratique, on peut considérer comme exacts les chiffres, d'ailleurs à peu près concordants, fixés par Fleischman, par Suitkine, par Emmet Holt, Morgan Rotch, etc., pour graduer les quantités de lait que le nourrisson prendra à chaque tétée.

Nous avons vérifié nous-même l'exactitude de ces données physiologiques durant l'expérience de quatre années que nous avons poursuivie, et nous avons cru utile de faire inscrire sur le verre du biberon les chiffres indiquant la graduation des tétées suivant l'âge des enfants.

Cet outillage nous a paru d'autant plus nécessaire que nous employons exclusivement le lait stérilisé industriellement, embouteillé dans des flacons de 1/2 ou 1/4 de litre; les mères ignorent absolument le prélèvement qu'il convient de faire sur ces flacons pour préparer chaque tétée et le biberon gradué peut au moins leur servir de guide. Il appartient aux membres du Congrès de juger cette instrumentation que nous leur soumettons, et de décider si elle devrait être imitée par les fabricants de biberons que nous livrent trop souvent des bouteilles bien imparfaites.

Depuis que nous avons à notre disposition un lait privé de germes morbides ou malsains, grâce à la stérilisation, on a pu étudier avec plus de précision dans quelle mesure le lait de vache devait être modifié pour être supporté par le nourrisson.

Autrefois on imputait sans doute au lait pur, à l'excès des substances protéiques, des accidents qui relevaient plutôt de l'impureté du lait. Néanmoins la grande majorité des médecins considèrent encore comme nécessaire la modification du lait de vache pour le rapprocher plus ou moins de la composition du lait de la femme: nos confrères américains fabriquent de toutes pièces dans les *milk laboratories* des laits artificiels en dosant, suivant l'âge de l'enfant, la caséine, le sucre de lait et la crème. D'après Morgan Rotch, le moindre excès de substance protéique serait nuisible dans les premiers temps de la vie. Le lait maternisé proposé par Gærtner répond aux mêmes préoccupations.

A défaut de ces laits modifiés, on a conseillé des *coupages* de lait de vache avec moitié, un tiers ou un quart d'eau bouillie, suivant les circonstances. et avec addition de lactose ou de saccharose. ou même d'un peu de crème de lait.

M. Budin et ses élèves, en employant le lait stérilisé dans des appareils Soxhlet, et nous-même en recourant au lait stérilisé industriellement. sommes arrivés à nous former une opinion un peu différente. Le lait *pur* ne nous paraît pas aussi redoutable pour les nourrissons qu'on le pense assez généralement; la plupart des enfants, à partir de six semaines ou deux mois. le supportent bien : ils se développent et s'accroissent normalement; j'ai vu pour ma part plusieurs centaines de nourrissons élevés heureusement au lait pur, additionné d'une faible quantité de sucre ordinaire.

Le tube digestif des jeunes enfants présente une souplesse et une puissance d'adaptation plus grande qu'on ne le croirait.

Quoi qu'il en soit. nous pensons que c'est bien plutôt par l'observation clinique que par des raisonnements plus ou moins séduisants que l'on pourra faire progresser nos connaissances dans cette question si complexe de l'allaitement. Le nourrisson est après tout le meilleur réactif physiologique de la valeur nutritive d'un lait et s'il est bien établi par les faits. comme nous en avons la certitude, qu'il prospère avec le lait de vache pur. c'est que cet aliment lui convient.

Les coupages au tiers ou au quart avec de l'eau bouillie à laquelle on ajoute un peu de sucre ordinaire de saccharose nous ont paru suffisants soit dans les deux premiers mois de la vie, soit pour les enfants qui ne supportent pas le lait pur avant cinq ou six mois.

La simplification du coupage du lait et la tolérance des nourrissons pour le lait pur ont une importance pratique de premier ordre, quand on envisage l'allaitement artificiel dans la classe populaire où la mortalité infantile est si élevée. Jusqu'à présent les laits modifiés et en particulier le lait maternisé de Gœrtner est d'un prix peu abordable : il ne faut pas songer à en généraliser l'emploi; d'autre part. il est préférable de donner le lait pur aux enfants du peuple dès que cela est possible, car on évite ainsi les coupages avec des mixtures fermentescibles et malsaines.

Les consultations hebdomadaires de nourrissons avec distribution de lait stérilisé. — Dans l'art de l'allaitement artificiel. comme dans les autres, il ne suffit pas d'avoir une méthode. il faut l'appliquer bien, et pour cela surveiller les enfants et conseiller les mères. La consultation de nourrissons nous permet d'atteindre ce double but. Chaque semaine. dans les premiers mois de la vie. les enfants sont apportés au dispensaire, sont déshabillés et pesés dans une pièce bien chauffée l'hiver, les variations de poids sont inscrites sur une fiche et le médecin, d'un coup d'œil, en inspectant l'enfant et en contrôlant sur la fiche les indications fournies par la balance, constate si la croissance est normale : il donne des conseils pour la graduation des tétées, pour les coupages du lait, s'il y a lieu ; il recherche les fautes commises par les mères, tâche d'en prévenir le retour, encourage les unes, blâme les autres, etc.

La consultation de nourrissons est une institution née en France, sous les auspices de M. Budin, et qui nous a déjà rendu d'inappréciables services ; elle est applicable aussi bien aux enfants sains qu'aux enfants atrophiques, elle permet aux mères de conserver leurs enfants auprès d'elles, au lieu de les confier à des nourrices mercenaires en province.

En effet, la consultation de nourrissons a comme corollaire nécessaire une distribution de lait stérilisé, soit tout à fait gratuite pour les indigents, soit à prix réduit pour les nécessiteux. Les mères viennent chaque matin chercher leur provision de lait ; j'ai déjà dit que le lait stérilisé industriellement se prête mieux à ces distributions en grand que le lait préparé dans des appareils de Soxhlet ; il nous faudrait chaque jour au dispensaire de Belleville un millier de petites bouteilles, pour les 150 enfants dont nous surveillons l'élevage, au lieu que nous distribuons très aisément 500 bouteilles de 1/2 de litre stérilisées industriellement.

Avant d'exposer les *résultats obtenus*, il importe d'écarter une objection assez grave faite à l'emploi du lait stérilisé industriellement pour l'allaitement artificiel.

On a dit que c'était là un aliment de conserve capable de produire le scorbut infantile, la maladie de Barlow, autrement dit. Bien des faits de ce genre ont été publiés dans tous les pays ; en France ces accidents ont paru plus exceptionnels, et mon collègue M. Netter n'a pu en relever que quelques cas sur des quantités innombrables d'enfants nourris au lait stérilisé. Il serait puéril de vouloir nier que le surchauffage du lait n'ait quelques inconvénients ; mais on doit se demander aussi si l'on n'a pas attribué au lait stérilisé des méfaits dont il est innocent. Il y a lieu d'abord de distinguer les laits modifiés et spécialement ceux fabriqués par synthèse dans les *milk laboratories* américains, des laits stérilisés purs et normaux. Ces laits modifiés sont vraiment des produits artificiels rappelant plus ou moins d'autres mixtures alimentaires dont les effets nocifs sont indiscutables. Aussi, avant d'affirmer que le lait stérilisé lui-même est en cause dans la production d'accidents plus ou moins graves, convient-il de pousser une enquête rigoureuse, de s'informer si des mixtures alimentaires, des conserves autres que le lait, n'ont pas été administrées à l'enfant.

Les enquêtes de ce genre ne sont pas toujours aisées, car les mères n'avouent pas volontiers leurs fautes : quant aux nourrices mercenaires, elles les cachent autant qu'elles peuvent et n'hésitent pas à tromper le médecin.

Quoi qu'il en soit, nous pouvons déclarer qu'en France le scorbut infantile est très exceptionnel.

M. Budin, depuis dix ans, sur un très grand nombre de nourrissons élevés au lait stérilisé avec des appareils de Soxhlet, n'en a pas observé un seul cas, et nous-même en quatre ans sur plus de 800 enfants nourris exclusivement au *lait stérilisé industriellement*, nous n'en avons pas rencontré un seul exemple bien que nous eussions l'esprit en éveil.

Maintenant nous allons passer sommairement en revue les avantages et les inconvénients du lait industriel dans l'allaitement des jeunes enfants sains, aussi bien que des atrophiques.

Si l'on envisage les enfants sains, les résultats les plus satisfaisants sont obtenus à partir de six semaines ou deux mois chez ceux qui ont reçu jusque-là le sein de leur mère ; la courbe de développement est également normale chez ceux qui reçoivent l'allaitement mixte peu de temps après leur naissance. Néanmoins avec une surveillance stricte, en graduant bien les tétées, en évitant soigneusement la suralimentation, on parvient très bien à élever les nouveau-nés par l'allaitement artificiel exclusif : dans cette première période de la vie, les échecs sont plus à craindre dans la classe populaire, à cause des négligences ou de la mauvaise volonté à suivre les règles prescrites. A partir de deux ou trois mois, il est rare que nous perdions des nourrissons allaités artificiellement et bien soignés, par suite de troubles gastro-intestinaux.

Les accoucheurs, auxquels échoit spécialement la surveillance des enfants sains, ont depuis longtemps mis en lumière les beaux résultats fournis par la stérilisation avec les appareils de Soxhlet : nous pouvons ajouter que les avantages du lait industriel, dans ces conditions, sont à peu près les mêmes.

Il appartenait aux médecins de montrer que le lait stérilisé était, en même temps qu'un aliment, un véritable médicament pour les enfants souffrant de troubles gastro-intestinaux. M. Comby, il y a plusieurs années, a déjà traité heureusement par le lait industriel un certain nombre d'enfants atteints de gastro-entérites plus ou moins graves.

Nous avons repris cette étude sur plusieurs centaines d'enfants au dispensaire de Belleville et nous avons suivi, la balance à la main, les effets du lait industriel chez les enfants devenus plus ou moins atrophiques à la suite de troubles gastro-intestinaux prolongés. Sauf pour les vrais athrepsiques de Parrot, c'est-à-dire pour ceux dont le degré d'atrophie est extrême, nous avons réussi généralement à arrêter d'abord les troubles gastro-intestinaux, et plus tard à faire croître régulièrement ces enfants.

Le docteur Battino (de Corfou) et le docteur Paul Ignard (Thèse de Paris 1898 : Le traitement de l'atrophie infantile par le lait stérilisé) ont dépouillé les nombreuses fiches du dispensaire de Belleville relatives aux enfants atrophiques. Ils sont arrivés tous deux, comme nous-même, à constater que l'atrophie infantile est généralement curable par le lait industriel, que la croissance jusque-là retardée, reprend un cours à peu près normal, mais que, jusqu'à un an et plus, les enfants conservent une diminution de poids un peu inférieure cependant à leur degré d'atrophie initiale. Leur aspect général devient satisfaisant, ils sont simplement retardés dans leur développement jusque vers l'âge de un an, où le processus nutritif prenant une activité plus grande, ils rattrapent généralement le temps perdu.

On ne saurait trop insister sur ces résultats acquis, car autrefois, en France, du moins, on considérait toute cette classe d'enfants atrophiques comme uniquement justiciable de l'allaitement au sein : dès qu'un enfant présentait une perte notable de poids, on s'empressait de recourir à la nourrice mercenaire.

Les enfants sains, non plus que les atrophiques nourris au lait industriel, ne sont presque jamais rachitiques.

Il est vrai que nous ne faisons usage des bouillies farineuses qu'à l'apparition des premières dents, même chez les atrophiques. On nous apporte parfois des enfants déjà rachitiques ; nous les traitons exclusivement par le lait stérilisé, auquel nous ajoutons volontiers du jaune d'œuf ou du jus de viande ; les tuméfactions épiphysaires diminuent, puis disparaissent assez rapidement sous l'influence de cette alimentation. Il est utile de rappeler ici que notre lait industriel contient plus de 4 pour 1000 de phosphate terreux.

À côté de ces avantages bien établis, voyons maintenant les inconvénients réels, il faut le reconnaître, du lait industriel. Il arrive que quelques bouteilles, dont la stérilisation ou le bouchage auront été défectueux, sont gâtées. Cette éventualité rare (une bouteille sur cent environ pendant l'été) impose aux mères ou aux nourrices le devoir de goûter chaque bouteille avant de charger le biberon. Mais une mère ou une nourrice, assez peu soigneuse pour ne pas s'assurer si le lait n'a pas de mauvais goût, pourrait commettre la même négligence avec un **autre lait, quel qu'il soit.**

Lorsque le lait embouteillé a été conservé pendant quelque temps avant d'être consommé, l'émulsion des globules graisseux peut être légèrement troublée et des grumeaux de beurre viennent flotter à la surface. Il est préférable d'enlever ces grumeaux avant de charger le biberon, quoique l'ingestion d'une petite quantité de beurre liquéfié quand on fait tiédir le biberon ne saurait incommoder sérieusement l'enfant.

On a dit que le lait contenu dans des flacons de 1/2 litre ne restait pas stérile pendant le temps nécessaire à sa consommation, c'est-à-dire pendant quelques heures ; qu'après avoir été débouché il pouvait être contaminé par des germes malsains et fermenter comme le lait ordinaire. Si cette crainte était fondée, il faudrait embouteiller le lait dans des flacons de contenance moindre, de 1/4 de litre ou même de 100 grammes. Jusqu'à présent il ne nous a pas paru que le prélèvement du lait pour charger les biberons compromît pratiquement la stérilisation, pourvu qu'on rebouche la bouteille à chaque fois, ce qui est vraiment bien facile.

Il est vrai qu'à l'époque des grandes chaleurs les nourrissons allaités artificiellement sont plus sujets aux flux intestinaux ; mais cette remarque s'applique aussi bien à ceux qui reçoivent le lait dans les petites bouteilles de Soxhlet qu'à ceux qui prennent le lait industriel ; bien plus, nous savons que les enfants nourris au sein ne sont pas à l'abri des diarrhées estivales.

Mais les catarrhes gastro-intestinaux qui apparaissent en rapport avec les hyperthermies saisonnières n'ont que peu de gravité chez les enfants nourris au lait stérilisé. Nous pouvons déclarer spécialement que les diarrhées survenant chez les enfants qui reçoivent du lait industriel sont bénignes en général, et cèdent en quelques jours sous l'influence de la diète hydrique, et de la réduction des tétées ; exception doit être faite pour les atrophiques, qui, ne recevant que trop tard le lait stérilisé, sont emportés en grand nombre. L'immense majorité des enfants sains résiste très bien à la diarrhée estivale quand ils en sont atteints.

Un accident beaucoup plus fréquent que la diarrhée est la constipation qui est parfois assez opiniâtre chez les nourrissons qui reçoivent le lait industriel.

La constipation cède quelquefois, mais non toujours, lorsqu'on mouille le lait d'un tiers d'eau bouillie; ce n'est donc pas seulement l'excès des principes protéiques qui intervient pour produire l'inertie de l'intestin.

On a signalé chez les enfants alimentés au lait stérilisé une anémie plus ou moins profonde avec bouffissure des téguments. M. Marfan a attribué ce trouble nutritif à l'action du lait pur, mais il se retrouve aussi chez ceux qui prennent le lait stérilisé coupé d'eau. Quelle part faire à l'allaitement et aux conditions d'hygiène défectueuses dans lesquelles vivent la plupart des enfants du peuple, pour expliquer le processus de déglobulisation qui se manifeste par une pâleur plus ou moins prononcée des téguments?

La question n'est pas aisée à résoudre, mais il est cependant certain que cette anémie est bien moins fréquente chez les enfants allaités au sein. L'usage précoce et régulier du jus de viande crue nous a donné de bons résultats pour combattre cette anémie.

Malgré ces inconvénients, les avantages de l'allaitement au lait stérilisé restent évidents: la découverte de la stérilisation, comme tous les médecins compétents se plaisent à le répéter, a fait subir à l'art de l'allaitement artificiel un progrès décisif; le biberon chargé de bon lait et bien aseptisé ne peut plus être considéré comme un instrument néfaste. On doit donc s'efforcer de vulgariser cet admirable progrès, de répandre le lait stérilisé dans la classe populaire pour limiter la mortalité infantile qui, ces jours derniers, faisait encore de terribles ravages à Paris.

Le lait industriel nous donne la même sécurité que le bon lait préparé dans des appareils de Soxhlet, et il est bien plus maniable pour les distributions gratuites ou à prix réduit, faites dans la classe populaire.

Dans nos maternités, ces distributions de lait commencent à fonctionner régulièrement. Que n'en est-il de même dans nos hôpitaux d'enfants de Paris où l'on apporte un grand nombre de nourrissons allaités artificiellement pour y être hospitalisés. Il ne faut pas séparer ces jeunes enfants de leurs mères, car l'hospitalisation nous donne une mortalité extrêmement élevée.

La comparaison du lait stérilisé industriel et du lait stérilisé ordinaire nous a paru intéressante à soumettre au Congrès de pédiatrie. De grands progrès peuvent être subordonnés à des modifications techniques dont l'expérience et le temps seuls dévoileront toute la portée.

B. — Discussion à propos des rapports
sur l'allaitement artificiel et le lait stérilisé.

M. le professeur d'Espine (Genève). — Le rapport de M. Variot m'a intéressé vivement et particulièrement à deux points de vue. Le premier est la rareté, pour ne pas dire l'absence de la maladie de Barlow à Paris. C'est la même chose à Genève. Tout au plus, peut-on rapprocher du scorbut l'anémie spéciale que j'ai observée chez des enfants nourris trop longtemps au lait stérilisé industriel. Le second point est le coupage. Le lait pur est le but auquel il faut arriver le plus vite possible par tâtonnements. Il n'y a pas de danger à tenter l'expérience avec le lait stérilisé pur pourvu qu'on l'arrête immédiatement s'il n'est pas digéré. Mais l'expérience m'a démontré que les enfants n'ont pas tous le même estomac et que, dans la majorité des cas, ils ne digèrent pas bien le lait pur avant trois mois révolus, et parfois seulement beaucoup plus tard.

M. Marfan (Paris). — Je voudrais présenter quelques observations qui me sont suggérées par les remarquables rapports que nous avons entendus.

M. Heubner pense qu'on ne peut établir des règles d'alimentation pour les nourrissons bien portants d'après ce que nous observons chez le nourrisson malade.

J'ai le regret de ne pas partager complètement son avis. La pathologie nous a souvent appris la physiologie; ce sont les faits morbides qui nous ont fourni des éclaircissements sur les localisations cérébrales et sur les fonctions du corps thyroïde. En matière d'allaitement, nous devons la connaissance de certaines règles à la constatation des bons effets thérapeutiques de la diminution de la quantité de nourriture ou de l'éloignement des repas dans un très grand nombre de cas.

M. Monti attache une grande importance à la distinction de l'albumine soluble et de la caséine. Je ne suis pas chimiste, et je le regrette; mais, quand je vois des hommes comme M. Duclaux se refuser à distinguer deux sortes de substances albuminoïdes dans le lait, je ne puis croire que l'on doive tenir compte de cette distinction dans la comparaison du lait de femme et du lait de vache.

En ce qui concerne la dilution du lait stérilisé, je crois que le désaccord entre M. Variot et moi n'est pas bien profond. M. Variot dilue le lait dans les premières semaines; je conseille la dilution jusqu'au quatrième ou cinquième mois. Mais, tous les deux, nous reconnaissons que les préceptes généraux doivent être modifiés dans nombre de cas particuliers. En tout cas, je juge indispensable de fixer par des chiffres des points de repère qui serviront pour les tâtonnements nécessaires dans chaque cas.

M. Variot distingue l'atrophie simple de l'athrepsie. J'accepte cette distinction. Il y a une atrophie simple, pondérale, sans état maladif qui résulte soit d'une insuffisance de nourriture, soit d'une maladie antérieure guérie; il y a une atrophie cachectique, avec des signes morbides variés. Dans l'atrophie simple, le lait stérilisé peut donner de bons résultats; dans l'atrophie cachectique, on n'en retire rien. Cependant cette distinction entre l'atrophie simple et l'athrepsie ne doit pas être radicale; car entre les deux états, on observe tous les intermédiaires.

En terminant, je désire déclarer, d'une manière plus nette et plus précise que je ne l'ai fait déjà, que, quelle que soit la méthode employée pour l'allaitement artificiel, jamais l'enfant qui y est soumis exclusivement ne ressemble entièrement au nourrisson alimenté exclusivement de lait de femme. Parmi les nourrissons qui n'ont jamais reçu celui-ci ou qui en ont été privés de bonne heure, il y en a plus des trois quarts qui offrent, plus ou moins marqué, le gonflement de l'extrémité antérieure des côtes que l'on désigne sous le nom de chapelet rachitique.

M. Concetti (Rome). — Je suis tout à fait d'accord avec le professeur Monti quant au rôle défavorable que l'acidité du lait exerce sur la digestion des nourrissons. J'ai trouvé très souvent, même dans l'allaitement naturel (par la mère ou par une nourrice), que la cause des troubles digestifs observés était une acidité anormale du lait et qu'on pouvait y remédier par les alcalins, qui restaient sans effet dans des cas où le lait n'offrait qu'une faible réaction d'acide.

Pour ce qui est de l'allaitement artificiel, je vois que, malgré toutes les études et toutes les tentatives pour se rapprocher le plus possible des conditions de l'allaitement naturel, on en est encore à discuter sur la question et à proposer des méthodes nouvelles ou des modifications aux méthodes connues. Cela démontre qu'au moins, jusqu'ici, l'allaitement artificiel ne remplace pas efficacement l'allaitement naturel et qu'il offre toujours de sérieux inconvénients. C'est un peu ce que l'on voit avec les maladies incurables : ce sont celles en effet qui comptent le plus grand nombre de remèdes plus efficaces les uns que les autres!

Ce qu'il faut considérer, — et il convient d'y attacher une grande importance, — c'est le pouvoir digestif individuel des enfants. Il y a des laits de femme qui se prêtent admirablement au développement de certains enfants et qui ne sont pas digérés par d'autres enfants. Chaque enfant a sa faculté digestive, qui lui est propre, et là est la raison pour laquelle l'allaitement maternel sera toujours le meilleur, parce que dans le lait de sa mère l'enfant trouve un aliment qui lui est approprié par un fait naturel héréditaire comme étant la continuation de l'alimentation qu'il venait de recevoir par la circulation placentaire avant la naissance. C'est pour cela que je voudrais qu'au lieu de formuler des vœux pour la diffusion de l'allaitement artificiel, nous en fissions tous pour la propagation de l'allaitement naturel, soit par la mère, soit par une bonne nourrice, rigoureusement surveillée, bien entendu.

Il ne faut accepter l'allaitement artificiel que comme une nécessité malheureuse qu'il faudrait réduire aux cas où on ne peut faire autrement et peut-être comme un aide de l'allaitement maternel, quand une mère n'a pas tout à fait assez de lait ou quand par nécessité elle doit pour quelques heures s'éloigner de son enfant (allaitement mixte).

Quant à ce qui est de la stérilisation du lait, je crois que la stérilisation du commerce, qui est à haute température et que préconise M. Variot, est la plus dangereuse et la moins adaptée à la bonne digestion des enfants. Il faudrait la réserver seulement pour les grandes villes où il est impossible de stériliser le lait tout de suite après la traite. Mais dans les petites villes, dans les campagnes, quand on peut avoir les vaches, comme on dit, sous la main, il est préférable de pratiquer la stérilisation à la maison, afin d'avoir le lait pour les 24 heures, naturellement en de petits flacons pour chaque repas de l'enfant.

M. Viola (de Constantinople) s'accorde avec M. Variot pour penser que le lait stérilisé dans l'industrie est supérieur au lait préparé à la maison avec le Soxhlet; mais c'est à la condition que les établissements qui le fabriquent soient surveillés par les autorités compétentes, qui doivent contrôler la réalité de la stérilisation, et la qualité du lait employé; il faut aussi que les bouteilles n'en contiennent pas plus d'un demi-litre, pour une tétée ou deux. Mais le lait bien stérilisé peut encore déterminer des accidents gastro-intestinaux, que fait disparaître le coupage.

M. le professeur BAGINSKY (Berlin). — Les exposés de MM. les rapporteurs présentent une telle quantité de choses intéressantes qu'il devient difficile d'entrer dans les détails de toutes, et de définir nettement la position qu'on occupe soi-même en présence de chacune d'elles.

Avant tout, je signalerai comme intéressantes les questions sur lesquelles s'est étendu M. Heubner, parce que ces questions paraissent ouvrir une voie à des considérations nouvelles.

Si toutefois nous jetons un regard en arrière sur le chemin que nous avons parcouru en physiologie, nous trouvons qu'il y a cinquante ans environ il était le même que celui que tout récemment M. Rubner et, sous sa direction, M. Heubner, s'appliquent à suivre. C'est la voie de la conception physique des processus vitaux et en particulier de la nutrition.

Quelque admirables que soient les progrès accomplis sous l'influence des considérations physico-chimiques, nous avons dû cependant faire cette expérience, et nous la faisons à présent tous les jours davantage, qu'il existe dans les processus physiologiques certaines relations biologiques particulières que les conceptions purement chimiques et physiques sont insuffisantes à expliquer. Je n'ai qu'à rappeler les faits les plus récents mis en lumière sur ce même sujet et ayant trait aux relations du lait de la mère avec les nourrissons.

S'il en est ainsi, comment est-il à craindre que la voie qui, étant physique, devrait être suivie par nous, nous amène encore à plus d'erreurs et de déceptions que la voie chimique ne nous en a déjà données?

L'évaluation en calories des substances alimentaires, et le fait d'exprimer en calories l'énergie latente contenue dans les aliments, constituent des moyens thérapeutiques auxiliaires excellents. Lorsque l'on veut contrôler la nutrition des enfants ainsi que je l'ai fait chez des enfants plus âgés, il y a certainement quelque avantage, après les avoir alimentés d'une façon qui leur convient, de pouvoir déterminer, en s'entourant de toutes les garanties scientifiques exigées dans les recherches sur les échanges nutritifs, les calories utilisées par ces derniers lors de leur développement parfait. On fait alors évidemment bien d'évaluer séparément les substances grasses et azotées, de même que les sucres. Seulement, il ne faut pas vouloir renverser le problème et se servir du nombre de calories pour en déduire le genre et la quantité de nourriture. On s'apercevrait alors, non sans regret, qu'on avait suivi une voie complètement erronée et que les enfants dépérissent, malgré le chiffre normal de calories.

Si ensuite M. Heubner ne se contente pas du chiffre seul de calories, mais pense que par des coefficients déduits de l'accroissement du corps et du chiffre de calories il puisse arriver à faire reposer l'absorption sur des bases plus certaines, je puis, sans calculer, lui dire d'avance que fatalement il ne peut rien trouver d'autre que ce qu'il a eu, à savoir que les enfants nourris le mieux et avec le plus de calories présenteront le coefficient le plus élevé. Mais cela veut-il dire autre chose, sinon que ces enfants précisément ont bien prospéré ?

Je veux bien consentir que le chiffre est un complément agréable trouvé par le calcul, qui permet d'avoir un aperçu général plus facile. Mais rien, absolument rien de plus. Avant tout, rien n'est acquis pour la question de l'alimentation elle-même par ce fait de posséder quelques chiffres. Avec cela on obtient à peine quelque chose de plus que ce que peut nous révéler la constatation *de visu* de l'état de bonne nutrition des enfants. Si dès à présent on voulait, en se basant sur les chiffres, se mettre à établir une alimentation particulière, on s'apercevrait bien vite que l'organisme ne s'y prête pas, mais poursuit le chemin qui lui est propre.

Messieurs, je suis d'accord avec M. Heubner que chaque enfant a son mode d'assimilation particulier ; qu'ici essayer vaut mieux qu'étudier, et quoique ce soit bien attristant, que, malgré les études si étendues sur l'alimentation, force nous est de nous contenter de résultats si minimes ; nous devons cependant considérer ces résultats comme les mêmes qu'autrefois on obtenait en agissant inconsciemment, tandis qu'aujourd'hui nous y apportons une compréhension plus claire.

En résumé, je ne crois pas que le calcul, si intéressant qu'il soit, puisse nous amener plus loin, car dans les recherches biologiques les chiffres — comme aussi celles des statistiques, par exemple — ne tiennent pas toujours.

Si, à présent, je me tourne vers les travaux des autres rapporteurs, j'avoue que les communications de M. Variot sont très encourageantes ; néanmoins je voudrais ajouter que je ne puis pas confirmer les faits qu'il vient de décrire, — au moins en ce qui concerne des enfants malades nourris avec du lait stérilisé.

Dans cette question il y a deux côtés à considérer :

1) L'alimentation avec du lait stérilisé pur (non coupé) depuis la naissance ;

2) L'alimentation en général, avec du lait stérilisé.

En ce qui concerne l'alimentation, il se peut qu'il existe des différences entre les enfants des diverses nationalités relativement à leur nutrition de même qu'il existe des enfants qui, dès le premier moment, ingèrent tout ce qu'on leur donne et prospèrent néanmoins. Mais ce sont des exceptions, et je ne puis, de par ma propre expérience, dire autre chose que ceci : lorsque, faute de mieux, on est obligé d'avoir recours à l'allaitement artificiel, les enfants prospèrent encore le mieux lorsqu'on commence à les nourrir avec du lait stérilisé, *coupé*, et chez lesquels on passe lentement et progressivement au lait stérilisé *pur*.

Quant au fait que le lait soit stérilisé, vous savez combien j'ai combattu en sa faveur depuis longtemps. Au point de vue de l'expérimentation et de l'observation à ce sujet, je me trouve dans les meilleures conditions que l'on puisse jamais imaginer. En effet, j'ai à ma disposition une étable avec des vaches, le tout très minutieusement entretenu; le lait, obtenu dans des conditions de la plus extrême propreté, est trait trois fois par jour, refroidi et envoyé de suite à l'hôpital des Enfants où sa stérilisation est effectuée avec les précautions les plus rigoureuses. Et, malgré tout cela, je ne peux point affirmer avoir jamais eu des résultats aussi favorables que ceux que décrit notre collègue M. Variot. Il est vrai que je n'ai presque pas affaire à d'autres enfants qu'à des enfants malades.

Je ne peux ici que corroborer l'opinion de M. Marfan, à savoir que le résultat est essentiellement différent selon les conditions dans lesquelles on applique l'allaitement par le lait stérilisé, et que tout dépend de l'état des enfants. Je dois aussi ajouter que j'ai vu deux cas absolument certains de maladie de Barlow dus uniquement à l'usage de lait stérilisé.

Messieurs, en somme, vous voyez que les travaux de ces dernières années sur l'alimentation des enfants n'ont certainement pas été inutiles; mais que, quand même, ils nous ont seulement amenés à nous rendre bien évident que *tout ne convient pas à tous*, et que, malgré nos nombreux travaux, bien des choses existent que les anciens connaissaient déjà fort bien.

M. Escherich de Gratz. — Le lait artificiel n'est bien supporté que par des enfants bien constitués ou à partir d'un certain âge. Le lait maternel contient sans doute des substances-ferments, adaptées aux besoins de l'enfant, que ne renferme pas le lait de vache; plus tard ces substances ne sont plus nécessaires.

J'ai constaté par des expériences que dans les premières semaines l'enfant n'a besoin que d'une petite quantité de substances albuminoïdes pour son développement; et le nombre des calories qu'on doit lui fournir est peut-être inférieur à celui qu'a indiqué Heubner. Je me propose de revenir sur ces points dans une communication.

M. Sevestre. — Il est très certain que l'allaitement maternel constitue pour les enfants l'alimentation idéale; mais on ne peut toujours le réaliser et, dans ces conditions, la stérilisation du lait nous rend des services considérables, et je connais un certain nombre d'enfants nourris de cette façon, soit dans les premiers mois, soit même dès la naissance et qui ont pu être élevés sans accident et ont présenté une croissance régulière.

Je ne pense pas que chez les enfants tout jeunes le lait stérilisé doive être donné pur et sous ce rapport je me sépare de certains de nos collègues et de la plupart des accoucheurs, ayant vu plusieurs fois des troubles digestifs chez des enfants allaités au lait stérilisé pur. Je crois utile de faire à cet égard une remarque. J'ai vu plusieurs fois des enfants suivis pendant deux ou trois semaines par l'accoucheur et mis par lui à l'usage du lait stérilisé pur. Vers ce moment, ou au bout de huit jours, ils présentaient quelques troubles gastriques qui cédaient en général, après que l'on avait coupé le lait avec un tiers ou un quart d'eau.

Quant à la question de savoir s'il faut employer le lait stérilisé industriellement ou le lait stérilisé chaque jour d'après la méthode de Soxhlet, je dois dire que j'ai obtenu en général avec ce dernier des résultats plus satisfaisants. D'ailleurs, lorsque le lait doit être coupé, cela permet d'ajouter l'eau avant la stérilisation, ce qui est toujours préférable.

C'est d'après ces principes que sont nourris les enfants dans un Établissement dirigé par un Comité médical dont j'ai l'honneur d'être le président. Je veux parler de l'établissement de la Pouponnière de Porchefontaine (près de Versailles), où se trouvent réunis 100 à 120 enfants, et qui sont nourris les uns au sein, les autres au lait stérilisé. Les résultats obtenus sont, en général, très satisfaisants, ainsi que vous pourrez vous en convaincre, si vous voulez bien aller visiter l'établissement.

M. SEITZ (Munich). — Comme médecin de la ville de Soxhlet, où cette méthode est très généralisée, j'ai vu par an entrer 5000 à 3000 enfants qui sont nourris artificiellement; pendant cinq années, j'ai vu seulement quatre cas de maladie de Barlow, je ne peux donc pas constater une relation entre la méthode Soxhlet et la fréquence de cette maladie. Au point de vue du rachitisme, je n'ai pas une connaissance personnelle de sa fréquence avant l'époque de Soxhlet ; mais on dit qu'elle était aussi grande.

Je ne crois pas que nous puissions abandonner la stérilisation modifiée (pendant 10 à 15 minutes), après ce que nous avons appris par Escherich, Heubner, Marfan, du rôle nocif des microbes pathogènes dans l'étiologie de certaines formes de gastro-entérite. Dans les grandes villes on peut donner du lait stérilisé industriellement ; mais pour le plus grand nombre de cas, il faut choisir un lait aussi bon que possible — avec crème et eau sucrée et bien stérilisé — jusqu'au temps où nous aurons une production aseptique du lait.

M. HEUBNER (Berlin) répond aux objections de Marfan qu'il ne peut se départir de sa rigueur et qu'il faut étudier l'alimentation artificielle sur des enfants sains. Il ne faudrait pas compliquer inutilement une question déjà si difficile et embrouillée. C'est ce qui arrive quand on s'adresse pour étudier la question à des cas pathologiques.

Il répond à Baginsky qu'il n'a pas saisi l'esprit de sa communication, ce qui peut-être tient à ce que les idées exprimées, tout en étant un peu en dehors de ce qu'on admet généralement, ont dû être résumées brièvement. Mais il voit qu'Escherich l'a bien compris. Il renvoie Baginsky à ses autres publications et se contente ici d'insister sur deux points. Il n'a nullement établi un coefficient d'apport d'énergie et de croissance, comme Baginsky le pense, mais simplement un coefficient du poids du corps. Ce sont là deux choses différentes. Avec cela il a obtenu une quantité qui peut servir de mesure à différents point de vue, par exemple pour mesurer la croissance corporelle. En outre, il n'a pas voulu avec ce nombre, ainsi que le croit Baginsky, doser la nature et la quantité de nourriture, mais il demande, étant donnée une certaine alimentation chez un enfant en bonne ou en mauvaise santé, quel est le coefficient d'énergie de cette alimentation pour l'enfant en question, et il voit d'après cela mieux que la composition chimique et le volume, si avant tout l'enfant reçoit une quantité suffisante d'énergie (ou peut-être une trop forte).

M. SCHLOSSMANN (de Dresde) pense qu'il existe dans le lait des substances inconnues douées de propriétés spécifiques : le lait renferme sans doute des ferments solubles adaptés à chaque espèce, que l'analyse chimique ne décèle pas encore, mais dont le rôle est de première importance dans l'allaitement.

M. GRAANBOOM d'Amsterdam a étudié la valeur du lait non coupé. Il en a une expérience assez grande, étant le premier qui ait fait cette étude. Plusieurs centaines d'enfants âgés de six semaines à une année dont une partie était tout à fait normale, l'autre partie souffrant de maladies des voies digestives, ont servi pour l'expérience. Les résultats ont été que les enfants bien portants et ayant un tube digestif normal supportaient bien le lait non coupé. D'un autre côté, l'expérience lui a montré que la deuxième partie, c'est-à-dire les enfants malades du côté du tube digestif, généralement ne le supportaient pas.

Quant au point de vue émis par le professeur Heubner, le docteur Graanboom est d'avis que la voie physique où nous mène la théorie du professeur Heubner ne nous satisfera pas. Chaque praticien a vu des cas où un nourrisson étant nourri avec le nombre de calories exigées par la théorie de Heubner, reste au-dessous du poids normal, tandis que d'autres, auxquels on donne un nombre de calories inférieur au nombre exigé par Heubner, atteignent un poids normal et même le dépassent.

M. JACOBI de New-York. — Quand le lait est dilué avec une décoction de céréales, la caséine se précipite en fins grumeaux. Il existe dans la salive un ferment sécrété par la parotide, dès la naissance, qui transforme les matières amylacées ; on n'a donc pas besoin d'attendre six mois ou un an pour donner des amylacés à un enfant : le lait est au contraire plus digestible, s'il est coupé avec une solution de céréales (orge, etc.) qu'avec de l'eau pure.

C. — Communications sur l'allaitement.

A PROPOS DES NOURRICES GOITREUSES

par M. le docteur BÉZY,

Chargé du cours de clinique infantile à la Faculté de médecine de l'Université de Toulouse,
Médecin des Hôpitaux.

La question que je désire poser devant le Congrès, sans avoir du reste la prétention de la voir résoudre immédiatement, est la suivante : lorsqu'une femme est présentée comme nourrice à l'examen d'un médecin, celui-ci doit-il la refuser par le seul fait qu'elle est goitreuse ?

Pour le moment, et jusqu'à plus ample informé, j'estime, quant à moi, qu'une nourrice goitreuse doit être refusée. Je me hâte d'ajouter que cette appréciation a pour base la prudence et non une certitude absolue ; aussi serai-je heureux de voir discuter mon opinion soit par ceux qui m'entendent, soit par ceux qui voudraient bien étudier plus tard la question.

Je demande la permission d'exposer les motifs qui m'ont amené à formuler cette opinion après examen des faits cliniques et pathologiques.

Le premier malade qui frappa mon attention fut la petite Berthe L.... âgée de six mois, que je vis dans ma clientèle, en avril 1897. Cette enfant était nourrie au sein par sa mère, jeune femme très bien portante, lorsqu'elle fut subitement prise de raideur musculaire. J'avoue que je pensai d'abord à des phénomènes convulsifs d'origine intestinale, avec d'autant plus de raison qu'elle avait eu un vomissement deux ou trois jours avant. Ce vomissement, attribué au trop grand rapprochement des tétées, n'avait pas reparu, la mère ayant pris des habitudes plus régulières. L'intestin fonctionnait du reste très bien.

En présence des accidents convulsifs qui débutent le 5 avril 1897, je m'enquiers des antécédents de famille et j'apprends que ma malade avait une sœur de cinq ans, bien portante, ayant été nourrie elle aussi par la mère et ayant eu une légère crise convulsive pendant l'allaitement. Un petit frère que la mère avait essayé de nourrir et qu'elle avait dû cesser d'allaiter pour cause de fatigue est mort de méningite (?) à trois mois.

Ne trouvant aucune autre cause à ces accidents que l'infection possible de l'appareil digestif, je dirige dans ce sens un traitement qui reste sans effet; les essais de sédation du système nerveux n'eurent pas de meilleurs résultats; les accès de convulsions devinrent rapidement de la contracture généralisée. Cet état persista pendant quinze jours, en s'aggravant, et l'enfant succomba sans avoir rien présenté qu'un peu d'œdème des membres inférieurs quelques heures avant sa mort.

Cette observation m'avait frappé : et je me demandais quelle pouvait être la pathogénie de cette tétanie sans pouvoir trouver une réponse satisfaisante. Rien, du côté d'aucun organe, ne me fournissait d'indication; mais il est à noter, et j'y reviendrai, que la mère était atteinte de la maladie de Basedow.

J'avais souvent pensé à cette petite malade et j'étais mécontent de mon diagnostic incomplet, lorsque quelques mois après, le 15 novembre 1897, je suis appelé auprès de la petite Marcelle F.... âgée de sept mois, qui présenta des accidents analogues. Voici en quelques mots son observation : père et mère bien portants, une sœur bien portante, un frère bien portant plus âgé de quinze mois que notre petite malade. Détail intéressant, la même nourrice a nourri les deux frères du même lait, sans interruption : cette nourrice a été presque toujours réglée, et le premier enfant qu'elle a nourri n'a jamais été malade. Aucun des deux nourrissons n'a été très régulièrement alimenté, mais aucun des deux n'a jamais présenté de phénomène intestinal.

Le 15 novembre 1897, la petite Marcelle étant fatiguée, je l'examine et reconnais une congestion pulmonaire qui disparaît en deux ou trois jours sous l'influence d'enveloppements humides du thorax. Je l'avais laissée en très bon état le 19 au matin, lorsque je suis rappelé le soir pour une crise convulsive que rien n'expliquait, ni dans l'état local, ni dans l'état général. Ces crises prennent le même aspect de contracture permanente que dans le cas précédent, tout traitement est inutile et l'enfant succombe après trente-cinq jours de maladie.

La nourrice n'avait pas de goitre aussi avéré que pour mon premier malade, mais son corps thyroïde était un peu développé, présentait des battements, et il y avait un certain degré d'exophtalmie.

Je fus frappé de ce fait dans lequel, comme pour mon premier malade, rien ne m'expliquait bien clairement cette tétanie ; mais je ne pus m'empêcher d'observer que les deux nourrices présentaient du basedowisme et de me demander s'il n'y avait pas là une relation de cause à effet.

Mon attention était éveillée sur ce point, lorsque je vis mon troisième malade en octobre 1898. Voici son observation résumée : père et mère bien portants, s'étant mariés jeunes (24 et 16 ans) et étant restés 20 ans sans avoir d'enfants. Georges L... naquit après une grossesse normale, mais un accouchement laborieux avec application du forceps le 27 octobre 1898. Il était beau et fut nourri au lait stérilisé pendant huit jours : il fut ensuite allaité par une nourrice bonne mais malpropre, à laquelle il fut retiré au bout de deux mois. A ce moment, il reprit du lait stérilisé pendant un jour et eut un fort vomissement. Remis en nourrice dès le lendemain, le vomissement ne reparut plus. Le lait de la nourrice avait huit mois quand elle prit l'enfant qui se développa mal pendant un mois, mais n'eut pas le moindre trouble digestif. A ce moment, l'enfant qui avait trois mois fut pris de convulsions qui se transformèrent immédiatement en contractures généralisées avec signe de Trousseau. Cet état dura environ quarante jours, et l'enfant succomba, malgré le traitement (bains, bromure, etc.).

Depuis lors, un nouvel enfant est né, il a environ trois mois, est nourri par la mère et se porte très bien.

Je souligne que la nourrice du petit Georges était porteuse d'un goitre et que la famille n'avait pas cru devoir suivre le conseil que j'avais donné de ne pas la garder.

Telles sont mes trois observations. Comme je l'ai dit, lorsque j'eus observé mon premier malade, je demeurai longtemps perplexe sur la question du diagnostic pathogénique. Lorsque j'eus observé le second, je ne pus m'empêcher de le rapprocher du premier, les manifestations cliniques étant identiques, et les nourrices ayant présenté toutes deux, la première très nettement, la seconde d'une façon plus douteuse, des manifestations de la maladie de Basedow. A dater de ce moment, je me promis, dès que l'occasion se présenterait d'étudier un nouveau cas de tétanie chez un nourrisson, d'examiner le corps thyroïde de sa nourrice. L'occasion ne se présenta qu'en octobre 1898. Ce cas de tétanie ne pouvant s'expliquer par d'autres raisons que la présence d'un goitre très net chez sa nourrice vint confirmer mes soupçons, et c'est depuis lors que, sans oser être absolument affirmatif, je n'ai plus accepté de nourrices goitreuses ; et voilà pourquoi je désire soumettre cette opinion à l'appréciation des membres du Congrès.

Avant de nous livrer à quelques considérations spéciales sur nos trois malades, nous devons, semble-t-il, répondre à trois questions générales : 1° la tétanie qui reconnaît des origines assez variables chez l'enfant (intoxications intestinales, hystérie, etc.) peut-elle être d'origine thyroïdienne ? 2° les phénomènes de thyroïdisme ou d'athyroïdmie, comme a proposé le D' Davel[1] sont-ils transmissibles par le lait de la nourrice au nourrisson ? 3° pourquoi ces accidents donnent-ils plutôt lieu à de la tétanie qu'à du myxœdème chez le nourrisson ?

1re QUESTION. — *La tétanie peut-elle être d'origine thyroïdienne ?* — Nous savons que la tétanie peut être d'origine thyroïdienne ; cette étiologie est signalée par Combe (de Lausanne) dans le chapitre myxœdème du *Traité des maladies de l'enfance*, récemment publié en France, et par Escherich (de Graz) dans le chapitre tétanie du même traité[2]. Je sais bien que ces faits ont été surtout signalés dans le myxœdème opératoire, mais il est permis d'admettre qu'ils peuvent se produire dans toute manifestation thyroïdienne.

J'invoquerai, à l'appui de cette manière de voir, le cas de Calabresse[3] : Un enfant atteint d'un myxœdème, qui présentait d'ailleurs quelques particularités cliniques, fut soumis avec succès au traitement thyroïdien ; mais ce traitement dut être suspendu à plusieurs reprises parce qu'il produisit des phénomènes de thyroïdisme qui disparurent chaque fois que le traitement fut interrompu. Or, parmi ces phéno-

---

1. *Société médicale argentine*, 31 juillet 1899.
2. *Traité des maladies de l'enfance*, sous la direction de GRANCHER, COMBY, MARFAN, chez Masson, 1898.
3. Acad. de Naples. *In Gaz. degli assed.*, 17 sept. 1898, p. 1190.

mènes, l'auteur cite le tremblement et les secousses musculaires, il est logique de supposer que, si le traitement avait continué, ces secousses musculaires auraient pris une intensité qui aurait rapproché ce cas de ceux de nos trois malades.

Je crois donc pouvoir tirer cette conclusion que la tétanie du nourrisson peut être d'origine thyroïdienne.

2ᵉ QUESTION. — *Les phénomènes de thyroïdisme sont-ils transmissibles par le lait, de la nourrice au nourrisson?* — Si cette première conclusion est admise, il faut nous demander maintenant si les phénomènes d'athyroïdémie de la nourrice peuvent être véhiculés par le lait de la nourrice au nourrisson.

Ici nous possédons des faits assez précis pour nous permettre d'être affirmatifs.

Mossé (de Toulouse) et Cathala (de Castillon) ont rapporté le fait d'un nourrisson atteint de goitre congénital qui se montra excessivement sensible au traitement thyroïdien suivi par la mère qui le nourrissait au sein [1]. D'autre part, Byrom Bramwel insiste sur les propriétés galactogogues du suc thyroïdien, mais il ajoute que ces propriétés ne peuvent être utilisées à cause de leur influence sur le nourrisson. Cet auteur rapporte un cas non douteux de ce genre dans lequel un nourrisson présenta des phénomènes d'intoxication chaque fois que la mère, atteinte de goitre exophtalmique, fut soumise au traitement thyroïdien [2]. Les rapports entre les phénomènes thyroïdiens de la nourrice et ceux du nourrisson semblent nettement établis, et il est probable qu'en appelant l'attention sur ces faits nous provoquerons de nouvelles observations.

3ᵉ QUESTION. — *Pourquoi les accidents donnent-ils plutôt lieu à de la tétanie qu'à du myxœdème chez le nourrisson?* — Il semble impossible de répondre à cette question, dans l'état actuel de la science. Y a-t-il à invoquer la susceptibilité du système nerveux et son affinité pour certains poisons à cet âge? Y a-t-il à faire intervenir le rôle du thymus, celui des organes hématopoïétiques dans la croissance [3]? Tout cela est possible, mais nous ne croyons pas devoir nous exposer à nous égarer sur cette question dans le domaine des hypothèses et des inconnues.

Si ces données générales sont admises, quel profit pouvons-nous en retirer pour tirer des conclusions particulières à nos trois malades?

La malade de la seconde observation est, je le reconnais, peu pro-

---

1. Académie de médecine, 12 avril 1898.

2. *The Lancet*, 1899, p. 162.

3. LANCEREAUX. Les glandes vasculaires sanguines: leur rôle pendant la croissance. (*Semaine médicale*, nᵒ 4, 1895.)

bante ; mais elle a cependant une certaine valeur. La nourrice a des phénomènes bien peu apparents, presque discutables : elle a nourri du même lait un frère aîné, qui n'a jamais rien présenté d'anormal. Mais il est permis de se demander si le lait qui a nourri notre petit malade, et qui avait 15 mois de date au moment de la naissance de celui-ci, n'était pas un bon véhicule pour le poison thyroïdien. De plus, ce petit malade relevait d'accidents pulmonaires quand il a été atteint. Or, Charrin[1], Jacob, etc., ont démontré que l'ablation du corps thyroïde rendait les animaux moins résistants aux infections. Le germe qui a produit les accidents pulmonaires n'a-t-il pas pu devenir plus virulent, sous l'influence du lait de la nourrice atteinte de goître? Nous savons enfin que des accidents tétaniques ont été produits sur l'animal par la thyroïdectomie[2].

L'observation du premier malade me semble un peu plus probante. Je sais bien que l'enfant, ayant été nourri par sa mère et non par une nourrice étrangère, il y a lieu de se poser la question de la part à faire à l'hérédité. Je sais bien aussi que la mère a nourri ses deux enfants et qu'un seul a présenté des accidents. Il n'en est pas moins vrai que, dans ce cas, rien ne peut nous expliquer la cause de cette tétanie à forme lente et grave, et que nous ne connaissons en aucune façon le mode de résistance du nourrisson à l'empoisonnement thyroïdien, question qu'il faudrait bien connaître pour avoir une opinion ferme. Mais n'est-on pas bien tenté, au point de vue clinique, d'établir un parallèle entre cette maladie à marche continue et cette cause, continue aussi, qui serait une intoxication quotidienne par un poison constamment véhiculé par le lait?

Quant au troisième malade, mon attention étant éveillée, je l'ai suivi avec grand soin, et je n'ai pu trouver aucune cause à cette tétanie qu'un empoisonnement thyroïdien, la nourrice étant franchement goitreuse, et non, comme les deux autres, atteinte de maladie de Basedow. Pour ce dernier cas, j'oserai être beaucoup plus affirmatif que pour les deux autres, et, depuis que je l'ai observé, je me suis imposé vis-à-vis des nourrices goitreuses une réserve dont je ne me départirai que lorsqu'il m'aura été démontré que je me trompe. Je suis très disposé à me rendre, le jour où cette démonstration serait faite.

Nous ne sommes point arrivés à cette opinion sans nous être fait une

1. *Revue des sciences générales pures et appliquées.* 1895. p. 564. Poisons de l'organisme. (*Encyclopédie des aides mémoire.*)
2. V. à ce sujet le Rapport de Mossé au Congr. de méd. int. Montpellier. 1898 (partie physiologique par Abelous).

objection qui vient peut-être aussi à l'esprit de nos auditeurs, et à laquelle il est bon de répondre : c'est la suivante. Dans nos régions du Midi, beaucoup de nourrices sont goitreuses et les accidents de ce genre sont rares chez les nourrissons. Je réponds à cela que nous ne sommes pas aussi bien renseignés que nous paraissons le croire. Outre que l'attention n'a pas encore été appelée sur ce point, peut-être y aurait-il lieu de vérifier de plus près beaucoup de décès de nourrissons qui sont inscrits sous la rubrique « convulsions ».

Mais, même en admettant que la communication du thyroïdisme de la nourrice au nourrisson soit rare, bien des éléments nous manquent pour apprécier cette rareté : étant donnée une nourrice goitreuse, savons-nous exactement quelle est la valeur de son corps thyroïde ? Sommes-nous suffisamment renseignés sur la valeur de ses glandes thyroïdiennes accessoires qui peuvent suppléer l'organe malade[1]? A un point de vue général, pouvons-nous, en présence d'un goitre, en affirmer la nature exacte et son coefficient toxique, si je puis ainsi m'exprimer? les résultats du traitement thyroïdien, si utiles dans beaucoup de cas, nous réservent souvent des surprises, jusqu'à présent inexplicables[2]. La Clinique de son côté nous montre des faits qui nous imposent la plus grande prudence. Je n'en veux pour preuve que les idées disparates qui règnent au sujet du goitre exophtalmique, ce qui doit, à notre humble avis, s'expliquer par la diversité des cas. Voici, en effet, le Dr Pader qui, à l'instigation de M. le professeur Debove, cherche à établir une parenté étroite entre le goitre exophtalmique et l'hystérie[3]. Par contre, Paul Courmont a récemment rapporté un cas de goitre exophtalmique, coïncidant avec des troubles de myxœdème[4]. Ces faits, joints à ceux que chacun peut se rappeler dans sa pratique personnelle, aux résultats très variables du traitement thyroïdien, aux formes différentes du myxœdème fruste, nous prouvent qu'au milieu de toutes ces inconnues il faut se contenter d'exposer les faits, en attendant que nous puissions les interpréter. Cela ne veut cependant pas dire qu'il faille rester muet en présence d'un fait clinique, sans chercher aucune explication.

C'est sans autre prétention que j'ai exposé ces faits sans attendre une démonstration physiologique, parce que, s'ils sont exacts, comme on est en droit de le supposer, ils ont une importance capitale. Pour

---

1. V. à ce sujet la thèse de doctorat de Verdun. Toulouse, 28 juillet 1897.
2. VAQUEZ. Les étapes historiques de l'opothérapie. (*Presse médicale*, p. 121, 10 mars 1900.)
3. PADER. Étude sur les rapports du goitre exophtalmique et de l'hystérie. *Thèse de Paris*, 1899.
4. Soc. des sc. médicales de Lyon, 6 décembre 1899.

le moment, je me contente de les résumer dans cette proposition : il
est bon d'étudier la question de savoir si une nourrice goitreuse doit
être refusée. Les accidents de tétanie survenus chez nos malades, la
facilité avec laquelle le traitement thyroïdien de la nourrice influence
le nourrisson, la sensibilité spéciale du jeune âge à ce traitement,
engagent à les refuser par prudence, jusqu'à ce qu'une connaissance
plus complète de la question permette d'avoir une opinion ferme,
favorable ou non à cette manière de voir.

LES DOCTRINES DE L'ALLAITEMENT ARTIFICIEL ; LAIT DE FEMME
AGISSANT COMME FERMENT

par M. le professeur ESCHERICH,

de Graz.

L' « allaitement artificiel », qui a été choisi par le Comité de la
Section comme première question d'étude, est tout à la fois le chapitre le plus important et le plus difficile de la pédiatrie.

Bien que le lait de la mère nous offre le type qu'il s'agit d'atteindre, et bien que dans le lait de vache nous possédions un aliment
de composition très similaire et, en outre, très aisément modifiable
par l'adjonction de certaines substances, nous sommes néanmoins
encore bien loin d'avoir résolu la question. La raison de cet échec
est probablement en ceci, que nous ne savons pas quels sont exactement les éléments constituants du lait de femme qui, dans l'allaitement, font sa supériorité bien connue sur le lait de vache. Il est
naturel qu'en premier lieu l'attention se soit portée sur les différences
quantitatives des matières nutritives contenues dans ces laits. Bie-
DERT a eu le mérite incontestable d'avoir, le premier, insisté sur les
différences, sur la concentration plus marquée et sur la digestibilité
plus difficile de la caséine du lait de vache. De nombreux auteurs ont
essayé d'effacer les différences qui existent dans les proportions res-
pectives de chacun des principes nutritifs contenus dans ces deux
laits, de même qu'ils ont essayé d'en corriger la qualité. La proposition émise aujourd'hui par M. Monti est née de la même idée.
Cependant aucun de ces auteurs n'a réussi jusqu'à présent à obtenir
un aliment qui soit l'équivalent du lait de mère. Cette constatation
est d'autant plus faite pour nous surprendre que, d'après les recherches les plus récentes, il paraît vraisemblable que dans certaines

limites la résorption des principes nutritifs du lait de vache n'est pas notablement inférieure à celle des éléments constituants du lait de femme. Au contraire, les résultats de toutes les recherches s'accordent en ceci que les enfants soumis à l'allaitement artificiel ingèrent une quantité trop abondante de nourriture et qu'il n'est pas rare que cette alimentation ne devienne chez eux la cause d'accidents graves et même mortels. Les recherches sur les échanges nutritifs démontrent que ces enfants absorbent et éliminent une quantité d'azote alimentaire dépassant de beaucoup leurs besoins.

L'échec de l'alimentation artificielle ne peut donc pas être entièrement attribué à l'apport insuffisant ou à la digestibilité imparfaite de la nourriture : il s'ensuit que toutes les tentatives ayant pour but de supprimer cette difficulté hypothétique par la digestion préalable ou par la substitution d'autres éléments ont également échoué.

Cet échec, qui suit comme leur ombre toutes les propositions émises dans le domaine de l'allaitement artificiel en vue d'améliorer les conditions de ce dernier, aurait dû avoir pour effet qu'on se posât la question si la voie de recherches suivie déjà depuis 50 ans peut réellement conduire au but : si, à côté des corps nutritifs et des sels sur lesquels, jusqu'à présent, on s'est borné à fixer exclusivement l'attention, il n'y a point d'autres éléments qu'on doive prendre en considération et qui, sans contribuer directement à la constitution de l'organisme ou à sa réserve d'énergie, sont néanmoins d'une importance capitale pour la prospérité du nourrisson.

Depuis peu nous connaissons un tel corps dans le *nucléon* découvert par Siegfried. Ce nucléon existe dans le lait de femme en quantité bien plus grande que dans le lait de vache. Je dois, de plus, rappeler l'existence des substances que l'analyse chimique ne parvient pas à déceler, et qui pourtant sont actives au point de vue physiologique, substances qui, du sang, passent dans les produits de sécrétion des glandes mammaires. Grâce à leur solubilité, ces substances pénètrent dans l'organisme de l'enfant où, bien qu'en quantité minime, ils arrivent à produire des effets puissants. La preuve scientifique de ce fait, déjà connu depuis bien longtemps des profanes, est fournie par l'expérience classique d'Ehrlich sur l'immunité des nourrissons et tout spécialement par l'expérience connue du changement de nourrice. En ce qui concerne le lait de femme en particulier, la preuve de l'existence de l'antitoxine diphtérique dans ce lait a été démontrée à ma clinique par MM. Schmid et Pfланz. Je présume aussi que c'est sur des raisons semblables que doit reposer la capacité de résistance frappante que les enfants nourris au sein offrent

contre les infections par les cocci pyogènes et qui est si différente de
celle des enfants nourris au biberon.

Il n'est pas facile de décrire en quelques mots les phénomènes que
nous voyons apparaître à la suite de l'allaitement artificiel. Je fais
abstraction des modifications subies par les évacuations alvines et de
la prédisposition beaucoup plus grande des enfants nourris au biberon, pour les maladies, celles-ci pouvant dépendre de causes diverses.
Je me bornerai à la description des phénomènes morbides d'ordre
général.

Ce qui est le plus frappant, c'est le fait que ces phénomènes n'apparaissent point chez tous les enfants soumis à l'allaitement artificiel
et qu'ils affectent, selon le sujet, une manière d'être et un degré d'intensité différents. La supériorité du lait de la mère devient surtout
évidente pendant les premières semaines de la vie et chez les enfants
atteints de faiblesse congénitale ou nés avant terme. La privation de
l'alimentation naturelle se manifeste alors par l'augmentation insuffisante d'abord, puis par la diminution de poids du corps; par la disparition du panicule adipeux, par l'affaissement, par le décubitus dans
un état de somnolence. Tôt ou tard on voit s'y associer des troubles
digestifs, fréquemment aussi des processus septiques jusqu'à ce que
la mort survienne, presque insidieusement, par arrêt progressif de
toutes les fonctions. Toutefois, même chez la plupart des enfants
robustes et nés à terme, de poids normal au moment de la naissance,
lorsque même on réussit à écarter tout trouble morbide, la courbe du
poids présente précisément pendant les premiers mois de la vie une
ascension plus lente que chez les enfants nourris au sein et élevés
dans des conditions identiques. C'est plus tard seulement que ces
enfants rattrapent le poids qui leur manque, et peuvent alors même
dépasser les enfants au sein. Dans nombre de cas ce retard de la
courbe du poids peut pourtant faire défaut, les enfants soumis à
l'allaitement artificiel augmentant dès le début d'une façon normale.
Mais, en comparant ces enfants modèles avec les enfants nourris au
sein, on constate qu'ils peuvent présenter pendant la première
période ou pendant toute la durée de la première année de leur vie,
et même après, une certaine pâleur des joues et des muqueuses, le
teint légèrement jaunâtre, moins de fraîcheur, moins d'activité, moins
de force musculaire, des chairs plus molles, le panicule adipeux
restant normal ou développé en excès.

En ce qui concerne la question tant discutée du rachitisme, celui-ci
est, d'après mon observation personnelle, à peine moins fréquent
chez les enfants au sein que chez les enfants au biberon, seulement

chez ces derniers il atteint plus souvent ses degrés les plus graves. Quant au scorbut infantile (maladie de Barlow), je ne l'ai pas constaté une seule fois sur les milliers d'enfants allaités artificiellement au lait stérilisé qui ont passé sous mes yeux à Munich et à Graz.

En considérant l'ensemble de ces phénomènes, l'impression se dégage qu'il s'agit plutôt de troubles dans l'assimilation et l'accroissement de la substance propre du corps que d'une digestion et d'une résorption insuffisantes. Par suite du remplacement incomplet des substances propres du corps désassimilées, ces troubles d'assimilation peuvent, chez les enfants chétifs, amener un épuisement progressif et la mort, tandis que chez les enfants plus âgés ils déterminent un accroissement trop facile du poids du corps, un mélange anormal des humeurs et de l'emmagasinement. Bien que dans les premiers cas, surtout, la dyspepsie et les troubles digestifs soient de règle, il n'est point nécessaire de les considérer comme l'affection première, l'affection principale. Il est, par contre, aisé de comprendre qu'un organisme fonctionnant avec un bilan inférieur au bilan moral ne puisse plus fournir le travail digestif nécessaire à la digestion du lait de vache (CAMERER), sans même compter sur les dangers innombrables dont le menace la surcharge alimentaire et les bactéries qu'il guettent de tous côtés.

Quoi qu'il en soit, lorsqu'on se livre à des réflexions de ce genre, l'idée finit par s'imposer que chez les enfants allaités artificiellement, outre les difficultés qu'ils ont à vaincre dans les voies digestives, il existe des troubles dans l'assimilation et l'utilisation des matières nutritives absorbées, c'est-à-dire des troubles dans des échanges nutritifs intermédiaires qui, selon leur gravité, aboutissent à une extinction progressive de la vie ou engendrent des troubles de la vie végétative. Ceci nous conduit à une théorie nouvelle du mode d'action du lait de femme.

∴

A mesure que nous pénétrons plus avant dans la connaissance des processus des échanges nutritifs, nous apercevons plus nettement que leur évolution normale est liée à la présence de certaines substances de la nature des ferments, que les organes glandulaires fournissent par la voie des sécrétions internes. Ces substances sont déversées dans les humeurs de l'organisme pour y faire subir aux principes nutritifs les transformations nécessaires afin de les rendre assimilables. Ces substances-ferments existent en excès dans l'organisme adulte. Il en est tout autrement chez le nouveau-né, le nourrisson. Nous voyons qu'en dotant celui-ci la nature a procédé avec une parcimonie extrême. En effet, au moment de la naissance, les fonctions ne sont développées que juste autant qu'il est absolument indispensable à la conservation et à la continuation de la vie extra-utérine, sous réserve de conditions particulièrement favorables. L'exactitude de cette remarque ressort d'une façon très nette quand on considère les sécrétions glandulaires qui représentent le travail le plus élevé et le plus compliqué de la vie végétative. Les recherches de ZWEIFEL ont les premières attiré l'attention sur la pauvreté du tube intestinal de l'enfant en ferments digestifs, ce qui établit la différenciation la plus caractéristique de son processus de digestion avec celui de l'adulte. Les observations de l'*École de Breslau*, de même que les recherches de PFAUNDLER sur le ferment oxydant du foie (sujet de sa communication au congrès) parlent en faveur de l'hypothèse qu'un état de choses analogue doit régner dans le domaine des sécrétions internes. Bien que nous n'ayons que des notions restreintes sur ces processus, spécialement chez les nourrissons, il est néanmoins permis de tirer des conclusions par analogie et d'admettre, comme pour tous les autres actes fonctionnels, que dans le domaine des échanges nutritifs il existe également des oscillations individuelles congénitales ou des états d'affaiblissement par des maladies qu'on reconnaît à l'assimilation et à l'accroissement insuffisants ou défectueux, au point de vue qualitatif de la substance propre du corps.

On devra s'attendre à noter ceci, surtout chez les enfants qui, nés avant terme ou présentant à la naissance un poids très inférieur à la normale, sont désignés comme *retardés* dans leur développement. La nature compense l'absence physiologique des sucs digestifs chez les nouveau-nés en élaborant pour eux le lait de femme de façon qu'il soit apte à être résorbé presque sans l'action de ferments. Mais à quoi leur sert-il d'avoir une nourriture digestible s'ils ne possèdent pas la capacité d'utiliser les éléments nutritifs, résorbés, de manière à les transformer en nutriments contribuant à l'accroissement du corps?

Il faut nous rappeler maintenant que, dans le lait de femme, il existe, en dehors des principes nutritifs sécrétés par la glande mammaire, des corps qui lui sont cédés par le sérum du sang : les antitoxines et certainement aussi les substances chargées d'entretenir l'assimilation que je nommerai tout court les ferments d'échanges nutritifs. Absorbés avec les matières nutritives ils pénètrent dans les humeurs de l'organisme infantile, où, comme dans l'organisme de la mère, ils régularisent les échanges nutritifs et suppléent ainsi à l'absence éventuelle (par suite du développement insuffisant du système glandulaire) de ces ferments dans l'organisme même de l'enfant ; leur quantité minime et leur composition de nature très complexe les feront encore pendant longtemps échapper à l'analyse chimique. Ce sera une tâche nouvelle et intéressante de déceler leur présence expérimentalement, à l'instar de celle des antitoxines, par l'étude de leurs effets physiologiques.

Nous savons déjà, à l'heure qu'il est, que des corps de ce genre sont contenus dans le lait de femme : je parle du fait découvert par Bouchut, et tout récemment confirmé à ma clinique par Moro, que le lait de femme renferme des quantités assez notables de ferment diastasique. Envisagé au point de vue téléologique, ce fait semble un gaspillage de la nature, car les aliments du nourrisson ne renferment point de substances devant être rendues propres à la digestion par l'action du ferment diastasique.

Cependant, si nous réfléchissons que la fonction diastasique est une propriété des tissus vivants et des ferments, largement répandue, nous sommes obligés de ne plus l'envisager comme entité en soi, mais comme preuve de la présence, en général, de substances-ferments, dont la destination véritable reste encore à rechercher, mais qui se trouve peut-être en rapport avec les hypothèses énoncées plus haut. De plus, le fait que ce ferment diastasique est relativement abondant dans le lait de femme, tandis que le lait de vache en est à peu près, sinon totalement dépourvu, est d'un certain intérêt ; il démontre, en effet, qu'il s'agit ici de corps spécifiques uniquement propres au lait humain.

L'expérience journalière enseigne qu'il est très possible de nourrir les enfants avec du lait, et même avec du lait stérilisé, dans lequel toute vie organique et tous ferments sont détruits.

Il n'y a pas un médecin d'enfants qui ne connaisse des cas isolés de nourrissons élevés au lait stérilisé, et qui dès le début présentent un développement normal et même un état général florissant. Ces cas démontrent que, dans certaines conditions, l'organisme infantile peut être privé des corps albuminoïdes spécifiques et des ferments contenus dans le lait de la mère (Bordet), sans en éprouver de dommage, c'est-à-dire lorsque les élaborations fonctionnelles de l'organisme infantile ont atteint un développement assez marqué pour pourvoir par eux-mêmes à la résorption et à l'assimilation de la nourriture. Il s'agit alors généralement d'enfants nés à terme, de poids initial normal ou au-dessus de la normale, ce qui prouve déjà qu'ils sont des sujets vigoureux et parfaitement développés.

A l'encontre de cela, nous voyons des enfants nés avant terme, atteints de faiblesse congénitale, affaiblis par la maladie (athrepsie) prospérer peu ou pas et présenter les phénomènes énoncés plus haut. Si avec cela on compare le développement d'un enfant en des conditions identiques, mais nourri au sein, on est tenté de parler d'une réaction spécifique de l'organisme que ces enfants offrent à l'apport du lait de la mère. A notre crèche où, malheureusement, nous n'avons à notre disposition qu'un nombre restreint de nourrices, nous avons assez souvent eu l'occasion de nous convaincre de l'effet pour ainsi dire merveilleux, produit par l'allaitement naturel exclusif ou même mixte. Nous n'avons jamais été capable d'obtenir les mêmes résultats par les soins les plus dévoués, ni par des modifications de la méthode d'alimentation, ni par l'administration de l'albumine soluble ou préalablement digérée. Au point de vue clinique, on acquiert comme une impression que le lait de femme doit contenir des substances stimulantes et tonifiantes, dans le sens le meilleur du mot, et que c'est dès ce moment seulement que la nourriture profite réellement à l'enfant et contribue à l'accroissement de sa substance propre.

C'est l'observation réitérée de ce fait qui m'a amené à croire que pour ces enfants le lait constituait à la fois une source d'alimentation et une source de forces contribuant à l'utilisation parfaite de ce qu'ils ingèrent.

C'est alors pour faciliter la compréhension de ces faits que s'offre tout naturellement à notre esprit l'hypothèse des ferments d'échanges nutritifs cités précédemment et dont nous pouvons bien admettre la présence dans le lait de femme ; ferments qui peut-être font défaut chez ces enfants par suite d'un retard de développement ou d'une production insuffisante. L'organisme infantile devient ainsi, pareillement à ce qui a eu lieu lors de la circulation placentaire, une sorte de circuit collatéral interposé dans les échanges nutritifs de la mère, de sorte que la secousse violente qu'il éprouve par sa séparation de l'organisme maternel se trouve en partie atténuée. Il nous est ainsi possible de comprendre que le lait de femme qui est si indispensable et que rien ne peut remplacer pour les enfants atteints de faiblesse congénitale, puisse, pour les enfants vigoureux et plus âgés, ne plus constituer qu'un aliment de bonne qualité et spécialement bien adapté aux organes digestifs, aliment dont ils peuvent être privés sans dommage particulier et auquel on peut substituer le lait de vache. De telle façon nous nous trouvons par une autre voie encore amenés à nous convaincre combien merveilleusement l'allaitement naturel répond à son but et à reconnaître combien sont vaines toutes les tentatives de rendre le lait de vache, par des mélanges et des modifications de ses éléments constituants, équivalent au lait de femme.

Il s'agit ici d'une hypothèse qui naturellement doit être vérifiée par des observations ultérieures. Des recherches dans ce sens sont en cours à notre clinique, et j'espère avoir l'occasion d'en communiquer les résultats.

La justification de cette hypothèse est en analogie avec l'immunité des nourrissons démontrée par Ehrlich et en concordance avec les observations cliniques sur les indications et l'utilité du lait de femme. Je cite ici encore un autre fait d'observation : le nombre restreint de nourrices que nous avons à notre disposition à la crèche nous oblige de répartir la petite quantité de lait de femme disponible entre le plus grand nombre possible de nourrissons nécessiteux, et de compléter leur ration journalière avec du lait de vache modifié (lait gras de Gaertner). La majorité de nos enfants nourris au sein est, en somme, soumis à l'allaitement mixte avec prépondérance notable de l'alimentation artificielle. Malgré cela, ces enfants, tout en présentant des matières alvines du type propre aux enfants alimentés avec du lait gras de Gaertner, se développent aussi bien et, quant à leur accroissement, ne diffèrent presque pas des enfants nourris au sein. Ce fait ne serait pas compréhensible si la supériorité du lait de femme résidait uniquement dans la digestibilité plus facile de ses principes nutritifs et surtout de l'albumine ; le bénéfice de l'allaitement au sein devrait alors décroître proportionnellement à la quantité de lait de femme remplacé par le lait de vache. Ce n'est pas le cas d'après nos observations, et d'autres auteurs aussi recommandent, pour la première période de la vie, précisément, l'allaitement mixte par adjonction même de minimes quantités de lait maternel. L'hypothèse de l'existence d'une substance-ferment excitant les échanges nutritifs, douée d'activité même dans de minimes quantités de lait de femme, nous fournit une explication naturelle de ce fait d'observation. Évidemment cela fait de nouveau reculer bien loin l'espoir qu'on réussisse jamais à trouver un aliment parfaitement équivalent au lait de femme utilisable précisément pour les êtres qui en ont le plus besoin.

Toutefois, reconnaître les difficultés, c'est déjà un pas de fait pour les vaincre. C'est pourquoi je me suis cru autorisé à présenter ici, à la suite des questions en discussion, cette hypothèse qui m'occupe depuis très longtemps.

L'incertitude qui règne encore à l'heure actuelle sur les différences principales entre le lait de femme et le lait de vache devient évidente lorsqu'on envisage quel grand nombre de propositions et de méthodes, ayant pour but de faire disparaître cette différence, ont été proposées autrefois et encore aujourd'hui.

En opposition aux systèmes fondés sur une base théorique, je considère comme méritant le plus de confiance la voie simple et sans artifice que j'ai suivie dès 1886 en adoptant ma méthode volumétrique : Recherches sur les quantités ou volumes de nourriture ingérée par les enfants nourris au sein, avec indication en chiffres de quantités correspondantes de lait de vache modifié et étendu d'eau. Je constate avec plaisir que Monti s'est servi de la même méthode dans le tableau qu'il donne de l'allaitement par le lait coupé de petit-lait.

La fixation du nombre des repas du nourrisson et de la quantité de nourriture de chacun de ces repas me semble être, jusqu'à présent, une chose des plus importantes dans l'alimentation de tout jeunes enfants; je suis persuadé que les résultats étonnamment favorables qu'obtient M. Variot par l'administration de lait de vache non coupé ni stérilisé sont dus à la façon très rigoureuse dont il restreint les quantités ingérées à chaque repas.

Je dois d'ailleurs avouer que, si justifié qu'il paraisse et qu'il soit, le fait de s'appuyer sur les conditions de l'allaitement au sein, pour établir une alimentation scientifique des nourrissons, ne constitue pas le but définitif à atteindre.

En faisant abstraction des différences qualitatives des deux genres de lait, on pourra toujours objecter que la suralimentation si habituelle chez les enfants nourris artificiellement peut tout autant exister chez les enfants nourris au sein. Les anciens essais de Biedert pour établir la nourriture minima ainsi que les expériences connues faites par Heubner conjointement avec Rubner sur l'assimilation et les échanges nutritifs chez les enfants nourris artificiellement doivent être considérés comme les premières tentatives faites pour établir les principes propres de la doctrine de l'alimentation artificielle en la délivrant de l'imitation servile de l'allaitement au sein. Les efforts de Cammerer et de Heubner pour faire concorder la doctrine des échanges nutritifs des nourrissons avec les lois découvertes par Rubner ont ouvert une voie nouvelle que nous saluons comme pleine de promesses pour arriver à la solution du problème. Ce progrès ne doit pas toutefois nous faire oublier ce qui dans les anciennes doctrines sur l'alimentation a fait ses preuves comme étant exact et utilisable, ainsi que c'est le cas, pour les qualités propres et la valeur différente des différents principes nutritifs contenus dans les divers laits. Malgré les mérites éminents de M. HEUBNER, je ne puis pas le suivre lorsqu'il veut évaluer la nourriture uniquement d'après sa valeur en calories. Il fixe le chiffre de 100 calories par kilogramme d'enfant comme chiffre type. Je crois que dans le total de ces chiffres il ne faut pas négliger la répartition des calories représentées par chacune des substances nutritives; de même ce chiffre type n'est pas applicable aux nourrissons d'âges différents, car il constitue plutôt la résultante de la méthode d'alimentation en usage que celle du besoin physiologique. Pour confirmer ce que je viens de dire, je joins à la fin de ce travail quelques chiffres recueillis à ma clinique par M. le Dr ADAM (assistant volontaire) relatifs aux quantités de nourriture prise par les nourrissons soumis à l'alimentation artificielle et qui répondent aux demandes qui nous ont été adressées dans ce sens par M. HEUBNER.

Les sujets d'observations sont pris parmi les pupilles de l'asile des Enfants trouvés de Styrie qui, en partie par suite de faiblesse congénitale, en partie à cause de quelque maladie externe n'altérant pas l'état général, ont dû être retenus à l'hôpital. Ces enfants furent nourris uniquement avec du *lait gras de Gaertner*, stérilisé à la laiterie et souvent même coupé d'eau. Ces enfants furent pesés très exactement tous les jours, et la quantité d'aliments donnée fut, comme pour tous les nourrissons de la clinique, exactement déterminée quant à sa quantité et à sa composition. De plus, à certains jours, le médecin fit lui-même des vérifications pour contrôler l'exactitude des pesées et mensurations; de même on procéda plusieurs fois à la pesée des matières alvines et à l'analyse de contrôle du lait gras de Gaertner. Pour faire ces calculs on a choisi des nourrissons qui depuis plusieurs semaines ou plusieurs mois n'avaient présenté absolument aucun trouble dans leur développement et qui dans leur accroissement ne restaient pas en dessous des chiffres établis par CAMMERER pour les nourrissons de cet âge et basés sur le poids à la naissance. C'est ainsi qu'on a pu réussir à établir approximativement, pour un chiffre de dix nourrissons à développement normal, la quantité de nourriture ingérée entre la deuxième et la douzième semaine de la vie. Cette époque est précisément la plus importante au point de vue physiologique et pratique, et nous ne possédons jusqu'ici sur elle que très peu de pesées.

TABLEAU COMPARATIF

des calories et des quantités de substances alimentaires prises par les enfants observés et de celles qu'ils auraient reçues
en suivant les données de **Biedert** et de **Heubner**.

AGE (en semaines)	III			IV			V			VI			VII			VIII			IX			X			XI			XII			XIII		
POIDS de l'enfant	3500			3800			4000			4500			4500			4700			4900			5000			5100			5250			5300		
AUTEURS	Biedert	Heubner	Observat. personnelle	Biedert	Heubner	Observ. pers.	Biedert	Heubner	Observ. pers.	Biedert	Heubner	Observ. pers.	Biedert	Heubner	Observ. pers.	Biedert	Heubner	Observ. pers.	Biedert	Heubner	Observ. pers.	Biedert	Heubner	Observ. pers.	Biedert	Heubner	Observ. pers.	Biedert	Heubner	Observ. pers.	Biedert	Heubner	Observ. pers.
Calories par kilog. d'enfant — Albumine	6.0	14.0	4.8	5.8	12.2	5.4	5.8	14.4	7.6	5.8	15.4	7.0	5.8	12.8	6.5	5.8	14.5	6.6	5.9	15.7	7.7	5.8	15.5	8.9	5.8	15.2	8.6	5.8	12.9	8.5	5.8	12.5	8.0
Calories par kilog. d'enfant — Graisse	15.5	52.6	21.9	14.7	51.0	25.0	14.7	51.5	51.5	14.7	51.9	51.5	14.7	50.4	29.5	14.7	56.9	29.9	14.9	56.0	51.8	14.8	55.5	40.5	14.7	51.6	58.8	14.8	54.0	57.5	14.8	57.2	56.0
Calories par kilog. d'enfant — Sucre	51.8	49.4	28.5	52.6	42.6	50.2	51.4	49.8	40.0	51.4	46.5	58.1	52.2	44.5	55.9	51.1	50.0	55.8	51.8	48.4	54.2	51.5	47.1	55.4	50.8	46.2	54.0	51.8	45.7	52.7	54.0	45.6	51.4
Calories par jour	175	325	182	242	325	224	207	599	512	225	591	551	257	594	519	242	179	529	247	179	577	239	179	425	281	179	425	271	179	425	275	179	425
Quantité de nourriture par jour	650	600	540	750	600	600	800	750	760	860	750	780	900	750	800	940	900	800	980	900	800	1000	900	800	1020	900	800	1050	900	800	1080	900	800

Les valeurs de nourriture exprimées en calories, après avoir été déterminées séparément pour chaque substance alimentaire, montrèrent que pour cette période d'âge le chiffre type de 100 calories par kilogramme fixé par Heubner n'était pas atteint, et même que les quantités de substances nutritives, surtout de l'albumine, restent pendant le premier mois de la vie notablement au-dessous du chiffre de nourriture minima établi par Biedert. Dans le tableau ci-après nous avons représenté en calories les quantités moyennes de substances nutritives par septenaires, trouvées par nous empiriquement ; à côté se trouve placée, pour la comparaison, l'indication des quantités de lait que le même enfant aurait reçues s'il avait été nourri d'après les méthodes de Biedert (1/5 de lait) ou de Heubner (2/5 de lait).

On voit au premier coup d'œil que ces deux méthodes, surtout celle de Heubner, prescrivent des quantités de nourriture bien plus grandes que celles absorbées par nos enfants dont l'accroissement a néanmoins été brillant. La valeur de ces chiffres pour la fixation des bases scientifiques de l'allaitement artificiel est évidente et elle a été très exactement mise en lumière dans le discours de M. Heubner.

J'engage ceux de mes auditeurs qui s'intéressent particulièrement à cette question d'aller visiter à l'Exposition la section autrichienne du groupe XVI (Hygiène) qui se trouve placée dans une pièce latérale du pavillon Pasteur. Là ils pourront voir la représentation graphique de la courbe du poids des nourrissons, celle des quantités et volume de nourriture absorbés par eux et exprimés en calories par kilogramme d'enfant: la comparaison de ces courbes avec celles obtenues par d'autres méthodes d'alimentation. Ils y verront aussi le plan et la photographie de la couveuse fabriquée d'après nos indications (chambre-couveuse), ainsi qu'un modèle des boîtes destinées à la crèche et qui doivent contenir tous les objets usuels pour chaque nourrisson (biberon, tétine, thermomètre, etc.).

LA CLINIQUE DES NOURRISSONS A DRESDE
SON ORGANISATION, SES PROCÉDÉS ET SES RÉFORMES
DANS L'ALIMENTATION

par **M.** le docteur **FLACHS**,

de Dresde.

La mortalité des nourrissons est un des plus grands fléaux de l'humanité. Je n'attirerai pas votre attention sur des faits déjà tant de fois discutés. J'essaierai seulement de vous montrer combien une institution consacrée spécialement aux nourrissons peut être utile pour combattre le mal. Mais je vous rappellerai que M. le professeur Biedert, de Hagenau, a depuis longtemps insisté sur l'utilité et même la nécessité d'un établissement destiné à des recherches concernant l'alimentation générale (*Versuchsanstalt für Ernährung*).

L'année dernière, à Munich, au Congrès des naturalistes et des médecins allemands (section de pédiatrie), il a publié ce qu'il a nommé lui-même son testament sur cette matière.

Le programme qu'il a proposé comprend l'alimentation générale — nourrissons, enfants, adultes, — à l'état de santé et de maladie, — programme étendu s'il en est et qui demandera beaucoup de temps pour sa réalisation.

C'est ce qui nous a donné l'idée, à M. le Dr Schlossmann et à moi, de mettre en pratique une partie de ces idées, en établissant à Dresde une clinique spéciale pour les nourrissons.

Il y a quelques années, le Dr Schlossmann avait fondé une policlinique pour les enfants, qui fut la base de notre institution. En 1898, une société fut instituée (*Kinderpoliklinik in der König Johann Vorstadt mit Säuglingsheim*) pour créer la clinique des nourrissons tout en gardant la policlinique. L'établissement, qui possédait d'abord 12 lits, en eut plus tard 18; aujourd'hui, nous pouvons au besoin prendre 25 nourrissons. Jusqu'à présent nos ressources n'ont pu encore nous permettre d'avoir un bâtiment spécial, ce que nous espérons pouvoir obtenir plus tard.

Pour le moment, la clinique occupe le premier étage d'une maison privée, comprenant : trois salles consacrées aux enfants et aux nourrices, une autre comme salle d'isolement pour des cas spéciaux, un cabinet de consultation, une chambre pour la sœur, une petite salle où le lait est préparé le matin, enfin cuisine et dépendances.

Dans la plus grande salle se trouvent quatre couveuses (modèle de

Lion simplifié). Au rez-de-chaussée sont installés le laboratoire de chimie et la policlinique (médecine interne et chirurgie).

Dans la clinique ne sont admis que les nourrissons malades, jusqu'à l'âge d'environ un an; les cas contagieux et ceux de chirurgie ne sont pas acceptés.

A la tête de la clinique sont deux docteurs en chef qui s'occupent également de la médecine interne de la policlinique. Le service de la policlinique comprend aussi un chirurgien, un oculiste, un spécialiste pour les maladies de la peau et des oreilles, et un dentiste. Tous ont leurs heures de consultation pendant lesquelles ils ont à leur disposition l'interne de la clinique.

La sœur supérieure a sous sa direction trois ou quatre élèves qui s'occupent des soins à donner aux enfants. L'engagement de ces jeunes filles doit durer un an. En entrant, elles doivent déposer une caution de 100 marks qui leur sera rendue à la fin de leur engagement. Si elles partent plus tôt, une certaine somme est retenue suivant la durée de leur stage. Après leur année de service, elles subissent un examen pour obtenir leur certificat de garde-malade; ces gardes-malades sont toujours très recherchées auprès des enfants. Nous n'avons pu répondre à toutes les demandes qui nous ont été adressées.

Pour le traitement des nourrissons, le lait maternel étant la meilleure nourriture, nous avons tout naturellement des nourrices. Grâce à l'amabilité de M. le professeur Léopold, de la Maternité à Dresde et au grand intérêt qu'il nous a témoigné, les nourrices nous sont envoyées directement de là. Après un examen très minutieux, elles sont acceptées avec leurs enfants à titre gratuit. D'abord elles nourrissent leurs enfants, tout en allaitant les nourrissons malades. Peu à peu elles commencent à sevrer leurs propres enfants qui se trouvent à merveille de cet allaitement mixte. De cette manière les enfants sont mieux préparés pour l'alimentation artificielle, s'ils quittent la maison, soit que la mère reprenne ses occupations habituelles, soit qu'elle entre comme nourrice dans une maison privée (ce qui a lieu quand nous pouvons nous passer d'elles). Pour des cas imprévus, nous tâchons tous d'avoir des nourrices en réserve, les bonnes nourrices étant recherchées à Dresde comme partout ailleurs.

Si le séjour de la nourrice se prolonge, elle reçoit un salaire de 40 marks par mois. Quand elle s'en va, son enfant est confié à une des mères-nourrices qui demeurent dans le voisinage de la clinique. Toutes les semaines elles doivent apporter les nourrissons au contrôle de la policlinique. Ainsi, en ne perdant pas les enfants de vue, nous pouvons jusqu'à un certain point empêcher cet infanticide légal des mères-nourrices qui coûte tant de vies à l'État.

Nous avons commencé à envoyer les enfants à la campagne. Il est des cas bien difficiles à guérir dans une clinique, pour lesquels un changement d'air est plus efficace que tout autre remède.

Quoique l'allaitement par une nourrice soit bien supérieur à l'allaitement artificiel, tous les bébés ne peuvent être nourris au sein. Il faut donc veiller à ce que l'allaitement artificiel soit réglé d'une manière consciencieuse. Pour des enfants en bonne santé, un régime bien suivi peut parfaitement remplacer l'allaitement naturel.

Il va sans dire que le lait vient de vaches saines qui ont été inoculées avec la tuberculine. Le plus grand soin est apporté en ce qui concerne le trayage et le transport du lait. Au laboratoire, sa densité et son degré d'acidité sont contrôlés (lessive de soude normale et phénophtaléine); plus tard on dose la teneur en beurre (méthode de Gerber : acide sulfurique, centrifugation, etc., — ou de Soxhlet : extraction au moyen de l'éther). Plusieurs fois par semaine, on dose aussi la teneur du lait en glycose (méthode de Fehling) et en matières azotées (procédé de Kjeldahl). Dans la plupart des cas, nous employons un mélange de crème et d'eau dans les mêmes proportions que celles du lait maternel. Les avantages de la crème sur le lait ordinaire sont : une plus grande propreté (nettoyage par la centrifugation) et une teneur plus constante en beurre, qui fait que la nourriture reste chaque jour la même.

Dans une petite salle spéciale, la nourriture est préparée dans les proportions voulues. Les mélanges sont alors distribués dans des flacons soigneusement nettoyés et stérilisés dans un appareil de Soxhlet. Les bouteilles sont fermées par une sorte de capsule en caoutchouc avec un anneau au goulot. Deux petits trous à l'anneau laissent sortir la vapeur. Une fois le flacon refroidi, les trous se ferment d'eux-mêmes et la fermeture est hermétique, ce qui est indiqué par la dépression de la capsule. Les flacons sont alors placés dans l'appareil de Soxhlet qui renferme quatre casiers, pouvant contenir chacun 80 bouteilles. L'appareil a une paroi double dont l'intervalle est rempli d'eau. Cette eau est mise en ébullition au moyen du gaz jusqu'à 97 degrés, ce qui s'annonce par une sonnerie électrique. L'ébullition est maintenue pendant 5 à 10 minutes, durée suffisante. Les flacons ainsi stérilisés que nous avons exposés à une température constante de 57 degrés n'offraient aucune décomposition pendant les trois premiers jours.

Un certain nombre de flacons sont réservés à l'usage de la clinique;

la plupart sont distribués soit à des familles privées qui les payent,
soit à la clientèle de la policlinique, à un prix très modéré ou même
à titre gratuit. Un mark doit être déposé pour les bouteilles. On vient
les chercher tous les jours entre une heure et trois; les flacons vides
sont rapportés le lendemain. Les mères n'ont qu'à chauffer les flacons
avant de les donner aux enfants et à remplacer l'obturateur par une
tétine. Cet arrangement vaut beaucoup mieux que toutes les prescriptions indiquées jusqu'à présent pour la préparation du lait à domicile.

Quant aux observations cliniques, j'ai peu de chose à ajouter à
ce qui est déjà connu de tous. Je désire seulement insister sur ce fait
que, le traitement des nourrissons étant basé uniquement sur un
diagnostic objectif, les observations et les études les plus minutieuses
peuvent être de la plus grande utilité pour la pathologie et la thérapeutique infantile.

La température, le pouls, le poids, sont représentés sur un tableau
par des tracés; la qualité et la quantité de la nourriture sont notées,
le lait maternel en rouge, l'autre nourriture en noir. La quantité du
lait que l'enfant tète est aussi notée; les selles sont examinées (couleur, forme, densité, contenu en microbes, etc.), de sorte que le
tableau peut rendre compte, autant que possible, de l'état de l'enfant.

Les différentes méthodes que nous avons appliquées, les expériences
que nous avons pu faire et les résultats obtenus pendant les deux
dernières années seront publiés dans les *Archives de Pédiatrie* (Baginsky et Monti).

Messieurs, dans l'alimentation des enfants, surtout dans l'allaitement artificiel, il y a très peu de choses absolument fixes. Étant donné
que l'absence de microbes dans le lait est indispensable, le problème
chimique suscite d'importants travaux. La même substance agit d'une
façon bien différente dans l'estomac de l'enfant ou dans une éprouvette; le mélange de laits rappelant le plus possible le lait maternel ne
sera jamais qu'un produit artificiel, et nous prônerons en vain les
avantages d'un nouveau succédané du lait maternel, s'il n'est pas à la
portée de toutes les bourses.

Ce n'est pourtant pas une raison pour se décourager. En raison de
tous les moyens que nous fournissent si largement les sciences naturelles, en raison des observations consciencieusement recueillies dans
les cliniques, nous arriverons au but. Le chemin à parcourir nous est
indiqué. On a travaillé partout. Mais, pour combattre avec succès la
mortalité des nourrissons, des cliniques spéciales, dans le genre de
celle que j'ai essayé de décrire, sont indispensables. En unissant la

pratique à la théorie, les cliniques des nourrissons nous fournissent un terrain sûr, propre à fructifier les résultats de la science. Ces cliniques sont devenues un réel besoin de la vie actuelle.

DE LA VALEUR DU LAIT DE CHÈVRE DANS L'ALIMENTATION DES ENFANTS

RAPPORT

par M. le docteur BARBELLION,

de Paris.

Historique. — De tout temps on a reconnu les inconvénients de l'allaitement artificiel, on a cherché à trouver un lait qui, soit *naturellement*, soit *artificiellement*, se rapproche de la composition du lait de femme.

1° *Naturellement* : on s'est vite aperçu des inconvénients du lait de vache. Celui-ci, outre qu'il est difficile de l'obtenir frais à Paris, est un lait trop riche en caséine et trop riche en beurre, donnant un caillot compact.

On a cherché dans les espèces animales voisines : la chèvre et l'ânesse ont été expérimentées.

La chèvre a joui pendant très longtemps d'un très grand renom ; elle était employée au siècle dernier et, en 1825, Richard, de Nancy, faisait connaître les bons résultats de l'emploi du lait de chèvre dans les hôpitaux de Lyon. Plus près de nous, le professeur Fournier préconisait la chèvre-nourrice comme la sauvegarde des nourrissons syphilitiques.

Au moment de l'établissement de la nourricerie des Enfants-Assistés, on se servit de la chèvre, puis celle-ci fut détrônée par l'ânesse.

Le lait d'ânesse est un lait très léger, plus léger même que le lait de femme, puisqu'il ne contient que 95 grammes de résidu sec au lieu de 125 par litre, 17 de caséine au lieu de 19, et 15 de beurre au lieu de 45 (analyses d'Armand Gautier).

On s'accorde généralement, à l'heure actuelle, pour dire que le lait d'ânesse est un lait extrêmement léger qui peut servir aux nourrissons débiles mais dont l'emploi est assez limité.

2° *Artificiellement :* on a cherché à remédier par des procédés mécaniques ou chimiques aux inconvénients du lait de vache. Ce qui rend ce lait indigeste, ce sont l'excès et les qualités de la caséine. On a donc cherché à décaséiner le lait de vache et on connaît 4 procédés :

a) Celui de Winter et Vigier, de Paris, qui a tout simplement pour effet de précipiter de la caséine avec la présure.

b) Celui de Gaertner, de Vienne, qui se sert d'un appareil ayant pour but d'amener par la centrifugation l'élimination d'une partie de la caséine.

c) Celui de Backhaus, qui soumet le lait à une digestion artificielle partielle par la pancréatine.

d) Celui de Budin et Michel, à peu près semblable au précédent.

Tous ces procédés artificiels n'ont jusqu'à présent donné que des résultats relatifs. Sans méconnaître leur mérite, on peut dire que le lait ainsi manipulé a perdu une partie de ses qualités propres, que sa correction ne s'adresse qu'à un de ses éléments constitutifs, la caséine, en laissant de côté les autres éléments, le beurre en **particulier**. Celui-ci reste en plus petite quantité que dans le lait de femme, ou bien, si l'on veut obtenir des laits gras comme dans le procédé de Gaertner, une partie du beurre n'est plus émulsionnée et **surnage** dans le liquide.

Enfin nous ajoutons que ce lait ne peut être obtenu à l'état frais, qu'il séjourne dans des flacons, condition qui, malgré la stérilisation, est peut-être d'une importance plus grande que celle que l'on suppose.

État actuel de la question. — Il est nécessaire de voir à l'heure actuelle si un retour ne pourrait pas être fait vers la recherche du lait naturel se rapprochant le mieux du lait de femme. Chose singulière, les analyses faites sur ce sujet datent de plus de dix ans, au bas mot.

Il nous a donc semblé intéressant de reprendre l'étude de l'analyse chimique du lait de chèvre à présent que la zootechnie a su acclimater en France, à Paris même, des espèces inconnues jusqu'à présent et fort différentes entre elles, comme on va le voir.

Le lait de chèvre a été condamné sur des analyses peu nombreuses, faites avec un lait recueilli on ne sait où et provenant véritablement des seules chèvres connues à l'époque (chèvres de la Corrèze, du Poitou, etc.).

On ne s'est pas occupé des conditions d'existence de ces bêtes, on a trouvé leur lait trop riche en caséine, pauvre en sucre, et cela a suffi pour que l'habitude soit prise de considérer le lait de chèvre comme un lait lourd, impropre à l'alimentation des nouveau-nés. — Si on se rapporte aux analyses du professeur Armand Gautier (*Chimie appliquée à la Physiologie*), il est facile de constater cependant que le lait de chèvre est le seul (malgré les mauvaises conditions du lait expérimenté) qui, par sa densité. le poids de son résidu sec, son beurre. se rapproche du lait de femme.

Moyennes établies par M. le professeur Gautier. d'après les observations recueillies par lui chez différents auteurs :

	FEMME.	ANESSE.	VACHE.	CHÈVRE.
Densité	1031.5	1035	1031.8	1032.5
Eau.	877	907	865	876
Résidu sec	123	95	155	124
Caséine.	19	17	56	57
Beurre	65	15.5	40.5	42
Sucre	55	58	55	40
Matières extraites et sels.	1.8	5	4	5.6

Quant à sa faible teneur en sucre. c'est évidemment un bien faible défaut auquel on remédie facilement par l'addition de lactose.

Les résultats que nous ont donnés les analyses faites avec la plus rigoureuse exactitude nous ont montré que certaines races de chèvres acclimatées en France. sélectionnées. soumises à une alimentation rationnelle et très étudiée. présentent des différences considérables entre elles. Les proportions du sucre, du beurre, de la caséine, des sels mêmes varient suivant que l'on s'adresse à des chèvres des Pyrénées. de Murcie, de Suisse, de Malte ou des Alpes. et suivant que l'on prend le lait de lactation ancienne ou de lactation nouvelle. Nous sommes arrivés ainsi à rétablir une gamme extrêmement précise de produits à composition constante, se trouvant facilement à Paris depuis la création d'une Chèvrerie-Modèle. Chose considérable, nous sommes arrivé à posséder *un lait naturel. peu coûteux. à composition constante. moins riche en caséine que le lait de vache, plus riche, par contre, que le lait d'ânesse et dont la composition se rapproche beaucoup plus sensiblement du lait de femme que tous les produits naturels ou artificiels dont on a fait usage jusqu'à présent.*

Les données fournies par la chimie ont été contrôlées par l'expérimentation et par la clinique : nous avons soumis à l'Académie de Médecine (séance du 10 juillet) les résultats de nos recherches de laboratoire, tandis que M. Boissard. accoucheur à l'hôpital Tenon, publiait dans le *Journal des Praticiens* du 30 mai les résultats cliniques obtenus à l'hôpital par l'emploi systématique du lait de chèvre. Ces résultats sont excellents.

114 MÉDECINE DE L'ENFANCE.

Depuis notre communication à l'Académie, nous avons poussé plus loin nos recherches et nous sommes aujourd'hui en mesure de les faire connaître dans les détails.

A. Recherches chimiques. — Elles sont résumées dans le tableau suivant.

	N° 1. Grosse chèvre des Pyrénées LACTATION ANCIENNE	N° 2. Chèvre de Murcie LACTATION ANCIENNE	N° 3. Chèvre de Murcie LACTATION NOUVELLE	N° 4. Chèvre suisse LACTATION ANCIENNE	N° 5. Chèvre suisse LACTATION NOUVELLE	N° 6. Chèvre de Malte	N° 7. Lait provenant de 60 chèvres alpines	N° 8. Ensemble de la traite	N° 9. Mélange des laits n°s 1 et 5 (par moitié)	N° 10. Mélange des laits n°s 3 et 5 (prop. de 3 à 2)
Réaction.	Neutre.	Légèr. alcaline.	Faibl. alcaline.	Neutre.	Faibl. alcaline.			Neutre.		
Densité.	1051.5	1052	1050	1052.5	1027	1055	1025.5	1050	1050	1028
Résidu sec.	159.75	128.75	129	115.5	100	146.5	102.5	152.5 p.l.	120	111.6
Eau	891	905	901	917	926	"	"	897.5	908	916
Sels	7.50	7.50	7.20	8	6	8.10	7.45	7.85	7	6.48
Partie organique. . .	152.22	121.80	121.25	107	94.5	"	"	124.65	115.56	105.42
Beurre.	50	56.50	11	26	24	44.85	54.40	59.6	37	50.80
Sucre de lait.	54.02	55.66	47.97	52.78	46.74	46.50	44.50	49	50.58	47.25
Caséine.	27.80	28.40	51.55	28	22.76	56.62	24.10	54.5	25.50	26.18
Lactoprotéine et d.. .	0.45	0.68	1.50	0.72	6	"	"	1.55	0.70	1.20

B. Recherches expérimentales. — I. *Propriété du coagulum.*

Le lait de chèvre ne s'est pas relevé jusqu'à présent d'une expérience faite il y a quinze ans sur son mode de coagulation. Ayant soumis ce lait à l'action de l'acide acétique, on trouva que le coagulum formé était au même titre que le lait de vache, à tel point compact, que l'on pouvait renverser l'éprouvette sans le faire tomber. Cela a suffi à faire condamner sans retour le lait de chèvre et pourtant rien n'est moins exact.

Nous avons soumis nos laits à l'action lactique à 2 pour 100, de l'acide chlorhydrique, de l'acide acétique, ces acides étant seuls ou associés. Toutes ces expériences, que l'on trouvera relatées en détail dans la thèse du Dr G. Lefort, nous ont prouvé que :

a) Le caillot du *lait de vache cru* forme un bloc compact, dense, rétractile et adhérent, ferme, se divisant par l'agitation en grumeaux peu solubles;

b) Le caillot du *lait de vache bouilli* présente les mêmes caractères que le précédent, mais ces caractères sont plus marqués, les grumeaux sont moins solubles;

c) Le caillot du *lait de vache stérilisé* est pris en masse moins compacte, moins dense, molle, se divisant par agitation en grumeaux assez solubles;

d) Le caillot du *lait de vache maternisé* est floconneux, presque homogène, très mou, très soluble ;

e) Le caillot du *lait de chèvre alpine cru* forme de très petits flocons légers, mous, très friables et très solubles, comme ceux du lait de femme et du lait d'ânesse ;

f) Le caillot du *lait de chèvre de Murcie cru* présente les mêmes caractères que le précédent ; les flocons sont un peu moins ténus, mais ils sont très friables et très solubles.

Pour ces deux dernières sortes de lait, la cuisson ne change en rien l'aspect du caillot, mais elle diminue sa solubilité.

Le caillot du lait de femme, du lait d'ânesse, du lait de chèvre, du lait maternisé, après agitation se précipite très lentement et incomplètement. Le caillot du lait de vache cru, bouilli ou stérilisé, se précipite très rapidement ; le sérum se sépare et redevient limpide immédiatement.

II. *Digestibilité*. — Soumis à l'action du suc gastrique de chien (gastérine du Dr Frémont), de la pepsine associée à l'acide chlorhydrique, de la pancréatine, nous sommes arrivés aux résultats suivants :

Tandis que le lait de femme, d'ânesse et de chèvre suisse ou alpine donnaient, au bout de 20 heures, une légère couche crémeuse et un liquide limpide et homogène, le lait de vache (qu'il fût stérilisé, cru ou bouilli) donnait un caillot compact, adhérent, de dissociation difficile ; au bout de 60 heures, le lait de vache stérilisé présentait encore un caillot égal aux 3/4 de la hauteur totale, le lait de vache bouilli égal à la 1/2 de la hauteur et le lait de vache cru égal au 1/5.

Traités ensuite par l'éther, les laits de femme, d'ânesse et de chèvre, laissaient très peu de résidus, tandis que le lait de vache conservait des flocons caséeux en assez grande abondance. Par contre, les résultats obtenus avec les laits des chèvres alpines ou suisses différaient des digestions artificielles obtenues avec le lait des chèvres de Corse et de Corrèze. Le lait de ces dernières races offrait des caractères de digestibilité bien moins grands que les premières.

D'une manière générale, il est facile de conclure que les digestions artificielles faites concurremment démontrent la supériorité manifeste du lait de certaines races de chèvres sur le lait de vache et l'équivalence de la digestibilité pour le lait des races en question avec le lait de femme et d'ânesse.

Accessoirement, il nous est apparu que, d'une manière générale, la digestibilité du lait cru est plus grande que celle du lait bouilli ou stérilisé et ceci nous a montré que l'on pourrait peut-être dans certains cas (toutes précautions d'asepsie observées) se servir du lait de chèvre cru, puisque cet animal est, comme on le sait, un des plus réfractaires à la tuberculose.

III. *Recherches cliniques*. — Ces recherches ayant été faites par M. Boissard, accoucheur à l'hôpital Tenon, nous ne saurions faire mieux que d'y renvoyer (*Journal des Praticiens, 30 mai 1900, De l'alimentation des nouveau-nés par le lait de chèvre*).

Conclusions. — En somme, il nous a semblé intéressant de reprendre l'étude d'un lait qui était méconnu et oublié. Nos recherches, entreprises sans aucun parti pris, ont été couronnées de succès, puisqu'il nous semble démontré que, à condition de se servir de certaines races de chèvres, on obtient un produit alimentaire naturel, de composition constante, dont l'excellence a été montrée théoriquement par l'analyse chimique, pratiquement par des digestions artificielles et les essais de M. Boissard.

Le lait des chèvres alpines et suisses est un lait léger que l'on peut donner aux nouveau-nés normaux de préférence au lait d'ânesse trop léger et au lait de vache trop lourd. Le lait des chèvres de Murcie et des Pyrénées est encore préférable au lait de vache pour des enfants à appareil digestif intact. Le lait des chèvres maltaises et nubiennes conviendra après le sevrage. Les richesses du lait de chèvre en sels en fera toujours un aliment de choix pour les rachitiques, les tuberculeux et les adultes débilités.

Enfin, il est une considération sur laquelle nous tenons à insister, c'est que, contrairement à l'opinion admise, *le lait de chèvre n'a pas d'odeur, ni de goût spécial*. Seules, certaines races présentent cet inconvénient. Le beurre tiré du lait de chèvre est d'une densité très faible, il est, en outre, constitué par des globules graisseux d'une finesse extrême, ce qui explique sa grande digestibilité.

Nous dirons en terminant que la chèvre est d'un prix peu élevé et d'un entretien facile, alors que la vache est d'un prix élevé et d'un entretien onéreux. *D'autre part, contrairement aux idées admises, la chèvre a une lactation abondante et de longue durée; elle donne du lait en toute saison.* Une fois la lactation terminée, il est facile de la transporter dans un lieu d'élevage pendant une nouvelle gestation. La chèvre est propre, alors que la vache ne l'est pas, malgré les soins les plus minutieux, *ce qui a son importance au point de vue de l'asepsie de la traite. La chèvre s'accommode parfaitement du séjour à Paris, tandis que la vache y contracte fatalement et rapidement la tuberculose.* D'ailleurs il est facile de soumettre la première comme la seconde à l'épreuve de la tuberculine.

Les conséquences de ces considérations sont les suivantes : la possibilité d'avoir à un prix très abordable un lait *frais, léger, vivant,* qui, trait aseptiquement, donnerait toutes les garanties exigées par l'hygiène.

LE LAIT COMPLET

par M. le docteur de PRZEDNIEWICZ

Après avoir rappelé les décisions de la Commission de 1857 et du Laboratoire municipal de Paris au sujet de l'écrémage, déplore la malhonnêteté du commerce du lait dans les grandes villes et dit que les dosages des éléments exigés par les autorités ne sont pas assez élevés et prêtent merveilleusement à la fraude. Elle cite différents chiffres d'analyse à l'appui de ses assertions. Ensuite elle critique l'introduction des laits stérilisés analogues qui sont la cause de tant d'accidents dont l'enfance est la première victime. Elle a voulu elle-même se rendre compte de la composition de ces sortes de laits ; elle en a recueilli des échantillons qu'elle a fait analyser par le chimiste A. Thézard.

D'après les résultats obtenus, elle conclut que ces laits ne constituent qu'un coupage malsain vendu très cher et qu'il y aurait lieu de les interdire.

Elle donne une indication de la façon dont les mères de famille devraient préparer le lait de vache destiné aux enfants et propose les vœux suivants :

1° Que les laits écrémés ne puissent plus être mis dans le commerce sans porter la mention « lait écrémé »;

2° Que tout lait qui n'aura pas au moins la composition suivante :

         Résidu fixe 151
         Beurre   40
         Caséine   50
         Albumine . . . .   9 à 10
         Matières minérales . . . . . .   6 à 7

dont au moins 2 grammes d'acide phosphorique, ne soit pas admis;

3° Que les laits stérilisés ou analogues soient entièrement interdits comme très nuisibles, étant donné le nombre d'accidents que nous avons chaque jour à enregistrer;

4° Qu'une circulaire indiquant aux mères de famille le meilleur moyen de préparer le lait d'animaux qu'elles destinent à leurs enfants soit envoyée dans toutes les villes et les villages.

LA MORTALITÉ DES ENFANTS AU-DESSOUS D'UN AN EN NORVÉGE

par M. le professeur Axel JOHANNESSEN

On a eu, depuis ces cinquante dernières années, l'attention attirée sur les rapports statistiques entre les enfants nés vivants et les enfants morts avant l'âge d'un an.

Il ressort immédiatement que la proportion est très différente pour les divers pays, mais que les variations des diverses années sont relativement peu sensibles dans un même pays.

Il semble, en conséquence, que l'on pourrait être autorisé à conclure que cette différence de la mortalité chez les divers peuples peut dépendre de certaines caractéristiques dominantes.

Depuis la moitié de ce siècle, la statistique s'est occupée de plus en plus de la mortalité infantile et il semble que l'on ait partagé l'opinion que la différence de la mortalité des nourrissons dépendait premièrement de la différence d'altitude du pays ou du lieu au-dessus du niveau de la mer et des conditions météorologiques [1].

Cependant cette opinion fut bientôt réfutée et l'on se rallia à d'autres manières de voir.

C'est ainsi que l'on reprit la conception à laquelle Casper [2] était arrivé en 1825, à la suite de ses comparaisons bien connues entre les familles princières et comtales et les familles de mendiants de Berlin, à savoir que le paupérisme est la grande et principale cause de la mortalité des nourrissons [3].

On a encore cherché les raisons de la variabilité de la mortalité chez les enfants de cet âge dans les fléaux calamiteux qui assaillent les états : famine, guerre, cherté des denrées, etc., dans les particularités caractéristiques des races et des coutumes, dans la nature des professions des parents (travail dans les fabriques, aux champs), dans la fécondité des populations en ce que la mortalité est au prorata des naissances et enfin dans l'influence que l'âge des parents peut avoir sur la vitalité des enfants (Körösi).

Mais, néanmoins, si quelques-unes de ces circonstances peuvent être susceptibles d'avoir une certaine importance pour l'enfant, il

---

1. Voir PFEIFFER. Die Kinder-Sterblichkeit. Gerhardt. *Handbuch der Kinder krankheiten*, W. I. Abth. I. 1881, p. 268.

2. Ueber die Sterblickkeit der Kinder in Berlin. *Beiträge zur medic. Statistik*, 1825.

3. NEEFE. Ueber den Einfluss der Wohlhabenkeit auf die Sterblichkeit in Breslau. *Zeitschrift f. Hygiene*, v. 24. 1897, p. 247.

paraît cependant plus sûr que ce sont les soins et l'allaitement de l'enfant qui jouent le rôle prépondérant dans la mortalité infantile. — Cette opinion (énergiquement soutenue, vers 1870, en France par Monot et Vacher, et en Allemagne par Hoffmann, Cless), est à présent victorieuse sur toute la ligne[1].

Autour de cette question fondamentale : « Les mères nourrissent-elles leurs enfants elles-mêmes? » se sont groupées d'autres questions qui découlent de cette dernière.

On a envisagé l'influence du climat, de la température et de l'humidité de l'air. Ces facteurs peuvent, évidemment, avoir quelque importance pour l'enfant nourri artificiellement, car la qualité et la composition du lait de vache, sa teneur en bactéries, en dépendent. On a encore considéré l'état de santé et la constitution de la mère. Mais toutes ces influences sont soumises, uniquement au plus ou moins grand pouvoir qu'a la mère de donner à son enfant une substantielle et abondante nourriture. Il en est de même du travail des parents, de leur aisance et de leur condition sociale, et aussi soit que la mère ne puisse allaiter elle-même son enfant parce qu'elle est occupée dehors, soit que l'alimentation artificielle, à cause de la pauvreté, du manque de culture, etc., soit effectuée en des conditions peu rassurantes.

Et quelles peuvent être les causes de la mortalité des enfants de cet âge?

En première ligne, il faut citer les maladies qui proviennent de certaines conditions particulières de l'alimentation, comme les affections gastro-intestinales, les atrophies, et ensuite les maladies des organes de la respiration qui les accompagnent très souvent. Mais à côté de ces éléments essentiels, il s'en présente encore d'autres, bien que jouant, dans l'ensemble, un rôle relativement moins important.

---

1. Voir WÜRTZBURG. Die Sauglingssterblichkeit im Deutschen Reiche während der Jahre 1875 bes. 1877 Arbeiten aus dem Kaiserlichen Gesundheitsamte. V. 2. 1887. V. 4, 1888.

ERÖSS. Ueber die Sterblichkeits verhältnisse der hengeborenen und Sauglinge. *Zeitschrift f. Hygiene* V. 19, 1895.

SCHLOSSMANN. Studien über Sauglingssterblichkeit. *Zeitschrift f. Hygiene* V. 24. 1897.

PRESL. Ueber die Sterblichkeit in den einzelnen Lebensclassen nach den Resultaten der Valkszählungen in den Jahren 1880 und 1890. *Internat. Hygiene Rundschau*, 1894, n° 49.

G. V. MAYR. *Statistik und Gesellschaftslekne.* V. 2, 1897.

PRINZING. Die Entwichetung der Rindersterblichkeit in den europäischen Staaten. *Jahrbücher für Nationalockonomie und Statistike* III Folge. V. 17, 1899. p. 577.

BIEDERT. Die Kindernährung im Sänglingsalter. 1897.

c'est la grande série des maladies infectieuses depuis la tuberculose et la syphilis jusqu'à la rougeole et la fièvre scarlatine.

Je donne ici un court tableau des taux de la mortalité des enfants de la première année dans les différents pays de l'Europe. (Ces renseignements statistiques ont été puisés dans les travaux de Prinzing et de Mayr déjà cités.)

PAYS	ANNÉES	TAUX DE L'ANNÉE servant de point de départ	TAUX LE PLUS ÉLEVÉ	TAUX DE LA DERNIÈRE ANNÉE
France	1840-95	15.95	18.40	16.80
Prusse	1816-95	16.90	20.82	20.52
Saxe.	1852-95	27	28.66	28.05
Bavière	1825-95	28.40	52.70	27.22*
Wurtemberg	1812-95	52.06	56	25.40
Bade	1852-95	26.12	27.89	22.25
Autriche.	1851-95	25.49	26.59	24.62
Italie	1865-96	22.58	22.49	18.55
Suisse.	1871-96	19.54	18.80	15.14
Belgique.	1841-95	15.05	17.41	16.39
Pays-Bas	1878-94	18.77	20.88	16.47
Russie.	1855-75	26.54	26.67	27.05
Finlande	1812-94	22.45	21.65	14.92
Serbie.	1881-95	15.71	15.69	18.02
Bulgarie.	1886-95	9.52	15.69	
Roumanie.	1876-92	22.04	19.54	22.04
Espagne.	1878-82	19.17		
Angleterre et p^r de Galles.	1858-94	15.50	15.70	14.80
Écosse	1855-94	11.21	12.72	12.45
Irlande	1866-94	9.52	9.90	10.08
Danemark.	1855-94	14.59	14.40	15.94
Suède.	1851-95	20.46	21.61	10.28

* Dans quelques districts comme Oberbayern et Schwaben la mortalité a atteint, en certaines années, plus de 40 p. 100; dans quelques villes comme Ingolstadt et Ebersberg, elle a été de 50 p. 100.

Le bureau statistique norvégien de Kristiania m'a complaisamment fourni les renseignements suivants sur la mortalité des enfants au-dessous d'un an, en Norvège.

Cette mortalité (voir tableaux 1 et 2) a atteint, dans les années 1876-1897, le taux de 9,76 pour 100 en moyenne chez les enfants de 0 à 1 an.

Ce pour cent apparaît comme le plus bas de tous les pays de l'Europe. La cause peut d'abord être attribuée à l'habitude très répandue qu'ont les mères d'allaiter elles-mêmes leurs enfants, mais on peut aussi ajouter que même lorsque les enfants sont placés en nourrice et nourris artificiellement, ils sont ordinairement bien soignés : une particularité du caractère norvégien est d'aimer les enfants et de tenir à honneur de les bien traiter.

Quant à la répartition de cette mortalité (voir tableau 2) elle est de 8 1/2 pour 100 dans les arrondissements ruraux, tandis que dans les villes, elle atteint 15.08 pour 100 en moyenne. Il est cependant évident que dans ces chiffres de grandes variations se peuvent produire, si l'on regarde les taux de quelques arrondissements particuliers.

En comparant les taux de la mortalité des différentes communes pour les années 1881 à 1885 et 1886 à 1890 (tableau 5). on trouve les résultats suivants :

Mortalité des enfants au dessous d'un an. en Norvège (années 1881-1890).

TAUX	1.49 2.49	2.50 4.99	5 7.49	7.50 9.99	10 14.99	15 19.99	20 22.88
1881-1885 :							
Nombre de communes rurales.		12	144	206	112	18	3
Nombre de communes urbaines.		1	5	56	56	5	1
1886-1890 :							
Nombre de communes rurales.	1	54	171	176	99	10	4
Nombre de communes urbaines.		1	6	19	50	5	

On voit ainsi (par cette comparaison) que le taux de la mortalité d'une petite commune de la préfecture de Söndre Trondhjem est de 1,49 pour 100 et quelques autres communes présentent un taux variant entre 2 1/2 et 5 pour 100.

La plupart des communes ont un taux de mortalité entre 5 et 10 pour 100 (mais les communes montrant un taux de 5 à 7 1/2 pour 100 sont montées de la première à la deuxième période, tandis que celles accusant un taux de 7 1/2 à 10 pour 100 sont descendues dans la même proportion).

Le plus grand nombre des communes urbaines entre dans les groupes de 7 1/2 à 10 pour 100 et de 10 à 15 pour 100.

Dans le dernier groupe sont placées les plus grandes villes comme

Bergen et Trondhyem. Kristiania est descendue de 19,90 pour 100, en 1878-1879, à 14,8 pour 100, en 1898.

Les communes qui présentent un petit taux, comme 2 1/2 à 5 pour 100, sont situées dans les districts agricoles de l'est du pays et en quelques autres de l'ouest et aussi dans le Nordland.

Les taux élevés, comme 15 à 20 pour 100, se rencontrent principalement dans les districts pauvres de l'ouest et du nord du pays, et au delà du cercle polaire. Les plus hauts taux, c'est-à-dire dépassant 20 pour 100, se voient seulement dans cette partie septentrionale de la Norvège où la vie et les conditions climatériques sont rudes et en laquelle la population est, en grande partie, composée de Lapons nomades.

Tant qu'à la différence de la mortalité chez les deux sexes le tableau n° 2, montre qu'en Norvège, comme dans les autres pays, la mortalité est plus grande parmi les garçons que parmi les filles. Pour ceux-là, elle est de 10.6 pour 100 et pour celles-ci de 8,9 pour 100.

L'opinion n'est pas encore d'accord jusqu'à quel point une naissance légitime ou illégitime peut avoir d'importance au point de vue des recherches statistiques sur la mortalité chez les enfants au-dessous d'un an.

Dans quelques villes comme Berlin, par exemple, la mortalité est (suivant Eröss) chez les enfants illégitimes le double que chez les légitimes: à Paris, elle est un peu plus élevée: à Vienne et à Prague, elle est (suivant Fischl), au contraire, considérablement moindre.

Les causes de ces grandes variations[1] — qui diminuent la sincérité des taux — ont été cherchées dans certaines particularités dont l'importance est essentielle pour l'enfant.

Il peut d'abord arriver que chez les enfants illégitimes les décès soient moindres que les naissances, parce que la mère contracte mariage dans la première année de la vie de l'enfant; de ce fait, l'enfant devient légitime et, en cas de mort, il est inscrit comme tel. Ensuite, les enfants illégitimes changent fréquemment de lieu, soit qu'ils naissent dans une maternité ou en tout autre lieu de la ville et sont placés après en nourrice, à la campagne, soit qu'ils naissent au domicile de la mère, à la campagne, et envoyés plus tard en nourrice dans la ville même où les mères exercent leur profession ou cherchent du travail.

On peut certainement faire, en Norvège, les mêmes remarques sur la valeur des taux qui montrent l'importance des naissances légi-

____

1. MAYR a. st. 281 et SCHLOSSMANN a. st. p. 98.

times ou illégitimes dans l'ensemble de la mortalité. Il faut cependant remarquer que dans notre pays le rapport entre les enfants légitimes et illégitimes, au point de vue des naissances comme des décès, est très homogène.

Les naissances sont montées (de 1876 à 1897) de 59 066 à 65 517 par an; dans ce total les illégitimes entrent pour 4552 à 4956.

Pour les décès, ils ont été chez les enfants légitimes de 9,25 pour 100 et chez les illégitimes de 15,55 pour 100. Cependant les taux de la mortalité parmi les premiers sont tombés, en certaines années, de 9,75 à 9 pour 100 et parmi les seconds sont, au contraire, montés de 12,4 à 17,22 pour 100. Ce taux de mortalité est surtout dû aux enfants illégitimes des villes.

La mortalité chez les enfants légitimes qui est, dans les arrondissements ruraux de 8,54 pour 100 en moyenne, est tombée de 8,8 à 8,05 pour 100 et celle des villes, qui est de 11,89 en moyenne, est tombée de 12,87 à 11,41 pour 100, tandis que la mortalité des enfants illégitimes, qui est dans les arrondissements ruraux de 11,59 pour 100 en moyenne, est montée de 10,25 à 12,62 pour 100 et celle des villes, qui est de 24,58 en moyenne, est montée de 18,79 à 26,8 pour 100.

Ces chiffres ont un intérêt assez considérable en ce qu'ils se rapportent à une situation sur laquelle l'attention a déjà été attirée[1].

On a trouvé chez nous que le nombre des enfants illégitimes des villes répond à peu près à celui des enfants nourris artificiellement, de même que le taux de la mortalité peut donner, dans l'ensemble, une certaine idée de la mortalité chez les enfants qui reçoivent une alimentation artificielle.

Il est intéressant de regarder, à cet égard, la liste du tableau 2, qui montre la mortalité chez les enfants de la première année dans les différents mois.

Pour le premier mois de la naissance, le rapport des taux est, dans les arrondissements ruraux, entre les enfants légitimes et illégitimes comme 1 : 1 1,2 (5,26 : 5,04); dans les villes, il est comme 1 : 2 (5,24 : 6,84). Pour le deuxième mois, ce rapport est également, dans les districts ruraux, comme 1 : 1 1/2; dans les villes, il est, au contraire, comme 1 : 5. (Pour le troisième mois, la proportion est la même que celle pour le premier mois. Pour les mois suivants, elle reste à peu près pareille.)

L'accroissement considérable qui se manifeste dans la proportion

---

1. Berner a. st. p. 49. Beretning om Sundhedstilstand i Kristiania for 1895, p. 50.

des décès pour le deuxième mois est, probablement, dû, entre autres causes, à celle-ci : qu'une grande partie des enfants illégitimes qui, jusqu'à ce moment, tétaient leurs mères, sont alors mis en nourrice.

Une autre preuve assez intéressante qui montrera le rôle que joue l'alimentation est fournie par le chiffre des décès de la première année (tableaux 3 et 4), placés en regard des mois.

Contrairement aux autres pays qui subissent une élévation de la mortalité pendant les mois d'été, la Norvège n'enregistre, à cette même époque, presque aucune augmentation de décès.

Les taux moyens pour chaque mois sont les suivants :

Janvier	— neuf	9.05	Juillet	— neuf, cinq	9.55
Février	— neuf	9.05	Août	— neuf, un	9.12
Mars	— neuf, quatre	9.42	Septembre	— six, neuf	6.98
Avril	— huit, six	8.61	Octobre	— sept, deux	7.24
Mai	— huit, quatre	8.45	Novembre	— six, neuf	6.02
Juin	— sept, neuf	7.96	Décembre	— sept, six	7.66

Tant qu'aux arrondissements ruraux, on ne peut trouver, soit pour les enfants légitimes ou illégitimes, la moindre augmentation dans les mois d'été.

Dans les villes, au contraire, les mois de juillet et d'août présentent, relativement, les plus hauts taux de mortalité (12,01 et 10,8 pour 100).

Cette élévation est due, en grande partie, aux décès chez les enfants illégitimes.

La mortalité, chez ces derniers, est, à cette époque, à peu près deux fois plus élevée que dans les mois de décembre les plus favorables. Autrement dit, la décomposition si dangereuse du lait, qui se produit pendant l'été, semble n'avoir une influence nocive que pour cette classe d'enfants qui, chez nous, représente les enfants artificiellement nourris, c'est-à-dire les enfants illégitimes des villes.

Conséquemment, je me permettrai, en quelques mots, de donner les résultats obtenus à l'hôpital des maladies de l'enfance de l'Université de Kristiania.

De 1893 à 1899, il a été traité 272 enfants au-dessous d'un an. Sur ce nombre, 123 sortirent guéris, soit 45,2 pour 100; 149 moururent, soit 54,8 pour 100.

La répartition des décès pour chacune des années ci-dessus se décompose ainsi :

Année 1893	— cinquante-huit	0/0 — 58.8 0/0
» 1894	— cinquante et un	0/0 — 51.5 0/0
» 1895	— soixante-trois	0/0 — 65.1 0/0
» 1896	— soixante-trois	0/0 — 65.2 0/0

Année 1897   cinquante-quatre 0/0   54.1 0/0
  »   1898   quarante-deux   0/0 - 42.5 0/0
  »   1899 - cinquante et un   0/0   51.5 0/0

Si du nombre total des décès on retranche 25 cas de mort dus à des maladies telles que : tuberculose, syphilis héréditaire. etc., la mortalité (dans les 126 autres cas), soit 46.5 pour 100. a été causée par les maladies du tube digestif et des organes de la respiration.

Parmi les garçons, le taux de la mortalité a été de 60 pour 60 et chez les filles de 47.5 pour 100.

Chez les enfants au-dessous de 6 mois. ce taux a été de 65 pour 100 et de 44,4 pour 100 chez les enfants au-dessus de cet âge.

Tous ces enfants sont entrés à l'hôpital dans un état de santé très précaire, 29 d'ailleurs moururent le jour même ou le lendemain de leur admission.

Parmi ceux sortis guéris. 92 ont montré une augmentation de poids, 21 n'ont accusé aucune variation.

Chez les décédés. 106 ont présenté une diminution de poids, 27 sont restés à l'état stationnaire. Chez 26 autres, le poids n'a pu être enregistré qu'une seule fois, la mort étant survenue le jour même ou le jour suivant de leur entrée.

Sur le total, 25 étaient, avant leur admission à l'hôpital, nourris au sein, le reste avait reçu une alimentation mixte ou était nourri entièrement au lait de vache ou avec des farines.

Les patients étaient couchés, en partie dans une salle de malades comprenant 8 à 10 lits. et en partie parmi d'autres enfants plus âgés dans une seconde salle.

Il va sans dire que tous les soins qui étaient en notre pouvoir furent prodigués.

Dans les dernières années, les taux de la mortalité ont considérablement diminué. Cependant, même un taux de 42.5 pour 100 est encore trop élevé. il est nécessaire de chercher les moyens qui peuvent faire cesser ce pour cent chez les nourrissons soignés dans les hôpitaux.

SUR QUELQUES POINTS DE LA LOI ROUSSEL

par M. le docteur BÉZY,

Chargé du cours de clinique infantile à la Faculté de médecine de l'Université de Toulouse,
Médecin des Hôpitaux.

La loi qui porte en France le nom de l'éminent médecin philanthrope, Théophile Roussel, a pour but, chacun le sait, de protéger l'enfant placé en nourrice loin du domicile de ses parents. Promulguée le 23 décembre 1874, cette loi a rendu d'immenses services. Aujourd'hui, après vingt-cinq ans d'exécution, il est juste, après avoir rendu hommage au zèle du sénateur qu'il nous est agréable de traiter de confrère, le Dr Roussel, de nous demander si cette loi a donné tout ce qu'elle pouvait donner, et si cette expérience de vingt-cinq ans ne nous permet pas de demander des améliorations.

Toute loi humaine est perfectible, et les nombreux travaux publiés sur la loi Roussel pour en demander le remaniement prouvent combien cette loi a su éveiller les sympathies et l'admiration de tous.

De très nombreux travaux ont été publiés sur ce sujet, examinant à des points de vue très divers les améliorations qu'il faudrait apporter à la loi Roussel. En juin 1898, un de mes élèves, le Dr Amans, demandait, dans une thèse, soutenue devant la Faculté de Toulouse, qu'il y eût un peu plus d'énergie dans la défense de l'enfant, que la surveillance de l'enfant fût plus étendue, que les bureaux de placement fussent supprimés, et surtout que le médecin prît, dans la surveillance de l'enfant, un rôle prépondérant sur celui de l'administrateur, à cause de sa compétence.

Pendant tout le courant de l'année 1899, la question a été étudiée surtout par la Société du Concours médical. C'est au sein de cette société qu'a été nommée une Commission dont faisaient partie MM. Théophile Roussel et Léon Labbé et qui a eu pour mission d'étudier cette question. On trouvera les noms de ses membres dans le journal le *Concours Médical* du 15 janvier 1899, et, dans les n°s 2, 4, 7, 9, 11, 12, 38, 40, 41, 45, 48, du même journal (année 1899), l'intéressante enquête, et le remarquable rapport du Dr Gassot, sur cette importante question.

On trouvera un bon résumé de cette question avec un parallèle entre la loi actuelle et les propositions de réforme, par le Dr Barthés, dans les *Annales de médecine et de chirurgie infantiles* du 15 mars 1900.

Enfin, tout récemment la question a été tranchée dans les réunions des médecins-inspecteurs de l'Assistance publique.

Il serait intéressant de reprendre en détail tous ces travaux. C'est ce que fait, en ce moment, un de mes élèves qui prépare sa thèse sur ce sujet. Mais cela sortirait des limites des communications faites à ce Congrès.

Je me bornerai donc, laissant absolument à part le côté administratif de la loi, à étudier simplement quelques points du côté médical des réformes à introduire, et encore n'insisterai-je que sur les points qui peuvent intéresser les enfants de tous les pays, n'oubliant pas que nous sommes réunis ici en Congrès international. On trouvera dans les excellents travaux que j'ai cités tous les renseignements nécessaires à une étude complète.

Quatre points principaux m'ont paru, d'après ma pratique personnelle, mériter des modifications importantes. Je vais les énoncer rapidement.

1° Les notions de médecine et d'hygiène infantiles exigées des médecins des circonscriptions ne sont pas suffisantes. Ces médecins très exacts et très méritants, du reste, sont nommés par le préfet qui ne peut avoir la compétence nécessaire pour apprécier leurs qualités. Je ne me permettrai certainement pas de juger les capacités d'un confrère : mais il m'est permis de regretter, aujourd'hui surtout que la pédiatrie est devenue une partie importante des sciences médicales, qu'on ne s'assure pas des capacités d'un médecin de circonscription avant de le nommer. Parmi les moyens qui pourraient concourir vers ce but, il en est un qui aurait mes préférences et que j'ai du reste indiqué ailleurs. Je voudrais voir créer, dans nos universités régionales, des certificats spéciaux (non seulement pour la pédiatrie mais pour les différentes branches de l'art de guérir) qui ne seraient accordés qu'après des études et des épreuves sérieuses. Le certificat de pédiatrie serait exigé des médecins qui seraient candidats à une circonscription[1]. C'est dans le même ordre d'idées que l'on a demandé, à juste droit, je pense, que l'inspecteur départemental soit toujours un docteur en médecine.

2° Les visites faites par le médecin au nourrisson ne sont pas suffisantes. Cette visite, en effet, n'est que mensuelle : de telle sorte que le médecin a le droit d'aller inspecter le nourrisson le 1ᵉʳ du mois et de n'y revenir que le 50 du mois suivant, c'est-à-dire de laisser écouler entre ses deux visites un intervalle de soixante jours. De tous côtés des plaintes se sont élevées dans ce sens et je n'y insisterai pas.

---

1. Cela a été fait dans une certaine mesure en Italie. Voir à ce sujet la communication du Dᵣ Luigi Concetti au Congrès de Budapesth, reproduit in *Archives de médecine des enfants*, septembre 1899, p. 716.

me contentant de répéter que ces visites doivent être beaucoup plus répétées surtout au début de l'allaitement. Elles devraient être au moins hebdomadaires le premier mois.

Mais l'important serait surtout que le médecin soit obligé de revenir voir, aussi souvent que cela serait nécessaire, l'enfant mal soigné et surtout malade. Il faudrait, dans ce cas, que le médecin soit assuré d'une rémunération suffisante de la part de la famille. Au Comité départemental de la Haute-Garonne, nous avons émis le vœu que la nourrice soit responsable de cette dette. Notre but est que la nourrice se fasse donner d'avance par la famille des garanties qu'un médecin ne saura jamais prendre.

3° Je suis étonné que l'on n'ait pas songé à rendre obligatoire pour la nourrice la déclaration d'une maladie contagieuse contractée soit par le nourrisson qu'elle a en garde, soit surtout par un de ses propres enfants. J'avoue que je n'avais pas pensé moi-même à cela, lorsque j'ai vu, cet hiver, conduire à la consultation de ma clinique deux enfants de la même famille atteints de diphtérie consécutive à la rougeole. La mère de ces deux enfants avait un nourrisson en garde. Il faudrait que, dans ces cas, la gardeuse soit responsable et passible d'une pénalité (sans quoi elle se gardera bien de faire une déclaration qui lui ferait enlever son nourrisson), si elle ne fait prévenir immédiatement le médecin.

4° Enfin peut-être serait-il bon de stimuler le zèle des uns et des autres soit en affichant la loi chez les intéressés, soit en publiant dans les localités les résultats obtenus par les nourrices et gardeuses de la région, soit en faisant mieux connaître à qui de droit les instructions de l'Académie à ce sujet, soit enfin en réunissant plus souvent qu'une fois par an les comités départementaux qui auraient ainsi des rapports plus étroits avec l'inspecteur de l'Assistance publique, et dont les membres pourraient causer entre eux des résultats de leur surveillance.

Je tiens à répéter en terminant que, si je n'ai pas repris tous les points récemment étudiés, c'est que cela eût été trop long, et que le court aperçu auquel je me suis arrêté m'a été surtout inspiré par des faits de ma pratique personnelle.

DISCUSSION

M. VARIOT (de Paris) ajoute encore quelques observations au sujet de la loi Roussel. Il montre que la visite mensuelle du médecin est insuffisante et inefficace, et il voudrait que les enfants placés chez des nourrices soient visités par un médecin une fois par semaine.

DIE GESETZE DER ALLTAEGLICHEN UNBEDINGT NOETHIGEN HYGIENISCHEN ANFORDERUNGEN SOLLEN DEM ELEMENTAR-UNTER RICHTE IN DEN ELEMENTAR-SCHULEN EINVERLEIBT WERDEN

von Dr LYNBOMIR NENADOVICS,

Bezirks-arzt in Pancsova.

Der Werth der hygienischen Fortschritte, sowol für das physische Wohl des Einzelnen als des Allgemeinen, ist von allen civilisirten Staaten anerkannt worden, und mit Recht hat die Gesetzgebung auch einen grossen Theil der leicht ausführbaren hygienischen Verbesserungen aufgenommen. Doch ist es zu erwägen, dass es sich mit den hygienischen Vorschriften, in vielen Punkten, in ähnlicher Weise, verhält, wie mit der öffentlichen Sittlichkeit.

Die Gesetzgebung ist wol in der Lage grobe moralische Ausschreitungen zu ahnden, sie wird jedoch nicht im Stande sein, allein jenen Grad von Gesittung der Bevölkerung aufzudrängen, welcher nothwendig ist, um die ganze Thätigkeit des einzelnen, auf eine moralische Grundlage, zu stellen.

Gerade so wie die Moral und anderweitige Tugenden, durch mehrere Generationen von Eltern und Lehrern, anerzogen werden müssen, um dauernd einen integrirenden Bestandtheil des Charakters zu bilden, müssen auch die Grundbegriffe der Hygiene, als welche Reinlichkeit, Desinfection und Entfernung aller Gesundheitsschädlichen Factoren zu betrachten sind, dem Volke durch die Schule, als von dem gewöhnlichen unzertrennlichen Begriffe, eingeimpft zu werden.

So lange die Hygiene nur unter den Fittigen des Gesetzes ihre Macht ausübt, wird eine heilbringende Wirkung derselben, wenn auch nicht eine fragliche, so dann doch eine beschränkte bleiben, erst wenn das Volk die gegebenen Vorschriften, durch die Schule, als die zu seinem physischen Heil unerlässlichen Anforderungen erlernen wird, werden auch dem idealen Ziele näher gerückten Erfolge zu gewärtigen sein.

Die Nothwendigkeit hygienischer Massnamen muss demnach dem Volke durch die Schule anerzogen werden. Jung gewohnt alt gethan.

Die Erziehung des Volkes für die Hygiene obliegt dem Lehrer und dem Aerzte.

Die hygienische Section des Pariser internationalen medicinischen Congress möge beschliessen : Die Regierungen der an dem internationalen medicinischen Congresse theilnehmenden civilisirten Na-

tionen seien aufzufordern, die Gesetze der alltäglichen unbedingt nöthigen hygienischen Anforderungen durch Einverleibung in den Unterricht in den Elementarschulen zur allgemeinen Geltung zu bringen,und zwar : über die Reinlichkeit im Allgemeinen und Körperreinigung insbesondere, über die Verhütung und Ausbreitung der Infectionskrankheiten, über die Schädlichkeit des Aufenthaltes in feuchten ungelüfteten Wohnungen, über die Behandlung der Sputa, u. s. w.

LES ENFANTS ABANDONNÉS EN HONGRIE

par M. le docteur Maurice SZALARDI

Directeur de la Maison des Enfants trouvés, à Budapest.

Mon rapport a deux buts : faire connaître la cause des enfants abandonnés en Hongrie et mentionner avec reconnaissance les institutions de la France, auxquelles nous devons en effet, d'avoir pu, en Hongrie aussi, nous occuper de la cause de ces enfants. Il y a quelques années, j'étais épouvanté de la mortalité immense des enfants en Hongrie, et, étant effrayé des expériences faites dans les endroits où l'on soigne de tels enfants assistés, j'ai poursuivi la chose, pour qu'on vienne en aide à ces enfants, lorsque, dans des endroits compétents on a prétendu que les institutions qui existent dans l'intérêt des enfants abandonnés, ne suffisent pas à leur tâche sans cela, ne diminuant en rien la mortalité des enfants, et que, d'un autre côté, elles avaient une influence déplorable sur les mœurs. A cette occasion, nous avons cité la France, nous avons donné en exemple ses institutions semblables, nous avons prouvé, que dans ces institutions, il ne meurt proportionnellement pas plus d'enfants que dans tout le pays; au contraire, que par eux la vie des enfants abandonnés, voués à la destruction, a été assurée. D'un autre côté, nous avons mentionné le fait que malgré des institutions existant depuis des siècles, le nombre des enfants illégitimes n'a plus augmenté en France, et n'était pas plus grand que dans d'autres pays.

Avec de tels et semblables arguments, nous avons réussi à vaincre les obstacles et commencer notre tâche de sauvetage d'enfants.

La cause des enfants trouvés, en Hongrie, courtement décrite, est la suivante :

Contre les avortements, les meurtres d'enfants et le délaissement des enfants, il y a d'anciennes lois; pour le fait et la punition de l'avortement, nous avons des dispositions du temps du roi Koloman, puisque, dans le premier livre, le cinquième article des lois du roi Koloman dit : *Mulieres partum suum necantes archidiacono allatæ penitentiam agant.* Mais dans les siècles suivants, on a très sévèrement puni les avortements, comme nous pouvons le voir, dans l'œuvre publiée en 1751, à Presbourg, de Mathias Bodo « *Jurisprudentia criminalis secundum praxim et constitutiones Hungaricas* », et dans la seconde partie, article LXI. « *De iis, quæ abortum studiose procurant* » et la punition à mort joue un rôle.

Du meurtre d'enfants, le paragraphe 68 de la loi de 1656, et le premier point de la loi de 1725 disposent clairement : ici le meurtre d'enfants est aussi puni par la mort; dans les cas particulièrement cruels, elles permettent aussi la torture.

Contre l'abandonnement des enfants, nous n'avons aucune instruction, dans nos lois avant le dix-neuvième siècle : ici aussi, Bodo peut servir de source; d'après lui, l'abandonnement de l'enfant, suivi de sa mort est puni par la mort; si l'enfant reste vivant, le châtiment est d'être battu de verges.

De l'entretien des enfants abandonnés dispose le douzième point du livre des lois de 1756, comme suit : *Infantes expositi vel in hospitalibus ad id deputatis, vel in eorum defectu, a magistratu locati sunt educandi.* Cette disposition, dont l'essentiel est que l'enfant trouvé est à élever et à soigner par la commune, reste jusqu'à nos jours, et seulement en 1845, on a ajouté la disposition de l'allaitement et sa surveillance sévère; de cela c'est aussi la commune qui a été chargée. De cette façon, jusque dans ces dernières années, c'était le devoir de la commune de prendre soin des enfants abandonnés, trouvés, ou orphelins et de tous les gens qui n'étaient pas en état de s'entretenir eux-mêmes; mais les communes ont seulement pris soin des enfants abandonnés d'une manière coupable, trouvés dans les rues, et seulement jusqu'à ce qu'on ait retrouvé la mère. Comme cela, on n'a pas aidé à la cause en question, dont l'essentiel est de sauver les enfants illégitimes et de ceux dont les parents n'ont pu prendre soin. L'État s'est exceptionnellement occupé des enfants Hongrois nés à l'étranger, dans des maisons pour les enfants assistés, en chargeant aussi la Commune compétente pour les frais.

En 1895, le Ministre de l'intérieur a investi l'Association de la Croix-Blanche, déjà établie, du droit de recueillir des enfants abandonnés et de les élever aux frais des communes compétentes.

Déjà, au commencement de ce siècle, des gens bienfaisants ont formé le projet de la solution de la cause des enfants trouvés. En 1805,

Stephan Tandor a légué 10 000 florins pour un asile des enfants assistés, à fonder à Budapest; en 1848, l'Hôpital des enfants a voulu donner asile aux enfants trouvés et même, en 1868, on a fondé une association d'asile d'enfants, mais le ministre n'en a pas permis le fonctionnement, motivant que c'était nuisible à la Société; enfin, en 1885, la Société de la Croix Blanche a pris naissance et elle a mené à la solution la cause des enfants trouvés, de degré en degré. En 1898, le ministre lui-même a décidé d'arranger la cause des enfants trouvés; pour ce but il a créé un impôt tel que chacun paye au-dessus de ses impôts directs 5 pour 100 de ces impôts, et que la somme gagnée de cette façon soit pour les frais des hôpitaux et des maisons d'enfants trouvés. Outre cela, jusqu'à ce qu'il entreprenne lui-même l'arrangement de la cause, il a chargé la Société de la Croix-Blanche et l'Asile des enfants, d'accepter et de soigner les enfants trouvés, abandonnés et les orphelins. Aux frais du fond cité plus haut, on élève jusqu'à l'âge de sept ans, non seulement les enfants trouvés, les orphelins et les enfants dont les parents sont malades, mais tous ceux aussi dont les parents obligés à les entretenir, parents ou grands-parents ne sont pas capables à pourvoir à leurs besoins.

D'après cela, la cause des enfants trouvés, diffère du système français en cela, que l'enfant est seulement accepté s'il y a une nécessité matérielle.

Cette disposition peut avoir pour motif que la mère ne veut pas avoir recours à l'assistance de l'État et elle détruit ou laisse périr plutôt l'enfant; là, par exemple, ou les recherches faites dans l'arrondissement compétent de la mère peuvent la compromettre. Dans ce cas, la Société de la Croix Blanche aide de la manière, qu'elle aide de sa propre fortune, la mère à élever l'enfant. En France, la mère qui a confié son enfant à l'assistance de l'État est obligée à tout révéler sur l'origine de son enfant, et elle ne connaît même pas l'endroit où on a donné son enfant à soigner, et l'enfant ne peut lui être rendu avant qu'elle ait remboursé les frais occasionnés par lui, ce qui arrive bien rarement, pendant que chez nous, le lien entre l'enfant et la mère n'est jamais interrompu. Ordinairement, nous acceptons la mère avec l'enfant, et si cela est possible, nous le faisons allaiter par elle-même; dans ce but nous avons des colonies où nous plaçons la mère avec l'enfant, et nous avons soin d'entretenir aussi la mère avec l'enfant; bref, la mère est la nourrice payée de son enfant. C'est sûrement à cela que nous devons le succès obtenu, en ce qui concerne la diminution de la mortalité des enfants, qui comme la statistique ci-dessous le montrera est plus favorable encore, que celui des maisons exemplaires, des enfants trouvés de Paris.

Nos systèmes concernant les enfants trouvés diffèrent encore d'une chose et cela est, que tandis qu'en France la recherche de la paternité est interdite, chez nous, elle est non seulement permise, mais la Société prête encore l'assistance d'un avocat à la mère, pour forcer le père naturel à entretenir l'enfant. D'après nos lois, il est obligé d'en avoir soin jusqu'à l'âge de 12 à 14 ans.

La Société de la Croix-Blanche.

La Société de la maison des enfants trouvés de la Croix-Blanche a commencé ses fonctions en 1885. Elle a ouvert un Institut où elle a donné asile aux mères et aux enfants, sans domicile; en outre, elle a donné aux pauvres enfants malades, le secours du médecin et des médicaments gratuits. Au commencement, elle fonctionnait dans une maison louée; en 1891 elle pratiqua dans sa propre petite maison, renfermant 50 lits, la bienfaisance, jusqu'à ce qu'en 1895 le ministre, lui ait enfin accordé le droit d'accepter les enfants abandonnés, aux frais des communautés. A présent, l'Institut possède une grande maison à deux étages, où il fonctionne de la manière suivante :

D'après la loi, l'Institut est obligé d'accepter tout enfant au-dessous de 7 ans et il dispose de la sorte que chez les enfants à la mamelle, la mère reste aussi à l'Institut; si la santé de la mère et celle de l'enfant le permettent, on les envoie, aux colonies de l'Institut servant à ce but. L'établissement a maintenant 94 colonies, où nous envoyons l'enfant avec la mère. Dans ces villages, des médecins payés pratiquent la surveillance; en outre, chaque enfant est visité, au moins 4 fois par an, par des médecins contrôleurs, délégués par l'Institut central. Les enfants malades sont soignés à l'Institut. Pendant l'année passée et cette année, l'Institut principal a fondé, en 7 endroits différents, des sociétés filiales qui fonctionnent de la même manière. Voilà les filiales en fonction jusqu'à présent : Arad, Szombazhely, Rimaszombat, Kassa. Puesvar, Gyula et Szeged. Nos tendances sont de faire établir dans chaque arrondissement de semblables institutions.

Le tableau, ci-dessous, montre le succès surprenant, que nous avons obtenu jusqu'à présent par nos efforts, qui démontre clairement que nous avons atteint brillamment le but que nous nous étions proposés, concernant la diminution de la mortalité des enfants. Pendant la dernière année, la mortalité des enfants au-dessous d'un an, donnés en nourrice n'était que de 11 pour 100. Si nous ajoutons à cela, le pourcentage des enfants morts à l'Institut même, la mortalité est encore moindre que celle des enfants de Budapest, malgré que la mortalité des enfants de Budapest soit plus petite que dans toutes les villes d'Europe, excepté de Paris.

TABLEAU I.

La mortalité des enfants (0-1 année) dans les grandes villes de l'Europe en 1898.

	NAISSANCES VIVANTES	MORTS	0/0
Saint-Pétersbourg	52.847	10.192	51.0
Madrid.	15.465	5.710	25.9
Berlin	46.684	10.521	22.5
Liverpool	22.490	4.464	19.8
Rome	11.566	1.284	19.6
Vienne.	50.028	9.696	19.5
Hambourg.	20.742	5.892	18.7
Varsovie.	23.461	4.260	18.1
Birmingham	18.607	5.370	18.1
Bruxelles.	15.240	2.584	18.0
Londres	153.840	22.199	16.6
Budapest.	25.061	8.809	16.0
Paris.	58.795	6.747	11.5

Si la mortalité des enfants est si petite actuellement à Budapest, tandis que cette ville était sous ce rapport il y a 25 ans, à l'exception de quelques villes allemandes, à la dernière place, ce succès, la Société peut se l'approprier de droit, parce qu'elle a non seulement préservé la vie des enfants abandonnés par ses actions humanitaires, mais elle a montré en même temps, le bon exemple des soins à donner aux enfants. L'objection, que la mortalité des enfants a diminué parce que nous avons envoyé les enfants en province, est réfutée par le tableau publié ci-dessus, d'après lequel, la mortalité des enfants a aussi bien diminué dans les arrondissements où nous envoyons nos enfants.

J'espère que si dans les autres parties du pays, aussi notre institution fonctionne régulièrement, non seulement à Budapest, mais dans toutes nos autres villes et dans tous les pays, nous réduirons également la mortalité des enfants.

TABLEAU II.

Mortalité des enfants (0-5 années) dans les Comitats : Tejér, Tolna, Szolnok et Pesth (1891-1898).

COMITATS	1891		1892		1893		1894		1895		1896		1897		1898	
	MORTS	0/0	MORTS	0/0	MORTS	0/0	MORTS	0/0	MORTS	0/0	MORTS	0/0	MORTS	0/0	MORTS	0/0
Tejér	5.698	46.0	5.595	45.9	5.269	40.8	2.618	54.4	2.692	54.1	3.050	58.1	2.664	55.5	2.584	28.8
Tolna	4.850	52.8	5.284	60	5.657	59.4	2.969	55.1	3.068	54.6	2.882	55.1	2.772	52.4	2.750	51.5
Szolnok	6.750	47.8	6.805	47.5	5.614	59.5	5.595	59.7	6.147	45.7	5.224	56.5	4.752	55	5.205	56
Pesth	14.125	48.5	14.454	58.2	15.945	45.5	15.717	45.4	15.047	40.8	12.859	59.4	10.769	51.9	11.876	55

TABLEAU III.

ANNÉES	RECUEILLIS À L'INSTITUT	MORTALITÉ des enfants aux frais de l'État (0-1 année).	MORTALITÉ des enfants aux frais de l'État au-dessus d'une année.	MORTALITÉ des enfants aux frais de l'État (0-7 années).	MORTALITÉ des enfants aux frais de l'Institut (0-1 année).	MORTALITÉ des enfants aux frais de l'Institut au-dessus d'une année.	MORTALITÉ des enfants aux frais de l'Institut (0-7 années).	MORTALITÉ À L'INSTITUT	MORTALITÉ DANS LES COLONIES
1895	648	18.50 0/0	5.50 0/0	17.05 0/0	14.15 0/0	10.52 0/0	11.11 0/0	5.54 0/0	14.07 0/0
1896	745	58.05 0/0	9.01 0/0	21.47 0/0	18.85 0/0	4.09 0/0	11.47 0/0	4.62 0/0	16.47 0/0
1897	892	17.74 0/0	14.11 0/0	15.56 0/0	14.47 0/0	10.91 0/0	12.69 0/0	5.25 0/0	14.02 0/0
1898	1.588	16.19 0/0	9.00 0/0	14.55 0/0	14.45 0/0	10.18 0/0	15.25 0/0	5.08 0/0	15.80 0/0
1899	2.254	15.58 0/0	7.54 0/0	11.57 0/0					

COMPTE RENDU DE L'HOPITAL SAINT-GEORGES POUR ENFANTS MALADES

par M. le docteur VIOLI,

de Constantinople.

Du premier juillet 1895 au 30 avril 1900, nous avons soigné à l'hôpital international de Saint-Georges, 10 555 enfants, de nationalités diverses.

Parmi ceux-ci, 6915 étaient atteints de maladies internes : 1519 de maladies chirurgicales ou des yeux ; 856 de maladies de la tête (gorge, nez, oreilles), 262 de maladies nerveuses, paralysies, malformations du squelette, 507 de diphtérie avec ou sans croup, 486 de maladies de la peau, 127 d'affections dentaires ; 105 d'affections non diagnostiquées.

Fièvre typhoïde. — Parmi les maladies infectieuses aiguës, nous avons eu à soigner 194 enfants, âgés de 10 mois à 11 ans, atteints de fièvre typhoïde, dont le diagnostic, malgré la première réaction de Widal, n'a pas été toujours facile à cause de la marche irrégulière de la maladie ; 37 convalescents ont rechuté probablement par écart de régime ; de ceux-ci, deux sont morts des suites d'une perforation intestinale ; des premiers, un est mort de marasme.

Le traitement a consisté en bains, ou ablutions froides, à l'extérieur et à l'intérieur ; limonades, de l'eau en abondance, additionnée ou non d'une boisson alcoolique.

Les complications bronchiques, broncho-pulmonaires, encéphaliques ont été soignées selon les circonstances.

Coqueluche. — Des 453 enfants affectés de la coqueluche, 113 ont été soignés avec des injections de sérum de génisse immunisé contre la variole. De cette médication hypodermique j'ai déjà parlé aux Congrès de Moscou et de Turin.

Le calme des accès a été obtenu, en général, 8 à 12 heures après la première inoculation chez 135 enfants.

Les inoculations faites avec du sérum, antidiphtéritique ou non, ont été pratiquées en trop petit nombre (18 enfants) pour pouvoir en tirer des conclusions.

Chez les autres enfants, nous avons suivi un traitement symptomatique, conseillant spécialement le changement d'air.

Cinq sont morts à la suite de broncho-pneumonie, deux de tuberculose pulmonaire et trois de méningite *tuberculeuse*.

Varicelle. — Nous avons eu 57 enfants malades de la varicelle. Nous l'avons vue transportée dans des familles par des personnes qui,

17 à 20 jours auparavant, avaient eu leurs enfants malades de la varicelle ; chez des enfants habitant le même toit, nous avons vu se manifester la maladie dans un intervalle de 8 à 45 jours. Et la maladie a
éclaté soit chez des enfants récemment vaccinés, soit chez des enfants
en évolution vaccinale, soit chez des enfants non encore vaccinés, ce
qui montre une fois de plus que la varicelle est une affection très
indépendante de la variole. Quinze enfants inoculés avec de la sérosité recueillie sur des pustules de varicelleux n'ont manifesté aucune
réaction locale ou générale : 5 de ceux-ci ayant été placés dans une
chambre non désinfectée habitée auparavant par des malades ont eu
la varicelle dans l'espace 9 à 18 jours.

Vaccination. — Parmi les 4797 vaccinations et revaccinations
pratiquées à l'hôpital et les 7675 pratiquées dans les écoles à la
municipalité de Péra, nous n'avons jamais eu à constater de complication.

Les animaux vaccinifères dont l'état de santé était préalablement
constaté, ont été soumis, avant l'inoculation du vaccin, à une injection de 1 cm. c. de tuberculine au 10ᵉ, et après la récolte du vaccin ont
été autopsiés. Les manipulations ont été exécutées avec une rigoureuse
asepsie. Le vaccin employé dans les *vaccinations* avait été récolté
dans la quinzaine, conservé aseptiquement, et il a donné 98 pour 100
de résultats positifs. Dans les *revaccinations* on s'est servi de celui qui
avait été récolté deux ou trois jours auparavant ; il nous a donné
67 pour 100 de succès.

Nous avons choisi, en plusieurs séances, parmi les enfants à vac-
ciner, 214 sujets qui se trouvaient approximativement dans les mêmes
conditions d'âge et de santé, et nous les avons inoculés la moitié avec
du vaccin recueilli depuis 8 à 15 jours, et l'autre moitié avec du vaccin
conservé depuis 2 ou 3 mois. Chez ces derniers, nous avons eu seulement 85 pour 100 de succès ; parmi ces derniers enfants vaccinés avec
succès, 102 revaccinés après un mois, avec de vaccin récemment
recueilli (une semaine), 13 ont de nouveau donné sur le point inoculé
des pustules typiques, tandis que la même expérience exécutée sur un
égal nombre de sujets déjà inoculés avec du vaccin frais n'a donné
que chez deux enfants des pustules typiques du vaccin. Dans la revac-
cination des enfants des écoles, nous avons eu, sur 525 enfants revaccinés avec du vaccin recueilli deux semaines auparavant, 42 pour 100
de résultats : les enfants non réussis dans cette expérience, revaccinés
à nouveau avec du vaccin frais, ont donné 19 1 2 pour 100 de succès,
tandis que chez les enfants déjà revaccinés avec du vaccin frais et sans
succès, nous n'avons pu constater que 2 1 4 pour 100 de succès.

Le nombre des pustules pratiquées sur les enfants a été proportionné, à leur âge et à leur constitution : dans nos expériences ce n'a pas été la quantité des pustules qui a préservé l'enfant, mais la qualité du vaccin provenant d'animaux vaccinifères inoculés avec du cowpox d'origine primitive récente.

Les vaccinations et revaccinations ont été pratiquées par des incisions faites avec un vaccinostyle à double tranchant, ayant eu soin que, soit l'instrument, soit la partie sur laquelle on inoculait le vaccin, fussent parfaitement aseptiques.

Péritonite tuberculeuse. — Parmi les maladies infectieuses chroniques nous avons eu des enfants atteints de péritonite tuberculeuse. De ceux-ci, 22 dont la péritonite était accompagnée d'ascite, sans autres manifestations tuberculeuses, ont été laparotomisés et ont guéri par première intention.

L'examen microscopique et les cultures de parcelles des péritoine ont confirmé le diagnostic. Neuf des opérés présentaient des traces de dégénérescence des ganglions mésentériques, des adhérences aux anses intestinales. 7 enfants opérés depuis 9 mois et demi à 2 ans, que nous avons pu suivre, vivent et sont en bonne santé, 5 sont morts, par tuberculose généralisée.

Nous avons préféré opérer dans le cas de péritonite ascitique, vu que dans les familles pauvres et dans les hôpitaux en général on n'a pas les conditions d'hygiène requises pour obtenir la guérison avec le traitement médical qui, suivi longtemps, n'a fait que laisser épuiser nos malades. En tout cas, l'opération n'a fait qu'améliorer les conditions du malade en facilitant ainsi sa guérison.

Appendicite. — Chez 21 enfants souffrant d'appendicite, nous avons eu 19 guérisons avec le traitement purement médical. Deux enfants venus *in extremis*, aux 6ᵉ et 7ᵉ jours de la maladie, laparotomisés à cause de la péritonite généralisée, ont succombé quelques heures après l'opération.

Diphtérie et croup. — Les 507 enfants, souffrants de diphtérie avec ou sans croup, ont été soignés, soit avec un simple traitement interne à base tonique, aidé d'un traitement local, désinfectant, soit en réunissant à cette thérapeutique les inoculations antidiphtériques.

Depuis que nous avons abandonné les injections faites avec des petites doses de sérum et que nous traitons les diphtéries graves, simples, ou compliquées, même de croup, avec une dose minimum de 20 ou 40 cm. c. de sérum par séance, selon l'âge de l'enfant, nous avons vu s'abaisser la mortalité de 14 à 7 1/2 pour 100. Et, en

général, avec une seule dose massive de sérum nous avons eu raison
de la maladie.

Nous avons dans les sténoses croupales, qui ne disparaissaient pas
avec une forte dose de sérum, en recours à l'intubation avec
80 pour 100 de bons résultats. Une seule fois, il nous est arrivé que
nous avons dû conserver à l'enfant le tube pendant trois semaines : et
comme on ne pouvait le supprimer, nous avons dû recourir à la trachéotomie. L'enfant soigné à la maison avec la canule est mort. deux
mois après. d'asphyxie.

Quand on nous a transporté à l'hôpital des enfants agonisants. nous
avons eu recours à la trachéotomie ; mais si le lendemain l'état du
malade s'améliorait. nous avons pratiqué l'intubation afin de rendre
plus facile la guérison de la plaie et diminuer les chances d'infection.
Dans la trachéotomie nous avons eu 61 pour 100 de succès.

Constipation. — La constipation chez 180 de nos enfants de quelques
semaines à 10 mois n'a pas été engendrée par malformation congénitale, mais par la mauvaise alimentation. En effet, la mère, la nourrice ont souvent l'habitude de trop nourrir leurs bébés. A chaque fois
que l'enfant pleure, elles ne se contentent pas de donner le sein. le
biberon, pour le faire boire, mais elles recourent aussi à des soupes, à
des panades, etc.

Cette suralimentation a donné lieu à des accidents de toute sorte.
Ces enfants ont perdu le sommeil, la tranquillité, ils n'ont fait que
pousser des cris déchirants à chaque instant ; ils ont eu des convulsions, même des dermatoses. Quelquefois une médication opiacée
donnée par un pharmacien complaisant est venue augmenter encore
la constipation.

Dans ces cas. la régularisation du régime, un purgatif léger répété
le plus rarement possible, le massage et l'électrothérapie nous ont
donné des résultats satisfaisants. Mais si la constipation a continué,
nous avons eu des dilatations d'estomac, du côlon, avec la dyspepsie
consécutive. Soit que la constipation dérive de ce qui précède, soit de
l'exagération des inflexions de l'S iliaque. nous avons trouvé un véritable soulagement et même la guérison de nos malades avec l'usage
prolongé du massage du ventre. Seulement celui-ci a dû être pratiqué pendant un ou plusieurs mois. selon la chronocité de la constipation.

Entérites. — Chez 816 enfants souffrant de gastro-entérite aiguë.
entérite cholériforme. entérite chronique, dysenterie. nous nous sommes
bien trouvé en faisant suivre à nos malades une diète hydrique très
rigoureuse. plutôt que de recourir seulement à des remèdes en usage,

Bronchite chronique, asthme. — Chez 77 enfants affectés de bronchites chroniques et asthme, le traitement aérothérapique accompagné de la gymnastique suédoise et de la masso-hydrothérapie nous ont donné des résultats satisfaisants.

Végétations adénoïdes. — Sur 856 enfants, souffrant des maladies de la gorge, du nez et des oreilles, nous avons vu ces maladies 254 fois provoquées par les végétations adénoïdes. Nous avons opéré même 7 enfants nouveau-nés souffrant d'accès de suffocation pendant qu'ils tétaient, et, après le grattage, nous avons vu disparaître tout à fait ces accès ainsi que des accès de laryngospasme dont d'autres enfants souffraient.

Syphilis. — La syphilis soit congénitale, 155 cas, soit acquise, 75 cas, joue un rôle de certaine importance parmi les malades que nous avons soignés. Avant la fondation de l'hôpital, très rarement nous rencontrions dans notre pratique privée des cas de syphilis.

Les frictions mercurielles, le sirop de Gibert, les injections hypodermiques de sublimé, nous ont bien réussi dans le traitement de la maladie. La mortalité a été de 28 pour 100 dans le cas de syphilis congénitale.

Tuberculoses. — Les enfants souffrant de tuberculose pulmonaire (17 malades) ont été améliorés ou guéris quand ils nous sont arrivés dès le commencement de la maladie, et nous avons pu les mettre dans de bonnes conditions hygiéniques. L'igazol du professeur Cervello, employé en inhalations, a contribué à améliorer l'état de nos enfants.

Les périostites, ostéites tuberculeuses, l'ostéomyélite ainsi que les tumeurs blanches (166 cas) ont souvent été améliorées, quelques-unes guéries radicalement, en ajoutant au traitement local un traitement ioduré à l'intérieur et en mettant le malade dans les meilleures conditions d'hygiène possibles.

Mall de Pott. — Dans le mal de Pott (21 cas), la méthode de CALOT ne nous a pas donné les résultats que nous espérions.

Même dans le cas de mal de Pott dorsal où le redressement a été facile, nous n'avons pas pu obtenir la guérison du petit malade qui avait été gardé plus d'une année dans les corsets plâtrés.

Dentition. — Nous avons observé chez 187 enfants, des symptômes que nous n'avons pas pu attribuer à autre chose qu'à la dentition. Il est évident qu'il ne faut pas considérer l'influence de la dentition comme un facteur de tout premier ordre dans la pathologie infantile ; mais il nous est arrivé d'observer chez les enfants qui avaient les gencives rouges, très enflées, douloureuses à la pression, qu'ils perdaient de leur versatilité, de leur gaîté ; qu'ils étaient pris parfois d'insomnie. d'assoupissement. de spasmes, de méningisme : ces phénomènes étaient quelquefois accompagnés de dérangements gastro-intestinaux, symptômes dus certainement à une auto-intoxication, laquelle cependant ne s'était point manifestée avant la période de dentition, bien que le mode d'alimentation des enfants fût le même. Et la preuve que la majorité de ces souffrances était due à la difficulté de la sortie des dents, nous l'avons eue lorsque nous avons vu en grande partie disparaître ces phénomènes après avoir pratiqué une incision ou le grattage des gencives afin de faciliter la sortie des dents.

Il nous a donc été impossible de nier la part que la dentition a prise dans l'apparition de certains de ces symptômes morbides que nous avons observés. En tout cas, en prenant en considération l'état congestif des gencives et en facilitant l'éruption des dents, si nous n'avons pas pu constater toujours la disparition totale des souffrances de l'enfant, nous avons pu néanmoins, par exclusion, nous mettre en état de mieux préciser le diagnostic de la maladie.

Lombricose. — De même pour la lombricose. Chez 151 enfants présentant comme symptômes : de l'insomnie, des convulsions, des vomissements, des maux de tête, des dérangements intestinaux, nous avons vu disparaître souvent ces symptômes par l'emploi d'un vermifuge qui, en améliorant l'état de l'enfant, permettait par l'expulsion, dans les selles des enfants, des ascarides, ou par l'examen microscopique de ces selles, de bien constater qu'on ne s'était pas trompé en attribuant l'état anormal de l'enfant à la lombricose.

Système nerveux. — Chez 262 enfants atteints de maladies du système nerveux, nous avons eu à soigner des affections du cerveau, de la moelle, des nerfs périphériques, des affections musculaires, des névroses. C'est l'électricité, le massage, la gymnastique suédoise. qui nous ont donné les meilleurs résultats dans le traitement de ces affections.

Diphtérie. — Parmi les maladies des yeux, nous avons à signaler deux enfants qui, ayant reçu une blessure dans l'œil droit pénétrant dans le vitré, se voyaient menacés d'énucléation de l'œil. Avec une séance de galvano-caustique intraoculaire, toute crainte d'infection est passée, et ils ont parfaitement guéri. Dans la rougeole, pendant l'éruption sur quelques enfants. nous avons observé une kératite ponctuée superficielle. siégeant de préférence au centre de la cornée. kératite qui a disparu avec l'éruption.

Pour abréger je ne parle pas d'autres maladies que nous avons eu à observer et à traiter : mais je me réserve de publier, dans quelques semaines, un compte rendu détaillé de l'hôpital qui viendra compléter cet exposé.

En attendant, j'ai l'honneur de soumettre au Congrès ces conclusions :

1° Qu'il est nécessaire d'avoir dans chaque ville un hôpital d'enfants, ou dans les hôpitaux de la ville une section destinée à l'enfance afin de voir diminuer la mortalité infantile ;

2° Qu'il faut avoir des hospices marins où seront soignées avec plus de chances de succès les manifestations externes de la tuberculose infantile ;

3° Que, dans les maladies de l'enfance il ne faut pas négliger la dentition et la lombricose, qui jouent parfois un rôle important dans le développement et l'entretien de certains états morbides des enfants ;

4° Que les végétations adénoïdes causent souvent des otorrhées et la surdité, entretiennent les maladies chroniques des bronches, les accès de laryngospasme ; et, dans beaucoup de cas, favorisent le mauvais développement du squelette ;

5° Que dans la péritonite tuberculeuse ascitique, lorsqu'elle n'est pas compliquée d'autres lésions tuberculeuses et qu'il est difficile d'assurer aux malades des conditions hygiéniques en rapport avec leur maladie, il est préférable de procéder à la laparotomie, plutôt que de perdre un temps précieux dans une médication peu efficace et facilitant l'affaiblissement du malade ;

6° Que dans l'appendicite, il est préférable de suivre le traitement médical si l'enfant n'a pas de symptômes de péritonite généralisée ;

7° Qu'avec l'hygiène et l'hydrothérapie, les auxiliaires les plus puissants dans la thérapeutique des enfants affaiblis ou souffrant de maladies chroniques, sont les injections de sérum artificiel, la massothérapie, la gymnastique suédoise et l'électrothérapie ;

8° Que dans le traitement de la diphtérie grave ou du croup, il faut recourir à des doses intensives de sérum, à la trachéotomie si l'enfant souffrant de la sténose laryngée est agonisant, autrement, à l'intubation. Le lendemain de la trachéotomie, on pourra intuber l'enfant afin d'obtenir plus rapidement la guérison de la plaie et diminuer les chances de complications ;

9° Que les vaccinations doivent être pratiquées avec du vaccin provenant d'une génisse inoculée avec du cow-pox spontané recueilli une ou tout au plus deux semaines avant l'opération ; les revaccinations. avec du vaccin recueilli dans la même semaine, afin d'obtenir des résultats positifs et une probabilité plus grande de préservation de la variole;

Que si la récolte du vaccin et l'inoculation ont été faites avec une asepsie rigoureuse, on n'aura à se plaindre d'aucune complication. soit dans les vaccinations, soit dans les revaccinations.

Tel est le résumé de notre pratique et de l'enseignement clinique que trouvent à l'hôpital Saint-Georges, les étudiants arrivés au terme de leurs études et qui veulent s'initier à la médecine infantile.

II

AFFECTIONS GASTRO-INTESTINALES
DES NOURRISSONS

1. — Rapports sur les infections
et les intoxications gastro-intestinales chez les enfants
du premier âge.

LE ROLE DES MICROBES DANS LES MALADIES GASTRO-INTESTINALES
DES NOURRISSONS — INFECTIONS ET INTOXICATIONS ECTOGENES

RAPPORT

par M. le professeur ESCHERICH,

de Graz.

Le Comité a voulu me confier le rapport sur les infections et intoxications d'origine ectogène. Suivant les règlements du Congrès, il n'y a que vingt-cinq minutes à ma disposition, ce qui me rend impossible de faire dans ce temps, un rapport complet de cette question encore si peu élucidée. Aussi, je crois que ces rapports n'ont pas le but ni de ramasser tout ce qu'on a écrit sur un certain chapitre, ni de décider des discussions scientifiques par un jugement catégorique. Le charme et la valeur de ces congrès internationaux sont plutôt pour les uns de donner l'occasion de développer sa manière de voir devant des collègues éminents réunis de toutes les parties du monde, pour les autres la possibilité d'entendre l'avis authentique de l'auteur et de s'éclairer par quelques questions sur les points obscurs, ce qui autrement nécessiterait de longues discussions littéraires.

J'ai l'impression que le comité partage cet avis, car il choisit comme rapporteurs des personnes qui sont placées au milieu de la lutte et dont les noms sont d'eux-mêmes un programme scientifique.

Si l'on m'a accordé ce rôle distingué, je crois le devoir à ce que je m'occupe depuis le commencement de ma carrière pédiatrique de ces questions et qu'il convient, à l'intention du comité, que je vous donne un tableau sommaire de ce que moi et mes élèves avons étudié sur le chapitre des maladies gastro-intestinales des nourrissons.

Donc, je demande pardon d'avance, si je me rattache spécialement aux travaux de ma clinique. Le bref délai de temps qui est à ma disposition ne me permet pas d'indiquer ici plus que les points de vue dont nous sommes partis et les résultats les plus importants où nous sommes parvenus.

La route nouvelle, sur laquelle nous essayons à attaquer le problème ancien de la pathogénie des maladies digestive des nourrissons, est la recherche et la différenciation des bactéries trouvées dans les selles de malades.

Elle m'était prescrite par mes travaux antérieurs sur les bactéries de l'intestin. En 1885, j'ai fait voir que la flore intestinale du nourrisson sain est caractérisée par une uniformité et une simplicité surprenantes.

D'un autre côté, il était facile de voir que, dans les selles des enfants atteints des gastro-entérites, se trouvent des bactéries bien différentes et en plus grand nombre. A première vue, il semble impossible de distinguer dans ce chaos les bactéries pathogènes des autres. Mais pourtant il fallait l'essayer. Ce que M. Koch avait trouvé, le bacille virgule du choléra asiatique, dans les selles de l'adulte, prouve qu'on ne doit pas désespérer d'en venir à bout dans les conditions beaucoup moins compliquées du nourrisson.

Toutefois, il faut se rappeler que cette méthode ne peut donner des résultats qu'en recherchant les cas aigus et tout à fait récents. à un moment où l'on peut encore soupçonner que l'agent nuisible n'a pas encore quitté l'intestin. Le nombre des cas convenables pour une telle recherche n'est pas grand, et je crois que souvent on a été trop peu scrupuleux dans le choix des cas, et que cela a produit bien des erreurs et des malentendus. Je déclare donc expressément que je ne parle ici que des maladies primitives aiguës d'origine bactérienne et que je laisse de côté toutes les formes qui n'entrent pas dans ce cadre, spécialement les maladies subaiguës chroniques ou secondaires.

Au temps où j'entrai dans ces études, on avait, au moins en Allemagne, formulé des conceptions assez précises sur la pathogénie de ces maladies. M. Baginsky avait attiré l'attention sur les deux phénomènes les plus incontestables d'épidémiologie : 1° la plus grande morbidité et la mortalité des enfants artificiellement nourris: 2° l'exagération de ces mêmes faits, parallèle avec l'élévation de la température.

L'explication qu'il avait donnée. et qui paraissait alors très bien établie, était que ce sont les fermentations ou la putréfaction favorisées par la chaleur, soit dans le lait. soit dans le contenu intestinal qui causent une intoxication de l'organisme et finissent par produire des altérations anatomiques de la paroi intestinale.

C'est suivant ces idées, alors généralement acceptées, que j'entrai dans mes recherches et commençai à étudier la végétation et les fermentations du lait. J'arrivai à la division des fermentations ectogènes et endogènes, ce qui me semble important encore aujourd'hui. La forme la plus fréquente et la plus typique des fermentations ectogènes est représentée par les diarrhées d'été, qui sont favorisées par la chaleur excessive de l'atmosphère. Les Américains ont décrit les premières sous le nom de choléra infantile, et, je crois entrer dans leur manière de voir, quand je propose de réserver ce nom pour les troubles digestifs qui sont produits par une intoxication du lait causée par la grande chaleur. Quoique ce soit une des parties qui sont les plus facilement accessibles aux recherches chimiques et bactériologiques, nous ne savons que très peu de choses de ces processus. Du reste, j'ajoute qu'à mon avis, ce n'est qu'une partie relativement petite des diarrhées d'été qui peut être réellement attribuée à telle intoxication alimentaire. Il y en a d'autres qui ont plutôt l'apparence des infections rapides: peut-être y a-t-il encore d'autres facteurs, qui jouent dedans un rôle et qui ne sont pas encore connues.

L'étude des fermentations endogènes est naturellement plus difficile et moins complète encore. Ils feront le sujet spécial du rapport de mon éminent collègue et ami Marfan. Je remarque seulement que ce qu'il entend par les troubles digestifs d'origine endogène ne coïncide pas avec ma définition. Pour ma part, j'appelle endogène, suivant le sens du mot, tout ce qui passe à l'intérieur du corps. Marfan fait une restriction en ne parlant des fermentations endogènes que dans le cas où elles sont produites par les bactéries habitant normalement l'intestin, qui ont subi peut-être une exagération de virulence. En présence de l'infection continuelle qui se produit dans le tractus intestinal du nourrisson, par la nourriture, par la salive, etc., on n'est pas obligé — à mon avis — de poser une telle hypothèse pour expliquer des fermentations endogènes. Il suffit de *savoir* qu'il y a des bactéries qui ne trouvent les conditions du développement qu'à l'intérieur de l'intestin, par exemple les anaérobies.

Je crois donc que la plus grande partie des fermentations anormales de l'intestin sont d'origine ectogène, produites par des bactéries introduites avec la nourriture.

Je ne nie pas qu'il y ait des cas où la nourriture introduite est stérile, comme chez les enfants à la mamelle et où cette nourriture est infectée dans l'estomac, ou dans l'intestin par des bactéries qui s'y trouvent ; mais, même dans ce cas classique de fermentation endogène, les bactéries sont venues du dehors, elles n'appartiennent pas à la flore normale et je me sers maintenant dans ces cas, pour éviter des erreurs, du terme plus précis de *infection du contenu intestinal* ou de *Chymus infection*.

Si réellement les fermentations anormales de l'intestin jouent un aussi grand rôle dans la pathogénèse des troubles intestinaux qu'on le suppose, on pouvait espérer réussir à isoler par les méthodes éprouvées dans l'étude des fermentations les agents provocateurs, les étudier expérimentalement et les comparer avec celles qui se passent en dehors du corps. Cet espoir ne s'est pas rempli. Malgré les efforts d'un grand nombre d'auteurs, nous ne connaissons que quelques données générales, montrant que la fermentation est acide dans la partie supérieure, alcaline ou fétide dans la partie inférieure de l'intestin.

Je ne connais que très peu de cas, où il semble y avoir une fermentation typique causée par le bacterium lactis ou le bacille butyrique, le proteus ou des levures (muguet). Dans la plus grande majorité, la décomposition se produit par un mélange des bactéries normales de l'intestin et des bactéries saprophytiques, mêlées par hasard et sans prédominance de l'une sur l'autre. Les recherches chimiques, exécutées surtout par Baginsky, n'ont prouvé rien d'extraordinaire ; il a trouvé de l'ammoniaque, des produits des putréfactions ordinaires, etc. Il en résulte que : *ou que les méthodes, dont nous nous servons, en ce moment, pour étudier les infections du chyme, sont absolument insuffisantes, ou bien ces infections et intoxications ne sont ni si fréquentes ni si dangereuses que l'on avait cru jusqu'ici.*

En effet, les résultats insuffisants de ces recherches, les observations des épidémies de diarrhées dans les hôpitaux (Heubner), enfin les constatations histologiques de M. Booker ont eu le mérite d'attirer l'attention des cliniciens allemands vers un groupe jusqu'ici trop peu étudié ; c'est le *groupe des maladies intestinales de nature infectieuse*. Il faut dire que l'école de Prague, avec von Ritter, Epstein et ses élèves Czewy et Fischl, qui se fondaient sur une nourriture très spéciale des nourrissons à la mamelle, avait toujours défendu la nature infectieuse de ces maladies. Mais ailleurs l'idée d'une origine infectieuse dans les maladies de l'intestin du nourrisson, analogues à celle du choléra asiatique et de la fièvre typhoïde, avait presque complétement disparu, sous l'empire des idées de fermentation et de la putréfaction. Pourtant, l'existence des épidémies de diarrhées infantiles prouve d'une manière assez démonstrative, qu'il y a de ces germes spécifiques. Il n'est pas même nécessaire de supposer toujours de maladies aussi typiques que le choléra.

Toutes les bactéries, qui sont douées de qualités pathogènes pour l'homme, sont capables de produire des irritations soit par leur présence, soit par leurs toxines.

C'est un fait connu que justement les muqueuses des nourrissons offrent une disposition spéciale vis-à-vis des bactéries pathogènes se trouvant sur le corps humain (manque de pouvoir protecteur). Je cite la muqueuse des voies respiratoires, qui nous donne le meilleur exemple de ce que j'appelle *catarrhe infectieux*. Malgré, ou grâce à réaction irritative de la muqueuse, les bactéries restent à la surface libre ; ce n'est que dans les infections graves et chez des individus peu résistants qu'elles entrent, à la faveur des lésions épithéliales, dans le tissu et produisent des altérations profondes, des ulcérations, et à la fin, l'infection générale de l'organisme.

Du reste, il faut dire que ce fait n'arrive pas si souvent que M. Czerny Moser le prétendent, qui l'acceptent comme un phénomène journalier et réservent à ces cas le nom de gastro-entérite.

Les maladies gastro-intestinales infectieuses sont, cela va sans dire, ndépendantes à un certain degré de l'alimentation, elles peuvent donc atteindre les enfants à la mamelle.

De même peuvent se répandre en épidémie et produire une endémie ans des hôpitaux encombrés dans les habitations, salles, etc. La théodes maladies infectieuses offre au point de vue épidémiologique mêmes lacunes que la théorie de la fermentation. L'hypothèse d'un processus infectieux concorde mieux avec le tableau clinique, le cours de ces maladies, l'absence de toxine et au contraire la constatation réelle des bactéries dans les selles des malades. C'est à ce point que commencent les travaux qui m'ont occupé pendant les dernières années.

En employant la méthode de coloration double, dont je me sers depuis longtemps, il est facile, dans certains cas, de distinguer des bactéries pathogènes, qui prennent le Gram et se différencient de la flore ordinaire qui se décolore.

De cette manière, on peut poser un diagnostic de telle ou telle infection par l'examen de la préparation à condition de considérer en même temps tous les symptômes.

Dans les hôpitaux, où ces infections se transmettent souvent d'un malade à l'autre, on a l'occasion d'observer les mêmes bactéries et certain symptômes identiques, sur tous les enfants atteints de la même infection, ce qui permet d'établir une classification étiologique de ces diarrhées.

Nous ne sommes pas encore allés bien loin dans cette voie. Cependant, nous avons fait connaître quelques-unes de ces infections, c'est celle due aux staphylocoques, aux streptocoques, au bacille pyocyanique, à certaines variétés de coli, du bacterium bleu ramifié, etc. Toutes ces bactéries sont connues comme pathogènes ; elles sont donc capables de produire des altérations inflammatoires lorsqu'elles sont en contact avec la muqueuse intestinale. Cela est prouvé par les produits de l'inflammation qui se trouvent dans les évacuations ; cela se prouve, dans certains cas, par la pénétration de ces bactéries dans le sang et dans l'urine; cela se prouve enfin, après la mort, par la présence de ces bactéries dans la paroi intestinale et quelquefois dans les organes. Pour quelques infections, existe des réactions du sérum qui font voir la réaction générale de l'organisme.

Dans tous ces cas, il s'agit probablement de l'infection ectogène, qui prend son origine, ou par le contact avec les bactéries pathogènes répandues dans l'entourage de l'homme, ou par la nourriture, spécialement le lait de vache.

Je ne peux pas entrer dans les détails cliniques ou bactériologiques, j'aurai peut-être l'occasion d'y revenir dans la discussion. Pour le moment, je n'insiste que sur l'existence et la séparation de maladies infectieuses à côté de la chymus infection, ce qui représente, à mon avis, le plus important progrès qui s'est produit dans ces dernières années dans le chapitre des maladies gastro-intestinales du nourrisson.

La division que j'adopte, fondée sur ces recherches bactériologiques, est la suivante :

Étiologie des troubles gastro-intestinaux aigus, primitifs d'origine bactérienne.

A. Intoxication ectogène : catarrhe toxique de l'estomac, de l'intestin : choléra infantum.

B. Infection du chyme : catarrhe dyspeptique d'origine alimentaire (D. catarrhalés (West). D. acide (Eichstadt).

C. Infections intestinales vraies : catarrhe inflammatoire D. inflammatoire (West).

Inflammation : gastrite ; entérite ; colite.

Si nous ajoutons, au commencement, les troubles fonctionnels (dyspepsie) et, à la fin, les maladies secondaires, cette division tirée des données bactériologiques, ressemble beaucoup à celle donnée par Marfan et encore à celle qui a été choisie par des cliniciens célèbres avant la période bactériologique. J'en tire l'espoir qu'elle aura non-seulement la valeur de vous faire voir mes idées, mais qu'elle correspond au groupement naturel des faits. Elle ne prétend pas du reste être complète puisqu'elle ne s'occupe que d'un certain groupe des affections intestinales, mais ce sont justement celles dont l'étude nous promet des renseignements propres à donner la solution du problème étiologique.

CONCLUSIONS. — I. — La question de l'importance des bactéries dans l'étiologie et la pathogénie des affections gastro-intestinales du nourrisson doit avoir pour point de départ, comme je l'ai fait dans mon travail sur les bactéries de l'intestin, paru en 1886, l'étude des conditions normales. Une série de travaux, sortis de ma clinique, ont établi les points suivants :

a) L'emploi de la méthode de coloration de la fibrine suivant le procédé de Weigert (recoloration à l'aide de la fuschine) donne une double coloration très utile à l'étude des fèces. Elle permet de différencier les bactéries qu'on trouve dans les selles des enfants au sein, du colibacille qui se décolore par le Gram. L'idée émise que cette particularité serait due à certaines conditions végétatives propres à l'intestin du nourrisson (présence de graisses. Schmidt, 1892) n'a pas été confirmée par les recherches ultérieures.

b) L'ensemencement sur milieux alcalins ordinaires (agar et gélatine en plaques) ne réussit que dans une mesure restreinte (5 à 10 pour 100) à faire développer les bactéries que montre l'examen microscopique (Eberle. 1894).

c) En employant certains milieux électifs, surtout acides (moût de bière acide). on voit que la multiplicité des germes qu'on trouve dans les selles normales du nourrisson est encore plus grande qu'on ne l'a admis jusqu'ici. Un fait particulièrement intéressant est la présence constante et abondante d'une variété de bactérie, colorable par le Gram, ramifiée. qui, morphologiquement, correspond aux caractères de la masse principale des bactéries présentes dans les selles normales, et que l'on peut identifier avec elles (Moro, Janvier. 1900).

d) En employant la réaction de Grüber-Vidal, on parvient à démontrer que les coli-bacilles présents dans les selles d'un nourrisson donné, même au bout d'intervalles de temps prolongés, sont dérivés d'une même espèce de coli. particulière. habitant le tube intestinal de cet individu. A l'aide de cette réaction on peut ainsi différencier un colibacille d'autres coli-bacilles, provenant d'individus différents, et par là même, des coli-bacilles introduits avec la nourriture, et cette propriété se conserve, sur les milieux nutritifs artificiels. pendant un assez long espace de temps.

II. — De ces recherches, il ressort que le développement des bactéries dans l'intestin du nourrisson, bien que celles-ci soient introduites en quelque sorte accidentellement, dans le méconium primitivement stérile, est soumis à certaines lois et est autochtone. Il en faut chercher les causes dans le fait de la composition chimique constante de la nourriture et du contenu intestinal, dans les conditions végétatives particulières où se trouve le microbe, enfin dans l'influence exercée par les fonctions vitales de l'organisme. La flore normale de l'intestin est l'expression et, en même temps, une des conditions du fonctionnement normal de l'intestin. Elle lutte pour maintenir tel ce fonctionnement et le rétablir lorsqu'il est détruit.

III. — La flore des selles, dans les conditions normales, est indépendante, dans une large mesure, de la variété et du nombre de bactéries introduites par l'alimentation. Toutefois, il suffit de très minimes modifications dans la composition chimique du contenu intestinal, dans les conditions de sécrétion et de résorption, dans l'état général ou dans le pouvoir de résistance de l'organisme, pour troubler les conditions de végétation de l'intestin au point que des bactéries d'une espèce différente ou d'origine ectogène par l'intermédiaire de l'alimentation peuvent s'y installer et s'y multiplier. La facilité toute particulière avec laquelle le lait s'altère, l'insuffisante protection qu'offre contre ces modifications l'estomac du nourrisson, font que ces infections ectogènes ont de nombreuses chances d'apparaître.

IV. — Toute une série de raisons, tirées tant de l'épidémiologie, que de l'observation clinique ou des recherches anatomo-pathologiques ou expérimentales, permettent de regarder comme très vraisemblable, que l'apparition dans l'intestin d'une nouvelle végétation bactérienne différente de la normale, surtout lorsqu'il s'agit de bactéries pouvant donner lieu à des fermentations ou ayant chez l'homme une action pathogène, suffit à déterminer pour son propre compte des phénomènes morbides. Bien plus, suivant les propriétés biologiques des bactéries en question, ou bien elles agiront sur les aliments et sur le contenu intestinal et, en les décomposant, donneront naisssance à des poisons (chymus infection) et auront ainsi une action purement toxique, ou bien elles seront de véritables agents infectieux, créant des processus inflammatoires sur la muqueuse intestinale et conduisant de là, par suite de la chute de l'épithélium, à l'infection généralisée (infection intestinale). Il n'est pas rare aussi que des produits bactériens toxiques, fabriqués en dehors de l'organisme (ectogènes), surtout à l'époque des chaleurs, donnent lieu à des phénomènes morbides. L'organisme de l'enfant est particulièrement sensible à ces influences comme d'une manière générale à toutes les infections bactériennes et intoxications.

V. — Il n'existe jusqu'ici aucune classification satisfaisante des affections gastro-intestinales du nourrisson.

Pour les affections dues à l'action des bactéries, il faut essayer de se conformer à leur étiologie.

Nous distinguons dans ce sens :

1º Les intoxications dues à une décomposition ectogène ;

2º L'infection du chyme (chymus infection) :

3º Les maladies infectieuses de l'intestin.

A la production des deux premiers groupes de troubles morbides peuvent concourir tous les saprophytes à multiplication rapide du lait et du tube intestinal, le bacterium lactis, les protéolytes, le proteus. Les agents de l'infection intestinale sont, d'une manière générale, tous les agents microbiens pathogènes pour l'homme. En ce qui concerne le nourrisson, il existe un certain nombre d'observations d'infections staphylococciques, streptococciques, coli-bacillaires ou à streptothrix (?), ou à bacille pyocyanique (?).

VI. — Étant donnés le mode d'infection et le terrain sur lequel elle se développe, il est facile de comprendre qu'il s'agit toujours d'une certaine quantité de microbes, si bien que les infections mixtes ou secondaires sont fréquentes. Celles-ci jouent un rôle important dans la pathogénie des complications et des suites éloignées de la maladie.

VII. — La croyance, admise sur la foi des statistiques, que plus de la moitié des cas de mort chez le nourrisson sont dus à une affection primitive du tube gastro-intestinal et que la fréquence va toujours en diminuant au fur et à mesure que l'on s'éloigne de la naissance, est en contradiction avec les résultats que nous donnent les documents personnels de l'examen clinique des nourrissons observés par nous.

VERDAUNGSSTÖRUNGEN IM SÄUGLINGSALTER
PATHOLOGISCH-ANATOMISCHES REFERAT, MIT DEMONSTRATION

RAPPORT

von Dr A. BAGINSKY,

a. o. Professor der Kinderheilkunde an der Universität Berlin,
Director des Kaiser und Kaiserin Friedrich Kinder Krankenhauses.

Als mir der ehrenvolle Auftrag von dem Vorstande der paediatrischen Section zuging, die gastro-intestinalen Erkrankungen des Säuglingsalters nach der Richtung der pathologisch anatomischen Veränderungen an dieser Stelle zur Erörterung zu bringen, war ich mir keinen Augenblick dessen unbewusst, dass ich kaum in der Lage sein werde Ihnen wesentlich Neues zu bieten. Ist doch durch die eingehenden Studien des letzten Jahrzehntes allein auf diesem Gebiete, bis auf im Ganzen wenige strittige Punkte, die Kenntniss der anatomischen Laesionen in so erfreulicher Weise vorgeschritten dass man, in Gegensatz zu den aetiologischen Fragen, die noch vielfach wesentlicher Aufschlüsse bedürfen, zu einem gewissen Ruhepunkte gelangt ist, und dass man wohl im Stande ist, eine einigermassen einheitliche Darstellung der vorliegenden Veränderungen zu geben.

Die hauptsächlichsten Differenzen, die noch bestehen, gehen, wie derjenige, welcher sich, dauernd und eingehend mit dem Material beschäftigt, weiss, ohne weiteres daraus hervor, dass nicht allen Bearbeitern das anatomische Material in der nöthigen Frische vorliegt und dass man Neigung gewinnt, sehr früh eintretende cadaveröse Veränderungen als *in vivo* entstandene pathologisch-anatomische Laesionen zu deuten. Die Zartheit der Objecte, die leichte Laedirbarkeit der Oberflächen insbesondere des Schleimhautepithels und der Drüsenschläuche führt wohl dazu, dass wenn nicht eine sehr rasche Fixirung *post mortem*, und zwar nach kaum mehr als 2. 3. 4 Stunden möglich ist, Alterationen des Gewebes sich kennzeichen. welche von den im Lebenden bestehenden Verhältnissen sehr wesentlich abweichen und doch mit den eigentlich krankhaften Veränderungen keinen unbedingten Zusammenhang mehr haben.

Ist man sich dessen einmal durch sorgliche Beobachtung und Vergleichung bewusst geworden. so kann es nicht fehlen. dass man geeignete Behandlung des Materials vorausgesetzt, an der Hand der vorliegenden, und mit den üblichen histologischen Methoden im

Ganzen leicht zu gewinnenden, anatomischen Bilder zu übereinstimmenden Ergebnissen gelangen kann. Freilich gehört eine gewisse Uebung und Ausdauer dazu, sich auch von besonderen Verhältnissen des Darmes, von Blähungszuständen oder starken Contractionen nicht täuschen zu lassen; indess ist doch auch dies im Ganzen leicht zu überwinden, und ich kann dem nicht zustimmen, dass man bei Studien am Magendarmkanal mehr als an anderen Organen Täuschungen unterliege. Was am meisten zu Täuschungen zu führen vermag, ist die trügerische cadaveröse Alteration und man muss es aussprechen, dass Befunde, welche an Leichen gemacht sind, die beispielsweise wie die von *Habel* studirten, 24 Stunden *post mortem*, oder noch später zur Section gekommen sind, für die vorliegenden Fragen als völlig unbrauchbar ausgeschaltet werden müssen. Was die Methode der Behandlung des Magendarmes betrifft, so verfährt man am besten so, dass man kleine Stückchen möglichst behutsam ausschneidet, dieselben ohne Zerrung auf festeren Unterlagen, wie Holzspahn, mit Nadeln befestigt und in 70 % Alkohol einbringt, nach etwa 2 Tagen dieselben dann in stärkeren Alkohol bis zum absoluten bringt, so völlig entwässert und schliesslich den Weg zur Einbettung in Celloidin, von dünnem bis zu concentrirtem, langsam und stetig durchführt, und so die Stücke für die Bearbeitung mit dem Mikrotom fertig stellt. Die vorsichtige und überwachte Lagerung ermöglicht es im Ganzen leicht Schrägschnitte zu vermeiden und sorgliche und gute senkrechte Schnitte zu erlangen. Die so vorbereiteten Schnitte sind mit Anilinfarben und mit Haematoxylin leicht und mit guter Differenzirung zu färben und gewähren einen vortrefflichen Einblick in die in der Magendarmwand vor sich gegangene pathologische Laesion.

Meine Herren! Von jeher hat man sich über die geringfügigen makroskopischen Veränderungen gegenüber den stürmischen, schliesslich zum Tode führenden klinischen Erscheinungen, zu verwundern gehabt, und so ist es dahin gekommen, dass man von der Ueberzeugung ausging, dass im Magendarmkanal weit mehr die direct toxischen oder anderweitig functionellen Störungen das Beherrschende in den deletären Prozessen seien, als die anatomische Laesion.

Es hat ziemlich lange gedauert, bis sich die Erkenntniss Bahn brach, dass die mikroskopische Untersuchung, sorgsam geführt, so schwere anatomische Veränderungen zu Tage fördert, wie nur je an irgend einem andern Organ und dass diese Veränderungen trotz der anscheinenden Dünne des Organs sich bei der Complicirtheit seiner Zusammensetzung dennoch nur auf einzelne Bezirke zu erstrecken vermögen; freilich ist hierbei nicht ausgeschlossen, dass die besonders schweren Veränderungen sämtliche Gewebe der Darmwand durchdringen.

Wenn ich, bevor ich an die Darstellung der pathologischen Prozesse herangehe, daran erinnern darf, dass die Magendarmwand im Wesentlichen aus vier Hauptstücken sich zusammensetzt, der eigentlichen Mucosa, der Submucosa, der Muscularis und der Serosa, so werden Sie sich gleichzeitig bewusst sein, dass die Mucosa unterhalb des zarten Epithellagers eine in ein bindegewebiges Substrat eingebettete Schicht von mit epithelialem Zellenlager ausgefüllten Schlauchdrüsen birgt, und dass zwischen den Schlauchdrüsen die Darmzotten des Dünndarmes von dem Epithelbelag bekleidet, sich über die Ausführungsgänge der Schlauchdrüsen säulenartig oder zitzenartig erheben. Am Fundus der Schlauchdrüsen zieht ein dichtes aus längsgestreiften Muskelfasern gebildetes Gewebelager, der so genannte Brückesche Muskel hin. (*Muscularis mucosae.*) Derselbe grenzt die Mucosa gegen die Submucosa ab, freilich nur so, dass Nerven, Lymphgefässe und Blutgefässe denselben durchdringen und auch bindegewebige mit reichlichen Zellen durchsetzte Züge das Zottengewebe bilden. Die Submucosa, von Hause aus bei jungen Kindern weit zellenreicher als bei Erwachsenen, wird aus einem lockeren Bindegewebe gebildet, in welchem Blutgefässe, Nervenplexus, Nervenzellen, eingebettet sind. Dieselbe geht in das doppelschichtige Muskellager der Darmwand über, zwischen welchem sich bei Kindern besonders deutlich hervortretende und nachweisbare Lymphgefässe (intralaminares Lymphgefässnetz) befinden. Die Serosa ist nach aussen, in lockeren meist Fettgewebe enthaltenden bindegewebigen Zügen der Muskelschicht aufgelagert.

Während dies die Hauptgewebsmasse der Magendarmwand ausmacht, begegnet man im Duodenum noch in der Submucosa eingelagerten Drüsenschläuchen mit hellem durchsichtigem schönem Epithellager, den Brunnerschen Drüsen, und weiter abwärts, den ganzen Dünndarm hindurch, theils einzelnen theils conglomerirt angeordneten Leucocytenreichen Follikeln, von denen die ersteren im Dickdarm besonders zahlreich und gross erscheinen. Man kann so unschwer zwei Hauptschichten (Hauptgewebsbestandtheile) von einander scheiden, die oberflächlichere dem Darmlumen zunächst zugewandte Mucosa mit ihrem Epithel, ihren Schlauchdrüsen und Zotten und die ganze darunter liegende Gewebsmasse, Submucosa mit eingelagerten Brunnerschen Drüsen und Follikeln, sammt den dazu gehörigen, Lymphgefässe einschliessenden Muskelschichten. Die Serosa steht mit diesem Gewebe der Darmwand functionell nur in wenig festen Zusammenhang.

Die entwickelungsgeschichtlichen Studien über den fortschreitenden Ausbau des wachsenden kindlichen Darmkanals, wie sie von mir und überdiess von *Toldt*, *Fischl* und ganz jüngst noch von *Cornelia de Lange* geführt worden sind, haben mit geringen Abweichungen über die Beschaffenheit der einzelnen wachsenden Gewebsbestandtheile, dennoch zu der übereinstimmenden Anschauung geführt, dass der gesammte kindliche Magendarmkanal des Neugeborenen keineswegs als vollkommen fertig und in der Entwickelung abgeschlossen betrachtet werden darf; vielmehr zeigt sich eine gewisse Unfertigkeit in allen Gewebsschichten, die sich aber ganz besonders auch in den drüsigen Gebilden, dem Hauptbestandtheile der Mucosa und in dem Follikelapparat markirt; in letzterem gleichsam im umgekehrtem Maasse als in dem ersteren, weil der Lymphapparat mit seinem enormen Zellenreichthum in der Submucosa eher eine Einschränkung als fortschreitende Ausbildung gelegentlich des weiteren Wachsthums erleidet. Immerhin geht aber aus der stetigen Wandlung ohne Weiteres hervor, dass pathologische Laesionen an den in solchem Zustande befindlichen Organe sehr leicht einen guten Boden finden, und dass die Verletzlichkeit der kindlichen Darmwand in dem biologischen Zustande derselben in den ersten Monaten nach der Geburt des Kindes gleichsam prädestinirt ist. Derselben unterliegen die stark sich verändernden Oberflächenschichten der Darmwand um so leichter, als sie am ehesten den mechanischen, chemischen und Infectionsinsulten durch die in den Ingesta geborgenen Schädlichkeiten ausgesetzt sind.

Wenn man sich nun im Einzelnen mit den Krankheitsprozessen beschäftigt, so kann man zunächst, von klinischer Beobachtung ausgehend, sich dem Eindruck nicht verschliessen, dass es Processe giebt, welche ohne wesentliche, wenigstens ohne andauernde anatomische Veränderungen einhergehen, dass vielmehr vielleicht nur hyperaemische Zustände diese, hauptsächlich functionellen Störungen begleiten.

Wenn ein Kind unter dem Einflusse einer nicht sehr aggressiven Noxe und der Ueberfüllung mit einem sonst wohl geeigneten, und nicht mit an sich schädlicher Substanz, welcher Art sie auch sei, versehenen Nährmaterial, plötzlich anfängt, unter Fieberbewegungen unruhig zu werden und diejenigen functionellen Störungen zu zeigen, welche wir unter dem Begriffe der *acuten Dyspepsie* zusammenfassen, die rasch, wie sie gekommen, ebenso rasch auch wieder vergehen, so werden wir wissen, dass irgend eine tiefer gehende anatomische Laesion der gesammten Organes kaum damit in Zusammenhang gebracht werden kann. Hier können nervöse Beeinflussungen der Drüsenabsonderungen, Veränderungen und Unregelmässigkeiten in der Verarbeitung der Ingesta, auch störende Beeinflussungen der Peristatik, Alles Vorgänge die in der physiologischen Leistung sich abspielen, das Wesentliche der Processe sein. Wir wissen doch aus der Physiologie der Verdauung, wie complicirt hier die Vorgänge sind, wie Absonderung und Leistung der Drüsenproducte, der Leber, des Pancreas und derjenigen der Darmwand selbst, mit den Leistungen der ungemein complicirten Nervenapparate des Darmkanals und viele andere, kaum noch erschlossene physiologische Vorgänge in einander zu greifen haben, um die Verarbeitung der Ingesta bis zur Chymisirung und Assimilation zu ermöglichen, und so die normalen Vorgänge zu gestalten und zu Ende zu führen. An jedem Theile kann eine Unterbrechung oder Schädigung entstehen, ohne dass die Organe selbst wesentliche Veränderungen sichtbarer Art erlitten haben und dennoch sind es markante ja schwerwiegende klinische Symptome, die hier in die Erscheinung treten können. So sehen wir bei diesen acuten dyspeptischen Processen, einmal Erbrechen von in fehlerhafter Weise veränderten, zersetzten Substanzen auftreten, nebenher Diarrhoeen oder auch wohl Obstipation mit Kolikschmerzen, gesteigerter Gasbildung und Auftreibung. Wir können an den fehlerhaften Ausscheidungen, die mit unverarbeiteten Resten des Nährmaterials oder fehlerhaft zersetzten Producten desselben überladen sind (Fett, Fettsäuren, fauligen intermediären Abbauproducten der Eiweisskörper bis zum Ammoniak) erkennen, dass die Assimilation und Resorption unterbrochen worden ist und fortlaufende Gewichtsbestimmungen, ebenso wie die Beobachtungen der Körpertemperatur belehren uns, dass die Ernährung darnieder liegt.

Indess Alles dies nur für kurze Frist, und vorübergehend. Nur wenige Tage vorsichtiger diätetischer Behandlung. Entziehung des Nährmaterials überhaupt, oder Zuführung nur des ausgesuchten, geeigneten und passenden, genügen den krankhaften Zustand vorbeizuführen — die dyspeptische Alteration zu beseitigen. Nichts desto weniger können nun aber doch diese dyspeptischen Vorgänge die ersten Erscheinungen und weiterhin die Begleiter aller der complicirten und schwerwiegenden anatomischen Laesionen sein, welche sich unter der Einwirkung feindlicher Noxen im kindlichen Darmkanal abspielen, ja es kann sicherlich der Verlauf und die weitere Entwickelung der Vorgänge so liegen, dass die störenden Producte der einmal eingeleiteten, dyspeptischen Zersetzung der Ingesta selbst, als die feindseligsten Mittel zur Anregung mehr oberflächlicher, oder tiefer liegender anatomischer Laesionen werden; weiss man doch aus dem Experiment, wie feindselig Producte wie die Ameisensäure, Essigsäure, Buttersäure auf der einen Seite, Indol, Phenol, Kresol, Amidosäuren bis zum Ammoniak auf der anderen Seite, dem zarten Epithelbelag der Magendarmschleimhaut und dem Epithellager der Lieberkühnschen Drüsen und vielleicht auch den Leucocytenmassen der Lymphfollikel zu werden vermögen.

Die Dyspepsie kann so den Ausgangspunkt der weitergehenden Störungen selbst abgeben, wie sie auf der anderen Seite nur als Begleiterscheinung und Ausdruck einer, von einer feindseligen Noxe eingeleiteten anatomischen Laesion aufzutreten und zu beharren vermag.

Es ist oben schon angegeben worden, dass immerhin die obersten, nach dem Lumen zu innerst gelegenen Schichten der Magen-Darmwand, in erster Reihe der Störung unterliegen müssen, weil in der weitaus grössten und überwiegenden Masse von Fällen in den Ingesta die Noxe mitgeführt wird und von der Oberfläche her zur Wirkung kommt: dabei ist freilich nicht ausgeschlossen, dass Einbrüche feindseliger Krankheitserreger auch von fernher in die Lymphbahn oder Blutbahn erfolgen können und dass von den Blutgefässen der Darmwand her jene und schwerwiegenden anatomischen Laesionen erregt werden können, die sich schliesslich bis zum schwersten geschwürigen und gangraenösen Zerfall zu steigern vermögen. Indess sind letztere Vorgänge immerhin nur seltenere, meist secundäre, und können wir hier, wo es sich um die Betrachtung der gewöhnlichen Enteritisformen der Säuglinge handelt, zunächst davon abstrahiren. Thatsächlich sind bei diesen die Oberflächeneinwirkungen der Schädlichkeiten die massgebenden.

Man kann nun unschwer zwei hauptsächliche Gruppen von primär entstehenden anatomischen Veränderungen unterscheiden:

1) Die Gruppe der katarrhalischen Veränderungen,
2) Die Gruppe der folliculären Veränderungen.

Freilich können und werden sich schliesslich beide bei den länger dauernden Processen mit einander verquicken, und es kann und wird dann schwierig anzugeben sein, wo der primäre Sitz der Erkrankung gewesen sei, — oder aber es kann schliesslich unter dem Einflusse der lang dauernden und stets fortschreitenden Alteration der immerhin doch nur aus dünnen Gewebschichten sich zusammensetzenden Darmwand eine so sehr schwere Läsion sich entfalten, dass die Veränderungen bis zum Verluste der gesammten normalen Gewebs-zusammensetzung vorschreiten.

Man wird sich, wenn man diese bezeichneten 2 Hauptgruppen von primären Erkrankungsformen annimmt, dem nicht verschliessen können, dass man, wie bei allen dergleichen Eintheilungen, einen gewissen Grad von Schematismus mit unterlaufen lässt, indess kann man sich doch bei sorgsamer Betrachtung der anatomischen Ver-hältnisse, und auch der diesen entsprechenden klinischen Krankheits-bilder, dennoch nicht davon losreissen, dass in der Grundlage die Eintheilung eine richtige sei.

Ich hoffe, wenn ich die anatomischen Bilder vor Ihren Augen vorüberzuführen die Ehre haben werde, Sie dann zu überzeugen, wie thatsächlich die Angriffspunkte der verschiedenen schädlichen Einwirkungen, welcher Art sie auch sein mögen, vorzugsweise sich in der bezeichneten Weise markiren, und wie, wenngleich Ueber-gangsformen zwischen den beiden besonderen und primären Laesio-nen vorhanden sind, und der Follikelapparat in letzter Linie sich immer gern auch bei den katarrhalischen Erkrankungen betheiligt, nichtsdestoweniger daran festgehalten werden kann, dass die beiden Hauptformen bestehen.

Der dyspeptische Katarrh geht am ehesten aus der einfachen dys-peptischen Störung (Functionsanomalie) hervor. Durchmustert man die Präparate, die gewonnen werden, wenn Kinder unter besonders ungünstigen Verhältnissen gelegentlich der ersten katarrhalischen Störung des Digestionstractus zu Grunde gegangen sind, so findet man die Oberfläche der Mucosa, des Magens sowohl wie auch der Darmschleimhaut mit grossen Haufen zelliger Gebilde (Lymphocyten) bedeckt (fig. 1); man findet weiter die Schlauchdrüsen erweitert, ihr Epithel verquollen, glasig geschwollen und gleichsam über die Ober-fläche hinausquellend; man findet dies ganz besonders auch in den unteren Abschnitten des Ileum und des Colon. In letzterem sieht man eine dicke Schleimmasse, die Mitte der Lieberkühn'schen Drü-sen einnehmend, während das gesammte Epithel-gross, verschleimt, glasig gequollen erscheint und den eigentlichen epithelialen Charac-ter eingebüsst hat.

Zumeist entsprechen diesen Vorgängen Anorexie, belegte Zunge, auch wohl Aufgetriebensein des Leibes, Erbrechen und meist wohl auch schleimige fadige dünnere oder klebrige grünliche Diarrhoeen. Vielfach findet man in den Stuhlgängen weissflockige Beimischungen, meist Nahrungsreste aus Fett und Eiweissresten bestehend und, wenn die Kinder mit Amylaceen genährt sind, auch noch zahlreiche mit

Iod sich blau färbende Amylumreste, Pflanzenbestandtheile (zellige Gebilde) und augenscheinlich dextrinisirte, mit Iod blauroth sich färbende gequollene schwer zu characterisirende Gebilde.

Repräsentirt dieses anatomische Bild also den mehr acuten oder auch wohl den recidivirenden leichteren subacuten Katarrh, so kann es immerhin aber zu jenen allerschwersten und rapid tödtlich verlaufenden Formen des *Katarrhus acutissimus*, wie man ihn von anatomischen Gesichtspunkten aus bezeichnen kann, oder der *Cholera infactum nostras*, wie man ihn klinisch nennt, hinüberführen. Thatsächlich ist die Cholera infantum, anatomisch genommen, nichts weiter als der intensivste katarrhalische Process der Darmschleimhaut, in seinem acutesten und am häufigsten tödtlich endenden Stadium meist ohne gerade sehr erhebliche Mitbetheiligung der Follikelapparate des Darmes.

Diese fehlt allerdings dann auch nicht, wenn mehrfach recidivirende leichtere dyspeptische Katarrhe den acuten Process vorbereitet haben.

s. Dann werden die foudroyanten Erscheinungen der Cholera infantum mit den Schlag auf Schlag erfolgenden Erbrechen und Diarrhoeen, den damit verbundenen rapiden Wasserverlusten und allen anderen, dieselben begleitenden Symptomen, wie Sklerem der Haut, Nierenhyperaemie und parenchymatösen Veränderungen des Nierengewebes, Bronchitiden und Lungenatelektasen, Anaemie des Gehirns u. s. w. eingeleitet.

Die Veränderungen der Mucosa bei der Cholera infantum sind auf weitere Strecken hin gerade zu colossal. Man beobachtet, selbst an frischesten, dem Cadaver entnommenen Darmstücken, Verlust des Epithels der Schleimhaut: die Zellen der Schlauchdrüsen des Darmes haben an Färbbarkeit und Gestalt eingebüsst und erscheinen als vielfach zusammengeflossene, kaum mehr als zellige Körper erkennbare Gebilde. Dieser schweren, weithin gehenden Laesion entspricht an vielen Stellen ein grosser Blutreichthum der Gefässe der Submucosa, und massenhaft etranaen sich lymphoide Zellen in der Mucosa, von der Submucosa her zwischen die Fundi der Schlauchdrüsen, dieselben gleichsam aus ihrem Lager hebend.

Die gleiche zellige Infiltration sieht man in den Zotten des Dünndarms, so dass die Zotten wie mit zellen vollgepfropft erscheinen. Dass bei einem so schweren Processe auch die folliculären Gebilde selbst nicht völlig unbetheiligt sein können, ist begreiflich: ihre rege Antheilnahme kennzeichnet sich schon an dem massenhaften Auftreten der lymphoiden Zellen auch in der Mucosa; indess kommt es des Weiteren, je nach der Länge der Dauer des Processes, zu Schwellungen. Verbreiterungen, Durchbrüchen und geschwürigem Zerfall, so dass Lücken in der Schleimhaut entstehen, die nach Verlust des Oberflächenepithels und nach Ausfall von Lieberkühn'schen Drüsen zu tief gehenden kraterförmigen Geschwürchen hinführen. In diesen so vorgeschrittenen Fällen findet man dann auch die intermusculären Lymphgefässe mitbetheiligt, das Endothel gequollen und auch hier in den Lymphgefässen selbst Anhäufungen von Rund zellen.

Ich gehe nicht besonders noch ein auf die schweren Veränderungen, welche gelegentlich dieses Processes auch die anderen Organe zeigen, und erwähne nur kurz, dass die ziemlich gross gewordenen Nieren bei ihrem im Ganzen blassen Aussehen parenchymatöse Alterationen zeigen, Zerfall des Harnkanälchenepithels auf weiten Strecken, Wucherungen und Vermehrungen der Glomerulusepithelien, hämorrhagische Ergüsse in die Bowmann'schen Kapseln und Verlust der Glomerulusschlingen. In einzelnen, meist länger hingezogenen Fällen findet man überdies multiple Eiterheerde in dem Nierengewebe. Eitriger Inhalt quillt aus den Nierenpapillen und den Nierenkelchen.

Hierzu kommen noch fettiger Zerfall des Lebergewebes in grosser Ausdehnung und zahlreiche bronchopneumonische Heerde mit Bronchitis und Verlegung der Bronchien durch Zellpröpfe.

Auch die Ohren sind verändert; gar nicht selten findet man Ansammlungen von Schleim und Eiter im Mittelohr. Nehmen Sie hierzu noch die gar nicht selten zu beobachtende, bis zur völligen Zerstörung vorgedrungene Neurose der unteren Cornealabschnitte, erythematöse und selbst nekrotische Zerstörungen der gesammten Hautgebilde, neben der insbesondere an Schenkeln, Unterbauchgegend und Nates zu beobachtenden derben (Sklerem) Beschaffenheit, die mikroskopisch sich durch nichts eigentlich Besonderes kennzeichnen lässt, so dürften Sie insgesammt damit die eigenthümlichen anatomischen Veränderungen bei der Cholera infantum erfasst haben.

Ich habe hierbei absichtlich noch nicht der Ansammlung von Microben gedacht. Man findet Coccen und Bacterien in der wie oben geschilderten, veränderten Mucosa; das Gleiche bis tief hinein in die Schlauchdrüsen, und ebenso in die Follic, largebilde; man findet Coccen und Bacillenanhäufungen in dem Parenchym der Nieren, zumeist in den Harnkanälchen; findet das Gleiche zumeist in den die Bronchioli erfüllenden Schleimpfröpfen und ebenso im Mittelohr. Wir werden alsbald weiter von diesen Microben zu handeln haben.

Charakterisirt sich so, wie gesagt, die Cholera infantum als

acutester, schwer zerstörender Katarrh mit den geschilderten secundären Veränderungen, so begegnen uns des Weiteren bei den Ver-
dauungsstörungen der jungen Säuglinge, je nach der Dauer und der
Schwere des Verlaufes, immer weiter vorschreitende und zu definitiver
Alteration, ja zur Verwüstung der Magendarmschleimhaut vorschreitende Veränderungen. Dieselben tragen, da sie an der Oberfläche der Darmwand in erster Reihe sich abspielen, entschieden
katarrhalischen Charakter, wie am besten auch noch daraus hervor-
geht, dass sie vielfach mit eigentlich einfachen unzweifelhaften katarrhalischen Veränderungen abwechseln. Nur dass sie zumeist auch,
entsprechend den auch an anderen Organen zu beobachtenden subacuten und chronischen Gewebsänderungen überhaupt, hyperplastischen Charakter anzunehmen im Stande sind. Neben Wucherungen und Quellungen der zelligen Gebilde, Anhäufungen von Rund-
zellen in den interstitiellen Lagern der Lieberkühn'schen Drüsen und
den Zottengebilden, neben all diesen findet man Wucherungen der
Schlauchdrüsen überhaupt mit gleichzeitiger Dilatation derselben und
einer weit ausgedehnten Verquellung und Verglasung der epithelialen
Gebilde. So nimmt denn die gesammte Darmoberfläche ein höchst
sonderbares Aussehen an (fig. 2, 5, 4), von hyperplastischen Zotten
und tief gehenden Schlauchdrüsenerweiterungen gebildet, was beides
zusammen schliesslich zu einer Verdickung der Schleimhaut und der
ganzen Darm and führt. Ich hoffe, Ihnen in den vorzulegenden Bildern
eine recht charakteristische Anschauung von diesen Veränderungen
zu geben, gleichzeitig aber dafür das Verständniss zu eröffnen, wie
diese sich überstürzenden Gewebshyperplasien von geringer Dauer
sind, wie unter der stetig weiter fortschreitenden katarrhalischen Ein-
schmelzung der epithelialen Gebilde, der gleichzeitigen, als Hyper-
aemie und Stase einhergehenden Circulationsstörungen und augenscheinlich unter den Einwirkungen chemisch in krankhafter Weise
bis zu fauligen Produkten veränderten Ingesta, schliesslich Zerfall,
Abstossung des flüchtig Neugebildeten eingeleitet wird und endlich
die ganze charakteristische anatomische Gestaltung der Darmwand
verloren geht und einem kaum mehr als Darmoberfläche erkennbaren
glatten zellreichen nahern narbigen Gewebe Platz macht (fig. 5, 6).

*Die Hyperplasie der Gebilde des chronischen Magendarmkatarrhs
führt in letzter Linie zu atrophischen degenerativen Gewebsverände-
rungen.*

Diese bisher noch immer ganz zu Unrecht angefochtene Thatsache
ist an der Hand sorgsamst bearbeiteter, von frischesten Cadavern
stammenden Präparate unweigerlich richtig, und wird sich bei allen

wirklich mit Sachkenntniss an die Bearbeitung herangehenden Arbeitern stetig mehr Anerkennung zu verschaffen wissen. — Nur muss man nicht von dem Gedanken beherrscht sein, dass die ganze Darmwand derartig schwere Läsion zeigt: es sind immer nur Strecken, wo man dergleichen findet: dazwischen begegnet man noch wohlgeformten Darmparthien, die freilich die Veränderungen des chronischen Darmkatarrhs, zellige Anhäufung im interstitiellen Gewebslager und den Zotten bei katarrhalischer Verschleimung der epithelialen Gebilde der Drüsen fast immer auch schon an sich tragen.

Alle diese im Magendarm in charakteristischer Weise vorgegangenen Veränderungen gehen mit intensiver Herabsetzung der Assimilation und Ernährung einher und mit, unter Bildung toxisch wirkender Produkte der Zersetzung, eingetretenem Darniederliegen der gesammten Vegetation der Kinder. Stetig fortschreitender Gewichtsverlust, tiefes Elendwerden der Kinder, Apathie, Diarrhoeen abwechselnd mit Obstipation, secundäre Erkrankungen der Nieren, der Bronchien, der Ohren, Furunculose, Decubitus und Sklerose der Haut. Alle diese Begleiterscheinungen sind nichts weiter als der Ausdruck der Wirkungen toxischer, vom Darm aus in die Blutbahn eingedrungener Substanzen, it Verbindung mit den Angriffen pathogener Microben von Aussen her, auf die durch Ernährungsstörungen wehrlos gewordenen Gewebe. Wo man unter solchen Verhältnissen danach sucht, vermag man auf die verschiedenartigsten Microben zu stossen, wovon alsbald noch die Rede sein wird.

Alles in Allem sehen wir also in den von der Oberfläche her vordringenden katarrhalischen Processen bis zur Verwüstung der gesammten Mucosa eine zusammenhängende Kette anatomischer Läsionen, welche den Follikelapparat mit der Länge der Dauer mit in den Bereich der Erkrankung reissen, welche füglich auch an Nerven, Gefässen und Muskelapparat nicht spurlos vorüber gehen, bei denen indess diese letztgenannten Gewebebestandtheile nur secundär betheiligt sind.

Meine Herren! ich hoffe unschwer Ihnen Alles dies in wenigen Anschauungsbildern, welche photographisch die Präparate wiedergeben, zur Klarheit zu bringen.

Ich wende mich nun der zweiten Hauptgruppe der anatomischen Läsionen des Darmtractus zu, den *folliculären Erkrankungsformen*.

Wir haben schon erfahren, dass Schwellungen der Follikel mit entzündlich hyperplastischer Vermehrung der lymphocytären Gebilde die katarrhalischen Krankheitsprocesse, sofern dieselben von einiger Dauer oder auch nur von grösserer Intensität sind, begleiten können (fih. 7) die chronischen katarrhalischen Zustände sind fast immer von Schwellungszuständen der Follikel und zwar der solitären sowohl, wie auch der gonglomerirten (Peyerschen Plaques) begleitet: ja es kann zu Durchbrüchen und Einschmelzungszuständen bis zur Geschwürbildung mit Kraterformen der Geschwüre kommen. Hier sind also die folliculären Veränderungen secundärer Natur, den katarrhalischen Formen folgend; ähnlich wie auch an anderen Schleimhäuten gelegentlich katarrhalischer oder entzündlicher Vorgänge, die den Lymphstrom aus den Schleimhäuten abführenden Lymphdrüsen, zu schwellen und entzündlich zu erkranken pflegen, wenngleich allerdings den lymphoiden Geweben der Darmwand eine ganz andere Stellung zukommt, als etwa irgend anderen mit einer Schleimhaut in Beziehung stehenden Lymphgefässen und Lymphdrüsen. Sind doch die Lymphdrüsengebilde anderer Schleimhäute als die Filter zu betrachten, in welchen sich die Noxen zu sammeln, zu stauen vermögen, und von welchen aus sie nicht selten aus dem Organismus eliminirt werden, um so den selben vor weiteren Schädigungen zu schützen. So selten nun eigentlich entzündliche oder infectiöse Lymphdrüsenerkrankungen sonst primär aufzutreten pflegen, — vielleicht thun sie dies überhaupt nicht, — so dass ich beispielsweise die als Drüsenfieber beschriebene Erkrankung als primäre Drüsenerkrankung nicht anzuerkennen vermag, so liegen im Darmkanal die Verhältnisse doch anders; in der Darmschleimhaut und der ganzen Darmwand sind die Lymphgefässe und follikulären Gebilde integrirende, zu der Function der Darmwand engstens in Beziehung stehende Gebilde, während die den anderen Lymphdrüsen an anderen Schleimhäuten entsprechenden Gebilde, in den visceralen Lymphdrüsen gegeben sind. Letztere sind es denn auch die am ehesten secundär erkranken. — Bei der Verbreitung und Ausdehnung der lymphatischen Gebilde in der Darmwand selbst, bei der Dünne der gesammten Darmwand und der engen Beziehung der Lymphapparate zur Resorption und Assimilation bleiben primäre Erkrankungen der Lymphapparate nicht aus und so sieht man Krankheitsvorgänge, bei welchen unter nur geringer und unwesentlicher Betheiligung der Oberfläche der Darmwand, die Lymphfollikel als die primär und eigentlich erkrankten Partieen erscheinen. Das ist so auffällig und so intensiv, dass die ganze Affection gleichsam nur in dem submucösen Lager zu verlaufen scheint, und dass mit der Quellung, Zellinfiltration und dem Durchbruch der Zellen nach oben, die Affection sich gleichsam als explosive, von unten nach oben dringende, die Schleimhaut von unten her alterirende darstellt (fig. 8). In der Regel verlaufen diese Processe mit hoher Schmerzhaftigkeit, mehr oder weniger heftigen Koliken, ziemlich lebhaftem Fieber, dick belegter Zunge, eingefallenem Leib und mit der Absonderung blutigflockiger, sehr zellenreicher kaum noch fäculenter Stuhlgänge, die eben unter Schmerzen und wenn die untersten Darmabschnitte, wie nicht selten, mit befallen sind, unter Tenesmen entleert werden.

Die Processe können als mehr leichte, nicht eigentlich infectiöse oder als schwerwiegende, den ganzen Organismus schwer betheiligende mit hoher Infectionsfähigkeit und mit Fieber einhergehende sich darstellen und man unterscheidet so die *einfache folliculäre Enteritis*, von der *eigentlich infectiösen, dysenterischen Form* (*Dysenterie*). Augenscheinlich spielt bei der Verschiedenheit und den Schwankungen der Grade der Krankheit die Verschiedenheit der Krankheitserreger, die Variation in der Virulenz derselben und ihren Stoffwechselproducten eine wesentliche Rolle.

Hat man doch gar nicht selten Gelegenheit bei den schwersten Formen selbst den Diphtheriebacillus als Krankheitserreger kennen zu lernen, und sind doch die erzeugten Geschwüre zuweilen mit pseudo-membranösen, echt nekrotisirend diphtheritischen Einlagerungen und Belägen versehen. Alle diese Processe können nun des Weiteren von secundären Erkrankungen anderer Organe, der Nieren, Bronchien und Lungen, der Ohren etc. begleitet sein, genau in demselben Maasse, oder noch mehr, als dies bei den katarrhalischen Processen der Fall ist.

Ich kann nicht unerwähnt lassen, dass gerade von französischer Seite, *Lesage* und *Guinon*, sich gegen diese Darstellung folliculärer Processe auflehnen und an ihrer Stelle die Mehrzahl der hier in Frage kommenden Processe unter den Namen der Enterocolites zusammenfassen. Dies ist deshalb nicht correct, weil mit dieser Bezeichnung « Colitis » nur die Localisation der Processe in den untersten Darmabschnitten betroffen wird, und so echt katarrhalische Processe mit den entschieden primären folliculären Entzündungen, um der Localisation willen, zusammengeworfen werden. Es giebt rein katarrhalische Colitisformen, die mit den folliculären Enteritiden gar nichts zu thun haben, während die folliculären Erkrankungsformen sehr wohl auch im Dünndarm vorzugsweise ihren Sitz haben können, und das Colon gänzlich oder nahezu, frei lassen; wenngleich gern zugestanden werden mag, dass die folliculären Erkrankungen vorzugsweise gern den Dickdarm und gerade das Colon descendens und die Curvatura sigmoidea der Kinder befallen. Das hängt damit zusammen dass die untersten Darmabschnitte (Colon und Curvatura sigmoidea) besonders

reich mit solitären Follikeln ausgestattet sind. Die folliculäre, Erkrankungen werden gern von stagnirenden Fäcalien aus erzeugt, was
begreiflicherweise bei der bekannten eigenartigen Gestaltung der
Curatura sigmoidea der Kinder, welche die Defäcation einigermassen
behindert, bei Kindern besonders leicht der Fall ist, augenscheinlich
weil hier die Noxen, welcher Art sie auch seien, am intensivsten zur
Geltung kommen. Man wird also nicht umhin können die Folliculitis
in ihrem leichten und schweren Grade als anatomisch wohl charakteristische und klinisch sich auch als eigenartig sich darstellende
primäre und selbstständige Erkrankungen anzuerkennen, dieselben
mögen nun im Dünndarm oder im Dickdarm ihren Hauptsitz haben.

Auch dies vermag ich wohl, an den wenigen hier vorzulegenden
Bildern Ihnen zur Anschauung zu bringen.

Meine Herren! Es giebt nun noch begreiflicherweise eine grosse
Reihe von anatomischen Läsionen, die man mit Fug und Recht in
das Bereich der Betrachtung zu ziehen hätte, wenn man ein voll-
ständiges anatomisches Bild der bei den Enteritiden der Säuglinge
vorkommenden Veränderungen entrollen wollte. Ich müsste der
mucös-membranösen Processe gedenken die mit Obstipation einher-
zugehen pflegen, gewisser geschwüriger Processe u. a. m.

Indess gehören dieselben doch nicht eigentlich in die Reihe der
gewöhnlichen mit Diarrhoeen eingehenden Darmerkrankungen der
Säuglinge im stricten Sinne — und so übergehe ich denn diese Processe an dieser Stelle, um mich noch mit einem anderen Theile der,
wie ich glaube, von den anatomischen Darstellungen gar nicht zu
trennenden Aufgabe, mit der Frage der Aetiologie und Pathogenese
der geschilderten Krankheitsformen zu beschäftigen.

Meine Herren! Ich muss das um so eher thun, als ich zu meiner
Ueberraschung gerade in der französischen Literatur bezüglich meiner
Auffassung der ätiologischen Vorgänge vielfach missverstanden worden bin, und gern Anlass nehme, in Kürze meinen von Anfang an
eingenommen, und seither nahezu nicht gewandelten und nicht geän-
derten Standpunkt klar zu legen. — Bei dem Umfange, den die hier
in Frage kommende Literatur angenommen, und über welche vor
Kurzem Herr College *Marfan* ein ebenso umfassendes, wie vortrefflich
kritisch gesichtetes Referat gegeben hat, bitte ich es nicht übel zu
nehmen und nicht als Eigenliebe zu deuten, wenn ich hier jetzt vorzugsweise auf meine eigene Arbeiten recurrire; kommen doch die
Auffassungen anderer Autoren bei den speciellen Berichten der
übrigen Herren Referenten noch genügend zur Geltung.

Ich will bemüht sein in gedrängtester Kürze einen Ueberblick über die fortschreitenden Untersuchungen, auf welche ich meine Auffassung gestützt habe, und sicher glaube stützen zu können, zu geben. In meiner ersten Publication über den Durchfall und Brechdurchfall der Kinder, in welcher ich im Anschlusse an die Mittheilungen von *Virchow* über die Sterblichkeitsverhältnisse Berlins, auf den Einfluss hoher Sommertemperaturen auf die Sterblichkeit der Kinder an diarrhöischen Erkrankungen hingewiesen habe, habe ich hervorgehoben, dass es sich, da der Einfluss der hohen Temperatur besonders an künstlich ernährten Kindern zu Tage trete, wesentlich um eine Wirkung von mit der künstlichen Nahrung eingeführter Gährungserregern (Keimen) handeln müsse, welche im Darmkanal der Kinder eine intensive Zersetzung des Nährmaterials zu Wege bringen und dabei giftige, schädlich wirkende Substanzen erzeugen. So fasste ich also den acuten Brechdurchfall als das Ergebniss eines im Darmkanal erzeugten Fäulnissvorganges auf, bei welchem die von aussen eingeführten Keime die Erreger und Unterhalter sind. — Ich ging hier also von der von *Escherich* später als *exogen* bezeichneten Infection aus, und diese Auffassung dass den exogenen Krankheitserregern bei den Gastro-Enteritiden eine Rolle zufallen, habe ich auch niemals verlassen. Ich erkenne auch heute noch eine *exogene* Infection an. — Als später durch die Untersuchungen *Escherichs* in die ganze Frage der Bacterienbefunde im kindlichen Darmtractus einigermassen Klarheit gebracht wurde und das constante Vorkommen der obligaten Darmbacterien des B. coli und B. lactis aërogenes erwiesen worden war, die chemischen gährungserregenden Wirkungen auf den Magen-Darminhalt durch *Escherich* selbst und durch *mich* aufgedeckt worden waren, wandte ich mich den naheliegenden Fragen zu : 1) in wie weit diese obligaten Darmbacterien vermöge der ihnen zukommenden biologischen Eigenschaften im Stande seien, selbst Schädigungen zu erzeugen, als deren Ausdruck die Enteritisformen zu Tage treten; 2) in wie weit überdies von aussen her eingeführte Bacterien hierbei mitwirken.

Ich konnte an der Hand weiterer Studien erweisen, dass die obligaten Darmbacterien-Formen mit anderen Formen (B. Proteus; Streptococcen, B. der rothen Milch, B. pyoceancus u. a. m.) zum Theil sogar in Conkurrenz treten, indem die einen als Säureerzeuger, die anderen als proteolytische Formen mit meist alkalischen Stoffwechselproducten bei dem Abbau des Eiweisses, bis zum Ammoniak herab, gegen einander zu wirken vermögen, dass indess in letzter Linie sowohl die eine, wie die andere vermöge ihrer Stoffwechselproducte direct, mechanisch und chemisch reizende und entzündungs-

erregende Wirkungen auf die Magen-Darmschleimhaut zu üben
vermögen.

Hier habe ich sonach neben den *exogen* auch die *endogen* feind-
lichen Wirkungen der Darmbacterien berücksichtigt und ätiologisch
mit herangezogen. Nachdem es mir dann noch des Weiteren, im
Verein mit *Stadthagen* geglückt war, eine toxische Substanz als
Stoffwechselproduct einer Proteusart zu ermitteln, habe ich in dieser
Zusammenwirkung wirklicher giftiger Substanzen mit den einfach
chemisch reizenden, die Bedeutung dieser ganzen Vorgänge erkannt.
Ich glaube bestimmt, dass auch die obligaten Darmbacterien insbesondere B. coli giftige Substanzen erzeugen können, und das eben-
sowohl diese endogenen Producte wie diejenigen der exogenen
Bacterien, soweit sie giftiger Natur sind, sich mit den einfachen
Producten der Gährung zur Schädigung der Darmwand und des
gesammten kindlichen Organismus vereinigen können und dass auf
diese Weise ebenso wohl die örtlichen wie die allgemeinen Erscheinungen der schweren Enteritiden zu Stande kommen. — Ich habe
mich hier, wie man erkennt, ebenso wenig auf das Ammoniak und
dessen feindliche Wirkung versteift, wie ich die Annahme einer
exogenen Infection verlassen habe, was beides fälschlicherweise
Lesage und *Lefèbre* in ihrem Berichte über meine Arbeiten angeben;
ich habe vielmehr, gerade weil ich dem Auftreten von reichlichen
Mengen Ammoniak in den Faeces Aufmerksamkeit schenkte, und
auch dieses abwechselnd mit Producten saurer Reaction erscheinen
sah, *Czernys* Auffassung und Hypothese der Säureintoxication des
Organismus mit Interesse aufgenommen, wenn ich sie gleich nicht
als begründet anzusehen vermag.

*Immerhin fasse ich, ob endogen oder exogen feindselig auftretende
Bacterien angeschuldigt werden, die ganzen sommerlichen Gastro-Enteritiden der Säuglinge als saprogene Krankheiten auf.*

Dabei habe ich stets, nachdem mir alles Suchen nach einem einheit-
lichen Krankheitserreger ergebnisslos blieb, die Auffassung vertreten, dass es sich nicht um einen specifischen Krankheitserreger
handle, sondern dass, sei es aus der Symbiose, also dem einfachen
Zusammenwirken einer grösseren Gruppe von Mikroben (Bacterien
und Coccen) oder dem Zusammenwirken ihrer Stoffwechselproducte,
die Enteritiden hervorgehen mögen; ja ich habe es direkt ausges-
prochen, es sei gar nicht unwahrscheinlich, dass nicht einmal überall
und allerotten dieselben Krankheitserreger wirksam sind, sondern
dass, je nach Klima, Ernährungsart und Lebensgewohnheiten der
Bevölkerung, verschiedene Bacterien als Krankheitserreger auftreten

mögen, die nur die eine gemeinsame Eigenschaft haben, saprogene Wirkungen auf die Eiweisskörper und die Kohlenhydrate der gereichten Nahrung zu üben, durch die chemische Action intensiv reizende Wirkungen auf die Schleimhaut auszuüben und durch die Erzeugung toxischer Substanzen eine Vergiftung der Organismus einzuleiten. — Ich habe dabei allerdings niemals ausser Augen gegeben, dass unter besonderen Verhältnissen gewisse besondere, nahezu spezifisch wirkende feindselige Mikroben, Enteritiden erzeugen und dieselben endemisch, in Anstalten, oder epidemisch in grösseren Kreisen machen können; ich habe einen solchen Mikroben beispielsweise selbst im B. pyocyaneus kennen gelernt, habe aber gerade diese durch einen specifischen Mikroben erzeugten Erkrankungsformen von den gewöhnlichen sommerlichen Gastro-Enteritiden jederzeit getrennt und sie aus einander gehalten.

Als mich die seither immer wieder aufgetauchte, bei einzelnen Autoren, wie *Epstein*, *Finkelstein*, *Lesage*, etc. immer wieder behauptete, und doch nicht erweisbare Auffassung der Specifität der Vorgänge und deren Erreger, zu erneuten Untersuchungen über die Aetiologie der Gastro-Enteritiden stachelte, konnte ich die Wahrnehmung nicht von der Hand weisen, dass man allerdings unter den obligaten Darmbacterien Escherich's, auf Bacterienstämme stosse, denen besonders virulente Eigenschaften anhaften, und *insbesondere konnte ich derartige schwer virulente Eigenschaften bei B. lactis entdecken*; indess waren es auch hier nicht specifische Wirkungen, auch war es nicht eine besondere Abart des B. lactis, sondern dasselbe auch sonst im Darmtractus gesunder Kinder vorkommende B. lactis, konnte unter besonderen Einflüssen, wie fehlerhafter Nahrungszufuhr nach Quantität (Suralimentation) und Qualität, namentlich bei sehr hoher Sommertemperatur, zu hoher Virulenz gesteigert werden, so dass es gewisse Eigenschaften annahm, die es für den Organismus besonders feindlich und gefährlich wirksam machte.

Ich durfte mich sonach auch nach der erneuten Untersuchung nur dahin aussprechen, das als *Krankheitserreger nicht specifische, sondern vulgäre saprophytische Bacterien des Darmkanals wirken, welche besondere Virulenz anzunehmen vermögen*. — Legte ich hier auf die endogene Entstehung besonderen Werth, so konnte ich doch an der Hand eigener mit Proteus und Pyocyaneusstämmen gewonnener Erfahrungen, und ebenfalls an der Hand der insbesondere von *Flügge* nachgewiesenen Wirkungen proteolytischer, hoch virulenter in der Milch enthaltener Bacterien, zu dem weiteren Satz gelangen, dass auch andere im Darmtractus ursprünglich nicht vorhandene Bacterien als Erreger der diarrhoeischen Erkrankungen auftreten können, womit also *neben den endogenen Einwirkungen von Mikreben der exogenen Infection ihr Recht gesichert wurde.*

Wogegen ich mich aber von Anfang aus bis heute, auf Grund aller dieser von mir ermittelten Thatsachen aussprechen musste, das ist gegen die Annahme, dass es sich bei den gewöhnlichen Gastro-Enteritiden um specifische Krankheitserreger handele.

Die Suche nach solchen ist bis in die jüngsten Tage gegangen und hierher gehören denn die von *Escherich* gemachten Angaben über eine specifischen Streptococcen-Enteritis, hervorgegangen aus der Einwirkung von Streptococcen und neuerdings über die specifischen Besonderheiten von B. coli-Stämmen, die sich angeblich durch ihr Färbeverhalten gegenüber der Weigert-Gramschen Färbung sollen differenziren lassen. — Herr College *Escherich* weiss es, und ich fühle das Bedürfniss dies diesem verdienten Forscher gegenüber offen hier nochmals auszusprechen, dass ich seine Arbeiten auf dem Gebiete der Verdauungsanomalieen der Kinder möglichst hoch veranschlage. Indessen darf mich diese Werthschätzung doch nicht davon abhalten ebenso aufrichtig meinen abweichenden Standpunkt kund zu geben, und nachhaltig zu vertreten.

Ich habe niemals geleugnet dass Streptococcen bei den Enteritiden der Säuglinge eine ätiologische Rolle mit spielen können, habe vielmehr frühzeitig auf das Vorkommen derselben, mit Bacillen gemeinsam bei den folliculären Enteritisformen, auch auf ihre Beziehungen zu den hyperplastischen Gebilden (Follikeln) hingewiesen, was ich aber leugnen muss, ist die specifische Wirkung und das specifische Gebundensein bestimmter Krankheitserscheinungen an ihre Anwesenheit. Man sieht sie vielmehr bei denselben Kranken ebenso wie andere Mikroben in schwankender Zahl auftreten und wieder verschwinden, ganz ohne dass ihnen eine specifische Bedeutung zukommt.

Daher ist der Name Streptococcen-Enteritis nicht gut gewählt, weil er Beziehungen präjudiciren kann, die nicht bestehen.

Wenn übrigens Streptococcen bei Enteritisformen der Säuglinge im mikroskopisch-bacteriologischen Fäcesbild besonders stark und überwiegend auftreten, so sind zwei Möglichkeiten ihres Eindringens in den Darmkanal vorhanden und wohl auch nachweisbar. Einmal können dieselben mittelst der mit Streptococcen beladenen Milch dem Kinde direct zugeführt werden; ursprünglich als saprophytäre oder besser gesagt vulgäre Microben auftretend, können sie im Darmkanal unter den gleichen Umständen wie auch andere Microben und gleichzeitig mit diesen virulent werden. Wir haben dann eine exogene Zuführung bei endogener Virulenz und es kann daraus sicher ein schweres Krankheitsbild hervorgehen.

Aber auch ein zweiter Weg der Infection der Darmwand ist gegeben, das ist der durch die Blutbahn, von fernliegenden Organen und deren Läsionen her: so habe ich gerade bei denjenigen Fällen, in welchen ich Streptococcen besonders reichlich in den Fäces nachzuweisen vermochte, grosse und zahlreiche Furunkel oder auch eitrige Otitiden, — bei welchen beiden Affectionen Streptococcen nachweisbar waren, — die schweren Darmerscheinungen begleiten sehen, so dass die Annahme erlaubt ist, dass ein Einbruch von der Haut her in die Blutbahn erfolgen kannte, und die Läsion der Darmwand mit den klinischen Symptomen, den Diarrhoeen, dem Herabkommen der Kinder und den gesammten Erscheinungen der Sepsis als der Effect secundärer Krankheitserreger bezeichnet werden durfte. — Man sieht, mit wie verschiedenen und complicirten Verhältnissen man hier zu thun haben kann.

Wie dies also bezüglich der Streptococcen variabel ist, so habe ich mich gelegentlich der eigenen Färbestudien nach den Angaben von Escherich, nicht von der Constanz der Färbeart, in Annahme der blauen oder rothen Farbe, je nach der mehr normalen oder krankhaften Beschaffenheit der Stuhlgänge überzeugen können. Auch hier sind wechselnde Verhältnisse vorhanden selbst bei ausgesprochenen diarrhoischen Affectionen. Alles in Allem kann ich auch nicht eine specifische Sonderstellung von Bacterien innerhalb des B. coligruppe anerkennen.

Wie es nun kommen mag, dass dieselben Bacterienformen so wesentlich verschiedene Virulenzgrade zu zeigen vermögen, wor ich gemüht, in einer besonderen Reihe von Versuchen, welche ich bisher noch nicht veröffentlicht habe, zu ermitteln. Ich habe eine Reihe von Bacterien über deren Virulenz Vorprüfungen und genaue Beobachtungen von mir gemacht wurden, symbiotisch zu cultiviren versucht, und ebenso verfuhrt die Culturen einzelner derselben auf den bakterienfreien Filtraten der anderen aufzubringen; beides in der Hoffnung so zu gesteigerten Virulenzen zu gelangen. — Ich habe ferner Streptococcen aus Fäces mit einem wenig virulenten B. colistamm zusammen cultivirt. — *Alles dies, ohne doch höher virulentere Wirkungen zu erreichen, als vorher.* — Ich habe alsdann B. Proteus mit B. coli zusammen cultivirt, auch die bacterienfreien Filtrate von B. Proteus dazu benutzt B. coli darauf anzubauen. *Es gelang nicht die Cultur virulenter zu machen als vorher.* — Ich habe weiter hin aus Milch gezüchtete Diplococcen auf nicht virulenten Filtraten von

B. Coli-Culturen cultivirt, ebenfalls ohne zu einem virulenteren Stamme von Milchdiplococcen zu gelangen.

Die Versuche, die in der Natur zu beobachtenden Virulenzsteigerung auf solche Weise zu erreichen, misslangen; freilich müssten dieselben wohl noch weiter unter Zusätzen von Darmsekreten oder Extracten der Darmschleimhaut fortgesetzt worden. Gewiss hat *Escherich* Recht, dass die einfach saprogene Auffassung der Gastro-Enteritis-formen der Säuglinge etwas Unbefriedigendes habe, und dass es unserm Verständniss zugängiger wäre specifische Bacterien als Krank-heitserreger ins Feld zu führen; indess muss man sich, wie die Frage bis zu diesem Augenblicke nach allen Versuchen noch liegt, damit zufrieden geben, und es wird der Sache nicht damit gedient, wenn man statt des noch Unaufgeklärten anderes nicht Stichhaltiges zu setzen versucht. — Es befriedigt uns schliesslich dies noch weniger und trägt auch nicht zur Klärung der Verhältnisse bei.

Während ich bis hierher und eigentlich in der ganzen Frage mit *Marfan* nahezu vollständig einer Meinung und in erfreulicher Ueber-einstimmung zu sein vermochte, da auch *Marfan* sich nicht zu der Annahme specifischer Erreger der Gastro-Enteritiden zu entschliessen vermag, so weiche ich nunmehr in der Auffassung und Erläuterung der die Gastro-Entéritiden begleitenden Allgemeinerscheinungen und secundären Erkrankungsformen nach mancher Richtung von ihm ab. *Marfan* glaubt auf Grund von, wie ich gern zugeben will, eingehenden und sehr sorgfältigen eigener Studien und auch kritischer Beleuch-tung aller der Arbeiten von *Sevestre*, *Nanu*, *Marot*, *Wurtz* und vielen Anderen, zu dem Schlusse berechtigt zu sein, dass die Allgemein-infection des kindlichen Organismus mittelst B. coli, in Folge von Durch- und Einbrüchen in die lymphatischen Wege und in die Blut-bahn zu einem gewissen Zeitpunkte der Erkrankung zu Stande kom-men. — Ich will dies keineswegs leugnen, wie ja es ohne Weiteres für solche Fälle zugegeben werden kann, wo schwere Läsionen der Darmwand, wie folliculäre Geschwüre, Abstossungen der Darmzotten, mit Blosslegung von nicht thrombosirten Blutgefässen etc. bestehen; indess wird eine derartige septische Invasion von B. coli vom Darm-kanal aus immer zu den selteneren Vorkommnissen gehören. Gerade die Darmwand ist mit einer Schutzwehr lymphatischer Gebilde und Leucocytenmassen ausgerüstet, wie kaum noch ein anderes Organ, und so am besten gerüstet, eindringende Bacterien abzufangen und zu vernichten. — *So kommt es denn, dass sich die meisten der als secundär bezeichneten Affectionen, Bronchitiden, Bronchopneumonie, Otitis, Furunculose, Pyelitis und Nephritis, etc., bei genauer Unter-*

suchung als echte ectogene entzündliche und Eiterungs-Prozesse erweisen. — So findet man bei Bronchitiden die Bacterien in den Bronchien, nicht in den Blutgefässen, ebenso bei Bronchopneumonien, wie ich dies ganz genau gerade hier zu erweisen vermochte und nachträglich auch *Spiegelberg* bestätigte. — So sind bei den nephritischen Erkrankungen die Bacterien nicht in den Blutgefässen, nicht in den Glomerulis sondern in den Harnkanälchen und interstitiellen Gewebe (fig. 9); ich will zugeben, dass dies nicht ganz streng beweisend ist: denn man kann diesen Befund auch in anderen Fällen als den gewöhnlichen Enteritiden haben, wo über den Einbruch des Bacterium in die Blutbahn gar kein Zweifel sein kann: so habe ich in dem von mir veröffentlichten Falle von Ecthyma pyocyanicum, in welchem der Einbruch in die Blutbahn von der Nasenschleimhaut her erfolgte, in den Nierenheerden das Bacterium nicht nur in den Gefässen, sondern auch im interstitiellen Gewebe und in den Harnkanälchen gefunden: freilich waren aber die Blutgefässe auch nicht frei. — So haben die Furunkel ihren Sitz meist und ursprünglich an derjenigen Stelle, wo die Haut zweist directlädirt wird, am Nacken und den Nates, oder wo bei unreiner Haltung der Badewanne durch das Baden die Haut inficirt wird[1], etc. — So schliessen Erysipelas und Meningitis an Otitis formen an. — Es handelt sich also hier überall um Einwirkungen von Bacterien und deren deletären Folgen an kranken die durch Enteritiden so herabgekommen sind, dass sie sich der feindseligen Angriffe von Bacterien ganz fremder Natur, von Bacterien, die im Darmkanal kaum je vorkommen (wie Pneumococcen etc.), nicht erwehren können, und wenn es, wie gesagt, auch für einzelne Fälle richtig sein mag, und wie ich gern zugebe, dass kreisende Streptococcen im Blute gefunden werden, und dass secundäre Streptococcen-Eiterheerde sich bilden, so ist doch festzuhalten, dass die Entstehung derselben weit eher die Folge ist von an anderen Orten erfolgten Einbrüchen, als gerade vom Darme her. — Die *allgemeine Sepsis der enteritischen Kinder ist keine intestinogene, oder wenigstens nur in den seltensten Fällen; sie ist eine nosoparasitäre ectogene, meist ärogene, hervorgegangen aus Angriffen von Bacterien auf in der Ernährung darniederliegende und der Schutzwehr beraubte Organe, bei hereinter genommenen kranken.*

Meine Herren! Ich habe versucht in kurzen Abrissen meine eigene Stellung zu der Frage Gastro-Enteritisformen der Säuglinge, soweit

1. Er ist ein sehr weit verbreiteter Missbrauch schmutzige Windeln und andere Wäsche un den Badewannen der Kinder aufzubewahren und auszuwaschen, so dass die Wannen inficirt ward.

es sich um die sommerlichen Erkrankungen und deren Folgezuständen handelt, klar zu legen. Gewiss ist Vieles in den Fragen noch dunkel, indessen hat doch der Weg der Forschung, der zurückgelegt worden ist, zu Ergebnissen geführt, die wohl geeignet waren zur Anbahnung einer verständigen, Leben und Gesundheit der jüngsten Altersstufen mehr als früher sichernden Prophylaxe.

(Folgt Demonstration pathologisch anatomischer Präparate mittelst diapositiver Photogramme.)

RÉSUMÉ DU RAPPORT

Au point de vue anatomo-pathologique, il convient de diviser les affections gastro-intestinales des nourrissons de la manière suivante :

I. TROUBLES FONCTIONNELS. — La *dyspepsie aiguë* ne s'accompagnant pas de modifications anatomiques importantes, sinon d'un léger degré d'hyperémie, relève de troubles des fonctions du tractus gastro-intestinal se présentant sous forme de : *a*) diminution des sécrétions digestives; *b*) viciation des actes digestifs, avec fermentations anormales; *c*) diminution de l'assimilation; *d*) vomissements et diarrhée; *e*) constipation et coliques.

Ces signes fonctionnels multiples sont parfois compliqués de symptômes généraux, tels que la fièvre, de symptômes nerveux, de modifications urinaires, etc., etc.

II. ALTÉRATIONS ANATOMIQUES. — 1) *Lésions anatomiques de nature catarrhale : a*) *catarrhe subaigu dyspeptique* avec hyperémie et gonflement œdémateux : infiltration cellulaire de la muqueuse : anomalies de la sécrétion : sécrétion catarrhale : *b*) *catarrhe suraigu, choléra infantile,* abrasion et destruction de l'épithélium gastro-intestinal sur de grandes surfaces. Cellules glandulaires gonflées et granuleuses, allant jusqu'à la nécrose. L'appareil folliculaire présente souvent du gonflement et de l'infiltration. Lésions secondaires de presque tous les organes, surtout du foie et des reins, mais aussi de l'encéphale, des poumons, de la rate, du péritoine, de la peau, des oreilles, des yeux, etc.: *c*) *catarrhe chronique gastro-intestinal*, infiltration de la muqueuse entière. Infiltration cellulaire et hyperémie. Hyperplasie des villosités intestinales et partiellement des glandes, lorsque le processus a duré longtemps. La participation de l'appareil folliculaire n'est pas rare, surtout dans le gros intestin. Altérations morbides des autres organes (broncho-pneumonie : néphrite : otite, etc.): *d*) *atrophie intestinale, cachexie intestinale, athrepsie*. Disparition partielle de l'appareil glandulaire de la muqueuse. Infiltration cellulaire et hyperémie partielle, souvent anémie grave de la muqueuse. La sous-muqueuse et la musculaire sont souvent amincies.

Tous ces processus de catarrhe (de *a* à *d*) sont accompagnés, dans la plupart des cas, de vomissements, diarrhée, coliques; la sécrétion de liquide et de mucosités est augmentée; l'assimilation est empêchée et les fonctions du foie et du pancréas sont troublées. Les déperditions aqueuses et le défaut d'assimilation déterminent des troubles profonds de la nutrition générale.

2) *Lésions anatomiques localisées à l'appareil folliculaire. Folliculite.* — Les lésions folliculaires sont fréquentes au cours des processus de catarrhe; mais elles peuvent aussi exister isolément: il en est ainsi dans : *a*) la *simple entérite folliculaire* : fièvre modérée, ténesme léger, coliques légères, sécrétion muco-sanguinolente. Les follicules sont infiltrés, proéminents, surtout dans le gros intestin; ils forment des saillies çà et là. Infiltration cellulaire; *b*) l'*entérite folliculaire infectieuse grave. Dysenterie.* — Infiltration de la muqueuse; destruction des follicules, avec formation d'abcès. Nécrose de grandes étendues de la muqueuse.

Dans ces deux catégories de faits, les autres organes sont atteints secondairement, surtout le foie, les poumons, les reins, les oreilles, etc.

III. *Causes des processus morbides gastro-intestinaux.* — Les troubles fonctionnels ainsi que les processus morbides graves liés à des altérations anatomiques ont pour origine : tantôt des infections ou intoxications *endogènes :* 1) l'action directe des microbes normaux de l'intestin, dont la virulence s'exalte dans des circonstances particulières (haute température, etc.) (B. coli; B. lactis, etc.); 2) l'action des produits toxiques se formant sous l'influence de ces microbes plus virulents aux dépens de la matière alimentaire; tantôt des infections ou intoxications ectogènes : 3) l'action des microbes saprophytes ou infectieux vulgaires introduits dans l'intestin avec les aliments et devenus virulents à la faveur de circonstances particulières (haute température, etc.); 4) les substances toxiques contenues dans les aliments et introduites dans l'intestin de l'enfant.

IV. Les processus morbides, par lesquels nous venons de résumer les affections gastro-intestinales des nourrissons et qui se développent le plus souvent sous l'influence de la chaleur de l'été, sont causés par des microbes saprophytes ou infectieux vulgaires de virulence exaltée et par leurs toxines; mais ces microbes ne sont pas spécifiques. Il existe toutefois une certaine prédilection des microbes pour telles parties de l'organe. C'est ainsi qu'on rencontre de préférence des bacilles dans les lésions des glandes de Lieberkühn, quoique des cocci puissent également les atteindre; mais les cocci préfèrent l'appareil folliculaire. C'est ce que montre l'entérite streptococcique, qui représente la majorité des entérites folliculaires; elle n'est pas spécifique.

V. Il existe sans doute aussi des gastro-entérites, déterminées, sous l'influence de conditions spéciales, par des microbes infectieux, qui autrefois n'habitaient pas généralement le tractus gastro-intestinal des nourrissons (B. pyocyaneus, etc.); mais elles sont à écarter du cadre des diarrhées d'été habituelles des nourrissons.

VI. La septicémie à point de départ intestinal est plus rare qu'on ne l'a dit jusqu'ici. On en a cependant observé des cas, avec localisation rénale surtout, où la suppuration et même la nécrose peuvent succéder à des infarctus. Cependant l'invasion du sang par les microbes venus de l'intestin est un phénomène exceptionnel et l'infection des organes éloignés est due plus souvent à un processus exogène, dans les gastro-entérites infantiles. Les organes affaiblis sont envahis par des microbes étrangers (pneumocoque, streptocoque, staphylocoque, pyocyaneus, etc.): c'est le noso-parasitisme des organes affaiblis.

Erklärung der Abbildungen.

Fig. I. — Dyspeptischer Magencatarrh.

Fig. II à III. — Wucherungen von Darmzotten beim chronischen Catarrh.

Fig. IV. — Wucherungen der Lieberkühnschen Drüsen beim chronischen Catarrh.

Fig. V à VI. — Zerstörte Mucosa bei Darmatrophie.

Fig. VII. — Folliculäre Enteritis.

Fig. VIII. — Folliculäres Darmgeschwür.

Fig. IX. — Bacterienhausen im Nierengewebe neben einem Glomerulus.

XIIIe CONGRÈS INTERNATIONAL DE MÉDECINE. PARIS 1900.

Section de Médecine de l'Enfance

Rapport de M. le Professeur BAGINSKY, de Berlin.

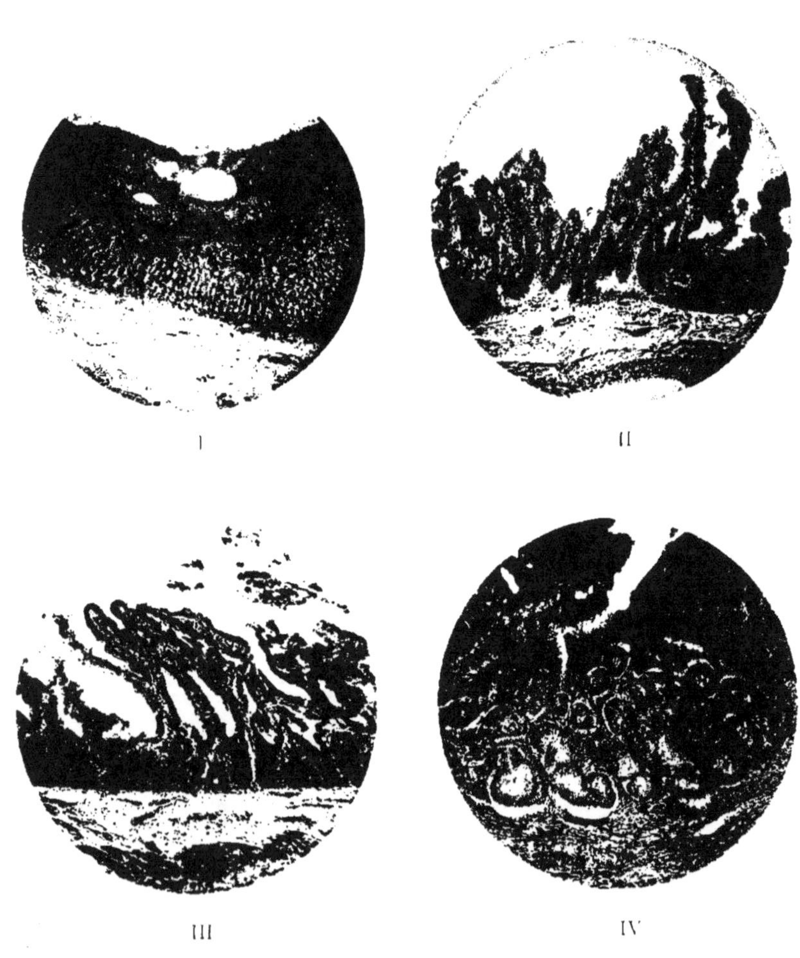

I   II

III   IV

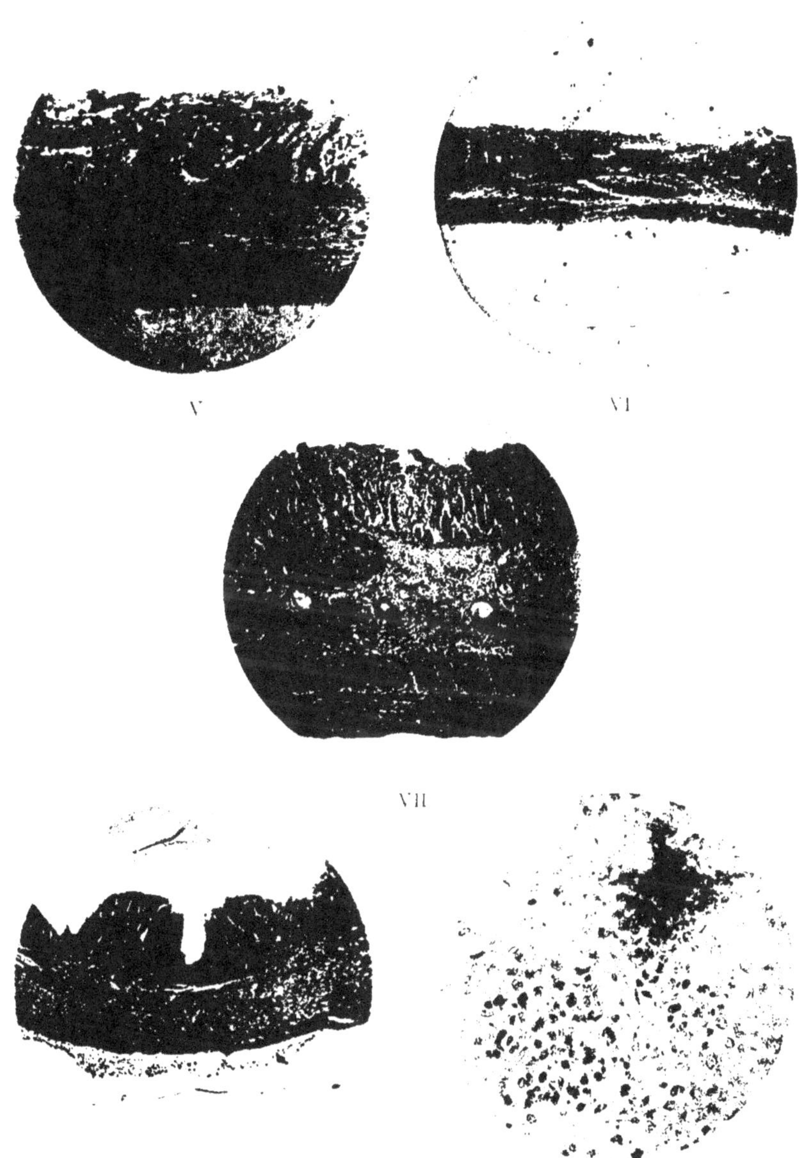

V

VI

VII

VIII

IX

INFECTIONS ET INTOXICATIONS GASTRO-INTESTINALES
DANS LA PREMIERE ENFANCE GASTRO-ENTÉRITES DES NOURRISSONS
ÉTIOLOGIE ET PATHOGÉNIE

RAPPORT

par M. le professeur Martinez VARGAS.

de Barcelone.

Chargé par le comité de Paris de faire un rapport sur ce point, je dirai d'abord que, dans les troubles gastro-intestinaux de la première enfance, l'étiologie et la pathogénie ont été radicalement transformées pendant ces dernières années. Tandis que la symptomatologie est la même qu'au commencement du siècle ou à peu de chose près, parce que les symptômes dominants, la diarrhée, la fièvre et les vomissements n'ont pas varié, les causes ont été l'objet de nombreuses investigations, d'heureuses découvertes qui sont venues détruire l'ancienne conception de la pathogénie et ont adapté cette dernière aux nouvelles idées de la microbiologie et de la chimie biologique.

Dans le temps, ces gastro-entérites semblaient être produites par des causes macroscopiques grossières, par l'excès d'alimentation, par les vers, par la dentition, par une alimentation impure, par l'accroissement de la chaleur pendant l'été, par le refroidissement durant l'hiver. Actuellement, sans déprécier l'influence de ces facteurs, ils ont été relégués au second plan, et quelques-uns ont dû être complètement repoussés. Ces titres, ces noms si suggestifs et si souvent employés, comme les diarrhées du sevrage, les diarrhées lientériques, séreuses, bilieuses et les catarrhes gastriques ou gastro-intestinaux infectieux ont perdu leur signification pathologique, leur hégémonie nosologique et doivent, par conséquent, être remplacés par d'autres noms plus en rapport avec la réalité et avec le progrès scientifique. En 1894, en faisant la classification des diarrhées infantiles à l'Académie royale de médecine de Barcelone, je signalais la nécessité de cette réforme pour en finir une fois pour toutes avec les erreurs de l'ancienne doctrine; car toute l'étiologie de ces troubles morbides de l'estomac et de l'intestin se trouve aujourd'hui réduite à l'action de certains microbes et des substances toxiques que ceux-ci élaborent, et ces combinaisons nosologiques si embrouillées ont été fondues en une simple *infection* ou *intoxication* qui, quand elles se réalisent dans l'intérieur de l'organisme, se nomment auto-infections et auto-intoxications intestinales.

De la sorte, nous nous rapprochons davantage de la classification étiologique, microbiologique et toxique de ces troubles et, malgré qu'aujourd'hui nous ne soyons pas encore arrivés à formuler une classification parfaite, nous sommes cependant bien près d'atteindre le but.

L'étiologie des gastro-entérites des enfants au sein ou de la première enfance comprend deux parties fondamentales : les causes primitives, essentielles, soit les microbes et leurs toxines, et les causes secondaires ou prédisposantes, soit la contagion, l'alimentation, la malpropreté, la chaleur, l'eau souterraine, le vent et les conditions urbaines.

Âge. — La question de l'âge intervient d'une manière très importante dans ce genre de troubles ; chez les enfants un peu grands déjà existent les mêmes microbes et les mêmes principes chimiques ; mais leur action morbide chez eux est limitée, et elle n'acquiert pas autant de violence que chez les tout jeunes enfants.

La clinique nous a démontré que le mal appelé choléra infantile, la diarrhée cholériforme, les diarrhées estivales qui produisent aussi leurs maux en hiver dans leur forme grave, sont particulières aux enfants qui n'ont pas plus d'un an ou d'un an et demi.

Ma statistique de Grenade, celle de Lewis Smith, celle de Holt, de Jeffries, enfin celle de Crandall, permettent de conclure que les enfants de un à douze ou dix-huit mois sont les seuls qui présentent les formes graves ou mortelles de ces diarrhées ou gastro-entérites ; et à de pareils résultats l'on arrive avec l'expérimentation, car le bacille pyocyanique engendre des troubles graves ou mortels chez les jeunes animaux seulement, et le bacille de Flügge qui, à peine s'il détermine la diarrhée chez les chiens déjà grands, produit sûrement la mort quand on infecte les tout jeunes chiens. Soit que la résistance organique soit moindre, soit parce que les épithéliums de l'intestin ne protègent pas autant, toujours est-il que la première enfance possède une prédilection spéciale pour ces troubles.

Microbes intestinaux. — L'action de plusieurs microbes dans la production de la gastro-entérite chez les nourrissons est aussi évidente qu'indiscutable. Quand bien même n'aurions-nous pas à ce sujet les révélations quotidiennes du microscope et des cultures, que nous pourrions le supposer ainsi, étant donné que les enfants exclusivement allaités par leur mère, c'est-à-dire qui consomment un aliment parfaitement stérile, arrivent à l'âge de 10 ou 12 mois sans avoir éprouvé aucun trouble digestif ; mais, si, d'un côté, il est impossible de nier l'intervention des microbes dans ces infections, par contre on ne peut encore affirmer quelle espèce de germe ou quel genre de microbe est le producteur de l'une ou de l'autre forme morbide; pas même dans les plus graves manifestations de l'infection ou de l'intoxication, ni dans la diarrhée cholériforme qui est capable de tuer un enfant dans l'espace de quelques heures, il n'a été possible d'isoler un germe qui, d'une manière constante et par lui-même, reproduisît le tableau clinique; si dans les maladies infectieuses typiques, on connaît le microbe spécifique, nous devons avouer qu'en ce qui concerne les gastro-entérites, nous n'avons pu arriver au même résultat, ce qui nous oblige à nous contenter à admettre que plusieurs microbes, moyennant une symbiose ou infection mixte, ou toute autre consécutive, engendrent la maladie.

L'enfant, en naissant, a son tube digestif complètement stérile; mais, après 4 à 6 heures, divers microbes viennent l'envahir à travers l'anus et la bouche, soit par l'air ou par les boissons, et à partir de ce moment-là ils commencent à pulluler dans l'estomac et dans l'intestin, pour ne plus en disparaître durant toute la vie. La microbiologie gastro-intestinale est très riche en variétés et en nombre; parmi ces variétés il existe deux espèces dominantes et saprophytes : le bacille lactéo-aérogène, qui vit habituellement et de préférence dans l'intestin grêle, et le bacillus coli communis, qui domine dans le gros intestin. Ces bacilles rendent des services très importants pour la digestion; mais à certains moments, au lieu d'être utiles, ils deviennent préjudiciables; ils se font ainsi pathogènes.

Au point de vue de l'infection gastro-intestinale, j'énumérerai seulement les germes qui, au moyen de l'investigation, ont été trouvés dans divers cas; par conséquent j'en exclurai les autres spécifiques qui peuvent se trouver dans le lait et dans l'intestin et sont producteurs des maladies indépendantes, savoir : le bacille typhique, le bacille tuberculeux, le diphtérique, le cholérique, celui de la fièvre exanthématique, l'aphteux, le dysentérique, pneumonique, malarique, etc. Pour les mêmes raisons, je m'abstiendrai de parler des microbes colorants du lait, des microbes du lait amer ou visqueux et des moisissures et levures qu'on peut trouver dans ce liquide.

Microbes des gastro-entérites.

Bacille lactéo-aérogène. — Il abonde d'une manière prodigieuse dans l'intestin grêle, après quelques heures seulement que l'enfant est né; par contre, il est assez rare dans le gros intestin; quelquefois dans les troubles infectieux on l'a trouvé circulant dans le sang. Dans le lait, en plein air ou dans l'estomac, il agit sur la lactose, développe la fermentation lactique et par conséquent produit l'acide lactique et des gaz; il détermine la coagulation. Son activité dépend de la quantité de lactose, et il peut vivre sans oxygène et au milieu de la fermentation. Injecté dans le sang des cobayes il détermine le collapsus et des lésions de catarrhe intestinal.

Bacillus coli communis. — Laissant de côté, pour le moment, sa ressemblance en forme et activité avec le bacille typhique et avec le bacillus enteritidis de Gärtner, il constitue une des bactéries les plus discutées sur le terrain clinique, par les diverses formes qu'il adopte et également par les divers troubles auxquels il prend part. C'est le saprogène du gros intestin, et on l'y trouve en grand nombre; c'est d'ailleurs dans le gros intestin qu'il réside habituellement. On peut le trouver aussi dans l'intestin grêle, dans la bouche et autres cavités, dans l'air, dans le lait et dans la terre. Szego l'a vu circulant avec le sang dans deux cas d'infection grave. Il est aérobie, mais il peut devenir anaérobie et vivre en pleine fermentation.

Il coagule le lait, fait fermenter la lactose, développant de l'acide lactique, toujours droit, de l'acide carbonique et quelque peu d'hydrogène et d'indol; dans les cultures il produit des toxines comparables à celles du bacille de Eberth.

Le point capital de ceci repose sur ce que l'on ignore comment le coli saprophyte se transforme en pathogène: on ne sait pas du tout si cette transformation s'opère par l'influence des phénomènes vitaux ou si c'est par l'action des corps de la série aromatique, comme l'indol, le scatol, le phénol ou le crésol. On a cherché à cultiver une race spéciale de coli; mais jusqu'à ce jour on n'a point obtenu d'uniformité dans les résultats, et pas davantage une variété qui corresponde constamment à une infection intestinale déterminée: on a voulu expliquer cette action pathogénique par l'abondance ou par l'exaltation de la virulence, ou bien par les deux facteurs réunis; mais il n'a pas été possible non plus d'obtenir à ce sujet une véritable démonstration expérimentale. Une fois découverte la qualité agglutinante du sérum, on a eu recours à ce procédé et l'on a pu se rendre parfaitement compte que le sérum des enfants malades avec infection gastro-intestinale n'a pas de pouvoir agglutinant sur les cultures du coli virulent, ou bien il l'a d'une façon si légère qu'il est à peu de chose près comme le normal: dans ces conditions, il serait impossible d'admettre l'existence d'une infection coli-bacillaire pure: on n'est pas non plus arrivé à séparer une race des infections coli bacillaires d'été. Nobécourt a inoculé des animaux avec des cultures de ces coli de diarrhées estivales, et il a pu se rendre compte que ce sérum agglutinait le bacille de l'animal même, mais était incapable d'en faire de même avec des bacilles coli recueillis chez d'autres individus attaqués de maladies analogues. Par conséquent, il est impossible d'affirmer qu'une variété de cette infection soit produite par le bacille coli. Peut-être faut-il faire intervenir son association avec divers autres germes; la clinique a démontré qu'en pareil cas il y a coïncidence entre le coli et le streptocoque, ainsi qu'avec le mesentericus, le pyocyanique, le proteus, la sarcine et le staphylocoque. La circonstance qu'il se trouve dans l'intestin en état normal quelques-uns de ces germes diminuerait un peu l'importance de leur pouvoir pathogénique; mais il n'y a point de doute que, dans les infections graves, l'association strepto-coli-bacillaire ou du coli avec le proteus est dominante.

Bacille pyocyanique (B. pyocyaneus). Considéré pendant longtemps comme saprophyte, il doit maintenant figurer parmi les microbes pathogènes, car l'ont ainsi démontré la clinique et Charrin avec ses expériences. Ses cultures ou ses produits toxiques injectés dans le sang produisent de graves lésions et même la mort chez certains animaux spécialement encore jeunes.

Le bacille de Gessard ou du pus bleu est le type le plus complet du polymorphisme; il est aérobie, mais il vit en dehors de l'oxygène, sans produire alors de pyocyanine; il se trouve dans l'air, dans la terre, dans l'eau, dans le lait et enfin dans nos cavités. Il produit deux sécrétions: une pigmentaire et l'autre toxique. La pigmentaire comprend 3 produits: l'un bleu (la pyocyanine); l'autre jaune (la pyoxantose) et la troisième vert fluorescent; la toxique possède 5 produits: les uns volatiles, qui s'obtiennent par distillation et qui diminuent l'excitabilité des nerfs moteurs et quelquefois parviennent à l'abolir complètement; et d'autres toxines protéiques insolubles dans l'alcool, pas dialysables, qui produisent de la diarrhée, amaigrissement, albuminurie et des hémorragies.

Baginsky l'a trouvé dans les déjections d'enfants avec diarrhée, et dans trois cas il a pu se rendre compte de la transmission de lit à lit, laquelle transmission dut s'opérer soit par l'air, soit par l'intermédiaire des infirmiers. Escherich l'a trouvé dans les déjections d'enfants avec une diarrhée caractéristique, soit la diarrhée concomitante, avec vésicules cutanées, hémorragiques et avec albuminurie; il ne put le découvrir dans le sang. Isolé en culture pure ou associé avec d'autres germes on l'a aperçu dans les selles diarrhéiques, dans la bouche, dans la sérosité des vésicules cutanées, dans les sécrétions nasales et laryngo-trachéales, dans le poumon, dans le pus de l'oreille moyenne ou de la pie-mère, dans le sac de la rate, dans les plaques de Peyer et dans le sang du cœur. Kossel, Salm et Hugo l'ont vu très abondant dans quelques déjections diarrhéiques où, avec son pigment, il donnait aux selles une couleur d'un vert intense.

Streptococcus. Il se trouve répandu un peu partout, sur le sol, dans l'air, dans la terre, dans l'eau, dans la bouche; Netter l'a trouvé dans le contenu intestinal. Dans les cas de mammite on peut l'apercevoir dans le lait. Quand l'investigation microscopique ne suffira pas pour le reconnaître, il sera indispensable d'avoir recours à la culture. Il est aérobie facultatif: mais il vit mieux sans oxygène; il est capable de coaguler le lait; la coagulation commence par le fond pour se propoger ensuite au reste. Il forme un acide qui diffère de l'acide lactique, oxalique et succinique et une toxalbumine qui est précipitable par l'alcool. Escherich l'a trouvé comme bactérie prédominante dans une diarrhée muco-sanguinolente et il put le découvrir dans les déjections, dans le sang, dans l'urine, dans les conduits lymphatiques et dans les organes.

Staphylococcus. Se trouve dans le milieu ambiant, dans le lait des femmes accouchées depuis peu et dans nos cavités, attendant le moment d'entrer en action, seul ou associé. Dans les infections diarrhéiques, on l'a découvert circulant avec le sang.

Il est aérobie facultatif; dans le lait il produit avec rapidité l'acide lactique, et à l'aide de ce dernier il produit la coagulation; développe dans les cultures une substance chromogène, mais pas constante, quelques diastases, une ptomaïne cristallisable, pas nitrogénée (flogosine de Leber) et des substances toxiques.

Proteus. Ils constituent un groupe représenté par le proteus vulgaire (Hausser), le mirabilis et le Zenkerü. Ce dernier se distingue des autres en ce qu'il ne liquéfie pas la gélatine et pas davantage le sérum. Ils sont anaérobies, vivent dans l'acide carbonique pur, se développent dans les composés albumineux, engendrent la putréfaction des tissus animaux et avec elle des gaz fétides et un poison énergique: ils sont constants dans les cas graves de diarrhée cholériforme, accompagnés de stupeur, collapsus, vomissements et déjections fréquentes, aqueuses et fétides. On ne le trouve pas dans les cas d'infection intestinale localisée, sans symptômes d'intoxication.

Cultivés en bouillon et gélatine liquide, et en faisant avec cette culture une injection dans la veine de l'oreille, il s'est produit une diarrhée grave avec assoupissement et accélération respiratoire; dans plus de la moitié des cas, l'infection veineuse a produit une hémorragie gastro-intestinale et une diarrhée des plus graves. Vaughan a

extrait de ces cultures une toxi-albumine qui, injectée sous la peau,
produit des vomissements, de la diarrhée et la mort.

Bacillus mesentericus vulgatus; *bacillus de Flügge et thyrothrix*.
Le mesentericus produit par fermentation la dissolution du ciment
intercellulaire des végétaux: il est pathogène quand il entre en
grande abondance dans l'intestin: sa culture injectée dans le sang,
dans le péritoine ou sous la peau, ne produit pas de grandes perturbations.

Par leur action sur la caséine on doit comprendre dans ce groupe
les bacilles de Flügge I, II et III et le subtilis, ainsi que le groupe
trouvé par Duclaux dans le fromage.

Le bacille I de Flügge seul agit sur la caséine; il respecte le
sucre ainsi que la graisse et il ne change ni l'odeur ni le goût du lait;
avec ses cultures, Lübbert a pu arriver à tuer les lapins en 24 heures,
et les jeunes chiens en 4 à 7 jours, produisant de l'inflammation et une
tuméfaction dans l'intestin. Deux centimètres cubes de ces cultures
injectés sous la peau, produisent chez les animaux des convulsions,
de la diarrhée, une hémorragie péritonéale et la mort; d'après Lübbert, ces effets sont produits par une toxine du corps même du
bacille. Le *bacillus subtilis* change sa qualité quand on le fait passer
par plusieurs animaux, ce qui exalte sa virulence et lui fait produire
des toxines très énergiques, presque mortelles.

Le *thyrothrix tenuis* est aérobie et suivant Lesage doit figurer
parmi les agents producteurs du choléra infantile.

Bacille butyrique. Contribue avec d'autres microbes à la fermentation butyrique des hydrocarbonées, manque dans l'estomac normal:
mais il existe lorsqu'il y a catarrhe gastrique ou gastro-ectasie. Dans
l'intestin il existe en état normal: son pouvoir pathogénique est très
faible; cependant en injectant dans le péritoine 12 centimètres cubi-
ques de lait infecté par ce bacille la mort s'est produite dans 24 heures.

Autres bacilles. E. Moro a isolé des déjections des enfants une bacille qu'il appele *acidophilus* parce qu'il prospère dans les milieux acides. Tissier en a isolé d'autres des mêmes selles avec cultures anaérobies: Thiercelin croit en avoir découvert un autre dans la diarrhée
cholériforme des enfants.

*Action des microbes intestinaux sur les principes alimentaires et
produits*. Ces microbes se trouvent dans l'estomac et dans l'intestin
en plus ou moins grand nombre et mis en contact avec les aliments
ils développent des actions fermentatives plus ou moins importantes
sur les protéiques, les graisses ou le sucre: les principales s'opèrent
sur la lactose et la caséine.

Sur la lactose agissent plusieurs microbes : le premier de tous est le lacto-aérogène : il produit par dédoublement la fermentation lactique, c'est-à-dire de l'acide lactique qui, lorsqu'il arrive à la proportion de 7 à 8 pour mille, coagule le lait avec développement d'acide carbonique ; produisent aussi quelque peu d'acide lactique, le bacillus mesentericus et le coli : une fois que la fermentation lactique est terminée, l'acide butyrique entre en fonction et se nourrissant d'acide lactique il développe la fermentation butyrique : avec ce dernier acide il donne au lait la saveur et l'odeur de beurre rance. Le bacillus butyricus est anaérobie et doit être considéré comme identique au bacillus *amylobacter* de Trecul et Van Tieghem et au *clostridum butyricum* de Prasmowsky.

Après la fermentation butyrique vient la propionique, l'acétique et la valérique : de ces fermentations diverses il en résulte une série d'acides et en plus le formique, l'acétone et l'alcool.

Sur la *caséine* agissent divers bacilles saprophytes, comme le subtilis, le mesentericus et ceux du groupe thyrothrix ; moyennant la formation de produits solubles, ils exercent une double action : en premier lieu par un ferment ayant de la ressemblance avec celui de la présure de l'estomac, ils coagulent la caséine sans acidifier le lait : et ensuite à l'aide d'un autre ferment, la *caséase* (Duclaux), ils liquéfient le coagulum de la caséine, le peptonisent et il en résulte la *caséone*.

La lactose s'oppose à la décomposition microbienne de la caséine et en quelque sorte elle empêche la putréfaction : mais comme ce sucre est décomposé et absorbé dans les premières portions de l'intestin grêle et que l'action sur la caséine s'opère plus tard, il est très rare de constater le développement de cette action. Même lorsque ces bacilles viennent à mourir dans l'estomac ils forment des spores qui traversent le pylore et se développent énergiquement dans l'intestin. Quand ces microbes abondent, il arrive, qu'en rendant assimilable la caséine pour s'être transformée en *caséone*, ils en profitent à leur propre avantage pour leur pullulation et alors ils détruisent la matière albuminoïdée produisant la putréfaction et avec elle les corps suivants : gaz (hydrogène, acide carbonique, ammoniaque, vestiges d'azote, hydrogène sulfuré et phosphoré) ; amides acides (complexes, leucine, tyrosine et quelquefois la créatinine) : acides gras (palmitique, caproïque, butyrique, formique, acétique, propionique et valérique) : substances analogues aux peptones fréquemment toxiques : alcaloïdes ou ptomaïnes (colidine, hydrocolidine, parvoline, conidine, cadavérine, mydaléine, neurine, etc.) : et des corps cycliques, phénol, indol, scatol, pyrrol et dérivés.

A part ces substances produites par fermentation endogène, nous devons en signaler une autre engendrée en dehors de l'organisme par fermentation exogène ou transmise directement au lait.

Dans ce groupe, la substance la plus importante de toutes est le *tyrotoxicon*. Décrite sous ce nom par Vaughan qui l'a trouvée dans le lait contenu dans les biberons ou dans les vases, on suppose qu'elle est produite par l'action du bacille butyrique ou autre semblable; elle peut également se produire dans l'estomac. C'est une substance formée par des aiguilles cristallines; expérimentalement on l'obtient en faisant agir l'acide nitrique sur la caséine du fromage. C'est un diazo-benzol qui possède une action semblable à la muscarine et qui résiste à des températures très élevées. Quand elle est ingérée dans l'estomac avec le lait, il provoque des sueurs, vomissements, diarrhée et amaigrissement; injecté à des jeunes animaux en quantité de 5 à 6 centigrammes, elle produit ces mêmes phénomènes ainsi que la mort.

Brieger a extrait du lait putréfié une substance qui produit des convulsions et à laquelle il a donné le nom de *spasmotoxine*.

Il convient d'ajouter que le lait de femme subit des altérations dues aux peines et autres émotions morales et de faire remarquer les qualités toxiques qui communiquent au lait de vache l'alimentation par les produits de distillation des céréales et des pommes de terre.

La seconde partie de l'étiologie des gastro-entérites comprend le groupe de causes secondaires, ou prédisposantes, c'est à dire ces facteurs qui favorisent l'infection ou qui sont les vecteurs de l'agent infectant

Contagion. Le moment de reconnaître et de déclarer le caractère contagieux et infectieux de ces affections intestinales est arrivé, surtout en ce qui concerne les enfants qui vivent en commun et du même âge, afin de lui opposer la prophylaxie convenable, de la même manière que dans la scarlatine, la rougeole, la fièvre typhoïde ou les angines. Nous voyons, tous les jours de façon pratique, que dans les familles où il y a plusieurs jeunes enfants, l'un des frères est attaqué d'une diarrhée de ce genre et peu de jours après un autre enfant est également malade et ainsi de suite les autres enfants. Holt rapporte un fait qui est démonstratif: On envoyait à une maison de campagne des enfants de la ville, malades de l'intestin, afin de pouvoir y jouir en général d'une santé complète. La femme chargée de laver leur linge de corps tomba malade et pendant qu'on lui cherchait une remplaçante les vêtements de ces jeunes enfants s'accumulèrent sérieusement, au point d'atteindre le chiffre de 200 à 500, placés dans de grandes cuves que l'on mettait dans une cour de la partie postérieure de l'édifice : dans l'espace d'un ou deux jours, avec la chaleur du mois de juillet, ces linges commencèrent à répandre une mauvaise odeur insupportable ; à peine eut-on le temps de s'en rendre compte et avant d'y avoir porté remède, que se développèrent en 56 heures deux cas de choléra infantile qui causèrent la mort de deux enfants ; l'un d'eux mourut athrepsique avec symptomes intestinaux, et apparurent des exacerbations chez plusieurs autres enfants qui souffraient de diarrhées et qui avaient commencé à se trouver mieux : le local une fois évacué et désinfecté, il ne vint se présenter aucun nouveau cas semblable. Il me serait facile de citer de nombreux cas du même genre.

Alimentation. Avec les aliments et les boissons arrivent dans le tube digestif tous les germes qui se trouvent éparpillés dans l'air, sur le sol et dans tout ce qui nous entoure ; c'est pour cela que la lactation artificielle est la source la plus abondante des infections gastro-intestinales.

Théoriquement, un enfant allaité par une mère saine et qui n'absorbe aucune boisson, c'est à dire, dont la nourriture exclusive se compose uniquement du lait du sein de sa mère, cet enfant ne doit pas avoir d'infection intestinale : même lorsque en pleine santé l'on a trouvé dans le lait récemment tiré des vaches ou de la femme quelques germes, l'investigation expérimentale a démontré que ces germes avaient gagné le conduit galactophore par l'extérieur ; après les premières extractions le liquide lacté est stérile : les épithéliums de la glande mammaire saine ne laissent pas passer dans le lait les germes du sang ; jusqu'à présent d'une manière expérimentale seulement on est parvenu à les faire traverser par la culture du bacille pyocyanique. Ceci explique la particularité que les enfants de quelques mois seulement, allaités exclusivement au sein, malgré leur susceptibilité à l'infection étant donné leur bas âge, n'en sont point atteints durant le premier été de leur vie, mais par contre sont fréquemment exposés à en être attaqués pendant le second été, quand ils font usage d'une alimentation mixte. Mais ceux de lactation maternelle exclusive sont exposés par l'effet du lait qu'on leur donne ou par celui d'autres boissons à base d'eau. J'ai eu l'occasion d'observer la diarrhée cholériforme chez un enfant de dix mois, allaité par sa mère. En général donc la lactation maternelle met les enfants à couvert de ces infections. Les statisques de Hoppe, Meinert et Ballard font voir que, parmi les enfants décédés à la suite de ces affections, trois pour cent seulement étaient alimentés par leur mère ou par une nourrice.

Quand l'enfant est sevré ou lorsque sans le sevrer on lui donne des aliments supplémentaires, le danger de l'infection existe à chaque instant, si l'on n'a pas le soin de stériliser rigoureusement l'aliment. L'impureté du lait est inévitable : par la mamelle de la vache, par les mains de la personne qui la trait, par la poussière de l'étable ; par les récipients où on le recueille, car ils sont souvent lavés avec de l'eau infectée ; par le transport, par les opérations domestiques. Il en résulte qu'il tombe dans le lait un grand nombre de germes qui se développent dans ce liquide ou ne peut plus nutritif, avec grande profusion. C'est pour tout cela qu'on s'explique qu'il y ait dans chaque centimètre cube de lait de 5 à 6 millions de bactéries. Dans l'espace de 25 heures, Miquel a pu compter 5 600 000 bactéries par centimètre cube. Quand on fait la séparation de la crème c'est cette dernière qui contient le plus grand nombre de bactéries ; dans un échantillon de lait, on a vu que pendant que la crème contenait 4 250 bactéries par centimètre cube, le sérum en contenait 56 ; dans une autre, la proportion était de 18 000 pour 175.

Malpropreté. Le manque de propreté tant pour le biberon que pour la cuiller, les linges ou serviettes, les vases etc., qui interviennent dans la préparation de l'aliment est une puissante cause d'infection intestinale ; aucune mère ne doit se mettre à préparer l'aliment sans être bien sûre de la parfaite propreté de tous ces objets ni sans s'être soigneusement lavé les mains.

Chaleur. Etant donné qu'il a été observé depuis des siècles que pendant l'été ces infections sont plus fréquentes et non seulement plus fréquentes, mais aussi plus graves, on leur a donné le nom de *diarrhées estivales.* La chaleur atmosphérique qui favorise la pullulation des germes partout, et qui fomente les fermentations est une des causes les plus puissantes. En examinant les causes de mortalité diarrhéique indiquées par Borobio de Saragosse, par Seibert, Baginsky et Meinert, on remarque qu'elles ont une certaine relation avec les courbes thermiques et que de même que celles-ci elles subissent une descente en hiver et une grande élévation en été, surtout en juillet et août.

La chaleur intervient dans la production des gastro-entérites, dans la transformation épidémique de celles-ci, et dans la mortalité infantile ; mais cette relation n'est ni constante ni absolue ; car des villes ou villages jouissants de températures moyennes égales, offrent une mortalité très forte, si on n'y pratique pas l'allaitement naturel et, d'autre part, ce ne sont pas les très jeunes enfants plus fragiles et plus sensibles qui souffrent le plus des mauvais effets de la chaleur, mais bien les enfants compris entre six et dix-huit mois, époque à laquelle ont lieu les essais ou l'établissement de l'alimentation artificielle.

Eaux souterraines et du sous-sol. Les eaux souterraines exercent peu d'influence sur l'invasion des gastro-entérites des nourrissons : par contre celles du sous-sol ont une certaine influence ; c'est du moins ce que dit Ballard de Leicester. Les maisons bâties sur le roc ferme présentent une mortalité de peu d'importance ou presque insignifiante, malgré que les autres conditions hygiéniques soient défavorables ; mais c'est le contraire qui arrive avec les sols poreux perméables à l'eau et l'air où la mortalité a considérablement augmenté, pour ne pas dire démesurément.

Vent. Dans les villes modernes avec leurs rues larges et droites, ni la direction ni la vitesse du vent ne paraissent avoir aucune influence sur la morbidité et la mortalité : dans tous les cas cette influence serait très légère : par contre dans les anciennes villes avec leurs carrefours et leurs rues étroites on observe que la direction du vent est indifférente ; mais son intensité influe beaucoup sur la morbidité gastro-intestinale et sur la mortalité ; une température modérée sans vent est accompagnée de beaucoup plus d'invasions que lorsque la chaleur est élevée et le vent très fort. Les cas les plus nombreux et les plus graves sont ceux qui se développent pendant les jours de grande chaleur et de grand calme atmosphérique.

Conditions urbaines et sociales. Les villes ou faubourgs populeux accroissent la morbidité avec leurs quartiers compacts de rues étroites sans être pavées et sur la surface desquelles coulent des ruisseaux d'eau noirâtre provenant des maisons, où l'on mêle des détritus de de végétaux avec des dépouilles d'animaux et où viennent satisfaire leur voracité des légions de mouches ; le danger est moins grand par la densité de la population que par le manque de drainage des eaux et de bonne ventilation.

Dentition. Pendant plusieurs siècles, on a cru que la dentition avait une influence pathogénique puissante sur les affections gastro-intestinales et diverses autres affections ; plus encore. car on était arrivé à croire qu'en été il convenait de respecter ces diarrhées à déjections visqueuses. afin d'éviter de sérieuses complications. Il n'existe point une telle influence morbide de la dentition ; la physiologie et la pathologie nient son existence et nient également deux faits d'observation journalière ; savoir : que ces *diarrhées de dentition* n'apparaissent pas en hiver. la dentition fut-elle très en retard et qu'en été un enfant avec de la diarrhée et les dents avec éruption, guérit de cette diarrhée du moment qu'on le transporte soit au bord d'une plage, soit à un endroit frais et même si le nombre de ses dents va en augmentant ou qu'il s'en annonce de nouvelles dans ses gencives. A combien d'enfants on aurait pu éviter la mort, si l'on n'avait pas jugé de façon erronée cette diarrhée et si on l'avait combattue dès le commencement de la maladie!

Pathogénie. Les divers microbes que j'ai énumérés antérieurement vivent dans le tube gastro-intestinal, et s'ils ne produisent pas la maladie d'une manière constante, c'est par suite de l'ensemble des *défenses* que l'organisme oppose à chaque instant et qui lui permettent de triompher de ces agents : cette protection dépend de la digestion normale, de l'intégrité des épithéliums, des sucs gastro-intestinaux, des organes lymphoïdes, du foie et du sang.

Une digestion normale évite une longue permanence des résidus alimentaires dans l'intestin : l'enfant allaité par sa mère ou par une nourrice a dans son estomac de l'acide chlorhydrique et consomme une caséine qui est complètement modifiée dans l'estomac et absorbée sans difficulté ; cette absorption rapide favorise l'antisepsie intestinale ; au contraire, l'enfant allaité avec du lait de vache ou avec des aliments mixtes ne possède pas autant d'acide chlorhydrique libre ; la caséine n'est pas transformée dans l'estomac, mais elle a besoin du concours de la trypsine du contenu intestinal ; laissant presque toujours un résidu indigestible qui est la paranucléine ; c'est pour cela, que pendant que la caséine reste dans l'intestin sans avoir été digérée, elle constitue un danger pour la santé, car elle offre un aliment aux microbes intestinaux et donne les éléments pour la putréfaction : ceci explique les différents caractères physiques des déjections procédant d'enfants allaités par la femme ou alimentés avec du lait de vache.

L'épithélium manifeste son activité protectrice en deshydratant les peptones et transformant les graisses quand une fois dedoublées elles le traversent, et il s'oppose à l'implantation de colonies microbiennes.

Même lorsqu'on a vu que les microbes peuvent traverser les épithéliums normaux, aussi facilement que les substances minérales, dans ces conditions ils ne conservent pas suffisamment de puissance pour engendrer une maladie. L'acide chlorhydrique du suc gastrique, la bile spécialement si elle agit dans un milieu acide, sont de puissantes défenses ; le manque d'oxygène dans l'intestin rend en outre difficile la vie des aérobies et même en supposant que les microbes ou leurs toxines aient vaincu ces premières difficultés, il reste encore d'autres moyens de protection organique : contre les toxines se trouve le foie qui a un pouvoir colossal pour les retenir ou les transformer.

comme cela est démontré par la fistule de Eck : et contre les microbes se trouvent les organes lymphoïdes qui permettent la phagocytose. En dernier lieu le sang reste avec son pouvoir bactéricide, par le sérum, par sa pression, par sa mobilité et par les leucocytes. Il faut ajouter à tout ceci les émonctoires : rénal, intestinal et cutané. C'est pour ces motifs que les microbes intestinaux traversent le tube digestif ou y vivent sans produire habituellement aucun trouble morbide.

Maintenant, quand la perturbation digestive empêche la transformation physiologique de la lactose, de la caséine ou de la graisse et qu'il s'opère une absorption insuffisante, il reste des produits qui servent de pâture, de moyens de culture pour les microbes et ces dernières se reproduisent prodigieusement ; quand un aliment impur introduit d'un seul coup dans le tube digestif un grand nombre de microbes, et quand en plus de ces derniers la substance alimentaire contient quelques principes chimiques comme le *tyrotoxicon* il s'établit une lutte entre ces agents et les défenses organiques. Les acides depuis le lactique jusqu'au propionique et valérique développent une action irritante sur les épithéliums et de cela nous avons la meilleure preuve dans l'érythème qui se forme à la marge de l'anus et aux fesses, du moment où ces déjections anormales se mettent en contact avec la peau : après l'inflammation apparaît le trouble de l'épithélium, sa dégénération, sa chute ; l'hypérémie intestinale conséquente fournit l'oxygène qui alimente les microbes aérobies : si en plus de la lactose vient à se décomposer la caséine, les produits de la putréfaction apparaissent ; et si, enfin, quelque germe pathogène agit, comme le staphylococcus ou le streptococcus, il se produit une toxi-albumine. La muqueuse intestinale dépourvue plus ou moins de l'épithélium est propre à une absorption facile des substances volatiles et fixes de l'intestin ; les microbes l'envahissent et la traversent avec facilité et si le foie n'est capable de détruire ou d'emmagasiner tous les principes chimiques anormaux et si les phagocytes ne fixent pas les microbes, ceux-ci, de même que les produits de la fermentation et de la putréfaction intestinales, arrivent jusqu'au sang, s'y implantent et circulent dans tout l'organisme. Alors les microbes et leurs poisons donnent naissance à des manifestations morbides de deux genres : les unes primitives d'un caractère plus ou moins transitoire, passagères, avec légère lésion, d'évolution rapide comme tout empoisonnement ; savoir : les vomissements, la fièvre, la lourdeur de tête, l'assoupissement, le soubresaut des tendons, les convulsions, la diarrhée abondante, ou la constipation, paralysie vaso-motrice, l'insuffisance rénale, les toxidermies ; d'autres plus lentes à se produire mais plus stables, d'évolution lente, avec lésions viscérales plus ou moins accentuées ; en un mot, les infections consécutives : les pneumonies, les méningites, les méningo-encéphalites, les néphrites et la furunculose, etc.

Si les énergies organiques aidées par une puissante élimination intestinale, rénale ou cutanée, ne résistent pas à l'œuvre de destruction de ces poisons, l'organisme est appelé à succomber tôt ou tard.

Un mot sur la classification : les troubles gastro-intestinaux aigus des enfants à la mamelle, pourraient se diviser d'après cette base étiologique et pathogénique en :

1º Indigestion ;

2º Infection gastro-intestinale (symptômes locaux et fièvre avec légère diarrhée) ;

3º Infection gastro-intestinale toxique (symptômes d'empoisonnement, forte diarrhée, convulsions, diarrhée cholériforme) ;

4º Infection gastro-intestinale toxique et compliquée (phénomènes locaux, empoisonnement du sang et des viscères, néphrite, pneumonie, méningo-encéphalite, etc.).

L'ÉTIOLOGIE ET LA PATHOGÉNIE DU CHOLÉRA INFANTILE

RAPPORT

par M. le docteur A.-B. MARFAN,

Agrégé, médecin des hôpitaux.

Ayant été chargé de présenter un rapport sur l'étiologie et la pathogénie des gastro-entérites des nourrissons, j'ai eu d'abord l'intention d'exposer l'ensemble du sujet à un point de vue critique et synthétique. Mais je me suis aperçu que je dépasserais ainsi les limites qui me sont assignées, ce que je désire éviter, car, en ma qualité de secrétaire, je sais combien vos séances vont être remplies et combien vos instants sont précieux. J'ai donc résolu de me cantonner dans l'étude de la mieux caractérisée parmi les formes de troubles digestifs du nourrisson : *le choléra infantile*. Même en resserrant la question dans ces limites, elle est encore assez vaste et permet d'envisager par un grand nombre de faces le problème de l'étiologie des gastro-entérites[1].

1. Le travail d'ensemble dont je voulais d'abord faire mon rapport au Congrès a été écrit ; mais il était beaucoup plus long que ne le comportait le règlement. Il a été publié en brochure sous le titre : *Les Gastro-entérites des nourrissons* (étiologie, pathogénie, prophylaxie). Paris. Masson. 1900.

Je définis le choléra infantile : une maladie des nourrissons (c'est-à-dire des sujets âgés de moins de deux ans), ayant son maximum de fréquence pendant l'été, caractérisée par un catarrhe gastro-intestinal suraigu accompagné de phénomènes généraux graves qui rappellent ceux du choléra asiatique.

Un tableau clinique sommaire me permettra de mieux préciser : un enfant âgé de moins de deux ans, ordinairement nourri au biberon, sujet à des troubles dyspeptiques, est pris brusquement de vomissements et de diarrhée. Quelques heures après (deux jours au plus tard) apparaissent des phénomènes généraux graves, témoignant d'une intoxication profonde : les principaux sont l'algidité périphérique, la cyanose et le collapsus : leur durée est courte : elle peut être de quelques heures; elle ne dépasse pas trois jours. Ce syndrome toxique se termine par la mort, ou par la guérison. ou par la substitution aux phénomènes cholériformes de symptômes révélant l'existence d'une complication secondaire : colite folliculaire, broncho - pneumonie, méningite, néphrite, phlegmon et gangrène de la peau, etc.

Quand la mort survient pendant la phase cholérique, la recherche des bactéries dans les humeurs, tissus ou organes des cadavres frais donne très souvent des résultats négatifs ; il est assez rare qu'on y puisse découvrir des microbes. Au contraire, quand la mort survient plus tard, dans la période de réaction et de complications secondaires, les recherches bactériologiques, pratiquées sur des cadavres frais, démontrent presque toujours la présence de microbes auxquels il est permis d'attribuer les accidents consécutifs : le plus souvent on trouve le bacterium coli et le streptocoque, isolés ou associés; plus rarement on rencontre le staphylocoque et le pneumocoque.

Ces résultats, rapprochés des caractères cliniques et anatomiques, conduisent à séparer et à opposer les deux phases de la maladie : la première, cholériforme. est une phase toxique; la seconde, dite de réaction typhoïde ou de complications secondaires, est une phase infectieuse. et les infections qui la constituent étant dues à des microbes qui habitent normalement l'organisme, il y a lieu de penser qu'elles sont d'origine endogène.

La première phase semble due à l'imprégnation de l'organisme par un poison venu de l'intestin. Si l'organisme résiste à cette intoxication, la guérison n'est pas assurée pour cela; à la faveur des altérations créées par le poison, des infections endogènes peuvent se développer en divers points, se combiner, donner naissance à des septicémies. à des complications métastatiques qui peuvent emporter le malade.

L'étiologie et la pathogénie doivent donc se proposer de déterminer l'origine, et, s'il se peut, la nature du poison générateur de la maladie.

C'est dans les deux premières années de la vie que s'observe le choléra infantile. Durant cette période la courbe de morbidité et de mortalité présente deux maxima : le premier occupe les trois ou quatre premiers mois : le second se place vers le douzième mois. Pour expliquer le premier, on peut invoquer la faible résistance que le très jeune enfant oppose à l'intoxication ; pour le second, le sevrage que beaucoup de mères pratiquent vers la fin de la première année.

En tout cas, il est certain que le choléra infantile se produit souvent au moment où l'enfant, jusque-là exclusivement élevé au sein, reçoit pour la première fois un aliment autre que le lait maternel.

Le choléra infantile est beaucoup plus fréquent dans la classe pauvre que dans la classe riche, ce qu'explique facilement l'ensemble de toutes les conditions étiologiques.

Des troubles digestifs antérieurs constituent une puissante prédisposition au choléra infantile. Quand on dit que le début de cette maladie est brusque, presque foudroyant, on ne veut pas dire par là que l'enfant est toujours surpris par la maladie en pleine santé. Contrairement à Trousseau, j'ai vu les accidents graves du choléra infantile éclater habituellement chez les nourrissons déjà atteints de troubles digestifs ; parfois, ils apparaissent chez des enfants qui ont de la dyspepsie chronique, ailleurs, ils sont précédés d'accidents de de catarrhe simple. Dans le dernier de ces cas, on peut supposer qu'il s'agit de troubles prodromiques. Mais dans les autres il semble bien que les troubles digestifs antérieurs ont favorisé l'action des poisons cholérigènes. Quoi qu'il en soit, il n'est pas rare de voir une dyspepsie chronique se terminer brusquement par une attaque de choléra infantile.

Mais l'étiologie du choléra infantile est dominée par deux grands faits : 1° cette maladie atteint presque exclusivement les nourrissons soumis à l'allaitement artificiel : 2° elle est infiniment plus fréquente pendant le temps des fortes chaleurs qu'aux autres époques de l'année.

Pour ma part, je n'ai jamais observé un véritable cas de choléra infantile chez un enfant exclusivement nourri au sein. Je ne nie pas l'existence de la maladie chez un nourrisson qui ne reçoit que le lait de sa mère ou de sa nourrice. Mais l'extraordinaire rareté des faits de ce genre permet de n'en pas tenir compte pour la pathogénie[1].

1. Les cas de cet ordre qui ont été rapportés manquent souvent de détails cliniques suffisants pour qu'on puisse se faire une opinion à leur sujet.

Le choléra infantile atteint presque toujours des nourrissons allaités au biberon, et le nom que les médecins américains lui ont donné : *Feeding bottles disease*, est, à ce point de vue, caractéristique. Les auteurs qui se livrent à l'étude des statistiques disent que, chez les enfants nourris au sein, la maladie s'observe dans la proportion de 2 pour 100. Mais il n'y a pas de statistique qui nous apprenne si ces enfants nourris au sein ne recevaient pas, en même temps que le lait maternel, un autre aliment. Or, là est la question. Je répète encore que, pour ma part, je n'ai pas observé un véritable cas de choléra infantile chez un enfant exclusivement nourri au sein.

Le choléra infantile est surtout une maladie d'été (*Summer's disease*). On peut le rencontrer durant toute l'année. Mais pendant l'automne, l'hiver et le printemps, les cas sont rares, isolés, sporadiques. Dès que la période des fortes chaleurs arrive, la maladie devient fréquente, meurtrière, et revêt la forme épidémique. Elle sévit surtout après huit ou dix jours de chaleur persistante : le nombre des cas diminue quand la pluie vient rafraîchir l'atmosphère.

Maladie des enfants au biberon, maladie d'été : telles sont les deux grandes notions de l'étiologie du choléra infantile.

Quant à la pathogénie, toute l'histoire clinique, anatomique et même bactériologique du choléra infantile fait présumer que cette maladie est liée à une intoxication dont la source se trouve dans le tube digestif. Sur cette conception générale, presque tous les auteurs sont d'accord. Mais ce poison cholérigène, quel est-il? Se forme-t-il dans le tube digestif ou y est-il apporté du dehors? Comment agit-il?

A ces questions, malgré des recherches nombreuses et intéressantes il n'est pas possible, à l'heure présente, de fournir une réponse ferme. Il y a là-dessus trois opinions. Nous allons les examiner et rechercher dans quelle mesure elles sont d'accord avec les données étiologiques fournies par l'observation.

Les uns pensent que ce poison prend naissance dans le tube digestif lui-même, sous l'influence des modifications que les fortes chaleurs lui font subir : c'est la théorie de l'*intoxication endogène*.

D'autres avancent que le poison est élaboré dans le tractus gastro-intestinal, mais par un microbe qui vient du dehors : c'est la théorie de l'*infection ectogène*.

D'autres enfin avancent que ce poison se produit dans le lait avant son ingestion, sous l'influence des hautes températures : *intoxication ectogène*. Examinons les arguments fournis en faveur de chacune de ces théories.

Intoxication endogène. — L'influence des hautes températures atmosphériques sur le tube digestif est incontestable; la pathologie des pays chauds en démontre la réalité. La chaleur diminue ou modifie les sécrétions digestives et hépatiques; elle augmente la soif et provoque l'ingestion, en quantité plus ou moins considérable, de liquides divers qui peuvent être la cause de troubles dyspeptiques. On peut donc supposer que ces conditions favorisent la production d'une toxi-infection endogène du tube digestif. Après avoir soutenu que le choléra infantile résulte d'une infection ectogène, M. Lesage, ayant ensuite vérifié un fait que j'ai avancé le premier, à savoir que des enfants nourris de lait stérilisé sont susceptibles de contracter la maladie, M. Lesage en est arrivé à penser qu'elle est la conséquence d'une toxi-infection endogène, prenant naissance dans le tube digestif modifié par les fortes chaleurs.

Il ne me paraît pas douteux que ces modifications préalables constituent une prédisposition au choléra infantile; il me paraît probable qu'elles expliquent, à elles seules, la plus grande fréquence, pendant l'été, des troubles digestifs vulgaires qui s'observent chez tous les nourrissons, aussi bien chez ceux qui sont nourris au sein que chez les autres. Mais il me paraît impossible de considérer ces modifications comme la cause efficiente du choléra infantile. Si elles étaient suffisantes pour engendrer la maladie à elles seules, on devrait observer le choléra infantile à peu près aussi fréquemment chez l'enfant nourri au sein que chez l'enfant nourri au biberon. Or, je le répète, chez le nourrisson qui ne reçoit pas d'autre aliment que le lait de sa mère ou de sa nourrice, le choléra infantile véritable est exceptionnel; pour ma part, je n'en ai pas vu d'exemple. La théorie de l'infection ou de l'intoxication endogène me semble donc devoir être rejetée.

Infection ectogène. — Divers microbes ont été accusés de produire par infection ectogène le choléra infantile : le bacterium coli commune ou une de ses variétés, le streptocoque et l'entérocoque, certaines bactéries protéolytiques, enfin le proteus vulgaris. Pour aucune de ces espèces, la preuve n'a pu être faite.

Les ferments lactiques qui se trouvent constamment dans le lait de vache appartiennent à la famille du bacterium coli. On a supposé que, dans certaines circonstances, le lait non stérilisé avait introduit dans le tube digestif un bacterium coli, devenu accidentellement virulent et cholérigène. On a supposé encore que, dans les crèches et les hôpitaux, le bacterium coli virulent qui se trouve dans les selles de la plupart des nourrissons diarrhéiques, pouvait se transmettre à des enfants sains par les mains des infirmières, des tétines, des biberons, etc., devenir ainsi l'agent d'une véritable contagion et provoquer de la gastro-entérite. Mais, s'il est démontré que le bacterium coli, hôte de l'intestin normal, est fréquemment un agent d'infection secondaire endogène. il est encore douteux qu'il puisse être un agent d'infection ectogène, particulièrement en ce qui concerne le choléra infantile[1]. On peut en dire tout autant de l'entérocoque de Thiercelin.

Il paraît bien prouvé qu'il existe des gastro-entérites dues à une infection ectogène par le streptocoque ; mais il est à peu près sûr que le véritable choléra infantile n'a pas de rapports avec ces formes à streptocoques.

Le lait de vache renferme presque toujours des microbes qui attaquent surtout la caséine, que M. Duclaux appelle *ferments de la caséine* et Flügge *bactéries protéolytiques*. Ces microbes appartiennent aux espèces, assez voisines les unes des autres, du *Bacillus subtilis*, du *Bacillus mesentericus vulgaris*, du *Tyrothrix tenuis*. Ces espèces ont comme propriété particulière de donner naissance à des spores qui résistent à des températures supérieures à 100 degrés et qui, par suite, subsistent dans le lait qui n'a subi qu'une stérilisation incomplète (ébullition, pasteurisation, chauffage au bain-marie à 100 degré). Comme on a pu observer le choléra infantile, ainsi que je le dirai dans un instant, chez des enfants nourris avec du lait stérilisé incomplètement. Flügge et Lübbert en ont conclu que, très probablement, les microbes du choléra infantile appartenaient aux bactéries protéolytiques; ils ont appuyé leurs conclusions sur des recherches expérimentales ; mais ils n'en ont jamais donné une preuve clinique. Il est vrai que M. Lesage a pu accuser, dans quelques cas très rares, le B. mesentericus et le Tyrothrix tenuis d'être les agents de gastro-entérites graves. Mais, depuis, le rôle des bactéries protéolytiques dans les gastro-entérites n'a pu être mis en évidence (Spiegelberg). Or, ces microbes se cultivent facilement et, par suite, il est probable qu'ils n'auraient pas échappé aux observateurs si vraiment ils étaient des agents de gastro-entérite grave.

D'après W. Booker, parmi les diarrhées des nourrissons, celles qui revêtent le type cholériforme seraient dues le plus souvent au *proteus vulgaris*. Le proteus que Booker a isolé dans les diarrhées d'été coagule le lait à la manière de la présure, décompose ensuite la caséine et les matières protéiques en donnant naissance à des produits très

---

1. Pour la discussion détaillée de tous ces points, je renvoie aux deux mémoires que j'ai publiés là-dessus : 1° Rôle des microbes dans les gastro-entérites des nourrissons : *Revue mensuelle des maladies de l'enfance*, 1899; 2° Étiologie, pathogénie et prophylaxie des gastro-entérites des nourrissons (Paris. Masson. 1900).

toxiques. Vaughan a cultivé le proteus de Booker sur la viande stérilisée ; il a constaté qu'il produisait une substance albuminoïde qui n'avait pas les caractères des peptones et qui, injectée dans les veines des chiens et des chats, provoque rapidement la mort de ces animaux. De son côté, Baginski a trouvé dans les selles cholériques, associée au Bacterium coli et au Bacterium lactis, une « bactérie blanche liquéfiante » qui n'est autre qu'une variété de proteus ; ce microbe coagule le lait, puis dissout le coagulum. Il est un agent énergique de destruction putride des albuminoïdes. Avec Stadthagen, Baginski l'a cultivé aussi sur de la viande de cheval ; il a isolé de la culture un corps probablement identique à un de ceux que Brieger a retirés de la viande de cheval en putréfaction. Une solution aqueuse de ce corps ressemblait à une solution de peptone ; inoculée sous la peau d'une souris, elle amena la mort de l'animal en deux ou trois jours ; l'autopsie montra de l'hyperémie généralisée, mais surtout marquée au niveau de l'intestin grêle. Cette bactérie, cultivée dans le lait, donne également un produit semblable à une peptone. Ajoutons que Tito Carbone a isolé plusieurs ptomaïnes de la culture du proteus vulgaris sur bouillie de viande (choline, éthylène diamine, gadinine, triméthylamine). Le caractère habituellement pathogène du proteus, sa propriété d'engendrer des produits très toxiques, donnent une certaine valeur aux assertions de W. Booker. Mais on n'est nullement autorisé à considérer ce microbe comme l'agent pathogène ordinaire du choléra infantile. En premier lieu, le proteus n'a presque jamais été retrouvé dans le lait ; par contre, il peut se rencontrer accidentellement dans les matières fécales du nourrisson en bonne santé. En outre, une grande obscurité règne sur le groupe du proteus qui renferme probablement des espèces diverses (les unes prenant le Gram, d'autres non ; les unes liquéfiant la gélatine, d'autres non). En somme on peut conclure que rien n'est encore démontré en ce qui concerne le rôle du proteus dans la genèse du choléra infantile.

Malgré l'insuffisance des preuves fournies jusqu'ici, certains auteurs continuent à admettre que divers microbes d'infection banale deviennent capables d'engendrer le choléra infantile lorsque sous l'influence des chaleurs de l'été, ils ont pullulé dans le lait et acquis peut-être une virulence spéciale. Il est certain que le tableau clinique de la maladie est assez variable et il est possible qu'on arrive un jour à établir des variétés ayant chacune leur caractéristique clinique et bactériologique. Mais, à l'heure présente, une pareille hypothèse ne s'appuie sur aucun fait. On a supposé encore que l'action cholérigène dépend de la symbiose de plusieurs microbes communs, symbiose qui se réaliserait plus facilement pendant les chaleurs de l'été. Les recherches de M. Metschnikoff sur le choléra asiatique permettent de poser la question : mais rien n'autorise encore à appliquer cette notion au choléra infantile.

Faut-il admettre enfin qu'il n'y a qu'un seul microbe pathogène du choléra infantile, mais que ce microbe est encore inconnu? Pour répondre affirmativement, on ne pourrait guère se fonder que sur la notion de contagiosité de la maladie ; or, cette notion n'est nullement prouvée ; les médecins d'enfants, si préparés à l'accepter, sont à peu près unanimes pour la repousser. Le choléra infantile est, pendant l'été, une maladie épidémique, mais non habituellement contagieuse ; un cas de choléra infantile ne provient pas en général d'un autre cas semblable. Ce que nous savons de l'étiologie de la fièvre typhoïde ne permet évidemment pas de considérer ce dernier fait comme un argument défavorable à la théorie de l'infection ectogène ; cependant, il plaide plutôt en faveur de celle de l'intoxication ectogène.

Intoxication ectogène. — C'est la théorie qui me paraît le plus vraisemblable, celle qui s'adapte le mieux aux faits cliniques et étiologiques. On peut la formuler comme il suit. Au moment de la traite, le lait animal, quelle que soit sa provenance, est toujours souillé par des microbes. Lorsqu'on l'abandonne ensuite à lui-même, les germes qu'il renferme se développent et altèrent sa composition. Pendant les fortes chaleurs, les fermentations s'opèrent avec une extrême activité et une très grande rapidité. Le poison du choléra infantile se forme dans le lait du fait de ces fermentations estivales ; il est produit soit par les microbes habituels du lait qui, sous l'influence des hautes températures, acquièrent une vitalité et des propriétés particulières, soit par des bactéries spéciales qui ne se développent que dans des conditions créées par l'été.

Je dois dire que nous ignorons la nature de ce poison. Est-il soluble dans l'alcool, comme le suppose Baginski, ou dans l'eau, comme l'avancent Roger et son élève Robert? Est-il identique au tyrotoxicon de Vaughan? Nous ne le savons pas. Tout ce qu'on peut supposer, c'est qu'il se développe aux dépens de la caséine, car, dans un travail récent, Vaughan et Clymonds[1] ont montré que, pendant l'été, les fromages putréfiés déterminent souvent chez l'homme de la gastro-entérite cholériforme, et que lorsqu'on inocule ces fromages aux animaux, ceux-ci succombent ordinairement avec des accidents analogues.

1. V. Vaughan et J.-T. Mac Clymonds. Some bacteriological poisons in milk and milk products. *Festchrift di Jacobi.* New-York, 1900, p. 108.

Mais j'ai été conduit à me rallier à la théorie de l'intoxication ectogène par deux ordres de faits : 1° la possibilité de voir apparaître le choléra infantile chez des nourrissons alimentés avec du lait stérilisé ; 2° les examens histo-bactériologiques de la muqueuse intestinale.

1° Je ne relaterai pas de nouveau les faits de choléra infantile que j'ai observés chez des nourrissons qui ne recevaient que du lait stérilisé ; on les trouvera dans mes publications antérieures[2]. Comment peut-on les interpréter ? D'abord par la théorie de l'intoxication endogène ; mais je viens de montrer qu'elle était incapable d'expliquer la genèse du choléra infantile. Ensuite, on peut supposer que le lait était stérilisé incomplètement. Le plus souvent, en effet, dans les cas auxquels je fais allusion, les enfants avaient été alimentés avec du lait traité par l'appareil de Soxhlet, traitement qui laisse subsister les spores des bactéries protéolytiques. Mais il n'est pas sûr que celles-ci soient nuisibles et, en tout cas, il est à peu près prouvé qu'elles ne sont pas la cause du choléra infantile. D'autre part, le lait stérilisé, ingéré par les enfants qui furent ensuite atteints de choléra infantile, avait été consommé moins de vingt-quatre heures après un chauffage prolongé ; il est difficile d'admettre que les microbes ou les spores qu'il renfermait n'avaient pas été notablement atténués par la chaleur et avaient gardé leur virulence.

Dans les faits que j'ai observés, ce qui m'a frappé, c'est que le lait avait été stérilisé longtemps après la traite (treize à seize heures). C'est ce qui m'a conduit à l'interprétation suivante. Lorsque, entre le moment de la traite et celui de la stérilisation, l'intervalle est trop grand, les microbes du lait pullulent, *surtout pendant l'été*, et peuvent parfois élaborer des toxines que la chaleur ne détruit pas, et qui sont peut-être la cause du choléra infantile. Durant l'hiver, la fermentation marchant beaucoup moins rapidement que pendant l'été, il est probable que le lait stérilisé tardivement est beaucoup moins nuisible et n'est pas la cause d'accidents aigus graves.

Jusqu'ici, mon hypothèse n'a pas reçu une démonstration expérimentale. M. Lesage a essayé de la vérifier sans réussir. Mais je remarquerai que des expériences destinées à prouver la toxicité du lait stérilisé trop tard doivent être multiples et variées ; qu'on doit les exécuter en diverses saisons, en divers lieux, dans des conditions très différentes. Celles que j'ai faites sont encore trop peu nombreuses et trop uniformes pour que je veuille en tirer une conclusion. Cependant j'en dirai un mot, puisque la question est soulevée. J'ai donc fait traire

1. *Traité de l'allaitement.* Paris, 1899, p. 105 et suivantes. — *Les gastro-entérites des nourrissons* étiologie, pathogénie, prophylaxie. Paris, 1900.

du lait dans une vacherie d'Issy, et le lait a été recueilli dans de grands ballons stérilisés. Ceux-ci étant bouchés à la ouate, le lait a été abandonné à lui-même, à la température ambiante (juin 1898), pendant un temps variable (douze, vingt-quatre, quarante-huit heures); au bout de ce temps, il était stérilisé à 115 degrés pendant deux minutes. On l'injectait ensuite dans le péritoine de cobayes. Dans le plus grand nombre de cas, ce lait ne s'est pas montré toxique; mais avec un lait stérilisé après quarante-huit heures, l'injection était suivie de mort. Cela prouve tout au moins que, dans certaines conditions, il peut se produire dans le lait des toxines que la chaleur ne détruit pas. Quant à l'objection tirée de ce que c'est une propriété générale des toxines microbiennes d'être détruites par la chaleur, je répondrai qu'il y a des exceptions à cette loi ; il me suffira de citer certaines toxines de la tuberculose, qui sont contenues dans la première lymphe de Koch.

Des faits qui viennent d'être exposés et discutés, j'ai déduit les préceptes suivants en ce qui concerne le choix d'un procédé de stérilisation ; ces préceptes contiennent pour moi la principale règle prophylactique pour défendre les nourrissons contre le choléra infantile.

« Êtes-vous dans le voisinage d'une source de lait qui vous offre toutes les garanties désirables, et pouvez-vous soumettre le liquide à l'action de la chaleur quelques instants après la traite ? Usez alors de la méthode de Soxhlet, ou employez l'ébullition, qui est presque aussi bonne, si vous assurez la parfaite propreté des vases, des biberons et des tétines ; dans les deux cas, que le lait soit consommé dans les vingt-quatre heures.

« Mais êtes-vous éloigné de la source du lait et ne pouvez-vous soumettre le liquide à l'action de la chaleur que plusieurs heures après la traite, repoussez la méthode de Soxhlet, repoussez l'ébullition. Alors, la seule ressource possible, c'est le lait stérilisé dans l'industrie. Ce lait, soumis au surchauffage aussitôt après la traite, se conserve bien pendant plusieurs jours. »

2° Nous avons recherché, avec M. Léon Bernard, la présence des microbes dans la muqueuse intestinale des nourrissons atteints de gastro-entérites. Les résultats que nous avons obtenus ont été les mêmes pour toutes les formes de gastro-entérites que nous avons pu étudier ; ils s'appliquent, en particulier, au choléra infantile. Dans les unes comme dans les autres, la présence des microbes est fréquente, mais non constante. Les microbes qui envahissent l'intestin appartiennent presque toujours à deux espèces : 1° des bâtonnets longs, moyens ou courts, se décolorant en général par le Gram, et représentant sans doute le plus souvent des variétés de colibacilles ; 2° des coques, le plus souvent en diplocoques, très rarement en streptocoques, qui résistent, en général, à la décoloration par l'iode et qui paraissent appartenir à un parasite normal de l'intestin (*diplococcus intestinalis* de Tavel, *entérocoque* de Thiercelin). D'autre part, les lésions habituelles des gastro-entérites communes des nourrissons — transformation mucoïde de l'épithélium des glandes tubulées, infiltration de l'espace interglandulaire, inflammation des follicules solitaires — ne semblent pas en rapport avec la présence des microbes. En effet, on voit souvent des glandes qui ont subi la transformation mucoïde complète, des espaces interglandulaires très agrandis et très infiltrés, des follicules lymphoïdes très gonflés et parfois ulcérés, sans qu'on y puisse constater la présence des bactéries. Mais il se pourrait que certaines lésions plus rares soient la conséquence de la présence des microbes; car, si nous ne les avons pas trouvées partout où il y a des microbes, nous ne les avons constatées que là où ceux-ci se rencontrent. Ces résultats nous ont conduit à penser que dans la plupart des gastro-entérites des nourrissons, et particulièrement dans le choléra infantile, les lésions ordinaires de la muqueuse digestive sont probablement dues à l'action de substances chimiques toxiques ou irritantes, quelle qu'en soit d'ailleurs l'origine. Quand ces agents ont altéré la muqueuse, à la faveur de ces altérations certains microbes du contenu gastro-intestinal peuvent envahir la paroi digestive. *Cet envahissement est un fait pathologique, mais c'est un fait secondaire, non pas un fait primitif; c'est un phénomène « conséquence », non pas un phénomène « cause ».* Ce phénomène « conséquence » pourra devenir cause à son tour, créer des lésions nouvelles de la paroi gastro-intestinale et devenir le point de départ d'une septicémie secondaire. En somme, les choses se passeraient comme dans l'empoisonnement par l'arsenic ou le tartre stibié ; seul le poison générateur est différent [1].

Dans le choléra infantile, ce poison paraît se former dans le lait, sous l'influence des fermentations et putréfactions qui commencent aussitôt après la traite *et qui, pendant l'été, sont particulièrement actives et rapides*. Il est probable que ce poison n'est pas détruit par la stérilisation et que celle-ci ne sera vraiment bienfaisante que si elle est effectuée presque aussitôt après la traite (deux ou trois heures au plus tard, pendant les fortes chaleurs) [2].

1. Marfan et L. Bernard. Sur la présence des microbes dans la muqueuse intestinale des nourrissons atteints de gastro-entérite. *Presse médicale*, 15 novembre 1899, n° 91, p. 289.

2. Dans cet exposé étiologique, j'ai considéré surtout le lait en tant qu'agent cholérigène. Il y aurait lieu de se demander si, pour les nourrissons qui appro-

B) Discussion à propos des rapports sur les infections et les intoxications gastro-intestinales dans la première enfance.

M. Marfan. — La classification proposée par M. Escherich est très rationnelle au point de vue théorique. Mais dans quelle mesure est-elle applicable dans la pratique? Il me semble qu'au point de vue clinique, de même qu'au point de vue bactériologique et anatomique, il sera bien difficile de tracer la limite entre une infection pariétale et une infection du contenu de l'intestin (Chymus Infection de M. Escherich). Il est d'ailleurs fort probable qu'une infection du contenu peut aboutir et aboutit fréquemment à une infection pariétale; le microbe qui a pullulé dans le chyme finira par envahir la paroi.

Pour ma part, je suis porté à employer le terme gastro-entérite pour désigner l'ensemble des troubles digestifs du nourrisson, parce que ce terme ne préjuge en rien la nature réelle de ces troubles et qu'il a le grand avantage de ne pas impliquer de théorie.

J'y ferais même rentrer les troubles qu'on a coutume de ranger sous la rubrique de « troubles dyspeptiques » parce qu'il est difficile de tracer la limite entre le catarrhe et la dyspepsie. Il est probable que ces troubles dyspeptiques ont un substratum anatomique, une lésion légère, superficielle, de l'épithélium et des glandes, comme toute albuminurie, si légère et si passagère soit-elle, correspond à une altération des glomérules. Je me croirais donc autorisé à désigner sous le nom de gastro-entérite l'ensemble des troubles digestifs non spécifiques des nourrissons (je dis non spécifiques pour écarter la fièvre typhoïde, la dysenterie vraie, le choléra asiatique, la tuberculose et la syphilis intestinales). Ceci dit, voici la classification que j'adopterais pour la clinique; elle est assez analogue à celle de M. Baginski.

Formes anatomo cliniques des gastro-entérites des nourrissons.

I. Gastro-entérites aiguës ou subaiguës.
- 1° Avec prédominance des lésions épithéliales (catarrhales).
  - Gastro-entérite simple { légère. / intense.
  - Choléra infantile.
- 2° Avec prédominance des lésions lymphoïdes (folliculaires): souvent consécutives aux formes catarrhales.
  - Forme typhoïde.
  - Forme dysentéroïde { bénigne. / grave.
- 3° Formes mixtes.

II. Gastro-entérite chronique : en général avec prédominance des lésions épithéliales (maladie du gros ventre).

III. Cachexie atrophique d'origine gastro-intestinale : peut succéder aux formes précédentes (formes chroniques, formes aiguës graves, formes simples à récidives) et peut survivre à la disparition des troubles digestifs.

chent de la fin de la seconde année et qui ne reçoivent pas exclusivement du lait, d'autres aliments, les fruits passés en particulier, ne peuvent pas être l'origine de diarrhées estivales. Mais nous rentrons ici dans la question du choléra nostras des adultes et des grands enfants.

M. Escherich ne croit pas sa division aussi théorique et aussi difficile à appliquer en pratique que M. Marfan semble le dire. L'infection du chyme se reconnaît surtout par l'absence de fièvre, par les caractères de la diarrhée de nature acide, par les selles contenant du mucus, mais pas de sang, pas de desquamation épithéliale, pas de pus. Les infections pariétales sont différentes et faciles à reconnaître en clinique. On a ici tout au contraire, de la fièvre, du pus, du sang, des microbes en abondance et une abondance exagérée de cellules, marquant l'intensité du processus destructif au niveau même de la paroi.

M. Marfan. — Je suis heureux d'avoir suscité les explications de M. Escherich. En somme, son infection du chyme répond à peu près aux formes dyspeptiques et catarrhales, tandis que l'infection pariétale répond aux formes folliculaires. Mais est-il bien sûr que dans les formes catarrhales il n'y ait jamais infection de la paroi? En tout cas, je constate avec satisfaction que M. Escherich, M. Baginski et moi-même nous reconnaissons les mêmes formes cliniques de troubles digestifs des nourrissons. Pour arriver à une entente désirable, je désignerai, si l'on veut, la forme simple légère de gastro-entérite sous le nom de dyspepsie gastro-intestinale passagère, la gastro-entérite chronique (maladie du gros ventre) sous le nom de dyspepsie gastro-intestinale chronique, et la cachexie atrophique sous le nom de catarrhe intestinal chronique, bien que sur ce dernier point, je fasse des réserves expresses sur la théorie de M. Baginski qui rattache l'atrophie infantile exclusivement au catarrhe chronique de l'estomac et de l'intestin.

M. Alvarez, au sujet du rapport de M. Marfan, dit avoir observé des cas de choléra infantile bien que le lait ait été stérilisé immédiatement après la traite. Aussi croit-il qu'il y a d'autres raisons pour expliquer la présence des microbes. En fait deux points sont certains : 1° l'enfant au sein n'a jamais de choléra infantile; 2° le choléra est d'autant plus fréquent que le lait est moins pur.

La véritable différence entre le lait de femme recueilli directement par l'enfant et le lait donné au biberon, c'est que le premier est un liquide vivant, conservant toutes ses propriétés biologiques, tandis que le lait du biberon est au contraire un liquide mort, c'est pour mieux dire, « un cadavre » dont chaque moment à partir qu'on l'éloigne de la traite, hâte la décomposition organique.

M. Martinez-Vargas. — Je désire insister sur la nécessité de rayer des cadres nosologiques le mot *choléra infantile*, parce que son étiologie est tout à fait différente de celle du choléra asiatique et, parce que, comme c'est pendant l'été que ces deux maladies se produisent, il peut en résulter des confusions dangereuses dans la prophylaxie publique et dans les familles. On devrait y substituer le mot *diarrhée cholériforme*. M. le professeur Marfan nous a parlé d'une façon si claire et brillante qu'on ne peut faire mieux; je partage son opinion dans beaucoup de cas, mais je crois qu'il y en a d'autres dans lesquels sa théorie ne peut pas se soutenir, à savoir, dans ceux où les enfants sont allaités au sein; j'ai eu occasion de voir une fillette de 10 mois, nourrie par sa mère, et qui, malgré cela, eut la diarrhée cholériforme; la mort survint en dix-huit heures, nonobstant tous les moyens thérapeutiques employés. Là on ne peut invoquer l'empoisonnement par le lait de vache, puisque le bébé n'en prenait pas ; mais la cause probable fut une soupe qu'on donnait tous les jours comme alimentation supplémentaire.

Ici on a dit qu'on peut observer des cas de diarrhée cholériforme en hiver ; pour ma part, je puis assurer que je n'en ai pas vu de cas en dehors de l'été, nonobstant que l'hiver soit à Barcelone tempéré ; tous les cas que j'ai eu occasion de voir se sont développés du mois de juin au mois de septembre. Il va sans dire que les autres formes d'infections intestinales, je les ai observées pendant l'hiver comme pendant l'été et bien plus fréquemment dans cette dernière saison.

A propos de la contagion, je ne crois pas que ces diarrhées soient si contagieuses que la rougeole ou la scarlatine, mais il n'est pas possible de nier une certaine influence de contagion dans la propagation, ou dans la production de nouveaux cas. Moi-même j'ai vu dans quelques familles qui ne sont pas des modèles de propreté, se développer 3 ou 4 cas successivement ; Baginsky a pu constater le fait et il me fait des signes affirmatifs ; Köplik a vu dans un grand dispensaire que les enfants attaqués de cette infection, guérissent beaucoup mieux dans le plein air (ambulatory) que dans les salles d'hôpital.

Quant à la classification, je suis d'avis que celle que je viens de proposer, de trouble fonctionnel (indigestion), infection simple, infection avec intoxication, infection et intoxication compliquée (pneumonie nephritis, etc.), met en union l'étiologie, la pathogénie, la clinique et l'anatomie pathologique.

M. Hutinel (de Paris). — Je crois que, dans toutes ces questions d'infections gastro-intestinales, nous sommes séparés par une question de mots plutôt que par une question de faits. Nous voyons trop la lésion et pas assez la cause. Celle-ci doit être cherchée dans le contenu de l'intestin, dans les germes et dans les ferments sécrétés par eux et capables de transformer les aliments en poisons. Il y a une première phase, dans laquelle se forment dans l'intestin des substances toxiques qui altèrent l'épithélium et modifient la circulation de la muqueuse. Ces troubles peuvent être passagers. Mais si l'infection s'accentue, entretenue par une mauvaise alimentation, on entre dans une deuxième phase, où apparaissent des lésions plus profondes de la paroi intestinale, avec pénétration des microbes dans son épaisseur et détermination de types cliniques et anatomiques plus ou moins caractérisés. Ainsi donc, ce ne sont là que des étapes successives.

M. d'Espine (de Genève). — Je ne crois pas qu'on puisse séparer l'infection de l'intoxication. Les maladies digestives des nourrissons sont dues à des fermentations anormales, qui sont fonctions de germes, lesquels peuvent exister dans l'intestin ou venir du dehors. Pour nous en tenir au choléra infantile survenant à la suite de l'ingestion de lait stérilisé, j'ai toujours constaté, dans les faits que j'ai observés, soit que les bouteilles avaient été laissées débouchées un certain temps, soit, en dehors de ces cas, que l'enfant était soumis à une suralimentation évidente.

M. Escherich s'élève contre la manière de voir de M. Baginski qui attribue quelque chose de spécifique aux diarrhées survenant en été et semble porté à admettre que sous l'influence de la chaleur le coli-bacille est susceptible d'acquérir une virulence plus grande. Il regarde l'augmentation de virulence et le rôle du coli-bacille dans ces cas, comme tout à fait problématique. L'idée d'une infection par l'un des germes pathogènes répandus autour de nous et auxquels l'organisme du nourrisson est si sensible, est beaucoup plus vraisemblable. Les bactéries conservent même après leur passage dans le canal intestinal leur réaction spéciale aux méthodes de coloration; et M. Escherich insiste sur l'utilité de sa méthode de coloration des selles, dont la valeur a déjà été confirmée à plusieurs reprises.

La division proposée par l'auteur contient les groupes admis par Baginsky, Marfan et autres. Nous ne différons, dit il, que par l'importance accordée à chacun de ces groupes. La distinction entre infection du chyme et infection vraie n'est pas seulement théorique mais pratique : l'infection du chyme réclame la suppression de l'alimentation lactée, les purgatifs, la diète hydrique, l'infection vraie nécessite l'isolement.

M. A. BAGINSKY. — Messieurs, la marche suivie jusqu'à présent dans la discussion sur les affections intestinales dans l'enfance m'oblige avant tout à rectifier un point qui apparemment n'a pas été compris selon sa portée exacte par M. Escherich. Ayant eu, dans ma dernière communication, à me prononcer d'une façon quelque peu contradictoire par rapport aux travaux de M. Escherich, j'ai eu à cœur de commencer mon discours d'une façon très courtoise en insistant sur les mérites de mon très honoré collègue. Cette expression de courtoisie, M. Escherich l'a considérée comme une *excuse*. Je regrette qu'il ne m'ait pas compris d'une façon plus conforme à ma pensée.

Je n'ai pas eu, le moins du monde, l'intention de m'excuser devant M. Escherich, et je considère comme un devoir pour ma situation de le déclarer hautement.

Quant au sujet de la discussion, je m'aperçois que, en raison de la différence fondamentale dans notre manière de concevoir toute cette question, il nous sera à peine possible d'arriver à une entente satisfaisante. J'ai eu ici, aujourd'hui, l'occasion de parler des facteurs étiologiques des affections gastro-intestinales accompagnées de diarrhée et de vomissement; il résulte nettement de mon exposé que j'ai en vue particulièrement les diarrhées estivales des enfants, les diarrhées qui déciment les enfants d'une façon si meurtrière, qui débutent au printemps, dès les premiers mois de chaleur, en subissant une exacerbation à mesure que la température atmosphérique s'élève et pouvant se prolonger, pour quelques cas retardataires, jusque dans la saison plus froide, bien que, dans la majorité des cas, elles disparaissent habituellement vers la fin d'août ou dans le cours du mois de septembre. — ces diarrhées estivales qui dans les grandes villes, telles que Berlin, Londres, New-York, etc., en raison des conditions climatologiques, sont devenues endémiques et qui, dans ces grandes villes, dominent dans le tableau de la mortalité des enfants du premier âge.

Je me suis appliqué à rechercher les facteurs étiologiques de ces diarrhées et j'ai, chaque fois, insisté sur ce point que ces formes morbides ne présentent étiologiquement aucun rapport avec les affections diarrhéiques qui sont capables de faire leur apparition, d'une manière plus ou moins sporadique et, parfois aussi, endémique, dans les hôpitaux, crèches, cliniques, etc.

Pour ces diarrhées estivales j'ai décrit, comme causes pathogènes, les miasmes introduits dans l'organisme avec une nourriture avariée sous l'influence des grandes chaleurs de l'été. Je ne vais pas si loin que M. Marfan pour accuser, comme cause pathogène unique, une substance toxique contenue dans la nourriture, car la grande quantité d'organismes vivants les plus divers (microbes) qui est introduite, peut aussi jouer un certain rôle. Mais, en thèse générale, j'ai depuis bien longtemps soutenu cette même notion que M. Marfan a largement développée ici aujourd'hui au point de vue étiologique, en insistant particulièrement sur la maladie désignée sous le nom de choléra infantile. Tant qu'on persiste à vouloir séparer ces formes morbides qui n'offrent rien d'infectieux ni de contagieux, mais sont plutôt, si l'on veut bien, de nature miasmatique, si l'on veut les séparer des diarrhées survenant endémiquement dans les hôpitaux, cliniques et parfois même dans les familles, il n'est pas possible qu'une entente s'établisse entre les auteurs.

Pour ces dernières affections endémiques, je ne veux pas nier la présence des facteurs pathogènes doués de propriétés spécifiques; moi-même j'ai assez écrit sur ce sujet. — Quant à leur rôle dans les autres formes morbides, je le rejette absolument aujourd'hui comme autrefois.

Si donc M. Escherich, en se basant sur des constatations isolées dans une clinique, revient toujours à ces formes morbides particulières et en partant de ce point, entend la généraliser à toutes les autres formes morbides de ce grand groupe des plus importants, il est impossible de nous entendre.

Ce qui rend si nuisibles les notions conçues par M. Escherich, c'est le fait que n'ayant à se baser que sur un nombre restreint d'observations, il ne cesse d'insister sur la contagiosité de l'affection.

Cette notion paralyse l'effort général tendant à réaliser le progrès en hygiène; elle entrave la réalisation des améliorations dans la production du lait, de la modification dans la totalité des conditions de vie des jeunes enfants.

Si à présent j'approfondis un peu les recherches de M. Escherich, je me vois obligé de revenir au reproche déjà formulé que ni moi ni mes assistants nous n'avons pu réussir à obtenir les résultats signalés par M. Escherich lui-même et par d'autres, paraît-il. La raison de notre insuccès serait notre instruction technique, insuffisante quant à la méthode de coloration introduite par M. Escherich. Ceci, messieurs, est le reproche le plus grave qu'on puisse adresser à un auteur travaillant sur les mêmes sujets que M. Escherich depuis de longues années.

Peut-être aurais-je pu glisser rapidement sur ce reproche, et simplement vous renvoyer à la liste de mes travaux ayant trait à la question. Je préfère pourtant entrer dans quelques détails, autant qu'il le faut pour faire ressortir le fait suivant : même lorsque nous observions d'une façon absolument stricte les instructions relatives au procédé de coloration indiqué par M. Escherich, nous arrivions constamment à des résultats totalement différents des siens. Il est impossible que ce soit de notre faute : c'est uniquement la faute d'une méthode infidèle dans les résultats que M. Escherich désire prouver. Il en résulte que l'auteur lui-même est forcé de chercher toujours de nouveaux subterfuges afin de faire tenir debout les affirmations posées au début et dont l'instabilité est décelée ensuite. Enfin, assez sur la méthode de coloration et la technique de M. Escherich.

Permettez maintenant, messieurs, que j'aborde la question de la division des affections intestinales, division proposée par M. Escherich. Même après les explications qu'il vient de donner à ce sujet à M. Marfan, je ne suis pas du tout fixé. En présence de l'idée peu nette que nous associons à tout ce qui a trait au chyme, que devons-nous penser d'une infection du chyme et qu'est-ce que le professeur de clinique ou le médecin praticien doivent faire de cette assertion hypothétique? Que doivent-ils se figurer sur l'infection du *chyme* par opposition à l'infection de *l'intestin?* Comment peut-on séparer la notion d'un chyme infecté de celle d'une paroi intestinale qui ne l'est pas? Cependant, où le chyme reste-t-il sinon au contact de la paroi intestinale? Tout cela ne tient pas debout devant la critique. Il en est tout autrement lorsque, tout en tenant compte des notions acquises en bactériologie et des considérations étiologiques en général, la division anatomo-pathologique claire et certaine se trouve maintenue ayant à sa base des phénomènes cliniques. Tout médecin peut bien comprendre que c'est un catarrhe et le déterminer cliniquement; et de même une entérite folliculaire accompagnée de déjections sanguinolentes et muqueuses, vu que des lésions tout à fait positives sont corrélatives du tableau clinique — ce qui permet d'édifier là-dessus une thérapeutique bien raisonnée.

Messieurs, les notions communiquées par M. Escherich ne sont pas faites pour élucider les circonstances si complexes des affections gastro-intestinales; elles ne peuvent que contribuer à augmenter les difficultés et l'obscurité qui les entourent encore.

Quelque désagréable qu'il me soit personnellement de critiquer aussi à fond la communication de M. Escherich, dans l'intérêt même de la chose, je n'ai pas cru devoir m'y soustraire.

M. Concetti (de Rome) regrette que son chef de clinique, M. le docteur Valagussa, ne soit pas présent. Il l'avait chargé d'étudier certaines affections aiguës de l'intestin des enfants, et il aurait pu donner des renseignements plus détaillés sur les nombreuses expériences faites dans son service à propos de la colite dysentériforme qui s'observe chez les enfants, surtout en été. Concetti rappelle les recherches du professeur Celli directeur de l'institut d'hygiène de l'Université de Rome, qui a isolé, des selles des dysentériques très graves, une variété spéciale de B. coli à laquelle il a donné le nom de dysentériforme. Par des inoculations sous-cutanées, à de jeunes chats, des cultures virulentes de ce bacille, il reproduit les lésions caractéristiques et donne la preuve clinique de la colite hémorragique dysentériforme.

Il a isolé la toxine en la précipitant par l'alcool; et les inoculations de cette toxine ont reproduit les mêmes formes, les mêmes lésions. Il a essayé de s'en servir pour immuniser des animaux, mais il n'a pas réussi complètement. Alors il s'est servi des toxi-protéines de ce B. coli dysentériforme extrait par la méthode de la trituration, de la dilution et de la centrifugation de ces cultures. Avec ces protéines très actives il a réussi, en pratiquant des inoculations progressivement plus fortes, à immuniser des animaux de grande taille (ânes) qui ont fourni un sérum très actif contre les bacilles virulents de la colite dysentériforme.

C'est avec ce sérum, dit l'orateur, que nous avons conduit nos expériences sur les enfants de la clinique pendant l'année dernière et pendant l'année courante. Nous avons expérimenté sur plus de 40 cas, avec les meilleurs résultats qu'on puisse espérer. Après une injection de 10 à 20 cent. c. de sérum dès les premières 24 heures, on voit disparaître la plupart des phénomènes généraux, surtout les phénomènes nerveux, l'abattement, la fièvre, etc. Les selles cessent d'être sanguinolentes, leur fréquence diminue et le ténesme douloureux cesse. Ensuite, parfois après une seconde ou une troisième inoculation à un intervalle de 24 à 48 heures tous les autres phénomènes s'atténuent et cessent jusqu'à la guérison complète en peu de jours. Dans quelques cas où le résultat restait négatif, nous avons trouvé que la colite était déterminée par une infection streptococcique : ce qui démontre que le sérum a une action tout à fait spécifique et non générale. Nous avons trouvé aussi que ce sérum n'a jamais eu d'action sur les autres formes aiguës de l'appareil digestif (gastro-entérites, entérites catarrhales) non dysentériformes : c'est là une preuve de la spécificité de cette variété de coli à produire exclusivement les formes dysentériques. En effet, la réaction Gruber-Widal nous a montré que le sang de nos enfants, tandis qu'il avait une action agglutinante sur les bacilles isolés des selles dysentériformes, ne possédait pas cette action sur les B. coli isolés des autres enfants, bien qu'ils fussent atteints d'autres affections aiguës de l'appareil gastro-intestinal. M. le docteur Valagussa publiera très prochainement les résultats de ses expériences dont l'importance n'échappera à personne.

C) Communications concernant les troubles digestifs des nourrissons.

RECHERCHES
SUR LA FLORE INTESTINALE NORMALE ET PATHOLOGIQUE DU NOURRISSON
par **M. H. TISSIER,**

de Paris.

Nous désirons exposer au Congrès le résultat de nos recherches faites depuis 4 ans dans le laboratoire de la clinique des Enfants-malades, sous la haute direction de M. le professeur Grancher et de son chef de laboratoire le docteur Veillon.

Il nous a semblé qu'il était important, avant d'aborder l'étude des gastro-entérites des nourrissons, de reprendre complètement la question, en étudiant à nouveau, aussi complètement que possible, la flore intestinale normale des nouveau-nés. Les résultats obtenus jusqu'ici par les bactériologistes nous semblaient obscurs et contradictoires. Les méthodes employées étaient, de l'avis de beaucoup d'entre eux, imparfaites. Elles consistaient en milieux aérés, plaques ou boîtes de Petri, à la gélatine ou à l'agar ordinaire. Ces milieux sont peu nutritifs et s'infectent facilement. De plus, dans un milieu privé d'air comme l'est l'intestin, ces méthodes, même avec l'addition de plaques de mica ou de couches surajoutées de gélatine, conduisaient les auteurs aux conclusions suivantes : il n'existe pas d'anaérobies dans le tube digestif du nourrisson, et les microbes aérobies ou facultatifs constituant la flore intestinale sont nombreux et variés. Ce sont : le B. coli, le B. lactis aerogenes, le proteus, le subtilis, le streptococcus coligracilis, le B. liquefaciens fluorescent vert, le B. liquéfiant jaune, le Schleiev-bacillus, le B. fluorescent vert non liquéfiant, le streptococcus coli-brevis, le staphylocoque blanc, le staphylocoque jaune, le micrococcus ovalis, le porcellancoccus, la sarcina ventriculi, la levure blanche, la levure rouge, la levure encapsulée, la honilia candida, le B. mesen-tericus, le Wurtzelbacillus, etc.

En un mot, dans des cas comme chez le nourrisson au sein normal où le microscope ne révèle qu'une ou deux espèces, ces méthodes donnent 14 espèces, et dans des cas de gastro-entérites où l'examen direct montre des espèces variées, elles ne donnent qu'une ou deux bactéries et quelquefois même le B. coli à l'état pur; de plus, les auteurs non seulement ne voient aucune différence entre les selles normales d'un enfant au sein et d'un enfant au biberon, mais même entre des selles normales et des selles pathologiques.

Tel était l'état de la question au moment où nous avons commencé nos recherches.

Il nous fallait donc trouver une autre méthode, une méthode générale permettant d'isoler aussi facilement des anaérobies stricts, des facultatifs ou des aérobies obligés. Nous avons choisi la méthode de VEILLON, qui, entre les mains de cet auteur, puis de ZUBER. RIST, COTTET, GUILLEMOT, avait déjà donné de si remarquables résultats. Nous ne pouvons la décrire ici, nous renvoyons aux travaux de ces différents auteurs.

Nous avons ainsi d'abord étudié les selles d'enfants bien portants rigoureusement au sein, à différents âges; puis nous avons fait de même pour les enfants alimentés au lait de vache, et ce n'est qu'après de nombreuses recherches que nous avons abordé l'étude des selles pathologiques.

Contrairement aux idées jusqu'ici admises, nous avons pu voir qu'il existait une différence notable non seulement entre la flore normale et pathologique, mais encore entre la flore de l'enfant au sein et celle de l'enfant au biberon.

Nous allons d'abord étudier la *flore intestinale normale* chez l'enfant au sein ; elle s'établit d'une façon régulière : après une première phase aseptique, qui dure depuis la naissance jusque vers la 10ᵉ ou la 20ᵉ heure les micro-organismes infectent progressivement le tube digestif.

Dans cette seconde phase d'infection croissante, avant toute alimentation, apparaissent, en même temps ou après une débâcle épithéliale de cellules plates ectodermiques d'origine buccale ou pharyngienne, de petits cocci, le B. coli (variété commune) et un petit bacille grêle. Après la première alimentation on voit successivement apparaître de gros bacilles, puis le B. de Bienstock, et le B. bifidus communis. Cette infection semble plutôt venir par la bouche ; seul le coli peut venir par la voie anale ; vers le milieu du 5ᵉ jour elle est à son maximum.

Dans une troisième phase, ou phase de transformation de la flore, l'aspect microbien se simplifie ; une espèce se substitue aux autres. Cette espèce est un anaérobie strict que nous avons décrit en 1899, le bacillus bifidus communis. Cette modification est sous sa dépendance. Sa durée. son début, dépendent de l'apparition de cette bactérie dans les selles.

Vers la fin du 4ᵉ jour, la flore normale est d'ordinaire constituée.

Depuis cette époque jusqu'au sevrage, l'aspect des selles d'un nourrisson au sein, bien portant, restera constant, invariable. Nous y trouverons toujours les mêmes espèces. Tout d'abord en nombre absolument prépondérant et presque uniquement le B. bifidus. A côté de lui en nombre extrêmement restreint le B. coli (variété commune), le streptocoque d'Hirsch-Libbman et le B. lactis aerogenes. Parfois il peut s'y joindre des espèces de passage, espèces anormales ne pouvant séjourner dans le tube digestif. Elles ne se trouvent pas dans les cas absolument normaux ; elles ne se montrent que dans des conditions déterminées : écart de régime, malpropreté, mauvaise hygiène.

Comparons maintenant à cet aspect bactérien si simple celui des selles d'un enfant alimenté au lait stérilisé.

Dans ce cas la phase d'infection croissante est plus longue, plus intense. Les espèces sont encore plus variées. Elle atteint son maximum vers le 4ᵉ jour. La phase de transformation est beaucoup plus lente, plus tardive et à peine marquée. Très peu d'espèces sont éliminées. Il ne se produit pas de substitution d'une espèce prépondérante. La flore normale ne semble être que la continuation de cette phase d'infection croissante. Les bactéries sont nombreuses, elles semblent même varier d'une selle à une autre; on trouve en effet le bacillus acidophilus de Moro, l'entérocoque de Thiercelin, que nous avons identifiés au micrococcus ovalis d'Escherich, le bacterium coli (variété commune), le B. lactis aerogenes, le streptocoque, d'Hirsch-Libbmann, le bifidus, une espèce nouvelle, le B. exilis, anaérobie facultatif, des sarcines, le staphylocoque blanc. Aucune espèce n'est absolument prépondérante.

Tel est l'aspect bactérien complexe des selles d'un nourrisson soumis à l'allaitement au lait stérilisé. Chez les enfants nourris à l'allaitement mixte, l'aspect de la flore rappelle beaucoup celui de l'enfant au sein ; mais tout dépend de l'âge où l'enfant est mis à cette alimentation. Quand il y est mis dès la naissance, l'aspect des selles rappelle celui de l'enfant au biberon. Quand il y est mis d'une façon tardive et que jusque-là il a été nourri au sein, l'aspect microcoscopique se rapproche de celui de l'enfant au sein.

Chacun des types que nous venons d'étudier est si défini qu'un examen direct des selles suffit pour faire le diagnostic du mode d'alimentation auquel est soumis le nourrisson.

Il est donc possible de surveiller par ce moyen l'alimentation du nourrisson au sein ; mais il est, par contre, impossible de différencier ainsi les selles d'un enfant nourri au lait stérilisé des selles d'un enfant nourri au lait ordinaire.

Examinons maintenant le rôle physiologique des microbes de l'intestin.

Chez l'enfant au sein, la digestion est complète, les déchets qui en proviennent sont pauvres en substances fermentescibles.

Le bifidus, qui forme à lui seul la presque totalité de la flore, agit sur la glucose, mais reste sans action sur la lactose. Il ne peut agir que sur les composés ultimes qui proviennent de l'hydratation des albuminoïdes. Les microbes fermentatifs de la lactose, le B. coli, le B. lactis, le streptocoque d'Hirsch-Libbmann sont en quantité si minime que leur action ne peut être très importante.

Ainsi chez le nourrisson au sein les fermentations microbiennes sont très accessoires, et les produits qui en résultent ne sont probablement que peu utiles à l'organisme.

Chez l'enfant au biberon, la digestion est incomplète, les déchets digestifs plus riches en substances fermentescibles, c'est ce qui explique la présence dans les selles du grand nombre des espèces agis sant sur la lactose avec ou sans production de gaz, comme le coli, le B. lactis aerogenes, le streptocoque intestinal, le staphylocoque blanc, le bacillus exilis, l'acidophilus.

Les protéolytiques sont donc extrêmement rares.

Nous allons maintenant étudier la *flore pathologique*. Si déjà à l'état normal nous avons constaté des différences entre les diverses variétés des nourrissons, à l'état pathologique ces différences ne font que s'accentuer. Les gastro-entérites légères, moyennes ou suraiguës sont loin d'avoir le même caractère de gravité chez l'enfant au sein que chez l'enfant au biberon. Les statistiques du reste en font foi. Celles de M. Lesage, celles de M. Donnon, curé d'Hermé en Seine-et-Marne, et celles de l'été de 1900 nous montrent que le nourrisson au sein semble jouir d'une véritable immunité, tandis que le nourrisson au biberon présente au contraire un véritable état de réceptivité.

Nous devons donc étudier séparément les selles pathologiques des deux grandes catégories de nourrissons. Mais, pour arriver à un résultat, il est nécessaire de procéder avec beaucoup de méthode. Nous devrons d'abord étudier une diarrhée dont nous connaîtrons la cause et quand ces effets nous seront connus, quand nous aurons vu les modifications d'une flore normale dans des conditions définies, nous pourrons alors aborder l'étude de la cause dans les cas où elle nous est inconnue, comme les diarrhées dites infectieuses.

Ainsi chez un enfant au sein, bien portant, nous cherchons à modifier l'aspect bactérien des selles par l'ingestion de calomel ou par des lavages de l'intestin ; nous constatons que l'espèce dominante B. bifidus diminue et présente des formes de souffrance; par contre, les espèces facultatives, B. coli et streptocoque d'Hirsch-Libbmann, prolifèrent. La prédominance de l'une ou de l'autre est la règle. Ce fait dépend simplement de leur nombre respectif antérieurement à l'expérience. Cette modification commence sept heures après l'ingestion, est à son maximum vers la 24e heure et disparaît 40 heures après.

Or dans les selles pathologiques, dans les gastro-entérites légères ou graves de l'enfant au sein, on constate toujours une semblable modification dans la forme et le rapport des espèces, mais on trouve presque toujours, en plus des bactéries ordinaires, des espèces que nous *n'avons pu retrouver dans des selles normales*.

Chez le nourrisson au biberon maintenant, le calomel, les lavages de l'intestin produisent une modification de la flore analogue à celle que nous venons de décrire chez l'enfant au sein ; mais elle est plus profonde, plus lente à disparaître. Elle débute vers la 7e heure, est à son maximum à la 24e et ne disparaît que 60 heures après.

Dans les gastro-entérites aiguës, on constate également cette modification et à côté d'elle il existe également des espèces *anormales*.

Dans les gastro-entérites chroniques, dans la selle du début on trouve des espèces différentes de celles que l'on rencontre chez l'enfant bien portant; dans les poussées successives de diarrhée on retrouve la modification liée à ce symptôme, c'est-à-dire prolifération des B. coli et du streptocoque de Hirsch-Libbmann.

Dans l'athrepsie ou cachexie intestinale, le type de la flore est spécial. Les bactéries sont peut-être moins abondantes, mais très variées. Les spirochètes apparaissent dans l'intestin, dans ces maladies chroniques, comme elles apparaissent dans les ulcérations chroniques de la bouche. On retrouve enfin les espèces anormales que l'on voit dans les diarrhées aiguës.

Les espèces anormales que nous avons rencontrées dans les gastro-entérites sont des espèces nouvelles dont nous avons donné la description dans notre thèse inaugurale. Ce sont le diplococcus griseus liquefaciens, le cocco-bacillus anaerobius perfœtens, le streptocoque décoloré par le gram de Cottet et Tissier, le B. anaerobius minutus et le B. coli, variété typhimorphe d'Hermann et Wurtz. Pour cette dernière espèce nous devons cependant dire que nous l'avons rencontrée chez un enfant bien portant au biberon, mais qui avait présenté des troubles digestifs 10 jours auparavant.

On peut donc, d'après ce que nous venons de dire, faire le diagnostic d'une selle pathologique; mais à l'examen direct il faudra toujours joindre les cultures. La durée, l'intensité de la modification de la flore, de même que la présence des spirochètes pourront servir à établir le pronostic.

Quelle est maintenant l'étiologie et la pathogénie des gastro-entérites du nourrisson?

La cause déterminante paraît être presque toujours une infection. Les espèces que nous avons décrites ne seraient-elles pas pathogènes que leur présence seule est importante, puisqu'elle indique une pénétration d'espèces anormales dans le tube digestif. La modification de la flore causée par le symptôme diarrhée est secondaire : on peut la reproduire artificiellement, et une substance comme le calomel ne peut agir sur le B. coli et le streptocoque d'Hirsch-Libbmann qu'en modifiant le milieu. Nous avons pu également nous rendre compte qu'elle ne se produisait qu'après l'apparition d'espèces anormales. La pullulation de ce coli et de ce streptocoque n'est pas indifférente, puisque leur virulence s'accroît et qu'en cas de lésions de la muqueuse ils peuvent pénétrer dans la circulation et de là dans les organes. Leur action n'est, en tout cas, que secondaire. Existe-t-il des entérites? Ce fait semble prouvé par l'action de certains poisons. Mais les substances produites par les saprophytes ne sont pas assez connues pour qu'on puisse leur attribuer une action primitive.

Tant que nous trouverons dans les selles des espèces anormales, ou tant que nous verrons que nous n'avons pas isolé toutes les espèces, il ne nous semble pas possible d'admettre l'action pathogène d'un saprophyte habituellement inoffensif, ce que l'on a voulu désigner sous le nom d'infection endogène. Les causes prédisposantes présentent un grand intérêt. Cette *immunité* de l'enfant au sein nous paraît due : 1° à l'état chimique de son contenu intestinal, milieu peu favorable à la croissance d'autres espèces ; 2° à la flore intestinale elle-même, qui contient une espèce empêchante en culture, le bifidus, et enfin des bacilles comme le B. coli et le B. lactis aerogenes qui, comme l'a démontré BIENSTOCK, s'oppose par simple force antagoniste aux fermentations putrides.

La *réceptivité* si particulière de l'enfant au biberon tient : 1° à l'état chimique de son contenu intestinal beaucoup plus riche en substances fermentescibles ; 2° à sa flore intestinale moins résistante à l'action des poisons et qui contient des espèces neutralisant l'action des empêchants, comme semble le faire l'acidophilus, et enfin des favorisantes comme certaines variété de sarcines.

DISCUSSION

M. ESCHERICH félicite M. Tissier de son grand et beau travail. Je connaissais, dit-il, les lacunes de mon premier travail, et je suis heureux de les voir remplies en partie. Les travaux récents de notre clinique concordent très bien avec les recherches de M. Tissier.

SUR LES EFFETS EXPÉRIMENTAUX DES INOCULATIONS
DES EXTRAITS DE MATIÈRES FÉCALES DES NOURRISSONS
A L'ÉTAT NORMAL ET PATHOLOGIQUE

par **M. P. HAUSHALTER**,

Professeur agrégé à la Faculté de médecine de Nancy

et par **M. Louis SPILLMANN**,

Ancien interne des Hôpitaux de Nancy.

Dans les gastro-entérites aiguës ou chroniques des nourrissons, les symptômes sont suivant les cas attribués en partie plus ou moins grande à la perte d'eau, à l'insuffisance de l'assimilation, à l'infection générale, aux infections secondaires du poumon, de la peau, etc. Une partie des symptômes revient à l'intoxication, c'est-à-dire à l'action des poisons fabriqués et résorbés dans l'intestin, poisons normaux que l'épithélium intestinal altéré arrête insuffisamment et que le foie neutralise incomplètement, poisons anormaux, produits des fermentations diverses, albumines toxiques ou alcaloïdes, fabriqués en quantité excessive par les microbes saprogènes habituels ou par les microbes pathogènes virulents venus de l'extérieur. C'est à l'action de ces poisons que l'on attribue dans les gastro-entérites et la diarrhée des enfants, les troubles du système nerveux, les altérations du foie, des organes hématopoiétiques, de la moelle osseuse, des os même dans le rachitisme, etc. Cette intoxication est admise comme très probable plutôt que rigoureusement démontrée. On la prouve indirectement et expérimentalement en montrant que le coli-bacille, agent habituel des diarrhées, fabrique à l'état virulent, des produits toxiques très actifs. L'étude chimique directe des poisons dans les différentes portions de l'intestin ou dans les matières fécales à l'état normal ou pathologique est entourée de difficultés pratiques insurmontables.

La méthode, *a priori* la plus simple, pour rechercher la richesse toxique des matières fécales est l'étude expérimentale de leur toxicité, la détermination de la toxicité ne pouvant renseigner d'ailleurs sur la nature des poisons intestinaux si complexes et si variés, mais uniquement sur la qualité toxique globale d'une matière fécale donnée. Elle ne renseigne même pas sur la quantité de poisons fabriqués puisqu'une partie des poisons normaux ou anormaux a pu, dans l'intestin malade, être résorbée en quantité plus ou moins forte avant d'arriver dans la dernière portion du gros intestin. Théoriquement il faudrait pouvoir évaluer la toxicité dans les différentes portions du tube digestif, recherches très imparfaites et très limitées puisqu'elles ne peuvent être pratiquées que sur le cadavre.

La détermination de la toxicité des matières fécales ne peut que renseigner sur la quantité de poisons éliminée; reste à savoir si cette portion éliminée est proportionnelle à la quantité de poisons fabriquée et à la quantité de poisons résorbée.

L'étude de la toxicité de matières fécales données peut être comprise à deux points de vue : on peut, d'une part, chercher à évaluer sa toxicité complète, c'est-à-dire la quantité nécessaire pour tuer dans les conditions voulues un kilogramme d'animal, de même que l'on recherche la toxicité d'une urine: on peut, d'autre part, par l'injection de doses fractionnées et rejetées à plus ou moins longs intervalles, rechercher leur action à longue échéance et les altérations plus ou moins profondes qu'elles peuvent amener.

L'étude du pouvoir toxique immédiat est entourée de réelles difficultés, surtout en ce qui concerne les matières diarrhéiques des enfants.

Tout d'abord il serait utile de posséder un point de repère, savoir quelle est la toxicité moyenne de matières fécales de poupons normaux: or, ce jalon nous paraît très difficile à poser, cette toxicité étant, comme nous le verrons, sujette à de fortes variations; d'autre part, il faut dans chaque expérience, autant que possible, étant donné que la toxicité des matières diarrhéiques peut varier d'une émission à l'autre, opérer, pour un animal, avec la quantité d'une seule émission, ou au plus avec l'émission d'une journée. Or, comme nous avons pu nous en assurer dans les diarrhées, les quantités émises chaque fois sont souvent très faibles et on ne possède généralement pas, à un moment donné, venant d'un seul enfant, une masse de matières dont l'inoculation puisse amener la mort immédiate ou même rapide de l'animal. Pour obvier en partie à cet inconvénient, nous avons choisi des animaux jeunes, des lapins dont le poids variait de 400 à 1800 grammes; le plus grand nombre était d'un poids de 500 grammes. D'après le procédé employé par Robert[1] dans sa thèse faite sous l'inspiration de Royer sur le rôle de l'intoxication dans les gastro-entérites des adultes, les matières, dans un délai aussi rapproché que possible de leur émission, étaient recueillies dans les langes à l'aide d'une spatule et diluées

____

1. ROBERT. *Thèse de Paris*, 1898.

dans une quantité d'alcool représentant 2 ou 3 fois leur volume. Le tout était filtré, la solution alcoolique évaporée à siccité au bain-marie et le résidu repris par une certaine quantité de sérum artificiel ou plutôt de solution saline stérilisée à 7 pour 1000 : on avait ainsi l'extrait alcoolique des matières ou mieux les poisons solubles dans l'alcool. Les matières restées sur le filtre étaient séchées aussi vite que possible, le résidu sec repris par du sérum artificiel et filtré; on avait ainsi l'extrait aqueux des matières ou plutôt les poisons solubles dans l'eau.

Dans tous les cas, nous avons opéré de cette façon pour rester toujours dans des conditions analogues, sans avoir la prétention de croire que ces extraits alcooliques et aqueux contiennent tous les poisons et les matières diarrhéiques. L'inoculation était pratiquée avec le mélange de l'extrait aqueux et de l'extrait alcoolique des matières provenant d'un cas donné. 15 inoculations ont été faites avec des extraits de matières normales, 28 avec des extraits de matières diarrhéiques.

L'inoculation a toujours été faite aussi aseptiquement que possible sous la peau ou dans les veines. Dans les infections intra-veineuses, la quantité de sérum inoculé a été en moyenne de 10 grammes par kilogramme d'animal; on n'a, par conséquent, à tenir aucun compte de l'action nocive du sérum véhicule.

I. — INOCULATIONS D'EXTRAITS DE MATIÈRES FÉCALES DE POUPONS BIEN PORTANTS.

A. *Inoculations sous-cutanées.*

1° *Inoculations des extraits de matières fécales d'un nouveau-né de 5 jours élevé au sein.*

3 lapins variant du poids de 460 grammes à 550 grammes sont inoculés : le premier avec des extraits de 14 grammes de matières par kilogramme (mort au bout de trois jours); le second avec les extraits de 17 grammes par kilogramme (mort au bout d'un mois; le troisième avec des extraits de 43 grammes par kilogramme (mort au bout de onze jours).

2° *Inoculations des extraits de matières fécales d'un poupon normal de 8 mois soumis à l'allaitement mixte avec prédominance de lait maternel.*

5 lapins variant du poids de 400 à 500 grammes sont inoculés : le premier avec les extraits de 22 grammes de matières par kilogramme (dépérit un peu, et est sacrifié au bout d'un mois); le second avec les extraits de 42 grammes par kilogramme (mort au bout de dix-neuf jours); le troisième avec les extraits de 44 grammes par kilogramme (normal encore au bout d'un mois); le quatrième avec les extraits de 55 grammes par kilogramme (normal au bout de cinq semaines); le cinquième avec les extraits de 55 grammes par kilogramme (mort au bout de deux jours).

B. *Inoculations intra-veineuses.*

1° *Inoculations des extraits de matières fécales d'un nouveau-né de 10 jours.*

Un lapin pesant 1160 grammes est inoculé avec les extraits de

5 grammes de matières par kilogramme (normal encore au bout d'un mois).

2° Inoculations des extraits de matières fécales d'un poupon normal de 8 mois, nourri à l'allaitement mixte avec prédominance du lait maternel.

5 lapins variant du poids de 500 à 1400 grammes sont inoculés : le premier avec les extraits de 8 grammes de matières par kilogramme (mort immédiate avec convulsions); le deuxième avec les extraits de 25 grammes par kilogramme (mort immédiate avec convulsions); le troisième avec les extraits de 44 grammes par kilogramme (mort immédiate avec convulsions).

3° Inoculations des extraits de matières fécales d'un enfant de 2 ans nourri avec laitages, panades, purées.

Un lapin pesant 1400 grammes est inoculé avec les extraits de 22 grammes de matières par kilogramme (dépérit un peu, vit encore au bout d'un mois).

A l'inspection de ces chiffres on est frappé de constater combien les effets obtenus sont peu en rapport avec les quantités d'extrait inoculées. En ce qui concerne les injections sous-cutanées, nous voyons des quantités faibles amener la mort en peu de jours et des quantités fortes laisser les animaux tout à fait intacts ou au contraire les tuer rapidement. Ces différences d'action ne peuvent s'interpréter par des fautes de technique ni par l'inoculation de produits plus ou moins septiques.

D'ailleurs, dans aucun cas, l'autopsie des animaux ne nous a révélé de lésions capables de s'expliquer par une infection générale; tout au plus, au point d'inoculation sous-cutanée, existait-il chez les animaux qui moururent comme chez ceux qui survécurent une infiltration diffuse, coïncidant avec la présence d'un exsudat fibrineux compact, constant dans presque tous les cas, malgré l'asepsie la plus rigoureuse avec laquelle était pratiquée l'inoculation.

Pour les inoculations intra-veineuses des extraits, nous voyons des différences tout aussi bizarres : avec des extraits d'un même enfant, chez 2 lapins de 500 grammes, la mort survient après l'inoculation de l'extrait de 8 grammes par kilogramme chez l'un, et de l'extrait de 44 grammes par kilogramme chez l'autre, les matières étant d'ailleurs d'aspect normal et identique.

A en juger d'après ces chiffres, il faudrait conclure que la richesse toxique des matières fécales d'un nourrisson bien portant, peut varier suivant les émissions dans des proportions très considérables. La richesse toxique des matières du nourrisson nourri exclusivement de lait n'est pas forcément non plus inférieure à celle d'un enfant dont la nourriture est plus variée. Comme nous venons de le voir, l'inoculation intra-veineuse de l'extrait de 22 grammes par kilogramme des matières fécales d'un enfant de 2 ans, nourri de semoule, laitage, pu-

Inoculation des extraits de matières fécales d'enfants atteints de gastro-entérite.

AGE DE L'ENFANT	NATURE DES SELLES	POIDS DE L'ANIMAL	POIDS RÉEL DES MATIÈRES	QUANTITÉ D'EXTRAIT inoculé par kg. d'animal	RÉSULTATS
		Grammes.	Grammes.	Grammes.	
6 mois.	Diarrhée verte liquide.	450	8	18	Mort au bout de deux jours.
4 mois.	Gastro-entérite.	450	10	22	Dépérissement; vit au bout d'un mois.
18 mois.	Selles vertes mastic.	450	10	22	Mort au bout de huit jours.
2 mois.	Diarrhée verte.	465	11	25	Mort au bout de six jours.
10 mois.	Entérite aiguë récente.	590	10	25	Mort au bout de deux jours.
4 mois.	Gastro-entérite chronique.	400	10	25	Dépérissement; vit au bout d'un mois.
6 mois.	Diarrhée verte.	400	10	25	Dépérissement; vit au bout d'un mois.
6 mois.	Diarrhée verte.	590	12	50	Mort au bout de deux jours.
22 mois.	Diarrhée verte.	450	20	44	Normal au bout d'un mois.
4 mois.	Diarrhée verte.	500	25	50	Dépérissement; vit au bout d'un mois.

B. Inoculations intra-veineuses.

Inoculation des extraits de matières fécales d'enfants atteints de diarrhée.

AGE DE L'ENFANT	NATURE DES SELLES	POIDS DE L'ANIMAL	POIDS RÉEL DES MATIÈRES	QUANTITÉ D'EXTRAIT inoculé par kg. d'animal.	RÉSULTATS
		Grammes.	Grammes.	Grammes.	
5 mois.	Diarrhée verte.	1150	5	4	Normal au bout d'un mois.
1 an. .	Diarrhée liquide à odeur acide.	1200	7	5	Dépérit un peu, mais survit.
6 mois.	Diarrhée verte.	1100	8	7	Normal au bout d'un mois.
4 mois.	Id.	1400	22	15	Mort avec convulsions pendant l'inoculation.
5 mois.	Id.	2150	56	16	Mort avec convulsions pendant l'inoculation.
7 mois.	Id.	1740	50	17	Normal au bout de dix jours.
2 mois.	Id.	1750	40	22	Mort avec convulsions pendant l'inoculation.
5 mois.	Diarrhée cholér. suivie de mort.	1400	55	26	Dépérit mais survit.
5 mois.	Diarrhée verte.	500	18	56	Mort au bout de onze jours.

rée, panade, n'a pas tué l'animal, mais l'a rendu simplement cachectique. D'après cela, on pourrait se demander s'il n'existe pas dans les matières fécales du nourrisson un élément variable qui contribue, pour une forte part, à modifier la toxicité des matières fécales et dont l'élimination, sinon la fabrication, est irrégulière, sans d'ailleurs que cette irrégularité soit en rapport avec des troubles de la santé. Nous ne voulons pas, pour le moment, pousser plus loin le problème ; nous nous contentons, aujourd'hui, d'énoncer simplement des faits.

II. — Inoculations d'extraits de matières fécales d'enfants atteints de gastro-entérite.

Les expériences furent toutes pratiquées avec des extraits de matières diarrhéiques provenant de nourrissons atteints de gastro-entérite aiguë ou chronique.

A. *Inoculations sous-cutanées.*

1° *Inoculations des extraits de matières d'un enfant de 11 mois atteint de gastro-entérite aiguë.*

2 lapins, pesant 1200 grammes sont inoculés, le premier avec les extraits de 10 grammes de matières par kilogramme (mort au bout de deux jours); le second de 24 grammes par kilogramme (mort au bout de trois jours); 3 lapins du même âge et du même poids (450 gr.) sont inoculés : le premier avec des extraits de 44 grammes par kilogramme (mort au bout de quatre jours); le second avec les extraits de 22 grammes par kilogramme (mort au bout de seize jours); le troisième avec des extraits de 11 grammes par kilogramme (mort au bout de un mois).

2° *Inoculations des extraits de matières fécales d'un enfant de 16 mois atteint de gastro-entérite chronique avec rachitisme au début et prurigo.*

4 lapins variant comme poids de 420 à 1200 grammes sont inoculés : le premier avec les extraits de 23 grammes de matières par kilogramme (mort au bout de deux jours); le second avec les extraits de 23 grammes par kilogramme (mort au bout de quatre jours); le troisième avec les extraits de 23 grammes par kilogramme (mort au bout de cinq jours); le quatrième avec des extraits de 37 grammes par kilogramme (mort au bout de trois jours).

En résumé :

1° Nous voyons à la suite des *injections sous-cutanées d'extraits*, mourir en moins de 10 jours, 12 lapins qui avaient reçu une fois l'extrait de 10 grammes par kilogramme, une fois l'extrait de 18 grammes, 7 fois l'extrait de 22 à 25 grammes, une fois l'extrait de 30 grammes, une fois l'extrait de 37 grammes et une fois l'extrait de 44 grammes ; mourir au bout de 16 jours un lapin qui avait reçu l'extrait de 22 grammes par kilogramme, au bout de 30 jours un autre qui avait reçu l'extrait de 50 grammes par kilogramme ; 3 encore vivants, mais cachectiques.

furent sacrifiés ayant reçu 25 grammes par kilogramme et 2 autres
tout à fait normaux un mois après l'inoculation, furent sacrifiés ayant
reçu l'extrait de 44 grammes et de 11 grammes par kilogramme. Chez
tous, soit qu'ils fussent morts à des délais rapprochés dans un état
d'amaigrissement plus ou moins accentué, soit qu'ils fussent devenus
cachectiques ou demeurés normaux, il existait au point d'inoculation
un empâtement diffus déterminé par la présence d'un exsudat fibrineux
compact; à l'autopsie les organes ne présentèrent aucune lésion appréciable chez ceux qui succombèrent.

Nous n'avons pu aucunement constater un rapport entre les effets
observés à la suite de l'inoculation, la forme aiguë ou chronique de la
gastro-entérite et l'aspect des selles. Nous voyons des quantités très
variables de matières, soit amener une mort rapide, soit permettre la
survie avec cachexie ou avec état normal. Nous voyons d'une part
l'extrait de 10 grammes par kilogramme tuer en 2 jours; d'autre part,
l'extrait de 44 grammes par kilogramme laisser l'animal normal, alors que
dans le premier cas il s'agissait d'un lapin de 1200 grammes et dans le
second d'un lapin de 450 grammes, ce qui ruine l'hypothèse de différences de résistance des animaux tenant à la question d'âge. En d'autres
termes, les effets des inoculations sous-cutanées présentent des variations suivant les individus, suivant les émissions, beaucoup plus que
suivant la dose, la forme clinique des diarrhées et l'aspect macroscopique des selles.

Les matières recueillies chez un même enfant atteint de diarrhée
peuvent à plusieurs jours d'intervalle conserver la même toxicité;
ainsi, dans un cas, la mort fut amenée dans un intervalle de 2 à 5 jours
chez 4 lapins, après inoculation d'extraits de matières dont le poids
variait de 25 à 55 grammes par kilogramme et qui avaient été émises
en 2 jours différents.

D'autre part, chez un même enfant, la toxicité des matières peut
varier dans de très fortes proportions dans des jours successifs et suivant des chiffres énoncés plus haut, les extraits des matières d'un
même enfant, tuèrent à 2 jours d'intervalle et en l'espace de 2 à 5 jours,
à la dose d'extraits de matière de 10 grammes et de 24 grammes par
kilogramme; par contre 5 jeunes lapins de même âge, de même poids
(450 gr.), inoculés en même temps avec les extraits de matières du
même enfant provenant d'une même émission, l'un à la dose d'extraits
de 44 grammes par kilogramme, l'autre à la dose de 22 grammes par
kilogramme, le troisième à la dose de 11 grammes par kilogramme.
subirent des effets tout à fait proportionnels à la fraction de matières
inoculées; le premier mourut au bout de 4 jours, le second au bout

de 16 jours et le troisième ne présenta aucune manifestation et survécut ; ce fait démontre d'une façon péremptoire que les effets de l'inoculation d'extraits de matières données, émises à un moment donné, ne dépendent nullement de la quantité absolue des matières mais de leur richesse toxique à ce moment, cette richesse toxique variant d'ailleurs suivant les individus et suivant les moments.

2° Nous voyons à la suite des *inoculations intra-veineuses d'extraits*, mourir avec convulsions, au cours de l'inoculation, 5 lapins qui avaient reçu : l'un 15 grammes par kilogramme, l'autre 16 grammes par kilogramme, l'autre 22 grammes par kilogramme ; mourir cachectique au bout de 11 jours un lapin qui avait reçu l'extrait de 56 grammes par kilogramme ; 2 encore vivants mais cachectiques furent sacrifiés au bout d'un mois et de 15 jours, l'un ayant reçu l'extrait de 5 grammes par kilogramme, l'autre l'extrait de 26 grammes par kilogramme, de matières diarrhéiques d'un enfant qui mourut le lendemain de diarrhée cholériforme ; 3 autres tout à fait normaux, l'un 10 jours, les deux autres un mois après l'inoculation furent sacrifiés ayant reçu les extraits de 17 grammes, de 4 grammes et de 7 grammes de matières diarrhéiques. .

Chez les animaux morts ou sacrifiés cachectiques n'existait aucune lésion appréciable des organes.

Ici encore les effets ne sont pas en rapport absolu avec la quantité d'extraits de matières inoculées, car, si nous voyons des animaux demeurer normaux après l'inoculation d'extraits de 4 grammes et de 7 grammes, quantités faibles, nous en voyons un devenir cachectique avec l'extrait de 5 grammes, 5 mourir immédiatement avec l'extrait de 15 à 22 grammes par kilogramme, un demeurer normal avec l'extrait de 17 grammes par kilogramme, et un autre mourir au bout de 10 jours après l'inoculation de 56 grammes par kilogramme.

Les effets ne nous ont pas paru proportionnels non plus avec la forme clinique de la diarrhée ; ainsi, l'inoculation de l'extrait de 26 grammes de matières diarrhéiques dans un cas de gastro-entérite cholériforme terminée par la mort permit une survie de 15 jours.

En somme, qu'il s'agisse d'inoculations sous-cutanées ou d'inoculations intra-veineuses, pratiquées avec des extraits de matières normales ou avec des extraits de matières diarrhéiques, on observe suivant les moments, suivant les cas, sans que rien les fasse prévoir, les effets les plus variables. Suivant les émissions, les extraits de matières normales peuvent être plus ou moins toxiques que les extraits de matières diarrhéiques. En général, lorsque l'inoculation produit des effets rapprochés, ces effets sont semblables pour les matières normales ou pour les matières diarrhéiques; en général aussi, la richesse toxique des matières diarrhéiques ne paraît pas dépasser la richesse toxique des matières du poupon normal, au moins dans les conditions dans lesquelles nous nous sommes placés, car il se peut qu'il y ait des poisons qui ne soient pas repris par les procédés que nous avons employés. Il est vrai qu'on pourrait arguer que dans les matières diarrhéiques, les poisons sont dilués alors qu'ils sont concentrés dans les matières normales, mais ceci n'explique pas les écarts considérables de toxicité de matières normales ou de matières pathologiques d'une même provenance ou d'aspect semblable.

Les résultats auxquels nous sommes arrivés, et qui demandent à être corroborés, n'ont pas la prétention d'être définitifs; ils sont loin de venir à l'encontre de l'hypothèse qui attribue une origine toxique à une série de symptômes ou de lésions, observés dans la gastro-entérite aiguë ou chronique; ils prouvent simplement ou bien que la détermination de la toxicité des matières fécales est complexe, ou bien que la quantité de poisons éliminés par les fèces diarrhéiques n'est pas en rapport direct avec la quantité de poisons élaborés ou résorbés dans l'intestin.

Ils prouvent surtout que l'intensité et la forme de l'intoxication dans les gastro-entérites de l'enfance ne dépendent pas seulement de la richesse toxique et de la nature des poisons intestinaux, mais beaucoup plus peut-être de l'état fonctionnel et surtout de l'état anatomique des tissus et des organes auxquels est dévolu le pouvoir de modifier, de neutraliser ou d'emmagasiner les poisons ; l'altération de ces organes dont les plus importants sont la muqueuse intestinale et le foie, pouvant dépendre aussi bien des formes suraiguës que des formes chroniques de la gastro-entérite. On sait l'importance du rôle de protection dévolu à l'épithélium intestinal; or il a été démontré en particulier par Baginsky et par Marfan que cet épithélium est altéré même dans les cas de diarrhées infantiles rattachés autrefois aux formes simplement catarrhales dues soi-disant à des troubles fonctionnels de la muqueuse. Ne faut-il pas attribuer un rôle aussi très important à la présence de microbes démontrés par Marfan dans les coupes de la muqueuse intestinale au cours de nombre d'entérites de l'enfance? On peut admettre que ces microbes fabriquent, *in situ*, des poisons dont la majeure partie est reprise par la circulation sans passer par la cavité intestinale. Enfin, au point de vue de l'intoxication intestinale, il faut tenir compte encore de la susceptibilité individuelle, en particulier de la susceptibilité du système nerveux vis-à-vis certains poisons qui laissent d'autres enfants indifférents.

Une partie intéressante dans l'étude de l'intoxication intestinale de l'enfance serait la recherche des effets éloignés obtenus à la suite d'inoculations à doses répétées et fractionnées des extraits de matières fécales normales ou pathologiques, une partie des symptômes et des lésions de la cachexie infantile, de l'anémie des nourrissons, de l'athrepsie, du rachitisme, étant actuellement attribuée par nombre d'auteurs à l'intoxication chronique d'origine intestinale.

Les recherches que nous avons ébauchées à ce sujet ne sont pas assez complètes pour être rapportées ici.

ALTÉRATIONS ANATOMO-PATHOLOGIQUES
DE LA MUQUEUSE GASTRO-INTESTINALE DANS L'ATROPHIE PRIMITIVE
ARTIFICIELLEMENT PRODUITE SUR LES PETITS CHIENS

par M. le professeur F. FEDE

Il regrette que dans plusieurs Traités on ne trouve pas un chapitre, sur cette importante maladie, meurtrière, très discutée, même dans certain Traité récent.

Il montre la nécessité de bien distinguer l'athrepsie primitive, laquelle dérive de l'allaitement insuffisant, mauvais, irrégulier et prématuré, artificiel au biberon, surtout quand il y a des causes prédisposantes : enfants nés avant terme, ou incomplètement développés, atteints de faiblesse congénitale, saison chaude, encombrement dans des salles ni vastes, ni bien aérées, ni propres.

L'autre athrepsie est secondaire, elle est causée par la tuberculose ou des altérations profondes de l'appareil digestif; par la syphilis héréditaire; et aussi par les diverses maladies cachectisantes, c'est-à-dire qu'on la doit considérer comme une cachexie conséquence des conditions spéciales locales ou générales.

On ne peut pas accepter les deux groupes d'enfants de BAGINSKY : les uns presque morts de faim, qui, dit-il, ne méritent pas d'être rangés parmi les athrepsiques, qu'il regarde peut-être comme des enfants presque sains, et plusieurs viennent des faiseuses d'anges : et les autres vraiment malades, qui montrent bien des perturbations du tube gastro-entérique, diarrhée, vomissement, diminution du poids, dénutrition et enfin atrophie. Pour l'auteur les uns et les autres ont les mêmes symptômes et les mêmes altérations de l'appareil gastro-intestinal, surtout de la muqueuse.

Et ce sont justement les altérations du tube gastro-entérique qui constituent la partie principale de cette communication.

Dans l'athrepsie du Parrot plusieurs ne reconnaissent pas une vraie entité morbide, et la regardent comme une syndrome des conditions pathologiques différentes, une cachexie variée dans les divers cas, un aboutissant; pendant que l'auteur la considère comme une vraie maladie spéciale.

D'un autre côté il y a des pédiatres qui n'admettent pas dans le tube gastro-entérique d'altérations importantes; et d'autres qui veulent y voir constamment des altérations profondes, c'est-à-dire la destruction à grands traits des glandes et des villosités, opinion vivement soutenue spécialement par Baginsky.

Depuis longtemps l'auteur, par des publications, des communications aux congrès et aux académies après des recherches suivies, exécutées par ses élèves, sur le tube gastro-entérique de plusieurs enfants morts athrepsiques dans leurs premiers mois pour une insuffisante et mauvaise alimentation, a prouvé qu'on ne trouve pas les graves lésions gastro-intestinales indiquées par les auteurs susdits, comme il montra aussi au congrès de Moscou, en présentant des figures et des préparations microscopiques avec intégrité des glandes et des villosités.

Mais on continue à soutenir qu'on rencontre toujours ces altérations, et il a voulu essayer la voie expérimentale, c'est-à-dire observer ce qu'on trouve dans l'atrophie des petits chiens rendus artificiellement atrophiques. Pendant l'année courante, dans son institut, il a fait dans une série de cinq expériences, différemment alimenter des petits chiens de peu de jours pour obtenir une atrophie égale à celle des enfants nouveau-nés, en recherchant après les altérations gastro-intestinales.

Des petits chiens fils de la même mère: un premier a été nourri régulièrement comme témoin; un deuxième avec du bon lait de vache stérilisé, mais en très petite quantité; un troisième avec du lait en quantité mais mauvais, altéré, acidifié, datant de deux ou plusieurs jours; un quatrième avec alimentation pas adaptée et prématurée, pain et farine de Nestlé.

On observa ces petits chiens jusqu'à la mort, en étudiant les perturbations des fonctions gastro-entériques, la diminution du poids, l'atrophie consécutive et après la mort ou le meurtre dans l'agonie furent faites les recherches macroscopiques et microscopiques sur tout l'appareil gastro-entérique.

Eh bien! toujours dans les cinq séries d'expérience, les résultats obtenus ont été constamment les mêmes. En comparant, comme montrent les figures et comme peut le voir qui veut dans les préparations microscopiques, les sections des mêmes traits intestinales, estomac, intestin grêle, gros intestin du petit chien témoin qui montre la parfaite intégrité des parties, et des petits chiens atrophiques, sauf l'amincissement des parois et une atrophie des tissus, une diminution du protoplasma cellulaire d'où un certain espace entre glandes et villosités, on n'a pas trouvé absolument la destruction à traits des glandes ou des villosités.

Et il est important d'observer que les petits chiens rendus atrophiques de quelque manière que ce fût, c'est-à-dire, par alimentation insuffisante, morts donc presque de faim, et par abondante mais mauvaise alimentation ou pas adaptée, qui seraient les vrais atrophiques de Baginsky, tous étant vivants ont montré les mêmes altérations, les perturbations digestives, la diarrhée, la diminution du poids jusqu'à l'atrophie : et tous après mort conservent dans l'estomac et dans les intestins les glandes, et dans leurs intestins grêles les villosités. A tout cela on ajoute que constamment, si dans les petits chiens tués dans leur état d'agonie, glandes et villosités se sont observé bien conservées : dans ceux que l'on a laissé mourir, on a trouvé villosités et glandes moins intègres, comme les montrent les figures, ce qui est assurément causé par la putréfaction cadavérique.

Ces recherches confirment ce que l'auteur soutient depuis plusieurs années : — et dans l'atrophie infantile ou athrepsie du Parrot on rencontre seulement l'amincissement, et des fois les processus catarrhaux du canal intestinal, mais jamais destruction à traits des glandes et des villosités. Dans les cas où ces destructions furent trouvées par divers observateurs et dernièrement par le Dr Cornelia de Lange, il s'agissait d'effets de graves processus pathologiques, surtout par ulcération de la muqueuse intestinale, c'est-à-dire d'atrophie secondaire et non pas primitive, et d'autres fois les lésions qui apparaissent sont produites par la putréfaction cadavérique.

RECHERCHES SUR LA PATHOGÉNIE
DES GASTRO-ENTÉRITES DES NOURRISSONS
par M. JEMMA.

de Gênes.

De nombreuses recherches sur les conditions de la stérilisation m'ont conduit aux conclusions suivantes :

1° Le lait contenant les cadavres des microbes qui se trouvent communément dans ce liquide (*B. coli, B. acidi lactice, B. butyraens, B. protéolytiques*), produit de graves désordres gastro-intestinaux chez les animaux qui en sont alimentés. Ces troubles sont caractérisés par des diarrhées graves, l'amaigrissement jusqu'à une vraie cachexie, et finalement la mort quand cette alimentation est continuée longtemps. Lorsque, après un certain temps (12, 15 jours), on la suspend et qu'on la remplace par une alimentation avec du bon lait stérilisé ou même l'allaitement maternel, les animaux survivent, mais restent dans un état cachectique plus ou moins accusé jusqu'au moment où ils meurent après un temps plus ou moins long. A l'autopsie, on trouve les lésions de la gastro-entérite chronique avec la dégénérescence graisseuse du foie. Ceux qui survivent restent maigres, ne se développent pas, et, sacrifiés après 2 ou 3 mois, on les trouve atteints histologiquement de gastro-entérite chronique avec foie dégénéré.

2° Le lait contenant seulement les cadavres du bacille coli produit sur les jeunes animaux des troubles et des lésions moins graves que celui renfermant les cadavres de toutes les bactéries habituellement contenues dans le lait.

3° Le lait contenant les cadavres des bacilles protéolytiques produit rarement des troubles ; ceux-ci sont légers et ne s'accompagnent pas de lésions graves.

RECHERCHES EXPÉRIMENTALES SUR LES TOXINES DU COLIBACILLE
par M. Giuseppe Antonio PETRONE.

de Naples.

Tous les auteurs, qui ont recherché les toxines du colibacille, ont constaté que ce microorganisme sécrète une toxine peu active dans nos milieux de culture.

Ainsi, pour citer quelques exemples, M. Gilbert a trouvé que, pour produire la mort d'un lapin, il faut lui injecter dans les veines 57 à 94 centimètres cubes par kilogramme du filtrat des cultures; MM. Cesaris Demel et Orlando, en injectant 20 à 25 centimètres cubes du filtrat de cultures très virulentes dans le péritoine des cobayes du poids de 450 à 500 grammes, en obtenaient difficilement la mort; Haushalter et Spillmann, injectant 15 centimètres cubes dans le péritoine, obtenaient la mort des cobayes après plusieurs jours par cachexie.

C'est pour cette raison que M. Celli, pour éviter d'injecter aux animaux de grandes quantités de liquide, s'est servi de la méthode de la précipitation alcoolique pour obtenir les toxines du colibacille coli-dysentérique, et non pas de la filtration à la bougie de porcelaine.

Seul Roger a obtenu naguère une toxine bien active d'un coli-bacille, qu'il a isolé des selles d'individus atteints de dysenterie. Ce colibacille, cultivé dans le bouillon, donnait une toxine capable de tuer un kilogramme de lapin par injection endoveineuse à la dose de 2 centimètres cubes : et cultivé dans un milieu composé de bouillon et de sérum sanguin de bœuf à parties égales il donnait une toxine capable de tuer un lapin, en 24 à 48 heures, à la dose de 10 gouttes, c'est-à-dire d'un demi-centimètre cube. Pour préparer cette dernière toxine il stérilisait la culture par le chloroforme, dont il se débarrassait ensuite par la décantation et l'évaporation.

Moi-même, qui ai fait, il y a deux ans, une première série de recherches sur ce sujet, je n'ai pas pu obtenir de toxines bien actives, bien que je me sois servi de différents échantillons de colibacille.

Devant ces résultats, différentes questions se présentent spontanément à notre esprit.

1° Le bacille d'Escherich trouve-t-il dans les milieux artificiels de culture le terrain propre au développement de ses toxines, ou bien celles-ci se produisent-elles presque exclusivement dans l'organisme animal?

2° Les milieux de culture employés jusqu'à présent, sont-ils les plus favorables au développement des propriétés toxigènes du colibacille, ou bien y en a-t-il d'autres plus propres?

3° Les toxines du colibacille jouent-elles le rôle principal, sinon unique dans l'action pathogène de ce microrganisme?

4° Ont-elles les propriétés fondamentales des toxines jusqu'ici mieux connues, savoir de la toxine tétanique et de la toxine diphtérique?

II

Avant de commencer l'exposition de mes recherches je tiens à déclarer que j'ai employé d'abord quatre échantillons de colibacilles typiques, dont trois isolés des selles d'enfants atteints de gastro-entérite et un des selles d'un enfant bien portant. Ensuite, j'ai borné mes recherches à celui qui m'avait donné au commencement les meilleurs résultats.

J'ai eu soin aussi d'en exalter la virulence par des passages répétés dans les cobayes, jusqu'à obtenir un colibacille capable de tuer un cobaye du poids de 500 grammes, à la dose d'un cinquantième de centimètre cube.

1re Question. — Le colibacille trouve-t-il dans les milieux artificiels de culture le terrain propre au développement de ses toxines, ou bien celles-ci se produisent-elles presque exclusivement dans l'organisme animal?

Pour la solution de cette question on peut, selon moi, employer deux moyens : ou rechercher et étudier la toxicité des tissus et des humeurs d'animaux injectés avec des cultures virulentes de colibacille, comme l'a fait M. Sidney Martin pour le bacille typhique (The Brish. méd. journ. 1898, p. 1569 et 1644): ou se servir de la méthode employée par Methschnikoff pour la recherche de la toxine du bacille du choléra, c'est-à-dire introduire dans la cavité péritonéale des animaux des sachets de collodion plein de bouillon ensemencé de colibacille.

J'ai suivi, en partie, pour le moment seulement la première méthode, en recherchant la toxicité du filtrat de l'exsudat péritonéal de beaucoup de cobayes injectés dans le péritoine avec de cultures virulentes de colibacille; et j'ai constaté que la toxicité de cet exsudat n'est pas supérieure à celle du filtrat des cultures en bouillon.

Je me réserve de faire ensuite des expériences avec la méthode de Metschnikoff.

2e Question. — Y a-t-il des terrains de culture plus propres que ceux employés jusqu'ici pour le développement d'une toxine plus énergique?

Avant de passer à l'étude de cette question, j'ai cru convenable de déterminer la durée qu'il faut donner à la culture pour obtenir le maximum de toxicité.

J'ai ensemencé dans ce but plusieurs matras de bouillon peptonisé et je les ai tenus au thermostate à 37°: et puis j'en ai essayé tous les deux jours la toxicité, toujours avec filtration préalable à la bougie de porcelaine. J'ai constaté que le maximum de toxicité se produit entre le cinquième et le huitième jour.

Et maintenant voici les milieux de culture que j'ai employés pour obtenir une toxine assez active.

1° Au bouillon ordinaire de viande de bœuf, peptonisé à un ou deux pour cent j'ai trouvé préférable le bouillon peptonisé à deux pour cent.

2° Bouillon de viande de bœuf, préalablement digéré avec solution à un pour cent de pepsine Merk à écailles d'or et d'acide chlorhydrique, pendant 24 heures à 39°. Cette méthode a été empruntée à celle que M. Louis Martin a employée pour la toxine diphtérique, avec la différence que je n'ai pas employé l'estomac de porc pour la digestion. J'ai trouvé que ce milieu de culture donne aussi pour les produits toxiques du bacterium coli de meilleurs résultats, que l'ordinaire bouillon peptonisé. Par exemple, la toxine obtenue avec ce milieu de culture, introduite dans le péritoine d'un cobaye de 500 grammes, le tue dans 12 à 18 heures à la dose de 4 c.c. ½, tandis que celle obtenue avec le commun bouillon peptoné au deux pour cent tue un cobaye du même poids à la dose de 6 centimètres cubes.

3° Bouillon de rate de bœuf digérée, comme dans la méthode précédente. On sait que Chantemesse a obtenu une toxine typhique assez énergique, en employant comme terrain de culture une solution de peptone de rate préparée selon la méthode de Martin; et qu'il a été porté à employer ce milieu par la considération que le bacille d'Eberth se développe très abondamment dans la rate et y vit longtemps.

Connaissant l'affinité qui existe entre le bacille d'Eberth et le colibacille, j'ai voulu moi aussi employer le bouillon de rate digérée, mais j'ai obtenu une toxine, dont l'activité n'est que peu supérieure aux précédentes, car elle tue un cobaye de 500 grammes à la dose de 3 à 4 centimètres cubes en 12 à 18 heures.

4° Bouillon de moelle osseuse digérée. La même considération m'a conduit à employer ce bouillon, mais il ne m'a pas donné de bons résultats.

5° Bouillon de cerveau digéré. On sait par les recherches de MM. Thoinot et Masselin que c'est dans le bulbe et dans la moelle épinière qu'il faut rechercher le colibacille, quand il est disparu des autres organes ; c'est pourquoi on doit supposer qu'il trouve dans la substance nerveuse des conditions de vie plus favorables qu'ailleurs. C'est pour cette raison que j'ai été conduit à employer le bouillon de cerveau digéré, comme Chantemesse avait employé le bouillon de rate pour le bacille d'Eberth. J'ai constaté que le colibacille se développe rapidement et richement dans ce terrain, de façon que ce milieu est fort propre pour un diagnostic bactériologique rapide, mais que les toxines qui s'y produisent sont peu supérieures, sinon égales, à celles qui se développent dans le bouillon de rate.

6° Bouillon de foie. Ce n'est pas un terrain propre, car il donne vite naissance à une réaction acide très prononcée.

7° Sérum de lait. Ce n'est pas non plus un bon terrain.

8° Sérum de sang absolu ou dilué avec une solution de chlorure de sodium à 0,75 pour cent. Il ne donne pas non plus de bons résultats.

9° Milieu composé de bouillon de rate ou de bouillon de cerveau, 4/5, et de sérum de sang ou liquide ascitique 1/5. C'est le meilleur des milieux que j'ai employés. Il n'est pas à conseiller d'ajouter une plus grande quantité de sérum ou de liquide ascitique, car le liquide, à cause de sa grande densité, se laisse filtrer très difficilement à la bougie de porcelaine.

J'ai obtenu de la sorte une toxine capable de tuer en 24 heures un cobaye de 500 grammes à la dose de 2 centimètres cubes par injection péritonéale, et un lapin de 950 grammes à la dose d'un centimètre cube et demi par injection endoveineuse.

10° Bouillon de viande de cheval peptonisée au 2 pour cent. J'ai constaté que c'est un très bon terrain pour le développement de la toxine du colibacille, supérieur au bouillon de viande de bœuf. Je me réserve de faire d'autres expériences avec le bouillon de viande de cheval digérée.

Enfin 11° Décoction de maïs absolue ou mêlée avec du bouillon de cerveau à parties égales. M. Lenti, considérant que la diversité de l'alimentation contribue notablement à la virulence des microbes intestinaux, spécialement du bacterium coli, a employé différentes substances alimentaires comme milieux de culture pour le coli-bacille, et il a trouvé que la décoction de maïs fait développer un coli-bacille très virulent et toxique. Mes résultats ne sont pas trop satisfaisants à ce point de vue, soit avec la simple décoction de maïs, soit avec le mélange de cette décoction et du bouillon de cerveau.

De façon que les terrains de culture qui m'ont donné les meilleurs résultats quant au développement de la toxine du coli-bacille, sont le bouillon de rate digéré et celui de cerveau aussi digéré, avec l'addition d'un peu de sérum de sang de bœuf ou de liquide ascitique.

Je n'ai pas expérimenté avec le sérum de sang humain.

Les animaux que j'ai employés, c'est-à-dire les cobayes et les lapins, étant injectés avec de fortes doses, tombent vite dans un état d'abattement qui s'accentue toujours plus jusqu'à la mort de l'animal, qui arrive souvent au milieu de convulsions, d'abord cloniques et puis tétaniques. Il se produit promptement un abaissement de la température qui augmente jusqu'à la mort, et un amaigrissement considérable. Les petites doses produisent au contraire une légère élévation de la température, qui revient bien vite au normal si la dose n'est pas mortelle, ou bien s'abaisse considérablement si la dose est mortelle. Les injections sous-cutanées donnent lieu à la formation d'abcès aseptiques.

C'est un fait remarquable que, même les petites doses qui ne semblent pas mortelles, produisent souvent une lente et progressive cachexie qui tue les animaux après plusieurs jours.

L'examen microscopique des organes des animaux morts après 12 à 48 heures permet de voir une considérable hyperémie dans le foie, les reins et les capsules surrénales, la rate, l'intestin grêle, et souvent aussi les poumons. Il n'y a pas de liquide dans les cavités séreuses, excepté si l'injection a été faite dans le péritoine, dans lequel cas celui-ci se montre fort rougi et avec une sérosité trouble plus ou moins abondante.

3e Question. — Cette toxine joue-t-elle le rôle le plus important, sinon unique, dans l'action pathogène de la bactérie qui l'a produite ?

C'est la même question qui a été faite à propos de la pathogénie du charbon, de l'infection staphylococcique, streptococcique et d'autres infections septicémiques.

Je crois que, même dans l'infection coli-bacillaire, et peut-être aussi dans les autres, dont je viens de parler, l'action principale est due aux produits toxiques qui, s'ils ne sont pas bien actifs, doivent par compensation se former en grande quantité, étant donné l'immense multiplication et diffusion des bacilles dans tout l'organisme. Mais je crois aussi qu'il ne faut pas négliger les autres facteurs, qui ont été invoqués isolément par les auteurs, mais qui, selon moi, exercent tous ensemble leur action sur l'organisme : j'entends parler de la soustraction d'oxygène et de matériaux nutritifs de la part d'un nombre si énorme de germes, de l'action mécanique sur les tissus et des embolies et des thromboses multiples auxquelles ils donnent lieu.

4e Question. — Quelle est la nature de ces produits toxiques ? Peut-on les comparer à la toxine diphtérique et à la tétanique ?

Comme le disent bien MM. Guinard et Artaud, le mécanisme d'action des toxines microbiennes peut se manifester de trois manières différentes.

1e Avec quelques toxines on observe des manifestations immédiates qui rappellent plus ou moins les symptômes de la maladie déterminée par le microbe qui les a sécrétées, ou bien elles n'ont aucun caractère spécifique et sérieux : un exemple pour le premier cas, c'est la toxine du choléra aviaire ; pour le deuxième, les produits solubles du b. pyocyanique, du staphylocoque pyogène, etc.

2° Il y a des toxines, comme celles du bacille diphthérique, qui introduites dans une veine ne produisent rien de bien apparent et d'important immédiatement après l'injection, mais qui, après une phase silencieuse de durée variable, provoquent des troubles plus ou moins graves qui s'exagèrent progressivement et produisent souvent la mort de l'animal.

3° Il y a enfin d'autres toxines qui produisent immédiatement des modifications fonctionnelles, coïncident avec leur introduction dans la veine ; mais ces effets immédiats disparaissent après une durée relativement brève, pour faire place à une période de calme, pendant laquelle l'animal semble complètement rétabli. Mais bien souvent il ne s'agit que d'un rétablissement apparent, car après quelques heures il apparaît des phénomènes toxiques différents des premiers par quelques-uns de leurs caractères, mais spécialement par leur marche. Ces dernières toxines agissent donc comme poisons et comme ferments. Or, étant donné la complexité de la composition et la diversité des produits solubles élaborés par les microbes, sur lesquelles bien des auteurs ont insisté, on a le droit de supposer que ce ne sont pas les mêmes éléments chimiques de la même élaboration totale qui ont la double action de poison et de ferment, mais que dans une même toxine il peut exister soit un poison direct, soit un ferment, soit l'un et l'autre à la fois. A cette dernière catégorie appartiennent, selon les auteurs les toxines du pneumo-bacillus liquefaciens bovis et la malléine.

Voilà ce que disent les auteurs que j'ai nommés.

Or, pour la deuxième catégorie de toxines, comme la diphtérique, il faut ajouter au caractère qu'elles ont d'agir après une période d'incubation, deux autres propriétés importantes, c'est-à-dire la propriété d'agir à très petites doses et celle de provoquer, quand elles sont injectées d'abord à doses petites et atténuées et puis à doses plus fortes, l'ainsi dite immunité active dans les animaux injectés et la formation d'antitoxines dans leurs humeurs.

Dans laquelle de ces catégories devons-nous placer la toxine colibacillaire que j'ai obtenue ?

Il lui manque la propriété d'agir à petites doses, car un coli-bacille qui tue un cobaye de 500 grammes à la dose d'un cinquantième de centimètre cube m'a donné, dans le bouillon de cerveau mêlé avec du liquide ascitique, une toxine capable de tuer en 24 heures un lapin de 950 grammes à la dose d'un centimètre cube et demi.

Il semble manquer, à ce que j'ai pu juger par un examen superficiel, la période d'incubation, car les animaux que j'ai injectés avec des doses mortelles tombent tout de suite dans un état d'abattement dont ils ne se relèvent plus.

Et il semble manquer aussi le troisième caractère. En effet, beaucoup de cobayes et trois lapins que j'ai injectés avec des doses croissantes de toxine sont tous morts à la suite d'une considérable cachexie, et le sérum d'un lapin ainsi traité ne m'a montré ni des propriétés préventives, ni des propriétés antitoxiques *in vitro*. Ce sérum, inoculé à la dose de 2 centimètres cubes à un cobaye, ne l'a pas préservé de l'action léthale d'une dose mortelle de toxine que je lui ai injectée après deux heures, et mêlé avec la toxine dans la proportion de 2 pour 5, n'a pas détruit l'action de cette toxine.

Peut-être en employant tout le temps (deux ans) que M. Chantemesse a employé pour immuniser un cheval contre la toxine typhique, et en faisant les injections à de longs intervalles, comme il l'a fait, on pourra arriver à obtenir un sérum antitoxique, comme disent l'avoir obtenu, même avant les expériences de Chantemesse sur le bacille typhique, MM. Cesaris-Demel et Orlando, Salvati et de Gaetano, Albarran et Mosny.

Mais cela est réservé à des expériences ultérieures.

En tout cas, s'il est permis de tirer des conclusions des résultats que j'ai obtenus jusqu'ici, il faut dire que les produits toxiques du coli-bacille ordinaire de l'intestin humain n'appartiennent pas à la catégorie de la toxine diphtérique, mais qu'ils sont des poisons variés à action immédiate.

L'étude de leurs propriétés physiques et chimiques pourra apporter beaucoup de lumière sur leur nature.

Des expériences ultérieures pourront démontrer s'il y a des colibacilles spéciaux qui, outre à posséder des propriétés toxigènes très prononcées, comme celui isolé dernièrement par Roger, produisent des toxines agissant comme de véritables ferments.

J'exprime la plus vive gratitude à M. le professeur Fede, qui m'a donné le moyen de faire ces expériences dans son laboratoire.

RECHERCHES EXPÉRIMENTALES
SUR LE ROLE PROTECTEUR DU FOIE CONTRE QUELQUES ALCALOIDES CHEZ LES ANIMAUX JEUNES ET ADULTES

par M. le docteur Giuseppe Antonio PETRONE,

de Naples.[1]

Il résulte des recherches de nombreux observateurs, spécialement de celles de M. Bouchard et de son école, que l'organisme humain est continuellement menacé d'intoxication par des substances nuisibles, qui proviennent du monde extérieur ou qui se produisent chez lui; substances qui en altéreraient certainement l'intégrité anatomique et fonctionnelle, s'ils ne pouvaient opposer à leur action des moyens énergiques de défense.

Nous pouvons dire, en général, que ces moyens de défense agissent par deux mécanismes fondamentaux : soit par la transformation des matières toxiques en produits inoffensifs ou utiles, soit par leur élimination. Ainsi, pour citer quelques exemples, la thyroïde et les capsules surrénales exercent leur action de défense en transformant les substances toxiques, tandis que le rein nous représente le type des organes éliminateurs, quoique quelques auteurs lui aient attribué aussi une sécrétion intérieure antitoxique.

Entre ces deux catégories d'organes nous devons placer le foie, qui joue sans doute un rôle très important dans la défense de l'organisme contre les intoxications, et dont l'action s'exerce par des mécanismes variés.

En effet, il arrête et transforme beaucoup de poisons d'origine alimentaire, comme les peptones et les savons; il arrête et rend inoffensifs plusieurs produits de la putréfaction des albuminoïdes, comme l'indol et le phénol, en les transformant en acides sulfo-conjugués; il retient les bromures et les iodures, les sels de fer et ceux de cuivre; il protège l'organisme contre d'autres produits de la putréfaction, notamment contre les ptomaïnes et, selon MM. Charrin et Cassin[2], contre ceux des produits toxiques des bactéries pathogènes, qui sont solubles dans l'alcool, tandis que M. Padoa[3] admet une action pro-

---

1. Travail de l'Institut de la Clinique des enfants de l'Université royale de Naples, dirigée par M. le prof. F. Fede, communiqué au XIIIe Congrès international de médecine, tenu à Paris du 2 au 9 août 1900.

2. CHARRIN et CASSIN. Des fonctions actives de la muqueuse de l'intestin dans la défense de l'organisme. *Arch. de phys.*, 1896.

3. PADOA. Sul diverso modo di agire della tossina tifica e della difterica a

tectrice même contre une véritable toxine, la toxine diphtérique ; enfin il agit sur les sels ammoniacaux et sur les produits azotés intermédiaires de la désassimilation organique, en les transformant en urée, qui, comme l'on sait, est une substance non seulement inoffensive, mais même utile à l'organisme par son action diurétique. Ainsi, comme le dit M. Roger[1], le foie est aussi le collaborateur de la fonction urinaire.

Ce même auteur[2] a démontré, d'autre part, que le foie exerce aussi une action de défense contre quelques microorganismes, comme celui du charbon et le staphylococcus aureus, et, dans un récent travail[3], il dit avoir constaté cette même action contre un coli-bacille spécial, qu'il a isolé des selles d'individus atteints de dysenterie et contre ses toxines.

M. Lemaire[4] croit, en outre, à l'action protectrice du foie contre le coli-bacille ordinaire, qui serait englobé et détruit par les endothéliums des vaisseaux hépatiques, tandis que Roger a trouvé que d'autres coli-bacilles qu'il a employés subissent une augmentation de virulence en traversant le foie.

Comme l'on voit, la fonction de défense du foie est très importante, puisqu'elle s'exerce soit contre les poisons provenant du tube alimentaire, qui, comme on le sait, est la source la plus abondante de matières toxiques pour l'organisme, soit contre ceux qui se produisent au sein des tissus, et en outre aussi contre quelques bactéries.

Cette fonction, pour ce qui concerne les poisons, est en partie une fonction d'élimination, comme celle du rein, en ce qu'une partie des poisons qui traversent cet organe sont éliminés avec la bile ; en partie c'est une fonction purement mécanique, en ce que le foie ralentit le passage dans la circulation générale de toutes les substances qui le traversent, et en ce qu'il en arrête plusieurs pour les reverser ensuite peu à peu dans la veine cave ; enfin, c'est une fonction chimique, en ce que le foie transforme en des produits inoffensifs ou utiles une partie des poisons qu'il a retenus.

Roger[5], d'autre part, a constaté un étroit parallélisme entre la fonction protectrice du foie et son contenu en glycogène. Ainsi elle

seconda che siano iniettate nella vena porta e nella vena gingulare. *Rev. méd.*, III, 1899.

1. Roger. Les intoxications. *Traité de path. gén.* de Bouchard, 1895.
2. Action des organes sur les microbes. *Soc. de biol.*, 12 mars 1898.
3. Le colibacille de la dysenterie. *Presse méd.*, 1900.
4. Lemaire. Rôle protecteur du foie contre le genre colibacillaire. *Arch. de méd. expér.*, 1899.
5. Roger. Action des organes sur les microbes, *loc. cit.*

manque dans le foie des embryons avant la formation du glycogène : elle diminue ou cesse entièrement dans le foie des animaux auxquels vient à manquer le glycogène pour une raison quelconque, comme dans l'inanition ; elle augmente, lorsque le contenu du glycogène croît, comme à la suite de l'administration du sucre à petites doses.

Or, tous les expérimentateurs qui ont étudié cette importante question se sont servis, pour leurs recherches, d'animaux adultes ou pas trop jeunes.

Il se pose donc la question suivante : Le foie de la première période de la vie exerce-t-il une action protectrice manifeste contre les poisons ?

Cette action est-elle égale, inférieure ou supérieure à celle du foie des adultes ?

Si nous considérons que cette action est exercée par la cellule hépatique, et que dans l'enfance la cellule hépatique n'a pas encore atteint son complet développement anatomique et fonctionnel, nous devrions dire *a priori* que la fonction protectrice du foie des enfants est inférieure à celle des adultes.

Mais, d'autre part, si nous tenons compte du volume de l'organe, qui est beaucoup plus grand chez l'enfant que chez l'adulte, comparativement au poids du corps ; de la vascularisation, qui, dans le foie de l'enfant, est plus riche, et de la sécrétion biliaire, qui chez lui semble plus abondante, nous devrions dire, au contraire, que la fonction protectrice du foie est supérieure chez l'enfant à ce qu'elle est chez l'adulte.

L'expérimentation peut seule résoudre cette question, qui certainement doit être considérée comme très importante, si l'on réfléchit, d'une part, que dans l'organisme infantile il y a une formation très abondante de produits toxiques, soit qu'ils proviennent du tube alimentaire, soit qu'ils proviennent de la vie cellulaire, si active en eux ; et, d'autre part, que les faibles tubes digestifs et la muqueuse intestinale, encore incomplètement développée, et peut-être les reins mêmes, ne peuvent pas exercer une action énergique de défense. J'ai dit même *les reins*, car il résulte des recherches de MM. Dastre et Loye[1] que, tandis que les reins des adultes, comme un filtre parfait, expulsent de l'organisme tout l'excès de solution physiologique de chlorure de sodium, que l'on introduit dans la masse sanguine, les reins des jeunes animaux ne possèdent pas à un égal degré cette fonction éliminatrice. Il en est donc peut-être de même pour d'autres substances.

Je passe à présent à l'exposition des premiers résultats des expé-

---

1. Dastre et Loye. Lavage du sang. *Arch. de phys.*, 1888, p. 95. — Sur l'injection de l'eau salée dans les vaisseaux. *Ibid.*, 1889, p. 255.

riences que j'ai entreprises pour la solution de la question sus-énoncée.

II. — Les auteurs qui ont étudié la fonction protectrice du foie ont suivi des voies différentes.

Quelques-uns ont supprimé la fonction hépatique, ou par l'extirpation de l'organe aux animaux (batraciens), ou par la ligature des vaisseaux hépatiques (*idem*), ou par l'injection d'une solution très diluée d'acide sulfurique dans la veine porte, ou par l'abouchement de la veine porte dans la veine cave inférieure ; et ensuite ils ont étudié, chez les animaux ainsi traités, l'action des poisons, aussi bien de ceux qui se produisent dans l'organisme même, que de ceux que l'on pouvait y introduire artificiellement.

D'autres ont tâché de résoudre cette question, en étudiant les différences de toxicité entre le sang de la veine porte et le sang des veines sushépatiques.

D'autres ont étudié l'action du foie sur les matières toxiques, hors de l'organisme ; et dans ce but, ils ont fait circuler artificiellement des solutions de substances toxiques dans des foies détachés du corps de l'animal, ou bien ils ont trituré des morceaux de foie et les ont mêlés avec les solutions toxiques.

D'autres, enfin, ont étudié l'action de défense du foie, en injectant les solutions toxiques, chez quelques animaux, dans une veine périphérique, et chez d'autres dans un rameau de la veine porte.

J'ai préféré, pour mes recherches, cette dernière méthode, car, avec certaines précautions, elle réalise mieux que les autres les conditions qui se vérifient dans les intoxications ordinaires, notamment de la part du tube gastro-intestinal.

Les poisons qui, dans les conditions normales ou pathologiques, passent dans la circulation porte, y entrent sans doute très lentement, à doses fractionnées et répétées, de façon qu'ils subissent une forte dilution dans la masse sanguine porte, et le foie a tout le temps nécessaire pour exercer sur eux son action.

De là la nécessité de faire des solutions très diluées des poisons à injecter et de faire l'injection très lentement, si l'on veut que l'expérimentation se rapproche autant que possible de ce qui se produit spontanément dans l'organisme.

Il faut, en outre, prendre d'autres précautions, si l'on veut éviter différentes causes d'erreur, c'est-à-dire il faut que l'injection soit faite sous une pression uniforme et constante, que la température du liquide soit égale à celle de l'animal à injecter, et que la dilution de la substance toxique et la rapidité de l'injection soient telles que l'injection soit terminée avant qu'il se produise une élimination considérable du poison. C'est seulement de la sorte que nous trouverons, avec la plus grande approximation possible, le vrai équivalent toxique expérimental, c'est-à-dire la quantité minime de poison qui, contenue dans la masse sanguine, est capable de produire la mort immédiate de l'animal.

Nous nous sommes donc guidé, dans la technique opératoire, par les résultats des expériences de MM. Dastre et Loye[1], suivant lesquelles, si l'on injecte de la solution physiologique de chlorure de sodium dans les veines des chiens avec une vitesse de 0,7 à 1 centimètre cube par minute et par kilogramme d'animal, et dans les veines des lapins avec une vitesse de 5 centimètres cubes sous une pression constante et à une température égale à celle du corps, on obtient une légère élimination du liquide, seulement après que la quantité du liquide injecté a atteint le quart de la masse sanguine de l'animal; et la quantité du liquide qui s'élimine par les reins est égale à celle que l'on introduit au fur et à mesure dans la veine, quand la quantité d'eau injectée a atteint le volume de la masse sanguine.

Avec ces règles présentes à l'esprit, nous pourrons très bien doser le degré de dilution à donner aux poisons que nous voulons employer, en tenant compte de leur pouvoir toxique.

III. — Mes expériences se sont bornées jusqu'ici à deux alcaloïdes végétaux : la strychnine et la morphine; et j'ai employé, comme animaux d'expérience, des chiens adultes et de petits chiens âgés de 20 à 70 jours, ayant toujours soin d'en prendre soit le poids du corps, soit celui du foie.

J'aurais dû faire aussi des recherches sur le contenu de glycogène du foie des petits chiens à l'âge de ceux que j'ai employés, car, autant que je sais, il n'existe pas de semblables recherches : mais je me réserve de les faire plus tard.

J'ai tâché, en outre, autant que possible, d'éviter les causes d'erreur dépendant de la diversité de race, de poids et d'âge, et quelquefois j'ai pu expérimenter à la fois sur des chiennes mères et sur leurs petits.

J'ai eu soin aussi de mettre tous les animaux dans les mêmes conditions opératoires, en ouvrant la cavité abdominale même à ceux qui étaient injectés dans la veine jugulaire; et j'ai cherché à éviter soit les pertes de sang, soit le refroidissement des intestins, qui est si nuisible notamment chez les jeunes animaux, chez lesquels, ainsi qu'il

1. DASTRE et LOYE (loc. cit.).

résulte des recherches de MM. Dastre et Loye, l'appareil régulateur thermique ne fonctionne pas encore d'une manière parfaite.

Comme les autres auteurs, qui ont fait de semblables expériences, j'ai recherché ce qui a été appelé par Joffroy et Serveau[1] la « toxicité expérimentale », et non pas la toxicité vraie, et cela pour avoir des résultats plus immédiats ; et j'ai tâché en même temps d'augmenter la valeur de mes résultats par la multiplicité des expériences.

Pour la strychnine, j'ai choisi la solution de sulfate à 1 sur 50 000 ; pour la morphine, la solution d'hydrochlorate au centième. Ces substances provenaient de la fabrique Merk.

La vitesse de l'injection a été de 1 centimètre cube par minute et par kilogramme.

Voici maintenant les tableaux d'ensemble de mes expériences :

Expériences faites avec la morphine.

	POIDS DU CORPS Gr.	POIDS DU FOIE Gr.	POIDS DU FOIE par kil. du corps Gr.	VEINE dans laquelle a été faite l'injection.	DOSE MORTELLE absolue. c. c.	DOSE MORTELLE par kilog. c. c.	RAPPORT
A. — Jeunes chiens.							
I. — Petit chien âgé de 55 jours.	970	51	52	v. jugul.	58	39	1 : 1.73
Petit chien frère. .	850	54	56.8	v. porte	62	67.56	
II. — Petit chien âgé de 60 jours.	1280	75	58.59	v. jugul.	48	37.49	1 : 1.62
Petit chien frère. .	1548	70	51.1	v. porte	82	60.76	
III. — Petit chien âgé de 70 jours.	2070	95	45.89	v. jugul.	80	38.6	
Petit chien frère. .	2000	96	48	v. porte	40[1]	20	
B. — Chiens adultes.							
I. — Chienne, mère des petits chiens n° I.	6470	256	57.49	v. jugul.	198	50.5	1 : 1.40
Chienne, mère des petits chiens n° II.	7000	245	55	v. porte	500	42.88	
II. — Chien adulte. . . .	4600	171	52.82	v. jugul.	128	29	1 : 1.62
—	4870	176	56.15	v. porte	250	47.23	
III. — Chien adulte. . . .	5200	199	58.26	v. jugul.	150	37.49	1 : 1.51
—	5400	217	40	v. porte	255	60.76	

1. Ce petit chien a subi de grandes pertes de sang pendant l'opération.

1. Joffroy et Serveau. Considérations générales sur la recherche de la toxicité expérimentale et toxicité vraie. *Arch. de méd. expér.*, 1896.

Expériences faites avec le sulfate de strychnine.

	POIDS DU CORPS Gr.	POIDS DU FOIE Gr.	POIDS DU FOIE par kil. du corps. Gr.	VEINE dans laquelle a été faite l'injection	DOSE MORTELLE absolue, c. c.	DOSE MORTELLE par kilog. c. c.	RAPPORT
A. — Jeunes chiens.							
I. — Petit chien âgé de 25 jours.	800	56	44	v. jugul.	18	22.5	1:5.1
Petit chien, frère du précédent. . . .	840	40	47.5	v. porte	60	71.4	
II. — Petit chien âgé de 25 jours.	955	51	55.5	v. jugul.	54	55.6	1:1.2
Petit chien frère .	840	48	57	v. porte	56	42.8	
III. — Petit chien âgé de 20 jours.	482	25	51.5	v. jugul.	7	14.5	1:5
Petit chien frère .	505	50.5	65.9	v. porte	22	45.5	
IV. — Petit chien âgé de deux mois. . . .	1585	75	54.1	v. jugul.	15	10.9	1:2.07
Petit chien frère .	1497	70	46.8	v. porte	54	22.6	
V. — Petit chien âgé de 50 jours.	740	51	68.8	v. jugul.	14	18.91	1:1.89
Petit chien frère .	780	50.7	60.4	v. porte	28	55.89	
VI. — Petit chien âgé de 45 jours.	755	52	68.87	v. jugul.	14	18.5	1:0.98
Petit chien frère .	655	41	62.59	v. porte	12	18.2*	
VII. — Petit chien âgé de 70 jours.	1500	100	66.66	v. jugul.	22	14.67	1:1.75
Petit chien frère .	1654	80	48.56	v. porte	40	25.59	
B. — Chiens adultes.							
I. — Chien adulte. . . .	4060	190	46.7	v. jugul.	142	54.9	1:1.22
—	5660	116	51.6	v. porte	155	42.8	
II. — Chienne adulte mère des petits chiens V.	4520	185	40.4	v. jugul.	60	15.28	1:1.56
Chienne adulte, mère des petits chiens IV.	4790	190	59.6	v. porte	100	20.8	
III. — Chien adulte. . . .	5000	190	57.5	v. jugul.	67	15.50	
—	4000	161	40.25	—	62	15.5	
—	5900	210	55.59	—	78	15.22	1:1.96
Chien adulte.	4450	155	54.5	v. porte	155	50.56	
—	4740	180	57.9	—	114	24.05	
—	3850	122	51.5	—	106	27.8	

Quelles conclusions pouvons-nous tirer de l'examen des expériences exposées dans les tableaux précédents?

1° En examinant les résultats des expériences faites avec la strychnine, on voit clairement que l'équivalent toxique expérimental de ce poison, c'est-à-dire la dose mortelle par kilogramme d'animal, varie beaucoup d'un animal à l'autre, notamment chez les animaux très jeunes, et cela soit chez ceux injectés dans la veine jugulaire, soit chez ceux injectés dans la veine porte. *En général*, cependant, *il est plus élevé chez les chiens très jeunes que chez les chiens adultes.*

En effet. — *a*) Chez les petits chiens injectés dans la veine jugulaire, l'équivalent toxique est représenté par les chiffres suivants :

$$10.9 - 14,5 - 14,67 - 18,5 - 18,9 - 22,5 - 55,6$$
$$\text{moyenne} \quad 19,55 :$$

b) Chez les petits chiens injectés dans la veine porte :

$$17.2 - 22,6 - 25,59 - 55,89 - 42,8 - 45,5 - 71,4$$
$$\text{moyenne} \quad 57,11 :$$

Le rapport entre les deux moyennes, représenté par l'équation $19,55 : 57,11 :: 1 : x$, est de $1 : 1,90$.

c) Chez les chiens adultes injectés dans la veine jugulaire :

$$15,28 - 15,28 - 15,50 - 15,5 - 54,9$$
$$\text{moyenne} \quad 18,04 :$$

Comme on le voit, chez ces chiens, si l'on exclut le dernier chiffre, très élevé. les résultats ont été plus uniformes.

d) Chez les chiens adultes injectés dans la veine porte :

$$20.8 - 24,05 - 27,8 - 50,56 - 42,8$$
$$\text{moyenne} = 29.2 :$$

Le rapport entre ces deux moyennes, représenté par l'équation $18,04 : 29.2 :: 1 : x$, est de $1 : 1,61$.

Cette variabilité. remarquable notamment chez les petits chiens, dérive, à mon avis. en grande partie, de la diversité d'âge des petits chiens et peut-être aussi de la diversité de leur nutrition, dépendant de l'allaitement maternel. Malgré cela, les résultats ne perdent pas de leur valeur, car, comme on l'a vu, chaque expérience a été faite, chez les petits chiens. sur des individus qui étaient nés de la même mère et qui étaient du même âge et à peu près du même poids.

Les résultats des expériences faites avec la morphine sont, au contraire, plus uniformes : et cela dépend, selon moi, soit du nombre plus restreint des expériences, soit de la différence plus petite dans l'âge des jeunes chiens, soit enfin du soin plus grand que j'ai pris dans le choix des animaux pour cette deuxième série d'expériences.

Voilà les chiffres représentant l'équivalent toxique de ce poison :

a) Chez les petits chiens injectés dans la veine jugulaire :

$$37,49 - 58,6 - 59$$
$$\text{moyenne} \quad 38,56 :$$

b) Chez les petits chiens injectés dans la veine porte :

$$60,76 - 67,56 - 20$$
$$\text{moyenne} = 64,06.$$

Il ne faut pas tenir compte du dernier chiffre, car il représente la dose mortelle par kilogramme d'un petit chien qui, pendant l'opération, eut de grandes pertes de sang.

Le rapport entre les deux moyennes, représenté par l'équation
$$58,56 : 64,06 :: 1 : x, \text{ est de } 1 : 1,67.$$

c) Chez les chiens adultes injectés dans la veine jugulaire :

$$29 - 50,5 - 57,49$$
$$\text{moyenne} = 52,25.$$

d) Chez les chiens adultes injectés dans la veine porte :

$$42,88 - 47,22 - 60,76$$
$$\text{moyenne} = 50,29.$$

Le rapport entre ces deux moyennes, représenté par l'équation
$$52,25 : 50,29 :: 1 : x, \text{ est de } 1 : 1,55.$$

Comme on le voit, *aussi pour la morphine l'équivalent toxique est plus grand chez les chiens très jeunes que chez les adultes.*

On n'observe pas la même chose dans la clinique, car, au dire de la plupart des cliniciens, la morphine est beaucoup mieux tolérée dans l'âge adulte que dans l'enfance. Mais peut-être est-il hasardé d'établir ici une comparaison entre les résultats de mes expériences et ceux de la clinique, car, comme je l'ai dit, j'ai recherché chez mes animaux la toxicité expérimentale et non pas la toxicité vraie.

2° Si nous examinons soit les rapports qui existent, pour chaque couple d'animaux, entre l'équivalent toxique chez les chiens injectés dans la veine jugulaire et l'équivalent toxique chez ceux injectés dans la veine porte, soit le rapport existant entre les moyennes de ces équivalents toxiques, nous devons dire que *l'action protectrice du foie contre les deux alcaloïdes que j'ai employés est assez énergique chez les chiens très jeunes, et elle est même un peu supérieure à celle que l'on rencontre chez les chiens adultes.*

En effet, nous avons eu, avec la strychnine, les résultats suivants :

a) Des petits chiens injectés dans la veine porte, deux sont morts avec une dose de poison triple de celle qui a tué les chiens injectés dans la veine jugulaire (rapports = 1 : 3 — 1 : 3,1), un est mort avec une dose supérieure au double (rapport = 1 : 2,07), deux avec une dose peu inférieure au double (rapports = 1 : 1,89 — 1 : 1,75) et deux avec une dose presque égale (rapports = 1 : 1,2 — 1 : 0,98). Dans ces deux derniers cas, il s'agit probablement plutôt d'une résistance particulière de l'animal au poison (résistance exceptionnellement élevée chez le premier petit chien du couple n° II, et exceptionnellement basse chez le deuxième petit chien du couple n° VI) que d'un défaut d'action protectrice du foie, car cet organe ne présentait aucune lésion ni à l'examen macroscopique ni à l'examen microscopique.

En moyenne, la dose de strychnine capable de tuer un kilogramme d'un petit chien injecté dans la veine porte est presque le double de celle qui tue un kilogramme d'un autre petit chien injecté dans la veine jugulaire (rapport = 1 : 1,90).

c) Au contraire, pour les chiens adultes, j'ai trouvé que la dose capable de tuer un kilogramme d'un animal injecté dans la veine porte est toujours inférieure au double de celle qui tue un kilogramme d'un autre animal injecté dans la veine jugulaire (rapports = 1 : 1,22 — 1 : 1,56 — 1 : 1,96), et, en moyenne, celle-là est un peu plus d'une fois et demie supérieure à celle-ci (rapport = 1 : 1,61).

Les résultats obtenus des expériences faites avec la morphine sont les suivants :

a) Pour les petits chiens, le rapport entre l'équivalent toxique chez les animaux injectés dans la veine jugulaire et l'équivalent toxique chez les animaux injectés dans la veine porte est dans un couple de 1 : 1,75. et dans un autre de 1 : 1,62. et en moyenne de 1 : 1,67.

b) Pour les chiens adultes, ce rapport est dans un premier couple de 1 : 1,40. dans un deuxième de 1 : 1,51 et dans un troisième de 1 : 1,62. et en moyenne de 1 : 1,55.

Quelles applications peuvent avoir les conclusions sus-énoncées dans la physiologie humaine?

Si nous retenons que la moyenne de la vie humaine est de 70 ans et celle de la vie des chiens de 10 ans, c'est-à-dire la septième partie, nous savons que les petits chiens employés dans mes expériences, qui étaient âgés de 20 à 70 jours, correspondent à la période de l'enfance comprise entre le 5° et le 18° mois. Or, il résulte des statistiques de M. Birch-Hirchfeld[1] que le poids du foie est, en moyenne, de 6.1 pour 100 du poids du corps dans le premier semestre, de 5,8 pour 100 dans le deuxième semestre et de 4,5 pour 100 dans la deuxième année, de façon que dans les deux premières années nous avons une moyenne de 5,4 pour 100, tandis que dans l'âge adulte la moyenne est de 2,7 pour 100. Donc, le rapport existant entre le poids du foie de l'adulte et le poids du foie de l'enfant des deux premières

---

1. BIRCH-HIRCHFELD. Maladies du foie. (Traité des maladies des enfants de Gehrard, vol. IV).

années de la vie, relativement au poids du corps, représenté par l'équation :

$$2.7 : 5.4 :: 1 : x.$$

est de 1 : 2.

Il n'existe pas le même rapport entre le poids du foie des chiens adultes et le poids du foie des jeunes chiens.

En effet, il résulte de mes statistiques que le foie des chiens adultes pèse, en moyenne, 5,7 pour 100 du poids du corps, et celui des petits chiens (âgés de 29-70 jours) 5,55 pour 100. Donc, le rapport existant entre les deux, représenté par l'équation :

$$5.7 : 5,55 :: 1 : x$$

est de 1 : 1,49.

Par conséquent, nous savons que chez l'homme le foie des premières périodes de la vie pèse le double du foie de l'âge adulte, relativement au poids du corps (rapport = 1 : 2), tandis que, chez le chien, le foie des premières périodes de la vie pèse seulement une fois et demie plus que le foie de l'âge adulte (rapport = 1 : 1,49).

Or, s'il est permis d'appliquer à l'homme les résultats de mes expériences sur les chiens, et si le volume d'un organe a une influence sur l'énergie de ses fonctions, il faut dire que *l'action protectrice du foie des enfants est plus énergique que celle du foie des adultes.*

En terminant, j'adresse ici l'expression de ma reconnaissance à M. le professeur Fede, qui m'a permis de faire ces recherches dans son laboratoire.

LA GLYCOSURIE ALIMENTAIRE DANS LA GASTRO-ENTÉRITE DES NOURRISSONS

par M. Eugène TERRIEN,

Ancien interne des Hôpitaux de Paris

J'ai eu à plusieurs reprises, dans le service de M. le professeur Grancher à l'hôpital des Enfants-Malades, l'occasion de rechercher la glycosurie alimentaire chez des nourrissons atteints de gastro-entérite. Or, les résultats qu'on obtient alors peuvent varier dans des proportions notables, suivant la nature du sucre employé, le titre de la dilution, la plus ou moins longue durée du temps d'absorption. Pour que ces résultats soient comparables entre eux, il est donc indispensable de suivre une technique toujours identique.

Et d'abord quel sucre employer? On a le choix entre trois substances : la saccharose, la glucose, la lactose. La saccharose ne nous a pas paru utilisable : elle n'est assimilable, en effet, qu'à la condition d'être transformée en lévulose et glucose. Que cette transformation soit troublée (ce qu'on peut craindre, puisqu'il s'agit ici de troubles digestifs), la saccharose passera dans l'urine sans modification ; or cette saccharosurie est de valeur nulle.

La glucose, à condition qu'elle soit pure (car la glucose impure donne des résultats tout différents) paraît tout d'abord être la substance de choix. En effet, chez le nourrisson à l'état physiologique, la tolérance du foie pour cette sorte de sucre est considérable, et l'on peut donner de fortes doses sans que la glycosurie apparaisse. Quand la fonction hépatique est troublée, au contraire, la glycosurie apparaît rapidement avec des doses faibles. Les écarts sont donc considérables, et par suite l'appréciation plus facile.

Voilà les avantages: mais il y a aussi les inconvénients : par suite de sa saveur très prononcée, la glucose est mal acceptée par les enfants; ils la refusent, ou ne prennent le biberon qu'en plusieurs fois (ce qui change les conditions de l'expérience) ou enfin ils vomissent après la tétée.

Avec la lactose, au contraire, les enfants vomissent rarement; ils prennent volontiers le biberon. Mais la méthode est moins sensible, pour ainsi dire. En effet le pouvoir d'assimilation du foie pour la lactose est moins élevé à l'état physiologique que pour la glucose, si bien qu'il y a ici beaucoup moins d'écart entre les doses qui provoquent la glycosurie alimentaire physiologique, et celles qui déterminent la glycosurie alimentaire pathologique

Quant au mode d'administration, il a toujours été le même : le sucre (lactose ou glucose pures) était ajouté au lait du biberon et absorbé dans un laps de temps variant entre dix et vingt minutes.

La recherche du sucre dans l'urine était faite au bout de trois à cinq heures au moyen de la potasse et de la liqueur de Fehling.

Quarante-deux examens ont ainsi été faits chez vingt et un enfants, âgés de moins d'un an, presque tous atteints de gastro-entérite à différents degrés, quelques-uns au contraire tout à fait sains. Chez ceux-ci, on déterminera la limite du *pouvoir d'assimilation* du foie normal vis-à-vis du sucre (lactose ou glucose); chez ceux-là on mesurera son abaissement dans l'état pathologique.

1. Achard et Weil, *Soc. méd. des hôpit.*, 10 mars 1898.

I. — René B.... 5 semaines : pèse 6270 gr. Enfant bien portant, prend des doses croissantes de glucose pure.

Février	glucose			
Le 7	12 gr.	soit 2 gr. par kil. du poids du corps : négatif		
9	18 gr.	3 gr.	—	
12	26 gr.	4 gr.	—	
15	30 gr.	5 gr.	—	
19	36 gr.	6 gr.		positif

L'enfant n'a à aucun moment présenté de diarrhée.

II. — Gustave B..., 5 semaines : pèse 4950 gr. Enfant bien portant. Prend aussi des doses croissantes de glucose pure.

Février	glucose			
Le 8	15 gr.	soit 3 gr. par kil. du poids du corps ; négatif		
12	20 gr.	4 gr.	—	
14	28 gr.	5 gr. 50	—	positif

L'enfant n'a pas présenté de diarrhée.

III. — H..., 6 semaines : pèse 5600 gr. Bien portant ; prend la glucose à doses progressives.

27 février prend 18 gr. de glucose, soit 5 gr. par kil. : négatif
5 mars — 22 gr. — 6 gr. —

L'enfant parti bien portant est ramené par la mère le 28 mars, amaigri (il pèse maintenant 5070 gr.), sans diarrhée.

28 mars prend 15 gr. de glucose, soit 5 gr. par kil. : négatif
5 avril — 22 gr. 7 gr. —
6 avril — 24 gr. — 7 gr. 50 — : positif

L'enfant est repris par la mère qui le ramène un mois plus tard ; enfant très émacié, aspect athrepsique, diarrhée.

2 mai prend 12 gr. de glucose ; soit 4 gr. par kil. : positif.

IV. — René B..., un an : pèse 6200 gr. Diarrhée à plusieurs reprises, bien qu'augmentant de poids (280 gr. en quatre jours). Foie gros.
Prend 20 gr. de glucose pure, soit 5 gr. 50 par kil. : positif.

V. — Enfant de un mois : pèse 2600 gr. Gastro-entérite depuis huit jours.
Prend 10 gr. de glucose ; soit 4 gr. par kil. : épreuve positive.

VI. — Émile C.... 9 mois : pèse 6900 gr. A eu de la gastro-entérite ; va bien actuellement, bien qu'il y ait encore un peu de diarrhée jaune.
Prend 21 gr. de glucose : soit 3 gr. par kil. : résultat négatif.

VII. — Auguste B.... 5 mois : pèse 4550 gr. Diarrhée verte très abondante depuis huit jours.
Prend 14 gr. de glucose : soit 3 gr. 10 par kil. : épreuve positive.

VIII. — André V.... 8 mois : pèse 6550 gr. A eu un peu de diarrhée actuellement guérie, mais encore des vomissements.
Le 15 mars prend 30 gr. de lactose, soit 5 gr. par kil : épreuve positive

Le 27 mars, la diarrhée est revenue, persistante ; l'enfant maigrit de 50 gr. par jour.

Prend 18 gr. de lactose ; soit 5 gr. par kil. ; épreuve positive.

IX. - James C..., 4 mois : pèse 4500 gr. A eu la diarrhée verte pendant 12 jours. Guéri, engraisse de 25 gr. par jour.

24 mars prend 18 gr. de lactose : soit 4 gr. par kil. : épreuve négative.
27 — 22 gr. 50 — 5 gr. — positive.

Le 5 avril, la diarrhée est revenue ; vomissements, a maigri de 60 gr.

Prend 18 gr. de lactose pure comme le 24 mars : cette fois épreuve positive.

X. — Raymond B..., pèse 4050 gr. Athrepsie sans diarrhée.

Prend 16 gr. de lactose ; soit 4 gr. par kil. ; épreuve positive.

XI. — Georges A..., 2 mois ; pèse 2800 gr. Gastro-entérite depuis dix-huit jours, amaigrissement.

5 mai, 8 gr. 25 de lactose ; soit 5 gr. par kil. ; épreuve positive.

Le 12 mai, la diarrhée a cessé, l'enfant devient athrepsique.

Prend 7 gr. de lactose : soit 2 gr. 50 par kil : épreuve positive.

XII. — Léon P..., 7 mois : pèse 4800 gr. Diarrhée depuis trois mois, verte depuis cinq jours. Le jour de l'entrée (27 avril) :

Prend 16 gr. 50 de lactose : soit 5 gr. 50 par kil. : épreuve positive.

Le 31, la diarrhée est arrêtée, l'enfant va bien.

Prend encore 16 gr. 50 de lactose ; épreuve négative.

Le 5 mai, l'enfant va bien, engraisse.

Prend 21 gr. 50 de lactose ; soit 4 gr. 50 par kil. : épreuve négative.

Le 12, la diarrhée a repris depuis trois jours, diminue de 150 gr. en trois jours.

Prend 20 gr. de lactose ; soit 4 gr. 50 par kil. ; épreuve positive.

XIII. - Raymond F..., 2 mois : pèse 5250 gr. Diarrhée depuis quinze jours. Devient athrepsique.

50 avril 15 gr. de lactose ; soit 4 gr. 50 par kil ; épreuve positive.
5 mai 10 gr. — 5 gr. — épreuve positive.

XIV. — Georges B..., 6 semaines ; pèse 2100 gr. Diarrhée verte pendant six jours, arrêtée depuis hier.

Prend 8 gr. de lactose : soit 3 gr. 50 par kil. : épreuve positive.

XV. — Maurice C..., 5 semaines : pèse 4800 gr. Diarrhée depuis huit jours. A maigri de 150 gr. : cependant l'enfant paraît en bon état.

Prend 18 gr. de lactose : soit 4 gr. par kil. ; épreuve négative.

XVI. — Jean C..., un mois et demi : pèse 2650 gr. Le 18 mai, diarrhée verte et vomissements depuis sa naissance.

Prend 8 gr. de lactose : soit 5 gr. par kil. : épreuve positive.

Le 22 mai, la diarrhée a cessé, le poids augmente (pèse 2980 gr.).

Prend 9 gr. de lactose : soit 5 gr. par kil. : épreuve positive.

XVII. — Robert G..., 4 mois : pèse 4800 gr., 18 mai, diarrhée verte très abondante depuis huit jours.

Prend 10 gr. de lactose : soit 2 gr. 65 par kil. : épreuve positive.

Le 22 mai, l'enfant va mieux : la diarrhée est arrêtée, il engraisse de 50 gr.

Prend 11 gr. de lactose : soit 5 gr. par kil. : épreuve positive.

XVIII. — Édouard M..., 5 mois : pèse 5400 gr. Diarrhée, vomissements pendant dix jours. Va bien depuis trois jours et engraisse de 570 gr.

Prend 17 gr. de lactose : soit 5 gr. par kil. : épreuve négative.

XIX. — Pierre J..., un mois : pèse 2520 gr. Diarrhée verte depuis neuf jours.

Prend 11 gr. de lactose : soit 4 gr. 40 par kil. : épreuve négative.

XX. — Albert D..., 7 mois : pèse 5750 gr. A eu de la diarrhée à l'entrée : n'en a plus et augmente de 90 gr. en quatre jours.

Prend 14 gr. de lactose : soit 4 gr. par kil. : épreuve négative.

XXI. — Édouard L..., 5 mois : pèse 5270 gr. Diarrhée verte depuis quelques jours.

Prend 12 gr. de lactose : soit 5 gr. 50 par kil. ; épreuve négative.

De tout ceci il résulte que : *avec la glucose pure* la glycosurie alimentaire n'apparaît chez le nourrisson bien portant que si l'on dépasse *cinq grammes* par kilogramme du poids du corps : dans trois observations, en effet, concernant des enfants sains (obs I, II, III), elle n'est survenue qu'avec des doses de 6 grammes, 5 gr. 50, 7 gr. 50 par kilogramme. On peut considérer comme pathologique une glycosurie survenant avec une dose de 4 grammes par kilogramme.

Avec la lactose l'écart est moins grand entre l'état normal et l'état pathologique, et partant l'appréciation plus délicate : le pouvoir d'assimilation physiologique est en effet manifestement moins élevé. Gross[1] l'estime à 5 gr. 50 environ par kilogramme d'enfant. Ce chiffre suivant nous est trop faible : peut être s'agissait-il dans ces cas de lactose impure[2]. Pour provoquer le glycosurie alimentaire *avec la lactose* chez un nourrisson bien portant il nous a toujours fallu donner une dose supérieure à 4 gr. 50 par kilogramme. A partir de 5 gr. 50 par kilogramme, et au-dessous, la glycosurie alimentaire peut être regardée comme pathologique.

Dans ces conditions la glycosurie alimentaire a été observée dans la moitié des cas environ de gastro-entérite. Elle a varié d'un jour à l'autre chez le même enfant, suivant l'intensité de la maladie, et a paru surtout en rapport avec ces deux facteurs : diarrhée, amaigrissement.

Une épreuve négative jusque-là chez un enfant bien portant peut devenir positive rapidement quand la diarrhée se déclare. (Observation III.)

1. *Jahrb. f. Kinderheilk.*, 1892, t. XXXIV, p. 85.
2. De même la glucose impure moins facilement assimilée par le foie donne plus rapidement naissance à la glycosurie alimentaire.

Les résultats de l'expérience suivent les fluctuations de la maladie, la glycosurie alimentaire apparaît avec la diarrhée, disparaît avec elle, reparaît quand elle revient (Observation XII.)

La glycosurie alimentaire peut persister avec des doses de 5 grammes de lactose et même moins par kilogramme d'enfant, alors même que la diarrhée a disparu dans les cas où l'enfant continue à maigrir (Observation XI.)

Peut-on de ces résultats tirer une conclusion, affirmer l'insuffisance fonctionnelle du foie? C'est là une question que nous ne voulons pas aborder, et il nous suffira d'avoir constaté ce fait : la fréquence de la glycosurie alimentaire dans la gastro-entérite des nourrissons.

ALTÉRATIONS DES ÉCHANGES NUTRITIFS CHEZ LES NOURRISSONS ATTEINTS DE MALADIES GASTRO-INTESTINALES

par M. PFAUNDLER,

de Gratz.

L'hypothèse de *Czerny* et *Keller*, qui prétendent que la cachexie des nourrissons atteints de gastro-entérite provient d'une intoxication acide ne doit pas être considérée comme démontrée, car les preuves données par ces auteurs, pour appuyer leur opinion, n'entraînent pas une conviction absolue. En effet l'élimination d'ammoniaque dans les urines des nourrissons, d'après mes recherches, est abondante dans la plupart des cas; cependant on trouve chez les nourrissons atteints de gastro-entérites et chez les nourrissons sains à peu près les mêmes taux. L'abondance de cette élimination est occasionnée en partie par un excès d'acidité physiologique des sucs organiques qui semble être en relation avec la grande quantité des substances grasses dans l'alimentation des nourrissons, mais tient probablement et surtout à un développement défectueux des fonctions oxydantes du foie dans le premier âge.

L'énergie du ferment oxydant hépatique a été précisée par des expériences faites sur le cadavre et dépend des changements anatomiques du foie malade.

RECHERCHES SUR L'ÉLIMINATION DES ACIDES SULFO-CONJUGUÉS
DE LA SÉRIE AROMATIQUE CHEZ LES ENFANTS

par M. le docteur Janvier GALLO de TOMMASI.

Assistant.
Clinique infantile de l'Université de Naples dirigée par le professeur E. De la

On a récemment démontré, par quelques travaux sur l'indicanurie, qu'il n'existe pas un rapport direct entre la proportion d'indican et la quantité totale des acides sulfo-conjugués dans l'urine. Par conséquent, en voulant exactement évaluer le degré de putréfaction de l'albumine dans l'organisme humain, il faut étudier *in toto* la quantité des substances de la série aromatique émises en vingt-quatre heures. Mais les observations de ce genre n'étant pas nombreuses dans la médecine infantile, et la question n'étant pas encore élucidée, j'ai cru nécessaire de fixer mon attention sur ce point, en l'étudiant surtout sous l'influence de l'âge, de l'état normal, de l'alimentation, de l'antisepsie intestinale et de certaines maladies des enfants. Dans mes recherches, j'ai employé la méthode de Baumann-Salkowsky; et mes résultats aboutissent aux *conclusions* suivantes.

1.) La quantité totale des acides sulfo-conjugués, éliminée dans les urines des vingt-quatre heures, en conditions physiologiques et à la suite d'une alimentation usuelle, varie beaucoup, non seulement d'un enfant à l'autre du même âge, mais aussi chez le même enfant d'un jour à l'autre. De plus, elle n'est jamais directement proportionnelle à son âge.

2.) D'après cette variabilité assez considérable, la quantité moyenne journalière n'a point de valeur diagnostique ou pathogénétique absolue. Néanmoins, je dois marquer que, chez les enfants de 4 à 6 ans, elle atteint en moyenne 0,0785 gramme, avec un minimum de 0.0571 et un maximum de 0,1471 gramme.

3.) A la suite du régime lacté, quoique en proportions variables, il s'est produit, dans tous mes cas une diminution de ce chiffre, jusqu'à descendre de 0,0558 gramme à 0,0078 gramme.

L'usage exclusif de viande, au contraire, apporte une augmentation plus ou moins considérable.

4.) Par l'usage médical du calomel, donné toujours à doses fractionnées (6-9 centigrammes *pro die*, répartis en trois prises dans la journée, pour éviter son action purgative), la quantité d'acide sulfo-conjugué, dans la plus grande partie de mes observations, est réduite ordinairement de 1 à 5 centigrammes dans les 24 heures.

5.) Quant aux modifications pathologiques de ces substances, il faut remarquer que dans quelques-unes des maladies en question, la quantité totale est augmentée (tuberculose osseuse et péritonéale, rougeole) tandis que pour d'autres elle n'a montré rien de remarquable (paralysie infantile, néphrite chronique, bronchite chronique, cirrhose hypertrophique du foie).

<hr>

L'ANTISEPSIE INTESTINALE CHEZ LES ENFANTS

par M. le professeur F. FEDE.

Directeur,

et par M. le docteur J. GALLO de TOMMASI.

Assistant.

Clinique infantile de l'Université de Naples.

L'antisepsie intestinale, essayée d'abord chez les adultes, dans la fièvre typhoïde, vient de prendre sa place même dans la thérapeutique médicale des enfants. Après une longue étude sur l'étiologie et les mauvais effets des troubles digestifs, qui jouent un rôle si intéressant dans la pathologie de la première enfance, elle commença par s'imposer impérieusement, toutes les fois qu'on voulait prévenir et empêcher l'empoisonnement de l'organisme humain. C'est bien pour cela qu'en toute occasion, les médecins usent des purgatifs, des lavements et des principaux agents pharmaceutiques, capables d'assurer la désinfection du tube digestif, dans tous les cas d'infection et d'intoxication gastro-intestinale. Mais les auteurs qui ont étudié cette importante question ne sont pas d'accord. Quelques-uns, tels que Albu, Bardet, Stern, Müller, pensent que cette méthode thérapeutique est sans aucune utilité, au contraire très nuisible; tandis que d'autres, parmi lesquels Petrescu, Strauss, Baginski, Escherich, Levery, Bouchard, Fürbringer, Descheemaecker, Riegner, Comby, Jacobi en font l'éloge, surtout à cause des bons résultats qu'on a obtenus par l'usage médical des divers antiseptiques chimiques, dans les intoxications et les infections gastro-intestinales.

Depuis longtemps, nous nous en sommes occupés au point de vue clinique et au point de vue expérimental, et nous avons déjà rapporté, au 5e Congrès italien de Pédiatrie (Turin, 1898), les effets satisfaisants, obtenus de la désinfection du tube digestif, par la voie de l'anus, tant chez les enfants de notre clinique que chez ceux des Réparts de l'hôpital « Incurabili » et de la pratique privée.

Or, nous avons voulu établir au juste point la valeur curative des antiseptiques intestinaux introduits par la bouche, en les employant également chez les malades de notre clinique des Enfants et Réparts de l'hôpital « Incurabili », et nous avons l'honneur de rappeler à ce Congrès les résultats obtenus par l'usage des trois substances suivantes :

Salol : 5-10 centigrammes à la fois, jusqu'à 0.50-1 gramme par jour.

Teinture d'iode : 10-15 gouttes, selon les différents âges, dans une potion gommeuse, une cuiller à café, toutes les deux heures.

Calomel, à doses réfractées : 5-12 centigrammes, répartis en trois prises dans la journée.

Dans nos recherches, nous avons jugé opportun de suivre ce mode opératoire :

En général, nous avons tenu les enfants en examen à l'alimentation usuelle de l'hôpital, en évitant tous les abus alimentaires, qui pouvaient causer quelques dangers aux malades et de faux effets pour nous. Nous opérons nos prélèvements, pour l'analyse, dans la partie centrale des fèces, avant la prise de l'antiseptique. Nous triturons soigneusement, dans un verre conique, 10 centigrammes d'excréments dans 10 centimètres cubes d'eau stérilisée.

Nous diluons 1 centimètre cube de cette solution dans 9 centimètres cubes d'eau stérilisée.

Enfin dans 9 centimètres cubes d'eau stérilisée, nous versons 1 centimètre cube de cette deuxième solution, en ayant ainsi une dilution au millième. Avec une pipette de 1 centimètre cube, nous ensemençons d'une seule goutte un tube contenant 5 centimètres cubes de gélatine fondue et le versons dans une boîte de Petri, en la mettant ensuite à l'étuve à 20°. Après quarante-huit heures, nous comptons exactement les colonies de micro-organismes développés. Cela, pendant trois jours. Au quatrième, nous donnions l'antiseptique et, dans la seconde journée de son administration, on répétait, dans les mêmes conditions, le mode opératoire que nous avons exposé. En outre, afin d'éviter toute erreur, qui pût résulter de l'incomplète démonstration de nos assertions, avant et après la désinfection de l'intestin, nous avons fait l'analyse des urines, en examinant avec la méthode de Baumann-Salkowski, la quantité totale des acides sulfo-conjugués, émise dans les vingt-quatre heures.

De même, nous avons aussi étudié les propriétés virulentes des excréments de ces enfants, en faisant l'inoculation, dans la cavité *des cobayes*, d'un centimètre cube de *culture en bouillon*, après le développement des germes contenus en eux-mêmes, pendant vingt-quatre heures.

Quant aux résultats obtenus, on ne peut pas relater ici les détails des expériences qu'on a faites, avec chacun de ces antiseptiques intestinaux; nous nous bornons seulement à dire, en résumé, que, par rapport à l'action microbicide et antifermentescible des divers antiseptiques, nos expériences ont montré la supériorité du calomel sur le salol et sur la teinture d'iode.

Par conséquent, nos résultats aboutissent aux *conclusions* suivantes :

1° Dans les infections et les intoxications gastro-intestinales, il est toujours utile d'employer quelques antiseptiques internes; et, à bien considérer les résultats que nous avons obtenus, il faut préférer, parmi ceux que nous avons employés, le calomel, qui a donné de grands avantages, le salol et la teinture d'iode n'ayant pas montré une valeur réelle microbicide et antifermentescible;

2° Pour mieux assurer l'antisepsie médicale, dans le cours de ces maladies et des troubles fonctionnels, il faut intervenir de bonne heure; c'est-à-dire lorsque les toxines n'ont pas encore envahi tout l'organisme, en empoisonnant notamment les centres nerveux et en troublant les fonctions organiques;

3° D'après ces principes, nous avons pratiqué l'étude des modifications au point de vue de la quantité des colonies microbiques constatées dans les milieux de culture, avant et après l'administration de ces substances. Il faut dire, par exemple, que nous en avons compté dans un cas 1050, avant l'usage du calomel, et 40 seulement, à la suite.

En même temps, nous avons observé, après l'emploi de cet agent pharmaceutique, la diminution de la virulence des cultures obtenues des matières fécales des enfants et la diminution des acides sulfo-conjugués également après l'administration de l'antiseptique.

BRONCHO-PNEUMONIES
CONSÉCUTIVES AUX INFECTIONS GASTRO-INTESTINALES
AVANTAGES QUE CETTE PATHOGÉNIE RAPPORTE A LA THÉRAPEUTIQUE

par **M**. le docteur Jean FREIXAS,

Médecin adjoint à l'Hôpital de la Sainte-Croix, de Barcelone.

L'infection gastro-intestinale et l'intoxication qui en résulte s'observent dans presque toutes les maladies. C'est grâce au bon fonctionnement des voies digestives et des différents émonctoires que l'organisme arrive à lutter contre leurs effets pernicieux. Aussi devons-nous favoriser cette lutte naturelle contre les infections d'origine gastro-intestinale, non seulement lorsque celles-ci dominent la scène pathologique, mais même lorsqu'elles sont atténuées. Cette pratique donne d'excellents résultats, en particulier dans les maladies exanthématiques. Au point de vue clinique, il faut distinguer trois éventualités :

1° L'infection gastro-intestinale est le phénomène prédominant ;

2° L'infection gastro-intestinale s'accompagne de déterminations secondaires importantes ;

3° L'infection gastro-intestinale est modérée ; les déterminations secondaires prennent une importance considérable.

Pour ce qui est de la broncho-pneumonie, voilà comment on peut établir la filiation des phénomènes : infection gastro-intestinale ; infection et intoxication sanguine ; création d'un foyer de congestion simple du poumon par l'intermédiaire du système nerveux ; modifications des sécrétions bronchiques ; intervention des micro-organismes des premières voies respiratoires (auto-infection) ou de l'extérieur (hétéro-infection).

Ainsi constituée, la broncho-pneumonie consécutive à l'infection gastro-intestinale n'affecte pas au point de vue clinique un type bien tranché. Elle revêt la forme de la congestion aiguë simple ou de la spléno-pneumonie, plus souvent celle de la broncho-pneumonie serpigineuse ; quelquefois elle reste latente. On ne rencontre que rarement les formes classiques. Mais ce qui la caractérise, c'est la relation de cause à effet entre l'infection digestive, phénomène primitif, et la lésion du poumon, détermination secondaire. La thérapeutique doit s'inspirer de cette pathogénie et viser surtout l'infection gastro-intestinale ; contre la broncho-pneumonie on dirigera le traitement symptomatique et général habituel.

UN CAS TRÈS GRAVE D'ATHREPSIE DU NOUVEAU-NÉ
ENCÉPHALOPATHIE — GUÉRISON

par M. le professeur L. BAUMEL.

Professeur de clinique des maladies des Enfants à l'Université de Montpellier.

et M. E. SCHEYDT,

Médecin de l'Hôpital de Cette.

« Certains troubles nerveux surviennent, dit Parrot, chez quelques malades, dans la période terminale de l'athrepsie.

« Ils sont de nature *comateuse* et *convulsive*. Plus rares, mais plus graves que les symptômes décrits jusqu'à présent, *ils annoncent toujours une mort prochaine* et coïncident avec l'extinction du cri, l'altération profonde de la face, la lividité de la peau et la diminution ou même la disparition des urines.

« Je propose, pour désigner leur ensemble symptomatique, la qualification d'*encéphalopathie athrepsique* [1]. »

C'est pour relever appel de ce jugement, souvent fort juste mais non irrévocable, porté par le parrain, nous pouvons dire par le père, de l'athrepsie, que nous avons cru devoir publier et faire connaître l'observation suivante.

Après sept ans de mariage et une fausse couche de trois mois Mme G... (de Cette) accouche, le 15 février 1899, d'un garçon, J. G..., qui pèse 2 kilos 670.

Le père est bien portant, âgé de 35 ans, et arthritique. La mère a 26 ans. Elle est chloro-anémique. Ni syphilis, ni tuberculose dans les antécédents.

Confié dès sa naissance à une nourrice, dans la maison, dont le lait avait cinq mois (tétées régulières chaque trois heures), l'enfant vomit à chaque tétée.

Le 20 février, nouvelle nourrice (son lait n'a que quinze jours). Les vomissements persistent. Le petit malade prenait de l'eau de Vichy et de l'eau seconde de chaux.

Le 28 février, il pèse 2 kilos 750.

Le 6 mars, tout le lait ingéré est immédiatement vomi. *Pendant dix-sept heures aucun lange n'a été mouillé.*

Le 8 mars, nouvelle nourrice dont le lait a quatre mois.

Le 9, l'enfant est mis dans la couveuse de Diffre.

---

1. J. PARROT. Clinique des nouveau-nés. *L'athrepsie*. Paris, Masson, 1877, p. 156.

Le 14, *convulsions*. Il en est de même le 16, le 17 et le 18.

Le 19, M. le professeur Baumel est appelé en consultation.

Ce jour-là l'état de l'enfant était le suivant : amaigrissement considérable; membres d'une gracilité extrême, réduits en quelque sorte au squelette; peau sèche, partout beaucoup trop ample; facies de vieillard absolument ridé; joues creuses; fontanelle antéro-supérieure très déprimée, recevant l'extrémité du pouce; vomissements, pas de diarrhée. Le corps tout entier, la face surtout, sont le siège de *convulsions* qui donnent à l'enfant un aspect horriblement grimaçant.

Une potion au chloral (15 centigrammes pour 60 de véhicule) arrête les convulsions, qui s'éloignent petit à petit et finissent le 22 mars. Une potion à l'eau de chaux (60 grammes) et teinture de musc (6 gouttes) est dirigée contre les troubles digestifs. Les vomissements continuent, mais l'enfant tète, dort par intervalles, urine et a des selles rares, presque insignifiantes et d'un vert foncé.

Le 25, il ne pèse que 2 kilos 269; des traces de *muguet* nécessitent des badigeonnages boratés (borate de soude, miel rosat, ā ā parties égales).

Le 27, il ne pèse que 2 kilos 255. Il a donc perdu 14 grammes en deux jours. *Les langes sont à peine mouillés; pas de selles depuis trente-six heures.* A l'aide d'un suppositoire à la glycérine solidifiée, on en obtient une petite, glaireuse.

Le 29, il a perdu 55 grammes; son poids n'est plus que de 2 kilos 200. Il tète difficilement, vomit toujours, ne va à la selle que par le moyen de suppositoires à la glycérine. Toute la cavité buccale est couverte du muguet.

Le 31, il pèse 70 grammes de moins, soit 2 kilos 130.

Le 4 avril, il a gagné 75 grammes. Son poids est de 2 kilos 205, mais la situation reste la même.

Le 7, il a perdu 10 grammes : 2 kilos 195. Il tète mal; se mouille peu; on n'obtient de selle que par le suppositoire. Il a souvent du hoquet.

Le 10, il a gagné 20 grammes : 2 kilos 215, mais toujours même état.

Le 11, la température axillaire est de 36°,1.

Le 14, il a gagné 15 grammes : 2 kilos 230; mais, le 18, il en perd 90 et retombe à 2 kilos 140. Toujours des vomissements en jet aussitôt qu'il a tété; souvent même une demi-heure après.

Dans les vomissements, avec le lait caillé on voit assez souvent des matières glaireuses (mucosités); le suppositoire provoque cepen-

dant des selles jaunes. et. le 22, il a gagné, en quatre jours, 60 grammes
(2 kilos 200).

De ce moment au 12 mai, il perd 120 grammes. Il ne pèse en effet
ce jour-là que 2 kilos 080.

Pendant une vingtaine de jours on l'a pesé journellement avant et
après les tétées. L'augmentation de poids, après celles-ci, a varié
entre 20 et 90 grammes: mais les vomissements ont été persistants,
les urines rares, les selles difficilement obtenues par les suppositoires; le sommeil, généralement de courte durée, est fréquemment
nterrompu par une agitation assez grande; le muguet, à peine disparu,
reparaît assez facilement.

Le 5, J. G... a eu une syncope au sein de la nourrice, qu'il ne se
décidait pas à téter, syncope qui passa lorsqu'il fut remis à la chaleur
de la couveuse.

Les jours suivants, on en constate de nouvelles, toujours au
moment où on le sort de la couveuse pour le faire téter, et l'on est
obligé de l'y remettre immédiatement.

Les *convulsions* reparaissent le 5 mai et continuent les 6, 7 et 8.
Elles cessent sous l'influence du chloral.

Le 12, nous prescrivons du benzo-naphtol (50 centigrammes dans
une potion de 60 grammes) et nous suspendons le chloral, pour ne le
reprendre que les 16 et 17 à cause de *nouvelles convulsions*.

A partir du 26 mai (l'enfant pèse ce jour-là 2 kilos 190), les vomissements sont moins fréquents et moins abondants; les convulsions
disparaissent, mais les selles restent difficiles : nous ajoutons, au benzo-naphtol. du salicylate de magnésie (ãã parties égales).

Le 2 juin, le poids a augmenté (2 kilos 540): toutefois les vomissements reparaissent trois jours après et le 9 juin le petit malade perd
encore de son poids et ne pèse plus que 2 kilos 185.

Les 10 et 11. surviennent des *convulsions*, enfin de petites ulcérations aux genoux et derrière les oreilles, qui se cicatrisent d'ailleurs
rapidement avec la poudre d'aristol.

Les *convulsions* deviennent *assez fréquentes* pour nous obliger à
doubler la dose de chloral (50 centigrammes).

Sous cette influence disparaissent peu à peu les convulsions: les
vomissements, même, diminuent sensiblement: d'autre part les selles
se régularisent. L'enfant pèse, le 16 juin, 2 kilos 500.

A partir de ce moment, la potion à la teinture de musc et à l'eau
de chaux est administrée alternativement dans la journée avec la
potion au benzo-naphtol et au salicylate de magnésie. Les badigeonnages boratés sont faits régulièrement trois fois par jour. Les *vomis-*

sements sont de moins en moins abondants, souvent même ils ont défaut après certaines tétées.

L'enfant gagne en poids tous les jours : le 20, il pèse 2 kilos 555; le 24, 2 kilos 460; le 28, 2 kilos 465; enfin le 2 juillet, 2 kilos 590.

Il y a eu, les jours précédents, des selles diarrhéiques; nous remplaçons le salicylate de magnésie par celui de bismuth, et à partir de ce moment nous avons recours tantôt à l'un, tantôt à l'autre de ces médicaments, suivant les indications fournies par les évacuations.

Les urines sont abondantes; le sommeil long, calme et régulier.

J. G... tète bien, souvent sans s'interrompre pour rejeter des gorgées de lait, contrairement à ce qui avait eu lieu jusque-là.

L'amélioration continue. Le 10 juillet le poids est de 2 kilos 845 et le 14 juillet de 3 kilos 100.

Cédant aux instances de la mère, nous permettons qu'on sorte l'enfant de la couveuse dans laquelle il est remis la nuit.

A partir de ce jour-là, la médication étant continuée, toutes les fonctions se régularisent et l'augmentation de poids est définitivement progressive.

Dès le 20 juillet, J. G... n'est plus mis, la nuit, dans la couveuse et couche dans son berceau. Les fenêtres de l'appartement, exposé au soleil, sont ouvertes dans la journée et, le 31, il est transporté à la campagne, à côté de Cette.

Courbe des pesées.

Le 18 juillet, la pesée donne. . . . . 3^k.210

22	—	—	3 590
26	—	—	3 540
30	—	—	3 780
3 août		—	3 880
7	—	—	3 925
11	—	—	4 025
15	—	—	4 100
19	—	—	4 205
23	—	—	4 545
27	—	—	4 550
31	—	—	4 640
4 septembre		—	4 810
8	—	—	4 965
12	—	—	5 090
16		—	5 260
20		—	5 470
24		—	5 650
28		—	5 825

Le 2 octobre, la pesée donne. 6 015
    6 —   —   6 195
    10 - -   —   6 550
    14 —   6 495
    18 —   —   6 620
    22 —   —   6 780
    26 —   —   6 940
    30 —   ---   7 050
    5 novembre   -   7 150

Ce jour-là, percent les deux incisives médianes inférieures.

    24 novembre, la pesée donne. 7 640
    1er décembre   —   7 850

Les dents du maxillaire supérieur provoquent de la fièvre.

    8 décembre, même poids. 7 850

néanmoins J. G... est vacciné.

    5 janvier 1900, la pesée donne. 8 215
    16 —   —   8 420
    19 issue des deux incisives médianes supérieures.
    25 janvier :   8 550

Jamais, pendant la maladie, aucune complication du côté des poumons.

L'état de l'enfant s'améliore graduellement de façon à rattraper le temps perdu.

Le 11 avril, il fait ses premiers pas. Actuellement il va aussi bien que possible.

L'observation précédente est, à notre avis, intéressante à plus d'un titre. Elle montre :

1° La *quantité notable de poids que peut perdre un nouveau-né*, sans que toutefois cette perte soit incompatible avec la vie (680 grammes dans le cas particulier. Voir la courbe ci-jointe);

2° La *longue durée* qui peut être celle de l'athrepsie (durée que l'on peut évaluer à trois mois dans notre observation, en ce qui concerne seulement la période d'état. et à plus de quatre, en y comprenant celles de la diminution primitive et de l'augmentation terminale du poids);

3° La possibilité, pour l'enfant. de *doubler* et même de *tripler les étapes* à un moment donné. c'est-à-dire de gagner en grammes non seulement la quantité propre à son âge. mais de réparer pour ainsi dire le temps perdu. comme l'indique, en particulier, l'augmentation du 10 au 14 juillet (62 grammes par jour pour un enfant de 6 mois, dont l'augmentation normale est en moyenne, à cet âge. de 20 grammes par vingt-quatre heures):

4° Enfin la *curabilité possible de l'encéphalopathie athrepsique* contrairement au jugement porté par Parrot lui-même.

C'est principalement pour ce motif, ainsi que nous l'avons dit plus haut, qu'a été communiquée par nous, au Congrès international. l'observation ci-dessus relatée.

DU TRAITEMENT DES ULCÉRATIONS ATHREPSIQUES ET GÉNÉRALEMENT
DES PLAIES ATONES DE L'ENFANT
PAR LE SOUS-CARBONATE DE FER EN APPLICATION EXTERNE

par **M**. le docteur R. SAINT-PHILIPPE,

Médecin de l'Hôpital des Enfants, de Bordeaux.

La peau des nouveau-nés et des nourrissons, par sa structure, l'insuffisance de sa circulation, la macération qu'elle subit avant l'accouchement, et d'autre part par la pression, les frottements et les adultérations auxquels elle est exposée, s'entame facilement et, une fois entamée, ne guérit pas vite. C'est aux talons, aux malléoles, sous l'occiput qu'on rencontre les petites plaies creusantes, que Parrot avait indiquées comme appartenant à l'athrepsie et qu'on trouve aussi chez les enfants chétifs simplement dystrophiques : mais on les observe aussi aux environs de l'anus. chez certains érythémateux. On les voit survenir à la vulve comme conséquence de l'herpès malin, de la varicelle, et ailleurs, un peu partout, comme suites de l'impétigo. de l'ecthyma, du pemphigus et aussi de la syphilis. Enfin le vésicatoire planté sur un mauvais terrain ou mal pansé peut laisser une plaie qui s'éternise. On peut donc dire que toute effraction de la peau constitue un danger chez l'enfant.

Autant de portes d'entrée, en effet, pour l'infection.

Chacun sait combien sont puissantes à cet âge les facultés d'absorption et de résorption. Les lymphatiques sont en travail permanent. et. sans parler de la gangrène, la septico-pyohémie. surtout dans les hôpitaux, survient avec une promptitude désespérante. se manifestant soit par des décharges dans le tissu cellulaire sous-cutané, soit par des lésions profondes. viscérales. qui mettent la vie en danger et. dans tous les cas, épuisent l'organisme et en font une proie facile pour les maladies qui passent.

Il y a donc un grand intérêt à guérir le plus tôt possible les lésions toutes petites, mais de grandes conséquences. La chose ne va pas aussi simplement qu'elle paraît. Ce n'est pas que les topiques manquent. L'antisepsie nous a dotés d'armes nombreuses. Mais les petits enfants supportent assez mal en général le mercure, l'acide phénique et ses dérivés, qui les empoisonnent plus promptement qu'on ne croit. L'acide borique est plutôt faible. L'iodoforme les empêche parfois de téter. L'aristol est irritant. Le sous-nitrate de bismuth est digérant, si je puis dire, et convient mieux pour les plaies à membranes diphtéroïdes. L'alun, le tannin font croûte. Ce sont des mordants qui dévorent les bourgeons exubérants plutôt qu'ils n'excitent la poussée de fermeture.

Après avoir essayé de tous les topiques, que je ne cherche pas à détrôner et qui peuvent avoir leurs indications, j'ai dû trouver mieux.

Le sous-carbonate de fer m'a donné, après de nombreux essais, de si remarquables résultats, surtout dans mon service hospitalier — résultats qui ont été rapportés dans la thèse de mon élève Raffin — que je n'hésite pas à le recommander à l'attention des praticiens. Ce produit est un mélange d'hydrate ferrique et de sous-carbonate de peroxyde de fer obtenu en précipitant du sulfate ferreux pur cristallisé par une solution de carbonate de soude cristallisé. Le précipité blanc verdâtre de carbonate ferreux est lavé à froid en agitant fréquemment jusqu'à ce qu'il ait pris une couleur rougeâtre. On le recueille sur une tôle et on fait sécher à l'air. C'est une poudre jaune rougeâtre, sans odeur et d'une saveur légèrement styptique.

Sous son action, on voit la plaie rougir très rapidement. Il y a là un travail irritatif qui se traduit par un appel de sang et une forte diapédèse. Le bourgeonnement apparaît presque tout de suite, pour devenir parfois excessif. En même temps, la plaie se rétrécit par la périphérie et la guérison survient en moyenne dans 8 à 15 jours.

Peut-être à cette action excitante peut-on ajouter une action antiseptique. D'après M. le Dr Barthe, agrégé de pharmacie à la Faculté de Bordeaux, la présence du sous-carbonate de fer empêcherait la pullulation des microbes pathogènes. C'est sur cette propriété que posséderait le fer et sur son aptitude à détruire, en la comburant, la matière organique que sont basés les procédés d'épuration de l'eau potable (Anderson, Pouchet, Buisine).

Enfin, il n'est pas interdit d'admettre que si l'organisme résorbe, même très peu, du topique appliqué sur la plaie, il en subsiste d'heureuses modifications dont bénéficie le sujet.

Le médicament est courant et d'un prix très modique. On peut en user *largo manu*. Il salit seulement un peu. Quant à la technique, elle est aussi simple que possible. Au lieu de laisser la poudre faire croûte à l'air libre — ce qui emmagasinerait le pus — je la dépose sur la plaie (que je bourre complétement) et je la recouvre d'un pansement humide de façon à ce que le mal baigne pour ainsi dire constamment dans cette crème de fer. Le pansement est renouvelé tous les jours, après lavage d'eau bouillie de noyer, de façon que du fer nouveau soit chaque jour apporté à la plaie languissante. Je n'ai jamais vu d'accident résulter de ce pansement, qui en vaut d'autres et certainement vaut mieux que beaucoup d'autres et qui pourrait être utilisé enfin, même chez les *adultes par exemple*, pour les ulcères variqueux.

III

TUBERCULOSE INFANTILE

.I. — Rapports sur la tuberculose infantile.

CONTAGION ET PROPHYLAXIE DE LA TUBERCULOSE INFANTILE

RAPPORT

par M. le professeur d'ESPINE,

de Genève.

Contagion.

Depuis que R. Koch a démontré la nature bacillaire de la tuberculose, on ne peut admettre que deux sources de la maladie chez l'enfant : la transmission du bacille tuberculeux par *hérédité* ou par *contagion*.

Mon savant co-rapporteur, le professeur Hutinel, s'est chargé de la question de l'hérédité. Il vous démontrera, mieux que je ne pourrais le faire, qu'il existe quelques cas prouvés de transmission du bacille de la mère au fœtus par effraction placentaire, mais que ce nombre est infime dans l'espèce humaine et absolument négligeable dans la pratique. Il vous parlera également de la transmission de la prédisposition, dont je n'aurai pas à m'occuper ici.

Pour mettre un peu d'ordre dans la question que votre Comité m'a fait l'honneur de me confier, j'étudierai successivement l'âge auquel se produit la contagion tuberculeuse chez l'enfant, puis les sources et les modes divers de cette contagion suivant les différentes portes d'entrée du bacille.

I. *Âge de la contagion.*

La statistique des autopsies démontre que la tuberculose est la cause de mort de beaucoup la plus fréquente dans l'enfance, et qu'on la rencontre en outre assez souvent sous la forme latente parmi des cadavres d'enfants qui ont succombé à d'autres maladies. Sur les 500 autopsies d'enfants de 0 à 15 ans, faites à Munich sous la direction de Bollinger, près de la moitié, soit 218 (45,6 pour 100), ont présenté des lésions tuberculeuses. Sur ce nombre, la tuberculose était la cause de la mort dans 150 cas (soit 50 pour 100), elle était latente dans 68 cas (15,6 pour 100), la mort étant survenue par le fait d'une autre maladie[1].

En étudiant la fréquence de la tuberculose infantile suivant l'âge, on voit, comme le montre Küss[2] dans sa remarquable thèse, se dégager une loi précise de pathologie infantile qui pourrait se formuler ainsi : *Le nombre des décès par tuberculose, à peu près nul dans les trois premiers mois de la vie, suit une progression lente, d'abord de trois mois à un an, puis plus rapide d'un à deux ans, pour atteindre son maximum entre deux et quatre ans.* Si, comme le dit Straus dans son livre sur le bacille de la tuberculose, la maladie remontait à une infection fœtale, la proportion des tuberculoses infantiles aux différents âges devrait être renversée.

Malheureusement la statistique mortuaire ne peut rien nous apprendre sur les formes bénignes de la tuberculose, dites scrofuleuses. Les statistiques de morbidité sont encore fragmentaires et ne tiennent pas compte surtout de l'âge où la lésion s'est produite. Ainsi, tandis qu'une statistique de Lebert[3], portant sur 557 cas de scrofule, n'en signale que 12 pour 100 dans les cinq premières années, et Rabl[4], sur 11 795 cas de scrofule observés à l'hôpital Elisabeth, à Hall, pendant 40 ans, en trouve seulement 6 pour 100 de 1 à 5 ans et 74 pour 100 de 6 à 15 ans, la proportion est renversée dans la statistique de Wohlgemuth[5], qui indique 47,4 pour 100 de cas de scrofule ganglionnaire de 0 à 5 ans, 20,8 pour 100 de 5 à 10 ans et 20 pour 100 de 10 à 20 ans. La même fréquence de la scrofule dans la première enfance ressort de la statistique de Lannelongue[6], qui porte sur 969 cas de tuberculose externe, dont 545, soit plus de la moitié, ont été observés chez des enfants de 0 à 5 ans.

Si l'on rapproche de ce fait la statistique des tuberculoses latentes trouvées à l'autopsie par Müller, où les trois quarts l'ont été chez *des enfants de 1 à 6 ans* (49 cas sur 68), on arrive à la conclusion que l'âge le plus dangereux pour la contagion tuberculeuse chez l'enfant est l'âge d'un à six ans, c'est-à-dire l'âge où l'enfant passe encore la

---

1. O. Müller. *Thèse de Munich*, 1896.
2. Küss. *Thèse de Paris*, 1898.
3. Lebert. *Traité pratique des maladies scrofuleuses*. Paris, 1849, p. 65.
4. Rabl. *Das Kaiserliche Elisabeth Kinderspital in Bad. Hall*, 1856-1896.
5. Wohlgemuth. *Arch. für Kinderheilk.*, 1890, t. IX, p. 555.
6. Lannelongue, cité in *Münch. med. Wochenschr.*, 1891, p. 498.

plus grande partie de son existence dans le milieu familial. Rien ne prouve d'ailleurs que les tuberculoses observées chez des enfants plus âgés ne remontent pas également à des formes latentes prises dans la première enfance.

II. *Sources et divers modes de contagion.*

Justifions d'abord le mot de contagion, qui nous a été imposé, et que l'on considère volontiers comme un épouvantail qui pourrait paralyser par la terreur les soins à donner aux tuberculeux. Notre vieille devise genevoise : *Post tenebras lux*, nous a rendu longtemps réfractaire à la peur de renseigner exactement les malades ou leur entourage sur les dangers qu'ils courent et le moyen de les conjurer.

Un germe microbien quelconque qui part d'un être vivant, que ce soit directement ou indirectement, et engendre une maladie chez un autre être vivant, détermine ce que la science médicale appelle contagion. Le mot est donc bien choisi pour la tuberculose, puisque nous ne connaissons comme source de l'infection que les produits rejetés au dehors par les foyers tuberculeux ouverts ou le lait des vaches tuberculeuses. Les infections par la viande tuberculeuse sont trop rares et trop faciles à prohiber pour entrer en ligne de compte dans la pratique.

Chaque maladie contagieuse a son mode spécial de transmission qu'il faut étudier avec soin pour la prophylaxie. Ainsi il y a autant de différence entre la contagiosité de la peste et de la tuberculose qu'il y en a entre celle de la variole et de la rage. Muselez tous les chiens et vous éteindrez la rage. Empêchez la dissémination des crachats ; obtenez leur désinfection ; ne permettez jamais de boire du lait cru, et vous aurez réduit au minimum le danger de contagion de la tuberculose.

Étudions successivement les deux sources principales de la contagion tuberculeuse, le *lait* et les *crachats* des phtisiques. Commençons par celle qui a la moindre importance, le lait des vaches tuberculeuses.

Chez l'enfant, la contagion par le lait est plus à craindre que chez l'adulte, puisque le régime lacté est exclusif ou prépondérant dans les premières années de la vie.

Le danger d'une infection par le tube digestif est indéniable, si l'on réfléchit que la proportion des vaches tuberculeuses est au minimum de 6 à 7 pour 100 suivant RÖCKL, et qu'en Allemagne, principalement dans l'Est et dans le Nord, cette proportion monte à 20 ou même

25 pour 100 pour les grands troupeaux, suivant Bollinger[1]. Il semble même que cette proportion est en voie de progression continue depuis les dix à vingt dernières années, comme le prouvent les statistiques de plusieurs grands abattoirs, celui de Leipzig par exemple[2].

Le lait de vache vendu en ville contient d'ailleurs souvent des bacilles tuberculeux. Obermüller en a constaté dans 8 échantillons sur 15 provenant de Berlin ; cette énorme proportion de 61 pour 100 tombe avec Petri à 10 pour 100, qui explique cette différence par la confusion possible du bacille de Koch avec un pseudo-bacille qu'on trouve souvent dans le beurre et qui a les mêmes réactions tinctoriales. Macfadyan[3] indique pour le lait d'Hacknay à Londres 22 pour 100. Par contre, Rabinovitch et Kempner[4], en tenant compte des observations de Petri, ont trouvé 10 fois des bacilles tuberculeux vrais sur le lait de 15 vaches ; ils ont démontré leur présence dans le lait, *même chez des vaches exemptes de tuberculose mammaire.*

Le beurre a été également incriminé. Le pseudo-bacille y a été trouvé plus fréquemment que le bacille de Koch (Weissenfeld[5]), et ce dernier ne semble y exister qu'en petite quantité; de sorte que le danger d'infection par le beurre n'est pas à comparer à celui qui résulte du lait cru.

Les expériences sur les animaux démontrent la possibilité de la tuberculisation par injection de lait bacillifère ou d'autres produits tuberculeux. Chauveau, le premier en 1868, Gerlach en 1869, puis toute une série d'expérimentateurs l'ont mis hors de doute. On sait aussi que l'infection intestinale se produit d'autant plus facilement *que le lait est plus riche en bacilles* et *que l'animal est plus jeune.* D'ailleurs il n'est pas nécessaire qu'il y ait ulcération intestinale pour déterminer une tuberculisation générale par cette voie ; les bacilles peuvent traverser la muqueuse sans lésion préalable (Dobroklonski[6]), et les leucocytes jouent un rôle important dans leur pénétration (Tchistovitch[7]).

Enfin il existe un certain nombre d'observations faites chez l'homme qui démontrent avec la précision d'une expérience de laboratoire la possibilité de la tuberculisation par ingestion. Vous avez encore pré-

1. Bollinger. Congrès de Berlin pour la lutte contre la tuberculose. 1899, p. 104.
2. Boysen. *Ueber die Gefahr der Verbreitung der Tuberculose durch die Kuhmilch.* Leipzig. 1900.
3. *Lancet*, 1899, t. II, p. 849.
4. *Deutsch. med. Wochenschr.*, 1899, p. 542.
5. Weissenfeld, *Berlin. Wochenschr.*, 1899, p. 1055.
6. Dobroklonski. *Arch. de méd. expér.*, 1899, t. II, p. 255.
7. Tchistovitch. *Ann. de l'Institut Pasteur.* 1889, t. III, p. 209.

sent à l'esprit le fait raconté par Brouardel, d'une grande institution de jeunes filles où cinq pensionnaires, ne présentant aucune tare héréditaire, moururent tuberculeuses dans l'espace de deux ans et où la vache qui fournissait le lait à la maison fut abattue et trouvée atteinte de tuberculose.

Ollivier, Bouley, Bung, Pruemers[1], etc., ont cité des cas analogues. Le seul problème difficile à résoudre est de savoir dans quelle proportion la contagion par le lait entre dans la statistique de la tuberculose infantile. L'anatomie pathologique démontre que dans l'immense majorité des cas, *c'est-à-dire dans 90 à 95 pour 100 de toutes les autopsies, les ganglions bronchiques sont le foyer tuberculeux le plus ancien et peuvent être considérés comme la porte d'entrée des bacilles.* Les autopsies de tuberculose primitive de l'intestin, des ganglions mésentériques et du péritoine absolument probantes sont rares. Ce qui est le plus fréquent, particulièrement dans les trois premières années de la vie, c'est de trouver à côté d'autres localisations, en particulier des ganglions bronchiques ou des poumons, une tuberculisation avancée et considérable des ganglions mésentériques. Mon père, Marc D'Espine[2], avait déjà constaté que la mortalité par tuberculose abdominale atteint son maximum chez l'enfant entre un et trois ans. Il est donc possible que ces cas mixtes soient également des cas de contagion par le lait, quoique, dans le cas des lésions broncho-pulmonaires ouvertes, on ne puisse exclure l'auto-infection par la déglutition des bacilles, puisque les enfants de cet âge ne crachent pas. Notre éminent secrétaire, le Dr Marfan[3], évalue la proportion des cas de tuberculose alimentaire chez les enfants d'un à cinq ans à 8 pour 100 de tous les cas de tuberculose observés à cet âge. C'est pour nous un minimum.

La source de contagion de beaucoup la plus importante pour l'enfance est toujours à chercher chez *un être humain atteint de tuberculose ouverte* et dans les produits bacillifères qu'il sécrète. A ce point de vue, les enfants sont infiniment moins dangereux que les adultes. Le pus des scrofules osseuses, cutanées ou ganglionnaires, est en effet beaucoup plus rarement le véhicule de la contagion que le crachat: il est d'abord beaucoup moins riche en bacilles et, secondement, les plaies sont aujourd'hui pansées avec des antiseptiques qui diminuent leur virulence. Quant aux crachats, ils ne sont expectorés que chez des enfants de plus de dix ans, excepté quand il y a des quintes de coqueluche.

1. Pruemers, *Hyg. Rundschau.* 1885, t. II, p. 525.
2. *Statistique mortuaire.* Genève, 1859.
3. *Traité des maladies de l'enfance,* article *Tuberculose,* 1897.

C'est le voisinage des *phtisiques adultes* qui explique la plupart des cas de tuberculose infantile. Comme on l'a très bien dit : *le crachat c'est l'ennemi.*

Comment se produit la contagion? Elle peut être *immédiate* par les baisers sur la bouche de l'enfant, ou encore, comme FLÜGGE l'a démontré expérimentalement, par les *postillons* (passez-moi l'expression, je n'en trouve pas d'autre) lancés par les phtisiques en parlant ou en toussant dans le voisinage immédiat des enfants. Les parents et les bonnes d'enfants phtisiques sont, en pareil cas, les agents ordinaires de la contagion.

Il est important de citer quelques exemples incontestables de cette transmission immédiate, sur laquelle les anticontagionnistes passent volontiers comme chat sur braise.

Ainsi REICH[1] raconte qu'une sage-femme de Neuembourg, manifestement phtisique et qui avait une expectoration purulente abondante, avait perdu dans sa clientèle dix nouveau-nés qu'elle avait accouchés et qui avaient succombé dans le cours de la première année à une méningite tuberculeuse. Elle avait l'habitude de les insuffler bouche à bouche, s'ils ne respiraient pas de suite. Elle mourut de phtisie quelque temps après. Les nouveau-nés accouchés pendant la même période par une autre sage-femme de Neuembourg, qui était bien portante, ne présentèrent rien de semblable.

Nous avons cité dans notre Manuel[2] une observation personnelle d'un enfant de sept mois sans antécédents héréditaires, qui était gardé et constamment embrassé par un frère de 19 ans, phtisique à la dernière période, et présentant les signes d'une grande caverne. Ce frère était né d'un autre père : la mère était saine et robuste. L'enfant mourut d'éclampsie et nous trouvâmes à l'autopsie des tubercules cérébraux ainsi que des ganglions caséeux plus anciens.

WASSERMANN[3] rapporte l'histoire d'un enfant né de parents absolument sains, qui mourut, à l'âge de dix semaines, de tuberculose pulmonaire caséeuse, constatée à l'autopsie. Il avait passé les neuf premiers jours de la vie en parfaite santé à la clinique d'accouchement de la Charité, et avait été recueilli pendant une semaine avec sa mère chez un oncle phtisique à crachats bacillifères. Depuis lors, l'enfant maigrit et dépérit.

L'inoculation de la salive bacillifère peut aussi se faire directement à une solution de continuité de la peau ou des muqueuses. Telles sont

1. REICH. *Berl. klin. Wochenschr.*, 1878, n° 57, 1879, p. 554.
2. D'ESPINE et PICOT. 6e édition, 1899, p. 578.
3. WASSERMANN. *Zeitschr. f. Hyg.*, 1894, t. XIX, p. 545.

les célèbres observations d'inoculation préputiale, au moment de la circoncision rituelle, due au procédé primitif d'hémostase consistant dans la succion de la plaie pratiquée par des rabbins phtisiques[1]. Tel est encore ce cas de lupus (cité par Leloir[2]) observé chez un garçon de six ans au niveau d'une plaie qui avait été pansée avec un morceau de taffetas d'Angleterre, mouillé par la salive d'une bonne phtisique. Le lupus d'ailleurs, qui est presque toujours primitif, commence, dans la majorité des cas, avant l'âge de quinze ans et ne peut s'expliquer que par une inoculation directe dont la cause échappe le plus souvent.

La tuberculose primitive de la conjonctive, qui est fort rare, s'explique de la même manière. Notre collègue, le professeur HALTENHOFF, en a observé un cas intéressant suivi d'adénite pré-auriculaire, puis cervicale et sous-maxillaire chez une fillette de trois ans et demi, qui était en rapports constants avec une personne phtisique à la deuxième période, ayant une expectoration abondante. L'ulcère conjonctival guérit par le curettage, la galvanocaustique et l'iodoforme ; trois ans après, la guérison locale s'était maintenue; mais les ganglions engorgés s'étaient tranformés en écrouelles persistantes et la santé générale de l'enfant semblait compromise.

La contagion immédiate peut se produire aussi par la déglutition de la salive de la personne atteinte, comme le prouve une observation de Demme[3]. Trois petits enfants sans tare héréditaire et confiés aux soins d'une nourrice sèche moururent, dans le cours de la première année, de tuberculose intestinale primitive, prouvée par l'autopsie. Comme un quatrième nourrisson élevé par la même femme mourut également, tout en étant nourri au lait stérilisé, et ne présenta à l'autopsie que des lésions tuberculeuses limitées à l'intestin et aux ganglions mésentériques, Demme fit une enquête et découvrit une fistule buccale venant de l'antre d'Highmore dont le pus était tuberculeux, comme le prouva l'inoculation du cobaye. La nourrice avait l'habitude de goûter chaque cuillère de la bouillie qu'elle donnait à l'enfant, pour s'assurer qu'elle n'était pas trop chaude.

La contagion immédiate par les poussières tuberculeuses provenant des crachats desséchés est chez l'enfant comme chez l'adulte le procédé d'infection le plus commun. La tuberculose infantile est une tuberculose d'*inhalation* dans l'immense majorité des cas. L'adénopathie bronchique en est le premier stade ; de là les bacilles peuvent

---

1. Voir la liste des cas in : d'Espine et Picot, 6e édition. 1899, p. 567.
2. Leloir. *Études sur la tuberculose* de Verneuil, 1892, t. III, p. 482.
3. Demme. 27e Rapport sur l'hôpital Jenner, pour 1899, Berne pour 1890, p. 11.

s'étendre de proche en proche au hile du poumon, à la plèvre, aux vaisseaux du voisinage, ou déterminer ainsi par embolie une généralisation aux méninges, aux os et aux viscères. C'est un des traits caractéristiques de la tuberculose infantile, que ces foyers ganglionnaires bronchiques qui peuvent rester latents pendant des années. Les maladies aiguës infectieuses de l'enfance, la rougeole et la coqueluche en particulier, ne sont tuberculisantes que parce qu'elles retentissent sur les ganglions bronchiques et libèrent les bacilles qui y étaient enfermés.

Les expériences de CORNET ont détruit la légende de l'ubiquité du germe de la tuberculose ; c'est *dans le voisinage immédiat des phtisiques* et principalement sur *le plancher de leurs habitations* qu'on trouve des bacilles, ceux qui sont rejetés en plein air perdant rapidement leur virulence sous l'influence de l'air et de la lumière solaire. On sait aujourd'hui qu'il y a des épidémies de maisons, d'ateliers, de chambres, qui s'expliquent par l'infection du plancher.

Or les habitations des familles pauvres principalement constituent, par leur exiguïté, le manque d'air et de soleil, l'encombrement, un milieu familial redoutable pour les enfants de phtisiques.

La tuberculose chirurgicale osseuse ou ganglionnaire a chez l'enfant une origine semblable à la tuberculose viscérale : elle est le plus souvent secondaire, l'autopsie démontrant en pareil cas un foyer primitif de contagion par inhalation dans les ganglions bronchiques. La tuberculose ganglionnaire cervicale, qui débute en général par les ganglions sous-maxillaires, dépend parfois d'une porte d'entrée bucco-pharyngée : l'infection tuberculeuse peut avoir comme point de départ une carie dentaire (STARK[1] a démontré deux fois la présence du bacille de Koch dans le contenu de l'alvéole), ou bien une tuberculose latente des amygdales (DIEULAFOY[2]), ou bien encore des végétations adénoïdes du pharynx (LERMOYEZ[3], SUCHANNEK[4]).

Enfin, il est possible que les dénudations de la peau, traumatiques ou eczémateuses, puissent être infectées directement par les poussières bacillifères, déposées à leur surface par les doigts et les ongles de l'enfant.

La contagion et la prédisposition de terrain s'unissent en pareil cas pour engendrer la tuberculose infantile, mais *le facteur essentiel est la contagion* ; séparez en effet les enfants de leurs parents phtisiques,

1. STARK in *Journal des médecins praticiens*, 1896, p. 852.
2. DIEULAFOY. *Bulletin de l'Académie de médecine*, avril 1895.
3. LERMOYEZ. *Presse*, 26 octobre 1895.
4. SUCHANNEK. *Zieglers Beiträge*, 1888, t. III, p. 51.

sortez-les du milieu familial, et vous les préserverez dans la grande majorité des cas. Bang[1] l'a prouvé expérimentalement pour la race bovine, en séparant dès la naissance tous les veaux nés de vaches tuberculeuses et en les faisant nourrir au lait bouilli. Une observation de Bernheim[2] équivaut pour la race humaine à une expérience de laboratoire. Trois fois il lui est arrivé d'accoucher de jumeaux vivants des mères tuberculeuses et d'obtenir dans les trois cas d'envoyer en nourrice à la campagne un des jumeaux, tandis que l'autre était nourri par une nourrice auprès de la mère. Ces derniers sont tous morts, tandis que les jumeaux envoyés à la campagne ont survécu. La rareté de la tuberculose constatée à l'autopsie des enfants assistés de l'hôpital de Prague est attribuée par Epstein[3] au fait que presque tous étaient séparés de leur mère dès les premiers jours et nourris au sein d'une nourrice saine.

Ne croyez pas, Messieurs, que je conclue de ces faits à la négation de la prédisposition. Le lymphatisme, la prédisposition spécifique qu'on appelle la scrofule, comme aussi toutes les détériorations de l'organisme, héréditaires ou acquises, jouent un rôle de premier ordre dans les succès des mesures prophylactiques qui ont pour but d'augmenter la résistance vitale de l'enfant. Mais, de même que les plus beaux champs du monde, ceux de la Beauce, par exemple, ne produiront pas de blé si on ne l'y sème, de même, pour la tuberculose, le terrain restera stérile si l'on éloigne la graine.

Les circonstances qui favorisent la contagion de la tuberculose infantile varient suivant l'âge. Exceptionnelle au berceau, où elle est due presque toujours à la transmission immédiate par une mère ou une bonne phtisique, elle est fréquente chez le petit enfant, parce qu'il vit par terre, touche tout avec ses doigts et porte la crasse parasitaire à la bouche ou sur les excoriations eczémateuses dont il est souvent affecté à cet âge. Cette contagion par la saleté a été bien exposée par notre collègue le Dr Comby[4] au Congrès de Montpellier. Dans le même ordre d'idées, Debecq[5] a insisté sur la fréquence des infections tuberculeuses chez les enfants onychophages.

Dès que l'enfant s'affranchit du milieu familial, dès qu'il va à l'école, c'est-à-dire à partir de cinq ou six ans, les infections tuberculeuses

1. Bang. *La lutte contre la tuberculose en Danemark*, trad. par Gosse. Genève, 1865, p. 58.
2. Bernheim. Congrès international de Rome, cité par Cornet. *Die Tuberculose*, Vienne, 1899, p. 272.
3. Epstein. *Vierteljahrsch. für prakt. Heilk.*, 1879, t. II, p. 102.
4. Comby. Congrès français de médecine, 4ᵉ session. Montpellier, 1899, p. 11.
5. Debecq. *La tuberculose infantile*, 15 février 1899.

deviennent beaucoup plus rares. *La décroissance de la mortalité par la tuberculose dans la seconde enfance est beaucoup moins marquée pour les filles que pour les garçons.* La statistique prussienne démontre qu'il y a peu de différence entre les sexes pour les deux premières années, mais qu'à partir de la 5ᵉ année la mortalité tuberculeuse des filles l'emporte sur celle des garçons et arrive à être, entre dix et quinze ans, presque deux fois plus forte chez les filles que chez les garçons. A l'âge adulte, au contraire, la proportion est inverse, ce que le professeur CORNET explique par le fait que les garçons s'affranchissent plus complètement du milieu familial que les filles, tandis qu'à l'âge adulte les hommes sont plus exposés que les femmes, par la vie dans les fabriques et les ateliers, à l'infection tuberculeuse.

Nous ne croyons guère au danger de contagion par l'*école* ou par es *hôpitaux*, pourvu que les principes de l'antisepsie et de la propreté y soient appliqués suivant les règles de l'hygiène. Nous n'avons trouvé dans la littérature qu'un seul cas de contagion scolaire, cité par Marius DUPONT[1], qui s'est passé dans une école primaire de la province de Tarragone où 90 à 100 enfants étaient entassés dans un local exigu sous la direction d'un instituteur atteint de phtisie avancée qui ne se faisait pas faute de cracher par terre.

En tout cas, la prophylaxie devra tenir compte du fait signalé par BROUARDEL[2] en France, où la statistique a démontré qu'un cinquième des instituteurs est atteint de tuberculose.

Prophylaxie.

Les mesures prophylactiques contre la tuberculose infantile ont pour but, les unes d'empêcher la contagion, les autres de diminuer la réceptivité de l'enfant contre le bacille en augmentant la résistance vitale. Nous serons très brefs sur les premières, les ayant exposées dans nos conclusions. La propreté, comme on l'a dit souvent, est la première condition d'une prophylaxie sérieuse. Les bains quotidiens et les ablutions froides ont non seulement pour résultat de fortifier l'enfant contre les intempéries de l'air, mais aussi de débarrasser la surface cutanée de germes nuisibles. Le lavage au savon et à la brosse des mains et des ongles, fait plusieurs fois par jour et en particulier avant chaque repas, diminuera dans une large mesure les chances d'infection.

1. DUPONT. *Archives de médecine des enfants*, 1899, t. II, p. 120.
2. BROUARDEL. *Œuvre de l'enseignement de l'hygiène et des sanatoriums maritimes*, n° 5, mai 1900, p. 10.

Des instructions détaillées données aux parents et aux instituteurs sur les dangers de la contagion tuberculeuse et sur les moyens de l'éviter devront être répandues partout.

L'usage toujours plus général du *lait stérilisé* pour les nourrissons a diminué certainement dans une large mesure les infections tuberculeuses par ingestion. Nous voudrions voir édicter par les pouvoirs publics l'épreuve par la tuberculine comme obligatoire pour toutes les vacheries urbaines et suburbaines, où les enfants vont boire du lait cru après traire. Genève possède un règlement de ce genre, édicté en 1896. « Il importe d'ailleurs. comme le disent Nocard et Leclainche [1], de combler les lacunes de la législation qui concerne la tuberculose et d'appliquer aux *suspects* un régime spécial. Devraient être considérés comme tels tous les bovidés qui ont cohabité habituellement avec un animal reconnu atteint, la suspicion pouvant être levée si l'animal résiste à l'épreuve de la tuberculine. De même que les malades, les suspects devraient être placés sous la surveillance sanitaire pour être livrés à la boucherie au moment jugé favorable par le propriétaire l'utilisation de leur lait ne devrait être permise qu'après constatation de la complète intégrité de la glande mammaire. »

Dans le grand-duché de Bade l'épreuve de la tuberculine est exigée pour les vacheries. Korn, qui a démontré la présence de bacilles tuberculeux virulents dans le quart des échantillons de beurre provenant du marché de Fribourg-en-Brisgau, réclame l'extension de cette mesure à tous les troupeaux servant à l'industrie laitière et l'interdiction d'employer dans cette industrie des personnes atteintes de phtisie.

Parmi les mesures prophylactiques hygiéniques, nous citerons en première ligne une bonne *éducation physique* et la *cure maritime*.

1. *Éducation physique.*

Pour l'éducation physique, nous répéterons ici ce que nous imprimions en 1877 dans la 1ʳᵉ édition de notre Manuel [2].

« La sollicitude doit être en éveil dès la naissance. Le choix d'une nourrice est d'une importance capitale. L'allaitement artificiel sera absolument proscrit.... Les plus grandes précautions seront prises au moment du sevrage. Plus tard, le régime de la viande crue peut rendre de grands services. Les substances grasses doivent entrer aussi pour une large part dans l'alimentation. Dès que l'enfant

---

1. Nocard et Leclainche. *Les maladies microbiennes.* Paris. 1896, p. 579.
2. D'Espine et Picot. 1ʳᵉ édition, 1877. p. 167.

commence à pouvoir marcher, courir, se promener, il faut l'habituer aux lavages froids le matin, à des sorties quotidiennes au grand air, et quand il a atteint l'âge de 10 à 12 ans, lui faire faire de la gymnastique ou de l'équitation.

« Pour les vêtements, le médecin se laissera guider par les circonstances et le climat. Il faut savoir prendre un juste milieu entre la méthode d'endurcissement à outrance et la méthode de préservation à outrance contre le froid extérieur, mais pencher plutôt pour la première. La principale préoccupation qui doit guider les parents dans l'éducation d'enfants prédisposés à la tuberculose est leur développement physique jusqu'à l'âge où ils pourront se livrer sans inconvénient à des études sérieuses. »

II. — *Les sanatoria maritimes.*

Tout le monde est d'accord aujourd'hui pour regarder la cure maritime prolongée comme l'agent le plus puissant que nous possédions pour guérir la scrofule. A plus forte raison, devons-nous la regarder comme l'agent prophylactique par excellence pour les enfants prédisposés à la tuberculose ou porteurs déjà de ces foyers latents d'où les bacilles pourront rayonner plus tard. Notre président d'honneur, le Dr BERGERON, ce maître vénéré de la pédiatrie française, a exprimé cette vérité dans des termes que j'aime à rappeler ici : « Si des individus déjà en puissance de scrofule peuvent être à ce point modifiés, que ne devrait-on pas attendre de la médication saline, si l'on pouvait soumettre à son action vivifiante les enfants chez lesquels des antécédents héréditaires suspects, certains états morbides aigus ou subaigus et l'ensemble de l'habitude extérieure, autorisent à soupçonner l'existence de la diathèse strumeuse et l'imminence de quelques-unes de ces manifestations ? »

C'est sous l'inspiration du Dr BERGERON qu'a été fondé par l'assistance publique l'hôpital marin de *Berck-sur-Mer*, le petit hôpital de 100 lits en 1861, le grand hôpital de 600 lits en 1869. Les résultats obtenus sont consignés dans la belle monographie du Dr CAZIN[2], dont j'extrais les résultats obtenus sur près de cinq mille enfants en 15 années.

La proportion des guérisons a atteint 70.7 pour 100 et celle des améliorations 5,2 pour 100 ; on peut donc admettre que près des

---

1. BERGERON. Du traitement et de la prophylaxie de la scrofule par les bains de mer. *Ann. d'hygiène*, 1868, t. XXIX, p. 241.
2. CAZIN. De l'influence des bains de mer sur la scrofule. Paris, 1885.

trois quarts ont bénéficié à des titres divers de la cure maritime.

Pour obtenir un pareil résultat, l'expérience a démontré qu'il fallait un séjour prolongé, d'autant plus long que la maladie était plus sérieuse : c'est ce que démontre la durée moyenne du séjour des enfants à Berck, qui a été de 425 jours.

Aujourd'hui l'œuvre des sanatoria maritimes, qui a commencé en Angleterre en 1796 par la formation de l'infirmerie royale de Margate, a pris de grandes proportions dans tous les pays. Ne pouvant les citer tous, je rappelle seulement en France l'hôpital Rothschild à Berck, la création du *sanatorium d'Arcachon*, de *Pen-Bron* au Croisic et de *Banyuls-sur-Mer* en 1887, ainsi que celle du sanatorium *Renée Sabran*, à la presqu'île de Gien en 1890.

L'*asile Dollfus*, plus modeste, avait été fondé à Cannes déjà en 1882 par Jean Dollfus de Mulhouse, et confié par la famille à la direction du Comité genevois des bains de mer à partir de 1886. Comme médecin du Comité, j'ai pu m'assurer moi-même du résultat obtenu dans la majorité des cas. La cure dure 9 mois, d'octobre à fin juin : la demi-cure de quatre mois et demi suffit pour les enfants légèrement atteints. Sur un total de 644 cures pour scrofule faites de 1882 à 1900, nous avons obtenu 548 guérisons (54 pour 100), 251 améliorations (59 pour 100), ce qui représente 95 pour 100 *de succès* ; 51 cas ont été stationnaires, 14 enfants sont morts, ce qui représente 7 pour 100 *d'insuccès*. Au point de vue prophylactique, les résultats ont été particulièrement brillants : sur 107 cas d'anémie lymphatique qui représentent surtout les prédisposés, nous comptons 70 guérisons et 37 améliorations[1].

En Allemagne, sous l'impulsion du professeur BENEKE de Marbourg, un grand sanatorium a été fondé en 1885, à l'île de Norderney ; il y en a d'autres aujourd'hui à Wyck sur l'île de Föhr, à Grossmüritz, etc. L'Autriche en a établi à Abbazia, la Hollande à Zandvoort, à Wykraam-Zee, la Belgique à Venduyne et à Middelkerke.

---

1. Voici la statistique pour maladies scrofuleuses soignées à l'asile Dollfus de 1882 à 1900 :

	Guéris.	Améliorés.	Stationnaires.	Morts.	Total.
Scrofule osseuse	125	111	15	10	261
Scrofule ganglionnaire externe	65	25	5	1	90
Anémie lymphatique	70	57	—	—	107
Scrofule de la peau et des muqueuses (yeux, nez, pharynx, oreilles)	49	45	7	—	101
Scrofule viscérale (ganglions bronchiques et mésentériques)	41	55	6	5	85
	548	251	51	14	644
	54 %	50 %	4.8 %	2.2 %	
	95 % succès		7 % insuccès		

L'Italie a créé presque dans chaque province un hospice maritime pour les enfants scrofuleux et rachitiques, où ils font des cures d'été.

Les *cures thermales* d'eaux salines et d'eaux mères ont été utilisées également pour le traitement gratuit des scrofuleux, soit en Allemagne où il existait 28 sanatoria aux bains d'eaux mères en 1894, soit en Suisse (Lavey, Rheinfelden), soit en France (Salins-Moutiers, Salies-de-Béarn, etc.).

L'influence altérante et reconstituante de la cure thermale saline est incontestable ; mais nous la considérons néanmoins comme inférieure à la cure marine dont l'agent le plus puissant est l'air de la mer imprégné d'effluves salins.

III. *Les cures d'altitude.*

Les succès remarquables obtenus dans la guérison des phtisiques adultes en Suisse à Davos (1550 mètres), depuis l'année 1866 ont amené la création de nombreux sanatoria d'altitude, soit en Suisse (Arosa, Maloja, Leysin, Montana-sur-Sierre), soit ailleurs.

Nous ne connaissons pas d'établissement spécialement destiné à la cure de la tuberculose infantile au-dessus de 1400 mètres, sauf les sanatoria scolaires pour garçons et jeunes filles de la classe aisée à Davos.

Un des fondateurs de la station à Davos, le Dr Spengler[1] attirait déjà en 1869 l'attention sur l'importance de la cure d'altitude pour la prophylaxie de la phtisie chez les enfants des tuberculeux.

Par contre, nous possédons en Suisse trois établissements d'altitude moyenne pour les enfants convalescents et en particulier pour les enfants scrofulo-tuberculeux, qui ont donné d'excellents résultats par une cure d'air comprimé hiver et été : c'est l'asile de *Langenbruck* dans le Jura bâlois, à 755 mètres, fondé par un comité bâlois, *Ægeri*, dans le canton de Zug, à 850 mètres, et *Schwäbrig* dans le canton d'Appenzell, à 1151 mètres, fondés par un comité zurichois.

IV. *Les asiles ruraux.*

Les asiles ruraux *d'Ormesson* et de *Villiers-sur-Marne* pour les enfants tuberculeux, fondés par l'OEuvre des enfants tuberculeux à Paris, ainsi que le Dispensaire ouvert à Paris et dirigé par le Dr Debrço, qui fournit gratuitement des médicaments à plus de cinq mille enfants

---

1. Spengler. *Die Landschaft Davos.* 1869. p. 40.

annuellement, rentrent plutôt dans le traitement que dans la prophylaxie de la phtisie. Néanmoins nous croyons devoir les signaler ici, ainsi que les colonies sanitaires de *Noisy-le-Grand* et de *Frémilly* qui en dépendent. De pareilles œuvres méritent d'être imitées parce qu'elles s'adressent à la population infantile des grandes villes qui fournit le plus grand contingent à la tuberculose sous toutes ses formes. Ajoutons que la cure d'Ormesson par l'aération et l'alimentation seules, portant sur l'ensemble des enfants de 5 à 12 ans admis depuis 10 ans, donne une proportion constante de guérisons de 34 pour 100 et de 50 pour 100 pour les enfants de 5 à 7 ans (Jaoul [1]).

Le Dr Derecq, dans son rapport sur la prophylaxie de la tuberculose infantile au Congrès de Berlin en 1899, a insisté avec raison sur la réceptivité vis-à-vis de la tuberculose des enfants convalescents de maladies aiguës. C'est ici que peut intervenir l'œuvre excellente des vacances.

V. *Colonies de vacances.*

Cette institution a été fondée à Zurich en 1876 par le pasteur Bion et s'est étendue aujourd'hui un peu partout. Commencée en Suisse avec 68 enfants, elle a fait bénéficier, en 1898, 2950 enfants répartis dans 85 colonies [2]. En outre, on a institué des *cures de lait* dans 55 colonies urbaines, consistant dans la distribution matin et soir de lait et de pain, ainsi que parfois dans des promenades combinées avec des jeux ; 6591 enfants pauvres et chétifs ont bénéficié de cette cure en 1898.

L'espoir de détruire la tuberculose est peut-être illusoire ; mais la statistique démontre que la lutte contre la tuberculose a déjà porté ses fruits. On a constaté, soit en Angleterre, soit en Prusse, une diminution réjouissante de la mortalité par la tuberculose.

L'Angleterre est le pays d'Europe où la mortalité par tuberculose est de beaucoup la plus basse. Cela tient, comme l'indique le professeur Brouardel [3], à ce que, depuis 1851, les prescriptions d'hygiène qui sont, sinon encore discutées, du moins à peine appliquées sur le continent, ont reçu une application méthodique. En effet, les statistique montrent que, pendant la période de 1851-1860, il mourut en Angleterre 2679 tuberculeux pour un million d'habitants ; en 1895, le chiffre de cette mortalité était tombée à 1465, et actuellement il n'est

1. Jaoul. *La tuberculose infantile.*
2. *Rapport sur l'hygiène publique en Suisse.* par le Dr Carrière, 15 avril 1900, p. 56.
3. Brouardel. *Œuvre de l'enseignement de l'hygiène,* n° 6, juin 1900, p. 8.

plus que de 1510, c'est-à-dire que *la mortalité tuberculeuse a diminué juste de moitié depuis 40 ans.*

En Prusse, d'après Cornet [1], la mortalité par tuberculose suit une décroissance continue depuis 1889 et a atteint aujourd'hui le tiers de sa fréquence primitive.

Je voudrais, en terminant, rappeler deux noms français, ceux du professeur Verneuil et du Dr Léon Petit, qui ont créé une vraie croisade contre la tuberculose et ont entraîné à leur suite toute une phalange de savants et de philanthropes. Leur nom mérite d'être cité parmi ceux des bienfaiteurs de l'humanité.

HÉRÉDITÉ DE LA TUBERCULOSE

RAPPORT

par M. le professeur HUTINEL [2]

S'il est un point bien établi par l'observation, c'est la fréquence de la tuberculose dans certaines familles : les enfants, nés de parents phtisiques, ont plus de tendance que les autres à devenir phtisiques eux-mêmes. Ce fait avait été noté par Hippocrate et, depuis des siècles, les médecins ont été unanimes à en reconnaître l'exactitude.

L'accord est moins facile quand il s'agit de l'interpréter. Pendant longtemps on l'a expliqué d'une façon qui semblait fort simple. La tuberculose, pensait-on, était le résultat d'une *diathèse* qui se transmettait par hérédité des parents à l'enfant.

Sous l'influence des découvertes de Villemin et de Koch, les idées se modifièrent. La tuberculose apparut comme le résultat d'une infection; la diathèse prit un corps, on connut son agent pathogène et on fut tout naturellement entraîné à considérer la maladie comme le résultat constant d'une transmission du germe par voie de contage.

La *contagion*, timidement acceptée jusque-là par quelques rares médecins, prit alors la première place dans l'étiologie de la tuberculose; au contraire, le rôle de l'*hérédité* s'effaça peu à peu. Pour ne pas la nier, on en vint à dire que les enfants, nés de tuberculeux, présen-

---

1. Cornet, *loc. cit.*, p. 476.
2. Ce rapport a été fait en collaboration avec le Dr G. Küss.

taient un amoindrissement de la vitalité qui favorisait la contagion, de la même façon que les autres causes banales de déchéance.

Cependant quelques médecins ne consentirent pas à reléguer à ce rang infime l'influence traditionnelle de l'hérédité. Sans contester l'importance du bacille, ni le rôle de la contagion, ils firent observer que le germe n'est pas tout, qu'il faut encore et surtout considérer le terrain sur lequel il doit pousser; et que, de toutes les causes qui modifient les aptitudes réactionnelles d'un sujet, il n'en est pas, en ce qui concerne la tuberculose, de plus importante que l'hérédité. C'était un retour aux idées des anciens.

Maintenant, nous nous trouvons en présence d'affirmations radicalement contradictoires. Certains auteurs n'admettent que la contagion; d'autres ne voient que l'hérédité. Il faut donc, ou faire un choix entre ces tendances opposées, ou chercher à les accorder.

La tâche est délicate. En effet, sans sortir du domaine de l'observation pure, dès qu'on cherche à préciser les affirmations des partisans de l'hérédité, on rencontre des contradictions flagrantes.

Pour les uns, la tuberculose est héréditaire dans le huitième des cas, pour d'autres (Leudet, Vallin, Hérard) dans la moitié; pour d'autres encore (Baumgarten, G. Arthaud), elle est presque fatale et constante.

Ces différences d'appréciation tiennent certainement aux conditions différentes dans lesquelles les observateurs se sont placés, aux faits qu'ils ont eus à leur disposition et aux idées théoriques qui les ont guidés.

Quelques-uns n'admettent que l'*hérédité directe* et se refusent à considérer comme héréditaires les cas dans lesquels un des ascendants, père ou mère, n'est pas notoirement tuberculeux; les autres, au contraire, étendent la notion de l'hérédité aux cas où les ascendants directs étant ou paraissant indemnes, les grands-parents ou les collatéraux sont tuberculeux: ils admettent ainsi l'*hérédité atavique* ou *collatérale*.

Et ce n'est pas la seule cause de divergence. Le diagnostic de tuberculose n'est pas posé avec la même facilité par tous les médecins. Les uns ne font entrer en ligne de compte que des tuberculoses avérées, indéniables: les autres reconnaissent ou soupçonnent des infections bacillaires, minimes, larvées, latentes ou torpides, et cela aussi bien chez les parents que chez les enfants.

Enfin, il est des cas où l'on parle d'hérédité, alors que l'influence héréditaire s'est exercée en sens inverse, les parents ayant été tuberculisés par leurs enfants

On rencontre donc des difficultés très grandes quand on se borne à examiner les faits, même sans chercher à les interpréter; ces difficultés augmentent encore quand on passe aux explications pathogéniques.

Trois hypothèses se présentent pour expliquer la tuberculose chez les rejetons des phtisiques :

1° La *contagion familiale*;

2° La transmission conceptionnelle ou utérine du germe tuberculeux des parents à l'enfant, c'est-à-dire l'*hérédité de graine*;

3° La transmission d'une prédisposition, ou l'*hérédité de terrain*, rendant plus efficaces les causes ubiquitaires de contagion.

La contagion est bien plus redoutable dans la famille du phtisique que partout ailleurs, et l'on ne voit pas comment l'enfant élevé par des parents tuberculeux, dans un local infecté, pourrait y échapper. Cette influence de la contagion familiale est indiscutable et rend très difficile à résoudre le problème de l'hérédité tuberculeuse. Seules, les observations d'enfants nés de phtisiques et séparés de leurs parents dès la naissance doivent entrer en ligne de compte. Si l'hérédité joue un rôle véritable dans la genèse de la maladie, ces enfants doivent se tuberculiser plus facilement que ceux qui vivent avec eux, dans des conditions identiques.

Les cas de ce genre sont d'ailleurs assez rares dans la littérature médicale et, chose curieuse, partisans et adversaires de l'hérédité les invoquent à tour de rôle à l'appui de leur thèse.

Au premier abord, la statistique des Enfants-Assistés ne semble guère favorable à la notion de l'hérédité tuberculeuse. Les enfants, issus de phtisiques pour une bonne part, et abandonnés très jeunes, sont élevés à la campagne. Ils s'y tuberculisent peu. Sans doute le contingent qu'ils fournissent à l'infection bacillaire est plus fort que ne l'indiquent ma statistique et celles de Stich et de Schnitzlein, car beaucoup de tuberculoses peuvent rester latentes ou méconnues. Mais, j'ai constaté dans ces dernières années un fait qui prouve que si ces enfants ne se tuberculisent pas, c'est faute d'occasion. Quand ils ont grandi, on les envoie dans les écoles professionnelles d'Yseure, de Villepreux, etc.; là ils trouvent des tuberculeux et ils sont décimés par la phtisie.

Cette observation vient à l'appui de celles de Zoppelius, de Landouzy, de Bang, de Sanson, de Marfan, etc., qui montrent que les enfants des phtisiques, même séparés de très bonne heure de leurs parents, présentent une facilité navrante à se tuberculiser.

G. Arthaud a suivi plusieurs familles qui, pour mettre leurs enfants à l'abri de l'hérédo-tuberculose, les avaient éloignés ; eh bien, malgré la séparation du milieu familial, toujours la tuberculose s'est développée ultérieurement.

Il m'est arrivé deux fois de noter des lésions tuberculeuses chez des enfants, nés d'une mère saine et d'un amant phtisique, alors que restaient indemnes les autres enfants, nés auparavant de la même mère et du père légitime, non tuberculeux.

Mais je n'insiste pas ; tout médecin connaît des faits qui mettent hors de doute l'influence de l'hérédité. Il reste à les interpréter.

Faut-il admettre la transmission héréditaire du germe tuberculeux ; doit-on invoquer une prédisposition spécifique ; ou bien faut-il se contenter de l'hypothèse d'une détérioration organique indifférente et banale, favorisant l'action des causes multiples d'infection bacillaire qui nous entourent ?

Cette question a un intérêt pratique de premier ordre. Si l'on admet l'hérédité du germe, l'enfant issu de parents phtisiques n'est pas seulement un candidat à la maladie, susceptible d'en être préservé ; c'est déjà un malade ; notion décevante, de nature à paralyser tout effort prophylactique.

L'idée de prédisposition et de contagion familiale est plus consolante : certes le péril est toujours menaçant, car le bacille de Koch est très répandu : mais la lutte est possible, si l'on peut se résoudre à envisager la situation comme elle doit l'être et à prendre les mesures draconiennes qu'elle comporte.

Cette raison ne peut et ne doit influencer en rien l'interprétation des faits. Quelle que soit la vérité, il faut la regarder en face.

Avant d'envisager les modes suivant lesquels l'hérédité peut se manifester, je dois justifier ce mot d'hérédité que j'appliquerai forcément à des choses qui n'ont rien à voir avec l'hérédité proprement dite. Il n'y a d'héréditaires, au sens absolu du mot, que les états pathologiques transmis à l'être nouveau dès son origine, dès la conception. Or, dans la tuberculose, comme dans les autres infections, ce n'est pas tant au moment de l'union du spermatozoïde avec l'ovule, que pendant la vie intra-utérine, que le rejeton se trouve exposé à la contamination.

Ce n'est pas là de l'hérédité vraie : c'est de l'hérédo-contagion ; et cependant l'habitude s'est établie d'étendre le mot d'hérédité à toutes les influences que la tuberculose des ascendants exerce sur les enfants.

I

La transmission héréditaire du *germe tuberculeux* a été particulièrement étudiée, et c'est sur elle que nous possédons les données les plus précises.

Nous connaissons assez bien ce germe et ses propriétés. Sans doute, au point de vue morphologique, il nous échappe souvent ; nos procédés de coloration ne suffisent pas toujours à le déceler ; et l'on peut se demander s'il ne se dissimule pas quelquefois, sous la forme de spores (ce qui est peu probable) ou de fragments difficiles à mettre en évidence ; mais, même dans ces cas, nous pouvons démontrer son existence à coup sûr, grâce à la méthode expérimentale. Aujourd'hui nous sommes en droit de repousser, comme dénués de valeur, les arguments théoriques par lesquels on prétendait autrefois démontrer l'impossibilité de l'hérédité tuberculeuse par infection conceptionnelle, mais, d'autre part, nous ne pouvons plus accepter l'idée d'une infection bacillaire que le cobaye, vrai réactif vivant, serait impuissant à révéler.

L'hérédité tuberculeuse est-elle possible par *infection ovulaire* ? *A priori* cela n'est pas absolument invraisemblable, puisque l'histoire de la pébrine et aussi celle de la syphilis nous fournissent des exemples d'infection transmises par l'ovule à des rejetons viables ; mais l'examen des faits rend cette hypothèse à peu près inacceptable.

Jamais on n'a trouvé de tubercules chez des fœtus âgés de moins de quatre mois, antérieurement à l'établissement de la circulation placentaire. En vain objectera-t-on que les lésions n'auraient pas pu se développer en si peu de temps ; il y a des observations qui prouvent que les bacilles se multiplient très activement dans les tissus embryonnaires.

Il n'est pas une seule observation de tuberculose congénitale qu'on ne puisse rattacher à une contagion intra-utérine. Les expériences d'inoculation de la tuberculose à des œufs de poule (Maffucci-Baumgarten) rentrent, en réalité, dans la catégorie des faits de contagion au cours du développement fœtal.

Les partisans de l'hérédité ont voulu tourner la difficulté en établissant l'existence d'une hérédité *parasitaire*, *d'origine paternelle*. Si cette hérédité était démontrée, l'existence d'une infection conceptionnelle deviendrait probable, rien de plus, car on pourrait encore soutenir l'hypothèse d'une infection utérine par le sperme et, secondairement à celle-ci, d'une contamination fœtale.

L'hérédité parasitaire d'origine paternelle implique d'abord une infectiosité démontrable du sperme des phtisiques. De nombreux travaux ont été publiés sur cette question. Sans citer ceux, déjà anciens, de Cavaquis, Landouzy et Martin, Salles, Sirena et Pernice, Aubeau, Carl Jani, il reste les recherches de Gœrtner, d'Albrecht, Dobroklonsky, Maffucci, Fure Spano, Westermayer, Walther, Jaeck, Nakarai, etc. Celles-ci démontrent que le sperme renferme des bacilles dans la tuberculose génitale et dans la granulie : mais elles ne résolvent pas la question de l'infectiosité du sperme dans les phtisies vulgaires, sans lésions génitales. En effet, si (pour Fure Spano et Nakarai) la virulence du sperme est habituelle chez tous les tuberculeux, Westermayer, Walther, Dobroklonsky, Albrecht ont eu constamment des résultats négatifs.

Même en admettant la présence fréquente des germes tuberculeux dans le sperme, il resterait à démontrer la possibilité de l'infection ovulaire.

Gœrtner a essayé vainement de réaliser l'infection conceptionnelle avec des lapins et des cobayes inoculés dans les testicules. Les résultats tout différents de Maffucci font partie d'une série d'expériences sujettes à revision, et l'on ne peut attacher qu'une médiocre importance à l'expérience unique dans laquelle Baumgarten, en 1892, aurait réussi à réaliser une tuberculose ovulaire d'origine paternelle.

En somme, les expériences de laboratoire ne résolvent pas le problème de l'hérédité parasitaire de la tuberculose d'origine paternelle. La clinique nous en apprend-elle davantage? Nous avons dépouillé à ce point de vue les observations publiées. Celles qui semblent les plus probantes peuvent toutes s'expliquer par une hérédo-prédisposition favorisant une contamination ultérieure. Laissons à l'avenir le soin de trancher la question; disons seulement, jusqu'à preuve du contraire, que l'infection tuberculeuse conceptionnelle nous semble problématique.

II

Si l'hérédité conceptionnelle n'est nullement prouvée, *l'hérédo-contagion transplacentaire* est absolument hors de doute.

De 1875 à 1900, on trouve dans la littérature médicale 15 cas de tuberculose humaine congénitale *avec lésions macroscopiques* et 11 observations d'infection bacillaire *sans lésions*. Les vétérinaires ont publié une cinquantaine de cas analogues, mais de valeur inégale, auxquels on peut joindre une trentaine de faits douteux. Il n'y a d'ailleurs aucun intérêt réel à faire le total des observations positives de tuberculose congénitale. Ce chiffre d'une centaine, auquel nous arrivons, est un nombre quelconque, indifférent, très éloigné du chiffre réel. La bacillose héréditaire ne s'est pas limitée dans ces vingt-cinq dernières années aux cas publiés. Beaucoup ont dû passer inaperçus, car la tuberculose héréditaire est compatible avec une survie plus ou moins longue.

Au lieu de compter les observations, il importe surtout de les classer, d'entrer dans leur détail et d'en tirer les enseignements qu'elles comportent.

En procédant de la sorte, on met en lumière quelques points que je tiens à préciser.

1er point. Les cas de tuberculose congénitale avec lésions macroscopiques sont extrêmement rares. Ce fait est établi par les nombreuses autopsies de nouveau-nés faites par les médecins et les vétérinaires de tous les pays. Cette rareté acquiert encore une signification plus grande quand on considère spécialement les enfants des tuberculeux, comme l'ont fait Royer, Walther, Kackel et Lungwitz, Ernst, Weichselbaum, Jani, Heller, Lehman. C'est là un point accepté par tout le monde; mais ce n'est pas, comme on a trop de tendance à le croire, un argument décisif contre l'infection tuberculeuse congénitale.

2e point. La bacillose fœtale peut, en effet, exister sans s'accompagner de lésions macroscopiques ni même histologiques. Landouzy et Martin ont mis ce fait en lumière en 1885 et il a été maintes fois vérifié depuis. Il peut s'expliquer de deux façons.

La première, qui semble la plus logique : c'est que la bacillose fœtale, sans lésions, répond à une infection intra-utérine des derniers jours de la vie qui n'a pas eu le temps de créer des tubercules visibles. Si on acceptait cette interprétation, le problème de l'hérédité parasitaire de la tuberculose serait jugé définitivement.

Aussi en a-t-on proposé une autre. La bacillose héréditaire sans lésions serait, pour quelques auteurs (Baumgarten, Landouzy, Kelsch), une forme tout à fait spéciale et quelque peu mystérieuse de tuberculose.

3e point. Les formes anatomiques de la tuberculose fœtale sont très variables. Ordinairement il s'agit de *granulies* plus ou moins généralisées, parfois très discrètes, plus souvent confluentes, atteignant la plupart des organes, notamment le foie, la rate, le poumon. Ce dernier organe est l'un des moins touchés quand l'enfant n'a pas respiré; au contraire, les lésions y sont plus accusées quand l'enfant a vécu quelque temps. La tuberculose fœtale n'est pas essentiellement une tuberculose pulmonaire. Quand, dans la vie intra-utérine, le bacille colonise dans le poumon, il a infecté antérieurement ou simultanément d'autres organes.

Lorsque l'infection bacillaire n'est pas suffisante pour créer une granulie, la tuberculose fœtale reste *localisée*. Souvent elle atteint le foie, en infectant simultanément les ganglions du hile et elle peut y rester cantonnée; ou bien elle s'étend aux organes voisins, notamment à la chaîne ganglionnaire médiastine; mais il n'est pas exact de dire avec Baumgarten, Bang, de Renzi, Hencke, etc., que le siège de prédilection de la tuberculose congénitale est dans les ganglions bronchiques. La tuberculose congénitale localisée ne se trouve pas nécessairement dans le foie et dans ses ganglions: elle a d'autres sièges de prédilection: la moelle des os, le système ganglionnaire et les capsules surrénales.

4e point. La tuberculose congénitale procède généralement d'une tuberculose miliaire ou d'une phtisie pulmonaire très avancée; cependant cela n'est pas constant.

Elle peut en effet survenir au cours de tuberculoses pulmonaires relativement bénignes, permettant une survie prolongée, **ou résulter** d'une tuberculisation de l'appareil génital interne. Le nombre des faits de ce genre doit même être plus grand que ne le feraient supposer les observations publiées.

5e point. Il est vraisemblable que la tuberculose maternelle se transmet au fœtus humain, surtout à la faveur de lésions placentaires tuberculeuses qui facilitent le passage des bacilles. Même dans les cas où le placenta se laisse forcer par la tuberculose, le rôle de défense qu'il exerce contre l'invasion bacillaire apparaît généralement.

6e point. La tuberculose fœtale est probablement compatible, dans quelques cas, avec un développement complet et une viabilité suffisante de l'enfant. Sans doute, dans la majorité des cas, elle n'est démontrable que chez des monstres, des fœtus morts avant terme ou des nouveau-nés peu viables: mais les cas dans lesquels la vie est possible sont précisément ceux qui doivent passer inaperçus.

III

Voyons maintenant ce que nous apprend la médecine expérimentale.

Un premier point semble établi : c'est l'excessive rareté, presque l'absence de tuberculoses congénitales avec lésions macroscopiques chez les petits de femelles rendues tuberculeuses. Cette rareté n'a rien qui nous étonne: en effet, les femelles sont généralement inoculées en pleine gestation, ce qui réduit à un délai très court l'espace qui sépare l'infection maternelle de la naissance souvent prématurée des petits.

L'hérédité bacillaire expérimentale n'a donc généralement été mise en évidence que par l'inoculation au cobaye des organes du fœtus. Les observations de ce genre ne sont pas nombreuses. Landouzy et Martin, Cavagnès, Calabrese, Ausset ont obtenu de cobayes ou de lapines tuberculisés quatre fœtus bacillisés, sur 19 séries d'expériences, Galtier a eu 15 fois des résultats négatifs et 4 résultats positifs. Sciolla et Poluueri ont également noté des faits positifs ; mais les expériences les plus importantes, sur ce point, sont celles de Gœrtner faites avec un luxe de précautions et une science si parfaite qu'elles défient toute critique. Gœrtner a pu réaliser la contagion intra-utérine une fois sur dix, en inoculant des lapines pleines par la voie veineuse. Tuberculisant des souris avant la fécondation, il obtint, une fois dans le dixième, une fois dans la moitié des cas (série 1 et 2 de ses expériences) des portées contenant un ou plusieurs petits bacillisés.

On ne peut donc pas contester la possibilité d'une hérédo-contagion, transmettant au fœtus soit des lésions tuberculeuses macroscopiquement appréciables, soit une infection bacillaire sans lésions.

La barrière placentaire peut être forcée par le germe de la tuberculose ; reste à savoir quelle est la fréquence de cette contagion intra-utérine.

Pour nous en rendre compte, nous devrons analyser quelques données qui, toutes, il est vrai, n'ont pas une égale valeur.

1° *La condition première de la contamination fœtale est l'infection sanguine de la mère.* Or, le bacille ne séjourne pas volontiers dans le sang ; il en disparaît vite comme l'ont montré Nocard et Gœrtner, et il ne se trouve pas dans la masse totale du sang d'un cobaye non encore arrivé à la période cachectique de la tuberculose (Kien). Mais, si le bacille ne séjourne pas dans le sang, il y passe certainement quelquefois. Les poussées de tuberculose miliaire hématogène, qui se rencontrent dans les phtisies vulgaires, démontrent ces passages, et le sang est assez virulent dans la granulie humaine. Il n'est donc pas impossible que, chez des tuberculeuses plus ou moins gravement atteintes, les bacilles arrivent au placenta ; mais, en dehors de la granulie et, sauf exception rare, ils ne peuvent y parvenir qu'en petit nombre.

2° Les bacilles, arrivés au placenta, se déposent-ils dans les sinuosités des espaces intervilleux, produisent-ils facilement des lésions, ont-ils des facilités plus ou moins grandes pour passer de la mère au

fœtus; on ne saurait le dire *a priori*. Il est vraisemblable que chez les
petits animaux de laboratoire : souris, cobayes et lapines, la barrière
placentaire se laisse franchir facilement par les leucocytes bacillifères
ou par les germes mobiles; au contraire, chez les ruminants et sans
doute aussi chez la femme la barrière semble plus forte et ne se
laisse probablement forcer qu'après la formation d'un tubercule qui
fait brèche. Or le placenta est peu favorable au développement des
tubercules ; même dans la granulie on ne les y rencontre guère et ils
sont toujours en petit nombre. Il y a donc là une particularité qui
semble peu favorable à l'hérédo-contagion; mais cette étude a besoin
d'être complétée.

5° Un renseignement plus important est fourni par le nombre élevé
des résultats négatifs obtenus dans la recherche méthodique des
bacilloses congénitales, spontanées ou expérimentales. Verchère,
Leyden, Chamberlan, Vignal, Hutinel, Loude, Strauss, Bolognesi,
Bugge, Doléris et Bourges, Mercier et Sicard ont inoculé sans succès
des fragments d'organes recueillis sur des fœtus nés de phtisiques
avancés.

Leyden, Nocard, Gallier, Jackh, Ausset, ont également échoué en
cherchant à déceler une tuberculose latente chez des petits nés de
lapines ou de cobayes tuberculisées. Sanchez Toledo, sur trente-cinq
portées de cobayes dont les mères avaient été inoculées avec de la
tuberculose aviaire, n'a jamais trouvé de bacilles dans le foie ni dans
la rate des fœtus.

Il ne faudrait pas cependant exagérer la valeur de ces expériences
négatives : elles démontrent que les infections congénitales généralisées sont rares, mais, comme elles ont consisté dans l'inoculation
d'une faible portion de la masse fœtale, elles prouvent peu de chose
contre la possibilité d'une tuberculose localisée. C'est probablement
pour cela que Gœrtner qui inoculait la presque totalité des organes
fœtaux, broyés et triturés, est arrivé aux résultats que l'on sait.

Mais ce que Gœrtner a vu, en opérant sur de petits animaux, n'est
peut-être pas absolument applicable à l'espèce humaine; nous venons
de dire pourquoi. D'autre part, il ne réussissait à tuberculiser les
fœtus qu'en donnant aux mères des tuberculoses extrêmement graves.

Si on étudie, chez l'animal, comme l'a fait Hanser, la transmission
d'une tuberculose commençante, aussi localisée que possible, on ne
se place pas davantage dans les conditions de la clinique humaine.
Les petits, exposés à la contagion placentaire, pendant une période
de douze à quarante-six jours (la tuberculose maternelle étant
minime), sont tous restés indemnes et ont pu survivre.

Chez la femme phtisique, des migrations bacillaires sont possibles, et cela pendant les neuf mois que dure la grossesse. Que la tuberculisation des enveloppes de l'œuf et du placenta soit rare, même dans ces conditions, nous sommes forcés de l'admettre; mais elle est possible. Sur ce point, l'expérimentation ne nous fournit donc pas l'argument décisif que nous cherchons.

4° Les autopsies des rejetons de phtisiques, pratiquées après une survie prolongée, offrent un peu plus d'intérêt. A vrai dire, les résultats sont surtout négatifs.

Robert Koch qui a eu dans son laboratoire beaucoup de femelles de cobayes, pleines au moment de l'infection tuberculeuse, ne les a jamais vues mettre bas des petits tuberculeux au moment de la naissance, et ces petits restèrent sains pendant de longs mois. Même remarque a été faite par Grancher, Strauss, Borrel, Jackh, Küss, etc.

5° Il faut, dans le même ordre d'idées, citer les injections de tuberculine pratiquée chez des descendants de tuberculeux. Nocard et Bang, ayant isolé les veaux nés dans des exploitations agricoles décimées par la tuberculose, ont pu, après quelques mois, les tuberculiser sans obtenir de réaction. Le même procédé peut être employé presque sans danger chez les jeunes enfants. Sur un petit enfant né d'une phtisique morte quelques heures après l'accouchement, je n'ai constaté aucune réaction après l'ingestion d'un dixième de milligramme de tuberculine.

Si nous passons en revue tous ces arguments nous voyons que la rareté des tubercules congénitaux et la difficulté de les déceler au moyen des inoculations partielles n'exclut pas la possibilité d'une bacillose limitée plus ou moins fréquente. L'absence de tuberculose chez des animaux nés de femelles tuberculeuses et gardées longtemps en vie, les résultats négatifs de la tuberculisation des bovidés ont une réelle valeur; mais tous ces faits ne peuvent pas être transportés intégralement dans la pathologie humaine.

Nous ne sommes donc pas trop surpris de voir que les partisans de l'hérédité parasitaire ne désarment pas; et il faut encore compter avec leur opinion.

Examinons les raisons sur lesquelles ils fondent leur conviction.

IV

L'analogie que l'on a voulu établir entre la syphilis et la tuberculose ne nous arrêtera pas. Ce que l'on observe dans la syphilis rend plutôt invraisemblable la fréquence d'une infection tuberculeuse héréditaire.

Les nouveau-nés hérédo-syphilitiques présentent des lésions très étendues de divers organes; les descendants du tuberculeux n'en ont presque jamais.

Les arguments cliniques ne méritent pas non plus, en thèse générale, la confiance qu'on leur a accordée trop souvent. Trop de causes s'associent, trop d'erreurs de diagnostic ou d'interprétations vicient l'emploi de la méthode d'observation clinique pour qu'on puisse accepter certaines conclusions souvent légèrement déduites.

Faisons une exception pour les cas de tuberculose qui atteignent des enfants soustraits dès leur naissance au contact de leurs parents. Doit-on expliquer ces faits par une contamination congénitale ou par une hérédo-prédisposition favorisant une contagion à laquelle l'enfant est exposé cent fois pour une après sa naissance? Les partisans de l'hérédité parasitaire pensent que l'hypothèse de l'hérédo-prédisposition ne s'accorde pas avec la fatalité du développement de la tuberculose. Si cette fatalité de l'héritage morbide était démontrée, elle ne serait guère explicable, en effet, que par une transmission du germe; mais elle ne l'est pas. La fatalité de la tuberculose héréditaire n'est pas soutenable; ce qui ne nous empêche pas de penser et de dire que dans les familles de tuberculeux les enfants sont presque tous touchés par la maladie, à des degrés divers. Beaucoup d'entre eux, heureusement, présentent des formes atténuées, bénignes et généralement méconnues, qui peuvent s'expliquer par la contagion à laquelle ils échappent difficilement.

1° Si nous consultons l'anatomie pathologique, nous trouvons un argument souvent invoqué par les partisans de l'hérédité parasitaire, à savoir : la grande fréquence de la tuberculose chez les enfants du premier âge; mais étudions de près cette fréquence. Un premier fait nous frappe : c'est qu'elle augmente avec l'âge; et, sur ce point, toutes les statistiques sont concordantes. Sur 100 autopsies, on compte un tuberculeux, dans les trois premiers mois de la vie: ce chiffre monte à 5 pour la première année: 24, de un à deux ans; 40, de deux à quatre ans. Il y a là, un gros argument à invoquer en faveur de la doctrine contagionniste.

2° Un deuxième fait; c'est la rareté, au-dessous de deux ans, de tuberculose vraiment latente. Il semble que les jeunes enfants résistent trop mal à l'action du bacille pour faire de ces tuberculoses; presque toujours ils présentent des formes graves, généralisées ou non. A partir de deux ans, les tuberculoses latentes ou en voie de guérison spontanée deviennent de plus en plus fréquentes. Comment faire remonter à une infection congénitale les bacilloses du jeune âge, puisque, entre la première enfance où l'on ne trouve jamais de tubercules et l'enfance proprement dite, il existe une période intermédiaire peu compatible avec l'existence de foyers latents. Nous ne nions pas que des tuberculoses précoces ou même congénitales, atténuées dans leur virulence ou survenant chez des sujets résistants, puissent s'arrêter et guérir : nous avons trouvé parfois des foyers calcifiés qui témoignent de cette évolution : mais ces faits sont rares et ne constituent qu'une exception.

5° Un troisième argument ressort de l'étude anatomique des lésions tuberculeuses du premier âge. La disposition des foyers initiaux impose presque nécessairement l'idée d'une contagion *post partum*.

Ces foyers ont leur maximum de fréquence dans les ganglions du médiastin. L'interprétation la plus plausible, c'est que les bacilles y parviennent par l'intermédiaire des voies aériennes. On a prétendu qu'ils pouvaient pénétrer tout aussi bien par la muqueuse nasale, par la bouche, n'importe où, pour aller se localiser dans le médiastin où ils trouveraient des conditions favorables à leur développement : et les partisans de l'hérédité ont affirmé que les bacilles étaient entrés dans le thorax, dès la vie intra-utérine, ou qu'ils avaient colonisé secondairement en cet endroit, en partant d'un foyer congénital situé en un point quelconque de l'économie.

Regardons les choses de près et ces hypothèses s'effondrent. La caséification des ganglions du médiastin n'est presque jamais la localisation unique de la tuberculose. Küss de Strasbourg l'avait pressenti dès 1850 et Parrot l'a démontré par ses belles recherches sur l'adénopathie similaire. Je l'ai vu moi-même et tous mes élèves ont pu le contrôler depuis bien des années. Le foyer caséeux du médiastin est presque toujours le reflet, l'image d'un foyer analogue et de même âge, situé dans le poumon. L'opinion inverse résulte de la difficulté et de l'insuffisance des recherches.

La loi de Parrot n'établit pas l'origine aérienne de la tuberculose médiastine, car la subordination des lésions des ganglions à celles du poumon existe, quelle que soit la provenance de l'infection pulmonaire ; mais si on étudie avec soin, comme l'a fait Küss, la disposition des lésions pulmonaires et médiastines, on constate que la disposition topographique des tubercules permet, dans presque tous les cas, d'éliminer une infection rétrograde, allant des ganglions au poumon ou une infection par voie sanguine d'un foyer latent et ignoré. Cette disposition des lésions est absolument superposable à celle des tuberculoses d'inoculation ; elle permet de suivre, dans ses étapes successives, la marche de l'infection bacillaire au sein de l'organisme.

Il nous est impossible de voir des tuberculoses congénitales dans ces tuberculoses pulmonaires et ganglionnaires. Elles nous apparaissent comme des exemples de tuberculose par inhalation.

Dans la grande majorité des cas, l'enfant s'infecte par les voies aériennes; dans d'autres cas plus rares, le bacille pénètre par la voie intestinale et envahit les ganglions du mésentère; mais n'insistons pas sur les différentes portes d'entrée de l'infection tuberculeuse.

Avec les notions que nous venons de résumer, il nous est facile de réfuter en quelques mots l'argumentation de Baumgarten qui reste, à l'heure actuelle, le dernier refuge des partisans de l'hérédité.

V

La doctrine peut se résumer ainsi : infection héréditaire de l'embryon, conceptionnelle le plus souvent; persistance du germe à l'état latent jusqu'à la naissance; puis, dans les premiers mois de la vie extra-utérine, formation de foyers tuberculeux qui, dans l'avenir, sont l'origine de la plupart des tuberculoses soi-disant spontanées et imputées à la contagion.

Cette théorie nous semble inacceptable. L'hypothèse d'une bacillose latente, chez le fœtus et le nouveau-né n'est pas compatible avec les faits déjà cités. D'autre part, les foyers tuberculeux dont elle invoque l'existence, sont généralement des lésions exogènes. Mais, s'il est impossible d'admettre l'origine congénitale de la plupart de ces foyers, on doit reconnaître, avec Baumgarten, qu'un grand nombre des tuberculoses de l'adolescence ou de l'âge adulte dérivent d'auto-infections ayant leur source dans des noyaux tuberculeux datant de la première enfance. On a tort de voir partout et toujours, dans une tuberculose qui éclate, la manifestation d'une contagion récente.

VI

Il nous semble démontré maintenant que l'hérédité tuberculeuse ne se manifeste qu'exceptionnellement par l'infection bacillaire du fœtus. Elle a d'autres façons de se révéler, plus habituelles et plus importantes cliniquement.

Tout d'abord elle se traduit par des *troubles dystrophiques*. L'existence de ces troubles est connue depuis les premiers âges de la médecine. Les rejetons des phtisiques ont souvent un habitus extérieur et une conformation qui constituent une véritable tare organique et qui sont pour eux comme un certificat d'origine. Toute maladie chronique, qui entraîne une déchéance chez le père ou chez la mère, les rend moins aptes à engendrer des enfants sains et physiologiquement normaux. C'est un fait d'observation que l'expérimentation a confirmé sans y rien ajouter.

Les enfants des phtisiques, médiocres au point de vue organique, peuvent, par leur valeur cérébrale, constituer des individualités utiles; mais leur amoindrissement dystrophique a pour résultat une tendance marquée à l'extinction de la race.

Il est essentiel de ne pas confondre ces tares dystrophiques avec l'*hérédo-prédisposition morbide*. Dystrophie et prédisposition héréditaire peuvent coexister; mais leur association n'est ni forcée, ni constante. Cette notion n'est pas nouvelle; et cependant une confusion regrettable s'établit souvent entre les dystrophiques héréditaires et les candidats à la phtisie. Tel sujet malingre et chétif résistera victorieusement à la tuberculose alors que d'autres, vigoureux en apparence, seront rapidement enlevés.

Est-il nécessaire maintenant d'énumérer les tares organiques des hérédo-tuberculeux? Ce sont là des données classiques. On note chez le fœtus, la multiléthalité, la gémellité et des monstruosités: chez l'enfant viable, des troubles de l'ossification, l'hippocratisme des doigts, des malformations thoraciques, une débilité allant jusqu'à l'infantilisme; enfin des malformations viscérales diverses.

A côté de ces tares, apparentes ou cachées, on a signalé des troubles biochimiques plus difficiles à saisir et peut-être plus intéressants. Malheureusement ce que nous savons sur ce point est bien peu de chose. Gaube a noté une déminéralisation calcique et magnésienne; Charrin a montré qu'au point de vue chimique les enfants des tuberculeux ont une vitalité fort réduite, et c'est tout.

Mais ces tares, organiques ou fonctionnelles, n'appartiennent pas en propre à la tuberculose. Elles peuvent être l'aboutissant d'états pathologiques variés : syphilis, alcoolisme, maladies nerveuses, cancer, vieillesse, déchéances diverses. Il n'en est pas moins vrai que certains indices, minimes parfois et cependant suffisants, permettent de dire d'un enfant : « Voilà un fils de tuberculeux ». Cette impression clinique, dont on a souvent peine à se défendre, résulte peut-être en partie de ce que la tuberculose, étant la plus commune des causes de dystrophie, est plus fréquemment que les autres retrouvée par l'analyse clinique.

VII

Nous arrivons maintenant à *l'hérédo-prédisposition*. Les descendants des phtisiques ne naissent pas tuberculeux, mais tuberculisables, a dit Peter. Personne ne nie cette prédisposition ; mais il importe de ne pas confondre l'aptitude que ces sujets ont à se tuberculiser avec celle qu'ils ont à faire une tuberculose plus ou moins rapide. Croire que les enfants des phtisiques sont destinés à devenir des tuberculeux incurables est une erreur clinique qui a trop longtemps régné en médecine.

Parmi les hérédo-tuberculeux, il en est un bon nombre qui présentent, à la fois, une réceptivité plus grande à l'infection et un terrain relativement résistant qui modifie l'évolution morbide. Les chlorotiques, Hanot l'a noté, sont souvent des filles de phtisiques ; et cependant la chlorose vraie n'aboutit guère à la phtisie. Les poussées tuberculeuses, pour Arthaud, s'atténueraient graduellement chez les descendants des phtisiques et la maladie tendrait à s'éteindre si la race parvenait à se perpétuer. Un exemple frappant de cette influence remarquable de l'hérédité tuberculeuse est fourni par les scrofuleux qui descendent si souvent de phtisiques et dont la tuberculose conserve pendant longtemps, parfois toute la vie, une allure torpide.

Mais, à côté de ces exemples favorables, il y en a d'autres, absolument inverses, qui justifient le vieil adage : *phtisis hereditaria omnium pessima*. Souvent on voit, à la puberté ou vers la vingtième année, éclore, chez les hérédo-tuberculeux, des phtisies aiguës ou subaiguës contre lesquelles on est désarmé.

Comment peut-on expliquer ces faits ?

Il serait facile, sans doute, d'invoquer une atténuation plus ou moins grande de la virulence des germes tuberculeux ; mais rien ne démontre cette atténuation. Si les ganglions scrofuleux ne suffisent pas à tuberculiser le lapin et ne donnent au cobaye qu'une tuberculose relativement bénigne, cela tient simplement à ce que les bacilles y sont peu nombreux. Vagedas, Kunla, Poupé et Vescley ont prétendu avoir isolé des races atténuées du bacille de Koch ; mais leurs résultats sont encore suspects, Auclair ayant prouvé l'identité de virulence des bacilles pris à des sources variées.

Nous pensons donc que l'influence du terrain est prépondérante.

Les modifications du terrain, chez les hérédo-tuberculeux, sont de deux ordres.

Les unes sont *banales*. Elles peuvent s'expliquer, chez les enfants issus de générateurs tuberculeux, soit par l'action cachectisante qu'exerce sur le rejeton la mauvaise qualité des cellules originelles, ovulaires ou spermatiques, soit par les conditions déplorables de nutrition que subit, pendant des mois, un fœtus porté par une mère gravement malade. Quelques-uns de ces enfants, qui sont une proie facile pour la première infection venue, échappent aux causes immédiates de mort; mais ils traînent une existence misérable jusqu'au jour où une tuberculose nouvellement acquise ou simplement réveillée vient à éclater chez eux.

Certains sujets, dont ni le père ni la mère ne semblent tuberculeux, sont pour la bacillose un terrain très propice. On accuse alors un grand-père, un oncle, une tante, avec qui ils n'ont parfois jamais vécu. Ce n'est pas là de l'hérédité : mais on est forcé de reconnaître que certaines familles sont plus tuberculisables que d'autres, de même que certaines espèces animales sont, plus que d'autres, sensibles à l'action du bacille.

A côté de ces prédispositions banales, il existe sans doute aussi une *prédisposition spécifique*, résultant de l'action sur l'embryon, à un stade quelconque de son développement, des produits solubles qui se forment dans l'organisme des tuberculeux, action qui se traduit, tantôt par une espèce de vaccination, tantôt par une influence absolument inverse. Mais gardons-nous de faire aucune hypothèse sur les aptitudes morbides des hérédo-tuberculeux; nous savons trop peu de chose sur les actions immunisantes ou prédisposantes qui s'exercent dans la bacillose pour avoir le droit d'en déduire quoi que ce soit.

Le terrain de l'enfant résulte à la fois de l'héritage paternel et de l'héritage maternel. Si l'un des ascendants est tuberculeux, l'autre pourra léguer au rejeton quelque chose de l'état réfractaire dont il est doué lui-même. On a dit (Beugnies) que, par le fait d'une véritable imprégnation, une femme ayant eu un premier enfant d'un mari phtisique transmet la prédisposition à la tuberculose aux autres enfants qu'elle a d'un mari absolument indemne.

L'éclosion des formes galopantes n'est pas toujours l'indice d'une prédisposition particulière; elle résulte le plus souvent d'une auto-infection, provenant de foyers caséeux latents depuis des années. On croit, dans ces cas, saisir un exemple frappant d'hérédo-prédisposition tandis qu'on se trouve en face d'un méfait à longue échéance de la contagion.

Parmi les membres d'une même famille, les uns semblent doués d'une immunité spéciale et résistent à l'infection bacillaire quand ils sont aux prises avec elle ; les autres succombent. Il se fait ainsi une sorte de sélection dont l'hérédité n'est pas le seul facteur.

D'autres héritages morbides que celui de la tuberculose peuvent modifier les aptitudes réactionnelles des enfants. Les uns confèrent une sorte d'immunité ; d'autres, au contraire, créent une réelle prédisposition ; mais il est impossible de ne voir dans l'hérédité tuberculeuse rien de plus qu'une diminution banale de la résistance cellulaire assimilable à ce qu'on observe dans ces derniers cas. Il y a dans l'hérédo-prédisposition créée par la tuberculose des ascendants quelque chose de spécial, sinon de spécifique, insaisissable encore dans sa cause et dans son essence, mais facile à observer dans ses effets.

CONCLUSIONS

Tout le monde est d'accord pour admettre que la tuberculose a une influence héréditaire considérable. L'hérédité tuberculeuse peut consister dans la transmission du germe, dans la transmission d'une prédisposition, ou se manifester par des troubles dystrophiques. Ces trois modes d'hérédité tantôt se superposent, tantôt existent isolément.

1° *Transmission du germe*. — A. La transmission du germe au moment de la conception constituerait au sens strict du mot la véritable hérédité. Cette transmission conceptionnelle n'est encore qu'une hypothèse dont aucun fait connu ne démontre la réalité et dont la vraisemblance même nous paraît problématique ; en particulier, la transmission parasitaire par le père n'est nullement prouvée.

B. Il est possible cependant qu'un fœtus naisse infecté par le germe tuberculeux : dans ce cas, il a été contagionné *in utero* par sa mère. Celle-ci est ordinairement atteinte d'une façon très grave : elle peut aussi ne présenter que des lésions peu étendues. La transmission se fait probablement à la faveur d'une lésion placentaire, parfois très localisée et facile à méconnaître.

C. La tuberculose congénitale n'a pas été rencontrée seulement chez des fœtus mort-nés ou des nourrissons succombant de bonne heure : elle a été vue également chez des enfants bien constitués et parfaitement viables : l'hérédo-contagion de la tuberculose est donc indiscutable et peut jouer un rôle dans la propagation de la phtisie.

D. Ce rôle paraît être très restreint. Pour affirmer l'extrême rareté de l'hérédo-contagion, on doit se baser, non pas sur le peu de fréquence des tubercules congénitaux (argument de médiocre valeur), ni sur la difficulté de mettre en évidence par les inoculations une bacillose congénitale (une infection limitée passant très facilement inaperçue); mais sur les arguments suivants :

I. *Rareté de la tuberculose chez les petits nés de femelles tuberculisées ou tuberculeuses et conservés en vie.*

II. *Impossibilité d'admettre une résistance particulière des jeunes sujets au développement du bacille*, ce que démontre : *a*. l'extrême rareté au-dessous de deux ans des tuberculoses vraiment latentes et momentanément silencieuses : *b*. l'évolution clinique de la tuberculose du premier âge.

III. *L'étude anatomique des formes initiales de la tuberculose infantile est tout en faveur d'une infection par contagion* post partum.

2° Hérédité hétéromorphe. - La tuberculose des ascendants influence les enfants d'une manière évidente, et presque nécessaire au point de vue du développement physique : les tares dystrophiques qui sont le fait de cette hérédité hétéromorphe ne doivent pas être confondues avec l'hérédo-prédisposition dont elles sont distinctes tout en pouvant coïncider avec elle.

3° Hérédo-prédisposition. — A. L'observation clinique démontre l'excessive fréquence de la tuberculose chez les enfants issus de générateurs tuberculeux, ou de familles dont certains membres sont tuberculeux.

Cette fréquence excessive est due, en partie tout au moins, à une hérédo-prédisposition ; mais elle est aussi attribuable, pour une certaine part, à un mode pathogénique, dont on néglige beaucoup trop l'influence dans la plupart des recherches sur l'étiologie de la tuberculose, nous voulons parler de l'auto-infection. Une grande partie des tuberculoses de l'âge adulte ou de la jeunesse sont la conséquence de foyers latents remontant au jeune âge, foyers qui relèvent presque toujours de la contagion : la tuberculose des ascendants a eu souvent pour rôle essentiel de créer cette contagion.

B. L'hérédité de prédisposition se traduit fréquemment par la gravité de la maladie : non seulement l'enfant est plus exposé à la tuberculose, mais souvent il lui résiste plus mal.

C. Par contre, la tuberculose héréditaire peut se présenter aussi sous une forme atténuée, comme si l'enfant était jusqu'à un certain point immunisé. On peut expliquer ces formes par une sorte d'hérédité mixte, les ascendants transmettant au rejeton une prédisposition à devenir tuberculeux en même temps qu'un état spécial de la résistance.

4° Prophylaxie. — Au point de vue prophylactique, le rôle du médecin est considérable : trois tâches s'imposent à lui :

1° La protection des enfants de tuberculeux contre l'invasion bacillaire, et particulièrement contre le danger redoutable du milieu familial infecté.

Cette protection est possible, puisque l'enfant de phtisique n'est presque jamais contaminé à la naissance : elle est réalisable, puisque nous savons de quelles manières on peut éviter à l'entourage d'un phtisique la contagion bacillaire ; elle est essentielle, puisque l'infection précoce de l'enfant détermine presque toujours la formation, soit d'une tuberculose immédiate à évolution rapide, soit d'une tuberculose larvée redoutable pour l'avenir.

2° Chez les enfants de phtisiques, un des dangers les plus sérieux consistant dans les foyers latents, sources des auto-infections ultérieures, on doit mettre en œuvre tous les moyens d'investigation capables d'en révéler l'existence : une exploration clinique minutieuse et répétée permettra souvent un diagnostic précoce, point de départ d'une thérapeutique efficace.

3° Enfin, on doit poursuivre chez les rejetons de phtisiques l'étude et le traitement de tous les troubles de l'évolution ou de la nutrition qui permettent de soupçonner une hérédo-prédisposition tuberculeuse.

FORMES CLINIQUES DE LA TUBERCULOSE DU PREMIER AGE
PARTICULIÈREMENT LES FORMES GÉNÉRALISÉES)

RAPPORT

par M. le professeur André MOUSSOUS.

de Bordeaux.

La grande fréquence de la tuberculose du premier âge, ses deux modes étiologiques (hérédité et contagion) ont été savamment exposés dans les rapports de M. Hutinel et d'Espine. Restent à envisager les expressions cliniques diverses de la maladie.

Pendant la seconde enfance la tuberculose revêt une grande variété de formes, affectant tantôt les allures d'une maladie locale, tantôt les allures d'une maladie générale. Citons (sans compter les tuberculoses d'ordre chirurgical) la phtisie pulmonaire vulgaire ou aiguë, la pleurésie, la péritonite tuberculeuse et le carreau, les tubercules cérébraux et la méningite tuberculeuse dite primitive, l'adénopathie trachéo-bronchique, la cirrhose cardio-tuberculeuse parmi les formes locales, la tuberculose miliaire aiguë et la typho-bacillose parmi les formes généralisées.

Cette multiplicité de formes n'existe pas dans la première enfance.

Ce n'est pas à dire qu'on ne puisse citer avant la troisième année quelques exemples classiques des différents types cliniques que nous venons d'énumérer, mais ces cas s'offrent plutôt à titre d'exceptions sur lesquelles nous ne pouvons nous arrêter une à une.

Dans la première enfance les formes thoraciques qui feront l'objet d'un rapport particulier et les formes généralisées dont je vais m'occuper sont de beaucoup les plus fréquentes et les plus importantes.

Telle devait être, vis-à-vis des formes généralisées, la conséquence forcée des constatations anatomo-pathologiques qui nous indiquent la tendance à la diffusion et à la généralisation des lésions tuberculeuses chez les jeunes enfants.

Au point de vue de sa provenance, cette tuberculose généralisée est *héréditaire* ou *acquise*.

Les quelques observations que nous possédons d'hérédité tuberculeuse réelle, hérédité de graine, sont toutes, comme on sait, des exemples d'hérédo-contagion par voie transplacentaire.

Bien rares sont les exemples d'enfants venus au monde porteurs de lésions tuberculeuses généralisées et ayant survécu. Après une alimentation sérieuse sept cas seulement me semblent rentrer dans cette catégorie, ce sont les faits de Sabouraud [1], Schmorl et Kockel [2], Holn [3], Ausset [4], Oustinoff [5], Auché et Chambrelent [6], Brudeau [7].

Les détails cliniques qui seuls devaient fixer mon attention manquent du reste d'une façon presque absolue dans ces différentes observations.

On s'est contenté presque toujours d'indiquer les signes de la débilité congénitale : les enfants étaient d'un poids inférieur à la normale, dépérissaient très rapidement et s'éteignaient au bout de quelques heures ou de quelques jours après avoir présenté ou non de la cyanose.

1. SABOURAUD. *Soc. de biologie*. 1891.
2. SCHMORL et KOCKEL.
3. Yvan HOLN. Ueber congenit. T. *Bull. du tera. der Kaises Franz. Joseph. Academie der Wissenschapten in Prague*. 1895.
4. AUSSET. *Bull. méd. du Nord*. 1898.
5. OUSTINOFF. *Gaz. hed.*. 25 sept. 1897.
6. AUCHÉ et CHAMBRELENT.
7. BRUDEAU. *Soc. obst. de Paris*. 1899.

Ces documents sont, comme on le voit, tout à fait insuffisants pour tenter à l'heure actuelle une description clinique des formes généralisées de la tuberculose héréditaire.

Mais ce n'est pas seulement par transmission du germe que la maladie des générateurs peut peser sur les rejetons.

Sans revenir en rien sur la question de l'hérédité tuberculeuse, indirecte, ou hétéromorphe, ni sur la question de l'hérédo-prédisposition, je dois cependant mentionner l'état de *dystrophie* observé chez nombre de nouveau-nés issus de parents tuberculeux.

« Dans ces cas, dit le Dr Landouzy[1], l'enfant n'arrive pas souvent à terme ou s'il y arrive naît rabougri, chétif, maigre, de faible poids, pour succomber en bas âge sans syndrome symptomatique éclatant, sans grand appareil anatomo-pathologique, en tous cas sans signe de grossière tuberculose, si bien que son décès est souvent classé sous la rubrique *débilité congénitale*. »

Tout en affirmant que cette hérédité dystrophiante n'avait rien d'original et devait être rapprochée de l'hérédité dystrophiante des alcooliques, des syphilitiques, des saturnins ou des vieillards, M. Charrin[2], en collaboration avec M. Bonniot et Guillemonat, a cherché récemment à traduire par des données positives tangibles les particularités par lesquelles ces nouveau-nés s'écartent du type normal. Il a noté, en dehors du manque de progression régulière du poids, un affaiblissement de la thermogenèse, une diminution dans l'acide carbonique et l'eau exhalés, une diminution dans l'élimination de l'urée, une hypertoxicité des urines, une utilisation incomplète des aliments, comme le démontre l'excès d'azote des matières fécales[3].

Si j'ai cru devoir rappeler cette dystrophie fréquente des fils de phtisiques avant d'aborder l'exposé clinique de la tuberculose acquise des enfants du premier âge, ce n'est pas que pour ma part je l'affirme spéciale, ce n'est pas que je la prétende plus que tout autre favorisante vis-à-vis de l'infection bacillaire. Je l'ai fait sous l'empire de considérations d'un autre ordre.

Le clinicien doit envisager les situations pathologiques dans la complexité que créent les conditions ordinaires de l'existence humaine.

S'il est vrai que nombre d'enfants nés de parents tuberculeux sont absolument normaux et sains, s'il est vrai que ceux qui sont venus au monde plus débiles ne sont nullement pour cela voués à la tuberculose et pourront en être préservés si l'on a soin de les soustraire immédia-

1. LANDOUZY. *Soc. méd. des hôpitaux.* 1886.
2. CHARRIN et RICHE. Compte rendu. *Soc. biolog.*, 1897.
3. CHARRIN. Congrès de la tuberculose. 1898.

tement au milieu familial infecté, il n'en est pas moins vrai aussi que ces notions connues d'un public médical éclairé ne sont pas encore assez répandues et assez bien comprises de tous pour avoir produit le fruit que l'on est en droit d'attendre de leur vulgarisation.

L'enfant procréé par des tuberculeux, venu au monde en état de débilité congénitale, reste la plupart du temps auprès de ses parents et va se trouver exposé à toutes les causes de contagion accumulées au foyer domestique.

Qu'il porte ou non en lui une prédisposition fatale, l'infection ne tardera pas à se faire et l'on va se trouver en face de deux états pathologiques superposés.

La maladie parasitaire sera greffée sur la dystrophie native.

La clinique ne peut faire abstraction d'une telle superposition.

Quelle que soit la porte d'entrée choisie par l'agent infectieux, que les bacilles pénètrent par la voie cutanée, pharyngienne, intestinale, ou qu'ils fassent effraction dans le parenchyme pulmonaire, lieu de pénétration que tous les travaux récents sur la tuberculose infantile montrent de beaucoup le plus fréquent, il s'écoule toujours, entre l'époque de l'inoculation et celle de la généralisation des lésions tuberculeuses qui vont donner lieu à des manifestations morbides appréciables, un temps plus ou moins long.

L'adénopathie en relation avec le chancre infectant s'établit silencieusement.

Par définition même il ne peut y avoir de symptômes cliniques de la *tuberculose latente*.

Les apparences de la santé sont conservées si la contagion atteint un enfant bien portant.

L'impossibilité où l'on est de déterminer le moment de l'infection ne permet pas d'apprécier la durée de *latence* de la tuberculose. Elle doit être de quelques semaines au moins, car il est bien rare de voir éclater chez les nourrissons les signes cliniques de la maladie acquise avant le troisième mois. Enfin la première étape de la tuberculose pour nous servir de la division établie par Kossel[1] peut n'être franchie que beaucoup plus tard, voire même jamais. On peut admettre que la tuberculose reste indéfiniment latente.

Lorsqu'elle entre *en évolution*, la tuberculose généralisée acquise prend tantôt une marche lente et apyrétique, tantôt une marche rapide et fébrile.

Nous distinguerons donc deux types cliniques :

1. Kossel. De la tuberculose chez les enfants en bas âge. *Zeitsch. f. hyg. u. infectionskz*, t. XXII, 1896.

a) La tuberculose généralisée chronique ;
b) La tuberculose généralisée aiguë.

Tuberculose généralisée chronique.

La *tuberculose généralisée chronique apyrétique*, pour nous servir de la désignation de M. Marfan, ou la *tuberculose diffuse des nourrissons*, pour employer l'application de M. Aviragnet[1] constitue le type le plus original et le plus fréquent de la tuberculose des enfants du premier âge. Cette modalité clinique assez vaguement signalée dans les ouvrages classiques de Rilliet et Barthez, Bouchut, Henoch, déjà mieux indiquée par Cadet de Gassicourt, a été surtout décrite par M. Marfan et Aviragnet[2], elle a été admise par le professeur Grancher[3] et par tous ceux qui depuis ont écrit sur la tuberculose des bébés. On en trouve de nombreuses observations dans les thèses de MM. Mutelet[4], Pascal[5], Potier[6], Constantinovitch[7].

On peut, avec Marfan, diviser son évolution en trois périodes : la période de début est très courte; la période d'état qui est souvent très longue et dure de longs mois; la période des accidents terminaux qui peut ne durer que quelques heures.

Le début est variable, il est très souvent marqué par une bronchite ou une broncho-pneumonie développées spontanément ou à la suite d'une rougeole, d'une coqueluche, d'une grippe ou bien par des bronchites à répétition. D'autres fois ce sont des troubles gastro-intestinaux qui entrent les premiers en scène, diarrhée fébrile légère, embarras gastrique fébrile, dans d'autres cas enfin le début est tout à fait insidieux.

Ces premiers accidents cèdent, ils cèdent même parfois vite ; mais, eux disparus, la fièvre tombée, la convalescence ne s'opère pas franchement. On s'aperçoit que l'état général est profondément troublé, que l'atteinte portée à l'organisme est disproportionnée aux conséquences habituelles d'une inflammation banale des voies respiratoires

1. AVIRAGNET. De la tuberculose chez les enfants. *Thèse de Paris*, 1892.

2. MARFAN. *Semaine médicale*, 1892. — Tub. diff. apyr. *Journal de clinique et thérapeut. infantiles*. 1894 et 1895. — *Abeille méd.*, 1895. — Épisodes et complications de la tuberculose généralisée. *Sem. méd.*, 1895.

3. GRANCHER. Clinique. *Journal de méd. et de chir. pratique*, 1891.

4. MUTELET. Contribution à l'étude de la tuberculose diffuse. *Thèse de Nancy*, 1898.

5. PASCAL. Contribution à l'étude de la tuberculose du premier âge. *Thèse de Paris*, 1892.

6. POTIER. *Thèse de Paris*, 1895.

7. CONSTANTINOVITCH. Essai sur les tuberculoses de la première enfance. *Thèse de Paris*, 1899.

ou gastro-intestinales : déjà se dessinent et s'esquissent les marques de la déchéance organique imposée par l'infection bacillaire.

Avec la période d'état, dès lors ouverte, l'aspect du petit malade devient tout à fait caractéristique. Il est amaigri, ses membres sont décharnés. La peau forme des plis et se colle sur les os, les téguments paraissent animés et parfois même ils offrent une teinte légèrement pigmentée.

Il y a un développement exagéré du système pileux, particulièrement à la face externe des bras, avant-bras, cuisses droite et gauche, ainsi que dans la région interscapulaire. Le visage est fatigué, les traits tirés, les yeux cernés, les cils particulièrement longs.

A cette apparence cachectique se joignent constamment trois symptômes dont la constatation offre une grande importance :

1º L'*hypertrophie de la rate* sur laquelle Angel Money, Landouzy, Gueyral, Médail, Manicatide, ont particulièrement insisté ;

2º L'*hypertrophie du foie* signalée par Aviragnet et qui paraît comme la splénomégalie en relation avec le développement de lésions tuberculeuses au sein du parenchyme hépatique ;

3º Enfin une tuméfaction généralisée à tous les petits ganglions lymphatiques sous-cutanés.

La *micro-polyadénopathie périphérique généralisée* sur laquelle Legroux a le premier appelé l'attention au congrès pour l'étude de la tuberculose en 1888 et qui a été étudiée depuis dans une série de travaux d'ordre clinique, anatomo-pathologique ou expérimental et qui sont dus à MM. Grancher et Hutinel, Marfan, Marinesco[1], Paul Simon[2], Pascal, Lesage[3], Potier, Pech[4], etc.

Les ganglions tuméfiés sont ceux qui occupent les parties latérales du cou, le creux inguinal, le creux axillaire, c'est-à-dire les *grands carrefours lymphatiques* pour employer l'expression de Legoux. Mais ceux du derrière de la tête et de la nuque, ceux des régions mastoïdiennes, parotidiennes, sous-maxillaires et sous-hyoïdiennes peuvent être également intéressés, voire même, mais beaucoup plus rarement d'après Marinesco, ceux des régions sus-épitrochléennes et poplitées.

A l'aine et particulièrement au cou, sous la minceur de la peau, lorsque l'enfant exécute un mouvement de torsion de la tête on peut apercevoir les petites saillies formées par l'induration ganglionnaire.

1. MARINESCO. *Thèse de Paris*, 1890.
2. Paul SIMON. Conférences sur la tuberculose, 1896.
3. PASCAL et LESAGE. *Polyadénite primitive*, 1892.
4. PECH. *Thèse de Toulouse*, 1897.

mais d'ordinaire, d'après la remarque du professeur Grancher, l'adénite périphérique est un symptôme peu apparent et qu'il faut chercher pour le trouver.

La palpation pratiquée de parti pris renseigne tout de suite. Si l'on explore les différentes régions sus-indiquées qui, en raison de l'amaigrissement, forment presque toujours de véritables dépressions, on sent sous la pulpe des doigts dans l'épaisseur du tissu cellulaire sous-cutanée de petites masses, dures, mobiles, qui roulent sous la peau comme des grains de plomb ou des petits pois.

Les ganglions indurés, toujours pris en grand nombre, sont sans adhérence entre eux, ils sont en général très faciles à sentir.

Cependant, dans certaines régions, la palpation doit être faite d'une façon méthodique.

Au creux axillaire ainsi que le conseille Potier, il faut avoir soin de refouler avec la pulpe du doigt la paroi inférieure de la région axillaire et la refouler en haut et en dedans contre le gril costal qui limite la région; on perçoit alors nettement les petits ganglions indurés disposés en chapelet qui roulent sous le doigt.

Pour trouver les ganglions iliaques, externes, très rarement pris du reste, il faut, d'après Marinesco, enfoncer les doigts sous l'arcade crurale.

Une des conditions qui favorise singulièrement la recherche des ganglions indurés, c'est leur indolence absolue. On peut les toucher, les presser sans provoquer la moindre douleur. Ce caractère d'indolence est constant, il est en outre durable comme toutes les autres particularités que nous venons de signaler. Les ganglions tuméfiés n'ont pas de tendance à s'enflammer, à contracter des adhérences entre eux ou avec les tissus voisins, et moins encore à suppurer.

Ces trois grands symptômes peuvent être l'unique cortège de l'état cachectique. A quelque moment que l'on examine l'enfant la fièvre fait défaut, la température est normale.

« La teinte cachectique, dit Marfan, l'amaigrissement, l'hypertrophie du foie, de la rate, la micro-polyadénopathie, l'apyrexie, tels sont les signes à peu près contants de la tuberculose généralisée chronique des enfants du premier âge. »

Toutes les autres particularités que peut révéler l'exploration clinique sont très inconstantes et n'ont par conséquent dans le tableau clinique qu'une importance de second ordre.

Signalons en particulier les râles de bronchite, les signes d'engorgement des ganglions trachéo-bronchique ou de congestion d'un des deux sommets, phénomènes d'ordinaire passagers et ne donnant lieu qu'à peu de troubles fonctionnels ; signalons aussi la possibilité de vomissements et de diarrhée.

Ces accidents gastro-intestinaux en particulier sont tout à fait rares ; en règle générale, les petits malades mangent beaucoup et bien, ils ont une voracité qui va jusqu'à la boulimie.

La cachexie, établie, s'accuse de jour en jour. La diminution lente et progressive du poids peut être constamment vérifiée. L'amaigrissement devient squelettique. L'œdème apparaît aux pieds et aux mains.

Si quelques faits semblent autoriser à penser que les amendements sont possibles, que des trêves plus ou moins longues peuvent être obtenues, en général il n'en est rien. Après un temps plus ou moins long survient l'issue fatale.

Lorsque la mort résulte des seuls progrès de l'état cachectique, elle s'effectue silencieusement. Les enfants s'éteignent sans souffrance apparente, sans réaction violente.

Sous le titre d'*épisodes et complications de la tuberculose chronique du premier âge*, Marfan a signalé les modifications qui peuvent être apportées aux grandes lignes de ce tableau clinique.

Ce sont tantôt des localisations prépondérantes de la tuberculose, mais n'enlevant rien à la marche chronique de l'affection telles que l'infiltration caséeuse localisée d'un poumon, le mal de Pott, l'adénopathie trachéo-bronchique, le carreau, tantôt des poussées fébriles liées à des infections secondaires.

Ces infections secondaires se localisent surtout du côté de l'appareil respiratoire ou du côté de l'appareil auditif.

Les bronchites et les broncho-pneumonies sont sans doute mécaniquement favorisées par l'adénopathie trachéo-bronchique. Quoiqu'elles soient dues à des agents microbiens vulgaires, leur relation avec la tuberculose chronique est incontestable.

Elles sont une des causes de mort les plus fréquentes et sont parfois cliniquement impossibles à différencier de l'infiltration tuberculeuse des poumons.

La pleurésie séreuse ou purulente peut être la conséquence de ces inflammations pulmonaires.

Les suppurations de l'oreille moyenne se rencontrent dans la moitié des cas. Cette otite est précédée de céphalalgie, d'agitation, souvent d'une élévation considérable de la température.

Enfin la fièvre peut s'éveiller sans que l'exploration la plus minutieuse puisse en faire découvrir la raison d'être ; elle est alors éphémère ou continue et semble uniquement relever du processus tuberculeux qui par instants pousse son œuvre d'une façon plus active.

La tuberculose diffuse telle que nous venons d'en retracer le tableau, y compris les accidents qui peuvent en modifier la marche, s'observe jusque vers l'âge de quatre à cinq ans : elle a son maximum de fréquence vers le quinzième mois. Lorsqu'elle s'établit plus tôt dès la première ou seconde partie de la première année, elle offre une marche plus rapide. Les troubles digestifs dont nous avons signalé la rareté relative tiennent au contraire une place très importante dans la symptomatologie. Il y a des vomissements et de la diarrhée habituels, le ventre est ballonné, parcouru de veinosités transparentes, l'amaigrissement donne aux bébés un air vieillot, fait chevaucher les unes sur les autres les différentes pièces de la voûte crânienne.

Tuberculose généralisée aiguë.

Dans la tuberculose diffuse où les lésions sont représentées par des foyers multiples et diffus, mais en somme relativement discrets, la plupart des effets nocifs subis par l'organisme semblent devoir être attribués aux différents poisons tuberculeux dont le rôle lentement cachectisant a été si nettement établi dans ces dernières années.

A côté de l'intoxication, l'infection semble reprendre ses droits dans la forme rapide et fébrile.

La tuberculose miliaire aiguë, cliniquement analogue à celle qui peut se manifester à tout autre moment de l'existence, semble implicitement admise chez les nourrissons par presque tous les auteurs. — Elle serait caractérisée par un état général grave, une fièvre intense, de la diarrhée, du ballonnement du ventre, de la tuméfaction de la rate, des sibilances disséminées dans les deux poumons, préludant aux accidents pulmonaires plus graves qui caractérisent la période terminale.

Mais, disons-le de suite, la tuberculose généralisée aiguë se présente très rarement chez les enfants du premier âge avec les allures classiques de la granulie.

Lorsque sur les cadavres de bébés on constate la granulose généralisée, le processus clinique dont on a été témoin a été fait de deux tronçons : une période fébrile avec des symptômes mal dessinés indiquant la souffrance de tout l'organisme, puis soit des accidents pulmonaires, soit des accidents cérébraux de haute gravité et entraînant rapidement la mort.

Tel est, du moins pour moi, le résultat qui se dégage de la lecture d'un grand nombre d'observations et des faits qui se sont déroulés sous mes yeux. Avant l'éclosion des accidents terminaux qui, par leur physionomie imposante et leur apparition très voisine du dénouement fatal, priment tous les autres symptômes et forcent la main sur l'étiquette définitive à donner à la maladie (broncho-pneumonie ou méningite), s'est écoulée une période plus ou moins longue caractérisée par quelques signes pulmonaires, quelques troubles digestifs, — ballonnement du ventre et diarrhée, un peu d'agitation, de l'hyperesthésie généralisée, parfois de la tuméfaction de la rate, du foie, voire même de la micropolyadénopathie, mais où, en somme, l'amaigrissement rapide coïncidant avec la fièvre a été le symptôme dominant.

Cette fièvre n'est du reste pas bien vive, le thermomètre monte seulement à 38°, 38°,5, 39° avec des rémissions plus ou moins marquées. Nous sommes en un mot en présence d'une *fièvre tuberculeuse infectieuse à forme atténuée*, mais qui au lieu de s'amender se termine d'une façon fatale.

L'élément fébrile n'est même pas dans les formes rapides un symptôme nécessaire et constant. Le lien qui unit la forme clinique à la forme anatomique semble n'avoir à cette époque de la vie rien d'absolu. Il est aujourd'hui parfaitement connu que des poussées granuliques généralisées peuvent s'effectuer chez le bébé sans solliciter le moindre appareil fébrile.

Ces constatations ont été souvent faites.

L'observation publiée par Audéoud en est, entre autres, un exemple probant.

En dehors de ces deux types il y a tel lieu d'admettre un processus beaucoup plus rapide décrit par Aviragnet sous le nom de *fièvre infectieuse tuberculeuse suraiguë* et qui aurait l'expression symptomatique d'une maladie générale dénoncée par la fièvre, les vomissements, la diarrhée, l'amaigrissement qui s'offrirait avec toutes les apparences d'un état typhoïde et ne s'observerait que chez les enfants très jeunes. Nous ne le croyons pas.

D'après les faits rapportés par Landouzy et Queyrat et l'observation analogue consignée par Aviragnet, l'autopsie n'a permis de découvrir que des lésions tuberculeuses rares et circonscrites, insuffisantes pour expliquer la mort. Dans le seul cas, celui d'Aviragnet, où la recherche des bacilles ait été méthodiquement poursuivie dans les différents viscères, cette recherche est restée négative, on ne peut donc admettre l'idée d'une infection bacillaire suraiguë.

Aviragnet avait du vivant du malade constaté les signes et porté le diagnostic de gastro-entérite aiguë, il est très vraisemblable que telle est réellement la maladie en cause, les lésions tuberculeuses n'ayant joué qu'un rôle accessoire.

La tuberculose généralisée des enfants est donc tantôt chronique et apyrétique, tantôt rapide et fébrile : les deux modalités cliniques ont entre elles des points de contact nombreux. Elles peuvent même présenter des combinaisons chronologiques telles que :

La forme fébrile peut préluder à la forme apyrétique ou inversement, la forme apyrétique peut être compliquée de périodes fébriles plus ou moins prolongées.

Elles ont surtout une tendance commune qui est d'aboutir le plus souvent l'une et l'autre à des accidents méningitiques, dont l'apparition soudaine et brutale a quelque chose de vraiment saisissant.

Cette *méningite des nourrissons*, comme on la désigne aujourd'hui, se présente sous deux formes : la *forme éclamptique* et la *forme hémiplégique*.

La première, de beaucoup la plus commune, se signale par des convulsions généralement précédées d'un ou deux jours de somnolence et de fièvre. Les phénomènes convulsifs font leur apparition d'abord d'une façon partielle intéressant les yeux, la face, un membre, puis se généralisent, la nuque se raidit, le strabisme s'établit, la fontanelle antérieure est tendue et bombée.

Entre les convulsions l'enfant ne reprend pas connaissance, puis le coma devient complet et définitif jusqu'à la mort.

Dans la *forme hémiplégique* surtout indiquée par M. Zappert[1] et dont M. Marfan[2] fournit également un exemple, aux phénomènes susindiqués se surajoute, dès les premiers jours, une hémiplégie persistante avec contracture et exagération des réflexes. La marche est également foudroyante.

En somme, comme le dit M. Marfan[3] : « Pas de prodromes ou prodromes insaisissables, céphalalgie impossible à apprécier, vomissements habituels, mais constipation et rétraction du ventre inconstantes, fièvre modérée, fontanelle tendue, nuque raide, puis convulsions avec ou sans hémiplégie, coma et mort, telle est la succession de la méningite des nourrissons ».

Le tout évolue en quelques jours, de deux à quatre.

Les conditions dans lesquelles se présente cette méningite qui n'est que l'aboutissant des autres manifestations de la tuberculose généra-

---

1. ZAPPERT. *Jahres. f. Kinderheilk.*, 1895, t. IX.
2. MARFAN. Article méningite tuberculeuse, *Traité des maladies de l'enfance*.
3. MARFAN. Article méningite tuberculeuse. *Traité des maladies de l'enfance*.

lisée aiguë ou chronique expliquent probablement cette évolution si rapide. En effet, dans les conditions inverses et lorsque la méningite se développe chez des bébés même très jeunes, mais dont l'état général n'est pas trop atteint, on la voit suivre une marche plus classique. Les thèses de Bosselut[1] et de Fournel[2] renferment beaucoup de faits de cette dernière catégorie.

Le caractère presque fatal de la tuberculose des enfants du premier âge, sa marche sournoise et rapide, qu'aucune médication ne semble susceptible d'enrayer, sa terminaison parfois si brutale au milieu de complications difficiles à prévoir; d'autre part, au contraire, le caractère moins sévère des affections dont elle prend le masque, l'efficacité de la thérapeutique dont certaines sont justiciables, voilà des raisons d'ordre majeur pour que tout clinicien soit désireux de pouvoir sûrement et rapidement reconnaître la terrible maladie. Rien malheureusement n'est plus difficile. Il n'est pas un auteur écrivant sur la matière qui ne se soit appesanti sur ce point, et si je voulais rapporter leur dire, j'aurais à les citer tous.

Depuis qu'en 1886, mon cher maître le professeur Landouzy, cherchant à vérifier l'ancienne affirmation de Trousseau, remarquait à la crèche de l'hôpital Tenon l'extrême fréquence de la tuberculose du premier âge et s'élevait de toute son éloquence contre l'opinion contraire qui régnait encore en maîtresse, tous ceux qui ont étudié à sa suite ont été unanimes à reconnaître la véracité de son dire. Mais, il faut bien l'avouer, la vérité s'est attachée plus à la lumière des constatations nécroscopiques que d'après des recherches d'ordre clinique.

Même après l'avertissement donné, même après les recherches confirmatives d'Aviragnet[3], de Froebelius[4], de Schwer[5], de Boltz[6], d'Hutinel[7], d'Haushalter[8], de Comby[9], etc., même avec le parti pris bien arrêté de rechercher la tuberculose au berceau des bébés malades, c'est à peine si nous savons aujourd'hui de temps à autre la reconnaître sous les apparences trompeuses qu'elle affecte.

Dans la seconde enfance comme chez l'adulte, en dehors des mani-

1. BOSSELUT. Méningite tuberculeuse du premier âge. *Thèse de Paris.* 1888.
2. FOURNEL. Méningite de la première enfance. *Thèse de Nancy.* 1896.
3. AVIRAGNET. *Loc cit.*
4. FROEBELIUS. *Jahrbuch für Kinderheilkunde,* 1885, t. XXIV.
5. SCHWER. *Inaugural dissertation* et *Allgmeine médicin. central. Zeitung.* n° 6. 1886.
6. BOLTZ. *Dissertation inaugurale.* Kiel. 1890.
7. HUTINEL. Congrès pour l'étude de la tuberculose. 1895.
8. HAUSHALTER. Congrès de Montpellier. 1898.
9. COMBY. Congrès de Montpellier. 1898.

festations symptomatiques en rapport avec les différentes formes cliniques de la tuberculose, il y a certains signes de premier ordre qui indiquent l'imprégnation de l'organisme par le poison tuberculeux : l'anémie, l'amaigrissement, l'asthénie neuro-musculaire, la tachycardie.

Hormis la tachycardie qui quelquefois notée par Bertheraud[1] se chiffrerait sans élévation du thermomètre par 150 à 150 pulsations, tous ces sujets sont chez les jeunes bébés d'une signification trop banale pour pouvoir être pratiquement utilisés.

Ils font même quelquefois totalement défaut.

Les exemples sont nombreux d'enfants mourant de tuberculose et conservant presque jusqu'au dernier moment les apparences d'une santé florissante. Il s'agit presque toujours de bébés nourris au sein qui conservent leur appétit et leur poids en dépit de l'évolution rapide du mal. En y regardant de près on pourrait bien remarquer qu'ils sont anémiques, que leurs chairs sont molles et flasques, que le foie et la rate sont tuméfiés, mais comme il y a loin de là à la consomption classique des tuberculeux !

Les liquides de l'organisme ont été interrogés avec l'espoir d'y découvrir un signe indirect de la bacillose.

Dans ce but l'étude histologique du sang a été dans les derniers temps poursuivie avec ardeur. Les conclusions qu'Holmes[2] croyait pouvoir tirer de ses modifications morphologiques sont généralement considérées comme exagérées. Ces recherches n'ont pas été du reste faites chez les bébés tuberculeux.

La presque impossibilité de recueillir les urines de vingt-quatre heures rend délicate l'appréciation des modifications quantitatives des différents éléments constitutifs de l'urine. On manque là d'une base précieuse pour apprécier le phénomène de déminéralisation qu'entraîne avec elle la tuberculose en évolution.

Quant aux indices qu'on croyait pouvoir retirer de la découverte de certains éléments anormaux, ils sont loin d'avoir la valeur qu'on leur supposait tout d'abord.

L'indicanurie, après avoir été indiquée par Hochsinger et Kahane[3] comme un signe révélateur de la tuberculose, a été depuis l'objet d'un très grand nombre de recherches poursuivies tant en France qu'à

1. BERTHERAUD. Diagnostic de la tuberculose pulmonaire des jeunes enfants. *Thèse de Paris*, 1889.

2. HOLMES. *Med. Record*, 1896.

3. HOCHSINGER et KAHANE. Ueber das Verhalten des Indicans bei der tuberculose des Kindesalters. *Beitrage Kinderheilkunde, aus dem œffentlichen Kinderkrankeninstitute in Wien*. Neue Folge. 11, 1892.

l'étranger: citons les travaux de Carlo Giarre[1]. Steffen[2]. Falm[3], enfin de Debary[4] et Zamfiresco[5].

Les conclusions qui se dégagent de toutes ces recherches sont que l'indicanurie, tout en étant fréquente chez les tuberculeux, ne se trouve pas chez tous, 60 pour 100 d'après Falm. Elle n'est pas, contrairement à l'affirmation de Hochsinger et Kahane, plus marquée dans la tuberculose étendue et grave que dans la tuberculose limitée et légère. enfin elle se rencontre dans une foule d'autres états pathologiques, et semble simplement dépendre, comme l'avait établi Albert Robin[6]. en 1876. de l'excès des fermentations intestinales.

Les espérances que l'on avait un moment fondées sur la signification de la micropolyadénopathie périphérique se sont aussi partiellement évanouies.

Après les premières recherches de Legroux et de Marinesco, on pensait cette micropolyadénopathie comme tellement unie à la tuberculose qu'on alla avec Pascal et Lesage jusqu'à la considérer comme pouvant être, dans certains cas, l'unique expression chez les jeunes enfants de l'infection bacillaire.

A la suite de ce premier engouement, les recherches de MM. Marfan. Potier, Bulius[7] ont enlevé à ce signe la valeur d'un symptôme pathognomonique.

On retrouve en effet la polyadénite. dans une foule d'états pathologiques de la première enfance, dans l'infection gastro-intestinale. dans le rachitisme, dans l'hérédo-syphilis. dans la convalescence des maladies graves. Signalée depuis longtemps dans la rubéole, Marfan et Bernard[8] l'ont retrouvée dans la rougeole. Pech[9] dans l'infection pneumococcique, enfin elle peut même être évoquée par des lésions cutanées très minimes comme celles que provoquent le prurigo. les affections parasitaires de la peau, les piqûres d'insectes : si l'identité n'est pas toujours complète entre ces diverses adénopathies, et celle des tuberculeux, il s'agit de nuances d'une appréciation bien délicate.

1. Giarre Carlo. Sul valore semeilogico nella indicanura nella tubercolosi infantili. *Lo Sperimentale*, anno XLVII.
2. Steffen. *Beitrage zur Indicanausscheidung bei Kind.*. Bd XXXIX. Heft I. Leipzig, 1872.
3. Falm. Ueber den diagnostischen Werth. der Indicanuria der Tubercul. im Kindesalter. *Jahr. f. Kind.*, 1894.
4. Debary. *Thèse de Bordeaux*. 1899
5. Zamfiresco. Albumine et indicanurie chez le nouveau-né et le nourrisson *Thèse de Paris*, 1898.
6. Albert Robin. *Essai d'urologie clinique : la fièvre typhoïde*. 1876.
7. Bulius. Documents sur la clinique et le diagnostic de la tuberculose dans les premières années de la vie. *Jahr. f. Kinderh.*, 1899.
8. Bernard. La rougeole aux Enfants-Malades. *Soc. méd. des hôpitaux*. 1897.
9. Pech. *Loc. cit.*

Les apparences cliniques sous lesquelles se dissimule la tuberculose sont variables suivant que l'on envisage la forme chronique apyrétique ou la forme fébrile.

La tuberculose diffuse peut être simulée par tous les états cachectiques du premier âge.

La *cachexie gastro-intestinale* des nourrissons se traduit par de la maigreur avec décoloration des téguments qui deviennent terreux, par des sueurs profuses, surtout à la nuque, par du ballonnement du ventre, de la tuméfaction du foie, parfois de l'induration des ganglions lymphatiques périphériques et les râles de bronchite. Malgré la constance des troubles digestifs, l'appétit peut persister, voire même être exagéré. En dépit de tous ces traits de ressemblance avec la cachexie tuberculeuse, il faut noter cependant l'antériorité des troubles digestifs sur tous les autres symptômes morbides, la fétidité constante des selles, l'absence de splénomégalie, et de ces petites nodosités que Widerhofer prétend avoir rencontrées en palpant le ventre des enfants tuberculeux et qu'il considère comme des indurations lymphatiques.

Si les troubles digestifs ont déjà conduit au rachitisme, celui-ci se manifeste par des douleurs ou des déformations osseuses.

La *cachexie syphilitique*, lorsqu'elle correspond à la forme viscérale, se traduit par de la maigreur, de la décoloration des téguments, un volume exagéré avec dureté du foie et de la rate, souvent des troubles digestifs et de la micropolyadénopathie. Enfin tuberculose et syphilis peuvent engendrer des lésions testiculaires. Malgré tous ces points de similitude, la ressemblance n'est pas absolue, il est rare que la syphilis ne se trahisse par quelques cicatrices des muqueuses ou de la peau, par de l'alopécie et que les ganglions indurés ne correspondent pas à des lésions récemment guéries.

L'état cachectique auquel peut conduire l'infection qui résulte de l'abondance ou de la continuité des petits abcès intra-dermiques que l'on observe souvent chez les nourrissons peut faire croire à un état plus grave, et comme l'exploration des différents organes reste ordinairement négative, c'est à la tuberculose que l'on songe. Dans cette *cachexie pyodermique*, pour nous servir de l'expression aujourd'hui courante, la tuméfaction des ganglions est presque constante, mais à côté des petites masses dures, rétractées, représentant l'adénopathie d'ordre toxique, on trouve des ganglions qui présentent tous les caractères de l'adénite inflammatoire et qui peuvent même s'abcéder ; enfin une thérapeutique rationnelle viendra vite dissiper les doutes.

L'*anémie pseudo-leucémique* s'accompagne d'un gonflement de la rate. En cas d'hésitation on devra pratiquer l'examen du sang.

Chez les très jeunes nourrissons enfin la tuberculose qui évolue sans fièvre et s'accompagne de troubles digestifs simule de tous points l'*athrepsie* : surtout si la tuberculose acquise vient se greffer sur un état de débilité congénitale. On ne pourra guère la soupçonner, que si les accidents gastro-intestinaux ont pris naissance sans faute d'hygiène alimentaire avérée et persistent en dépit d'une thérapeutique bien comprise.

La tuberculose généralement aiguë et fébrile peut être confondue soit avec la fièvre typhoïde, soit avec la gastro-entérite aiguë.

La fièvre typhoïde des nourrissons, par ses symptômes assez vagues comme début, par les troubles méningitiques qui y figurent si souvent : abattement, somnolence, raideur de la nuque accompagnée d'un peu de ballonnement du ventre et de diarrhée, par la fréquence de la broncho-pneumonie, est faite pour simuler la tuberculose aiguë, soit à prédominance cérébrale, soit à prédominance thoracique. La séro-réaction de Vidal qui réussit bien chez les enfants pourra être utilisée pour sortir d'embarras.

La gastro-entérite aiguë, par ses bizarreries d'allures, ses alternatives d'accalmie et de recrudescence, ses répercussions sur les organes thoraciques, sa facilité à éveiller le méningisme, enfin par son retentissement si rapide et si profond sur l'état général, se plie à toutes les apparences, à tous les groupements symptomatiques que peut provoquer la tuberculose généralisée aiguë.

L'importance des troubles gastro-intestinaux, leur entrée en scène généralement assez brusque sont les seuls détails à prendre sérieusement en considération dans ce diagnostic différentiel.

Mais s'il est délicat de savoir ce qui est tuberculose et ce qui n'est pas tuberculose, plus difficile encore est de reconnaître la combinaison de la bacillose et des différents états pathologiques que nous venons d'énumérer. Cette combinaison, il faut bien le savoir, est chose vulgaire.

La tuberculose s'associe aux différentes formes de la gastro-entérite, au rachitisme, à l'hérédo-syphilis, à certaines anémies, voire même à la fièvre typhoïde : enfin nous ne saurions trop le répéter, elle appelle toutes les infections secondaires. Nous avons déjà signalé la bronchite, la broncho-pneumonie, l'otite, la gastro-entérite. MM. Hutinel et Labbé[1] ont insisté sur les conditions favorables que le terrain des bébés tuberculeux offre aux infections cutanées staphylococciques.

Si l'on examine l'enfant à l'époque où une de ces inflammations surajoutées est en pleine activité, il ne faut pas laisser captiver son

---

1. HUTINEL et LABBÉ. Contribution à l'étude des infections staphylococciques. *Arch. gén. de méd.*, 1896.

attention par l'accident du moment, sous peine de méconnaître la tuberculose qui en a favorisé l'apparition.

Nous touchons heureusement à l'heure où tous ces problèmes de diagnostic, jusqu'à présent si difficiles, vont (nous l'espérons du moins) se trouver facilités.

Déjà deux méthodes de diagnostic indirect de la tuberculose sont entrées dans la pratique. Elles sont basées l'une et l'autre sur les réactions fébriles obtenues chez les tuberculeux, dans un cas par de simples injections hypodermiques de sérum artificiel (méthode de Sirol), dans le second cas par l'emploi de la tuberculine. Cette seconde méthode, qui n'est que l'application à la tuberculose humaine d'un procédé qui donne dans la médecine vétérinaire de si brillants résultats, a été particulièrement étudiée chez l'enfant par le professeur Hutinel[1]. Les travaux poursuivis dans son service par MM. Gaffié[2] et Bertherand[3] et dans celui du Dr Comby par M. Mettetal[4] ont, en réglant définitivement le *modus faciendi*, établi l'innocuité et la sincérité de ce moyen de diagnostic.

Sans entrer dans plus de détails, remarquons cependant qu'une condition est absolument nécessaire pour songer à l'utiliser. Cette condition est une apyrexie complète remontant à plusieurs jours déjà. Les cas fébriles lui échappent forcément. Si l'avenir confirme les espérances que semble nous offrir la séro-réaction tuberculeuse, cette lacune se trouvera comblée.

Depuis que MM. Arloing et P. Courmont[5] ont montré que le sérum et les humeurs des tuberculeux agglutinaient des bacilles mobiles de la tuberculose tout comme le sérum d'un typhique agglutine le bacille d'Eberth et ont indiqué le profit que l'on pouvait retirer de cette propriété agglutinante pour le diagnostic de la tuberculose, les résultats qu'ils ont énoncés ont été confirmés par MM. Dubard, Mongourd[6], Buard[7], Rothamel[8], Bendix[9]. Si quelques-uns les ont mis en doute,

1. HUTINEL. *Soc. méd. des hôpitaux.* mars 1895.

2. GAFFIÉ. Diagnostic de la tuberculose pulmonaire infantile. *Thèse de Paris.* 1895.

3. BERTHERAND. Le diagnostic de la tuberculose pulmonaire des jeunes enfants *Thèse de Paris.* 1899.

4. METTETAL. Valeur de la tuberculine dans le diagnostic de la tuberculose de la première enfance. *Thèse de Paris.* 1900.

5. ARLOING et COURMONT. Congrès de la tuberculose. 1898; *Bull. acad. des sciences,* 1898; Congrès Berlin pour la tuberculose. 1899; *Journal de phys. et path. gén..* 1900.

6. MONGOURD et BUARD. *Bull. Soc. de biologie.* 1898 et 1899; *Soc. d'anat. de Bordeaux,* 1898.

7. BUARD. De la séro-réaction tuberculeuse: Étude spéciale chez l'enfant. *Thèse de Bordeaux.* 1900.

8. ROTHAMEL. *Thèse de Bordeaux,* 1899.

9. BENDIX. *Bull. méd..* avril 1900.

ou semblent avoir montré peu d'empressement à les contrôler, je crois qu'il faut en accuser : la difficulté d'avoir et de conserver des cultures mobiles, la sensibilité variable de différentes cultures, le temps plus ou moins long pendant lequel elles sont utilisables, enfin l'atténuation ou mieux la disparition du pouvoir agglutinatif dans les formes graves et très rapides et dans les périodes trop avancées de la maladie. Tous points indiqués maintenant par MM. Arloing et Courmont, Rothamel, Bendix.

En tenant compte de toutes ces particularités, M. Buard a entrepris dans sa thèse l'étude de la séro-réaction tuberculeuse chez les enfants. Il a trouvé, suivant les cas, la réaction sensible à trois, deux, et une goutte de sérum pour quinze gouttes de culture.

Un certain nombre de faits l'autorisent même à penser qu'en dehors du procédé ordinaire on pourra utiliser deux manières de faire plus rapides et ne nécessitant pas de recourir à la piqûre directe de la veine pour se procurer du sang.

Ce sont :

1° La séro-réaction extemporanée faite sur une lame, à une goutte de culture on ajoute une goutte de sérum sanguin, on recouvre d'une lamelle, on borde à la paraffine et l'on examine immédiatement au microscope si la séro-réaction se produit et en combien de temps.

2° Cette même séro-réaction extemporanée faite avec du sang recueilli sur papier stérilisé, puis dilué au moment de l'emploi avec de l'eau stérilisée, une goutte d'eau pour une goutte de sang recueilli et deux gouttes de ce mélange pour une goutte de culture.

Les recherches de M. Buard ont été faites, il est vrai, surtout dans les cas de tuberculose avérée et rarement sur des bébés très jeunes. Pour poursuivre cette étude on ne pouvait tout d'abord s'attacher uniquement à des cas douteux et attendre les résultats plus ou moins lointains de l'autopsie. Leur caractère de précision permet d'attendre avec confiance le contrôle de faits nouveaux.

FORMES CLINIQUES DE LA TUBERCULOSE DU PREMIER AGE
(PARTICULIÉREMENT LES FORMES THORACIQUES)

RAPPORT

par M. le docteur H. RICHARDIÉRE,

Médecin de l'Hôpital Trousseau.

Dans les rapports qui vous ont déjà été présentés, MM. d'ESPINE et HUTINEL ont étudié les questions relatives à l'étiologie, à l'hérédité, à la contagion et à la prophylaxie de la tuberculose infantile. M. MOUSSOUS s'est réservé l'étude spéciale des formes cliniques de la tuberculose généralisée et les symptômes généraux de la maladie. La question ainsi délimitée, il me reste à exposer les formes cliniques de la tuberculose infantile, envisagées uniquement au point de vue de la médecine interne, spécialisée par convention à l'appareil broncho-pulmonaire (c'est-à-dire les déterminations bronchiques, pulmonaires, ganglionnaires, trachéo-bronchiques), avec l'étiologie spéciale à leur localisation et les difficultés de leur diagnostic.

Le diagnostic de la tuberculose des enfants du premier âge est, en effet, encore très embarrassant dans un grand nombre de cas. Bien souvent, en présence d'un enfant cachectique, soupçonné de tuberculose, ou d'un enfant présentant des signes évidents de bronchopneumonie, suspecte comme nature, nous devons rester dans la réserve et nous contenter d'émettre un diagnostic de probabilité et non de certitude. Aussi sera-t-il nécessaire, comme conclusion de ce rapport, de passer en revue les nouveaux moyens de diagnostic proposés dans ces dernières années, et de mettre en relief les procédés, utilisables en clinique, qui peuvent faciliter le rôle de médecin.

I

Si l'on prenait à la lettre l'énoncé de la question, la tuberculose des enfants du premier âge ne devrait être étudiée que dans la première année de la vie. Le premier âge étant l'époque de la vie qui s'étend depuis la naissance jusqu'au sevrage, seuls les nourrissons rentreraient dans le cadre de notre étude. Il a semblé toutefois que, pour la tuberculose, il y avait lieu d'étendre quelque peu les limites du premier âge et de les porter jusqu'à la fin de la deuxième année. En effet, dans la première année de la vie, la tuberculose est une maladie rare. Sur 102 autopsies d'enfants au-dessous d'un an, Hutinel, cité par Berthérand, n'a trouvé que 4 cas de tuberculose. Comby, sur 72 autopsies de 1 à 5 mois, aucun cas; 7,5 pour 100 de 5 à 6 mois, 22 pour 100 de 6 mois à 12 mois. Biedert sur 1508 de tuberculose infantile en trouve 6,8 pour 100 au-dessous d'un an. Hervieu sur 991 autopsies d'enfants n'a trouvé que 10 tuberculeux au-dessous d'un an. Froebelius sur 91570 nourrissons de 1 à 4 mois a vu 416 tuberculeux sur 18569 morts. Schiver, sur 690 enfants au-dessous d'un an, en a trouvé 44 tuberculeux. La statistique de Baltz donne pour le pourcentage de la tuberculose :

<pre>
0,89 pour 100 — de 5 à 6 semaines.
4,26   — de 5 à 6 mois.
9,22   — de 6 à 12 mois.
</pre>

D'autre part, après la première année, la tuberculose devient extrêmement fréquente. De 1 à 5 ans, un tiers des enfants autopsiés est tuberculeux (Hutinel, Comby, Goldschmidt, Kossel, Landouzi, Queyrat, Rillet et Barthez, Schiver).

Si la rareté de la tuberculose dans la première année de la vie et sa fréquence extrême dans la deuxième année ne justifiaient pas suffisamment l'extension donnée à la notion de premier âge, il conviendrait encore de faire remarquer que la tuberculose, au point de vue clinique, diffère peu en réalité dans la première et dans la deuxième année de la vie.

II

La tuberculose se présente chez les enfants du premier âge avec quelques caractères qui lui donnent une physionomie spéciale, et qui établissent entre la tuberculose infantile et la tuberculose des enfants plus âgés et des adultes des différences cliniques appréciables. Ces caractères sont d'autant plus accentués que les enfants sont plus jeunes: ils s'atténuent au fur et à mesure que la tuberculose frappe des sujets plus âgés. Ils n'existent, pour ainsi dire, plus chez les enfants qui ont passé la 10ᵉ ou la 12ᵉ année. A partir de cet âge, la tuberculose des enfants s'identifie cliniquement de plus en plus avec la tuberculose des adultes.

La tuberculose des jeunes enfants présente avant tout ce caractère important : d'être presque toujours une tuberculose généralisée. Tonnellé a montré, le premier, que cette tuberculose était presque toujours une tuberculose générale, et depuis, l'exactitude de cette observation a été vérifiée universellement. A l'autopsie d'un jeune enfant tuberculeux, la plupart des organes présentent des tubercules. Sur 125 autopsies de tuberculeux en bas âge, Schiver a noté des tubercules dans le foie (104 fois), dans les organes respiratoires (105 fois), dans le rein (85 fois), etc. Le poumon échappe rarement à l'infection, et il est exceptionnel qu'il soit seul malade.

Avec la généralisation des tubercules, la participation fréquente et grave du système lymphatique est un autre caractère important de la tuberculose du premier âge. Elle se manifeste par les adénopathies considérables qu'on observe si souvent à l'autopsie. Les ganglions thoraciques sont surtout atteints de lésions graves et avancées. Ils peuvent même être les premiers intéressés par l'infection tuberculeuse, et la propagation de leurs lésions tuberculeuses aux poumons est un fait fréquent, assez spécial à l'enfant (Weigert, Michaël).

Ces deux caractères (généralisation de l'infection tuberculeuse, importance du rôle joué dans la dissémination des bacilles et des tubercules par le système lymphatique) rapprochent la tuberculose des jeunes enfants de la tuberculose expérimentale, produite chez les animaux par l'inoculation de tubercules ou de cultures des bacilles de Koch.

Pourquoi l'enfant présente-t-il une tendance aussi marquée à la généralisation de la tuberculose?

Si on admet l'hypothèse que l'enfant est tuberculeux par l'hérédité du germe tuberculeux, et qu'il naît, portant dans son sang ou dans ses tissus les bacilles tuberculeux qu'il a puisés dans le sang de sa mère ou dans le placenta maternel, il est facile d'expliquer chez lui la généralisation ordinaire de la tuberculose. Dans cette hypothèse, la tuberculose propagée par le sang est une tuberculose toujours générale, comme la syphilis héréditaire est d'emblée une syphilis générale sans accident initial.

Cette explication n'est cependant pas le plus souvent acceptable. En effet, l'hypothèse de l'hérédité du germe n'est pas généralement admise. L'hérédité est plutôt une hérédité de terrain. L'enfant hérite de ses parents tuberculeux plus souvent de tissus facilement tuberculisables, peu résistants aux bacilles, que du germe tuberculeux lui-même. C'est plutôt dans le défaut de résistance des tissus qu'il faut chercher la raison de la généralisation de la tuberculose.

Chez l'enfant, tous les tissus sans exception, tous les organes, tous les appareils sont facilement accessibles à l'action des germes virulents.

Si ces germes pénètrent en quantité suffisante dans l'organisme (par les voies respiratoires ou par les voies digestives), chacun des organes qui les arrêtera deviendra un foyer de germination tuberculeuse.

Si l'infection se fait par l'air, les organes respiratoires seront la première étape du processus tuberculeux bientôt suivie de l'envahissement des organes plus éloignés du foyer de l'infection.

Dans la tuberculose par infection des voies digestives, le foie sera la première station d'arrêt des bacilles. Le foie, si fréquemment atteint dans la tuberculose infantile, sera encore un des premiers organes atteints dans la localisation des tubercules, provenant de l'infection du sang par le système lymphatique.

Une autre raison de la généralisation de la tuberculose peut encore être donnée. Quand la tuberculose se déclare chez un adulte, elle se manifeste chez un sujet qui vit depuis longtemps dans les milieux imprégnés des germes de la tuberculose. Si le sujet a résisté jusqu'au jour où il est atteint, c'est que ses tissus présentaient une résistance innée à l'action des bacilles. Le plus souvent, il n'est devenu tuberculeux que parce que son organisme s'est trouvé déprimé ou affaibli par les maladies, l'alcoolisme, le surmenage, la dépression morale, le chagrin. Avant d'être envahis par les tubercules, ses tissus se sont fortifiés dans leur résistance de chaque jour contre les bacilles. En dehors du foyer d'invasion primitive, ils pourront donc continuer à présenter une certaine résistance et, seul, l'organe infecté restera atteint pendant un temps plus ou moins long.

Chez les jeunes enfants, cette résistance acquise des tissus par l'accoutumance à l'infection n'existe pas. Les organes sont vierges de tout contact avec les germes tuberculeux. Si les enfants sont tuberculisables par hérédité de terrain, ils deviennent tuberculeux à la première invasion de l'organisme par les bacilles, et la généralisation de l'infection est d'autant plus rapide qu'aucun organe n'a pris l'habitude et n'a le pouvoir de réagir contre le virus tuberculeux.

D'autres causes physiologiques propres à l'enfant expliquent encore la tendance à la généralisation. Je ne puis que rappeler l'activité de la circulation, l'importance du système lymphatique, l'intensité des phénomènes nutritifs, la nécessité pour l'enfant d'entretenir ses réserves organiques et de les employer pour sa croissance.

III

Au point de vue clinique, les tuberculoses des enfants du premier âge peuvent être divisées, suivant leur marche, en *formes rapides* et en *formes lentes*.

Dans les *formes rapides*, une division a été proposée et semble devoir être conservée : c'est la division en *tuberculoses généralisées sans localisation spéciale* et en *tuberculoses généralisées à localisation spéciale* (presque uniquement à localisation broncho-pulmonaire).

Aux premières formes, aux tuberculoses généralisées sans localisation spéciale correspondent les tuberculoses dans lesquelles la propagation du virus se fait surtout par le sang. Ce sont les granulies et leurs variétés, dans lesquelles la maladie revêt la forme d'une maladie infectieuse, l'aspect d'une fièvre typhoïde le plus souvent.

Nous laisserons de côté ces formes cliniques étudiées par M. Moussous.

Dans les *formes lentes*, à marche chronique, la même division peut être faite en formes sans localisation spéciale et ses formes à localisation spéciale (presque toujours broncho-pulmonaire dans la première enfance).

A. — Tuberculoses généralisées à localisation broncho-pulmonaire spéciale, à marche rapide.

Ces tuberculoses sont les plus fréquentes dans la tuberculose infantile. Elles peuvent être observées chez les enfants indemnes de toutes maladies antérieures : souvent elles sont consécutives à la rougeole ou à la coqueluche. La rougeole et la coqueluche facilitent-elles l'infection tuberculeuse par les lésions broncho-pulmonaires qu'elles provoquent, ou donnent-elles seulement un coup de fouet à des lésions tuberculeuses préexistantes, latentes jusque-là ? Les deux opinions ont leurs partisans et peuvent être également défendues. Le fait certain est l'apparition fréquente de la tuberculose pendant le cours ou dans la convalescence de ces deux maladies infectieuses.

Dans les tuberculoses broncho-pulmonaires, il peut y avoir prédominance des symptômes de catarrhe, de broncho-pneumonie ou de dyspnée, suivant que les bronches, le parenchyme pulmonaire ou les ganglions trachéo-bronchiques sont plus particulièrement touchés. Cependant, il est rare que ces formes soient pures et que les lésions frappent uniquement telle ou telle partie de l'appareil respiratoire. Le plus souvent, toutes les parties sont touchées, mais à un degré inégal. C'est la prédominance des symptômes en rapport avec le catarrhe ou l'hépatisation qui seule détermine la forme clinique. Au point de vue anatomo-pathologique, les lésions sont presque toujours complexes.

1º Tuberculose généralisée à forme bronchitique à marche aiguë.

Cette forme de tuberculose est assez rare. Elle se voit à la suite et pendant la convalescence de la rougeole ou de la coqueluche. Elle peut aussi être primitive ; en pareil cas, la maladie débute et évolue pendant quelque temps comme une infection générale, aiguë ; elle simule une fièvre typhoïde, dans laquelle les symptômes thoraciques seraient prédominants.

Quel que soit le mode de début, une fois la maladie constituée, elle se manifeste de la façon suivante :

Avec des symptômes généraux sur lesquels nous reviendrons dans une description générale, car ils sont communs à toutes les formes, il existe des symptômes de bronchite, qui n'ont rien de caractéristique.

Il y a de la toux, plus ou moins fréquente, quinteuse parfois, quand les ganglions trachéo-bronchiques sont intéressés.

La dyspnée est généralement plus marquée que dans une bronchite ordinaire. Souvent la dyspnée est assez forte pour s'accompagner de battements des ailes du nez, et parfois de tirage (surtout latéro-costal). Quelquefois il y a de véritables accès de suffocation.

Dans quelques cas, plus caractéristiques, la dyspnée est assez intense pour amener des signes d'asphyxie (cyanose du visage et des extrémités, gonflement du système veineux du cou et de la tête).

La percussion du thorax ne donne pas de résultat, sauf s'il y a adénopathie trachéo-bronchique appréciable.

A l'auscultation, on perçoit des signes de bronchite, des râles disséminés sans localisation prédominante, variables dans leur siège et dans leur abondance.

En un mot, les signes locaux sont ceux d'une bronchite. Seuls les signes généraux permettent le diagnostic. Les bronchites (simple ou grippale) peuvent surtout être confondues avec cette forme de tuberculose. Si l'on ne tenait compte des symptômes généraux, on ne pourrait soupçonner la tuberculose qu'en s'appuyant sur l'absence de catarrhe nasal et sur l'absence du bacille de Pfeiffer dans le sang.

2º Forme asthmatique ou suffocante.

Dans cette forme, très rare, les symptômes sont ceux de la forme bronchitique, avec cette différence que la dyspnée y est portée à son maximum et les signes d'auscultation à leur minimum.

Il s'y joint un état asphyxique permanent avec des accès de suffocation, qui simulent l'obstruction du larynx, telle qu'on l'observe dans le croup diphtérique : les accès intermittents peuvent tuer l'enfant dans les premiers jours qui suivent le début de la maladie. Le diagnostic est surtout à faire avec le croup d'emblée.

3° *Forme broncho-pneumonique.*

Cette forme de tuberculose infantile est la plus fréquente de toutes. Elle s'observe surtout après un an et jusqu'à 4 ou 5 ans.

Elle débute quelquefois brusquement, comme une pneumonie ou une broncho-pneumonie primitive, en pleine bonne santé ou à la suite d'une infection quelconque (grippe, rougeole, coqueluche) : plus souvent, le début est lent : les symptômes généraux d'amaigrissement, de fièvre, de dénutrition existaient depuis quelque temps, lorsque l'auscultation de la poitrine fait constater pour la première fois des signes d'hépatisation ou de congestion.

Une fois constitué, le tableau clinique est celui d'une broncho-pneumonie. Les symptômes généraux sont ceux de la broncho-pneumonie avec les quelques signes que nous montrerons plus spéciaux à la tuberculose. Les signes locaux sont ceux d'une broncho-pneumonie, sans localisation spéciale, peut-être plus fréquente à la partie moyenne et aux bases qu'aux sommets.

Cette broncho-pneumonie est diffuse dans les premiers temps, puis, après quelques oscillations, les signes d'hépatisation deviennent plus fixes. Une fois fixés, ils restent perceptibles aux mêmes points jusqu'à la fin de la maladie. Les signes stéthoscopiques n'ont en eux-mêmes rien de caractéristique. Ce sont les râles, les souffles, voire même les signes cavitaires ou pseudo-cavitaires qu'on peut constater dans toute zone d'hépatisation pulmonaire. Dans l'évolution de la maladie, il y a lieu de considérer comme une probabilité en faveur de la tuberculose l'apparition de signes cavitaires succédant à des signes d'hépatisation.

Au point de vue de la marche de la maladie, on peut distinguer deux variétés : *a*) une tuberculose broncho-pneumonique, qui évolue rapidement en 5 à 6 semaines, et se termine au bout de ce temps par l'asphyxie, le collapsus, ou la cachexie; *b*) une tuberculose broncho-pneumonique à évolution beaucoup plus lente, qui procède par poussées successives et se termine seulement après 2 ou 3 mois comme la variété précédente, quelquefois aussi par tuberculose généralisée infectieuse (granulie) ou par méningite.

B. — Tuberculoses infantiles à marche lente.

Comme j'ai dû le faire remarquer à propos des tuberculoses à marche rapide, les formes lentes localisées que j'ai à passer en revue ne répondent qu'à des déterminations prédominantes sur tel ou tel organe. Presque toujours avec des tuberculoses locales prédominantes, on note à l'autopsie la présence de tubercules granuliques disséminés dans d'autres organes, et en particulier dans le foie et dans la rate.

Les tuberculoses lentes infantiles peuvent aussi prédominer dans quelques organes du système respiratoire ; localisée aux poumons, cette forme de tuberculose simulerait une phtisie pulmonaire commune.

Cette forme clinique, si tant est qu'elle existe, est extrêmement rare dans la première enfance. Pour ma part, je n'en ai observé aucun cas au-dessous de deux ans.

Presque toutes les descriptions qui ont été données de la phtisie pulmonaire vulgaire des enfants se rapportent à des enfants âgés de plusieurs années.

Dans la première enfance, les tuberculoses qui se rapprocheront le plus de cette forme sont des tuberculoses à forme broncho-pneumonique et à signes cavitaires, c'est-à-dire avec caséification et ramollissement du tissu pulmonaire. La marche, plus lente que celle de la forme broncho-pneumonique ordinaire, est toutefois encore assez rapide et presque toujours sans arrêt.

La localisation aux ganglions trachéo-bronchiques est plus fréquente et donne lieu à la phtisie bronchique. Cette forme est surtout une forme de début. Elle n'est et ne peut être une forme pure. Il est inévitable qu'à une certaine période les poumons d'abord, puis l'organisme tout entier, soient envahis par le bacille tuberculeux. Les symptômes en rapport avec l'adénopathie trachéo-bronchique qui donnent à cette localisation de la tuberculose une physionomie spéciale, sont la toux coqueluchoïde, les signes de compression intra-thoracique. Les signes stéthoscopiques bien connus sont : la matité interscapulaire, l'affaiblissement unilatéral du murmure vésiculaire, le souffle bronchique, etc.

La localisation aux séreuses (tuberculose pleuro-péritonéale) est tout à fait rare dans la première enfance. J'ai eu cependant l'occasion d'en observer un cas chez une enfant de deux ans.

La maladie débuta par une augmentation de volume du ventre

(par de l'ascite), avec développement de la circulation sous-cutanée abdominale. Rapidement la plèvre droite fut atteinte et devint le siège d'un épanchement qui dut être ponctionné. L'enfant succomba au bout de trois semaines de séjour à l'hôpital. A l'autopsie, il y avait de la tuberculose granuleuse généralisée avec semis tuberculeux extrêmement abondant sur le péritoine et la plèvre.

IV

Les symptômes généraux communs à toutes les formes de tuberculose infantile doivent être rappelés brièvement, car ce sont ceux qui, le plus souvent, font diagnostiquer la tuberculose ou permettent au moins de la soupçonner. Les signes locaux ne sont pas révélateurs en eux-mêmes; ils servent seulement, en clinique, à localiser la forme de la maladie générale.

Avec les symptômes généraux, les conditions étiologiques ont une réelle importance.

La tuberculose connue ou constatée chez les parents est un argument de grande valeur pour diagnostiquer la tuberculose chez les enfants du premier âge. Il en est de même du début de la maladie, dans le cours ou pendant la convalescence d'une des maladies infectieuses de l'enfant qu'on sait prédisposé à la tuberculose, ou rendre manifeste une tuberculose latente jusque-là.

L'aspect extérieur des enfants tuberculeux est quelquefois révélateur en lui-même. Ces enfants sont chétifs et malingres. Ils maigrissent rapidement, malgré la persistance ordinaire de l'appétit. Ils se nourrissent volontiers, parfois avec voracité. Ils digèrent sans diarrhée et néanmoins leur poids n'augmente pas. Souvent même, le poids diminue d'une façon régulière, malgré l'augmentation de la ration alimentaire quotidienne.

L'amaigrissement des enfants porte sur le tissu cellulaire et aussi sur les muscles (particulièrement sur les membres) qui s'atrophient. La peau paraît collée sur les os.

La peau a une coloration fréquemment bistrée, grisâtre, avec des taches de pigment plus marquées.

Le système pileux est généralement développé d'une façon anormale, particulièrement sur la peau de la région dorsale supérieure et de la face interne des jambes.

L'amaigrissement de l'enfant rend facilement appréciables certaines hypertrophies d'organes, l'hypertrophie du foie et de la rate, celle des ganglions lymphatiques périphériques.

L'hypertrophie généralisée des ganglions lymphatiques (micropolyadénie) a été signalée par LEGROUX et considérée par lui et par ses élèves comme un signe de tuberculose. Elle n'a pas une valeur absolue, car elle a pu être constatée dans d'autres infections générales (syphilis, entérite, rougeole). Elle garde néanmoins une réelle valeur quand elle est constatée chez un enfant soupçonné tuberculeux par d'autres symptômes généraux et locaux.

La température n'a elle-même rien de spécifique. C'est plutôt dans sa discordance avec le pouls qu'on peut trouver les éléments du diagnostic. Rappelons, d'ailleurs, que dans la tuberculose infantile, il peut y avoir de longues périodes d'apyrexie sans que la tuberculose doive être éliminée. Il pourrait même y avoir apyrexie complète, d'après MARFAN.

La dyspnée a plus d'importance. Elle est souvent, par son intensité, hors de proportion avec les signes constatés à l'examen stéthoscopique.

V

La difficulté du diagnostic de la tuberculose des enfants du premier âge a suscité, dans ces derniers temps, une série de recherches ayant toutes pour but de faciliter la solution du problème.

Parmi les différents moyens de diagnostic proposés récemment : injections de sérum artificiel, épreuve par tuberculine, examen radioscopique et radiographique, séro-diagnostic, etc., un seul a une valeur absolue : c'est la constatation, dans les crachats, des bacilles de la tuberculose.

Chez les enfants tuberculeux, comme chez les adultes, ce signe est pathognomonique. Malheureusement, il n'est pas facile d'obtenir des crachats des enfants tuberculeux. En effet, les enfants ne crachent pas, et d'autre part leurs tuberculoses pulmonaires, le plus souvent à forme broncho-pneumonique, sont souvent sans expectoration. Ce n'est guère que dans le cas de coqueluche qu'on peut avoir facilement les crachats.

Pour obtenir les crachats, on s'est efforcé de les trouver dans les selles (KOSSEL), dans l'arrière-gorge, dont KAUFFMANN et BULLER conseillèrent de racler les parois pour recueillir le mucus.

Ces procédés ne donnèrent que peu de résultats. C'est alors que HENRI MEUNIER proposa de recueillir, par la sonde gastrique, les crachats avalés par les enfants et de rechercher dans ces produits expectorés et déglutis les bacilles de Koch.

Le moment le plus favorable pour faire le cathétérisme gastrique est le matin, lorsque l'enfant, au réveil et encore à jeun, a eu les premières quintes de toux. On obtient ainsi les crachats presque purs, dont l'examen peut donner les renseignements les plus importants.

BERTHERAND, qui a mis en pratique le procédé de H. MEUNIER, n'hésite pas à en proclamer la grande valeur. Sur 50 observations, il a eu 21 examens de crachats positifs, confirmés par l'évolution clinique ou par l'autopsie; 9 examens ont été négatifs et également confirmés par la marche de la maladie, sa terminaison et l'examen *post mortem*.

B. — Communications sur la tuberculose infantile.

QUELQUES REMARQUES SUR LA TUBERCULOSE INFANTILE
A RIO-DE-JANEIRO

par M. le professeur MONCORVO,

Membre correspondant de l'Académie de médecine de Paris.

Jusqu'au commencement du xixe siècle l'étude spéciale de la tuberculose infantile n'avait point encore attiré l'attention des cliniciens. On peut citer Tonnelé, en France, comme étant celui qui s'en est occupé le premier, en 1825, pour démontrer la tendance du mal à se généraliser aux premières époques de la vie. Après lui Papavoine a fait voir la fréquence des lésions ganglionnaires sous la dépendance de la tuberculose dans le jeune âge.

Bientôt cet intéressant sujet attira progressivement l'attention des pédiatres; puis on vit apparaître de curieuses recherches sur la fréquence et les particularités de la bacillose des jeunes enfants.

De 1874 à 1885, Frœbelius enregistra dans la crèche de St-Pétersbourg 91 570 nourrissons dont 416 ont succombé à la tuberculose sur un total de 18 569, soit 4 pour 100 de la mortalité générale.

Schwer a dressé, en 1886, le tableau qui suit :

Parmi 94 natimorts aucun n'a été reconnu tuberculeux.

D'un jour à 4 semaines on a inscrit 169, dont tous se trouvaient indemnes.

De 5 à 9 semaines 125, dont l'un tuberculeux.

De 3 à 5 mois, 144 enfants dont 15 étaient atteints, soit 4 pour 100.

De 6 à 12 mois, 160 enfants dont 28 tuberculeux, soit 17,5 pour 100.

De 2 ans, 188 enfants dont 49 affectés du mal, soit 26 pour 100.

De 5 ans, 104, dont 47 affectés, soit 45,2 pour 100.

De 4 ans, 82 enfants, dont 27 tuberculeux, soit 52,9 pour 100.

De 5 ans, 55, dont 20 tuberculeux, soit 37,7 pour 100.

De 6 à 10 ans, 112 enfants, dont 40 affectés, soit 35,7 pour 100.

De 11 à 15 ans, 89 enfants, dont 28 tuberculeux, soit 51,5 pour 100.

En France, Landouzy a mis en relief la grande fréquence de la maladie dans l'enfance à partir du deuxième trimestre, et Queyrat, son élève, en a signalé la majeure proportion après la deuxième année.

Boltz, de Kiel, dans la période de 1875 à 1889, a relevé la mortalité de 89 pour 100 chez des nouveau-nés de 5 à 10 semaines, de 4,26 chez des enfants de 3 à 5 mois, de 9,22 chez d'autres de 6 à 12 mois, de 19,58 chez des enfants de 12 à 24 mois; ces chiffres donnant lieu à un pourcentage de 27,8 pour la première année et de 26,2 pour la deuxième.

Aviragnet, en 1890, en faisant l'autopsie d'un certain nombre d'enfants de la crèche de l'hôpital Tenon, compris entre l'âge de 0 à 2 ans, se trouva à même de constater une fois sur quatre l'existence de l'affection, ce qui fournit une proportion de 21,7 pour 100.

Ces petits sujets, au nombre de quinze, ont été répartis comme il suit :

De 0 à 1 an, 7	5 mois.	5
	4 mois et demi.	1
	10 mois.	2
	12 —	1
De 1 à 2 ans. 8	16 mois	1
	19 —	1
	21 —	1
	22 —	1
	23 —	1
	24 —	5

Barthez et Sanné ont consigné dans la 3e édition (1891) du Traité de Rilliet et Barthez le résultat de 525 autopsies chez des enfants décédés entre 1 et 15 ans, lesquelles ont révélé chez 514 l'existence de la tuberculose, ainsi répartis :

De 1 à 2 ans et demi	47
De 3 à 5 —	107
De 6 à 10 —	107
De 11 à 15 ans	55
	514

Les lésions tuberculeuses ont été de la sorte retrouvées à la proportion de 96,2 sur le total des autopsies.

Envisageant ce sujet en ce qui concerne l'Amérique australe, nous

nous trouvâmes dépourvus des documents qui nous autorisent à juger de la fréquence et de la mortalité par la tuberculose infantile dans les divers pays dont elle se compose, exception faite de la République Argentine et en quelque sorte du Brésil.

C'est ainsi que dans l'œuvre organisée sous le nom de *Patronage et Assistance de l'enfance* à Buenos-Aires, en s'occupant de la statistique démographo-sanitaire, le Dr Emilio Coni a signalé la proportion de la tuberculose infantile dans cette capitale par des chiffres équivalents à ceux de la syphilis.

Tout en associant pourtant au groupe de la tuberculose plusieurs autres entités morbides, telles que la méningite tuberculeuse, la scrofule, le carreau, etc., qui figurent dans d'autres tableaux démographiques dans la proportion de 801 cas, le démographe argentin a fait encore remarquer que cette cause mortuaire agissait dans une plus vaste échelle.

Jusqu'à 1886, les données démographo-sanitaires relevées à Rio-de-Janeiro en ce qui regarde la léthalité par la tuberculose n'offrent rien de profitable vis-à-vis des premières années de la vie. Ce n'est qu'à partir de cela que les décès par cette cause ont été classés d'après les différentes phases de l'enfance.

Nous sommes redevable à notre collègue et ami, M. le Dr A. Portugal, chargé de la statistique démographo-sanitaire municipale à Rio, d'un tableau dressé sous ce point de vue depuis 1886 jusqu'à la fin de 1890.

En les envisageant séparément pour chaque année on les aura répartis comme il suit :

1886
De 0 à 1 an   68 décès — 32,7 p. 1000 de la mortalité générale.
De 1 à 5 ans 114   —   — 54,8   —
De 6 à 15 —   77   —   — 37   —
                 259

1887
De 0 à 1 an   56 décès — 27,6 p. 1000 de la mortalité générale.
De 1 à 5 ans 183   —   — 90,3   —
De 6 à 15 —   55   —   — 27,1   —
                 294

1888
De 0 à 1 an   51 décès — 25,6 p. 1000 de la mortalité générale.
De 1 à 5 ans 126   —   — 76,2   —
De 6 à 15 —   45   —   — 22,6   —
                 222

1889
De 0 à 1 an   69 décès — 31,6 p. 1000 de la mortalité générale.
De 1 à 5 ans   169   —   — 67,6   —
De 6 à 15 -   78   —   — 35,8

                  ___
                  516

1890
De 0 à 1 an   56 décès — 25,4 p. 1000 de la mortalité générale.
De 1 à 5 ans   127   —   — 58,5   —
De 6 à 15 —   64   —   — 29   —

                  ___
                  249

Ces tableaux annuels peuvent se réduire au suivant qui comprend le total des décès par la tuberculose à chaque période de l'enfance :

De 0 à 1 an . . . . 500 (60 par an)
De 2 à 5 ans . . . . 721 (140   —   )
De 6 à 15 — . . . . 319 (55   —   )

Il en ressort un total de 1340 décès par la tuberculose pendant le laps de temps signalé, parmi lesquels on relève 609 cas appartenant à des enfants du sexe masculin et 731 à des fillettes, en laissant voir un excès de 122 du côté de ces dernières.

En recherchant dans ces tableaux officiels ce qui se rapporte aux localisations du mal en question, nous sommes arrivé à les répartir comme il suit :

Tuberculose généralisée :
De 0 à 1 an   1
De 1 à 7 ans   10
De 8 à 17 —   2
                                                           ___
                                                            13

Tuberculose pulmonaire :
De 0 à 1 an   20
De 1 à 7 ans 66
De 8 à 15 —   54
                                                           ___
                                                           140

Méningite tuberculeuse :
De 0 à 1 an   3
De 1 à 7 ans   7
De 8 à 15 —   2
                                                           ___
                                                            12

Tuberculose péritonéale :
De 0 à 1 an   29
De 1 à 7 ans 31
De 8 à 15 —   4
                                                           ___
                                                            64

Tuberculose d'autres viscères :

De 0 à 1 an	7
De 1 à 7 ans	15
De 8 à 15 —	2
	24

De ce qui précède nous nous croyons autorisé à conclure :

1° Qu'au cours des cinq années ci-dessus indiquées les petits sujets de 1 à 5 ans ont payé le plus grand tribut à la tuberculose (140 par an), venant après ceux de 0 à 1 an (60 par an) et enfin ceux de 6 à 15 ans (56 par an) :

2° Que la proportion de la mortalité infantile par la tuberculose n'a guère suivi de près celle de l'accroissement rapide de la population de Rio. Ayant atteint, en 1889, le chiffre le plus élevé (516), les décès par cette cause ont baissé, l'année suivante, à celui de 249 ;

3° Que le coefficient de la léthalité infantile par la tuberculose sur 1000 décès par la même cause est de 126,8 ;

4° Que le sexe ne semble guère exercer aucune influence étiologique sur la tuberculose infantile dans notre capitale ;

5° Que les statistiques officielles ne nous fournissent point d'éléments pour en connaître les rapports avec les races ;

6° Que d'après ces mêmes données, nous devons signaler la prédominance pulmonaire du mal sur leurs autres localisations (140 cas) retrouvées pour la plupart chez des enfants de 1 à 7 ans (60 cas) ;

7° Qu'après la localisation pulmonaire vinrent en ordre décroissant :

La localisation péritonéale	64 cas
La tuberculose généralisée	15 —
La tuberculose des méninges	12 —
Localisations viscérales mal définies	24 —

Cette classification émanée directement des causes des décès signalées dans les certificats s'éloigne en quelque sorte de celle appartenant aux tableaux démographo-sanitaires des divers autres pays. En gardant, par exemple, le silence sur les localisations du mal sur les différentes pièces du squelette, ces documents rapportent à sa détermination péritonéale le chiffre élevé de 64, évidemment en disproportion avec celui de 15, à compte de la tuberculose disséminée.

Étant données ces lacunes qui ne permettent guère de déductions positives en ce qui regarde le siège de l'affection qui nous occupe, il en ressort au plus qu'il faut retrancher du chiffre total des décès par la tuberculose un certain nombre de cas de cette nature qui figurent dans les tableaux statistiques sous des rubriques diverses, telles que l'athrepsie, la faiblesse congénitale, la bronchite, l'entérite, la fièvre typhoïde, etc.

On n'aura donc pas à discuter l'avantage qui proviendrait d'un accord fixé parmi les cliniciens dans le sens de porter avec la précision possible les diagnostics enregistrés dans les certificats de décès, sans quoi la statistique mortuaire ne se prêtera jamais à des conclusions utiles.

Pour se faire une juste idée de la fréquence, des caractères et des suites de la tuberculose infantile, il convient certes de se rendre compte de ce qui concerne sa morbidité. N'ayant à Rio d'autre source à consulter dans ce but que les archives de notre service, c'est pour cela que je reproduis ici le tableau ci-dessous concernant les petits tuberculeux y soignés au cours des trois dernières années (1897-1899) :

```
Total des enfants admis. . . . . . . . . . . . . . . . .  2 550
Enfants tuberculeux. . . . . . . . . . . . . . . . . . .    515
```

Ces derniers ont été ainsi répartis :

D'après l'âge :

```
De 0 à 1 an. . . . . . . . . . . . .    111 — 23,2 pour 100
De 1 à 2 ans . . . . . . . . . . . .    103 — 20     —
De 2 à 7 —  . . . . . . . . . . . .     218 — 42,3   —
De 7 à 15 —  . . . . . . . . . . . .      85 — 16,1   —
                                        ———
                                        515
```

D'après le sexe :

```
Garçons. . . . . . . . . . . . . .      272 — 52,8 pour 100
Fillettes . . . . . . . . . . . . .     243 — 47,2    —
                                        ———
                                        515
```

D'après la race :

```
Blancs. . . . . . . . . . . . . . .     379 — 73,5 pour 100
Métis. . . . . . . . . . . . . . . .    104 — 21     —
Nègres. . . . . . . . . . . . . . .      32 —  6.2    —
                                        ———
                                        515
```

D'après la marche et les localisations :

```
Tuberculose aiguë et subaiguë. . . .      56 — 10,8 pour 100
Tuberculose pulmonaire plus ou
   moins torpide. . . . . . . . . . .    213 — 41,3    —
Tuberculose pulmonaire avec des si-
   gnes marqués d'adénopathie tra-
   chéo-bronchique . . . . . . . . . .   168 — 32,6    —
Tuberculose ganglionnaire périphé-
   rique. . . . . . . . . . . . . . .     23 —  4.4
Tuberculose hépatique (type Hutinel).      1 —
Méningite tuberculeuse. . . . . . .        6 —  1.1
Coxo-tuberculose . . . . . . . . . .      23 —  4.4
Mal de Pott. . . . . . . . . . . . .      15 —  2,9    —
Arthrite du genou . . . . . . . . . .     10 —  1.9
                                        ———
                                        515
```

On a enregistré 20 décès, plusieurs autres enfants ayant succombé après leur sortie du service. Cette circonstance explique qu'il nous ait été impossible de fixer pour nos cas le chiffre précis de la léthalité.

Il ressort cependant des données qui viennent d'être consignées que 20,3 pour 100 de nos petits sujets laissaient apercevoir des signes et des symptômes d'une tuberculose.

L'examen du tableau comprenant les petits tuberculeux à chaque période de l'enfance permet de remarquer la proportion presque équivalente de la maladie au cours des deux premières années, rapportée pendant la première par le pourcentage de 25,2 et par celle de 20 pendant la deuxième.

Il en est aussi aisé de conclure que les deux premières années fournissent le plus grand contingent à la tuberculose; tandis que les chiffres globaux des cas signalés atteignirent la somme de 204, le total des petits malades annotés au cours de la deuxième phase (3 à 7 ans) n'excéda que de 218, ce qui montre un petit excès à peine de 14 cas sur celui du premier groupe.

Il en ressort au plus que, de la septième à la quinzième année, la maladie subit une diminution marquée, fournissant le pourcentage de 16,1.

Il y a encore à relever que la proportion des cas enregistrés au cours de la première année par rapport à chaque mois laisse voir qu'étant d'une extrême rareté pendant les six premiers mois, la tuberculose s'accroît progressivement au cours du deuxième semestre. Cela s'accorde du reste avec ce qu'on observe à ce propos dans les autres pays de l'Europe et de l'Amérique.

Pour ne point dépasser les limites de notre propre observation, nous y reproduisons un exemple prélevé sur nos statistiques. Prenant au hasard la période d'une année constituée par le deuxième semestre de 1898 et le premier de 1899, on aura ainsi répartis les petits tuberculeux amenés dans notre service n'ayant pas encore dépassé la première année.

De 0 à 1 mois.	0 cas
De 2 mois.	3 —
De 3 mois.	4 —
De 4 mois.	2 —
De 5 mois.	3 —
De 6 mois.	3 —
De 7 mois.	0 —
De 8 mois.	5 —
De 9 mois.	1 —
De 10 mois	4 —
De 11 mois	6 —
De 12 mois	15 —
	46

Ainsi donc, tandis que les petits malades entrés au cours du premier semestre ne dépassèrent pas le nombre de 15, le chiffre de ceux admis pendant le deuxième semestre s'éleva à 51.

L'excès de 29 cas sur le compte des fillettes atteintes du mal ne semble devoir attirer particulièrement notre attention, car le sexe n'exerce pas, dans le jeune âge, une influence étiologique appréciable sur l'acquisition ou la marche de la tuberculose.

75 pour 100 de nos petits sujets appartenaient à la race blanche, 21 pour 100 à la race mixte, 6,2 pour 100 étaient des noirs.

S'il est vrai que les nègres sont très frappés par la tuberculose dans certains régions des États-Unis du Nord ainsi que de la République Argentine, rien n'est moins exact que l'avis de certains auteurs, Bordier entre autres, d'après lequel ce terrible mal social aurait une prédilection pour les individus de race noire.

Pour ce qui est des localisations de la maladie, chez nos 515 petits sujets, il importe de relever que, malgré la tendance indéniable de la bacillose à la dissémination, dans le jeune âge, il n'est pourtant moins exact que les examens cliniques en ont bien souvent dévoilé la détermination pulmonaire et médiastinale, cela dans une proportion supérieure à la moitié des cas observés (581 sur 515).

Qu'il nous soit permis à ce propos de signaler l'erreur déplorable mais prédominante dans les tableaux démographo-sanitaires qui consiste à enregistrer un grand nombre de cas de tuberculose sous la rubrique de *tabes mésentérique*. Nous tâchons depuis bien longtemps d'éviter cette proportion exagérée de ces cas.

D'ailleurs, les symptômes par lesquels on a prétendu la caractériser n'offrent rien de particulier et sont bien au contraire analogues à ceux qui dénoncent des troubles divers du tabes gastro-intestinal tenant à des maladies générales infectieuses, au nombre desquelles la malaria occupe chez nous le premier rang.

Ce que nous venons de dire à l'égard du tabes mésentérique, dont je me suis occupé depuis longtemps dans mes conférences, a reçu dernièrement l'appui de M. Marfan dans le Traité de Grancher.

Pendant longtemps, dit-il, on a tracé de cette affection une description de fantaisie; pendant longtemps on en a fait la cause principale sinon unique du marasme infantile. On la désignait sous la dénomination de *carreau*. On lui attribuait des signes physiques très spéciaux et un grand cortège de symptômes fonctionnels et généraux.

En envisageant les signes physiques (intumescence abdominale, tumeurs perceptibles à la palpation, dilatation des veines, engorgement des ganglions sous-cutanés) ainsi que les symptômes fonctionnels (voracité, douleurs, diarrhée, accidents de compression), il arrive à cette conclusion qu'aucun de ces caractères n'appartient spécialement à l'entité morbide dont il s'agit, mais qu'ils sont communs aux diverses affections de l'appareil digestif.

Désireux d'enregistrer dans notre service tous les cas suspects ou avérés de ce mal de misère, et cela avant tout dans le but de nous rendre bien compte de sa fréquence et de son extension dans le jeune âge, nous nous sommes décidé depuis bien des années à l'examen rigoureux de chaque petit malade, quel que soit le motif de son admission, dans le but de rechercher l'existence d'une tuberculose qui échappe souvent encore à la connaissance des personnes de son entourage ou à celle du petit malade lui-même. Nous nous attachons donc à établir le diagnostic de la tuberculose précoce, qui constitue un premier degré précédant les trois autres phases classiques et consistant exclusivement dans une modification du timbre inspiratoire, lequel s'affaiblit ou devient rude ou soufflant. Ce fait important sur lequel nous avions dès longtemps appelé l'attention de nos élèves a reçu dernièrement la confirmation la plus complète de la part de M. le professeur Grancher.

L'invasion des ganglions médiastinaux suivant fatalement, d'après certains auteurs, celle du parenchyme pulmonaire, indique logiquement la valeur des signes qui révèlent la coïncidence de l'adénopathie trachéo-bronchique dans l'hypothèse en question.

Depuis quinze ans environ nous nous efforçons journellement de mettre en relief la coexistence fréquente de cette macroadénie, laquelle se dénonce parfois, en outre des signes classiques, par celui désigné par nos élèves sous la dénomination de signe de Moncorvo et qui consiste à provoquer un mouvement de toux plus ou moins accusé au moyen de la percussion du plan antérieur de la poitrine, notamment au niveau de l'articulation sterno-claviculaire droite. Très récemment notre vénéré collègue de l'Académie de médecine, M. Mesnet, a cru devoir appeler l'attention des cliniciens sur la valeur de l'association de l'adénopathie trachéo-bronchique pour le diagnostic de la tuberculose chez les adultes.

L'absence de l'expectoration aux premiers âges, même s'il s'agit d'un cas de tuberculose ulcérée, ne laisse point d'opposer quelque embarras au diagnostic du mal par l'examen bactériologique. Dans certains cas pourtant nous nous sommes trouvé à même de recueillir une quantité suffisante de mucosités pour cet examen en les prenant au moyen d'une pelote de ouate hydrophile insinuée dans la gorge entre les mors d'une pince courbe avant l'explosion provoquée ou spontanée de la toux.

Aussi, nous nous sommes élevé contre l'adoption de la tuberculine comme moyen révélateur d'une tuberculose infantile à diagnostic obscur. Après nos premiers essais et par suite de quelques accidents que nous avons eu à constater, nous nous sommes décidé à demander sur cela l'avis de notre regretté maître M. le professeur Henoch, de Berlin, ainsi que celui de notre savant maître et ami M. le professeur Gerhardt, aussi de Berlin, lesquels ne tardèrent guère à nous renseigner sur les conséquences évidemment fâcheuses qu'ils avaient eu à enregistrer à la suite de l'emploi de cet agent dénonciateur de la tuberculose dans le jeune âge. Leurs conclusions s'accordent avec celles de Grancher et Debove qui l'ont condamné pour le diagnostic des cas de cette nature.

Parrot, Warthin, Hocksing et d'autres cliniciens ainsi que plusieurs expérimentateurs qui avaient pratiqué des recherches sur des animaux laissèrent hors de doute la transmissibilité de la tuberculose maternelle au fœtus, alors qu'à une époque plus reculée l'hérédité était jugée presque partout le mode le plus commun de la contraction du mal. Les intéressantes recherches pourtant de Landouzy et de ses élèves vinrent bientôt mettre en lumière l'exclusivisme exagéré d'une telle conception pathogénique. Elles ont démontré, il est vrai, la réceptivité transmise par la mère à son enfant du mal, un régime bien réglé aurait pu les préserver.

L'enquête minutieuse à laquelle nous nous sommes livré par rapport aux antécédents familiaux ou personnels de nos petits tuberculeux nous engage à attacher la plus grande valeur à la contagion du mal.

Aussi avons-nous recherché à ce propos l'influence des autres facteurs pathogènes capables d'accroître ou d'exagérer la prédisposition morbide des petits sujets. En examinant sous ce point de vue nos 515 tuberculeux, nous nous trouvâmes à même de reconnaître que 205 d'entre eux portaient des stigmates plus ou moins avérés de l'hérédité syphilitique, c'est-à-dire 50,9 pour 100. D'un autre côté, 212 présentaient des symptômes de malaria, ce qui donne une proportion de 41,1 pour 100. Ce fait contribue une fois de plus pour annihiler la doctrine conçue et soutenue par Boudin de l'incompatibilité du paludisme et de la tuberculose.

Pour ce qui est de la séméiologie de la tuberculose infantile à Rio elle ne revêt guère de particularités dignes d'être notées: elle se révèle par les caractères propres à celle que l'on observe en Europe et dans l'Amérique du Nord.

Dans nos conférences nous nous sommes attaché à mettre en relief l'ignorance dominante dans notre public en général des notions les plus élémentaires d'hygiène, ce qui entrave en réalité la mise en pratique des mesures opposées à la propagation de ce mal social. Sans nous y arrêter nous rappellerons sommairement quelques pratiques usuelles dans notre vie sociale fort dangereuses d'ailleurs vis-à-vis de la contagion du mal.

Ainsi notre habitude de baiser les enfants sur les lèvres est très blâmable. Chacun le fait librement avec la plus parfaite insouciance de la part des familles, comme l'on voit souvent dans les promenades et les jardins publics.

Fort récemment encore et sous la direction de Flügge, professeur de l'Université de Breslau, Stecher, Laschtschenks, Heymann et Beninde se sont livrés à de nouvelles expériences au sujet de la transmission de la tuberculose, lesquelles leur ont permis de vérifier que lorsqu'on parle, on tousse ou on éternue, il s'échappe de la cavité buccale un nombre considérable de gouttelettes de salive, lesquelles, grâce à leur poids spécifique, flottent dans l'air, pouvant être de la sorte entraînées à longue distance par les courants aériens. D'autres recherches de ces observateurs leur laissèrent reconnaître que des germes introduits artificiellement dans la cavité buccale sont jetés à un mètre de distance quand l'individu soumis à l'expérience se met à parler.

Il y a aussi à signaler l'habitude dangereuse qui consiste à engager les petits sujets à se traîner ou à se frotter sur un parquet manquant absolument parfois de propreté. L'infection bacillaire s'effectue alors souvent par inhalation et par ingestion, étant donnée la tendance naturelle des petits enfants à porter à tout instant leurs doigts à la bouche.

On a généralement adopté chez nous l'usage d'un petit instrument pourvu d'une sorte de tétine en caoutchouc que les nourrissons maintiennent entre les lèvres en les suçant.

Ces instruments qui tombent à tout moment par terre sont immédiatement et sans la moindre désinfection préalable réintroduits dans la bouche en y portant toute sorte de germes avec lesquels ils sont mis en contact.

Nous les confisquons dans notre service à tous ceux qui s'en présentent pourvus, ce qui nous a permis d'en faire une belle collection.

Les jouets qui roulent sur les parquets ou sur le sol des jardins ou sur les trottoirs et que les bébés portent continuellement à leur bouche les exposent certes à de pareils dangers.

Il y a lieu ici d'incriminer l'absence de mesures réglementaires appliquées à l'allaitement mercenaire dans notre capitale. Nous avions rédigé, en 1875, un projet de réglementation des nourrices, mais ce fut en vain et nous ne réussîmes pas à le voir adopté.

Quelques ans plus tard nous parvînmes par notre initiative individuelle avec la collaboration d'un autre confrère à installer dans une des artères les plus centrales de Rio un bureau pour l'examen gratuit des nourrices: cette fois encore notre tentative échoua faute d'une loi municipale rendant obligatoire cette mesure hygiénique.

Enfin, dernièrement, la Préfecture municipale a créé par un décret l'installation d'un bureau d'inspection des nourrices: cette décision préfectorale pourtant figure à peine dans le répertoire des lois municipales.

Il en est de même en ce qui regarde l'inspection des vacheries ainsi que l'analyse du lait livré à la consommation publique.

Encore ici il nous faut rappeler que des règlements ont été décrétés également par la Préfecture analogues à ceux adoptés dans les capitales du vieil et du nouveau monde y compris l'emploi de la tuberculine pour le triage des animaux. Mais rien de cela n'a été mis en pratique jusqu'à l'heure qu'il est. Cette lacune est d'autant plus regrettable que d'autres capitales latino-américaines telles que Santiago de Chile et Buenos-Aires jouissent des bénéfices des règlements concernant l'inspection des nourrices et des vacheries.

Notre observation personnelle nous a laissé découvrir nombre de cas de tuberculose infantile tenant évidemment à cette condition étiologique.

Au nombre des causes qui favorisent le développement et la propagation du mal qui nous occupe, il y a certes lieu de relever celles qui tiennent à l'insalubrité des habitations. Cette condition pathogène, chez nous, joue un rôle des plus importants pour la contagion et la léthalité par la tuberculose. Les petits bébés en particulier en subissent les conséquences nuisibles.

Les domiciles des gens pauvres sont ici les plus défectueux, soit par le défaut d'aération, de lumière, de cubage des appartements, par l'humidité, soit encore en général par le manque de propreté. Les expériences de Franz Mignesco ont fait voir que la culture pure des bacilles de Koch exposée aux rayons solaires s'éteint dans un délai qui varie de quelques minutes à quelques heures, cela sans avoir recours à des rayons concentrés.

Le libre accès à la lumière solaire y devrait être secondé par la ventilation des appartements et la propreté des parquets. Dès 1887, alors que la désinfection des crachats devint obligatoire dans les prisons prussiennes, 70 000 individus ont échappé à la tuberculose jusqu'à 1895. Le Dr Mamerto Cadiz, délégué du gouvernement du Chili au quatrième Congrès pour l'étude de la tuberculose à Paris (1898), a relevé la salubrité notoire des habitations de la classe pauvre comme étant l'une des conditions les plus puissantes de la grande mortalité par la tuberculose à Santiago. Aussi s'est-il empressé d'ajouter qu'il y avait des petites habitations nommées *ranchos* que seul le feu serait capable de purifier.

L'isolement des contaminés dans des sanatoriums spécialement consacrés au traitement de la tuberculose devient aujourd'hui une ressource précieuse pour entraver la propagation du mal, au point que des philanthropes, des médecins et des gouvernements, frappés par les succès croissants de créations de cette nature ont pensé à en étendre les bénéfices aux classes déshéritées de la fortune.

Biehmer, Dellweiller, les initiateurs en Allemagne de ces bienfaisantes institutions, parvinrent bientôt à en démontrer les avantages considérables, et bref les sanatoriums populaires pour les tuberculeux furent jugés avec raison le *primum movens* parmi les moyens que nous possédons pour la lutte contre ce terrible mal social.

C'est par les *moralités* économiques, dit Brouardel, qu'imposent aux sociétés modernes les principes de solidarité sociale que le sanatorium populaire, instrument de prophylaxie et de cure de la tuberculose, est devenu, en Allemagne, le principal rouage de tout un système préventif et curatif mis aux mains des offices d'assurance contre la maladie, contre l'invalidité et la vieillesse, auxquels, depuis près de vingt ans, la loi fait aux ouvriers comme aux patrons l'obligation de s'affilier.

Il faut d'ailleurs se rappeler que la création et la multiplication de ces institutions humanitaires y reçoivent l'appui et le concours de toutes les classes sociales. L'état, la province, la commune, les compagnies d'assurance, d'industries, les associations coopératives, les particuliers, la croix rouge, les médecins apportent leur activité et leur contribution pour la réalisation de ce but.

Plus récemment, la Compagnie impériale d'assurance contre l'invalidité a décidé, dans l'intention d'arrêter la propagation de la tuberculose, la fondation des sanatoriums populaires, lesquels fournissent 20 pour 100 de guérisons et 60 à 65 pour 100 d'améliorations.

L'influence de l'Empereur, de l'Impératrice, ainsi que du Parlement n'a fait qu'augmenter le prestige de ces institutions du bien.

Il faut pourtant convenir que cette œuvre méritante réclame pour son exécution une activité, une énergie considérables et plus encore des sommes peu communes. Or, tous les pays ne se trouvent pas également doués de ressources suffisantes pour de pareilles entreprises. Notre pays est malheureusement de ce nombre d'autant plus que son étendue considérable crée de sérieuses difficultés à la multiplication de ces installations. Cela ne semble nullement exagéré quand on connaît ce qu'ont dû vaincre d'autres centres civilisés plus riches que le nôtre pour se mettre à l'œuvre.

Pour se faire une idée de la portée de telles créations, il suffira de lire ce que les délégués de l'Académie de médecine de Paris au Congrès pour la lutte contre la tuberculose à Berlin ont écrit à ce sujet.

M. le professeur Brouardel, rapporteur de la susdite commission, s'est exprimé ainsi : « Les notes des délégués de l'Académie ne laissent rien ignorer des difficultés de divers ordres ni de la complexité du problème qu'est, chez nous, l'organisation : d'un système protectionniste complet et efficace contre le mal de misère qu'est la tuberculose : d'un système complet d'assistance de nos légions de tuberculeux, de tout degré et de toute catégorie. »

Ces difficultés si franchement relevées pour son riche pays par l'éminent professeur parisien laissent prévoir ce que nous autres aurons à surmonter pour atteindre la réalisation d'un pareil désidératum.

Bien certain de tous les embarras à vaincre pour le but en question, M. le Dr Calmette, directeur de l'Institut Pasteur de Lille, a conçu l'heureuse idée d'un projet qu'il vient d'offrir à la commission extraparlementaire chargée d'étudier les moyens de combattre ce terrible fléau universel; lequel viendra, ce nous semble, combler une grande lacune dans le traitement prophylactique et hygiénique du mal. En admettant un centre industriel de 400 000 habitants renfermant 250 000 ouvriers, dont 15 000 tuberculeux à divers degrés, il reconnaît que 6 000 parmi ces derniers auraient obtenu une amélioration plus ou moins marquée en leur permettant de rentrer au sein de leurs familles. Il fait alors observer que si l'on avait eu recours pour un semblable résultat aux sanatoriums populaires, il faudrait avoir 60 établissements de cette nature pourvus chacun de 100 lits, dont l'installation aurait dû coûter 50 000 000 francs environ, somme que, même en France, il ne serait guère facile d'obtenir. Le Dr Calmette est aussi d'avis que l'éducation du peuple dans le sens de faire demander en temps opportun les sanatoriums, de même que le mouvement réclamé pour la propagation de créations analogues exigeraient environ un quart de siècle.

Après cela il propose la substitution de ceux-ci par la création de *dispensaires anti-tuberculeux* dont le nombre doit être réglé d'après les exigences de chaque arrondissement.

En découvrant à son début le mal à combattre, en prodiguant des conseils utiles pour sa prophylaxie, les ressources thérapeutiques et pécuniaires, les médecins chargés de ces dispensaires arriveront à soustraire à la misère et à la mort grand nombre de malheureux absolument désarmés pour la lutte contre un si terrible fléau. Au moyen d'une enquête soigneusement faite dans leur circonscription ils parviendront à découvrir les tuberculeux insouciants qu'ils prendront sous leur garde en leur prescrivant un traitement hygiénique approprié tout en préservant les personnes de leur entourage par des désinfections rigoureuses des appartements, du mobilier et des vêtements.

Rien donc de plus utile ni de plus pratique pour arrêter la propagation du mal, lorsque les circonstances spéciales d'une ville ou d'un pays ne comportent pas la fondation des sanatoriums populaires.

Nous sommes donc portés à croire qu'ils viendraient rendre un grand service dans notre capitale où la tuberculose fera de croissants ravages, si de sérieuses mesures hygiéniques ne lui sont opposées.

TUBERCULOSE INFANTILE A BUCAREST

par M. le professeur N.-C. THOMESCO

de Bucarest.

Permettez-moi de vous dire quelques mots sur certaines particularités de la tuberculose chez les enfants. Depuis que j'ai l'honneur de diriger, comme professeur, le service de clinique infantile de Bucarest, ces particularités de la tuberculose m'ont toujours frappé. Particularités qui ont une grande importance au point de vue de l'étiologie et de la prophylaxie de cette terrible maladie.

Je possède ici une statistique qui montre que, sur ces cinq dernières années, de 1895 à 1899 inclusivement, nous avons soigné dans notre service 5697 malades : sur ce nombre nous trouvons 505 tuberculeux, ce qui fait en moyenne une proportion de 8,82 pour 100. Cette proportion est au-dessous de la vérité car pendant les 4 mois d'été nous ne recevons presque pas de tuberculeux, notre service étant encombré par la gastro-entérite, en revanche, pendant les mois de printemps sur

100 malades il y en a près de 80 qui sont tuberculeux. En cherchan le chiffre des morts pour ces 5 dernières années nous trouvons sur 100 morts 22 provoquées par la tuberculose.

Voyons maintenant, sur les 505 cas de notre statistique, quelle est la moyenne entre la tuberculose pulmonaire et les autres localisations tuberculeuses. Nous trouvons 128 cas de tuberculose pulmonaire et 575 cas de tuberculose à autres localisations. D'autre part, la tuberculose pulmonaire ne commence à devenir fréquente qu'à partir de dix ans, elle est très rare avant un an. Parmi les autres localisations nous trouvons par ordre de fréquence : 129 cas de tuberculose généralisée, 81 cas de méningite, 75 cas de péritonite, 55 cas de tuberculose osseuse, etc. Ce qu'il faut surtout remarquer ici, c'est la fréquence relative de la tuberculose généralisée, de la méningite et de la péritonite par rapport à la tuberculose pulmonaire. Pourquoi ces formes sont-elles plus fréquentes dans l'enfance? C'est ici surtout que nous voulons attirer l'attention du Congrès sur les portes d'entrée du bacille de Koch chez l'enfant.

L'enfant devient plus facilement la proie de la tuberculose parce que la défense, chez lui, n'est pas encore bien organisée. La tuberculose qui se manifeste chez les adultes, a, en grande partie, son origine dans la vie infantile. La tuberculose étant une maladie à trêves morbides et à longues échéances, si elle ne s'est pas généralisée, l'enfant à plus de chances d'en échapper; mais elle se montrera plus tard chez l'adulte, sous une forme localisée.

Nous allons démontrer maintenant la manière par laquelle l'enfant devient tuberculeux.

Les grandes portes de pénétration du bacille de Koch dans l'organisme infantile sont :

1° Les voies respiratoires supérieures : le nez, la bouche, le pharynx avec les amygdales;

2° La voie digestive;

5° La voie cutanée.

De la bouche, du pharynx et des amygdales, les bacilles pénétrent dans les lymphatiques et arrivent aux ganglions du cou et aux ganglions trachéo-bronchiques et puis de là aux poumons; voilà le chemin le plus fréquemment suivi par le bacille. La tuberculose pulmonaire est avant tout, chez les enfants, une tuberculose ganglionnaire, trachéo-bronchique.

L'infection par la voie digestive se fait par les aliments, par la viande, par le lait, non pas tant celui des vaches tuberculeuses, mais celui souillé par le bacille de Koch, et la preuve la plus évidente est la distribution de la tuberculose en Roumanie où elle est très rare chez les bovidés, la proportion n'étant que de 5 pour 1000 dans l'abattoir de Bucarest ; tandis qu'en Allemagne et en Angleterre la proportion est de 25 pour 100, il en est de même en Amérique ; en Autriche seulement et surtout dans les abattoirs de Vienne, le pourcentage est de 2 pour 100, et cela provient de ce que le bétail est importé de la Hongrie où la tuberculose chez les bovidés est aussi rare qu'en Roumanie. Cependant je tiens à porter à votre connaissance que dernièrement le comité supérieur d'épizootie a décidé de soumettre à l'épreuve de la tuberculine tous les bovidés qui entrent dans nos abattoirs. Le danger par la viande n'est pas aussi grand et est en même temps plus facile à éviter ; il n'en est pas de même avec le lait, car chez les enfants il forme la base de l'alimentation.

Il me semble qu'on accuse trop le lait des vaches tuberculeuses au lieu d'incriminer plutôt le lait souillé par la traite et d'autres modalités possibles de contamination par le bacille, auxquels le lait est exposé. On a dit que le danger tenait à la consommation du lait cru ; de notre statistique résulte le contraire, car sur 505 cas d'enfants tuberculeux nous avons le nombre considérable de 75 cas de tuberculose péritonéale, et chez nous le pauvre comme le riche fait bouillir son lait.

On se tuberculise surtout par les mains, car tout le monde sait la mauvaise habitude qu'ont les enfants de se mettre les doigts dans le nez et dans la bouche, et comme les stomatites sont fréquentes chez eux.

Par conséquent, la tuberculose est rare chez les bovidés en Roumanie, mais nous avons une très grande proportion de tuberculose péritonéale chez les enfants et une très grande mortalité dans les villes par la tuberculose pulmonaire chez les adultes, mortalité qui atteint 55 pour 10 000 tandis que pour la campagne elle n'est que de 0,5 pour 10 000.

Cette petite mortalité à la campagne s'explique par le fait que notre paysan fait de l'aérothérapie en se couchant et passe la plupart du temps en plein air ; quant aux bovidés ils ne sont pas tenus enfermés et passent tout le temps au pâturage.

Nous trouvons aussi dans notre statistique en nombre considérable la méningite tuberculeuse : sa fréquence chez les enfants est remarquable : et elle est, le plus souvent la dernière étape d'une tuberculose généralisée. Si au point de vue clinique la méningite tuberculeuse a l'apparence d'une manifestation primitive, nous trouvons toujours, à la nécropsie un foyer quelconque dans l'organisme et presque toujours un ganglion trachéo-bronchique caséeux. Dans ces cas, il est difficile d'admettre que le bacille se transporte par la voie lympha tique du ganglion bronchique à la pie-mère, il est plus probable que le bacille qui se trouve dans les cavités nasales pénétrera plus facilement dans les méninges.

Quant au ganglion trachéo-bronchique caséeux, si l'enfant n'est pas tué par une méningite ou par une autre complication il reste dans cet état latent jusqu'à l'âge de la puberté ou adulte pour produire une tuberculose pulmonaire ou pleurale.

La grande fréquence de la généralisation de la tuberculose chez les enfants provient chez eux de la défense qui n'est pas bien organisée et surtout parce que toutes les portes d'entrée sont à la fois entr'ouvertes : *la porte respiratoire* par les grippes et les bronchites répétées, broncho-pneumonies, rougeoles et coqueluches; *la porte digestive* par les entérites, gastro-entérites et entérocolites, et *la porte cutanée* par les impétigos, les érythèmes fessiers. Ainsi assiégé de tous côtés l'organisme fléchit, le bacille sort de son habitat lymphatique et pénètre dans la circulation; voilà la généralisation.

En résumé, l'on doit prendre contre la tuberculose toutes les mesures que nous prenons contre les maladies contagieuses.

L'on doit appliquer des mesures d'hygiène et de protection de l'enfance contre la contamination par le crachat soit dans la famille soit à l'école.

Faire l'antisepsie de la bouche et du nez plusieurs fois par jour.

Installer dans les écoles, en dehors des crachoirs, des lavabos où les enfants puissent se laver plus souvent les mains, car c'est plutôt par les mains souillées par le bacille que la tuberculose se gagne.

Les jardins publics et les promenades sont les grands foyers d'infection où les enfants s'inoculent, car là, à côté des enfants, vont aussi les tuberculeux respirer du bon air, et crachent en même temps par terre ou sur une petite pierre avec laquelle l'enfant s'amusera ensuite en l'introduisant dans la bouche, ou les doigts salis dans le nez. Par conséquent nous devons diriger notre prophylaxie contre ceux-ci.

Répandre l'enseignement de l'hygiène dans les écoles de toutes catégories.

Créer des colonies scolaires pendant les vacances, et leur donner une plus grande extension là où elles existent.

Fonder des sanatoria pour les enfants lymphatiques, rachitiques et pour tous les prédisposés à la tuberculose.

Montrer aux parents par des conférences et des publications en quoi réside le danger pour qu'eux, à leur tour, deviennent des agents éclairés de la prophylaxie.

Enfin toutes les mesures prophylactiques préconisées chez les adultes doivent s'appliquer aussi chez les enfants, car la vraie prophylaxie de la tuberculose n'est que la prophylaxie de la tuberculose infantile, première étape de la tuberculose de l'adulte.

IV

MALADIES DES MÉNINGES ET DU SYSTÈME NERVEUX

I. — Rapports sur les méningites aiguës non tuberculeuses.

SUR LES MÉNINGITES AIGUËS NON TUBERCULEUSES CHEZ LES ENFANTS

RAPPORT

par **M** le professeur Luigi **CONCETTI**.

Directeur de la clinique pédiatrique de l'Université royale de Rome

Le présent rapport est fondé exclusivement sur mes observations personnelles, et repose sur 90 cas de méningites aiguës non tuberculeuses, et aussi 15 cas de polio-encéphalo-myélites aiguës récentes, que l'on devra, comme on le verra à propos de l'étiologie, considérer au même point de vue. Les 105 cas observés, soit dans ma clinique, soit à l'hôpital, soit dans ma clientèle privée, à l'exception de 18, ont tous été étudiés complètement, avec les ressources de la bactériologie et de la chimie, en me servant du liquide cérébro-spinal extrait par la ponction lombaire. Cette opération je l'ai pratiquée aussi dans 50 autres cas de maladies du système nerveux central ou de ses enveloppes (22 de méningite tuberculeuse, 14 d'hydrocéphalie chronique congénitale, 9 de tumeurs du cerveau ou du rachis, 7 de tétanie. 2 d'hydroméningocèle, 1 d'hématorachis). et j'utiliserai quelques notions que j'en ai retirées, pour des détails de comparaison en rapport avec le sujet qui nous occupe. En tout, j'ai ponctionné le rachis chez 159 enfants, de 1 à 55 fois; en tout, je compte que je n'ai pas pratiqué moins de 450 ponctions lombaires. Je me hâte de dire que. en aucun de ces nombreux cas, je n'ai eu à regretter le moindre accident du fait de cette opération, que je considère comme tout à fait inoffensive, bien que dans beaucoup de ces cas elle ait été pratiquée sur des malades allant et venant; deux fois seulement les enfants ont accusé un léger mal de tête tout à fait passager. Dans les formes aiguës de méningites, l'autopsie m'a donné des renseignements 22 fois: dans les autres cas. terminés par la mort. l'autopsie n'a pu être

pratiquée. Enfin dans le but d'élucider quelques questions de pathologie, je rapporterai des séries d'expériences pratiquées sur les animaux, surtout avec les matériaux qui m'ont été fournis par les cas
cliniques qui ont été l'objet de mes observations.

Sur les 90 cas de méningite aiguë non tuberculeuse, la recherche
de l'élément bactérique fait défaut en 18 cas, soit parce que le liquide
extrait était en trop petite quantité, soit par la raison que quelques-
uns de ces cas remontent à une époque antérieure à la pratique de la
ponction lombaire. L'élément bactérique pathogène a été isolé dans
29 cas. Dans les autres 45 cas, le liquide s'est montré tout à fait stérile:
mais il faut dire que, dans 24 de ces cas, la recherche a dû être faite
trop tard, c'est-à-dire lorsque le processus aigu étant passé, il n'en
restait que les conséquences (hydrocéphalie, amaurose, raideur de la
nuque, paralysies, convulsions, etc.): et dans ces conditions le résultat perd toute sa valeur, parce qu'on sait que la vie des microbes
ne dure pas, comme nous le verrons très longtemps. Au contraire,
dans les 27 autres cas on serait autorisé à affirmer que la méningite
a une origine non bactérienne, et qu'on a eu affaire à ces méningites
séreuses aiguës simples, comme en ont rapporté QUINCKE, MARFAN, et
moi-même, etc. En tout cas, c'est une question sur laquelle le dernier
mot n'est pas encore dit.

Sur les 29 cas de méningite d'origine bactérienne, 12 cas ont
donné le diplocoque lancéolé et encapsulé de Talamon-Fränkel,
10 fois à l'état de pureté, 1 fois associé au staphylocoque pyogène
doré et 1 fois au diplocoque intracellulaire (méningocoque) de Weichselbaum. Dans 5 de ces cas la méningite était associée à une pneumonie lobaire à diplocoques (méningite métapneumonique); dans les
autres la méningite était primitive. Dans 12 cas nous avons isolé le
diplocoque intracellulaire de Weichselbaum, 11 fois à l'état de pureté, et 1 fois, nous l'avons dit, associé au diplocoque de Fränkel,
chez un enfant d'un an convalescent de rougeole sans localisations
pulmonaires. Dans un autre cas la méningite fut suivie d'une broncho-pneumonie qui détermina la mort. Dans tous les autres cas, la
méningite était primitive. Dans 4 cas nous avons trouvé le bacté-
rium coli com., et dans un dernier cas le bacille pyocyanique, chez
un enfant convalescent d'une fièvre typhoïde.

La méthode que nous avons suivie dans nos recherches était la
suivante. Après avoir bien nettoyé la peau avec l'éther, et ensuite avec
une solution de sublimé, et encore une fois avec de l'éther, on pratiquait la ponction avec une grosse aiguille de platine iridié, flambée
à la lampe. Après avoir laissé écouler les premières gouttes de liquide,

le restant était recueilli dans les tubes stérilisés, ou était ensemencé dans des tubes sur agar et sur bouillon. Presque jamais je n'ai dû me servir de l'aspiration; et, en tout cas, le liquide aspiré n'était jamais réservé pour l'examen bactériologique, mais pour les autres recherches, en raison de la difficulté de bien s'assurer de la stérilité au cours des manœuvres nécessaires. Les tubes contenant les cultures étaient portés au thermostate à 35° ou 37°; quant aux autres, ou bien ils étaient laissés à la température ordinaire, ou bien ils étaient aussi placés dans l'étuve. Le liquide extrait était centrifugé, et les parties inférieures qui devaient contenir la plus grande quantité de bacilles servaient pour l'examen microscopique, pour les inoculations aux animaux ou pour faire d'autres ensemencements dans d'autres milieux de culture. Les animaux étaient inoculés aussi avec les cultures en bouillons, ou développées à la surface des tubes d'agar. Les animaux qui m'ont servi pour ces recherches ont été des cobayes, de petits lapins, des rats, de petits chats, de petits chiens. Les inoculations ont été pratiquées ou dans la plèvre, ou sous la peau, ou dans le péritoine, ou dans la cavité arachnoïdienne, soit par la trépanation du crâne, soit par la ponction lombaire. Souvent le microorganisme était de nouveau isolé de ces animaux et transporté sur d'autres terrains de culture, et sur d'autres animaux. Ce qui restait du liquide était utilisé pour les recherches chimiques.

La ponction lombaire était pratiquée en prenant comme point de repère la ligne tirée des deux épines iliaques postérieures et supérieures, et dans l'espace intervertébral qui se trouve sur cette ligne. L'enfant était placé dans la position latérale, et incliné sur lui-même de façon à former une courbure à grande convexité extérieure. Après avoir retiré l'aiguille on fermait la piqûre avec du collodion. Dans ces expériences j'ai été assisté avec le plus grand zèle par mes assistants les D' F. VALAGUSSA et A. LONGO, à qui j'adresse mes plus vifs remerciements.

I. Méningites aiguës bactériennes.

La pratique de la ponction lombaire, depuis QUINCKE, a beaucoup facilité l'étude des méningites, surtout chez les enfants, soit au point de vue du diagnostic, soit au point de vue de l'étiologie, comme aussi au point de vue de la thérapeutique. Avant ce temps, dans la plupart des cas on restait sur le terrain des hypothèses. Dans les cas légers, on parlait souvent de phénomènes éclamptiques, de l'irritabilité du système nerveux dans l'âge infantile, du méningisme, etc. Si par hasard le diagnostic de méningite venait à être formulé, il restait toujours sans une preuve évidente, et parfois il finissait par être retiré, parce que la méningite était considérée comme une maladie difficile à guérir au moins complètement, sans laisser de traces plus ou moins durables, quelquefois pour toute la vie (hydrocéphalie, amaurose, surdité, idiotie, etc.). Dans les cas graves, si la maladie aboutissait à la guérison, on était toujours incertain sur l'espèce microbienne en cause, et parfois on proclamait la probabilité d'avoir guéri des méningites tuberculeuses. Si au contraire la mort survenait après une durée plus ou moins prolongée, à l'autopsie on ne trouvait que les effets (hydrocéphalie, épaississement des membranes), et pas de traces d'éléments bactériques. Dans les cas enfin où l'autopsie pouvait être pratiquée dans la période aiguë de la maladie, cela se vérifiait surtout dans les formes les plus graves, à marche rapide, et que dans la plupart des cas nous verrons causées par le diplocoque lancéolé de Fränkel. Et c'est cette raison qui a fait croire jusqu'à ces derniers temps que ce micro-organisme jouait le rôle prépondérant dans l'étiologie de cette maladie, tandis que le méningocoque était plus rarement en cause; en effet, comme nous le verrons, les méningites méningococciques sont les plus faciles à guérir, et lorsqu'elles se terminent par la mort, celle-ci arrive à longue échéance, lorsque le microbe a épuisé sa vitalité et n'apparaît plus dans les essais de culture.

Action défavorable du liquide cérébro-spinal sur la vie des microbes.

En effet, depuis que, grâce à la ponction lombaire, dans toutes les formes de méningite, la recherche bactériologique est possible, même dans les cas les plus légers, et dès les premiers jours de leur manifestation, deux faits importants ont pu être démontrés : 1° la prédominance des formes méningococciques et leur bénignité vis-à-vis des formes pneumococciques; 2° la possibilité des formes simples, séreuses, amicrobiennes.

En vérité, pour ce qui regarde cette forme de méningite séreuse simple, il faut, comme je l'ai annoncé, faire des réserves, et ne pas conclure que si dans une méningite on trouve un exsudat stérile, elle n'a pu être déterminée par un agent microbien, surtout si la recherche a été pratiquée quelque temps après le début de la maladie, et si nous pensons que le liquide cérébro-spinal ne constitue pas un terrain de culture favorable à la vie des microbes. C'est pour cela que je crois nécessaire, avant de poursuivre mon rapport sur les méningites infectieuses, d'ouvrir une parenthèse sur ce sujet qui se prête bien à expliquer beaucoup de choses, comme nous pourrons le voir dans nos observations. Que le liquide cérébro-spinal soit un mauvais terrain de culture pour les microbes, je l'avais déjà démontré dans un travail publié il y a deux ans[1]. Il résulte évidemment de mes expériences que le streptocoque pyogène, que les staphylocoques pyogènes doré et blanc, que le diplocoque de Fränkel, que le bacterium coli com. ensemencés dans le liquide cérébro-spinal ou dans le bouillon mêlé en diverses proportions au liquide cérébro-spinal, montrent une moindre vitalité et aussi une moindre virulence, qui s'explique soit par le retard de la mort ou par la survie des animaux, soit par des lésions anatomo-pathologiques moins intenses. Ces expériences s'accordent bien avec l'observation clinique et expérimentale. En effet, soit dans les maladies infectieuses, soit dans les infections expérimentales, par rapport aux localisations très fréquentes dans les autres séreuses et dans les autres organes, les localisations au système nerveux et aux méninges sont extrêmement rares.

De nouvelles observations faites à l'occasion de ce travail ont conduit aux mêmes constatations à propos du diplocoque intra-cellulaire de Weichselbaum, comme il résulte d'un travail qui vient de paraître de mon assistant, le D* A. Longo. Un méningocoque isolé d'une très grave méningite cérébro-spinale chez un enfant de 5 ans, montrait un développement considérable non seulement sur l'agar, mais aussi dans la gélatine et dans le bouillon à la température ordinaire : au contraire, ensemencé dans le liquide cérébro-spinal, bien qu'assez riche en albumine (0,85 0/0), il ne s'y développa que très difficilement, et seulement après 5 jours de thermostat il donna un léger dépôt au fond du tube. Ensemencé ensuite dans d'autres terrains de culture, le développement apparut très faible dans l'agar et manqua dans la gélatine et dans le bouillon à 18°. Chez une petite fille de 5 ans qui nous fut amenée avec hydrocéphalie et amaurose résiduelles d'une méningite cérébro-spinale qui avait débuté 2 mois avant, on a pu à peine isoler un méningocoque chétif, épuisé, et qui ne fut pas capable de vivre longtemps, s'étant complètement épuisé au deuxième passage dans l'agar. Dans le cas de méningite, les ponctions successivement répétées après un court délai donnent une diminution progressive des micro-organismes, comme aussi une diminution de leur activité biologique et pathogène. Peut-être, faudrait-il admettre l'existence de

1. Chemische Untersuch. über die hydrocephalische Flüssigkeit, und über ihre Wirkung gegenguber pathogenen Bacterien. *Arch. f. Kinder heilk.*. XXIV. Bd 1898. — Ricerche chim. sol. liquido idrocefal. e sua azione contro alcuni batteri pathogeni. *Bull. della reale Accademia med. di Roma*, 1898. p. 2.

certaines conditions spéciales qui favorisent les localisations microbiennes dans les méninges. MARFAN, moi-même et d'autres avons démontré, combien dans le cours des toxi-infections gastro-intestinales sont fréquentes les manifestations méningées aiguës, et parfois avec constatation des microbes virulents et pathogènes dans le liquide cérébro-spinal. J'aurai l'occasion de vous le confirmer dans le cours de ce rapport. Lorsque le méningocoque vient d'être isolé dans ces conditions, par exemple, lorsque la ponction lombaire a été pratiquée dans des cas extrêmement graves, et, dès les premiers jours, j'ai constaté qu'il se présente avec le maximum de son activité pathogène. Après peu de jours il changeait ses propriétés avec une remarquable tendance à s'épuiser, pour les reprendre *ou* en dehors de l'organisme sur des terrains de culture plus favorables *ou* dans l'organisme humain lui-même, lorsque se reproduisaient les conditions primitives qui avaient provoqué la première atteinte. Je viens de dire, il y a un instant, que les toxi-infections intestinales présentaient fréquemment ces conditions, et j'y reviendrai tout à l'heure. Je pourrais aussi démontrer que ces mêmes conditions peuvent déterminer ce changement de virulence du méningocoque avec une aggravation de la maladie. Dans un cas de méningite cérébro-spinale traitée il y a peu de mois dans ma clinique chez un garçon de 7 ans, les trois premières ponctions donnèrent un méningocoque qui s'est montré tour à tour moins actif, moins virulent; et cela était en rapport avec une amélioration progressive et notable de la maladie. La quatrième et la cinquième ponction donnèrent un liquide stérile. L'enfant marcha vers la guérison. Un trouble digestif causa une vraie fièvre gastro-intestinale qui fut suivie d'une aggravation, d'un retour de phénomènes méningitiques très graves. À une nouvelle ponction lombaire le liquide extrait contenait d'abondants méningocoques doués d'une faible aptitude à cultiver.

Mon assistant, le Dr LONGO, qui a fait une étude minutieuse de ce micro-organisme[1], arrive à la conclusion que la note dominante dans sa biologie est une tendance marquée à la vie saprophytique, tandis que la vie parasitaire exerce sur lui une action défavorable. Le saprophytisme semble le fortifier, et lui donner des propriétés morphologiques et culturales qui lui font défaut après avoir vécu de la vie parasitaire. Selon moi, cela serait explicable par le fait que dans la vie parasitaire, c'est l'action défavorable du liquide cérébro-spinal qui produit des changements. En effet, dans certaines conditions, aussi dans la vie parasitaire, il montre une activité biologique et pathogène

1. Il policlinico. Rome 1900.

bien prononcée comme il arrive lorsqu'il est isolé des formes méningitiques très graves et très près de leur début. Eh bien! il suffit que l'on fasse passer ce micro-organisme si actif, si pathogène, une seule fois, à travers la dure-mère d'un lapin, pour qu'il perde complètement son pouvoir pathogène et qu'il offre une moindre activité biologique.

Méningocoque et pneumocoque.

Les diversités morphologiques, biologiques et pathogènes rencontrées par les divers auteurs, dans les différents échantillons de méningocoque isolés des diverses formes de méningite cérébro-spinale ont déterminé certains d'entre eux à croire à la possibilité d'avoir affaire à des micro-organismes différents, au moins à des variétés distinctes, mais bien délimitées. PFAUNDLER a fait une synthèse des diverses observations, et vient d'établir deux types de méningocoque bien séparés l'un de l'autre et qu'il appelle du nom des auteurs qui en ont donné la description : le premier serait le type WEICHSELBAUM, l'autre le type HEUBNER, que, pour être plus exact, il devrait appeler le type JÆGER-HEUBNER. Les caractères qui distinguent ces deux types seraient les suivants :

Type WEICHSELBAUM :	Type JÆGER-HEUBNER :
Groupement en tétraèdres : rarement courtes chaînettes.	Groupement en amas : souvent formation de chaînettes.
Se décolore avec le Gram.	Se colore avec le Gram, se développe vivement en donnant des pellicules plus ou moins épaisses.
Dans l'agar à 37° depuis 48 heures forme des colonies rares, comme des gouttelettes de rosée.	Se développe bien à la température ordinaire (18°) sur gélatine, sur bouillon, sur pommes de terre, dans le lait.
Ne se développe pas à la température ordinaire ni sur gélatine, ni sur bouillon, ni sur pommes de terre.	

Or, toutes ces différences, et d'autres aussi, nous les avons rencontrées dans le même méningocoque, isolé du même malade, selon les diverses conditions dans lesquelles il se trouvait placé. Par conséquent nous devons dire que le méningocoque est un type de microorganisme unique, mais qui offre des variétés selon les conditions de vie dans lesquelles on le considère.

Il y a d'autres auteurs, au contraire, qui ont cru devoir faire de ce micro-organisme une simple variété du diplocoque lancéolé et encapsulé de Talamon Frankel. Mais les différences entre les deux microbes sont telles, que beaucoup d'entre eux, même parmi les plus convaincus, sont revenus aux idées dualistes que nous soutenons.

Comme je l'ai dit déjà, avant la pratique de la ponction lombaire, le diplocoque lancéolé et encapsulé de Frankel était considéré sinon

comme l'unique, du moins comme le principal agent de la méningite
cérébro-spinale. La raison de cette croyance était fondée sur le fait
que les recherches bactériologiques étaient pratiquées seulement dans
les autopsies. Or nous savons que les méningites diplococciques sont
les plus graves, et sont celles qui se terminent le plus fréquemment
par la mort, donnant par conséquent, le plus souvent, la possibilité
d'étudier les lésions anatomo-pathologiques. Au contraire, les formes
méningococciques donnent une plus fréquente possibilité de guérison,
et échappent aux recherches anatomiques. D'autre part, aujour-
d'hui, on est tombé dans une exagération inverse : on tend à considérer le méningocoque comme l'agent spécifique sinon unique,
certainement prédominant, de la méningite cérébro-spinale, et les
méningites diplococciques sont considérées comme exclusivement
secondaires aux pneumonies relevant de ce microbe. Mais si cela est
vrai dans beaucoup de cas, on ne peut nier qu'il existe des méningites
cérébro-spinales diplococciques primitives, ou au moins indépendantes
de la localisation pulmonaire qui peut faire absolument défaut. Notre
statistique porte sur 12 méningites diplococciques, dont trois seulement se sont compliquées de pneumonie. Parmi les 9 autres, dans 1 il
y avait association microbienne avec le staphylocoque pyogène doré
et dans une autre avec le méningocoque. Tous ces cas se sont terminés par la mort. Les 7 autres étaient pures, 5 seulement se sont
terminés par la guérison. C'est-à-dire que sur 12 cas la léthalité a été
de 75 0 0. Ces chiffres démontrent : 1° l'existence de méningites diplococciques primitives (d'origine peut-être ou nasale, ou otitique, ou
septicémique) : 2° l'extrême gravité de ces formes.

Si, d'autre part nous considérons les méningites méningococciques,
nous avons la démonstration du fait déjà annoncé, de leur bénignité relative. Sur 12 cas nous avons enregistré seulement 3 morts :
dans un cas il y avait association avec le diplocoque, et la gravité
exceptionnelle doit être mise au compte plutôt du diplocoque que du
méningocoque : la maladie fut foudroyante, tumultueuse chez un
enfant de 1 an convalescent d'une rougeole normale, sans complications pulmonaires et qui fut emporté en 5 jours. Dans un autre cas,
chez une petite fille de 15 mois, rachitique, la méningite marchait
vers la guérison, lorsqu'une broncho-pneumonie très grave ralluma les
phénomènes cérébraux et causa la mort en peu de jours. Le troisième
cas fut le seul dans lequel on eut affaire à une forme pure très grave
terminée par la mort en 5 jours. En tout cas, la mortalité des méningites méningococciques est restée limitée à 25 0/0 : c'est la proportion
inverse de celle que nous avons eue dans les méningites diplococ-

ciques. Or, tous les cas de méningite méningococcique qui aboutissaient à la guérison (75 0/0). avant la pratique de la ponction lombaire, auraient échappé aux recherches bactériologiques; et par ce fait on peut avoir l'explication de la rareté avec laquelle elles étaient décrites. tandis que plus fréquemment on arrivait à avoir un résultat bactériologique positif en faveur du diplocoque de Fränkel. à localisations méningées presque toujours mortelles.

Comme vous le voyez, je base mon rapport surtout, presque exclusivement, sur les deux micro-organismes qui dans l'étiologie de la méningite cérébro-spinale occupent la place principale. Tout le monde sait, d'ailleurs, qu'ils ne sont pas les seuls. Dans la série de mes recherches j'ai trouvé quatre fois le bacterium coli commune; une fois le bacille pyocyanique chez un enfant en convalescence d'une fièvre typhoïde (réaction de Widal positive), et une fois le staphylocoque pyogène doré associé avec le diplocoque de Fränkel. D'autres auteurs enfin ont trouvé les streptocoques, les staphylocoques, le bacille d'Eberth, le bacterium lactis aerogenes (Escherich), certains streptotrix (Eppinger), etc.

Méningites diplo-pneumococciques.

Une première différence entre le diplocoque lancéolé et encapsulé de Fränkel (pneumocoque) et le diplocoque intracellulaire de Weichselbaum (méningocoque), se voit dans les diverses manifestations cliniques des deux méningites correspondantes. Il va sans dire que si nous considérons seulement les différences au point de vue du pronostic, il y a déjà une gravité extrêmement plus grande des premières que des autres. Les méningites diplococciques éclatent et évoluent d'une façon tumultueuse. leur forme est toujours très grave. leur marche très rapide, surtout s'il s'agit des variétés métapneumoniques. Les tracés ci-dessous (I, II et III) en donnent une démonstration évidente, pour ce qui regarde le début brusque. l'élévation de la température, la rapidité de la marche. Les phénomènes nerveux évoluent de la même manière. Les trois cas de méningite métapneumonique que nous enregistrons se sont tous terminés par la mort dans un délai de temps qui n'a pas dépassé 5 jours. La même forme rapidement fatale s'est montrée dans le cas d'association méningococcique chez un enfant de 1 an. en convalescence d'une rougeole normale (tracé IV).

De même dans les autres cas à localisation primitive et à issue fatale on voit prédominer la marche tumultueuse rapide. comme dans les tracés V et VI.

Une exception à la règle nous fut donnée par deux cas très bénins et
à issue favorable, mais toujours rapide, et qui méritent une descrip-

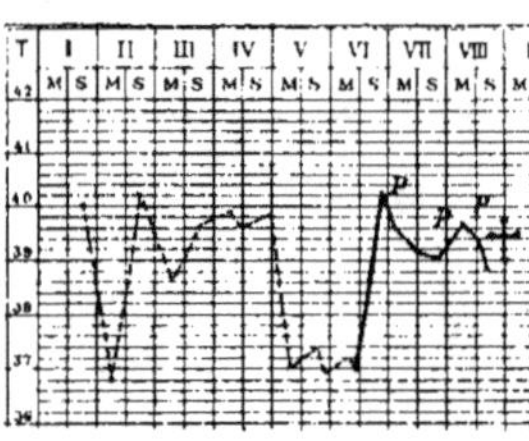

Pneumonie.   Méningite.

Tracé 1. — P. ponctions lombaires.

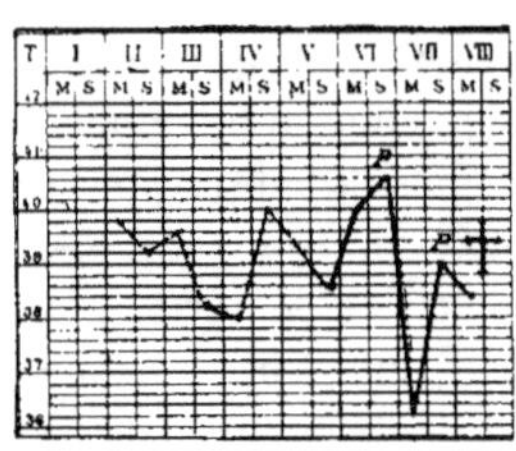

Tracé 2.

P. ponctions lombaires.

tion à part pour des considérations intéressantes aux points de vue
étiologique et pathogénique. Nous avons observé le premier de ces

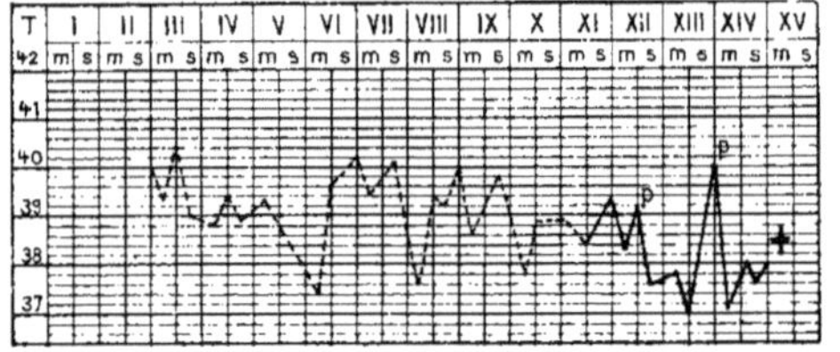

Bronchopneumonie.   Méningite.

Tracé 3.

Tracé 4.

P, ponctions lombaires.

deux cas chez une petite fille de 20 mois, à constitution et antécédents
amiliaux et personnels très mauvais. Hérédo-syphilitique, elle était

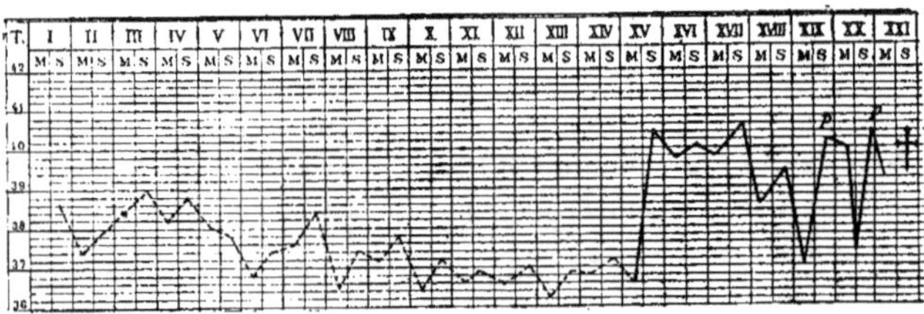

Tracé 5. — P, ponctions lombaires.

Toxi-inf. gastro-intestinale.   Méningite.

née avec une atrésie de l'anus pour laquelle elle dut subir l'opération de l'anus artificiel : quelques semaines après la naissance, elle
présenta une hydrocéphalie chronique qui fut heureusement traitée

par des préparations mercurielles et iodées et la ponction lombaire
plusieurs fois répétée. Malgré cela son crâne présentait les signes
d'une légère hydrocéphalie. Tous les symptômes d'une méningite
aiguë étaient évidents, mais d'une manière tellement atténuée que le
doute eût été justifié, sinon sur l'existence d'une méningite, du moins
sur sa nature diplococcique, si l'examen bactériologique du liquide
extrait par deux ponctions lombaires successives n'avait montré le
diplocoque lancéolé et encapsulé de Talamon-Fränkel (V. tracé VII).
Le deuxième cas de forme bénigne et à issue favorable nous fut présenté par un enfant âgé de 20 mois, qui 7 mois auparavant avait été
atteint d'une entérocolite grave avec phénomènes cérébraux aigus

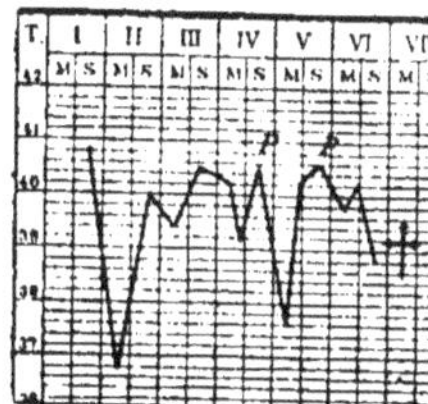

Tracé 6.
P. ponctions lombaires.

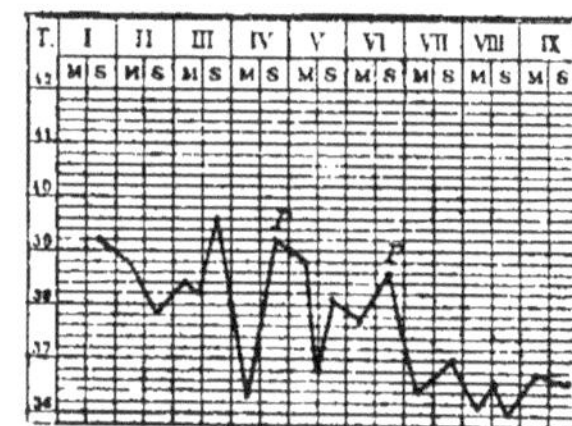

Tracé 7.
P. ponctions lombaires.

suivis d'une hydrocéphalie avec accroissement de 5 cm. de la circonférence crânienne en moins de deux mois. Le traitement mercuriel
suivi pendant quinze jours ne produisit aucune amélioration, le volume du crâne ne faisant que s'accroître. Les ponctions lombaires
furent suivies d'un résultat merveilleux. Le liquide extrait était stérile
et sans action sur les animaux ; il contenait une petite quantité d'albumine (0,05 pour 100). Or la méningite aiguë qui suivit à 7 mois de
distance présenta la même forme bénigne, atténuée, à brève évolution,
à issue favorable comme dans le cas précédent. Les ponctions lombaires pratiquées dès le deuxième jour donnèrent un liquide opales-
cent, trouble, qui par le repos forma un réticule distinct fibrino-
épendymaire, avec 0,70 pour 100 d'albumine et d'abondants lympho-
cytes et diplocoques de Fränkel.

Les injections sur les animaux montrèrent qu'ils étaient dépourvus
de toute action pathogène.

Ce qui est remarquable, c'est que ces deux seuls cas à forme exceptionnellement bénigne se sont vérifiés chez deux enfants qui, quelque
temps avant, avaient souffert d'hydrocéphalie, de laquelle il restait
encore les traces. Et du moment que nous savons que le liquide hydro-

céphalique constitue un mauvais terrain de culture pour les microbes,

compris le pneumocoque, je crois qu'il ne serait point absurde de penser que c'est à cette condition d'hydrocéphalie que doit se rattacher la bénignité de la maladie, la virulence amoindrie du diplocoque.

Dans deux autres cas nous avons constaté une forme atténuée de méningite diplococcique avec une évolution prolongée jusqu'à la troi-

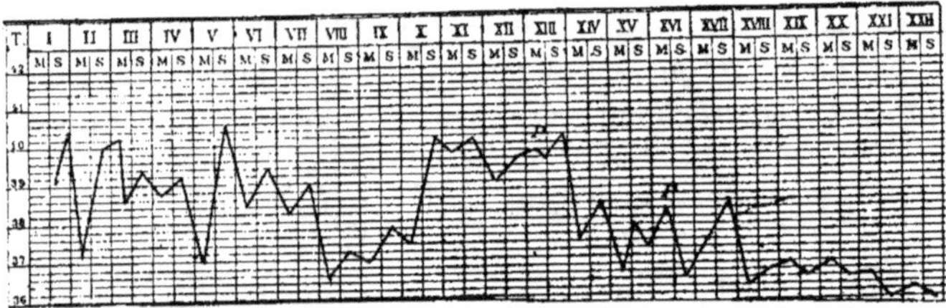

Tracé 8. — P. P. Ponctions lombaires.

sième semaine bien que la terminaison n'en ait pas été la même. Dans le premier cas, chez une petite fille de 7 mois le début fut tumultueux et menaçant ; mais, après, la maladie s'est montrée plus bénigne et s'est terminée par la guérison. (V. tracé VIII.) Le liquide cérébro-

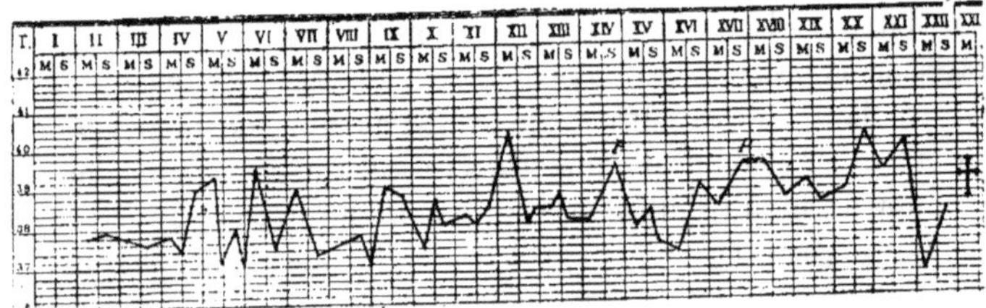

Tracé 9 — P. P. Ponctions lombaires.

spinal extrait après 15 jours était trouble et contenait 0,5 pour 100 d'albumine et d'abondants diplocoques lancéolés et encapsulés qui inoculés sur un lapin ont produit la mort au 25e jour dans un marasme très accentué. L'autre cas est survenu chez une petite fille de 15 mois qui souffrait d'un eczéma impétigineux de la figure avec écoulement purulent des narines. Le liquide cérébro-spinal était trouble et renfermait des diplocoques et des staphylocoques pyogènes dorés : les mêmes microbes furent isolés du liquide nasal. La marche se prolongea pendant 5 semaines, et finit par la mort. Il est admis que bien des méningites, soi-disant primitives, sont d'origine nasale (V. tracé IX).

Méningites diplo-méningococciques.

Ces formes de méningite à décours prolongé, nous l'avons vu, sont rarement observées dans les formes diplococciques. Au contraire elles sont fréquentes dans les formes méningococciques, dans lesquelles on observe très rarement la marche rapide, extrêmement grave, qui est caractéristique des formes diplococciques. Les méningites méningococciques peuvent éclater d'une façon tumultueuse, avec température initiale très élevée et manifestations nerveuses épouvantables; mais elles ont tendance à se prolonger, non seulement durant des semaines, mais des mois, parfois une année et plus. Elles commencent par prendre une allure intermittente avec des accès plus ou moins graves, d'abord très près l'un de l'autre, qui ensuite s'éloignent et deviennent moins graves jusqu'à la guérison. Dans les cas à terminaison fatale, il survient un amaigrissement notable, une cachexie profonde, les phéno-

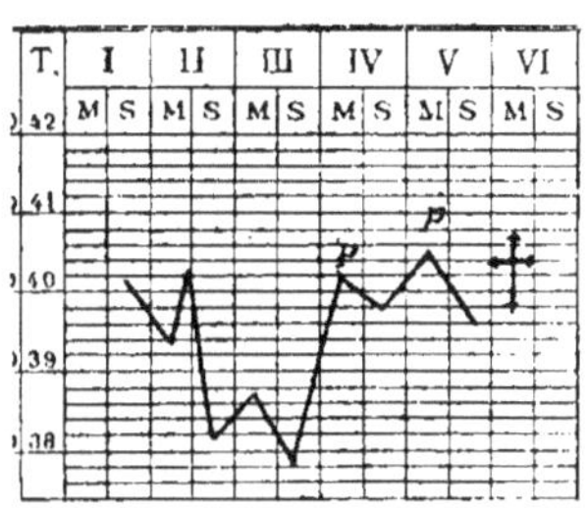

Tracé 10.

mènes nerveux reprennent leur gravité et se font plus fréquents, et la mort survient dans l'épuisement général de l'organisme. Dans deux cas seulement j'ai observé la forme tumultueuse, très grave, rapide, qui est propre aux méningites diplococciques mais dans la première il y avait association du diplocoque de Fränkel qui doit avoir joué le rôle principal dans l'évolution de la maladie (v. tracé 4°). De même dans le cas exceptionnel d'un enfant de 16 mois qui fut emporté entre le 5e et le 4e jour par la forme clinique caractéristique des méningites diplococciques (V. voir tracé X), dans le liquide cérébro-spinal nous avons trouvé en culture pure un méningocoque qui montrait une activité biologique et culturale des plus actives, comme nous le verrons mieux lorsque nous parlerons avec plus de détails de la biologie de ce micro-organisme. En tout cas, cette exception, comme aussi les exceptions que nous avons vues possibles dans les formes diplococciques, nous imposent la réserve de ne pas nous fier trop aveuglément aux différences cliniques, pour ce diagnostic différentiel entre les méningites diplococciques et méningococciques. La marche prolongée, la tendance à s'atténuer, à prendre une allure intermittente donneront de grandes probabilités en faveur de la forme méningococcique, qui pourront devenir peut-être des certitudes au delà des 3 semaines, parce que c'est la limite maximum pendant laquelle j'ai vu se prolonger les formes diplococciques. Au contraire la caractéristique clinique des formes méningococciques, c'est de se prolonger 1, 2, 3 mois et davantage. A ce propos je dois dire que depuis la pratique de la ponction lombaire répétée plusieurs fois dans un but thérapeutique, ces formes prolongées ne vont plus au delà de certaines limites comme il était facile de le voir avant cette pratique ; je dois dire aussi que jusqu'à présent, très rarement mes observations personnelles m'ont montré comme séquelles l'hydrocéphalie, ni l'amau-

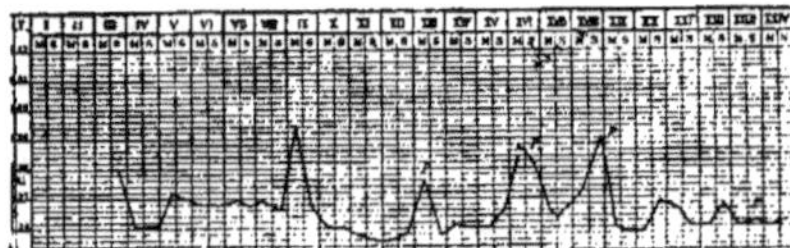

Tracé 11. — Malade depuis un mois chez elle.   P. Ponctions lombaires.

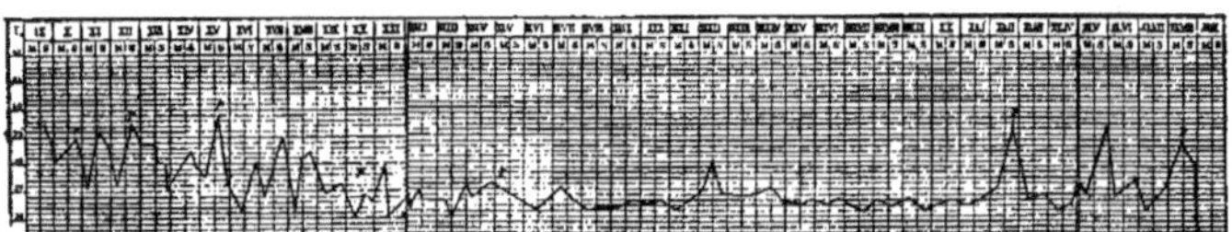

Tracé 12.

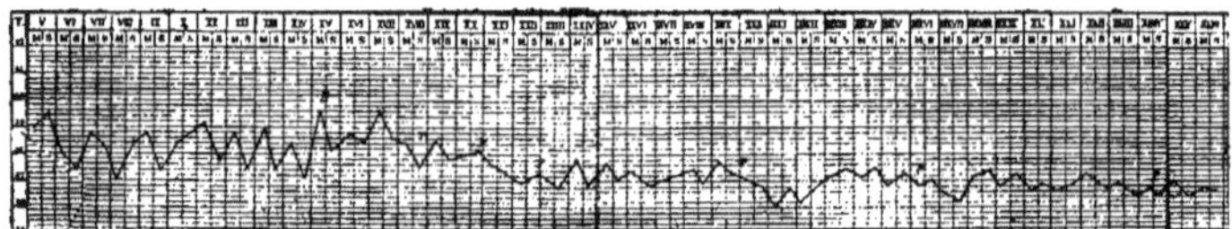

Tracé 13.

rose, ni la surdité, ni l'idiotie, ni les paralysies, ni la cachexie, comme il arrivait très fréquemment de le voir à l'époque antérieure.

Les tracés XI, XII, XIII représentent la forme clinique de trois cas typiques soignés à la clinique dans ces deux dernières années. Tous les trois sont sortis après guérison *complète* entre 45 et 50 jours. Seulement chez tous les trois la tendance a persisté à une production exagérée du liquide cérébro-spinal. C'est, comme le dit le professeur Mya, une espèce d'hyperhydrose cérébro-spinale, se produisant même après la guérison, après une ou deux semaines, et durant de quatre à six semaines, produisant des phénomènes de compression cérébrale (agitation, insomnie, sursauts musculaires, tête portée en arrière, etc.)

qui disparaissaient tout d'un coup après qu'on avait retiré 40, 60,
80 centimètres cubes de liquide cérébro-spinal tout à fait normal dans
sa composition. Or, ce fait nous explique bien la facilité de production
des hydrocéphalies résiduelles de ces méningites, et les conséquences
relatives, amaurose, paralysies spastiques, raideur de la nuque, etc.,
et comment le traitement par les ponctions lombaires peut réussir à
les éviter. Dans les dernières semaines de cette année il me fut
amené à la clinique une petite fille de 5 ans, qui deux mois avant,
avait eu une méningite cérébro-spinale avec hydrocéphalie et amaurose résiduelles. La ponction lombaire nous donna un méningocoque
très épuisé et qui mourut au deuxième passage sur agar. Après 5 à
6 ponctions lombaires elle commença à distinguer la lumière, et on
put constater une évidente réaction pupillaire[1]. Dans un autre cas
identique chez une petite fille de 8 mois, après 5 à 6 ponctions lombaires nous avons pu constater le retour complet de la faculté

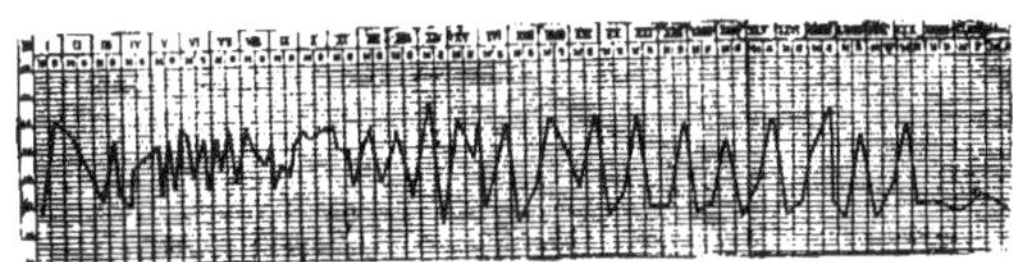

Tracé 14.

visuelle. La maladie datait de 5 mois, et le liquide extrait n'avait
montré nulle trace de micro-organismes. Dans la série de mes observations je compte encore d'autres cas de ce genre, pour trois desquels la guérison finit par être complète.

Or, si je reprends les notes cliniques des cas de méningite cérébro-
spinale observés dans la période de temps qui a précédé la pratique
de la ponction lombaire, j'en trouve enregistrés 14 avec tous les
signes caractéristiques de la forme méningococcique avec son allure
intermittente, d'une durée exceptionnellement prolongée, bien au
delà de ce qu'on observe actuellement, et avec une fréquence énorme
de suites résiduelles, comme : hydrocéphalie, opistothonos, amaurose,
contracture du rachis en arc de cercle, paralysies, surdité, convulsions, atrophie générale, décubitus, etc. Le cas le plus rapide n'a pas
duré moins de 52 jours et finit avec la guérison (Tracé XIV) : cas tout
à fait exceptionnel, et qui dénota une virulence spontanément amoindrie de l'agent pathogène. Dans d'autres cas aussi, à issue favorable,

1. Actuellement (septembre 1900) elle a regagné parfaitement le pouvoir visuel.

la durée de la maladie s'est prolongée jusqu'à 5, 4, 9 mois, et les derniers phénomènes à disparaître furent l'opistothonos, l'amaurose, la parésie des extrémités inférieures (Tracé XV). D'autres cas, après une durée qui s'est prolongée jusqu'à 4, 7, 10 mois se terminèrent par la mort. Depuis la première période aiguë, la maladie présentait une allure tout à fait irrégulière. La température variait de l'apyrexie complète et de l'hypothermie, aux degrés moyens, jusqu'aux hyperthermies rapidement ascendantes (40°-41°) et rapidement descendantes (Tracés XVI, XVII et XVIII) : accès à périodes irrégulières, de céphalée, de vomissements, de convulsions ; parfois amaurose, surdité, appétit vorace : presque toujours raideur de la nuque et du rachis, paralysies, ventre en bateau jusqu'à dessiner la colonne vertébrale au-dessous des parois abdominales extrêmement amoindries ; atrophie générale extrême, décubitus, intelligence parfois indemne, parfois abolie. A l'autopsie, les ventricules cérébraux étaient plus ou moins dilatés, quelquefois jusqu'à contenir 400, 500, 800 cmc. de liquide tout à fait limpide, et le cerveau réduit à une poche à parois épaisses n'ayant pas plus de 2 à 5 centimètres ; les membranes externes étaient opaques, épaissies, plus ou moins adhérentes à la substance cérébrale : çà et là on apercevait des épaississements fibreux, ou fibrino-purulents, qui, en un cas, s'étendaient de la face ventrale du cervelet jusqu'à la partie antérieure du bulbe, et, dans un autre cas d'amaurose, étaient limitées aux régions occipitales avec peu ou point d'hydrocéphalie ; en un cas j'ai constaté un ramollissement du cervelet : jamais trace de tuberculose.

Dans cette série de cas, la recherche bactériologique fait défaut ; mais si nous faisons une comparaison entre ces cas et les cas d'observation récente, je crois pouvoir sûrement affirmer qu'ils doivent être considérés comme de vraies méningites méningococciques. J'en trouve aussi la démonstration dans beaucoup de cas observés dernièrement à une époque assez éloignée du commencement de la maladie, c'est-à-dire lorsque notre intervention fut tardive. Quant je relaterai de ces formes de méningite aiguë ancienne qui nous furent amenées depuis quelques mois, avec hydrocéphalie, amaurose, etc., et dans lesquelles l'examen bactériologique donna un résultat négatif à cause de l'intervention trop tardive, nous trouverons en ces cas de vrais traits d'union avec les formes d'observation récente et à marche relativement rapide, et celles formées d'observation plus ancienne caractérisées par une évolution très prolongée, et par les lésions constatées à l'autopsie. Je suis convaincu que l'intervention thérapeutique active que nous avons rendue de pratique usuelle, peut bien donner l'explication de

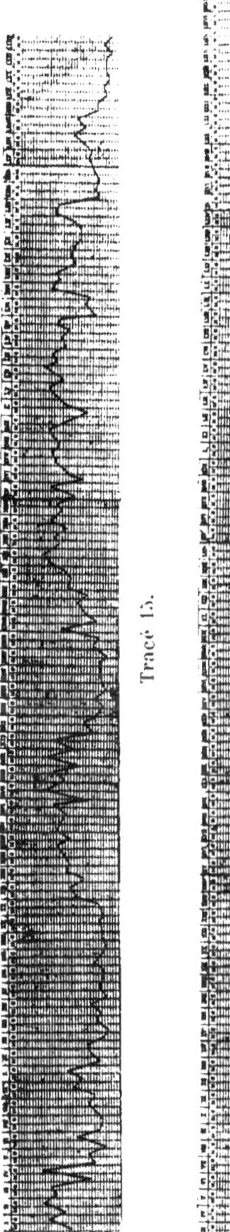

Tracé 15.

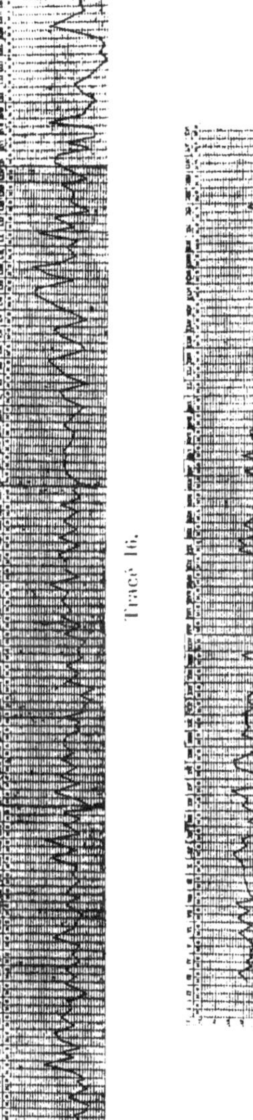

Tracé 16.

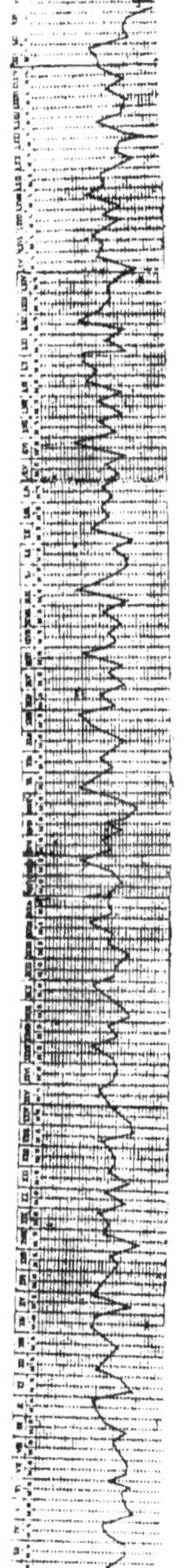

Tracé 17.

Tracé 18.

ces différences dans la marche, dans la forme clinique, dans la terminaison de cette maladie.

Conditions biologiques du diplo-méningocoque.

La caractéristique prédominante des méningites méningococciques à se prolonger est une démonstration que le méningocoque possède une virulence qui tend très vite à s'épuiser, si bien que la forme clinique persiste alors que le méningocoque a cessé d'agir depuis longtemps : il ne reste en vie que pendant quelques semaines, et ce sont les conséquences peut-être aussi de l'action persistante des produits toxiques qui prolongent la maladie. Dans les cas très graves, surtout si la recherche est pratiquée dès les premiers jours, le méningocoque se présente abondant, et avec le maximum de son activité biologique.

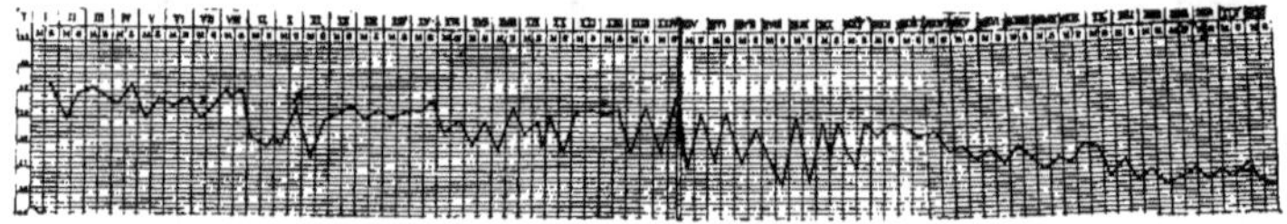

Tracé 19.

Dans l'exsudat prédominent d'une manière absolue les formes extra-cellulaires souvent disposées en chaînettes (Fig. A. 1). Dans les terrains de culture il se développe vigoureusement, même dans les conditions les moins favorables. Ensemencé en stric sur agar glycériné, à la température de 35°-37°, après 1 ou 2 jours, il forme des pellicules épaisses, humides, transparentes à la lumière artificielle, dues à la fusion des grosses colonies (Fig. A. 5): dans la gélatine et dans le bouillon, à la température ordinaire, on a aussi un notable développement. Par des passages répétés son activité végétative s'accroît, et dans ces conditions il peut rester en vie environ pendant 2 mois. Après quelques jours, dans les ponctions successives, surtout si la maladie marche vers l'amélioration, on commence à observer un épuisement du méningocoque : les formes endocellulaires se montrant de plus en plus fréquentes peuvent arriver à remplir les cellules avec 6, 8, 12 éléments et avoir l'apparence du pus blennorragique : il ne se dispose plus en chaînettes, mais en petits amas, en tétraèdres, en formes isolées (Fig. A. 2). Dans l'agar-agar le développement est lent, chétif ; rarement on observe les pellicules, mais plutôt les petites colonies isolées comme des gouttelettes de rosée (Fig. A. 4): à la tem-

pérature ordinaire il ne se fait plus aucun développement ni dans la
gélatine ni dans le bouillon, ni sur pommes de terre. Après quelques
jours encore les cultures restent stériles ou bien le méningocoque ne

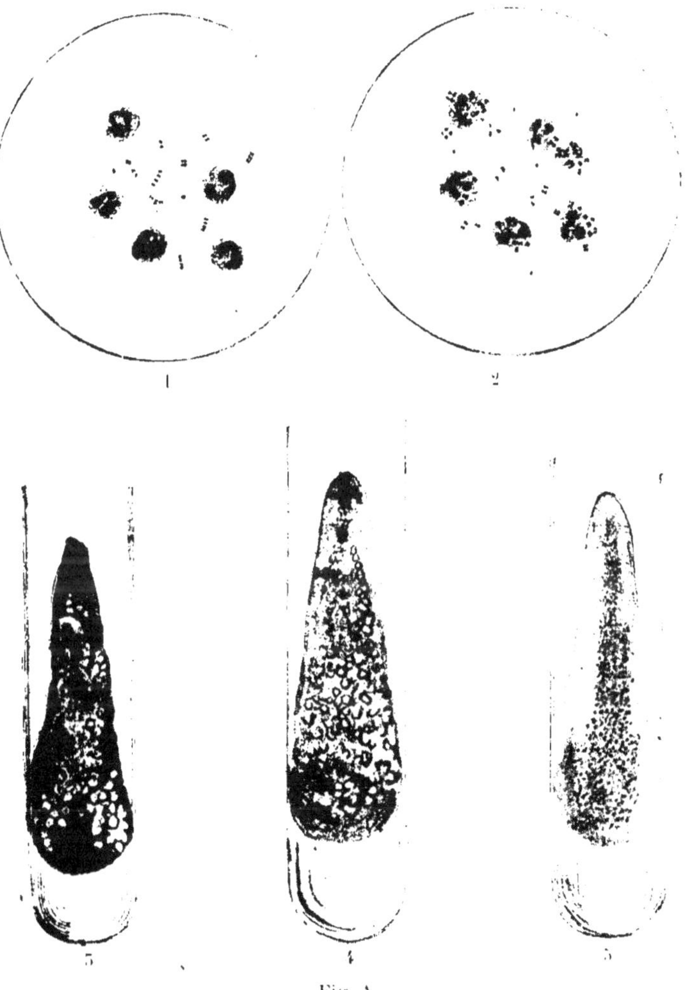

Fig. A.

se développe qu'après plusieurs jours de thermostate, en rares et
petites colonies, et rarement il résiste au deuxième passage (Fig. A. 5).
C'est ce qu'il arrive de voir déjà dans la deuxième ou dans la troisième
semaine. Dans un cas exceptionnel, il fut trouvé en ces conditions bio-

logiques au deuxième mois de la maladie chez une petite fille de 5 ans.
Dans un cas soigné dernièrement à la clinique, nous avons assisté à
cet épuisement graduel du méningocoque, jusqu'à ce qu'au 20e et au
25e jour les cultures restèrent stériles. A ce moment l'enfant eut une
fièvre gastro-intestinale causée par des troubles alimentaires, et les
phénomènes méningés empirèrent d'une façon notable. La ponction
lombaire nous a révélé de nouveau l'existence du méningocoque au
42e jour, mais en de mauvaises conditions biologiques, avec un développement peu important. tandis que, six jours après, les ponctions
successives donnèrent un liquide qui resta de nouveau stérile, et la
guérison fut définitive.

Ces manifestations de faible activité biologique, nous les avons
rencontrées avec le méningocoque dans deux conditions : 1o quand
l'examen bactériologique était pratiqué à une période avancée de la
maladie, surtout si elle tendait vers l'amélioration, comme dans le
cas exposé ci-dessus : 2o nous les avons trouvées dans les premiers
jours de la maladie, lorsque. d'après les premiers symptômes, on
pouvait porter un pronostic favorable, c'est à-dire dans les cas bénins. Dans le cas de méningite méningococcique à forme exceptionnellement rapide, grave, tumultueuse, je n'ai pu rencontrer dans
l'exsudat qu'une ou deux formes endocellulaires ; les autres étaient
toutes disposées en chaînettes ou en gros amas, ou isolées (Fig. A. 1),
le développement cultural était des plus vigoureux : en 24 heures
l'ensemencement en strie sur agar-agar donnait une pellicule épaisse,
pulpeuse, humide, translucide, etc. (Fig. A. 5). Ces particularités dans
l'aspect et dans le développement pourraient par conséquent être
précieuses, et donner un élément de prévision pronostique, jusqu'ici
méconnu.

D'après les expériences faites dans ma clinique par mon assistant
le docteur A. Longo, ces conditions différentes dans lesquelles peut se
montrer le méningocoque, peuvent se reproduire artificiellement dans
le laboratoire, selon qu'on l'oblige à vivre en saprophyte ou en parasite. Si d'un liquide cérébro-spinal on isole un méningocoque peu
actif, on peut exalter son activité par des passages successifs sur des
terrains de culture convenables. On peut passer, à travers plusieurs
agar-agar glycérinés, ensemencés en strie, du faible développement
en rares gouttelettes de rosée, aux pellicules épaisses, humides,
translucides à la lumière artificielle, au développement à la température ordinaire sur gélatine, en bouillon, sur pommes de terre : des
groupements en tétraèdres ou en formes isolées, aux gros amas, en
chaînettes, etc. Et tandis qu'un méningocoque à peine isolé d'un

exsudat méningitique s'épuise rapidement et meurt à bref délai au plus en 8-10 jours, depuis les passages répétés sur agar, le même méningocoque peut rester en vie dans un tube jusqu'au 25ᵉ jour. Le contraire arrive si on l'oblige à la vie parasitaire. Si on inocule une culture vigoureuse d'un méningocoque très actif dans la cavité sous-arachnoïdienne d'un lapin, on le retire de là en une condition d'épuisement marqué. Peut-être cela dépend-il de l'action délétère que le liquide cérébro-spinal exerce sur le micro-organisme. En effet, nous avons provoqué le même épuisement par un passage de l'agar en un liquide cérébro-spinal extrait d'un enfant hydrocéphalique, bien qu'assez riche en albumine (0,85 pour 100) : et dans les cas de méningite très grave, le méningocoque peut, dans le liquide cérébro-spinal, présenter les caractères d'une activité biologique très accentuée. Il est naturel que dans les cas très graves de méningite on doive penser à des conditions qui nous sont inconnues, et qui permettent d'expliquer l'activité biologique et pathogène du méningocoque sur les méninges, en réduisant au minimum l'action protectrice du liquide cérébro-spinal. Nous avons vu qu'il faut admettre que les toxi-infections gastro-intestinales peuvent jouer un rôle très important pour déterminer ces conditions spéciales, et il est fréquent de voir dans les cas de méningite une participation de l'appareil digestif.

De l'ensemble des faits que nous avons exposés, une conséquence absolument certaine découle, à savoir que le méningocoque est un micro-organisme unique, et que les différences, les types, les variétés qu'on en a voulu établir ne sont que des manifestations accessoires dépendant des diverses conditions dans lesquelles il vit, soit naturellement dans l'organisme, soit artificiellement dans les laboratoires. Le même micro-organisme peut passer d'une forme à l'autre et revenir à la première, quand ces conditions changent.

Le docteur Longo s'est occupé aussi de rechercher quelques-uns des produits de l'activité biologique du méningocoque. Dans le bouillon d'Abba il n'a pas trouvé la production de ferments soit diastasiques, soit émulsifs, soit inversifs. Seulement, avec un échantillon très actif, il a pu constater l'existence d'un enzyme diastasique. Dans la plupart des cas il a constaté un pouvoir acidifiant sur le lait avec coagulation secondaire : action qu'il a vu faire défaut avec un méningocoque très actif. Il n'a jamais pu avoir de production d'indol.

Virulence du diplo-méningocoque.

L'étude de la virulence du méningocoque nous a donné des résultats assez limités, mais intéressants en rapport avec les différences biologiques que nous venons d'exposer. La virulence du méningocoque s'épuise beaucoup plus précocement que son activité culturale. Lorsque la forme méningitique, bien que grave, est à la deuxième, à la troisième semaine ; lorsque la forme méningitique se présente comme devant être assez bénigne, de même lorsque le liquide est extrait dès les premiers jours ; lorsque l'apparence microscopique et culturale fait supposer un certain degré d'épuisement, toute tentative d'inoculation chez les animaux (sous-cutanée, péritonéale, pleurale, sous-arachnoïdienne, intraveineuse) donne un résultat négatif. Nous avons obtenu le même résultat avec les cobayes, les lapins, les rats blancs, les petits chiens, les petits chats. Chez deux lapins, nous avons fait précéder l'injection sous-arachnoïdienne de l'inoculation sous-durale d'une goutte de solution d'acide lactique à 25 pour 100 dans le but de diminuer la résistance locale, et toujours avec le même résultat. Nous avons injecté le liquide cérébro-spinal centrifugé soit immédiatement après l'extraction, soit après l'avoir gardé pendant 24-48 heures dans le thermostate, nous avons injecté les cultures en bouillon, les émulsions des cultures en strie sur agar, etc., et toujours avec le même résultat négatif. Et, ce qui est plus remarquable, avec ces injections, le méningocoque s'épuisait encore plus rapidement, au point qu'il était difficile de le reprendre pour le ramener de nouveau à la vie saprophytique. Sur ce point on doit accepter ce que dit le docteur Longo : que c'est la vie parasitaire qui s'oppose à l'exaltation biologique du méningocoque.

Au contraire, nous avons obtenu des résultats positifs, comme l'a rapporté le docteur Longo, avec le liquide très actif isolé des méningites très graves, et dans les périodes initiales. Mais faites avec ces liquides, les injections sous-cutanées, endopéritonéales et endopleurales chez les cobayes et chez les lapins n'ont également produit aucun effet pathogène. Au contraire, les injections sous-durales chez les lapins, après la trépanation des os crâniens, soit du liquide cérébro-spinal centrifugé, soit des cultures très récentes, ont donné quelque chose qui pourrait bien rappeler la forme méningitique. Quelques-uns de ces lapins sont morts au quatrième jour après avoir présenté des convulsions générales, des rigidités spastiques, surtout dans les muscles de la nuque et du tronc, jusqu'à porter la tête fortement contracturée sur le dos, des contractions rythmiques des muscles de la face, etc. A l'autopsie on a constaté une légère augmentation du liquide cérébro-spinal, une légère injection des méninges, et d'abondants méningocoques dans le liquide cérébral en position extra-cellulaire, en amas, en courtes chaînettes. Nous n'avons jamais pu constater ni purulence, ni trouble dans les méninges. Les méningocoques isolés de ces animaux montraient déjà des traces évidentes d'épuisement, et transportés sur d'autres animaux ils avaient perdu absolument leur virulence. En aucun cas nous n'avons pu constater d'action pathogène avec ces méningocoques repris d'autres animaux. C'est toujours le même effet dangereux de la vie parasitaire sur l'activité et sur la virulence du méningocoque.

Les autres lapins, qui survécurent à l'inoculation sans présenter de phénomènes morbides, ou en présentant seulement quelques légères contractions des muscles du cou et de la face, furent sacrifiés du 5e au 8e jour. Les méninges avaient une apparence tout à fait normale. Dans le liquide cérébro-spinal nous avons toujours constaté des méningocoques en culture pure, mais faible, lente, nullement pathogène pour d'autres animaux et qui rapidement s'épuisaient en vie saprophytique. Encore une fois, nous voyons se répéter le fait qu'un méningocoque vigoureux, et d'un léger degré pathogène, c'est-à-dire du type JÆGER HEUBNER, transporté en vie parasitaire, s'épuise et prend le type WEICHSELBAUM.

Le rapide épuisement des activités biologique et pathogène du méningocoque nous donne la raison des résultats négatifs dans les recherches bactériologiques, surtout lorsque celles-ci sont pratiquées à une période un peu éloignée du commencement de la maladie; et pourquoi selon la période dans laquelle elles sont pratiquées, on peut avoir l'un ou l'autre des types du méningocoque. doué d'une activité biologique et pathogène plus ou moins exaltée.

Quel peut être le temps utile pour obtenir un résultat positif dans la recherche bactériologique? Il n'est pas facile de le dire. Cela dépendra de la plus ou moins grande virulence primitive du méningocoque, et aussi des conditions de résistance personnelle. et de l'action plus ou moins défavorable du liquide cérébro-spinal sur le microorganisme. Il y a des cas dans lesquels on l'a trouvé complètement épuisé aux 20e et 25e jours, et d'autres dans lesquels il était encore vivant après sept mois. Chez une petite fille de quatre ans avec une forme classique de méningite cérébro-spinale méningococcique (forme prolongée, allure intermittente (tracé XIX). céphalée, raideur de la nuque. hyperesthésie. puis vomissements. signe de

Kernig, herpes labialis, convulsions, terminaison favorable), le liquide extrait aux 8e, 10e et 22e jours a toujours été stérile', si bien que dans les premières ponctions le liquide fut légèrement trouble et discrètement corpusculé. Or, je trouve difficile de devoir admettre une méningite simple, amicrobienne; je crois plutôt que le méningocoque s'était épuisé rapidement avant le huitième jour.

Or, cette propriété du méningocoque semble se trouver en opposition avec la longue durée de la maladie, avec les manifestations fébriles, avec l'amaigrissement notable. De l'examen de la forme clinique, et des observations faites dans les autopsies, il résulte que la condition anatomique plus fréquente est représentée par l'hydrocéphalie, parfois ancienne. Beaucoup d'amauroses, d'après ce que donne l'examen ophtalmoscopique, et d'après leur facilité à guérir, sont certainement en rapport avec l'hydrocéphalie. Celle-ci est l'effet d'une augmentation de sécrétion de liquide cérébro-spinal due à l'irritation inflammatoire de l'épendyme et des plexus choroïdiens, qui persiste pendant plusieurs semaines, comme nous l'avons constaté plus haut dans beaucoup de cas. Or, ce fait explique bien la fréquence des grandes hydrocéphalies avant la pratique de la ponction lombaire, surtout si nous considérons que les pouvoirs absorbants sont très limités. Du jour où j'ai fait de la ponction lombaire une méthode usuelle dans le traitement de ces méningites chez les enfants, j'ai constamment observé que l'évolution de la maladie était très abrégée. Tandis que autrefois elle était de plusieurs mois, à présent il n'est question que de semaines.

La ponction lombaire méthodiquement répétée, à brefs intervalles dans la période aiguë (chaque jour, tous les deux jours, même deux fois dans les vingt-quatre heures), puis à des périodes plus éloignées, doit expliquer son action favorable, aussi à un autre point de vue. Dans la période initiale surtout, nous pouvons, grâce à elle, évacuer des quantités notables d'éléments pathogènes (bactériques et toxiques), et avec cela nous diminuons cette irritation constante des méninges, et empêchons tous ces éléments de s'accumuler, de sorte que le processus morbide qui sans cela serait très grave, finit par devenir bénin. Nous devons aussi compter sur l'épuisement facile du méningocoque, de sorte que la maladie avorte. Nous devons aussi considérer l'action favorable exercée par la décompression sur la substance cérébrale et sur la circulation sanguine. Quelquefois c'est cette compression rapide qui est la cause de la mort, surtout à un âge plus avancé, lorsque les sutures et les fontanelles sont fermées. L'action sur la circulation sanguine doit s'opposer aux stases, et faciliter les pouvoirs absorbants comme nous le voyons à un degré plus accentué dans les épanchements pleuraux. Dans des cas d'hydrocéphalie récente j'ai pu constater, après une ou deux ponctions, une amélioration rapide et durable.

Mais quelquefois il y a des conditions anatomiques plus graves, et pour lesquelles le mécanisme de la guérison n'est pas aussi facile, et pour lesquelles la ponction lombaire ne peut exercer que peu ou point d'action. Dans un cas d'amaurose consécutive à une méningite cérébro-spinale, à l'autopsie je ne trouvai nulle trace d'hydrocéphalie, mais des stratifications fibrino-purulentes dans les circonvolutions occipitales avec altération profonde de la substance nerveuse correspondante. Dans un autre cas terminé par la mort, après trois mois et demi de maladie, une stratification semblable s'étendait de la face ventrale du cervelet jusqu'à la paroi antérieure du bulbe et de la moelle cervicale. Dans ce cas il faut penser à la possibilité d'une obstruction des voies de communication entre les cavités ventriculaires et les espaces sous-arachnoïdiens, de façon à déterminer une hydrocéphalie due à une rétention de liquide, comme il arrive fréquemment de voir dans certaines hydrocéphalies congénitales; et dans ces cas la ponction lombaire ne peut expliquer aucune action, et ne donne issue qu'à quelques gouttes de liquide spinal, parce qu'il n'y a plus de communications entre le sac méningé spinal et les ventricules.

De tout ce que je viens d'exposer il résulte nettement que le méningocoque intra-cellulaire de Weichselbaum peut être considéré comme un vrai agent pathogène de la méningite cérébro-spinale, et que l'étiologie et la pathogénie de celle-ci ont été clairement mises en lumière par les recherches bactériologiques, par la forme clinique, par l'anatomie pathologique, et par les expériences sur les animaux. Mais il ne faut pas, par une exagération inconsidérée, voir dans le méningocoque l'agent pathogène spécifique unique de la méningite cérébro-spinale. Nous avons déjà vu comment aussi le diplocoque capsulé et lancéolé de Talamon-Fränkel jouait un rôle important non seulement pour déterminer des localisations méningées secondaires à la pneumonie, mais aussi pour déterminer de vraies méningites aiguës primitives, d'origine peut-être ou nasale, ou otitique, ou pharyngée ou septicémique. Nous avons vu aussi les différences entre les méningites diplococciques et les méningococciques, au point de vue de la forme clinique, du pronostic, de la terminaison. Parmi les cas que j'ai observés, et constatés par l'examen bactériologique, la plus longue durée d'une méningite diplococcique fut représentée par trois semaines, et ceci constitue déjà une exception. Les formes communes ont une évolution rapide, tumultueuse.

Virulence du diplo-pneumocoque.

Il est intéressant d'étudier comment se comporte la virulence du pneumocoque en comparaison avec ce que nous venons de voir à propos du méningocoque. On sait que le diplocoque de Fränkel qui se trouve dans les crachats des pneumoniques est doué d'une extrême virulence pour certains animaux, surtout pour les lapins, et que cette virulence tend à s'exalter d'une façon énorme par des passages à travers d'autres animaux. Des quantités minimes de sang bien que desséché sont ainsi capables de produire les septicémies les plus graves. Nous avons injecté sous la dure-mère de petits lapins deux à trois gouttes de sang d'un lapin mort par septicémie diplococcique. Les lapins sont tous morts entre six et sept heures avec une septicémie intense sans traces de lésions méningées. Le même résultat, un peu moins foudroyant, a été obtenu en injectant, soit sous la dure-mère cérébrale, soit sous la dure-mère spinale (par la ponction lombaire) de petites quantités de crachats pneumoniques émulsionnés.

Cette double propriété du diplocoque, d'une part d'exalter sa virulence en vie parasitaire à travers les animaux, et d'autre part de s'épuiser rapidement dans la vie culturale, constitue un important caractère différentiel vis-à-vis du méningocoque, qui au contraire s'épuise en vie parasitaire pour s'exalter en vie saprophytique. Mais cette propriété de s'exalter par les inoculations sur les animaux, je ne l'ai pas trouvée dans le diplocoque isolé de nos cas de méningite. J'ai inoculé le liquide cérébro-spinal, tout de suite après son extraction, ou bien après vingt-quatre à quarante-huit heures de thermostate, toujours traité par la centrifugation; j'ai inoculé les cultures en bouillon ou les émulsions des cultures en strie sur agar-agar : les inoculations ont été pratiquées dans la plèvre, dans le péritoine, sous la peau, dans la cavité arachnoïdienne, chez les cobayes, chez les lapins, chez les rats, chez les petits chats. Une fois seulement j'ai pu constater la mort d'un lapin dans des conditions marastiques, vingt-cinq jours après l'inoculation sous-durale d'une culture en strie de pneumocoque sur agar. Or, il est connu que le pneumocoque perd rapidement sa virulence. Mais pour expliquer ce que je viens d'exposer, il faut dire que c'est toujours l'action défavorable que le liquide cérébro-spinal exerce sur le diplocoque qui est la cause de ce défaut d'action pathogène. Cette action défavorable du liquide cérébro-spinal est moindre envers le méningocoque. Lorsque le pneumocoque arrive à produire des méningites purulentes à stratifications épaisses et très étendues, il faut non seulement admettre une grande virulence du microorganisme, mais surtout des conditions de la part de l'organisme telles que ses pouvoirs de résistance surtout locale deviennent inactifs. Ces résistances peuvent varier d'un sujet à l'autre.

Chez un enfant d'un an une méningite aiguë éclata pendant la convalescence d'une pneumonie. La ponction lombaire confirma le diagnostic et révéla une quantité énorme de diplocoques. La mort survint après trois jours. A l'autopsie les méninges semblaient normales; seulement l'examen microscopique du liquide sous-arachnoïdien révéla des corpuscules blancs et d'abondants diplocoques qui furent isolés en culture pure. C'était donc, pouvait-on dire, plutôt une méningite bactérienne qu'une méningite anatomique, laquelle sans un examen attentif serait passée inaperçue, comme un cas de méningisme banal. Dans ce cas l'action protectrice du liquide cérébro-spinal s'est expliquée dans des limites de localisation en s'opposant à l'exsudation fibrino-purulente; tandis que le diplocoque très virulent agit surtout par ses produits toxiques sur la substance corticale du cerveau, et sur tout l'organisme, avec production de phénomènes nerveux et de la mort.

Méningites à B. pyocyanique, à streptocoques, à staphylocoques,
à B. d'Eberth, etc.

Comme nous venons de le voir, le méningocoque et le pneumocoque sont les deux microorganismes qui jouent le rôle principal dans la production des méningites aiguës. Mais il y a aussi d'autres microorganismes qui, soit à l'autopsie, soit par la ponction lombaire, ont été trouvés comme agents pathogènes de ces formes morbides. Je ne dirai rien sur les méningites à streptocoques, ni sur celles à staphylocoques, ou à bacille d'Eberth, ou à bact. lactis aerogenes, etc., par la raison que je ne les ai jamais rencontrées dans ma pratique personnelle. Dans un cas, et il est le seul, j'ai rencontré le bacille pyocyanique chez un enfant de six ans : les phénomènes méningitiques éclatèrent au déclin d'une rechute de fièvre typhoïde, avec réaction de Widal positive. La méningite à forme très grave amena la mort de l'enfant au huitième jour, avec vomissements, céphalée, raideur de la nuque, signe de Kernig, température intermittente avec accès très élevés (40°-40°5). Deux ponctions lombaires donnèrent issue à 40-45 centimètres cubes de liquide limpide, avec 1,15 0/00 d'albumine, et qui donna en culture pure le bacille pyocyanique. L'enfant n'avait pas paru souffrir des oreilles, ni du nez. L'autopsie ne put être pratiquée.

Méningites à B. Coli. Influence des infections intestinales sur la production des méningites.

Les méningites à bacterium coli constatées par nous sont au nombre de quatre, et je suis convaincu qu'elles devraient être assez fréquentes, si on les recherchait avec plus d'attention. On sait combien fréquentes sont les manifestations nerveuses, non seulement au commencement, mais aussi dans le déclin, et dans la convalescence des toxi-infections gastro-intestinales chez les enfants. MARFAN et moi, nous avons les premiers appelé l'attention des pédiatres sur certaines formes de méningites aiguës et d'hydrocéphalie chez des enfants atteints de ces affections aiguës de l'appareil digestif. Il est certain que de telles formes dépendent de l'introduction dans la circulation et de l'action sur le système nerveux des substances pathogènes qui ont leur origine dans l'appareil gastro-intestinal. Peut-être la plupart de ces substances sont-elles de nature chimique, comme on peut le démontrer par l'indicanurie, par l'augmentation de la toxicité urinaire, par les éruptions de la peau, etc. Ces substances qui sont le produit de la putréfaction intestinale et de la vie de beaucoup de microbes endogènes et exogènes, transportées par la circulation générale, après avoir franchi les barrières de l'épithélium intestinal et du foie, peuvent faire retentir leur action irritative sur les revêtements cérébraux et donner la forme clinique d'une méningite aiguë, avec hyperhydrose cérébro-spinale, jusqu'à la formation d'une vraie hydrocéphalie. En effet, dans ces cas, la ponction lombaire donne une quantité notable de liquide et un contenu albumineux un peu plus abondant qu'habituellement: mais le liquide est toujours limpide, toujours stérile, même s'il est extrait dans les premiers jours de la manifestation méningitique. Nous aurons l'occasion de revenir tout à l'heure sur ce point.

Mais en dehors des substances de nature chimique, il faut considérer aussi l'élément bactérien représenté dans la plupart des cas par le bacterium coli exceptionnellement virulent, et qui, lorsque la muqueuse intestinale est lésée, peut bien la franchir et déterminer des localisations à distance par exemple dans les poumons, dans les reins, etc. Dans des conditions analogues, ESCHERICH a constaté une broncho-pneumonie secondaire due au streptococcus enteritidis. Dans

les quatre cas dans lesquels j'ai trouvé le bacterium coli dans le liquide
cérébro-spinal, on avait affaire à quatre enfants qui, depuis une à trois
semaines, présentaient des formes aiguës d'infection gastro-intestinale, certainement non typhique (réaction de Widal négative). La
manifestation méningée avait éclaté d'emblée, dans le déclin de la
maladie primitive : fièvre élevée, convulsions, raideur de la nuque,
agitation, insomnie, cris aigus, vomissements, hyperesthésie, exagération des réflexes rotuliens, dans un cas amaurose. La ponction
lombaire pratiquée du deuxième au troisième jour donna issue à 40,
55, 70, 80 centimètres cubes de liquide sous forte pression, limpide,
d'un poids spécifique de 1005 à 1015, avec un contenu albumineux de
0,6, 1 0/00. L'examen bactériologique donna une culture pure de bacterium coli. Deux cas se sont terminés par la guérison et deux par la
mort. L'autopsie ne put être faite.

Les conséquences à tirer de ces observations sont que, dans le
cours d'une toxi-infection gastro-intestinale aiguë, le bacterium coli
peut franchir les parois intestinales et déterminer parmi les autres
localisations une méningite aiguë à forme très grave, souvent mor
telle. Dans les cas qui aboutissent à la guérison, comme nous l'avons
vu, comme dans les autres formes bactériennes, il peut persister une
hydrocéphalie, qui d'ailleurs pourra être évitée par les ponctions lombaires. L'influence des affections aiguës de l'appareil digestif sur la
production des méningites est un argument qui mérite la plus grande
attention de la part des pédiatres. Et tout d'abord il faut étudier l'influence directe des agents pathogènes de la maladie primitive pour
distinguer les formes purement toxiques des formes infectieuses
(bact. coli), aux points de vue étiologique, clinique, anatomo-pathologique et thérapeutique. En second lieu il faut étudier l'influence
indirecte que les toxi-infections digestives peuvent exercer sur la
production de toutes les autres méningites bactériennes en dehors du
bact. coli. Nous avons vu, surtout pour le méningocoque, cette
influence être en quelques cas réelle, non seulement pour les déterminer, mais aussi pour en déterminer les aggravations, les vraies
rechutes. Peut-être cette influence doit-elle être considérée comme
diminuant les résistances surtout locales, en préparant la localisation
des microorganismes, en modifiant la constitution du liquide cérébro-spinal, anéantissant son action protectrice que nous avons vue
constante envers presque tous les microorganismes.

II. **Méningites aiguës amicrobiennes.**

Nous avons vu comment dans la série de mes observations personnelles, dans quarante-trois cas, l'examen du liquide cérébro-spinal a donné un résultat tout à fait négatif. Il ne faut pas en conclure que toutes ces méningites doivent être considérées comme d'origine non infectieuse. Dans presque la moitié des cas (dans 21) les enfants nous furent amenés à une période avancée de leur maladie d'un minimum de un mois à un maximum de deux ans, la plupart de trois à huit mois. De ce qui nous fut rapporté par les parents dans un tiers des cas, sept fois, la maladie aurait éclaté, et aurait eu la marche d'une méningite aiguë; dans les quatorze autres cas la méningite aurait été précédée d'une grave toxi-infection gastro-intestinale, et les phénomènes nerveux auraient éclaté dans le déclin de la maladie. Les manifestations aiguës de la méningite se seraient par degrés atténuées; mais la note prédominante résiduelle était l'hydrocéphalie qui fut constatée dans seize cas sur vingt et un. Dans trois cas il y avait aussi amaurose complète; et dans presque tous il y avait raideur de la nuque, agitation, insomnie, paralysie des jambes, exagération des réflexes rotuliens, de temps en temps convulsions, et parfois fièvre. La ponction lombaire donna issue sous forte pression à des quantités notables de liquide, jusqu'à 70, 90, 120 centimètres cubes. Seulement, en de rares cas, la quantité de liquide était limitée à quelques centimètres cubes sortant par gouttes. Le liquide était limpide, le contenu albumineux variait entre 0,5, 1 et 1,5 0/0; ce qui nous donnait l'idée de la nature inflammatoire du liquide qui, dans les cas normaux, ne contient que 0,15 à 20 0/00 d'albumine. L'examen bactériologique ainsi que l'inoculation aux animaux de quantités abondantes (10 à 20 centimètres cubes) donnèrent toujours un résultat négatif. Tout cela on le comprend aisément, si on se rappelle ce que nous avons vu à propos des formes diplo et méningococciques dans lesquelles l'épuisement de l'élément bactérien est facile à vérifier dans un temps assez court. Certainement il faut supposer que les sept cas qui éclatèrent d'emblée comme des formes vraiment méningitiques doivent être rapportés aux formes bactériennes, et avec toute probabilité aux formes méningococciques. Et ces cas servent à compléter justement la description de cette maladie en les comparant aux diverses variétés que nous venons de voir, et donnent la démonstration de leur tendance à se prolonger, à se terminer par l'hydrocéphalie, par l'amaurose, etc.; et de l'heureuse influence de la ponction lombaire pour éviter surtout ces fâcheuses conséquences.

Pour ce qui est des quatorze autres cas, ils sont aussi une preuve évidente de la grande influence des toxi-infections gastro-intestinales dans la production des manifestations aiguës méningées. Que l'agent déterminant ait été toxique ou infectieux, que d'autres micro-organismes aient pu, par cette cause déterminante, se localiser sur les méninges, nous n'avons pas le moyen de le savoir, et ceci ne contredit pas notre thèse. Seulement, je le répète, il faut dire que c'est un argument qui mérite de nouvelles études, de nouvelles observations. Quelques-uns de ces vingt et un cas furent soustraits à notre observation depuis la première ou la deuxième ponction. Tous les autres furent traités par la méthode iodo-mercurielle et par les ponctions méthodiquement répétées. Dans les cas plus récents, 2 à 4 ponctions ont suffi pour amener une amélioration rapide, et ensuite la guérison complète. Dans les autres les ponctions furent répétées jusqu'à 18, 22, 55 fois.

Les guérisons constatées sont au nombre de cinq, et appartiennent aux cas plus récents, de un à deux mois ; dans un cas seulement, la maladie datait de six mois, avec amaurose, dont aussi l'enfant réussit à guérir. Des cinq cas sortis guéris, quatre appartiennent à la série des formes qui commencèrent comme de vraies méningites aiguës ; ce qui permet encore de croire à la nature méningococcique de la maladie. Des trois autres cas à début rapide, tumultueux, nous en avons perdu un de vue, le deuxième mourut après 22 ponctions par un accroissement fatal de l'hydrocéphalie ; mais il faut dire que le traitement commença un an après le début de la maladie, dans un état d'hydrocéphalie très marquée ; dans le troisième, nous avons dû nous contenter d'une simple amélioration qui, du reste, n'est pas peu de chose en raison des conditions dans lesquelles l'enfant nous fut amené. La maladie datait de deux ans ; il y avait hydrocéphalie, amaurose, paralysie spastique des jambes avec impossibilité de se tenir debout, raideur de la nuque, agitation, cris, etc. L'examen ophtalmoscopique révéla une cécité absolue et l'atrophie des nerfs optiques. Après les 6e et 7e ponctions, il commença à distinguer le jour de la nuit : à présent, après 55 ponctions, il est capable de voir en pleine lumière un objet qui lui passe devant les yeux sans toutefois en pouvoir distinguer les contours. Un nouvel examen ophtalmoscopique a pu faire constater qu'il y a une zone limitée de la rétine capable d'être impressionnée par les rayons lumineux, et de déterminer une contraction réflexe de l'iris. Du reste, il se tient debout, et peut aussi marcher avec un peu de soutien, il

est tranquille, etc. Je crois qu'il gagnera encore pour ce qui regarde
la déambulation (l'enfant a maintenant quatre ans), mais pour ce
qui regarde la fonction visuelle je crois qu'il n'a pas à espérer
davantage, et je suis certain que si le traitement avait été commencé
plus tôt, la guérison aurait pu être complète. Mais cela prouve que,
même dans les cas anciens, il faut tenter et poursuivre avec persévérance, non pas des semaines, mais des mois. Une notable amélioration aussi fut constatée par nous dans cinq autres cas. Dans un autre
cas la mort fut déterminée par un accès d'éclampsie, lorsque la maladie semblait marcher vers une positive amélioration, bien que le traitement n'eût commencé que sept mois après le début et que les ponctions pratiquées eussent atteint le chiffre de ¡dix-huit. Un troisième
cas se termina par la mort avec augmentation constante de l'hydrocéphalie. En tout cas, dans cette série de faits, on voit aussi, à l'évidence, l'heureuse influence de la ponction lombaire.

Dans les vingt-deux autres cas dans lesquels l'examen bactériologique me donna un résultat négatif, l'observation a pu être faite dans
un temps assez voisin du début de la maladie, de deux à vingt jours :
dans la plupart des cas de deux à cinq jours. De ces vingt-deux cas,
j'en ai enregistré un dont l'invasion avait été rapide, tumultueuse, en
pleine santé, comme dans les formes bactériennes communes; et
bien que le liquide fût extrait aux 3e, 4e, 5e jours il resta toujours
stérile. Le contenu albumineux n'a pu nous fournir un critère quelconque, parce que tandis que dans deux cas il n'y avait que des
traces d'albumine, dans les autres elle a varié de 0,5 à 1 0/00. Dans
très peu de cas nous avons pu constater la formation du réticule à
l'état de repos. Dans les treize autres cas, les phénomènes méningitiques éclatèrent dans le cours de toxi-infections intestinales qui dans
quelques cas dataient de six à huit semaines. La réaction négative de
l'épreuve de WIDAL nous assurait l'exclusion d'une infection typhique.
Dans ces cas encore, l'examen bactériologique du liquide extrait,
également dans les premières quarante-huit heures de la manifestation méningitique, fut toujours négatif. Le contenu en albumine
variait de 0,15 à 0, 80/00. Dans la plupart des cas, nous n'avons constaté aucune formation de réticule. Les ponctions lombaires ont été
répétées jusqu'à huit et dix fois avec des intervalles plus ou moins
voisins ou éloignés, selon que le cas était plus ou moins aigu. Les
résultats furent assez heureux, puisque sur vingt-deux cas nous enregistrons treize guérisons et neuf morts. Les guérisons furent toutes
complètes, sans hydrocéphalies, sans amauroses résiduelles, tandis
que nous avons vu avec quelle fréquence ces conséquences se véri-

fiaient dans les cas où l'intervention avait été trop tardive, ou avait fait défaut.

Pour ce qui regarde l'étiologie de ces formes, serons-nous donc autorisés à proclamer leur nature simplement toxique, à l'exclusion de tout élément bactérien? Le vouloir affirmer pour les vingt-deux cas serait peut-être trop hasardé. Il faut se rappeler la facilité avec laquelle beaucoup de microbes s'épuisent et meurent après avoir déterminé des formes de méningites très graves et que le temps qui s'écoule du commencement de la maladie à la mort des microbes ne dépasse jamais quelques semaines, et quelquefois peut être réduit à moins de huit jours. Or, parmi les vingt-deux cas appartenant à cette série, nous en avons dans lesquels la recherche a été pratiquée le 10e, le 15e, le 20e jour, espace de temps qui est très suffisant pour épuiser la vitalité et surtout la virulence de la plupart des microbes connus (diplocoques, streptocoques). D'un autre côté, il faut aussi considérer que, dans une méningite à localisation surtout cérébrale, le liquide qui se trouve surtout dans les parties inférieures du sac méningé spinal peut contenir peu ou point d'élément bactérien, qui par sa ténuité peut échapper à l'observation. Il y a des cas dans lesquels l'examen microscopique du liquide extrait renferme peu ou point de microorganismes, et où il faut pratiquer les cultures ou l'injection chez les animaux pour le déceler, tandis que, à l'autopsie, on trouve d'épaisses et étendues stratifications fibro-purulentes avec des quantités énormes de diplocoques. Il est vrai que dans nos observations nous n'avons jamais laissé de recourir à ces recherches, en ayant aussi la précaution de centrifuger le liquide. Dans deux cas, l'autopsie elle-même nous avait confirmé la nature amicrobienne de la maladie. Dans un cas la méningite éclata à la troisième semaine d'une infection intestinale : la ponction lombaire fut pratiquée le deuxième jour, et l'enfant mourut le jour suivant. L'autopsie releva une légère augmentation du liquide cérébro-spinal et une hyperémie des méninges avec œdème des espaces sous-arachnoïdiens. Les cultures faites avec le liquide endoventriculaire et des espaces sous-arachnoïdiens furent négatives. Le liquide cérébro-spinal renfermait presque 1 pour 100 d'albumine. Dans l'autre cas, une petite fille de dix mois présenta une forme méningitique complète et assez prolongée dans le cours d'un érysipèle (raideur de la nuque et du rachis, Kernig, strabisme, paralysies et contractures, trépidations musculaires, vomissements, etc.). Les ponctions lombaires furent toujours stériles. A l'autopsie on trouva une augmentation du liquide endoventriculaire, qui se montra stérile ainsi que le liquide sous-arachnoïdien.

Nous avons par conséquent des preuves assez concluantes pour pouvoir affirmer que les méninges peuvent quelquefois être stimulées, irritées, par des produits toxiques, soit d'origine gastro-intestinale, soit d'origine bactérienne à distance (érysipèle, pneumonie, etc.), jusqu'à donner la forme clinique complète d'une méningite aiguë, sans qu'à l'autopsie on trouve rien de plus qu'une production plus ou moins exagérée de liquide cérébro-spinal dépourvu absolument de tout élément bactérien. MYA a démontré cette hyperhydrose cérébro-spinale dans le rachitisme (intoxication lente intestinale?) et sous l'influence d'une intoxication pneumonique (pneumonie) sans que le pneumocoque se localise sur les méninges. Sous l'influence d'une intoxication gastro-intestinale, l'éclampsie, les crises méningitiformes ou de méningisme sont assez fréquentes en dehors de toute localisation bactérienne sur les méninges. Des faits du même genre peuvent se vérifier par l'action des autres éléments toxiques, par exemple, dans l'insuffisance rénale, avec œdème cérébral et augmentation du liquide sous-arachnoïdien et endoventriculaire. Il est par conséquent démontré que les méninges peuvent être irritées par des agents de nature chimique, toxique, non bactérienne : si cette action est limitée, transitoire, l'effet se bornera à de simples accidents éclamptiques, à de l'agitation, à du méningisme, etc. Si la cause agit plus profondément, d'une manière continue, à répétition, on pourra arriver à l'exsudation exagérée de liquide, à la vraie méningite séreuse aiguë simple, non infectieuse; et la terminaison pourra tendre vers la guérison plus ou moins rapide, à l'hydrocéphalie, à l'amaurose, aux paralysies, à la mort, selon l'intensité de l'agent pathogène, selon la résistance individuelle, et selon le traitement qui sera mis en œuvre, précisément comme nous l'avons vu dans les autres formes de méningite bactérienne. Et c'est à ces formes toxiques que je crois devoir réserver l'appellation de *méningite séreuse aiguë*. Aussi, dans les formes bactériennes on peut avoir un exsudat limpide; mais cette propriété n'est pas constante, tandis que dans les formes toxiques je n'ai jamais rencontré ni purulence ni trouble de l'exsudat. Je suis convaincu que dans la série de ces vingt-deux cas, sans la pratique de la ponction lombaire, la quantité de cas de mort aurait été beaucoup plus considérable et que les guérisons n'auraient pas été aussi complètes, mais que beaucoup d'entre elles auraient été entravées par des hydrocéphalies, par des paralysies, etc., comme nous l'avons constaté dans les autres séries de cas. Dorénavant, il faudra mieux fixer notre attention surtout sur les formes secondaires aux toxi-infections gastro-intestinales, parce que ce n'est pas seulement dans le sens que nous avons jusqu'ici indiqué qu'elles agissent.

C'est un nouveau chapitre qui découle de l'observation rationnelle des faits et qui nous transporte des lésions méningées aux lésions de la substance même du système nerveux sous l'action des mêmes causes pathogènes.

Encéphalomyélites aiguës.

Quelquefois j'ai pu observer que, dans des conditions étiologiques identiques, il survient des phénomènes très graves du système nerveux, mais tout à fait différents de ceux qui caractérisent les formes méningitiques. Depuis le premier début, la note dominante est représentée par une prostration, par une adynamie très grave, par une inertie flaccide des muscles, avec abolition de tous les réflexes, avec torpeur, inconscience, parfois des sursauts tendineux, pouls petit, accéléré, stase capillaire dans la peau, hypothermie, refus de se nourrir, etc. Chez les petits enfants la fontanelle était déprimée. La ponction lombaire ne donnait issue qu'à quelques rares gouttes de liquide, ou bien elle restait absolument blanche. Tous ces enfants sont morts, mais je ne possède aucune autopsie. Faut-il dire dans ces cas que l'agent pathogène, plus probablement toxique, s'est porté directement sur la substance grise du système nerveux jusqu'à l'abolition de sa fonction, plutôt qu'expliquer son action irritante sur les méninges? Marfan a observé des scléroses disséminées résiduelles, de la même manière que dans les autres cas il avait observé les hydrocéphalies. L'agent pathogène est unique : la localisation et les conséquences en sont diverses.

Et qui peut dire si, en recherchant aussi les autres formes morbides qui frappent d'une manière aiguë le système nerveux, on ne pourra pas arriver à la conclusion que beaucoup de processus pathogènes, qui jusqu'ici ont été considérés comme tout à fait distincts, doivent être réunis sous une unique conception pathologique? J'ai pratiqué la ponction lombaire dans dix cas de poliomyélite antérieure aiguë, et dans trois cas de poliencéphalite aiguë. Sur neuf de ces cas j'ai examiné bactériologiquement le liquide extrait, et dans deux cas j'ai isolé le diplocoque lancéolé et encapsulé de Talamon-Fränkel, et dans un cas le méningocoque intra-cellulaire de Weichselbaum. Les deux premiers cas furent observés, l'un du deuxième au troisième jour, l'autre au septième jour; les six autres cas à résultat négatif, à l'exception de l'un d'eux qui fut ponctionné le quatrième jour, le furent à une époque bien plus éloignée du commencement de la maladie : de huit à trente jours. Dans tous les cas la quantité de liquide extrait était supérieure à la normale, jusqu'à 50 à 60 centimètres cubes : le contenu en albumine variait de 0,4 et 0,5 à 1 0/00 : l'aspect était toujours limpide. L'inoculation chez les animaux a été toujours sans accidents.

Tout le monde sait avec combien de preuves on a cherché à démontrer la nature infectieuse des poliencéphalomyélites aiguës, qui par leur marche, par le fait de se présenter souvent sous la forme épidémique, la laissaient soupçonner déjà depuis longtemps. La rareté des autopsies dans la période initiale de la maladie en rendait difficile la démonstration. Or, la ponction lombaire nous offre des conditions favorables pour résoudre la question dès le premier jour de l'atteinte morbide, aussi bien dans les cas graves que dans les cas légers. Il est naturel que la condition la plus favorable soit en rapport avec la précocité de l'intervention, pour éviter que l'épuisement des microbes ne nous trompe dans les résultats, ou dans les appréciations. Les six cas à résultat négatif furent ponctionnés de huit à vingt-trois jours après le début de la maladie. Il est probable qu'à ce moment-là l'intervention a été trop tardive. On doit attribuer la même importance négative aux résultats négatifs obtenus après la mort dans l'examen de la moelle ou de la substance corticale du cerveau, lorsqu'il n'est pas pratiqué dans les premières périodes de la maladie.

Unicité étiologique et pathogénique des processus méningitiques et encéphalomyélitiques.

De la même manière que nous avons vu pour les processus méningitiques, aussi bien que pour les formes myélitiques et encéphalitiques, on ne peut nier que l'agent pathogène puisse être de nature chimique, toxique. Quelle que soit son origine, transporté dans la grande circulation, il peut produire des manifestations différentes selon la localisation, selon la part de l'organisme qui offre une moindre résistance à son action. Sur la peau il se bornera à produire de simples érythèmes; sur les méninges et sur les revêtements internes ventriculaires il produira les irritations méningées, les hydrocéphalies; sur les éléments cellulaires du système nerveux il pourra limiter son action à des altérations moléculaires passagères facilement réparables, ou arriver aux formes plus profondes, nécrosiques, en formant une gamme allant depuis la tuméfaction des granulations chromatophiles et de la chromatolyse jusqu'à la désintégration de la substance chromatique avec atrophie du noyau et de la cellule (Marinesco). Et à côté des lésions de la cellule nerveuse nous constaterons des dilatations vasculaires, de l'infiltration leucocytaire, une prolifération conjonctivale, ou pour mieux dire, l'irritation de la névroglie soit primitive de la part des agents inflammatoires, soit secondaire à la dégénération des éléments nerveux. En un mot nous arriverons à la constitution des vrais foyers myélitiques et encéphalitiques plus ou moins profonds, plus ou moins étendus, plus ou moins capables d'une *restitutio ad integrum*.

Comme on le voit, cette manière de considérer la pathogénie de tous ces processus aigus qui frappent le système nerveux central et ses revêtements nous porte à réunir plusieurs maladies qui jusqu'ici étaient décrites dans des chapitres différents de la pathologie infantile. Mais cet unicisme part d'un côté de la multiplicité de l'agent pathogène, pour aboutir d'autre part à une différenciation de processus, selon la localisation de la cause morbide.

Quant à l'agent pathogène, on peut le considérer comme unique sous la dénomination d'un élément toxi-infectieux, mais qui peut se diviser en éléments bactériens et toxiques, et ceux-ci à leur tour peuvent se diviser en éléments bactériens pneumococciques, méningococciques, streptococciques, etc., et en éléments toxiques de provenance ou gastro-intestinale ou pneumonique, ou de quelque autre espèce bactérienne. Et pour ce qui regarde la différenciation individuelle, on peut considérer la forme méningitique, poliomyélitique, poliencéphalitique, mixte, etc. Et d'ailleurs chaque forme présentera des variétés selon le pouvoir plus ou moins intensif de l'agent morbide, et du plus ou moins de résistance individuelle et locale. Mais en tous cas la conception fondamentale pathogénique reste unique.

Avec cette manière de concevoir ces processus morbides, on voit combien sont absolument inutiles et oiseuses toutes les discussions académiques sur le plus ou moins de spécificité du méningocoque pour produire la méningite cérébro-spinale, du moment que le même méningocoque comme aussi le diplocoque de Fränkel, ainsi que nous l'avons vu, peuvent déterminer les poliomyélites antérieures aiguës; du moment que presque tous les microbes pathogènes connus peuvent déterminer des méningites peu faciles à différencier entre elles; du moment que des méningites similaires peuvent être produites en dehors de tout élément bactérien, seulement sous l'influence des produits toxiques divers; du moment que le même diplocoque, que le même méningocoque sont capables de déterminer des formes abortives, simplement séreuses, à peine diagnostiquables sinon par la ressource de l'examen bactériologique, jusqu'aux formes à exsudat trouble, jusqu'aux stratifications fibrino-purulentes étendues et épaisses. Cependant, qu'une infection méningococcique se répande en une localité, en un hôpital, en un asile, et nous aurons la description d'une épidémie de méningite cérébro-spinale méningococcique. Mais le même fait on l'a observé avec le streptocoque, avec le pneumocoque, etc. Qu'une épidémie de toxi-infections gastro-intestinales éclate l'été, et sous certaines conditions spéciales du système nerveux, nous pourrons observer dans un délai de temps et des localités données de vraies épidémies de méningite séreuse aiguë, comme nous l'avons constaté à Rome pendant la saison d'avril à août de ces deux dernières années. Que des formes de ce genre se présentent isolées, et nous aurons les cas sporadiques de l'une ou de l'autre nature. C'est pour cela que je considère qu'il est inutile et oiseux de parler de différences entre les méningites cérébro-spinales épidémiques et sporadiques. Quant à ce qui est des formes diverses que prendra la maladie, c'est la raison individuelle, c'est la diversité de résistance locale qui nous expliquera la détermination de la forme poliencéphalitique, ou de la forme poliomyélitique, ou de la forme méningée, ou des formes mixtes. Comme il est facile de le voir, je vais beaucoup plus loin que les idées de STRÜMPELL qui identifiait sous la même raison pathogénique la poliomyélite avec la poliencéphalite.

Dans ces derniers temps on a beaucoup parlé des poliomyélites antérieures aiguës à période initiale très douloureuse. Ces formes-là, je les vois très souvent, surtout lorsque l'enfant nous est amené dès les premiers jours. D'autre part, il suffit d'interroger minutieusement les parents, et aussi les enfants s'ils sont plus âgés, pour rester convaincu que ces formes douloureuses ne sont pas rares. Or cette douleur en ceinture, qui parfois s'étend jusqu'aux jambes, qui augmente par la compression ou par les mouvements, n'est due qu'à la participation des méninges au processus irritatif qui a frappé la moelle épinière. Les proportions dans lesquelles les méninges peuvent participer au processus myélitique sont très différentes. En un cas j'ai vu la forme douloureuse prédominer absolument sur la forme paralytique : l'abolition des réflexes, un peu de flaccidité musculaire, une légère atrophie consécutive, la douleur limitée exclusivement à la région lombaire et qui manquait le long des nerfs, donnèrent la note prédominante, indicatrice de l'atteinte spinale ; mais la forme douloureuse était tellement accentuée qu'à peine on put arriver au diagnostic d'une paralysie spinale infantile.

Dans les myélites expérimentales aussi on a vu que dans presque tous les cas les méninges participaient à l'inflammation (Marinesco).

Dans certains cas on a dû admettre que les microbes arrivaient à la moelle par le liquide céphalo-rachidien et commençaient par former des colonies dans les méninges pour ne pénétrer que secondairement dans la moelle.

La conclusion qui découle de tout ce que je viens de dire est que l'on devrait commencer à faire un travail analytique de tous les cas qui s'offrent à l'observation, et qui devraient être étudiés complètement au point de vue clinique, étiologique, anatomo-pathologique et bactériologique. Ces observations recueillies, on devrait se livrer à un travail de synthèse rationnelle, en réunissant toutes les différentes manifestations qui, sous la forme aiguë, frappent dans l'âge infantile le système nerveux central et ses revêtements, en les considérant comme le produit d'un élément causal unique de nature toxi-infectieuse qui agit de la même manière et aboutissant aux mêmes conséquences. De cette conception unitaire on pourra ensuite se livrer à un nouveau travail analytique pour distinguer les diverses formes, soit au point de vue de l'élément causal, déterminant, exogène, comme on voudra l'appeler, soit au point de vue de l'élément individuel prédisposant, endogène, pour se rendre compte des différentes localisations et des différentes modalités cliniques et anatomo-pathologiques. Rien ne se prête mieux que le tableau suivant à donner une idée de cette conception synthétique et analytique qu'on doit avoir, je crois, à propos de la pathogénie de ces formes morbides auxquelles nous avons consacré ce rapport.

Pathogénie des méningo-encéphalo-myélites.

CAUSES EXOGÈNES, DÉTERMINANTES		CAUSES ENDOGÈNES, PRÉDISPOSANTES	
Toxi-infections aiguës	**Bactériennes.** — Méningococcus. Diplococcus pneumoniae. Bact. coli. Bacillus Eberthi. Streptocoques. Staphylocoques. Bac. pyocyanique. Bact. lactis. aerog. Etc.	**Méningitiques.** — Cérébrales. Spinales. Cérébro-spinales.	
	Toxiques. — Gastro-intestinales. Pneumoniques. Infections générales.	**De la substance nerveuse.** — Poliencéphalites. Poliomyélites. Poliencéphalo-myélites. Névrites.	
		Mixtes. — Méningo-encéphalo-myélites.	

Messieurs, c'est d'après ce plan que, je crois, on doit diriger dorénavant les recherches ayant pour but l'étude complète, rationnelle de ces formes morbides qui avec tant de fréquence, avec tant de gravité, frappent l'âge infantile. De cette étude nous pourrons tirer les plus grands avantages soit au point de vue prophylactique, soit au point de vue thérapeutique. Dans le cours de ce rapport nous avons fait voir jusqu'à l'évidence la part importante qui est réservée au médecin prévoyant et actif pour prévenir et pour guérir des ravages qui amènent la mort, ou des conséquences auprès desquelles la mort elle-même serait mille fois préférable. Et je croirais avoir bien mérité la confiance qu'a eue en moi le Comité directeur du Congrès en me faisant l'honneur de me confier ce rapport, si par cette contribution, je pouvais déterminer d'autres collègues plus savants à en faire le point de départ de leurs recherches, et contribuer à vulgariser davantage la pratique de la ponction lombaire.

MÉNINGITES AIGUËS NON TUBERCULEUSES

RAPPORT

par M. le docteur NETTER,

de Paris.

Les points sur lesquels je me propose d'attirer votre attention sont les suivants :

1° La fréquence relative de la méningite cérébro-spinale épidémique qui à l'heure présente est en voie d'augmentation non douteuse sur la plus grande partie du globe ;

2° Les renseignements précieux que fournissent au diagnostic la recherche du signe de Kernig et la ponction lombaire ;

3° Les méthodes de traitement les plus utiles.

I

En temps ordinaire les méningites aiguës non tuberculeuses sont presque toujours secondaires à des altérations de l'oreille, du nez, au traumatisme, aux maladies générales ou locales (pneumonie).

Les méningites aiguës primitives sont rares et ne s'observent qu'à intervalles assez longs.

De 1885 à 1886 l'existence de plusieurs foyers de méningite cérébro-spinale, en même temps que l'apparition de cas sus-indiqués plus nombreux de méningite cérébro-spinale, avait été signalée de divers côtés, en même temps qu'une recrudescence et une gravité plus grande des pneumonies. C'est ainsi qu'en 1886 Fraenkel, à Berlin.

Foa et Teffredozzi à Turin, Weichselbaum à Vienne, nous-même à Paris nous signalions simultanément l'existence de méningites suppurées à pneumocoques.

Du même moment la méningite revêtait l'apparence épidémique à Cologne (Leechbeult), dans le Danemark, la Suède, la Finlande.

Depuis 1890 et surtout 1893-1894, les foyers épidémiques étaient plus nombreux. On les signale à Copenhague, en Italie (Padoue, Bonini), et dans plusieurs villes de l'Allemagne du Nord et du Sud (Berlin, Hambourg, Stuttgart, Carlsruhe); en Autriche-Hongrie (Vienne, Budapest); en Amérique (New-York, Boston). L'étude de ces petites épidémies a été le point de départ d'acquisitions très précieuses pour la clinique, la bactériologie, l'épendymite.

Depuis ce moment la proportion des localités envahies a beaucoup augmenté.

On en a signalé un assez grand nombre en Allemagne (Hambourg, Brême, Kiel, Königsberg, Munich, etc.). En Autriche-Hongrie on peut citer une épidémie importante à Tripail. En Italie, des faits nombreux ont été recueillis par nos collègues.

La plupart des États de la Confédération américaine ont été plus ou moins éprouvés. A New-York, New-Jersey, Pensylvanie, Massachusetts, Maryland sont venus se joindre les États du Centre comme l'Illinois (Chicago, 1898), Ohio, Missouri, Zowa, Kansas; du Sud (Georgie, Texas); de l'Ouest (Colorado et Nouvelle-Californie). Le Klondyke, le Canada ont été également envahis par l'épidémie.

La France, depuis la grande épidémie de 1847-1848, avait été peu touchée en dehors de quelques petits foyers à peu près exclusivement relevés dans les casernes, à Aix, à Bayonne, à Cherbourg, etc. Depuis la fin de 1897 la méningite est devenue sensiblement plus commune.

C'est à cette date qu'il convient de faire remonter son apparition à Paris où les cas se multiplient à partir de mars 1898 sans que l'on puisse noter à l'heure actuelle une diminution sensible. La ville de Lille est envahie au même moment dans une proportion plus faible. Signalons la présence du mal dans un certain nombre de localités plus ou moins rapprochées de Paris, Versailles, Dreux, Poitiers, Angers. Depuis le commencement de 1900 les cas deviennent assez nombreux à Marseille où ils sont d'abord signalés par d'Astros et Engelhardt.

Il ne s'agit pas de cas très nombreux et il n'est pas aisé d'établir de connexion entre les cas apparaissant d'une façon en apparence irrégulière dans les divers points de la ville. Le fait n'a, du reste, rien de bien surprenant et nous le trouvons déjà signalé dans toutes les relations antérieures de méningite épidémique.

C'est ainsi du reste que la méningite va procéder dans les autres pays.

En Belgique, des cas sont signalés dans l'armée, d'abord à Anvers en 1895. 1 cas, puis à Bruxelles en 1896, dit Neef, 16 cas.

En 1900, Hendrix en rapporte 2 observations recueillies sur des enfants de Bruxelles.

En Hollande, Nolen signale l'existence de quelques cas à Leyde en 1897. De Bruin en publie 9 observations recueillies dans un hôpital d'enfants à Amsterdam en 1899 et 1900.

Notre ami le docteur Looft a observé un certain nombre de cas à Bergen en Norvège en 1900.

En Roumanie, Manicatide, en Grèce, Assymis ont vu des malades.

Une épidémie relativement importante a fait son apparition à Dublin, à la fin de 1899. Parons et Littldale en font connaître 5 cas, Drury 9.

On signale l'apparition d'un certain nombre de cas à Liverpool (Barr), à Bristol (Mitchell Clarke), à Glasgow, à Nottingham (Henry Handford). A Londres, on ne parle pas à proprement parler d'épidémie de méningite cérébro-spinale. Still, Carr Bahlow et Lees signalent en revanche la fréquence d'une forme spéciale de méningite simple, la « posterior basis meningitis » dans laquelle ils trouvent un microbe analogue à celui de Weichselbaum.

En Asie, la méningite est signalée dans l'Inde par Buchanan. En Afrique nous voyons par les communications du docteur Billet qu'elle sévit actuellement à Constantine, par celles de Marchow, qu'elle s'observe dans le Soudan. Des médecins anglais et allemands nous montrent son développement dans le sud du continent africain, tandis que des journaux politiques et médicaux signalent ses ravages, en 1899, à Omdurman dans la Nubie.

Des observations publiées dans la *Censtralasion medical Gazette* nous montrent que l'Océanie obéit à la règle générale.

Cette brève revue nous montre que nous avons bien raison de dire qu'à l'heure actuelle il existe un peu partout un réveil de la méningite cérébro-spinale épidémique et que les praticiens ne sauraient perdre de vue cette notion fort importante.

Nous n'avons nullement l'intention ici d'étudier plus particulièrement la méningite cérébro-spinale épidémique. Nous ne voulons mettre en avant qu'une particularité, la grande variation de son évolution. On aurait grand tort de croire que la méningite cérébro-spinale présente toujours des symptômes d'excitation très marqués, qu'elle s'accompagne régulièrement de fièvre vive et que sa marche très rapide en fasse une affection de courte durée, qu'elle se termine par la mort ou aboutisse à la guérison. La méningite cérébro-spinale présente souvent des cas de modalités très diverses. On peut y rencontrer tous les symptômes. La raideur de la nuque elle-même, qui en est le signe le plus constant, peut manquer. C'est la marche surtout qui montre le plus de différences. Si le début est habituellement assez brusque, la fièvre peut être à peu près nulle. La méningite peut présenter une durée des plus longues. Nous l'avons vue se prolonger quatre mois. Cette forme prolongée de la méningite cérébro-spinale interrompue ou non par des rémissions, a été signalée dans les premières épidémies; mais elle ne semble pas avoir assez attiré l'attention. Peut-être était-elle moins commune que de nos jours. Dans tous les cas, l'analyse des observations récentes montre qu'elle est fréquente.

Sur 207 observations dont 125 terminées par décès, nous en trouvons 77 dont la durée a dépassé un mois, et parmi celles-ci 51 dont la durée a dépassé deux mois. En ne prenant que les cas terminés par la guérison, 85, la proportion de méningites de longue durée s'élève encore. 57 ont duré plus d'un mois et 20 plus de deux mois.

II

Le diagnostic des méningites a de tout temps présenté des difficultés très grandes. Dans les cas terminés par la guérison on est toujours porté à se demander s'il s'agissait bien de lésions inflammatoires organiques des méninges, s'il ne s'agissait pas tout simplement des troubles inorganiques dynamiques de nature réflexe ou toxique.

Les mots de pseudoméningite (Bouchut), de méningisme (Dupré) ont été accueillis avec une grande faveur. Nous ne contestons pas la possibilité de troubles simplement dynamiques déterminant des symptômes méningitiques: mais il est évident que les altérations inflammatoires des méninges comme celles des séreuses en général, peuvent présenter des degrés très divers et qu'à côté des inflammations purulentes seules envisagées d'habitude il existe des altérations initiales moins marquées, qui sont susceptibles de rétrocéder avec une grande rapidité sans laisser la moindre trace.

L'histoire suivante à laquelle nous avons assisté dans le courant du mois d'avril nous en fournira un exemple.

Un malade âgé de 42 ans, de tempérament assez nerveux est pris d'une pneumonie lobaire grave. Le huitième jour la température s'élève, l'agitation devient plus marquée. Il existe un myosis notable. Le sujet est pris de mouvements incoordonnés aux membres supérieurs qui rappellent les mouvements de la chorée. Il existe un spasme pharyngé à type hydrophobique. Si l'on introduit un peu d'eau dans la bouche le malade ne peut ni la rejeter ni l'avaler.

La raideur de la nuque est très manifeste et le signe de Kernig très accentué. Ces symptômes nous font admettre l'existence d'une méningite pneumococcique à son début. Nous prescrivons les bains chauds et pratiquons la ponction lombaire; celle-ci nous permet de retirer 40 grammes d'un liquide clair, transparent qui paraît au premier abord être du liquide céphalo-rachidien normal. Les symptômes durent trente-six heures et cèdent, tandis que se produit une nouvelle poussée pneumonique dans le côté atteint au début.

Faut-il considérer un cas de ce genre comme se rapportant à une méningite vraie ou à du méningisme?

Si l'on envisage les apparences macroscopiques du liquide, la disparition rapide des symptômes, on est assez tenté d'accepter la dernière interprétation.

Il s'agissait cependant à n'en pas douter d'une méningite. En effet, le liquide qui paraissait du liquide céphalo-rachidien normal présente au bout de quelques heures de repos des flocons fibrineux à la vérité peu nombreux.

L'analyse chimique y révèle une proportion anormale d'albumine. L'examen bactériologique établit la présence du pneumocoque. Tous ces caractères prouvent que nous étions en présence d'une méningite séreuse.

Les cas de ce genre sont certainement nombreux et leur nature réelle reste aisément méconnue si l'on n'a pas recours à la ponction lombaire.

Nous avons eu maintes fois l'occasion d'insister sur les renseignements que peut fournir au diagnostic la recherche du signe indiqué par Kernig : l'impossibilité de redresser complètement le genou d'un sujet dont la cuisse est en flexion sur le bassin. Il n'est pas indispensable de faire asseoir le malade, le signe de Kernig peut être recherché en laissant le malade dans le décubitus dorsal pourvu que l'on ait bien soin de fléchir à angle droit la cuisse sur le bassin.

Avant nos communications, le signe de Kernig avait été un peu négligé en dépit des observations confirmatives de Bull, Henoch, Friis Blümm, Urban. Aujourd'hui son importance est reconnue de toutes parts et nous citerons tout particulièrement les communications de Herrick et d'Osler, en Amérique; Cippolina et Maragliano, en Italie; Dieulafoy, Astros, Billiet, en France; Buchanay, aux Indes et Sinclair, en Australie, etc.

Le signe de Kernig est un des symptômes les plus constants de la méningite.

Kernig le trouve dans 15 cas de méningite aiguë et 6 cas de méningite chronique.

Friis le constate 55 fois sur 60, soit 88,5 pour 100; Herrek. 17 fois sur 19, soit 89,4 pour 100.

Nous-même, en 1898, nous le trouvions 41 fois sur 46, soit 90 pour 100 et en 1899-1900, 60 sur 79, soit 85,5 pour 100.

Dans un relevé général, Roglet, qui a consacré une thèse fort intéressante à ce signe, arrive à une proportion de 179 sur 186, soit 85,5 pour 100.

Le signe de Kernig s'observe dans les diverses variétés de méningites.

Notre dernier travail nous le montre 28 fois sur 30, soit 95,5 pour 100, dans les méningites épidémiques 9 fois sur 9, dans les méningites secondaires 29 sur 40, soit 72,5 pour 100, dans les méningites tuberculeuses.

On ne saurait, en présence de ces chiffres, mettre en doute l'importance de cette recherche pour le diagnostic. Sans doute le symptôme peut n'apparaître que quelques jours après le début, il peut être intermittent pendant une certaine période. Je ne crois pas toutefois qu'il existe beaucoup de signes pathognomoniques que l'on enregistre avec une pareille fréquence.

Le signe de Kernig ne peut-il pas s'observer en dehors de la méningite? Les premières recherches semblèrent bien prouver que non et nous nous étions personnellement prononcé dans ce sens. Nous ne saurions aujourd'hui être aussi affirmatif. Les explications fort pauvres que l'on a proposées au sujet de la pathogénie du signe de Kernig ne permettent en aucune façon de dire pourquoi il serait exclusivement possible dans les cas d'inflammation des méninges.

On a cité des observations de méningite cérébro-spinale dans les hémorragies méningées, dans des abcès du cerveau (Klippel).

Il est deux maladies dans lesquelles les déterminations méningitiques sont relativement assez communes et dans lesquelles nous avons relevé le signe de Kernig avec une certaine fréquence : ce sont la fièvre typhoïde et la pneumonie.

Nous avons trouvé 44 fois le signe de Kernig sur 315 observations de fièvre typhoïde de 1898 à 1900, ce qui donne une proportion de 11,8 pour 100.

Dans environ la moitié de ces observations, le signe de Kernig coïncidait avec de la raideur de la nuque ou du tronc, des douleurs, des paralysies oculaires. La forme spinale méningitique de la fièvre typhoïde a été décrite par plusieurs auteurs. Nous ne saurions affirmer que dans tous les cas il y ait eu des lésions inflammatoires des méninges, mais dans nombre d'observations, nous en avons la preuve manifeste par les caractères fournis par le liquide recueilli par la ponction lombaire.

Les fièvres typhoïdes au cours desquelles nous avons trouvé le signe de Kernig sont sensiblement plus graves que les autres. Cette gravité s'affirme par la plus grande léthalité et la fréquence plus grande des rechutes. La proportion des décès a été de 20,5 au lieu de 7 pour 100, celle des rechutes de 45,6 au lieu de 16 pour 100.

Dans les pneumonies nous avons rencontré quelquefois le signe de Kernig. Le plus ordinairement le liquide donné par la ponction lombaire a été manifestement inflammatoire. Le fait a cependant subi quelques exceptions.

Je ne crois pas qu'il soit nécessaire ici d'insister sur l'importance de la ponction lombaire au point de vue du diagnostic.

Nous apprécions tous à sa valeur l'ingénieuse découverte de Quincke. Nous savons que la ponction lombaire est inoffensive à la condition de ne pas évacuer trop de liquide et surtout de ne pas l'aspirer avec trop de violence.

Le liquide recueilli fournit des indications très précieuses.

En général, dans les cas de méningite, il renferme du pus ou de la fibrine qui peut ne se séparer qu'après quelques heures. On y trouve une quantité plus ou moins marquée d'albumine. La culture dans des milieux appropriés donne naissance à des colonies de microbes pathogènes.

Aucun de ces caractères n'est absolument constant. C'est ainsi que la ponction dans des cas de méningite bactérienne avérée peut ramener un liquide tout à fait clair ne renfermant que des traces d'albumine et ne se développant pas dans les cultures.

III

Nous avons eu l'occasion de constater bien souvent les heureux effets du bain chaud dans le traitement des méningites aiguës. Ce procédé de traitement a été pour la première fois préconisé par Auprefit. Il a été employé d'une façon assez diverse par les auteurs qui l'ont appliqué.

Nous croyons que les bains doivent être assez nombreux, quatre ou cinq par jour, que la durée devra être d'une heure si possible, que la température sera de 38° à 40°.

Les bains chauds ont une action évidente sur la plupart des symptômes et en particulier sur les douleurs, les contractures et le délire. Ils ont de plus, semble-t-il, une influence directe sur la marche de la maladie.

Dans la méningite tuberculeuse elle-même, ils sont utiles en atténuant certains symptômes et nous ont paru rendre plus fréquentes les rémissions.

Dans les méningites non tuberculeuses et surtout dans les méningites cérébro-spinales, leur action est plus complète encore.

Nous avons enregistré personnellement dans ces dernières années 9 guérisons de méningite purulente sur 14 cas, soit 64,5 pour 100.

Nous avons été amené à considérer la ponction lombaire comme un élément très important du traitement des méningites cérébro-spinales. Nous croyons que sa principale utilité ne réside pas dans la réduction rapide de la tension du liquide céphalo-rachidien.

Elle a enlevé une petite quantité des agents pathogènes. Aussi est-il bon de répéter ces ponctions à plusieurs reprises dans le cours de la maladie.

Nous nous servons pour la ponction d'une aiguille de Pravaz ordinaire et nous avons pu dans plusieurs cas avec cette aiguille retirer un pus tellement épais, qu'on a peine à croire que l'aspiration en soit possible.

Conclusions.

1° Il existe actuellement sur tout le globe une fréquence insolite de la méningite cérébro-spinale. Bien que les cas soient souvent en apparence isolés, et sans relation apparente entre eux, on doit poser ici le diagnostic de méningite épidémique ;

2° Les meilleurs renseignements sont fournis par la ponction lombaire qui permet de reconnaître les qualités du liquide céphalo-rachidien ;

3° Le signe de Kernig peut fournir des renseignements utiles bien qu'il ne paraisse pas être absolument exclusif d'autre signification :

4° Les bains chauds répétés et les ponctions lombaires répétées sont des moyens de traitement précieux.

MÉNINGITES AIGUËS NON TUBERCULEUSES

RAPPORT

par M. le professeur MYA,
de Florence.

En prenant l'étiologie comme base plus rationnelle de la classification nosologique, on trouve d'abord le groupe très naturel et bien distinct des *méningites d'origine bactérienne*, dans lequel l'agent pathogène permet de distinguer quelques formes de méningites aiguës et subaiguës, qui étaient autrefois groupées artificiellement sous le nom de *méningites simples*, de *méningites purulentes*, d'après la nature de l'exsudat, ou bien distinguées en *méningites de la base*, *méningites de la convexité*, *méningites ventriculaires*, d'après la localisation prévalente de l'inflammation. Aujourd'hui, par contre, avec la connaissance exacte du micro-organisme pathogène, on comprend dans une étiologie identique, un nombre de formes apparemment diverses à cause de leur siège, de la nature de l'exsudat et, parfois, de la symptomatologie clinique, d'une manière analogue à ce qui a été fait pour les maladies inflammatoires d'origine infectieuse d'autres séreuses.

Le plus grand nombre des méningites dans la première enfance, en nous tenant aux observations faites surtout en Allemagne (JÄGER, HEUBNER, etc.), en Amérique, en Angleterre, ainsi qu'aux nôtres, est produit par le micro-organisme de WEICHSELBAUM (*meningococcus intracellularis meningitidis*), qui doit être absolument distingué du *diplococcus lanceolatus capsulatus* de la pneumonie (TALAMON-FRÄNKEL) par ses propriétés morphologiques et biologiques.

Les types cliniques déterminés par ce micro-organisme se réduisent essentiellement à deux (en ne tenant pas compte des nombreuses variétés) :

a) Le type aigu ou suraigu, avec les caractères ordinaires de la méningite cérébro-spinale épidémique, c'est-à-dire : raideur prononcée de la nuque, opisthotonos, vomissements, symptomatologie tétanique, fièvre élevée, etc. L'exsudat en pareil cas est très abondant, répandu sur toute la surface du myélencéphale, et éminemment fibrino-purulent. Le micro-organisme est abondant, souvent extra-cellulaire, dans la plupart des cas doué d'une action pathogène sur les animaux sensibles (souris, chèvres, par injection subdurale). La durée peut osciller entre 5 et 10-12 jours. La maladie est presque toujours mortelle ; parfois elle s'atténue dans la forme suivante.

b) Type subaigu, qui se prolonge parfois jusqu'à quelques mois. La forme illustrée par Caub sous le nom de *simplex basis posterior meningitis* appartient à cette catégorie. Il est plus commun chez les enfants en bas âge (nourrissons et première enfance).

Dans cette forme clinique, la symptomatologie tétaniforme prédomine aussi, mais plus atténuée que dans le type précédent. Le sensorium est généralement intact, la fièvre modérée. L'exsudat, moins abondant, moins purulent, peut être circonscrit à la région basilaire et postérieure pendant tout le cours de la maladie. Le liquide extrait par la ponction lombaire a souvent les caractères d'un exsudat séreux (méningite séreuse due au *diplococcus intracellularis*). Le micro-organisme, beaucoup moins abondant que dans la forme précédente, est parfois dépourvu d'action pathogène sur les animaux sensibles. Cette forme peut guérir radicalement, passer à l'état d'hydrocéphalie secondaire, ou produire la mort à la suite de maladies secondaires, ou de reprise aiguë et généralisation de l'inflammation, rentrant de cette façon dans le type précédent.

La bactérie méningitogène la plus commune chez les enfants en bas âge après la précédente est le *diplococcus lanceolatus capsulatus*. La forme clinique qu'il détermine a généralement un cours aigu, un pronostic très grave, et une symptomatologie polymorphe, beaucoup moins caractéristique que celle qui est déterminée par le *meningococcus* de Weichselbaum. L'exsudation est diffuse, presque toujours fibrino-purulente ; toutefois les formes circonscrites et à exsudation éminemment séreuse ne manquent pas. Pour ces méningites aussi, il faut se méfier des résultats de la ponction lombaire, spécialement en ce qui concerne l'aspect du liquide extrait, qui parfois est séreux, tandis que l'exsudat existant dans les tissus de l'arachnoïde est souvent fibrino-purulent. La méningite due au *diplococcus lanceolatus capsulatus* est souvent accompagnée ou précédée de pneumonie, d'otite ou de quelque autre localisation.

Les méningites due au *streptococcus pyogenes* s'observent plus rarement que les formes précédentes et sont généralement secondaires à une septicémie ou à une suppuration développée dans les environs de la cavité crânienne. On peut dire la même chose des formes dues aux staphylocoques.

Quant aux formes dues au coli-bacille, au bacille d'Eberth, et à d'autres micro-organismes plus rares, elles sont peu fréquentes chez l'enfant en bas âge, elles n'ont pas de symptomatologie spécifique et le diagnostic *intra vitam* est rendu possible seulement par l'examen bactériologique du liquide extrait au moyen de la ponction lombaire.

La voie que suivent plus communément les agents pathogènes pour arriver aux régions sous-arachnoïdiennes est représentée par la circulation sanguine (infection hématogène). L'infection méningitique peut aussi avoir lieu par une diffusion provenant de foyers situés dans les régions qui communiquent avec la cavité crânienne (infection d'origine otique, nasale, etc.).

Au groupe naturel des méningites bactériennes on oppose le groupe plus indéterminé des *méningites d'origine toxi-infectieuse et toxique*, connues sous les noms d'**hydrocéphalie aiguë, épendymite aiguë, de méningite ventriculaire, méningite séreuse non bactérienne,** etc. Il manquerait, pour quelques-unes de ces dernières, les caractères d'une véritable inflammation, puisque les caractères d'un vrai exsudat manquent dans le liquide céphalo-rachidien, ainsi que les traces d'une inflammation, passée ou actuelle, dans l'examen anatomo-pathologique des parois ventriculaires. Pour ces formes, qui s'associent parfois à des maladies infectieuses à localisation différente (pneumonie, fièvre typhoïde, maladies exanthématiques, gastro-entérites) et qui sont généralement caractérisées par une riche et imposante symptomatologie clinique, il serait bon de préférer l'appellation d'*hydrocéphalie aiguë*, d'*hyperhidrose cérébro-spinale*, à celui de méningite.

D'autre part, des observations exactes et nombreuses semblent avoir démontré que, si l'on se tient aux données de l'examen chimique et microscopique du transsudat, le qualificatif d'inflammatoire convient à certains épanchements séreux aigus dans les cavités cérébrales d'origine toxique.

Le mécanisme pathogénique dans ces formes est toujours très obscur, et l'on ne peut compter pour son interprétation que sur les quelques facteurs suivants :

a) Action probable irritante, lymphagogue et vasomotrice des toxines primaires et secondaires d'origine bactérienne.

b) Sensibilité spéciale, propre à la première enfance, du réseau capillaire sanguin cérébral aux actions toxiques que nous venons de mentionner.

Il est très probable, du reste, que le champ d'action principal des toxines bactériennes ou d'origine auto-toxique est représenté dans la symptomatologie clinique du méningisme par le système nerveux central, et que les variations quantitatives du liquide céphalo-rachidien ne sont qu'un épiphénomène d'une importance subordonnée, comme il résulte des observations toujours plus nombreuses de cérébropathie aiguë d'origine toxi-infectieuse ou auto-toxique.

B. — Discussion sur les méningites aiguës non tuberculeuses.

M. Henri Koplik (de New-York) dit qu'à son avis, en se basant sur une épidémie observée à New-York, il n'y a pas de différence entre la méningite sporadique et la méningite cérébro-spinale épidémique.

Il entre ensuite dans la distinction des différentes formes de méningite cérébro-spinale et reconnaît trois types :

A) Un type aigu caractérisé par son début soudain, la température élevée, le délire violent, la rigidité et les convulsions;

B) Un deuxième type ou forme comateuse qui se caractérise par l'absence des convulsions. Dans ces deux cas, la ponction lombaire donne toujours un liquide franchement purulent.

C) Le troisième type, ou subaigu, est marqué par l'atténuation de tous les symptômes, et par la tendance à l'opisthotonos. Ici la ponction lombaire donne parfois un liquide purulent, mais plus souvent séreux ou séro-purulent.

L'examen bactériologique montre la présence du diplocoque de Weichselbaum. M. Koplik insiste ensuite sur le diagnostic différentiel entre la méningite tuberculeuse et la méningite cérébro-spinale. Ce qui aide surtout au diagnostic, c'est que, dans la méningite tuberculeuse, les paralysies des membres ou des organes sensoriels sont plus fréquentes. Enfin M. Koplik insiste sur la valeur de la ponction lombaire et confirme complètement les résultats mis en relief par M. Netter. Il pense que la ponction précoce même dans la méningite tuberculeuse est susceptible d'amener un amendement. Dans la méningite cérébro-spinale, elle est susceptible d'amener la guérison complète, à la condition d'être répétée; et, grâce à elle, la guérison peut s'obtenir sans qu'on ait à redouter les phénomènes consécutifs à la guérison des méningites (cécité, surdité, émaciation).

M. Marfan demande à M. Netter ce qu'il pense de la fréquence du signe de Kernig dans la méningite tuberculeuse.

M. Netter répond que le signe de Kernig est assez fréquent dans la méningite tuberculeuse, mais qu'il manque cependant plus que dans la méningite cérébro-spinale. Il l'a trouvé 29 fois sur 40 dans la méningite tuberculeuse, 28 fois sur 50 dans la méningite cérébro-spinale et 9 fois sur 9 cas de méningites secondaires.

M. Marfan pense que le signe de Kernig est beaucoup moins fréquent dans la méningite tuberculeuse. Dans le semestre d'hiver de l'an dernier, à l'hôpital des Enfants-Malades, sur 15 cas de méningites tuberculeuses, il n'a pas trouvé une seule fois le signe de Kernig; il venait de remettre une note à M. Dieulafoy, constatant ce fait, quand vint à l'hôpital une petite malade atteinte de méningite tuberculeuse vraie, vérifiée par l'autopsie; elle présentait le signe de Kernig très nettement. Il pense donc que le signe de Kernig est assez rare dans la méningite tuberculeuse. Il rappelle l'hypothèse de M. Dieulafoy sur l'origine spinale de ce signe.

hypothèse qui est un peu en désaccord avec la fréquence relative des lésions spinales dans la méningite tuberculeuse.

M. NETTER est d'accord avec M. Marfan sur presque tous les points. Il n'y a là qu'une question de chiffres. Quant à la pathogénie du signe de Kernig, on ne peut faire que des hypothèses: il semble cependant qu'il relève d'une altération des nerfs de la queue de cheval.

C. — Communications sur les maladies des méninges et du système nerveux.

UN CAS DE MÉNINGITE TYPHIQUE SURVENU DIX JOURS AVANT LA DÉCLARATION D'UNE FIÈVRE TYPHOÏDE
CONSIDÉRATIONS IMPORTANTES AU POINT DE VUE DU TRAITEMENT

par M. le docteur HAGOPOFF,

de Constantinople.

J'ai soigné, il y a environ cinq mois, une petite fille âgée de quatre ans, dont voici l'histoire :

Son père, ancien albuminurique, était tuberculeux et est mort de bacillose intestinale. Sa mère, à peau vénitienne, emphysémateuse, a succombé à une péritonite par perforation au cours d'une fièvre typhoïde qu'elle avait contractée à la période de convalescence de sa fille. Celle-ci, qui fait l'objet de notre communication, a été élevée au sein, mais toujours souffrante, elle est sujette aux bronchites à répétition, à la micro-polyadénie; elle a eu des écoulements d'oreille, une adénite tuberculeuse au cou du côté gauche. Pas de maladies éruptives. Elle fut atteinte, le 8 mars dernier, d'une pneumonie franche du côté droit avec fièvre 39°.5; défervescence complète au bout de neuf jours.

Mais le vingt-troisième jour de sa pneumonie (quatorze jours après l'apyrexie complète (36° à 37°), la fièvre se ralluma (39°.4) avec des symptômes méningitiques au complet : constipation, vomissements, convulsions, irrégularité du pouls, raie vaso-motrice, raideur de la nuque et du dos, position en chien de fusil, respiration de Cheynes-Stokes, cris hydrencéphaliques, photophobie, ventre en bateau, léger ptosis; mais il n'existait ni le signe de Kernig, ni strabisme.

En présence de cette méningite, j'avais tout naturellement pensé à la tuberculose étant donné les antécédents de notre petite malade.

Mais voilà que le dixième jour, alors que les symptômes de la méningite s'étaient amendés malgré la persistance de la température, des taches rosées lenticulaires abondantes apparaissent avec tous leurs caractères. La fièvre typhoïde ainsi confirmée fit son cours normal et le quinzième jour la température descendit à 56°,7, et après de grandes oscillations (57° à 59°.5) arriva le vingt et unième jour à la sous-normale de la convalescence (56°.5). Guérison complète.

Ainsi qu'on vient de voir d'après ce qui précède, il s'agissait donc bel et bien d'une méningite éberthienne à la façon de méningites bacillaires ou à pneumocoques.

Quant à la question du traitement, voici ma conduite à tenir, d'ailleurs toujours la même, auprès d'un petit typhique : dès le commencement de la maladie, je prescris d'abord, dans le cas de constipation, un purgatif; puis, après effet, je fais donner de grands lavements froids à 15°. J'ai l'habitude, au lieu de l'eau bouillie simple, d'employer l'eau bouillie salée (sérum chirurgical) qui élève la tension vasculaire en même temps qu'elle alimente le typhique et active la phagocytose. Le nombre des lavements sera proportionnel au degré de l'hyperthermie (2 à 6 par vingt-quatre heures).

Si la diarrhée existe, je prescris, tout en continuant les lavements, une potion à parties égales de sous-nitrate de bismuth et de benzo-naphtol.

Quand la température vespérale dépasse 59°, je fais combiner aux lavements le drap mouillé (10 à 20 minutes de durée suivant l'âge).

Ce traitement fort simple suffit le plus souvent largement chez les enfants qui seront tout naturellement préparés aux bains froids lorsque leur indication s'impose.

Ceux-ci sont indiqués toutes les fois que la température vespérale rectale a tendance à monter et dépasse 40°,5 plus de deux jours de suite.

Au lieu de donner des bains froids d'emblée, je fais remplir la baignoire d'eau à la température de 50° à 52°, je fais refroidir l'eau progressivement au degré voulu. Je n'emploie les bains froids (à 22° et au-dessous) que très exceptionnellement : car lorsque je vois que les bains froids (à 25°) à eux seuls ne sont pas suffisants, je leur combine les lavements froids à l'intervalle des bains ou les nuits seulement. Et cela nous a toujours réussi à provoquer l'abaissement thermique.

J'ai traité, dans l'espace d'un an et demi, une vingtaine de petits typhiques avec la méthode que je viens de décrire, tous ont guéri. Je n'emploie, bien entendu, *jamais* les médications antithermiques.

TUMOR GLANDULÆ PINEALIS ET HYDROCEPHALUS CONGENITUS
SUR UN CAS TRÈS RARE D'HYDROCÉPHALIE CONGÉNITALE
CHEZ UN NOUVEAU-NÉ PAR DÉGÉNÉRESCENCE KYSTIQUE
DE LA GLANDE PINÉALE

par M. le docteur V. P. IOUKOVSKY,

de Saint-Pétersbourg.

La glande *pinéale (epiphysis cerebri)* est un organe appendiculaire développé sur la voûte du ventricule moyen; elle est située sous le bourrelet du corp calleux, en arrière et à l'entrée du troisième ventricule, dans le sillon sagittal qui sépare les tubercules quadrijumeaux antérieurs. C'est pour cela que les tumeurs de la glande pinéale peuvent comprimer l'*aqueduc de Sylvius* et la veine de *Galien*, fermer l'entrée de l'*aqueduc de Sylvius (aditus ad aquæductum Sylvii)*, compromettre le retour du sang veineux et entraîner une hydrocéphalie interne. Mais les tumeurs de la glande pinéale sont très rares chez les personnes adultes. En ce qui concerne les enfants, nous n'avons même trouvé aucune indication dans la littérature sur une telle localisation des tumeurs cérébrales; sans compter qu'il est en général bien rare de rencontrer des cas de tumeurs cérébrales congénitales.

L'hydrocéphalie congénitale, dans notre cas, atteignit des proportions si considérables, qu'elle avait presque entièrement détruit les hémisphères du cerveau, dont il n'y avait qu'un petit reste réuni à la pie-mère.

Néanmoins l'hydrocéphalie ne pouvait être diagnostiquée pendant la vie : le crâne n'était pas du tout agrandi et les dimensions se trouvaient normales, même les sutures et la grande fontanelle ne présentaient point de changements particuliers.

L'enfant naquit à terme, était bien développé et avait une bonne nutrition; il mourut au sixième jour de sa vie. Pendant la dissection du crâne. il s'écoula à peu près 500 centimètres cubes de liquide. La tumeur de la glande pinéale se trouvait devant les tubercules quadrijumeaux antérieurs et fermait entièrement l'*entrée de l'aqueduc de Sylvius*, il s'ensuivit l'hydrocéphalie.

Les détails cliniques de ce cas extrordinairement rare et les explications possibles des changements anatomiques seront fournis dans un mémoire détaillé (avec des planches).

LE RÉFLEXE DE LA PLANTE DU PIED CHEZ LES NOUVEAU-NÉS

par M. le docteur G. FINIZIO,

de Naples.

Qui parcourt les différents traités des maladies nerveuses ou des maladies des enfants, les plus récents y compris, peut facilement observer que nous manquons encore d'une étude organique sur la manière de se comporter des réflexes chez les enfants. Or, grâce à l'importante valeur sémiologique que l'étude des réflexes acquiert de plus en plus dans la neuropathologie; à présent qu'on n'étudie pas simplement leur absence ou leur présence, mais même l'intensité du mouvement provoqué. ainsi que sa forme et sa localisation, il ressort clairement que l'intérêt serait grand de l'évaluation exacte de ces symptômes objectifs.

Et cela spécialement chez les enfants, chez lesquels il n'est pas ordinairement permis d'étudier les symptômes subjectifs, et où quelquefois nous ne pouvons même pas bien apprécier les symptômes fonctionnels.

Mais pour réussir dans un tel but, il faut avant tout une connaissance exacte de la manière de se comporter des réflexes dans les conditions physiologiques. comment ils peuvent varier selon les différents âges de l'enfant, et quelles sont les modifications qu'ils peuvent subir dans les diverses aptitudes fonctionnelles que l'organisme en voie de développement acquiert de jour en jour. C'est certainement une étude vaste et difficile que j'ai seulement commencée. A présent je rapporte seulement l'étude sur le réflexe de la plante du pied faite sur 500 nouveau-nés à la *Maternità degli Incurabili*, où les enfants sont ordinairement soignés jusqu'au troisième jour pour passer ensuite dans l'asile de l'*Annunziata*.

Chez les nouveau-nés. il est fort difficile de bien observer ce réflexe, car il est difficile d'obtenir que les muscles du pied et de la jambe ne soient pas en état de contraction.

Pour exciter le réflexe, il faut patiemment attendre un moment où les muscles de la jambe et du pied soient en état de relâchement.

Comme Babinski l'a noté, il n'est pas indifférent d'exciter légèrement ou énergiquement, de chatouiller simplement ou de piquer la plante du pied. Cette dernière manière d'excitation ne provoque pas seulement des mouvements très vifs des différents segments des membres inférieurs, mais surtout provoque la contraction du membre, en sorte qu'une exacte évaluation du phénomène n'est pas possible. En outre, j'ai souvent observé que tandis que le chatouillement de la plante du pied produit la flexion des orteils, la piqûre, au contraire, produit l'extension des orteils.

Il faut donc bien considérer les deux modalités d'excitations, car cela pourrait expliquer les conclusions, non toujours uniformes, des différents observateurs.

Il est vrai que Babinski[1] dit seulement : « le chatouillement de la plante du pied provoque normalement chez le nouveau-né l'extension des orteils », mais il ne déclare pas si ce fait est constant. Muggia[2] dit seulement que chez les nouveau-nés tranquilles et sans autres stimulants, si l'on touche le côté intérieur du pied, on a généralement l'extension du gros orteil au lieu de la flexion. Giudiceandrea[3] soutient au contraire, que chez les nouveau-nés il n'a jamais pu observer un mouvement d'extension des doigts. Quelquefois il lui a paru voir un mouvement de flexion, mais à peine indiqué et très problématique.

Quant à moi, j'ai toujours employé le chatouillement avec un pinceau mou pour l'étude du mouvement des doigts du pied après l'excitation du réflexe de la plante. De la sorte j'ai pu constater que chez les nouveau-nés, du premier au troisième jour de vie, le réflexe de la plante manque 5 fois sur 100, apparaît d'une manière indécise 10 fois sur 100, provoque l'extension du seul gros orteil ou de tous les orteils 15 fois sur 100 : au contraire provoque la flexion des doigts 70 fois.

J'ai tâché d'étudier aussi avec le réflexe de la plante, proprement dit, les autres réflexes, qu'on peut considérer comme un appendice ou une modalité de ce réflexe. Ce sont le réflexe *antagoniste* de Schäffer[4], et le réflexe du *fascia lata* étudié par Brissaud[5]. Quant au réflexe antagoniste ainsi nommé par Schäffer, parce qu'il s'exerce sur les muscles antagonistes de ceux qui sont excités, voici ce que j'ai observé chez les nouveau-nés. Quand on saisit le tendon d'Achille au niveau de son tiers moyen et supérieur, entre le pouce d'un côté et l'index de l'autre et que l'on presse rudement, on constate que le nouveau-né donne des signes de souffrance et presque toujours fait une légère flexion du pied et parfois aussi du gros orteil. Piquant

1. BABINSKI. Du phénomène des orteils et de sa valeur sémiologique. *Semaine médicale*, 1898, p. 521.
2. MUGGIA. Del valore semeiotico del riflesso dell' alluce nei bambini. *Acad. de méd. de Turin*, 6 juillet 1900.
3. V. GIUDICEANDREA. Sul fenomeno delle dita del piede di Babinski. *Soc. Lausiriane des hôpitaux de Rome*, 1899.
4. SCHAEFFER. *Neurol. Centralbl.*, 15 novembre 1897.
5. BRISSAUD. *Gaz. heb. de méd. et de chirurg.*, 15 mars 1896.

ensuite la peau de la région du tendon d'Achille on observe que le
pied et les doigts font ordinairement le même mouvement. Lequel
est également identique à celui qui est noté, chez le même nouveau-
né, après l'excitation du réflexe de la plante, selon la méthode de
Babinski. Ces faits confirment l'opinion déjà exprimée par Babinski[1].
Le réflexe décrit par Schäffer n'est pas un réflexe *sui generis*, mais
bien le même phénomène du pied qui peut être provoqué non seulement en chatouillant la plante du pied, mais encore d'autres parties
de la peau. Il est vrai que la manière de se comporter du réflexe,
après les deux modalités d'excitation, n'est pas toujours identique.
Mais j'observe que, en se limitant à une seule modalité d'excitation,
comme en chatouillant la plante du pied, on voit des cas dans lesquels on provoque l'extension des doigts.

Brissaud déjà depuis 1896 a décrit sous le nom de réflexe du *fascia
lata* un réflexe particulier, qui, pour moi, n'est qu'une modalité du
réflexe de la plante. Il a observé parmi les adultes que quand on sti-
mule légèrement la plante du pied, on peut constater, presque toujours, une contraction des adducteurs et du couturier. Toutefois il
a constaté que la première contraction, presque toujours, est localisée
à l'extenseur du *fascia lata*. Moi aussi, après une légère stimulation,
j'ai souvent constaté l'adduction de la cuisse, mais je n'ai pas pu
vérifier si la première contraction s'était localisée au tenseur du *fascia
lata*. Très souvent, au contraire, j'ai observé que la stimulation énergique de la plante du pied donne lieu, outre l'adduction de la cuisse,
à des mouvements très vifs des divers segments du membre inférieur,
comme des doigts sur le pied, de celui-ci sur la jambe, de la jambe
sur la cuisse et de la cuisse sur le bassin. Quelquefois ces mouvements se sont propagés aussi au membre inférieur de l'autre côté,
avec un ordre de succession rappelant la loi des réflexes formulée par
Pflüger.

Enfin, quant à la manière de se comporter du réflexe de la plante
du pied en rapport avec les autres réflexes cutanés et tendineux, voici
ce que j'ai observé. Le réflexe de la plante du pied est parmi les réflexes cutanés celui qui s'observe le plus souvent. Au contraire, les
autres réflexes cutanés, comme l'épigastrique, l'abdominal, le fessier,
l'épinier manquent très souvent. Chez les nouveau-nés que j'ai examinés les réflexes cutanés ne présentaient pas cette vivacité que tout
le monde admet; au contraire, ceux-ci souvent manquaient tout à fait,
et je puis dire que l'existence du réflexe crémastérien est très rare.

---

1. BABINSKI. *Soc. de Neurol. de Paris.* 11 janvier 1903

Quand le réflexe de la plante manque, je n'ai observé la présence d'aucun autre réflexe cutané. Au contraire, le réflexe de la plante s'observe souvent chez les nouveau-nés, qui ne présentent aucun ou présentent seulement quelques-uns des réflexes cutanés. Dans des conditions semblables, quand le réflexe de la plante s'explique par l'extension des doigts, on observe plus constamment la présence des autres réflexes cutanés.

Le réflexe rotulien, comme le réflexe de la plante, s'observe toujours chez le nouveau-né[1]. Il y a nombre de cas où existe le réflexe de la plante et où manque le rotulien; mais plus rarement on observe le contraire. J'ai noté qu'il n'y a pas de rapport constant entre la modalité du réflexe de la plante et le réflexe du genou. Cependant la localisation du réflexe aux orteils coïncide avec le réflexe rotulien vif dans bien des cas. Le cas suivant mérite une mention particulière. Enfant né d'accouchement laborieux, qui présentait une céphalhématome. Un coup sec sur le tendon d'Achille ou encore en soulevant le membre inférieur par le gros orteil provoquait une série de mouvements du pied sur la jambe, une vraie trépidation épileptoïde : le réflexe rotulien était très vif : le réflexe de la plante du pied s'expliquait par la flexion des doigts. Ce cas rappelle quelques cas de maladie de Little, où également j'ai noté la flexion des doigts.

Mais ce cas est exceptionnel. Au contraire, dans la plus grande partie des nouveau-nés après l'accouchement laborieux ou avec l'aide des forceps j'ai noté, à côté du réflexe de la rotule vif, l'extension des doigts du pied. Dans quelques-uns de ces cas on pouvait observer même le réflexe tendineux du membre supérieur. Si l'on considère que l'accouchement laborieux et l'application des forceps peuvent produire des hémorragies dans les méninges et parfois aussi dans le cerveau, que ces conditions tiennent le premier rang dans l'étiologie de la maladie de Little, on comprend que ces symptômes soient dus, pour le moins, au dérangement fonctionnel des faisceaux pyramidaux.

J'ai noté l'extension des doigts du pied dans plusieurs cas de nouveau-nés en présentation irrégulière, tantôt de face, tantôt de sommet. Les deux cas suivants sont dignes de mention spéciale : 1º mâle de deux jours, né en présentation du sommet et avec application de forceps. Le réflexe rotulien est vif. Le réflexe de la plante présente à gauche flexion des doigts, à droite extension. Ayant examiné l'enfant le jour suivant, ces faits persistaient. 2º Garçon de deux jours.

1. Je l'ai trouvé chez 70 0/0 des nouveau-nés.

Né avec le secours des forceps pour accouchement prolongé. Le réflexe rotulien est normal. Le réflexe de la plante du pied provoque à droite la flexion des doigts et l'extension à gauche.

Il est très vraisemblable que ces faits dépendent de conditions particulières de la mécanique de l'accouchement, ou de l'application des forceps, qui ont produit une pression inégale sur les deux moitiés du crâne de l'enfant. Là où la pression a été plus intense la perturbation fonctionnelle des faisceaux pyramidaux s'est produite, et cela s'explique par l'extension des doigts du pied de côté opposé. A cet égard nous soutenons que Boeri pour le phénomène de Babinski, que Schäeffer pour son prétendu réflexe antagoniste ont proposé d'utiliser ce phénomène pour le diagnostic du côté de la lésion cérébrale.

Comme déjà Bednar, Babinski, Soltmann, Hochsinger, j'ai souvent observé chez le nouveau-né un certain degré de contracture musculaire, sensible particulièrement dans les membres inférieurs. Je crois fort vraisemblable que cette contracture consiste en une augmentation du ton musculaire par action réflexe, car j'ai souvent vu qu'il s'accentuait quand l'enfant pleurait ou était exposé au froid, ou si tout autre stimulant agissait sur la peau. Mais quel rapport existe-t-il entre ce réflexe particulier, qui constitue le ton musculaire (Muskense) et le réflexe de la plante du pied? Vraiment je n'ai pu apercevoir aucun rapport, car dans des cas semblables j'ai vérifié qu'il se produisait également l'extension de la flexion des doigts du pied. A cet égard je rapporte encore que chez les nouveau-nés, comme cela a été observé chez les adultes (van Geuschsten, Babinski, de Renzi et Toop), j'ai pu m'assurer qu'il n'y a pas de rapport non plus entre l'état du ton musculaire et celui des réflexes tendineux. Hochsinger[1] rapporte qu'il a observé des cas d'hypertonie des nourrissons avec contractures accentuées et toutefois avec réflexes tendineux et même cutanés très faibles. D'après cela, la *spasmophilie*, chez le nouveau-né, n'équivaut pas à la « disposition exagérée aux mouvements réflexes », au contraire de ce que Soltmann écrivait. Quand il y a hypertonie, les réflexes ne sont pas toujours exagérés.

De la même manière qu'il n'y a pas de correspondance entre les réflexes cutanés et les réflexes tendineux, ainsi il n'y a pas non plus de correspondance entre ces deux ordres des réflexes et celui qui constitue le ton musculaire.

1. Hochsinger. *Wiener medicinische Wochenschrift*, n° 7-12. 1900.

V

COMMUNICATIONS SUR LA DIPHTÉRIE

SUR UN ASPECT ACTINOMYCOSIQUE DU BACILLE DE LŒFFLER
DANS QUELQUES CONDITIONS DE SA VIE SAPROPHYTIQUE

RAPPORT

par **M**. le professeur Luigi **CONCETTI**,

Directeur de la clinique pédiatrique de l'Université Royale de Rome.

La différente morphologie dans laquelle peut se présenter le bacille de Löffler a été le point de départ de beaucoup de questions, et beaucoup de problèmes ont été posés sur le terrain de la discussion. Quelques-uns de ces problèmes regardent la valeur qu'on doit donner aux formes longues, clavées, enchevêtrées, vis-à-vis des formes petites, disposées parallèlement, ou à petits groupes, ou à V ou à L, etc. D'autres s'élèvent à des questions de nature plus haute, et se réfèrent aux traits d'union, aux affinités filogénitiques que le bacille de Löffler montre d'avoir avec d'autres bacilles similaires, par exemple celui de la tuberculose, celui de la morve, etc., et à la possibilité que ce groupe homogène des bacilles semble avoir avec un type d'origine commune représenté [par la famille des streptothrix, de laquelle ils seraient à considérer comme dérivés. Pour ce qui regarde la première question, je crois l'avoir résolue dans d'autres travaux précédents, et j'aurai l'occasion d'y revenir dans le cours de la discussion actuelle. Quant à l'autre, les difficultés sont bien plus graves, et jusqu'ici il n'y a que des observations isolées, incomplètes, et c'est par la réunion de ces observations qu'on a fondé une espèce de doctrine à laquelle néanmoins il faut encore une base plus solide qui jusqu'ici lui manque. C'est pour cela que je crois intéressant de porter à la connaissance de mes collègues un cas que j'ai eu l'occasion d'observer cette année dans ma clinique, non moins que les recherches auxquelles je me suis livré, et les résultats que j'ai obtenus. Et avant tout je viens en brefs traits à la description de ces cliniques.

La petite fille Starronelli Ada, 8 ans, me fut amenée le 1ᵉʳ février

1900. Les antécédents familiaux et personnels n'offrent rien d'intéressant. Il y a 15 jours, elle commença à se plaindre d'une laryngite qui s'est manifestée d'emblée avec une toux enrouée, aboyante, avec voilement de la voix, qui était elle aussi enrouée, et qui par degrés est arrivée à l'extinction presque complète. La respiration était difficile, peineuse, remouveuse, rude, et surtout pendant la nuit l'empêchait de dormir et l'obligeait à s'asseoir sur son lit pour s'aider avec tous les muscles auxiliaires de la respiration. La mère ne sait pas nous renseigner sur l'état de la température : mais il semble que la fièvre a manqué ou qu'elle fut très légère. La maladie, malgré une thérapie presque nulle, a eu un décours doux : la laryngite s'est prolongée en manière subaiguë. Toutefois tous les symptômes ont présenté une accentuation graduelle, surtout la sténose laryngée qui dans les trois derniers jours a pris le vrai caractère du tirage. L'examen de la gorge ne révéla qu'une légère hyperémie de la muqueuse. Du reste, pas de fièvre, par d'engorgements glandulaires. L'inspiration était rude, avec un bruit de scie qui s'entend à distance : on observa une légère rétraction du jugulum et de la base de la poitrine. Pas de cyanose. L'examen laryngoscopique releva une hyperémie avec exsudation catarrhale de la muqueuse, un léger œdème sous-coudal et une parésie des muscles crico-arythénoïdiens postérieurs.

Nous sommes tellement habitués à considérer le croup diphtérique comme une maladie essentiellement aiguë, que je trouve bien justifié le doute qu'en présence d'un cas pareil la plupart des médecins puissent avancer sur la nature diphtérique de ces formes de laryngite. Mais, d'autre part, je ne saurais oublier que la diphtérie peut bien présenter non seulement un décours subaigu, mais aussi chronique, et que le larynx est une localité qui depuis le nez a la propriété de se prêter à ce prolongement de la forme chronique (1). D'ailleurs nous nous trouvions en pleine épidémie de diphtérie ; de sorte que je me trouvais justifié de proposer à mes élèves le diagnostic de laryngite subaiguë de nature probablement diphtérique, sauf à attendre le résultat de l'examen bactériologique. Je pratique une injection de 1000 u. j. de sérum antidiphtérique, et fais appliquer des compresses froides autour du cou et inhaler deux fois par jour une solution de

1. CONCETTI. Un caso di difteria chronica. *Arch. di Pathol. infant. Napoli*, 1884. — Sulla difterite primitiva delle narici, éd. 1892. — Sur la difterite cronica del naso, *idem* 1892. — Studi clinici e ricerche experimentali sulla difterite, Roma 1894. — La difterite. Tratt. ital. di Patol. del Prof. Managliano. Milano 1896. — A proposito del prolungarii di alcuni forme difteriche nella laringe. *Bull. della Accad. med. di Roma* 1896. — Rendiconti della clinica Pediatrica di Roma 1894-1898.

formaline à 1-2 0 0. Dans le même temps j'ai recueilli les matériaux pour l'examen bactériologique.

Depuis deux jours (5 février) la respiration était moins rude, moins remouveuse : la voix et la toux gardaient les mêmes caractères : l'amélioration de la sténose a permis à la malade de dormir plus tranquille. On injecta en outre 2000 u. i. de serum. L'examen microscopique du tampon précédent a cependant décelé beaucoup de formes bacillaires colorables avec la méthode spécifique de Neisser. Nous reviendrons tout à l'heure sur la morphologie de ces formes bacillaires et sur leurs propriétés culturales. Pour le moment nous avions la certitude d'avoir affaire à une forme certainement diphtérique.

Le 5 février l'amélioration était plus notable pour la sténose laryngée qui la faisait dormir bien la nuit : la respiration était tranquille et à peine entendait-on un peu de bruit inspiratoire lorsque la petite fille se trouvait agitée, ou si elle voulait faire une inspiration forcée. Il n'y avait pas plus de vaintument du jugulum ni de la base de la poitrine. La toux et la voix étaient toujours un peu enrouées, bitonales, un peu voilées, mais à un moindre degré. On injecta encore 2000 u. i. et on poursuivit avec les inhalations de formaline. L'observation bactériologique donna pour la deuxième fois les mêmes formes bacillaires.

L'amélioration a continué d'une manière progressive, constante, bien que lente. L'examen bactériologique fait voir une diminution de l'élément bacillaire qui a disparu complètement depuis la deuxième semaine. Les urines ont été toujours normales.

En conclusion nous nous sommes trouvés en face d'une diphtérie laryngée, d'un croup diphtérique à décours subaigu, prolongé, de la durée de presque deux mois : une forme légère, sans phénomènes d'empoisonnement général, qui a pu rester pendant 15 jours sans aucun traitement, mais qui allait empirant progressivement. Le traitement spécifique sérothérapique a arrêté la maladie, mais pas tout d'un coup, mais par degrés, avec une extrême lenteur, jusqu'à la guérison. Le traitement local avec les inhalations de formaline a aidé le traitement spécifique. Et jusqu'ici le cas n'est pas destiné à susciter trop de merveilles, parce que, comme je l'ai dit, il n'est pas excessivement rare. Mais ce qui donne beaucoup d'intérêt au cas actuel c'est le résultat des recherches bactériologiques, comme nous le verrons tout à l'heure.

Comme il est connu par des publications précédentes (1), mon chef

1. VALAGUSSA. Contributo alla rapida diagnosi batteriologica della difterita. Roma 1897. Suppl. Policlin. — Idem, *ibid.*, 1900. — CONCETTI. Rasche Methode zur bacteriologischen Diagnose der Diphtheritis. *Wien. Medic. Woch.*, 1900, n° 10.

de clinique, le D^r Fr. Valagussa, a proposé une méthode très pratique pour le diagnostic bactériologique rapide de la diphtérie. Nous nous servons d'un tampon de coton hydrophile monté sur un bâton de verre, trempé en un terrain de culture composé de : agar, résine et glucose, et enfermé dans un tube, le tout naturellement bien stérilisé. Avec ce tampon nous recueillons les matériaux dans la gorge, dans l'ouverture du larynx, dans les fausses membranes, etc. ; et après l'avoir rapidement enfermé de nouveau dans le tube on met celui-ci dans l'étuve à 35-37 degrés. Après 4-5 heures on le retire, et on glisse légèrement, en le roulant, ce tampon sur un verre porte-objet bien lavé et stérilisé, on le dessèche, on le fixe à la lampe, et on le colore avec la méthode de Neisser, c'est-à-dire en premier temps avec une solution de bleu de méthylène avec acide acétique et alcool pendant 4-5 secondes, et ensuite avec une solution de vésuvine pendant 15-20 secondes. Toute la préparation, tous les microbes restent colorés en jaune, les bacilles pseudo-diphtériques aussi : les bacilles de Löffer au contraire présentent aux deux extrémités deux points fortement colorés en bleu foncé. Lorsqu'il y a de grands amas de bacilles, à première vue, on a l'impression de voir une masse de cocci très petits ; mais on voit aisément que ces points bleus sont tous disposés deux à deux, et on voit autour d'eux dessiné le bacille en jaune. Cela existe évidemment dans les bacilles isolés. Il n'y a que quelques sarcines qui prennent la coloration bleue, mais il est très facile de les distinguer. Ces préparations apparaissent très nitides et élégantes.

L'observation directe des matériaux recueillis nous a donné, comme je l'ai annoncé, des formes bacillaires parfaitement colorées avec le Neisser. Il y avait çà et là quelques rares petites formes, mais en général prédominaient les formes bacillaires longues, grosses, clavées, non colorables en toute leur extension, comme divisées en 3, 4, 10 segments bien colorés et comme tenus en place par la membrane externe du bacille ; quelques-unes étaient disposées en corne de cerf terminé par une grosse boule. On observait aussi des formes de cocci (staphylocoque pyog. doré), et quelques liquéfiants banals. Le résultat a été le même pour les quatre observations successives que nous avons faites.

L'examen cultural a donné des résultats tout à fait surprenants. Dans les cultures en plaques de agar en boîtes de Petri avec la méthode des trois dilutions, depuis 48 heures de thermostate, dans la première boîte la surface s'est recouverte d'une quantité énorme de petites colonies qui en se confluant ont formé une pellicule sèche, épaisse, compacte, croûteuse, d'une couleur jaune orange foncé.

Dans la deuxième boîte il y avait aussi une grande quantité de ces colonies jaunes, sèches, relevées, bosselées, croûteuses, adhérentes au substratum, à bords sinueux. Dans la troisième il n'y avait que trois de ces colonies. En plus on y voyait des colonies de staphylocoques, et d'autres pâles, d'un bacille liquéfiant. Ces colonies jaunes rappelaient exactement celles des diverses streptothrix, de l'actynomycose, de la tuberculose, etc. Le passage avec ensemencement en stries sur tubes de agar-agar donnait depuis 24 heures un développement de petites colonies qui rappelaient celles de la diphtérie normale ; depuis 48 heures elles tendaient à se réunir et à former une pellicule jaune orangé, sèche, qui devint de plus en plus épaisse, et se releva en tubercules durs, croûteux, mamelonnés. Sur sérum de Löffler elles présentaient les mêmes caractères, sans le liquifier. Les cultures sur pigrine en gélatine formaient à la surface une pellicule légère avec un bouton central au point d'enfoncement, bouton qui se ride et se durcit ; le long du canal de la pigrine se formaient des rubans terminés en un petit grain de millet ; la gélatine ne se liquéfiait pas. Dans le bouillon se formaient à la surface de petites colonies avec un point central plus foncé avec un alon plus clair, et depuis, un deuxième alon, jusqu'à former une pellicule qui tomba au fond sans troubler le liquide. Sur pommes de terre trempées en NaCl se formaient de petites colonies humides, d'un jaune pâle, peu adhérentes. Sur blanc d'œuf solidifié les petites colonies jaunâtres restaient isolées, minces, et aisément détachables, sans former pellicule.

Avec des passages périodiques, chaque 3-4 semaine, sur d'autres tubes d'agar on observait une diminution de l'activité culturale, avec pellicule moins épaisse, moins croûteuse, mais toujours sèche, plissée, ondulée, ratatinée, et une diminution du pigment.

Pour ce qui regarde la morphologie du microrganisme constituant ces cultures, les premières étaient formées presque exclusivement de bacilles très longs, filamenteux, à contenu grossièrement granuleux, clavés, etc. On avait la sensation de voir de longues chaînes de cocci ; mais il était facile de se convaincre qu'on avait affaire à la division en granulations du protoplasma du filament restées en disposition streptococciforme par les parois du filament moins bien colorées. Les granulations prenaient fort bien la coloration, tandis que les espaces intermédiaires ne se coloraient pas ; quelques traits du filament restaient aussi décolorés. Parfois on croyait voir des vraies ramifications. Les formes petites étaient fort rares à voir. Après trois ou quatre mois de passages on ne voyait au microscope que de grands amas de cocci, quelques-uns légèrement allongés en forme bacillaire ; il n'était pas rare de voir 2, 3, 5 de ces cocci encore disposés en petites chaînettes. Tout cela donnait l'idée que ces cocci, ces petits bâtonnets, ces gros bacilles à 2, 3, 5 granulations, n'étaient que la division, la fragmentation des longs filaments granuleux des premières cultures : n'étaient que les anciennes granulations qui avaient acquis leur liberté et leur individualité (spores) ; que tout cela n'était que l'effet de la segmentation, de la multiplication des gros et longs bacilles avec dégénération et résorption de la paroi externe, qui restait en quelques endroits à témoigner son existence. Si la culture en agar a cette apparence cocciforme on la passe en bouillon, après 24 heures on la trouve constituée de petits bacilles à l'apparence du vrai bacille de Löffler typique. Cet aspect bacillaire caractéristique de diphtérie on le trouve aussi sur les passages en pommes de terre. Il n'y a plus trace de filaments. Dans les cultures intermédiaires on observe des formes bacillaires petites, enflées : des formes en fuseaux, des claves, de grosses formes sphérulaires isolées ou réunies, et de rares filaments.

Toutes ces cultures se sont montrées tout à fait dépourvues de tout pouvoir pathogène. Aussi avec les injections endoveineuses : aussi avec les inoculations endopéritonéales n'avons-nous jamais pu observer la formation des productions nodulaires caractéristiques des espèces pathogènes de la famille des streptothrix (actinomycose).

A ce point, sachant que parmi les streptothrix les espèces les plus anaérobiennes sont celles qui se prêtent le mieux à la vie parasitaire, nous avons cherché d'essayer l'influence que la culture en anaérobiose pourrait avoir sur nos microrganismes. C'est pour cela que nous l'avons ensemencée en bouillon à l'abri de l'air et de l'oxygène. Après 8 à 10 heures nous avons constaté un développement évident, et après 24 heures la formation d'une pellicule assez épaisse, friable, qui tomba au fond du liquide. Transportée sur agar agar en strie, a donné de petites colonies pâles, et par leur confluence une pellicule mince, comme il arrive avec le vrai bacille de Löffler typique. Aussi la morphologie du microbe était celle du bacille diphtérique normal. Enfin sur les animaux a montré avoir gagné son pouvoir pathogène et toxinogène. En effet l'injection de 3-5 cmc. de culture en bouillon sous la peau des cobayes et des lapins très jeunes les tuait en 4 ou 6 jours avec infiltration hémorragique et œdème, parfois avec nécrose du tissu conjonctif au point d'inoculation, avec infiltration hémorragique des capsules surrénales, et parfois avec péricardite hémorragique et œdème pulmonaire. Les mêmes cultures filtrées et privées des germes ont donné les mêmes résultats. Et ce qui est plus intéressant, le sérum antidiphtérique a montré posséder une action protectrice contre les effets des injections de nos cultures et de nos filtrats.

C'est avec tous ces artifices que nous avons réussi à reconduire nos microrganismes du type actinomycosique, non pathogène, au vrai type du bacille de Löffler pathogène, toxicogène. Mais comment est-ce que nous devons considérer ces transformations?

Tout le monde connaît les affinités qui existent entre le bacille de la diphtérie, celui de la tuberculose, celui de la morve, et les relations pilogénétiques qu'on suppose avoir tous ces germes avec un type unique représenté par la famille des streptothrix. Au début on considérait les streptothrix comme de simples saprophytes. Plus tard on a rapproché d'eux certains organismes pathogènes (actinomycose, farcin de bœuf, pied de madura, etc.), et aujourd'hui tous ces cas forment un groupe bien homogène. Les bacilles de la tuberculose, de la diphtérie, de la morve peuvent présenter des éléments nettement ramifiés avec des caractères culturaux semblables. L'influence du changement de milieu, certains agents physiques peuvent déterminer des variations de forme, et des manifestations culturales et pathogènes. Il y a cependant une condition nécessaire pour bien apprécier ces variations, et c'est le retour constant à la forme primitive typique lorsque de tels éléments soient placés dans les conditions de vie normales. Le cas actuel me semble destiné à donner la preuve authentique de cette dérivation. Les recherches de Noeske (1) ont révélé que dans ces conditions exceptionnelles de l'organisme, et seulement dans ces conditions, le bacille de la tuberculose peut se montrer chez les lapins en une forme spéciale rayonnée semblable à l'actinomycose. La quantité énorme des cellules et des granulations éosinophiles qui se trouvent dans les tissus seraient l'indice de cette défense de l'organisme. Il y a beaucoup d'espèces microbiennes qui dans des conditions défavorables, en défaut de nutrition, présentent des changements de forme et de propriétés (b. acati, b. subtilis, b. antracis, b. piocianis, etc.), avec le retour complet et rapide à la forme normale que de tels éléments modifiés tératologiquement se trouvent placés dans le milieu habituel. J'ai trouvé que juste le bacille de Löffler dans des conditions défavorables (vieillesse des cultures, symbiose avec le streptocoque) peut prendre des formes anormales, en filaments, clavés, avec protoplasma qui se divise en grosses granulations, à disposition rayonnée avec diminution du pouvoir toxinogène, etc. (2) ; et je voyais en ces

<hr>

1. *Deut. Zeit. f. Chir.*, 1900, Bd 55, H. 5, n° 4.
2. CONCETTI e MEMMO. Sulla tossicita del bacillo di Löffler in rapporto ella sua morphologia. *Ann. di Igiène sperimentale*, 1898, VIII.

variations un trait d'union pilogénétique qui le réunissait au bacille
de la tuberculose, un rappel à la critique au type primitif de l'actynomycose, des streptothrix. Peut-être que l'organisme humain aussi
peut fournir lui-même des conditions défavorables analogues (leucocytes?) Quelquefois ces conditions défavorables pourront agir superficiellement, avec la possibilité d'un retour rapide, plus ou moins, aux
conditions primitives. Mais en maintes circonstances ces modifications pourront être profondes, et rester vraiment héréditaires, dans
les générations successives. Et alors il faut voir si on peut trouver
des expédients pour le reconduire au type primitif. Nous y reviendrons
tout à l'heure.

L'école française, d'après les conclusions de M. Martin, a prétendu
que les formes bacillaires grosses, clavées, enchevêtrées, du bacille
de Löffler soient à considérer comme les seules normales, vraiment
pathogènes, jusqu'à nier la nature diphtérique des formes petites,
jusqu'à proclamer l'abstention dans ce cas de l'intervention avec le
traitement sérothérapique. Je me suis plusieurs fois élevé contre ces
conclusions qui sont extrêmement dangereuses dans la pratique. J'ai
démontré jusqu'à l'évidence que la production de toxine est immen-
sément [plus active dans les formes petites, et qu'elle est minime
dans les formes grandes. J'en ai apporté aussi la preuve clinique, et le
cas actuel n'est qu'une démonstration en plus de ma thèse.

La formation des claves est pour la plupart des observateurs l'indice
d'une dégénération, d'une condition défavorable dans laquelle se
trouve le microrganisme. Nous l'avons vu pour la diphtérie, Noeske
pour la tuberculose, Hansen pour le b. aceti, etc. Même dans l'actinomycose la formation des claves représenterait une altération dégé-
nératrice qui commence dans les vieilles cultures par un renflement
des filaments, tandis que la formation de la clave ne commence qu'a-
près l'inoculation sur les animaux par l'action délétère des leucocytes (Benda). La clave ne représenterait qu'un élément dégénéré,
mort.

Il faut admettre qu'en beaucoup de cas, dans des conditions spéciales de résistance de la part de l'organisme (rôle des leucocytes?)
le bacille de Löffler peut se trouver dans des conditions telles qu'il
réduise à néant son pouvoir pathogène, et se montre dans le maximum des apparences actinomycosiformes (diphtéries bénignes). Quelquefois cette condition est transitoire. Mais en d'autres circonstances
elle peut avoir opéré profondément au point que ces variations peuvent persister, devenir héréditaires et se reproduire dans les générations successives, et porter l'observateur à se tromper, hors de la

bonne voie, et l'induire dans la persuasion d'avoir à faire avec une forme commune de streptotrix, et de lui attribuer un rôle diphtéroïde en écartant absolument le bacille de Löffler. Tout récemment le professeur Trambusti vient de présenter à l'Académie de médecine de Palerme (1) dans la séance du 19 avril 1900 un cas de stomatite diphtéroïde légère avec des formes bacillaires en longs filaments ramifiés, qui donnaient des coloris blanchâtres, dorés, rappelant les streptothrix. Plus récemment le professeur Silvestrini à l'Académie physicale de Fivense dans la séance du 27 juin 1900 a exposé avoir isolé d'une angine diphtéroïde des bacilles pyriformes avec des spirochaetes, se demandant s'ils ne pourraient représenter une condition spéciale d'être du bacille de Löffler. Mya dit avoir observé des formes analogues.

Dans nos cas nous avons eu une forme bacillaire qui, pour l'aspect morphologique, pour la qualité de ses propriétés culturales, pour la production de substance chromogène, pour le manque de pouvoir pathogène spécifique, et de toute production de toxine, donnait à croire qu'on avait affaire à une forme pure et simple de streptotrix. Les modifications dans les passages successifs reproduisent les modifications qui s'observent aussi dans ces microrganismes. Si nous nous rapportons à la description que Boström et Gasparini donnent de l'actinomycose, nous y lisons tout ce que nous avons observé dans nos recherches sur le notri-microrganisme. En effet les auteurs cités s'expriment ainsi : « L'actinomycose est un champignon filamenteux, ondulé ou en spirale : ramifications qui après se séparent, se divisent en filaments, en bâtonnets plus longs, en petits bacilles, en formes sphériques, en petits cocci. De ces cocci se forment de nouveau de petits bacilles, des bâtonnets qui s'allongent, se ramifient, et prennent quelquefois la forme clavée : les granulations sphériques, produit de la division des protoplasmes, sont maintenues en chaînettes par le résidu de la paroi micéliale ; granulations à qui on a donné le significatif de vraies spores. »

Si nous avions arrêté nos recherches à ce point-là, nous aussi aurions dû arriver à la conclusion que cette forme de laryngite subaiguë était en rapport causal avec un streptothrix. Mais nous avions la persuasion intime d'avoir affaire à une diphtérie aussi par la preuve favorable du traitement avec le sérum antidiphtérique. Seulement nous étions convaincus que les conditions défavorables qui devaient avoir agi sur nos microrganismes devaient avoir agi d'une

---

1. V. *Riforma Medica*, 5 mai 1900.
2. *Ibid.*, 24 juillet 1900.

manière profonde, de sorte à faire transmettre aussi dans les générations successives, d'une manière héréditaire, les modifications, les variations induites sur le bacille même. Dans ce cas il était nécessaire de rechercher quelles pouvaient être les conditions qui auraient pu le reconduire au type primordial. Nous avons choisi la culture en anaérobiose pour les raisons exposées auparavant ; et nous y avons réussi, jusqu'à obtenir le retour au pouvoir pathogène, à la production de la toxine.

En mettant en rapport les résultats de nos recherches bactériologiques sur le cas actuel avec tout ce que nous avons vu à propos des formes longues que nous avons isolées en d'autres cas cliniques et obtenues dans le laboratoire, il n'était pas absurde de penser que nos microrganismes actinomycosiformes ne pourraient représenter une manière spéciale d'être du bacille de Löffler durable et héréditaire. La culture en anaérobiose a été la condition qui l'a reconduit au type primitif normal avec ses propriétés morphologiques, culturales et pathogènes. C'est ainsi que nous avons pu l'étudier dans les deux conditions, et avoir la démonstration que sa vie saprophytique n'est qu'une variété de la grande famille des streptothrix. Jusqu'à ce moment-ci on en avait seulement une preuve d'induction fournie par les quelques apparences morphologiques. Mais on n'avait jamais, à ce que je sache, décrit des cas dans lesquels ces variations seraient en manière durable héréditaire de faire croire à une vraie forme actinomycosique, ou tout au moins de donner la démonstration de la dérivation de la forme actinomycoïde en la reportant à la vraie forme bacillaire typique du bacille diphtérique.

Si maintenant nous faisons une comparaison entre le bacille de Löffler en vie parasitaire et celui qui vit saprophytiquement en vieillissant dans les cultures, et la forme actinomycosique que nous venons d'étudier, nous pouvons noter les faits suivants : 1° Le bacille de Löffler à forme petite représente le premier degré d'une échelle dans laquelle nous voyons s'épuiser le pouvoir pathogène au fur et à mesure que des formes petites et moyennes on passe aux formes grandes, clavées, géantes; 2° Dans la forme actinomycosique les figures clavées, ramifiées représentent le maximum de l'activité culturale avec un pouvoir pathogène minime ou nul; c'est par degrés que nous venons (depuis la culture en anaérobiose) aux formes moyennes et petites où il reprend son pouvoir pathogène ; 3° Les formes grosses, clavées, représentent par conséquent le parasitisme de la forme actinomycosique (type primordial), tandis que les formes grosses des vieilles cultures représentent le saprophytisme de la forme parasitaire. La même chose s'avère dans la tuberculose qui, en exaltant son activité culturale, tend à perdre son pouvoir pathogène et à se transformer en formes grandes, clavées, rayonnées. La forme clavée qui pourrait représenter, si on peut le dire, le maximum du parasitisme possible de la forme actinomycosique, de l'autre côté, ne représente que le minimum de l'activité pathogène dans la forme parasitaire.

Or il faudrait étudier si parmi les sortes de variétés des streptothrix qui se trouvent dans l'air, dans les eaux, dans le sol, dans l'organisme lui-même, surtout dans la bouche et dans les premières voies respiratoires, et qui vivent en saprophytes, il n'y a pas des espèces qui, mises en conditions favorables, ne pourraient se transformer en espèces pathogènes, en formes diphtériques. Nous pourrons peut-être trouver l'application de tant de cas de diphtérie qui éclatent sous forme endémique à l'abri de tout foyer épidémique, et de tant de cas de latence de la diphtérie en certains endroits, où un cas de diphtérie pousse depuis 1 ou 2 ans après des autres. C'est une étude que je me propose de faire et qui pourra jeter une grande lumière sur tant de problèmes épidémiologiques.

REMARQUES SUR 1778 CAS DE DIPHTÉRIE

par M. le docteur H. RICHARDIÈRE,

Médecin de l'Hôpital Trousseau.

J'ai été chargé pendant les trois années 1897, 1898 et 1899 du traitement de la diphtérie à l'hôpital Trousseau, ou des hôpitaux d'enfants de la ville de Paris. Pendant ce temps, j'ai dû soigner 1778 enfants, tous atteints de diphtérie, vérifiée par l'examen bactériologique. Le traitement a consisté, dans tous les cas, sans exception, en injections de sérum antidiphtérique de Roux, fourni par l'Institut Pasteur de Paris. La plupart des enfants n'ont été injectés qu'une fois. Quelques-uns ont reçu deux injections. Exceptionnellement, trois injections ont été pratiquées.

Ce que je désire faire connaître à la section de Pédiatrie du Congrès international de médecine, ce sont les résultats fournis par la sérothérapie antidiphtérique dans ces 1778 cas de diphtérie et aussi les remarques que j'ai faites sur la diphtérie, sur ses complications, sur les associations microbiennes.

I

Statistique des 1778 cas de diphtérie.

Mes 1778 cas de diphtérie se répartissent de la façon suivante : 696 en 1897, 498 en 1898 et 584 en 1899.

En comprenant tous les cas sans exception, même ceux où l'enfant a été apporté mourant à l'hôpital, même ceux où il est mort au moment de son entrée avant toute intervention médicale, les 1778 cas ont donné 280 morts, soit une mortalité de 15.74 pour 100.

Si des 1778 cas, on déduit 75 cas de morts dans les vingt-quatre heures après l'entrée à l'hôpital, c'est-à-dire dans les conditions où le traitement n'avait pas encore pu faire sentir son action, il reste 205 morts, soit une mortalité de 11, 50 pour 100.

En rapprochant ces chiffres de la mortalité par diphtérie à l'hôpital Trousseau pendant les années 1890, 1891, 1892 où le traitement par le sérum antitoxique n'était pas encore institué, on juge immédiatement l'efficacité du traitement sérothérapique et on voit dans quelles proportions ce traitement a diminué la mortalité de la diphtérie.

En effet, pendant les années 1890, 91, et 92, il y a eu 5176 entrées pour diphtérie à l'hôpital Trousseau. Ces 5176 entrées ont donné 1544 guérisons et 1757 morts, soit une mortalité de 54,68 pour 100. Encore convient-il de faire remarquer que les 5176 comprenaient vraisemblablement un certain nombre d'angines et de laryngites admises par erreur à la diphtérie, le plus souvent moins graves que la diphtérie elle-même, et que dans notre statistique nous ne tenons compte que des cas vérifiés par la clinique et par l'examen bactériologique.

On peut dire actuellement qu'avec le traitement par le sérum le pronostic de la diphtérie ne nécessitant pas d'opération sur le larynx (tubage et trachéotomie) est devenu réellement presque bénin. En effet, sur mes 1778 cas, 1115 rentrent dans cette catégorie (diphtéries sans opération sur le larynx). Ce sont les angines avec ou sans autre manifestation diphtérique, les coryzas, les vulvites, les conjonctivites, les croups non opérés. Ils donnent 61 morts, soit une mortalité de 5,54 pour 100.

Il n'en est plus de même lorsque l'opération sur le larynx devient nécessaire. Sur 450 croups tubés une ou plusieurs fois, j'ai eu 116 morts, soit une mortalité de 27 pour 100.

Dans 27 cas, où la trachéotomie a été faite sans tubage antérieur, il y a eu 9 morts, soit une mortalité de 33,33 pour 100.

Enfin lorsque, le tubage étant insuffisant pour remédier à l'obstruction du larynx, il faut recourir à la trachéotomie après le tubage infructueux, le pronostic est très grave. Sur 141 trachéotomies secondaires, j'ai eu 84 morts, soit une mortalité de 59,60 pour 100.

II

Technique du traitement.

Je rappellerai en quelques mots seulement la façon dont ont été soignés mes malades, tous enfants, dont le plus jeune avait 4 mois et le plus âgé 16 ans.

Tous ont reçu au moins une injection de sérum antidiphtérique de Roux. La dose de sérum a été de 10 centimètres cubes pour les enfants âgés de moins d'un an, de 15 centimètres cubes entre 1 an et 2 ans. Au-dessus de 2 ans, tous les malades ont été injectés de 20 centimètres cubes.

Comme traitement local, on a fait de grands lavages de la bouche ou du nez, et, dans les cas de diphtérie de la peau ou de la muqueuse des organes génitaux, des applications locales avec une solution de permanganate de chaux à 1/4000ᵉ.

Les badigeonnages de la gorge n'ont pas été généralement employés. Il me semble qu'ils ont plus d'inconvénients que d'avantages. Les badigeonnages même pratiqués sans violence font souvent saigner la muqueuse et en ouvrant un certain nombre de capillaires sanguins et lymphatiques facilitent certainement l'absorption des toxines diphtériques et les injections secondaires par les micro-organismes qui pullulent dans la bouche. Ils sont, d'autre part, rendus difficiles par la résistance de la plupart des enfants. Les employer méthodiquement m'a paru supprimer un des avantages du traitement par le sérum, d'une simplicité si opportune chez les enfants.

J'ai réservé les badigeonnages pour les cas, rares à la vérité, où les fausses membranes auraient une tendance à se reproduire malgré les injections de sérum répétées plusieurs fois. En pareil cas, il me paraît hors de doute que des attouchements avec un topique tel que la glycérine ou sublimé au trentième ou l'eau oxygénée fraîchement préparée facilitent la chute des membranes et empêchent leur reproduction. J'ajouterai que je n'ai jamais vu ces cas de reproduction indéfinie des fausses membranes, ces cas de diphtérie chronique qu'on observait parfois avant l'emploi du sérum et que Cadet de Gassicourt avait décrits dans ses cliniques de l'hôpital Trousseau.

Accidents imputables au traitement par le sérum.

Les accidents imputables au traitement par le sérum ont été sans importance. Après plusieurs années de pratique du traitement sérothérapique, après des milliers d'observations de ce traitement, on peut proclamer hautement qu'il est inoffensif, autrement moins dangereux que l'emploi de la plupart des médicaments quelque peu toxiques, dont nous nous servons en médecine infantile.

Pour ma part, je n'ai observé aucun accident vraiment sérieux.

Voici ce que j'ai vu :

Sur plus de 5000 injections de sérum, j'ai observé 4 fois un abcès au niveau de la piqûre. L'abcès, dû certainement à un défaut d'antisepsie locale, était assez volumineux. Il renfermait une quantité abondante de pus fétide, avec des streptocoques en quantité énorme. Ces abcès ont été incisés. Après l'incision, les enfants ont guéri rapidement. Une fois, sans que j'aie pu savoir comment le fait pouvait être interprété, il y a eu simultanément un abcès au niveau de la piqûre, dans le flanc droit, et un autre abcès à distance dans la région de la cuisse droite.

Les accidents les plus fréquents ont été les éruptions sériques. Je les ai observées chez 198 enfants. Chose remarquable, elles se sont souvent produites par série. Nous restions plusieurs semaines sans en observer, puis brusquement plusieurs de nos enfants en étaient atteints simultanément. Il m'est arrivé à un certain moment d'en observer sur la moitié des enfants soignés dans les salles.

J'ai observé cinq variétés de types éruptifs :

1° Le type scarlatiniforme (140 fois) ;

2° Le type d'urticaire (52 fois) ;

3° Le type d'érythème polymorphe (16 fois) ;

4° Le type de roséole (8 fois) ;

5° Le type de purpura (2 fois).

Quelquefois, ces types ont existé simultanément ou se sont succédé chez le même enfant à quelques jours d'intervalle.

On a noté la date d'apparition de ces exceptions et on a trouvé que les éruptions scarlatiniformes s'étaient montrées :

Le 2e jour après l'injection	8 fois.
Le 3e —	18 —
Le 4e —	58 —
Le 5e —	54
Le 6e —	10 —
Le 7e —	8 —
Le 9e —	6 —
Après le 10e jour	12 fois.

Les deux plus tardives ont apparu le 15e jour.

Les exceptions à type d'urticaire ont eu le début suivant :

Le 3e jour.   2 fois.
Le 4e   —   6   —
Le 6e   —   2   —
Le 7e   —   4   —
Le 8e   —   2   —
Le 9e   —   2   —
Après le 10e jour. . . . .   10 fois.

La plus tardive a eu lieu le 14e jour.

Les éruptions à type d'érythème polymorphe se sont montrées toutes après le 10e jour, du 10e au 15e.

Des éruptions de roséole, 4 ont apparu avant le 10e jour, 2 après.

Les éruptions de purpura ont été les plus tardives de toutes. On les a observées le 16e et le 18e jour après l'injection.

Quelle qu'ait été la variété de l'éruption, les symptômes qui l'ont précédée ou accompagnée ont été à peu près invariablement les mêmes. L'éruption a été précédée de quelques heures par une légère élévation de température de 1 degré à 1 degré et demi. Puis, l'éruption est devenue appréciable, accompagnée le plus souvent d'une diarrhée assez abondante, d'odeur fétide.

Généralement l'éruption n'a pas duré plus de vingt-quatre à quarante-huit heures et a disparu rapidement avec la diarrhée qui l'a accompagnée.

Des accidents articulaires ont suivi quelquefois les injections de sérum (dans 15 cas).

Ils ont accompagné ou suivi les éruptions, jamais ils ne se sont montrés isolément.

Le plus souvent, ils ont consisté dans des douleurs articulaires, dans des arthralgies frappant diverses articulations des membres sans réaction inflammatoire des jointures. Les enfants se plaignaient de souffrir des jointures sans qu'il y eût ni rougeur ni gonflement des articulations.

Dans 5 cas seulement, il y a eu des arthrites vraies avec rougeur de la peau, gonflement des articulations et signes d'épanchement articulaire dans les genoux. Ces arthrites ont d'ailleurs cédé dans l'espace de quelques jours à des applications locales de salicylate de méthyle.

Les accidents que je viens d'énumérer sont les seuls que je puisse attribuer en toute certitude au sérum antidiphtérique.

Plus douteuse est l'influence du sérum dans deux faits que j'ai observés et que je crois peut-être dus à son action.

Ce sont deux cas d'hyperthermie, à forme intermittente, que j'ai notés dans les conditions suivantes.

Deux enfants ont eu en même temps que des éruptions urticariennes une température très élevée qui est montée le premier jour à 40 degrés et quelques dixièmes. L'éruption a pâli rapidement, mais la fièvre a persisté dans un cas huit jours et dans l'autre quatorze jours. La température était intermittente. Le soir, elle était très élevée, dépassant 39 degrés. Le matin, elle redevenait normale. Il n'y avait aucun symptôme autre que la fièvre, digne d'être relevé! Ces deux enfants ont guéri sans autre accident.

Le sulfate de quinine n'a eu aucune action sur la température.

Ces deux enfants habitaient Paris et n'avaient jamais eu d'accident d'impaludisme. Leur rate était normale.

III

Le pronostic de la diphtérie, telle que nous l'observons à l'hôpital Trousseau avec une mortalité totale de 15,74 pour 100 et réduite de 11,50 pour 100 est-il encore susceptible de s'améliorer ou devons-nous admettre que la sérothérapie ne puisse jamais de résultats encore plus favorables?

Pour répondre à cette question, il nous faut montrer quelles ont été les principales causes de la mort des enfants diphtériques.

Dans la grande majorité des cas, la mort a été due soit à la toxicité dans l'angine diphtérique, soit à la broncho-pneumonie dans le croup.

L'angine diphtérique toxique peut être toxique d'emblée ou devenir toxique.

Dans le premier cas, le moins fréquent, il semble vraiment que la sérothérapie soit impuissante. Il s'agit d'enfants profondément intoxiqués dès le début. On les amène à l'hôpital avec des symptômes généraux extrêmement graves (hyperthermie, albuminurie abondante, refroidissement des extrémités, collapsus cardiaque). Les symptômes locaux sont peu accentués, sauf le retentissement ganglionnaire. Chez ces enfants, le sérum antidiphtérique détermine, comme chez les autres, la chute des membranes. Mais les symptômes d'intoxication persistent et amènent rapidement la mort. Il y a certainement dès le début abondante production du poison diphtérique et absorption de ce poison par le sang. Le sérum paraît impuissant à neutraliser l'action du poison.

J'ai essayé vainement dans les diphtéries toxiques primitives de faire des injections répétées de sérum de Roux. (J'en ai injecté jusqu'à 100 centimètres cubes.) J'ai injecté le sérum dans les veines sans aucun résultat. Le pronostic a toujours été fatal.

Jusqu'à nouvel ordre, je considère ces angines toxiques primitives comme sans remède.

Les angines toxiques secondaires ont un pronostic moins inexorable. Ces angines deviennent souvent toxiques faute d'injections de sérum faites en temps voulu.

Les enfants qui en sont atteints ont eu une angine mal soignée ou même non soignée dans les premiers jours. On amène ces enfants à l'hôpital, lorsqu'ils commencent à présenter, après plusieurs jours de maladie, les signes de collapsus cardiaque, en rapport avec l'intoxication lente.

Ces accidents peuvent être prévenus, lorsque l'enfant est soigné en temps opportun, dès le début de l'angine. J'ai la conviction qu'ils diminueront de plus en plus de fréquence au fur et à mesure que la nécessité du traitement immédiat sera mieux comprise par les médecins appelés à soigner les diphtériques.

Une fois déclarés, les accidents toxiques secondaires sont très redoutables, presque toujours mortels. Contre ces accidents, il est inutile de recourir aux injections de sérum antidiphtérique.

Comme ils consistent essentiellement dans le collapsus cardiaque avec syncopes, troubles du rythme cardiaque, refroidissement des extrémités, de tout temps on a cherché à les combattre par les toniques du cœur. J'ai essayé tous ces toniques ou presque tous. Après bien des essais, j'y ai renoncé, après avoir reconnu leur inefficacité. Seul, le sulfate de spartéine m'a semblé non pas les combattre, mais en diminuer la fréquence et peut-être les empêcher de se produire, au moins dans quelques cas.

Lorsque j'avais des raisons de craindre qu'une angine grave ou qu'une angine traitée tardivement par le sérum antidiphtérique ne fût suivie d'accidents toxiques secondaires, je donnais aux enfants le sulfate de spartéine à la dose de 0,05 centigramme par année. Il m'a semblé qu'en employant ainsi ce médicament, le collapsus cardiaque secondaire devenait plus rare.

Je dois mentionner ici, dans un fait malheureusement unique (l'observation n'ayant pu être répétée), la très heureuse influence d'injections massives de sérum artificiel dans un cas de diphtérie toxique secondaire. Dans ce fait publié dans la *Gazette des maladies infantiles*, nous avons vu, mon interne Balthazard et moi, les injections de sérum artificiel produire une diurèse abondante avec élimination de toxine 7 fois supérieure à celle des urines, les jours où il n'y avait pas eu d'injections de sérum artificiel.

Cette observation montre que les injections de sérum artificiel favorisent l'élimination par le rein des molécules toxiques que renferme le sang. Elle me paraît devoir être renouvelée car elle concorde de tous points avec les recherches de Ruser et de Korangi, qui ont montré le rôle important que joue le chlorure de sodium dans l'excrétion rénale.

La broncho-pneumonie a été de beaucoup la cause de la mort la plus fréquente. Elle a été constatée plus de 160 fois à l'autopsie.

Comme chez les enfants atteints de croup, l'opération du tubage ou de la trachéotomie a toujours été pratiquée, même *in extremis*, l'asphyxie par obstruction du larynx n'a jamais été la cause directe de la mort. On peut dire que chez les enfants malades du croup, la broncho-pneumonie a été la cause de la mort dans l'immense majorité des cas.

A ce propos, je crois pouvoir dire que le tubage est rarement à mon avis une cause de broncho-pneumonie. On le constate, il est vrai, assez souvent chez les enfants tubés. Mais elle n'est pas rare dans les croups non tubés et, de plus, il est fréquent qu'elle soit constatée avant l'opération de tubage. J'ai la conviction que, dans un assez grand nombre de cas, la broncho-pneumonie est antérieure à l'opération sans que des signes puissent être mis en évidence. Si elle devient manifeste après le tubage, l'opération ne peut en être tenue pour responsable.

Le pronostic de la broncho-pneumonie du croup garde toute sa gravité et son traitement ne me paraît pas établi. Pour m'en tenir à la balnéation, je n'ai pas tiré de réel avantage de son emploi systématique. Avec des bains froids entre 20 et 25 degrés, j'ai eu 77 morts sur 100 et quelques cas de broncho-pneumonie. Avec des bains chauds à 58 et 39 degrés, j'ai eu 19 morts sur 50 cas. Dans une série de 65 malades traités par les ventouses sèches et la potion de Todd, j'ai eu 17 guérisons et 48 morts. On voit que, dans ces trois séries de malades, les résultats ont été sensiblement les mêmes et que c'est dans la série, où la balnéation froide a été systématiquement employée, qu'ils ont été les moins bons ! Les complications ont été assez fréquentes, rarement assez graves pour entraîner la mort.

Les complications le plus souvent notées ont été : la suppuration des ganglions maxillaires (50 fois). Dans deux cas, il y a suppuration des ganglions du médiastin, complication qui a entraîné la mort par septicémie.

Les otites simples ou doubles ont existé chez 62 malades. Deux fois seulement, elles se sont compliquées de mastoïdite. Dans les autres cas. elles ont guéri sans intervention chirurgicale quelconque. Les abcès de l'oreille se sont ouverts spontanément. Une fois ouverts, ils ont été traités par des injections antiseptiques dans les oreilles et des pansements antiseptiques.

Parmi les complications rares, je citerai l'œdème de la glotte (7 fois); la gangrène du larynx (5 fois); l'endocardite (2 fois); la méningite cérébro-spinale suppurée (2 fois); la pleurésie (5 fois); l'ictère avec polycholie (4 fois).

Trois enfants ont eu des crises d'éclampsie et ont succombé sans que l'autopsie fît découvrir aucune lésion appréciable à l'examen microscopique des centres nerveux.

J'ai observé 51 cas de paralysie diphtérique, le plus souvent limitée au voile du palais, quelquefois, mais rarement, généralisée. Comme je l'ai fait remarquer dans une autre communication ce chiffre de 51 paralysies doit être certainement considéré comme inférieur à la réalité. En effet, par suite de l'évolution rapide de la diphtérie traitée par le sérum, les enfants passent peu de temps dans nos salles. Des cas de paralysie peuvent donc se déclarer après leur sortie sans que nous en soyons informés.

Chez deux enfants. la paralysie était sous la dépendance de la diphtérie mais ne rentrait pas dans le cadre des névrites diphtériques. Il s'agissait de paralysie à forme hémiplégique. dans ces cas avec aphonie certainement due à une lésion cérébrale localisée, causée vraisemblablement par une embolie ou une thrombose de l'artère sylvienne.

Un certain nombre de mes malades ont été atteints de diphtérie, alors qu'ils présentaient une autre maladie infectieuse en voie d'évolution. La diphtérie s'est parfois trouvée singulièrement aggravée de ce fait.

C'est ainsi que la diphtérie frappant les enfants tuberculeux (pulmonaires ou osseux) est particulièrement grave. Sur 25 tuberculeux qui ont été atteints de diphtérie. 21 sont morts de broncho-pneumonie ou d'angine toxique. Dans 5 cas, la diphtérie a été l'occasion de poussées tuberculeuses généralisées à forme broncho-pneumonique.

Chez les rougeoleux. le croup diphtérique est également très grave. L'opération du tubage. comme nous l'avons montré Sevestre et moi, est possible chez les enfants. mais la broncho-pneumonie est particulièrement redoutable.

De toutes les maladies infectieuses. la coqueluche est la maladie qui assombrit le moins le pronostic de la diphtérie. Tous les coquelucheux atteints de diphtérie que j'ai gardés dans mes salles après les avoir isolés, ont guéri, sauf un seul qui a succombé à une angine toxique. Deux d'entre eux ont été atteints de broncho-pneumonie et ont cependant guéri. Plusieurs coquelucheux ont dû être tubés et ont généralement gardé leur tube malgré la violence des quintes.

Je ne voudrais pas, à propos de cette communication, soulever la question si importante et encore controversée des associations microbiennes dans la diphtérie.

Il me faut cependant dire quelques mots des résultats fournis par l'examen bactériologique dans 1778 cas de diphtérie.

Au point de vue de la recherche du bacille diphtérique sur sérum de Löffler, nous avons trouvé prédominants dans à peu près un quart des cas des bacilles longs, enchevêtrés, dont la présence implique immédiatement le diagnostic de diphtérie. Dans les trois quarts des autres cas, nous avons trouvé des bacilles moyens et courts. Les bacilles moyens sont incontestablement des bacilles diphtériques. Les cas dans lesquels nous les avons trouvés étaient, d'ailleurs, presque toujours des cas que la clinique seule aurait fait ranger dans la diphtérie.

Le plus ordinairement, les bacilles moyens étaient accompagnés de bacilles courts plus ou moins nombreux.

Quelquefois on n'a trouvé que des bacilles courts. Ces cas ne figurent pas dans notre statistique. Nous les avons éliminés. En effet, la virulence du bacille court ne nous paraît pas démontrée et jusqu'à nouvel ordre nous pensons que les malades, chez lesquels on les rencontre seuls, ne doivent pas être considérés comme diphtériques. Les angines, à bacilles courts, ne se comportent pas comme les angines diphtériques vraies. Elles peuvent être accompagnées de complications graves ; quelquefois même elles sont suivies de mort. Mais leurs complications ne sont pas celles de la diphtérie. Ce sont des septicémies générales ou pulmonaires, des broncho-pneumonies en particulier.

Je n'ai jamais vu les angines à bacilles courts, compliquées des accidents bulbo-cardiaque et des paralysies, qui sont les manifestations les plus évidentes de l'intoxication diphtérique.

En plus des bacilles diphtériques longs ou moyens, les examens bactériologiques ont fait constater la présence, on peut dire constante, des streptocoques. Quand les streptocoques n'étaient pas apparents sur le sérum, ils le devenaient par la culture sur gélose du prélèvement de la gorge.

La constance de la présence des streptocoques dans la gorge est un fait actuellement bien établi. Il n'y a donc rien d'extraordinaire à ce que ce micro-organisme puisse être constaté dans les examens bactériologiques de la gorge des enfants malades.

On ne peut déduire de cette constatation qu'une conséquence négative : c'est qu'elle ne signifie rien au point de vue du pronostic de la
maladie.

Pour que la présence des streptocoques dans la gorge puisse donner
quelques indications au point de vue du pronostic, il faudrait discuter
la valeur de sa présence, de sa plus ou moins grande abondance dans
les frottis des fausses membranes et dans leurs coupes (Procédé de
Sevestre et Méry). Il faudra aussi que la virulence des streptocoques
dans les mêmes conditions de temps et de milieu soit préalablement
établie.

Ces recherches, en admettant qu'elles donnent des résultats à l'abri
de toute discussion, ne sont plus du domaine des cliniciens. Elles
demandent un outillage approprié et nécessitent trop de temps pour
donner des indications pronostiques, au moment où il serait surtout
intéressant de les avoir. Quand les recherches du laboratoire sont
terminées, l'évolution de la maladie nous a renseignés depuis longtemps sur le pronostic.

DISCUSSION.

M. TRIBOULET (Paris) n'a pas entendu parler dans la communication
de M. Richardière [de complications rénales. Serait-ce que l'auteur n'en a
pas observé? Pour sa part, M. Triboulet a observé deux cas d'urémie
mortels à la suite d'injection de sérum.

M. RICHARDIÈRE. — J'ai rapporté tous les faits que j'ai observés. Ceux
qui ne sont pas mentionnés n'ont pas été vus. Pendant un certain temps,
j'ai fait doser l'albumine avant et après l'injection de sérum et je n'ai vu,
dans les cas où il y avait albuminurie, ni augmentation ni diminution.

M. BÉZY (Toulouse) confirme ce que vient de dire M. Richardière. L'injection de sérum, ainsi que l'a montré un de ses élèves, paraît sans influence sur l'albuminurie. Il répondra à M. Triboulet que, dans bien des
cas, il peut y avoir une néphrite latente, d'origine ancienne, qui peut-être
est cause des accidents graves observés parfois. Quant à ce qui est des
doses à injecter, M. Bézy se base, pour renouveler les injections, sur la
température et sur la présence des fausses membranes. Cette manière
de faire semble en désaccord avec ce que vient de dire M. Richardière ;
aussi M. Bézy demande-t-il ce qu'il faut penser des injections répétées.

M. HÉRON (de Tours) appuie l'observation de son confrère de Toulouse
et ne pense pas qu'une dose unique ou uniforme de sérum, suffise à tous
les cas et que son degré de force ait peu d'influence sur la marche de la
diphtérie dans les cas graves. A l'hôpital et dans sa pratique de ville, il a
pour règle de répéter une et deux fois l'injection, quand deux ou trois
jours après la première, la situation du malade ne s'améliore pas, soit au
point de vue de l'abaissement de la fièvre, soit au point de vue, surtout,
du détachement des membranes diphtériques. Il a injecté ainsi jusqu'à
50 et 60 grammes en trois jours chez des malades profondément atteints

et réfractaires à une ou deux injections, et l'intensité de l'intoxication comme la gravité de ces cas étaient telles, que dans trois d'entre eux, la guérison a été accompagnée ou suivie d'une paralysie de plus ou moins longue durée du voile du palais.

Il est donc bon et opportun, dans les cas graves, de répéter plusieurs fois l'injection et à dose variable selon leur degré de gravité.

M. VIOLI demande à M. Richardière : 1° si la dose de sérum injecté a toujours été la même dans les cas graves et dans les cas légers ; 2° si les enfants souffrant de diphtérie grave avaient une diphtérie grave parce que celle-ci était primitivement grave ou bien parce que le traitement a été commencé trop tardivement. En général M. Violi est partisan des doses massives d'emblée, mais sans répéter l'injection.

M. RICHARDIÈRE dit qu'en général une seule injection suffit. Cependant, dans certains cas, il peut être utile de renouveler deux ou trois fois la première dose. En tout cas, il ne faut pas se baser sur la température, car souvent l'injection de sérum amène une élévation thermique. Seule la persistance des membranes est une indication à renouveler l'injection.

M. GEFFRIER (d'Orléans) rapporte un cas semblable aux observations de M. Triboulet. Un enfant de huit mois, atteint de diphtérie oculaire bénigne, reçut presque à la fin de sa maladie, une injection de 10 centimètres de sérum. A partir de ce moment, anurie complète, puis mort cinq jours après. En tout cas, M. Geffrier pense que la dose de 10 centimètres est presque toujours suffisante.

INJECTIONS DE SÉRUM ANTIDIPHTÉRIQUE DANS UN BUT PROPHYLACTIQUE A DES ENFANTS ATTEINTS DE ROUGEOLE

par MM. NETTER et Nattan LARRIER

Étant donnés les bons résultats prophylactiques fournis par l'usage des injections de sérum antidiphtérique, j'ai pensé qu'elles pourraient donner des résultats satisfaisants dans la rougeole où les complications diphtériques sont assez fréquentes.

Pendant l'année 1899, nous avons été chargé à la direction du service de la rougeole à l'hôpital Trousseau où sont entrés 855 enfants.

Désireux de prévenir dans la limite du possible la production de cas intérieurs de diphtérie, nous avons soumis sans exception tous ces malades, le jour de l'entrée, à une injection de sérum antidiphtérique.

Le sérum injecté provenait de l'Institut Pasteur. La dose inoculée était de 10 c. c. Chez les nourrissons elle a été de 5 c. c.

Il y a eu dans le service 27 cas de diphtérie.

Dans 12 de ces cas la diphtérie existait au moment de l'admission.

6 de ces cas étaient des diphtéries oculaires.
4   —   —   laryngées.
1   —   pharyngées.

Dans un de ces cas, il s'agissait d'une enfant entrée avec une paralysie diphtérique.

Les 15 cas de diphtérie survenus après l'admission chez des enfants soumis aux injections préventives comprenaient :

12 diphtéries oculaires.
5 diphtéries laryngées.

Si nous envisageons le temps qui s'est écoulé entre l'injection et l'apparition de la diphtérie, nous trouvons qu'il a été :

1 fois de.	2	jours.
2 —	5	—
1 -	4	—
1 —	5	—
1 — moins de.	7	—
1 —	9	
1 —	10	—
1 —	11	—
5 —	15	—
1 —	16	—
1 —	21	—
1 — 2 mois et.	5	jours.

Il convient de défalquer les 5 cas survenus deux ou trois jours après l'injection et les cas survenus après 21 jours et 2 mois.

Il reste encore 10 cas de diphtérie éclatant dans la période au cours de laquelle l'infection de sérum exerce d'ordinaire une influence préventive.

Il semble donc que, chez les sujets atteints de rougeole, l'action préventive du sérum antidiphtérique soit moins efficace que chez les autres enfants, que le sérum prévienne moins les déterminations oculaires de la diphtérie.

Nous ajouterons que l'injection préventive ne semble avoir aucune action atténuante sur la diphtérie qu'elle ne peut prévenir. La très grande majorité de nos cas se sont en effet terminés par la mort.

Les bacilles diphtériques isolés chez les malades ne présentaient point de caractères particuliers.

Le nombre considérable d'injections pratiquées chez les malades retenus longtemps dans le service permet d'apprécier le peu de fréquence des accidents consécutifs aux injections.

Nous n'avons relevé que 9 cas d'éruption avec fièvre.

L'éruption a été notée 5 fois après 15 jours, 1 fois après 12 et 14 jours. Ce sont les intervalles le plus communément observés en dehors de la rougeole.

L'intervalle a été moins élevé chez 5 autres malades où il n'a été que de 8, 5 et 2 jours.

Il n'est pas indiqué dans la dernière observation.

Les éruptions ont été particulièrement peu nombreuses, 1,05 pour 100.

Deux ans auparavant, dans un service de scarlatine, elles avaient été de 12 pour 100.

Il s'est agi dans tous les cas d'enfants qui n'ont pas eu la diphtérie.

Les accidents de sérum ont été relevés en février, mars et avril. Après ce dernier mois on ne les constate que 2 fois. Peut-être convient-il d'attribuer leur rareté à ce fait que l'on inoculait du sérum recueilli après 5 ou 4 mois.

DISCUSSION.

M. HALLÉ demande à M. Netter si la virulence du bacille diphtérique a été recherchée.

M. NETTER répond que cette virulence a été vérifiée pour le plus grand nombre des cas.

M. MARFAN. — Puisque M. Netter nous a parlé de la diphtérie dans la rougeole, je crois utile de rappeler les faits suivants. Ayant été chargé du service de la rougeole à l'hôpital des Enfants-Malades, au commencement de la présente année, j'ai observé, dans les premiers jours, un enfant qui, pendant la période d'éruption, présenta de la raucité de la voix; la chose est assez banale et nous n'y attachâmes d'abord aucune importance, d'autant que la gorge ne présentait aucun exsudat blanchâtre; mais deux jours après, la laryngite s'aggrava et exigea le tubage; l'examen bactériologique des matières rejetées au moment de l'opération montra que la laryngite était diphtérique; on pratiqua une injection de sérum; mais il était trop tard, sans doute, l'enfant mourut; il avait d'ailleurs de la broncho-pneumonie. Ayant eu l'attention éveillée par ce fait, nous remarquâmes que, beaucoup plus souvent qu'en temps ordinaire, nos rougeoleux présentaient des symptômes laryngés; nous décidâmes d'injecter 20 centimètres cubes de sérum antidiphtérique à tous ceux qui auraient de la raucité de la voix un peu prononcée. Nous n'avons plus eu à déplorer de mort par laryngite, bien que l'examen bactériologique, fait après l'injection, nous ait montré que la plupart de ces laryngites étaient diphtériques.

Nous n'avons pas observé la diphtérie oculaire si souvent relevée par M. Netter.

M. VEILLON désire préciser quelques points au sujet du diagnostic bactériologique de la diphtérie. Les erreurs sont fréquentes. Dans nombre de cas, les recherches sont insuffisantes et n'ont de valeur que par l'inoculation. En particulier, dans certaines conjonctivites, on trouve très fréquemment un microbe qui présente tous les caractères du bacille diphtérique, mais que l'inoculation montre de nature absolument différente. Il est donc indispensable de savoir si le bacille en question a été inoculé.

M. **Netter** répond que la qualité du bacille diphtérique est incontestable dans les cas auxquels il a fait allusion. La preuve a été faite dans nombre de cas, et en particulier des vérifications ont été faites à l'institut Pasteur.

M. **Seitz** (de Munich) a vu, lors de la dernière épidémie de rougeole, un grand nombre de cas de croup, sans que l'examen bactériologique ait confirmé, pour le plus grand nombre, le diagnostic de diphtérie. Il semble qu'il y ait des conditions locales qui règlent cette association du croup et de la rougeole, d'ailleurs plus fréquente à l'hôpital. Quant à la valeur prophylactique du sérum, les cultures sont nécessaires pour l'établir nettement.

M. **Thomesco** (de Bucarest) dit que les laryngites sont fréquentes au début de la rougeole. On se trompe souvent en attribuant à la diphtérie ces manifestations. Le tubage, dans ces cas, est préférable au sérum qui peut être dangereux.

M. **Marfan**. — Je veux répondre un mot à M. Thomesco. Nous n'ignorons pas qu'il y a dans la rougeole deux variétés de laryngite: les unes, précoces ou tardives, superficielles ou profondes, ne sont pas diphtériques: les autres sont diphtériques. C'est parce que nous connaissions l'existence des premières qu'en présence de notre cas initial, nous n'avons pas pensé à la diphtérie, en quoi nous avons eu peut-être tort. Quant au tubage, il est bien entendu qu'il a été pratiqué quand la suffocation l'exigeait: mais, si la laryngite est diphtérique, il ne suffit pas: il faut y joindre l'injection de sérum. En somme, je trouve notre conduite légitime. J'ai d'ailleurs pour règle qu'en présence d'un cas de laryngite, si on soupçonne la diphtérie, même avant d'avoir la certitude de l'examen bactériologique, il faut injecter du sérum. Nous pouvons bien dire aujourd'hui que cette pratique n'offre aucun inconvénient et qu'elle a de grands avantages.

M. **Violi** (de Constantinople) demande à M. Netter quelle est la dose de sérum qu'il a inoculée.

M. **Netter** répond que cette dose a été de 10 centimètres.

M. **Violi** dit que, pour sa part, les inoculations préventives ne lui ont pas donné de résultats positifs. L'isolement et l'antisepsie lui ont paru les seuls moyens efficaces d'éviter la propagation de la maladie. Cependant il a eu recours au sérum dans certains cas de diphtérie compliquant la rougeole.

LE SÉRUM ANTIDIPHTÉRIQUE A MADRID

RAPPORT

par M. Jules ROBERT,

de Madrid.

L'auteur présente le tracé de la mortalité diphtérique, comprenant vingt années (1880-1899). Cette courbe en clocher, fort curieuse, démontre graphiquement que la diphtérie à Madrid a été jugulée par le sérum.

Les chiffres de mortalité la plus basse avant l'application du sérum furent de 199 et 196 décès annuels ; au moment de l'acmé épidémique, en 1886, la mortalité s'éleva à 1586 décès.

En 1893, l'emploi du sérum fit baisser le chiffre des décès au nombre de 159. Mais, en 1896, la mortalité remonte à 165, à 168 en 1897, et 276 et 265 pour les années 1898 et 1899.

Ce tracé indique qu'il y a tendance à une nouvelle poussée épidémique, ou bien qu'il y a un certain relâchement dans la pratique, et que l'on n'injecte pas toujours aussi vite qu'il le faudrait. C'est, du moins, ce qu'il a constaté à Madrid, et il présume qu'il en est de même ailleurs.

DISCUSSION

M. Moussous (Bordeaux) confirme la manière de voir de M. Robert.

RÉSULTATS OBTENUS DANS LE TRAITEMENT DU CROUP DIPHTÉRIQUE AVANT ET APRÈS LA SÉROTHÉRAPIE (STATISTIQUE PERSONNELLE)

par M. le docteur D. GALATTI,

de Vienne

Si je prends la liberté de poser comme sujet de discussion l'activité du sérum dans les cas de diphtérie observés dans ma pratique privée, et si, en face des chiffres géants cités par d'autres observateurs, je ne m'appuie que sur un nombre d'observations relativement petit, c'est parce que les matériaux restreints que je possède ont été

recueillis dans des conditions toutes spéciales qui leur donnent une valeur particulière. Je vais rapidement exposer ces conditions.

Presque toutes les statistiques sur l'action du sérum antidiphtérique, dès qu'elles reposent sur un nombre de cas quelque peu considérable, ont trait à des malades observés à l'hôpital. Les adversaires de la sérothérapie objectent toujours à nouveau contre la validité, comme preuve, des statistiques hospitalières favorables à la sérothérapie, la valeur inégale, au point de vue de la gravité, des cas soignés dans les hôpitaux avant l'ère de la sérothérapie et depuis celle-ci; ils allèguent que, depuis l'introduction du sérum dans la thérapeutique de la diphtérie, les hôpitaux reçoivent un nombre relativement plus grand de cas bénins. Cette objection réfutée de maints côtés, même en ce qui concerne les statistiques hospitalières, tombe dès qu'il ne s'agit que des malades de la clientèle privée.

Le transport à l'hôpital d'un enfant atteint de diphtérie dépend d'une multitude de facteurs, parmi lesquels la thérapeutique à mettre en vigueur entre en ligne de compte même pour les parents aisés. Quant au fait de mettre en traitement médical, c'est-à-dire de confier à un médecin de ville un enfant atteint de diphtérie, cela dépend uniquement du symptôme qui vient essentiellement inquiéter les parents. Comme ces premiers symptômes sont indépendants de la thérapeutique employée, quelle qu'elle soit, il n'existe aucune raison pour que, depuis l'introduction du sérum dans le traitement de la diphtérie, les cas bénins soient devenus plus fréquents qu'autrefois en clientèle privée, surtout lorsqu'il s'agit de sténose laryngée.

Il est encore une autre objection importante qu'on soulève contre les statistiques de sérothérapie tirées, soit des services hospitaliers, soit de la clientèle privée. On parle d'un changement du *génie épidémique*: on dit que l'évolution plus favorable, la mortalité plus faible de la diphtérie sous l'influence de la sérothérapie ne doivent point être attribuées à cette dernière, mais qu'elles sont en rapport avec le caractère plus bénin que la diphtérie a affecté depuis cette époque. Cette objection, qu'il est aussi facile de soulever qu'il est difficile de la soutenir, ne peut, en somme, être faite que là *où la totalité de tous les cas de diphtérie traités, cas graves autant que bénins, sont employés pour établir la statistique*. En règle générale, on va déjà à l'encontre de cette objection en groupant les observations selon la gravité des cas traités, et en attachant une importance essentielle à l'efficacité de la sérothérapie dans le traitement des cas graves. Pourtant le scepticisme est parfois si fort qu'on ne craint pas de juger avec un certain parti pris la gravité d'un cas.

La façon dont j'ai établi ma statistique a permis d'éviter toutes ces incertitudes. En effet, je ne donne pas une statistique globale de tous les cas de diphtérie que j'ai eus en traitement dans la clientèle; je donne seulement la statistique des cas compliqués de phénomènes de sténose laryngée. De plus, afin qu'on ne puisse croire que pour juger de la gravité des phénomènes de sténose laryngée mon opinion objective ait été seule décisive, je tiens à faire remarquer immédiatement que ma statistique ne comprend que les cas traités par d'autres médecins qui ne m'avaient appelé que pour pratiquer le tubage. Il n'existe aucune raison pour supposer que ces médecins, en jugeant la gravité des phénomènes morbides, eussent été influencés par la sérothérapie; il faut y ajouter que mon rôle a été, en quelque sorte, de réexaminer la détermination de mes confrères. Avant, de même qu'après l'introduction de la sérothérapie, non seulement je ne suis pas intervenu par le tubage dans *tous* les cas et *de suite*, mais j'ai bien souvent conseillé de temporiser, et cela avec juste raison, comme les faits l'ont démontré. *Cette façon d'établir la statistique offre, selon moi, la plus grande garantie possible quant à la valeur égale des cas communiqués, datant soit de la période d'avant, soit de la période d'après l'avènement de la sérothérapie.* Je me garde de parler d'une garantie *absolue*, parce que, nous le savons, des cas en apparence bénins se terminent par la mort, tandis que d'autres fois des cas paraissant très graves surprennent par leur évolution favorable. A propos de ces cas, je voudrais précisément faire ressortir qu'ils ne sont point aussi fréquents que les adversaires de la sérothérapie le prétendent. Ils présentent évidemment ce qui dans les statistiques se trouve rangé sous la rubrique des « erreurs du hasard ».

L'importance statistique de ces erreurs devient d'autant moindre que les éléments d'observation employés sont plus considérables.

La vraisemblance que les déductions de la statistique se rapprochent de la vérité augmente à mesure que s'accroît le volume des matériaux d'observation. Sous ce rapport, je crois que mes 61 observations, prises rigoureusement, bien qu'elles puissent paraître peu nombreuses aux statisticiens de profession, le sont assez au point de vue de la statistique médicale pour justifier la prétention que les déductions en soient considérées comme dignes de confiance.

Je passe à présent à la discussion des observations de diphtérie accompagnée de phénomènes de sténose laryngée, observations résumées dans les tableaux qu'on trouvera plus loin.

Les soixante et un cas de diphtérie dans lesquels j'ai été appelé en consultation pour pratiquer le tubage se répartissent sur plusieurs années, de sorte que le caractère moyen que la maladie aurait pu affecter n'entre pas en ligne de compte. Ce serait en général un hasard des plus remarquables. — je n'ose nullement nier ces jeux du hasard! — si juste le moment de l'avènement de la sérothérapie eût coïncidé avec une modification du caractère de l'épidémie!

De mes 61 observations, 29 datent de la période pré-sérothérapique, 52 de la période sérothérapique.

Comme je l'ai déjà dit, je ne procédais pas toujours immédiatement à l'opération. mais je conseillais parfois de temporiser. De cette manière le nombre total des tubages se trouva réduit à 41. Le temps d'attente était utilisé, lors de la sérothérapie, pour pratiquer une ou plusieurs injections de sérum. et à l'époque pré-sérothérapique pour recourir aux moyens de traitement usuels.

La proportion des cas opérés et non opérés s'établit comme suit :

Sur 29 cas de diphtérie avec sténose laryngée de l'époque pré-sérothérapique, il y a eu 6 cas guéris sans opération, donc 21 pour 100.

Sur 52 cas de diphtérie avec sténose laryngée de la période sérothérapique, il y a eu 14 cas guéris sans intervention, donc 44 pour 100.

La guérison des sténoses laryngées réussit par conséquent *sans opération* pendant la période de sérothérapie dans un nombre de cas deux fois aussi grand que dans la période précédente La sérothérapie n'est certainement pas capable d'empêcher l'apparition, dans la diphtérie, de tous les phénomènes de sténose laryngée ; elle n'est pas davantage capable de rendre toutes les sténoses assez insignifiantes pour que l'opération devienne superflue ; mais comme je puis l'affirmer en tant que première déduction résultant de ma statistique, elle est néanmoins en état de modérer et même de faire disparaître la sténose laryngée dans un nombre de cas assez considérable.

Ce résultat favorable ne peut pas être imputé à ce fait que dans la période de sérothérapie les cas de diphtérie, pour lesquels on m'avait appelé, aient été plus bénins que ceux de la période pré-sérothérapique. Une observation attentive des cas esquissés brièvement dans mes tableaux l'enseigne nettement. A ce propos, je voudrais fixer l'attention principalement sur la comparaison des cas non tubés de la période de sérothérapie avec les cas tubés de la période pré-sérothérapique. Cette comparaison démontrerait qu'aux observations de tubage de la période pré-sérothérapique correspondent des cas aussi graves de la période de sérothérapie, mais dans lesquels l'emploi du sérum a permis de s'abstenir du tubage.

La nécessité de procéder au tubage. devenue plus rare pendant la période de sérothérapie, ne peut pas être attribuée à la faveur d'une différence d'âge. On aurait pu croire que plus un enfant, atteint de diphtérie, était jeune, plus l'opération du tubage avec sténose laryngée fût imminente. Sous ce rapport, on constate, d'après mes tableaux, ce qui suit :

AGE	PÉRIODE D'AVANT LA SÉROTHÉRAPIE			PÉRIODE SÉROTHÉRAPIQUE		
	NOMBRE DE CAS	DONT NON TUBÉS	O O	NOMBRE DE CAS	DONT NON TUBÉS	O O
Jusqu'à 2 ans.	19	5	55 1 2	8	4	50
De 2 à 4 ans.	15	5	27	10	4	40
Au-dessus de 4 ans	7	—	—	14	6	42 5 4

A tous les âges, le tubage est devenu plus rarement nécessaire. Une translation dans la combinaison des années d'âge a pourtant eu lieu, dans ce sens que la supérieure de ces époques d'âge offre un contingent plus considérable dans la période de sérothérapie, alors que c'était justement à cet âge que, avant l'avènement de la sérothérapie, on ne pouvait, dans aucun cas, s'abstenir du tubage. Si donc on voulait revendiquer quelque influence en faveur de l'âge sur l'intensité de la sténose, — je ne dis point que je le fais — cette influence serait alors juste plutôt contraire à l'efficacité du sérum et non favorable.

De plus, nous n'avons point eu affaire à des cas plus bénins depuis la sérothérapie. En ce qui concerne les phénomènes locaux — sur les amygdales, le voile du palais, sur la portion visible de la muqueuse du pharynx — qui d'ailleurs ne peuvent offrir aucune mesure pour évaluer l'intensité de la sténose laryngée, nous trouvons que les cas *non tubés* de la période de la sérothérapie ne diffèrent point particulièrement des cas *tubés* de la période précédente. Dans trois cas de chacune de ces deux périodes, on ne constata plus d'exsudat diphtérique visible; dans d'autres cas l'extension de l'exsudat a été variable. Quant à la sténose laryngée, on voit, dans les cas *non tubés* de la période de sérothérapie, mentionnée dans quatre cas sa gravité; dans trois on insiste sur l'existence des accès de suffocation. *A la période pré-sérothérapique ces phénomènes n'ont pas conduit à l'opération; dans un cas seulement à la période de la sérothérapie on a pu s'abstenir d'opérer sept fois.*

Comparons à présent les succès du tubage. A la période pré-sérothérapique on a eu après l'intubation *une seule fois* recours à la trachéotomie: à la période du sérum *cinq fois*. Ceci démontre avec évidence combien graves étaient les cas arrivés en traitement. Sur les 25 cas de tubage de la période d'avant le sérum, il y a eu 11 morts = 47,8 pour 100. Sur les 18 cas de tubage traités par le sérum, il y a eu 1 mort = 5.5 pour 100. Cette mort, elle a peut-être été de ma faute, c'était le premier cas traité par le sérum, je n'en ai probablement pas injecté assez. N'ayant pas été au début favorablement disposé pour la sérothérapie, je craignais que l'injection de trop fortes doses n'entraînât quelques effets fâcheux pour la santé. J'ai donc pratiqué dans ce cas une seule injection de sérum de Behring n° 2, n'osant pas injecter davantage, tandis que plus tard, lorsque je le jugeais nécessaire, j'élevai la dose totale à 6000, 7500 et même 8000 unités d'antitoxines. C'est à cette circonstance que j'attribue mes bons résultats ultérieurs.

Et même si l'on met à la charge de la sérothérapie cet unique cas de mort qui en réalité incombe à mon inexpérience, la différence est quand même écrasante.

A une mortalité de 50 pour 100 des tubés sans sérum, nous avons à opposer une léthalité à peine d'un peu plus de 5 pour 100.

En d'autres termes, cela veut dire que grâce à la sérothérapie les dangers de la sténose laryngée menaçant les enfants atteints de diphtérie se trouvent presque complètement écartés. Nous avons ici affaire à des cas présentant des phénomènes locaux très graves. C'est dans ces cas précisément que la sérothérapie déploie sa plus grande efficacité.

Parmi les malades tubés qui ont succombé, nous constatons presque toujours une pneumonie, un catarrhe intense ou de l'adynamie cardiaque. On pourrait donc être d'avis que ce sont ces complications qui ont amené la mort. Cette opinion est fausse. Comme on le voit déjà de ce fait que cinq fois on a été obligé de pratiquer la trachéotomie secondaire, j'avais dans la période de la sérothérapie affaire à des sténoses laryngées extrêmement graves. Là réside déjà la preuve qu'il y avait aussi des complications du côté des poumons. Je tiens à faire ressortir d'une façon expresse leur existence, afin de détruire d'avance la raison d'être de toute objection sur ce point. Il est exact, toutefois, que chez les tubés traités par le sérum, ces complications n'ont pas atteint un degré mettant la vie en danger, bien qu'elles aient été déjà extrêmement prononcées avant l'injection. *Mais c'est par là que se manifeste encore le succès de la sérothérapie.* Elle a réussi à prévenir ce qui, sans elle, aurait pu amener la mort.

La sérothérapie paraît exerce une certaine influence sur la durée du tubage. Afin de développer ce point, j'ai rangé les matériaux des tableaux de la manière suivante : pour reconnaître son influence sur le tubage, comme tel, j'ai exclu de ma statistique tous les cas où l'on a été obligé de pratiquer la trachéotomie secondaire. Il reste alors pour la période pré-sérothérapique 22 cas, pour la période de sérothérapie 15 cas de tubages[1]. Pour ces tubages je calcule donc la durée du séjour du tube dans le larynx dans tous les cas de guérison et de mort. J'obtiens alors comme durée moyenne du tubage, exprimée en heures et par malade.

	Guérisons.	Morts.	Tubages sans trachéotomie secondaire.
A la période pré-sérothérapique	108 h.	45 h.	78 h. 1,2
A la période de sérothérapie	50 h.	48 h.	57 h.

Je n'insiste pas sur la différence de la durée moyenne du tubage chez les tubés morts, d'autant plus qu'elle n'est pas énorme et que pour la période de sérothérapie un seul cas entre seulement en ligne de compte; par contre, j'insiste sur la différence dans la durée moyenne hors des deux périodes, chez les malades guéris, et qui ne se fait pas moins remarquer pour le total des tubages sans trachéotomie secondaire. La durée du tubage, à la période de sérothérapie est à peine un peu plus de moitié de celle de la période d'avant le sérum.

Ceci n'est pas dû à ce que les cas traités à la période de sérothérapie sont plus bénins que ceux traités à la période d'avant le sérum. Abstraction faite des constatations de l'examen objectif qui sont contraires à cette opinion, l'impression subjective que j'ai ressentie était celle que les cas tubés lors de la période de sérothérapie ont été aussi graves, sinon plus graves, que n'ont été ceux traités à la période pré-sérothérapique. En tenant compte de cela, on peut dire que *le traitement par le sérum a fait diminuer de moitié la durée moyenne du tubage nécessaire.* Ceci est facile à expliquer. L'effet que la sérothérapie exerce sur la disparition des fausses membranes des muqueuses accessibles à nos regards s'étend également sur les membranes diphtériques des muqueuses du larynx et de la trachée. Outre la durée moyenne du tubage en général, il est intéressant de relever la durée moyenne du tubage pour chaque cas isolé. Celle-ci était à la période de sérothérapie : 50 heures, 56, 48, 50, 52, 65, 67, 68 79 heures, à la période pré-sérothérapique, 51, 52, 45 1 2, 48, 52, 56, 57, 84.

---

1. J'exclus de ce dernier chiffre l'observation 12, qui précède un tubage temporaire; de sorte qu'il reste 12 cas seulement.

108 1 2. 111, 258 et 454 heures. Le nombre des heures de la durée moyenne du tubage est beaucoup plus considérable pour la période pré-sérothérapique que pour la période de sérothérapie. La durée du tubage pendant la sérothérapie est beaucoup plus stable et produit l'impression comme si tous ces laps de temps se seraient groupés autour d'un nombre d'heures d'une certaine fixité. Sur moi — et peut-être aussi sur d'autres observateurs — ce fait produit l'impression comme si le progrès ultérieur de la durée du tubage et, par suite, de la durée de la sténose du larynx eût été limitée subitement. Cet arrêt a été déterminé dans la sérothérapie, et il a eu lieu le troisième jour environ (au bout de 65 à 79 heures). C'est aussi à peu près le moment où les injections de sérum développent leur plus grande action sur les exsudats visibles des muqueuses.

Les résultats de tout ce que nous venons de dire peuvent être résumés de la façon suivante :

1) Mes matériaux d'observations offrent la plus grande certitude possible quant à l'égalité de la valeur des cas de la période de la sérothérapie avec ceux de la période pré-sérothérapique ;

2) Par la sérothérapie on réussit souvent à rendre inutile l'opération chez des malades qui sans cela n'auraient pas échappé au tubage ;

3) La sérothérapie abaisse énormément la mortalité des malades tubés ;

4) La sérothérapie diminue notablement la durée même du tubage.

De ces propositions bien démontrées par mes observations, je conclus que les injections de sérum curatif dans la thérapeutique de la sténose laryngée diphtérique rendent des services inappréciables. Dans l'intérêt de l'enfance souffrante et au nom des parents accablés de douleur, je désirerais engager tout médecin à ne point tarder, comme cela arrive malheureusement encore trop souvent, lorsqu'il s'agit de pratiquer une injection de sérum dans le croup ainsi que dans les autres manifestations de la diphtérie. Je les engage de même à ne point s'arrêter à de petites doses de sérum, d'autant plus qu'aucun effet fâcheux n'est à craindre à la suite de l'injection du sérum.

Juin 1892-Octobre 1894.   **A. — Diphtérie avec sténose laryngée.**   *Période pré-sérothérapique.*

Nº d'ordre	NOM	AGE	EXSUDAT.	TUBAGE	TRACHÉOTOMIE	RÉSULTAT	OBSERVATIONS
1	Jeannette M.....	5 1 2 ans	Sur les amygdales et la paroi postérieure du pharynx.	48 heures		Guérison	
2	Irène S..........	6 ans	Diphtérie du pharynx en voie de guérison	52 heures		Guérison	Accès intenses de suffocation. La voix reste rauque pendant 2 mois.
3	Adèle Koz.......	15 mois	Sur la paroi postérieure du pharynx et sur les amygdales (exsudat en plaques).	44 heures 5 4		Mort	Pneumonie.
4	Anna Sch.......	2 ans	Pas d'exsudat.	56 heures		Mort	Pneumonie.
5	Paul Szensi.....	5 1 2 ans	2 petites plaques sur l'amygdale droite.	5 tubages. Durée totale 108 h. 1 2.		Guérison	Déglutition de deux tubes qu'on retrouve ensuite dans les matières.
6	Otto Sch........	5 1 2 ans	D'un jaune sale sur tout le pharynx.	52 heures		Guérison	Diphtérie nasale très intense. Bronchite.
7	Gisela R........	2 1 2 ans	Sur l'amygdale gauc.	45 1 2 heures		Guérison	Accès de suffocation intenses. Catarrhe.
8	Aloisia R.......	2 1 2 ans	Sur les 2 amygdales.	25 1 2 heures	Trachéot. secondaire.	Mort	
9	Anna B.........	25 mois	Plaques en îlots sur les amygdales.	4 tubages. Durée totale 258 heures.		Guérison	Rachitisme. Bronchite. Accès de suffocation. Faiblesse cardiaque. Apathie.
10	Fritz H.........	5 ans	Lardacé, couenneux, étendu, sur les 2 amygdales.	57 heures		Guérison	Mourant. Sténose intense. Phénomènes de collapsus pendant et après le tubage.
11	Rosa K.........	5 1,2 ans	Amygdale gauche et piliers.	84 heures		Guérison	Rachitisme prononcé. Anémie.

Juin 1892-Octobre 1894.   A. — Diphtérie avec sténose laryngée.   *Période pré-sérothérapique.*

N° D'ORDRE	NOM	AGE	EXSUDAT	TUBAGE	TRACHÉOTOMIE	RÉSULTAT	OBSERVATIONS
12	Olga Bl.........	5 1/2 ans	Étendu, d'un jaune sale, lardacé, sur tout le pharynx.	29 heures	Sans intervention	Mort	Diphtérie nasale. Catarrhe intense. Apathie pendant toute la maladie.
13	Leo W.........	20 mois	En arrière de l'amygdale g. Rougeur.	5 tubages. Durée 111 h.		Guérison	Catarrhe purulent très intense.
14	Fanny L.........	4 1/2 ans	Couennes, comme un haricot, sur les amygdales.	56 heures		Mort	Diphtérie nasale. Faiblesse constante du pouls.
15	Rosa Ob.........	9 1/2 ans	Sur la luette et les piliers.	28 heures		Mort	Pneumonie. Tempér.
16	Laise M.........	2 3/4 ans	En plaques isolées sur les amygdales.	49 1/2 heures		Mort	Bronchopneumonie.
17	Gisela N.........	9 1/2 ans	Très étendu sur la muqueuse pharyngée et sur l'épiglotte.	75 heures		Mort	Adynamie cardiaque.
18	Resi E.........	4 ans	Amygdales, luette, paroi postér. du pharynx.	51 heures		Guérison	Broncho. Après l'expectoration du tube, légers phénomènes de sténose laryngée. Guérison ensuite.
19	Félix Sch	5 ans	Étendu sur toute la muqueuse du pharynx.	51 heures		Mort	Croup descendant.
20	Ernst R.........	8 1/2 mois	Amygdales, paroi du pharynx, luette, épiglotte.	57 1/2 heures		Mort	Bronchite intense.
21	Carl R.........	20 mois	Exsudat constaté pendant 7 jours, puis pharynx détergé.	10 tubages, durée totale 436 heures.		Guérison	Huit jours après le dernier tubage, mort de rétrécissement laryngé cicatriciel du larynx.

Juin 1892-Octobre 1894.   **A. — Diphtérie avec sténose laryngée.**   *Période pré-sérothérapique.*

N° d'ordre	NOM	AGE	EXSUDAT	TUBAGE	TRACHÉOTOMIE	RÉSULTAT	OBSERVATIONS
22	Ernst S.........	10 mois	Pas d'exsudat.	58 heures	Sans inter-vention.	Mort	Pneumonie.
23	Hilda R.........	5 ans	Pas d'exsudat, rou-geur.	Au bout de 56 h. rejet du tube.		Guérison	Léger catarrhe. Après le rejet, respiration normale.
24	Hans H........	5 1/2 ans	En ilots sur les amyg-dales.	Sans inter-vention.		Guérison	Léger catarrhe. Pendant 24 heures de phénomènes assez intenses de sténose laryngée. Traitement homéopathique.
25	Rudolf R........	5 1/2 ans	Paroi postérieure du pharynx, les amyg-dales et la luette.	—		Guérison	La gêne respiratoire a duré 4 jours; la dépression épigastrique très accentuée par moments. Inhalations. Badigeonnages avec collutoire au sublimé.
26	Karl F..........	11 mois	Pas d'exsudat.	—		Guérison	Respiration sténosique laryngée pendant 24 heures.
27	Ernst K.........	11 mois	Id.	—		Guérison	Broncho. Respiration de sténose laryngée pendant deux jours. Au deuxième jour, début de scarlatine.
28	Paul N..........	18 mois	Id.	—		Guérison	Légère broncho. Accès de suffocation intense menaçant l'existence pendant plusieurs heures.
29	Minna G........	2 ans 3/4	Sur l'amygdale dr., petite plaque.	—		Guérison	Le 19 dans la nuit présente subitement des phénomènes de sténose et de suffocation. La respiration bruyante encore au bout de plusieurs jours.

Octobre 1894-Novembre 1899. **Diphtérie avec sténose laryngée.** *Sérothérapie.*

N° D'ORDRE	NOM	AGE	EXSUDAT	TUBAGE	TRACHÉOTOMIE	RÉSULTAT	OBSERVATIONS
1	Mitzi K.........	5 ans	Diphtérie du pharynx venant de se terminer.	48 heures		Mort	Injection Behring (1500 A. E.).
2	Heinrich Sch....	1 an	Exsudats étendus sur le pharynx et amygdales.	79 heures		Guérison	1 injection Behring n° 2 (1000 A. E.)
3	Robert S........	5 ans	En lentilles, sur les deux amygdales ; en stries sur le pharynx.	67 heures		Guérison	2 injections Behring (3000 A. E.).
4	Mizzi R.	18 mois	Exsud. lenticulaires sur chaque amygdale.	12 tubages, 7 auto-extubations. Durée 215 h.	Trachéot. secondaire.	Guérison	Décanulement difficile, rétrécissement cicatriciel. 5 inject. Behring. n° 1, 2 5 (5000 A. E.).
5	Ernst K........	5 ans	Amygdales, luette, paroi postérieure du pharynx.	65 heures		Guérison	Diphtérie nasale. Pas d'incident. 2 inj. Behring n° 2 (2000 A. E.).
6	Paul H.........	5 1/2 ans	Pas d'exsudat.	50 heures		Guérison	Après le détubage, légère gêne respiratoire. 2 injections Behring n° 2 (2000 A. E.).
7	Paula K.........	2 3/4 ans	Sur tout le pharynx exsudat gris sale.	48 heures		Guérison	4 injections Behring, 2 fois n° 2. 2 fois n° 3 (5000 A. E.).
8	Paul R.........	4 3/4 ans	Paroi postérieure du pharynx.	72 heures		Guérison	1 injection Paltauf (1000 A. E.) 2 inj. Behring II et III (2500 A. E.)
9	Friedericki W...	7 1/5 ans	Plaque d'exsudat mince jaunâtre sur l'amygdale gauc.	52 heures		Guérison	2 inject. Behring 2 et 5 (2500 A. E.).

Octobre 1894-Novembre 1899.   **Diphtérie avec sténose laryngée.**   *Sérothérapie.*

N° D'ORDRE	NOM	AGE	EXSUDAT	TUBAGE	TRACHÉOTOMIE	RÉSULTAT	OBSERVATIONS
10	Karl. O	5 ans	Exsudat sur les amygdales tuméfiées et sur la paroi postér. du pharynx.		Mourant. Trachéotomie après essai de tubage.	Guérison apr. 20 jours	Décan. au 8e j. Catarrhe des voies aériennes, exanthème dù au sérum. Évolution normale. Inject. (4500 A. E.).
11	Salomon M......	4 1/2 ans	Début avec angine et exanthème. Exs. sur amygdales et pharynx.	56 heures		Guérison	5 injections de sérum à 1500 A. E. (4500 A. E.) Behring.
12	Robert G.......	12 ans	Pas d'exsudat. croup bénin.	5 tubag. temp. (écouvillonnage). Rejet de 2 membranes.		Guérison	Des accès de suffocation répétés. Aphonie pendant quelques jours. Injection de 4500 A. E. Behring.
13	Robert D........	15 mois	Pas d'exsudat.	4 tubages. Durée totale, 77 heures	Trachéot. secondaire.	Amélioration	Impossibilité d'accomplir l'essai de décanulement Retubage. Nouvelle trachéotomie. L'enfant garde la canule Paltauf. Injection de 6000 A. E.
14	Robert C.......	5 ans	Exsud. diphtériques étendus sur la muqueuse du pharynx	2 tubages. Durée totale 68 heures		Guérison	Injection de 8000 A. E. Behring.
15	Fritz M.........	2 1/4 ans	Légers exsudats sur l'amygdale droite.	2 tubages, 75h. Auto-extubation.		Guérison	Trois accès de suffocation très violents. Gargouillement dans le tube. Bronchite. Exanth. Injection 1500 A. E.
16	Carl K.........	5 1/2 ans	Léger exsudat sur les amygdales.	50 heures auto-extubation.			Broncho. sténose laryngée très notable. Paltauf A. E. Injection de 4000 A. E.

Octobre 1894-Novembre 1899. **Diphtérie avec sténose laryngée.** *Sérothérapie.*

N° D'ORDRE	NOM	AGE	EXSUDAT	TUBAGE	TRACHÉOTOMIE	RÉSULTAT	OBSERVATIONS
17	Franz B.	5 1/4 ans	Pas d'exsudat.	7 tubages avec des intervalles de 15 à 8 h. Durée 119 heures	Trachéot. au bout de six jours.	Guérison	Décanulement au bout de 14 jours. Paltauf (7500 A. E.).
18	Erwa S.	15 mois	Exsudats étendus de couleur sale, sur la muqueuse du pharynx.	Tub. imposs. à cause de bourrage de membranes et de l'adynamie.	Trachéotom.	Guérison au bout de 5 semaines.	Sténose extrême. Injection 4500 A. E. Exanthème du sérum. Décanulement au bout de 6 jours.
19	Louise P.	5 1/2 ans	Rougeur, exsud. miliaire sur l'amygdale droite.	Sans intervention.		Guérison	Sténose intense. Gêne respiratoire. Injection Behring 2. Amélioration après.
20	Valérie P.	14 mois	La diphtérie du pharynx et des phénomènes laryngés vient de disparaître.			Guérison	Environ 6000 A. E. en injection. Accès de suffocation. Sténose.
21	Ferdinand F.	2 ans	A gauche dans la dépression amygdalienne.			Guérison	Respiration sifflante. Injection de Behring 2 et 3 (2500 A. E.).
22	Léopold Sch.	7 ans	Exsudats luisants blanchâtres sur la paroi postérieure du pharynx.			Guérison	A la suite de 1 injection Behring 5 (1500 A. E.). Amendement des symptômes de sténose intense et disparition rapide des exsudats.
23	Erna R.	4 ans	Sur les amydales, piliers et paroi postér. du pharynx.			Guérison	Les phénomènes de sténose ont duré 2 jours, plusieurs accès de suffocation. Injection de 6000 A. E. Behring.

Octobre 1894-Novembre 1899.   **Diphtérie avec sténose laryngée.**   *Sérothérapie.*

N° D'ORDRE	NOM	AGE	EXSUDAT	TUBAGE	TRACHEOTOMIE	RÉSULTAT	OBSERVATIONS
24	Mitzi R.........	6 ans	Piliers, luette, paroi post. du pharynx.	Sans intervention.	Sans intervention.	Guérison	Accès de suffocation. Raucité. Injection (de 5000 A. E.) Behring.
25	Thea Th.........	18 mois	Pas d'exsudat.			Guérison	Complication de bronchite. Deux accès violents de suffocation. Injection (de 5000 A. E.) Paltauf.
26	Wenzel L.......	2 1/2 ans	Il y a deux jours des exsudats formant voile sur les amygdales.			Guérison	Légers phénomènes de sténose laryngée; ensuite inspir. avec dépressions assez fortes. Injection de 2000 A. E.
27	Mitzi K.........	2 1/2 ans	Pas d'exs., rougeur de la muqueuse du pharynx.			Guérison	Accès de suffocation. Injection de 1500 A. E. Behring.
28	Robert St.......	5 ans	Sur les amygdales et la paroi postér. du pharynx.			Guérison	Pendant la toux, gêne respiratoire due à l'obstruction par membranes, paralysie post-diphtérique des muscles de l'œil. Inj. de 5000 A. E. Behring.
29	Valérie Z........	6 ans	Entre la luette et les amygdales.			Guérison	Bronchite. Gêne respiratoire. Inject. de 4500 A. E. Behring.
30	Paul Sp.........	14 mois	Luette et paroi post. du pharynx.			Guérison	Sténose intense. Inj. de 1000 A. E. Paltauf et 5000 Behring.
31	Léopoldine Sp...	4 ans	Paroi postérieure du pharynx.			Guérison	Sténose intense, dépressions inspiratoires, toux aboyante, 1 injection Paltauf 1000 A. E., 1 injection Behring 1500 A. E.
32	N. Fr...........	18 mois	Pas d'exsudat.			Guérison	2 injections Paltauf à 1500, 5000 A. E.

Résumé des deux tableaux A et B.

TABLEAU A.
Résumé.

29 cas. — 25 opérés avec 14 cas de mort.
6 cas sans intervention = 21 0/0 des cas de sténose laryngée.
Mortalité des opérés : 47,8 0/0.
Mortalité totale : 58,8 0/0.
Durée moyenne du temps d'intubation = 108 heures dans les cas de guérison et sans trachéotomie secondaire.

TABLEAU B.
Résumé.

52 cas. — 18 opérés avec 1 cas de mort.
14 sans intervention = 45 0/0 de cas de sténose laryngée.
Mortalité des opérés : 5,55 0/0.
Mortalité totale : 5,125 0/0.
Durée moyenne du temps d'intubation = 58 heures pour les cas de guérison et sans trachéotomie secondaire.

L'ÉCOUVILLONNAGE LARYNGO-TRACHÉAL DANS LE CROUP
PRÉSENTATION D'INSTRUMENTS

par M. le docteur GEFFRIER,

d'Orléans.

Au cours d'une épidémie de diphtérie qui sévit à Orléans pendant tout l'hiver de 1889-90, j'ai observé un certain nombre d'enfants trachéotomisés, chez lesquels des membranes abondantes se formant dans la trachée, sortaient difficilement par la canule malgré l'introduction répétée de quelques grammes d'un liquide tiède, tel que l'eau boriquée, suivant l'exemple de mes maîtres Labric et Archambault.

Pour faciliter le détachement des membranes fibrineuses et obtenir leur expulsion, j'imaginai d'opérer de la façon suivante :

1° Pulvérisation par l'orifice de la canule dans la trachée d'une solution chaude de benzoate de soude à 1/50. Je dis chaude et non tiède, parce que le liquide se refroidit brusquement par suite de la pulvérisation.

2° Introduction, par la canule, d'une plume d'oie longue et flexible, bien souple et intacte de sa pointe garnie de ses barbes, qui est portée rapidement jusqu'au niveau de la bifurcation de la trachée, puis vivement tournée entre les doigts pour tâcher d'envrillonner les mucosités et les membranes, enfin rapidement retirée, essuyée, puis réintroduite.

Cela à plusieurs reprises, jusqu'à ce que les barbes de la plume formant écouvillon, ne ramènent plus que le liquide de la pulvérisation qui est reprise à plusieurs fois pendant l'écouvillonnage.

5° Si pendant l'écouvillonnage à la plume, l'oreille perçoit le bruit de drapeau ou de clapet caractéristique d'une membrane à demi-détachée qui reste en partie adhérente, la pince à fausses membranes (modèle Collin) est introduite par la canule, puis largement ouverte, on attend une forte secousse de toux qui ne fait pas longtemps défaut quand on pulvérise la solution de benzoate de soude dans la canule ; on referme brusquement la pince au moment même d'une violente expiration due à la toux, puis on retire la pince fermée ; on recommence plusieurs fois cette manœuvre.

En procédant de cette façon j'ai pu fréquemment retirer des lambeaux parfois très étendus de membranes trachéales ou même bronchiques, qui n'arrivaient pas à être expulsées spontanément.

J'ai pu voir guérir ainsi des petits malades que le retour de la dyspnée après trachéotomie semblait vouer à une fin prochaine.

J'ai eu beaucoup plus rarement à mettre cette manœuvre en pratique depuis les remarquables succès de sérum antidiphtérique, grâce auquel on a pu revenir au tubage de Bouchut, délaissé depuis longtemps. Les trachéotomies sont en effet devenues beaucoup plus rares et les accumulations de membranes dans la trachée sont maintenant, au moins dans la région où j'exerce, tout à fait exceptionnelles.

Mais un nouveau genre d'écouvillonnage vint s'adapter aux nouvelles méthodes de traitement du croup diphtérique :

Le docteur Variot écrivit depuis 1895, dans le *Journal de clinique et de thérapeutique infantiles*, plusieurs articles pour démontrer l'utilité du tubage momentané, comme procédé d'écouvillonnage du larynx.

En 1897, parut un travail de Mlle Schultze, inspiré par le docteur Variot. Dans le très intéressant historique que fait Mlle Schultze de l'écouvillonnage du larynx, elle cite, à propos du croup spécialement, les tentatives de Dieffenbach, d'Horace Green, de Sérullaz, même de Dupuytren, mais surtout de Loiseau, qui exécuta l'écouvillonnage du larynx dans le croup un grand nombre de fois et inventa même à cet effet, une série d'instruments que j'ai eu le regret de ne pouvoir retrouver.

Pour le docteur Variot, le tube d'O'Dwyer, modifié par Bayeux, est le meilleur instrument d'écouvillonnage : il détache les fausses membranes, leur permet de sortir par l'orifice dont il est perforé et produit en même temps la dilatation de la glotte pour en combattre le spasme, comme l'avait déjà proposé Renou (de Saumur) qui opérait avec une pince courbe à polypes du larynx.

Pour ce qui est de cette dilatation, je n'en nie pas les avantages, mais pour le détachement des membranes et surtout pour leur expulsion, le tube me paraît insuffisant : l'orifice en est assez étroit pour que des membranes d'un certain volume n'y passent que difficilement et en risquant de l'obturer complètement.

De fait, les cas qui m'ont porté à admettre l'utilité de ce genre d'écouvillonnage ont trait à des enfants qui, après tubage, ne respiraient pas, et qui, immédiatement détubés, ont pu expulser une membrane trachéale, reprendre respiration et n'être pas retubés grâce à l'influence du sérum antidiphtérique qui s'opposait à la reproduction des membranes.

Relisant le premier mémoire de Variot, paru en 1895 dans la *Revue de clinique et de thérapeutique infantiles*, j'y ai constaté que sur quatre observations, dans la première seulement, la membrane est sortie par le tube qui a été enlevé ensuite de propos délibéré ; dans l'observation II le tube a été expulsé par l'enfant en même temps que la membrane ; dans l'observation III, le tube a été dégluti en même temps que la membrane était expulsée ; enfin dans l'observation IV, le tube a été spontanément expulsé dix minutes après la membrane dont le passage avait dû probablement le déplacer.

J'ai voulu essayer de faire mieux et, après de longs tâtonnements, j'ai fini par adopter l'instrument que j'ai l'honneur de vous présenter, et qui a été exécuté par M. Aubry.

Il consiste en un tube de petit diamètre qui a la courbure voulue pour pénétrer facilement dans le larynx : l'air peut passer librement entre ce tube et la paroi laryngo-trachéale.

Dans ce tube, se meut longitudinalement une tige terminée à l'extrémité laryngienne de l'instrument par un bouton mousse : entre ce bouton et l'extrémité ouverte du tube, la tige est garnie d'un faisceau de crins semblable à celui de l'instrument qui a été proposé pour retirer les épingles de la vessie ou de celui dont on s'est servi pour certains corps étrangers de l'œsophage.

Un petit ressort à boudin maintient ces crins tendus et appliqués le long de la tige conductrice, dans le larynx et jusque dans la trachée. Un mouvement du pouce de la main droite tire sur l'anneau qui correspond à la tige intérieure et fait saillir les crins en rapprochant leurs deux extrémités, le milieu de l'anse formée par chaque crin vient alors en contact avec la muqueuse trachéale, on retire doucement l'appareil en maintenant les crins dans la même position, on le nettoie dans de l'eau bouillie ou dans toute solution qu'on voudra employer, pourvu qu'elle soit bien supportée par la muqueuse et on recommence si cela paraît nécessaire.

Il n'est pas besoin de dire que l'introduction de l'instrument se fait exactement comme l'introduction du tube à tuber. avec le porte-tube.

Grâce au petit diamètre de l'instrument. il n'empêche pas le passage de l'air pendant toute la durée de son introduction. Pendant sa sortie, d'ailleurs toujours assez rapide. l'air peut encore passer à travers les anses de crin.

Cet écouvillon laryngo-trachéal a surtout son indication dans les cas où on a lieu de supposer l'existence de membranes épaisses à l'entrée des voies respiratoires, car il est clair qu'il ne combattra point le spasme glottique : c'est uniquement un extracteur de membranes; s'il ne les entraîne pas avec lui. il les détache suffisamment pour que l'effort de toux consécutif ait grandes chances de les expulser. Il réussira d'autant mieux que l'enfant sera plus âgé, l'influence prépondérante du spasme glottique par la production du tirage, diminuant ordinairement avec l'âge.

L'instrument que j'ai l'honneur de vous présenter, n'est encore qu'à la période d'essai et je ne me dissimule pas ses imperfections : je me propose de remédier à celles d'entre elles qui m'ont frappé à l'usage : ainsi, l'introduction de l'instrument dans l'orifice supérieur du larynx est rendue difficile par la flexibilité de la tige terminale. Il sera facile de rendre cette extrémité plus rigide en ne laissant le ressort à boudin que dans la partie courbée. De plus, les crins de Florence, quand ils sont à leur maximum de dilatation, sont un peu trop durs et raclent un peu trop vigoureusement la muqueuse : il faudra prendre des crins plus souples et plus fins. J'aurais préféré le caoutchouc au crin. des difficultés de construction s'y sont opposées pour le moment; le crin de cheval, ou toute autre substance analogue, pourrait être employé.

P.-S. — Au moment de faire ma communication, mon constructeur M. Aubry, me remet l'instrument avec les perfectionnements que je lui avais signalés : l'extrémité de la tige terminale a été rendue rigide et sera plus facilement conduite dans l'intérieur du larynx; les crins plus souples et moins serrés frotteront beaucoup plus durement la surface de la muqueuse, enfin il a été construit plusieurs modèles de l'instrument de dimensions variées, pour les différents âges.

DISCUSSION

M. Sevestre. — L'instrument de M. Geffrier est assurément très ingénieux, mais je me demande si le frottement des crins contre la muqueuse ne risque pas de produire des érosions de cette muqueuse et de favoriser ainsi les inoculations secondaires, ce qu'il faut toujours éviter dans la diphtérie. Aussi je préférerai toujours pratiquer de préférence le tubage.

D'ailleurs je crois que M. Variot a lui-même renoncé à l'écouvillonnage.

M. VARIOT. — Je n'ai pas renoncé à l'écouvillonnage, mais je pense qu'il ne doit pas être employé partout. On peut dire qu'il y a deux sortes de croup : ceux où l'élément spasmodique est à peine marqué ou absent, tandis que les membranes sont très abondantes; ceux au contraire où l'élément nerveux, le spasme domine.

Aux premiers convient souvent l'écouvillonnage. Chez un enfant de 4 ou 5 ans, pas trop nerveux, on peut pratiquer l'écouvillonnage et l'enfant s'en trouve mieux. Par contre cette pratique est tout à fait contre-indiquée chez les tout jeunes enfants. Nous avons fait des essais sur plus de cent enfants et nous avons eu des succès dans la proportion de un sur trois, ce qui nous a prouvé que l'écouvillonnage n'est pas toujours indiqué. Il est certain que le procédé le plus simple est toujours préférable. Or, à cet égard, peut-on dire que le tubage soit toujours plus simple que l'écouvillonnage? Aussi, tout en limitant ses indications, je ne sais pourquoi on y renoncerait.

A une question de M. Martin, M. Variot répond qu'il croit que l'écouvillonnage ne doit pas être répété.

M. MARTIN (de Paris) pense avec M. Variot qu'il faut distinguer deux cas : ceux où le larynx est dur, contracté, qui réclament l'emploi du tube, et ceux où il présente un certain degré de flaccidité, où l'on a la sensation d'une obstruction et c'est ici surtout, comme l'a bien distingué M. Variot, que convient l'écouvillonnage. M. Martin préfère toutefois, dans bien des cas, lorsque par exemple les membranes sont profondément situées, le procédé de M. Bayeux, suivi d'une injection d'huile mentholée.

Souvent l'introduction du tube et son rejet presque immédiat constituent un véritable écouvillonnage. C'est ce qui arriva lors du premier tubage fait par MM. Roux et Chailloux : l'enfant rejeta le tube, puis, à la suite, des membranes et guérit. En somme, l'écouvillonnage est souvent un procédé utile, mais à la condition de n'être pas répété.

Quant à l'instrument de M. Geffrier, M. Martin redoute l'emploi des crins de Florence.

M. VIOLI demande à M. Variot s'il a observé des infections secondaires à la suite de l'écouvillonnage.

M. VARIOT. — L'écouvillonnage n'expose pas à plus de danger que le tubage. Dans les deux cas, tout dépend de l'habileté de l'opérateur.

NOUVEAUX INSTRUMENTS POUR L'INTUBATION DU LARYNX DANS LE CROUP

par M. le docteur TSAKIRIS.

de Paris.

J'ai l'honneur de vous présenter les instruments dont je me sers pour faire en ville l'intubation du larynx dans le croup. Ces instruments diffèrent sensiblement de ceux inventés par O'Dwyer.

L'*ouvre-bouche* modèle Mathieu est basé sur le principe du cric : ses gouttières sont mobiles et ne dérapent pas.

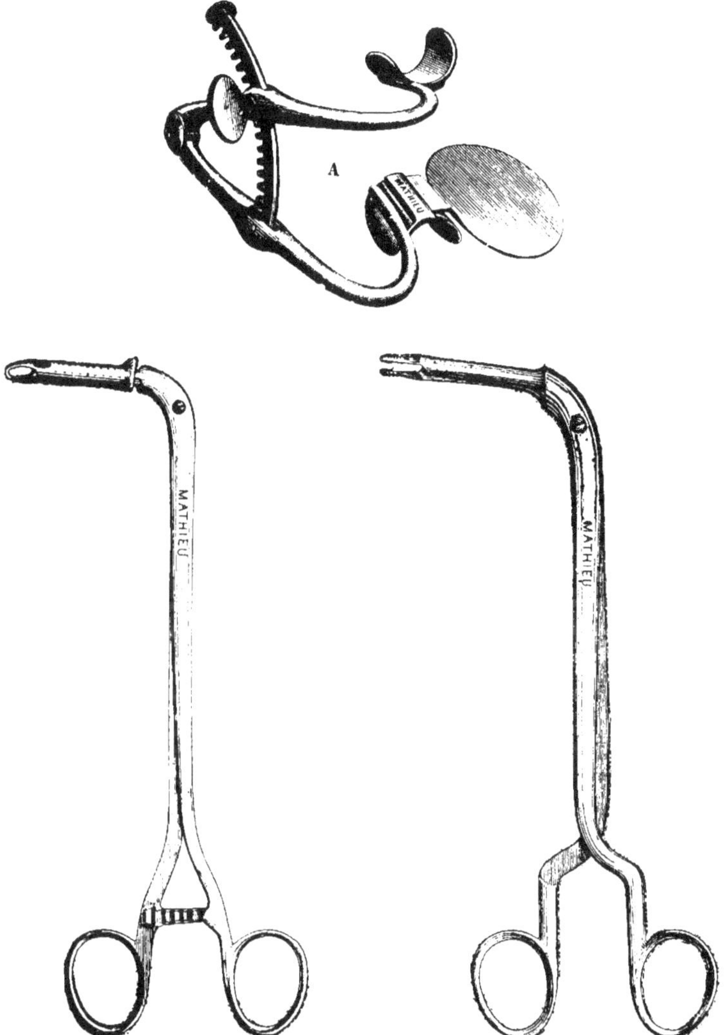

L'*introducteur* n'est qu'une simple pince : le mandrin est supprimé comme inutile.

L'*extracteur* est représenté également par une pince mais à mors plus longs.

Les *tubes* sont en aluminium et présentent la même longueur que ceux d'O'Dwyer; mais ils en diffèrent d'abord par leur extrémité inférieure qui se termine en arcade délimitant deux œillets. Cette arcade déjetée d'un côté est surmontée de deux orifices ovalaires; puis par leur extrémité supérieure ou tête dont la hauteur est moitié moindre.

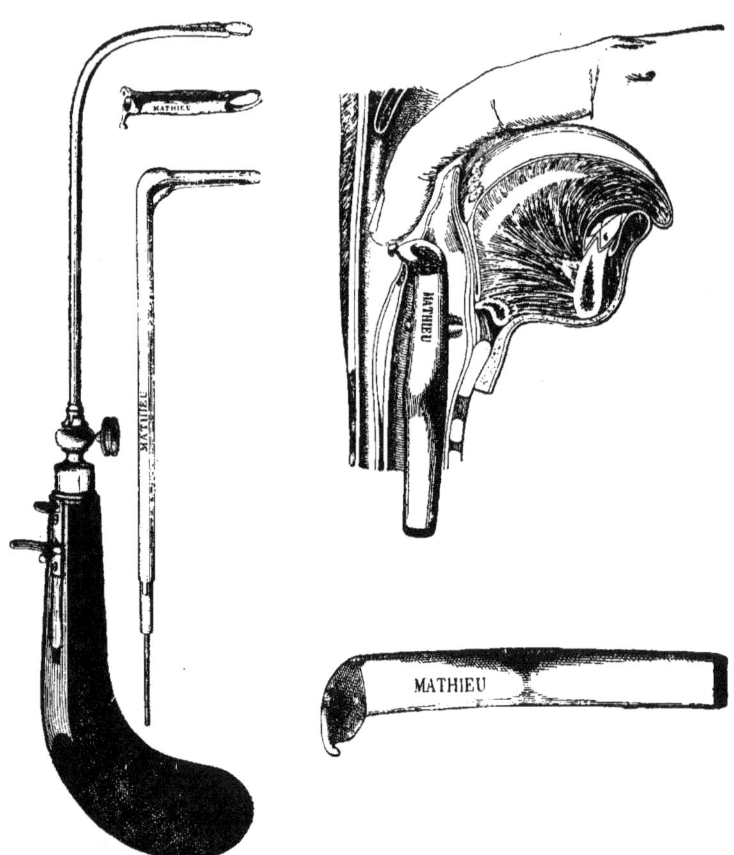

Ayant diminué la hauteur de la tête nous avons obtenu certains avantages, mais par contre nous avons rendu l'extraction plus laborieuse. C'est alors que nous avons eu l'idée d'employer le procédé de l'énucléation du tube procédé que nous avons décrit un des premiers en France (voir *Gazette des Hôpitaux de Paris*, 14 mai 1895 et notre *Thèse*. Paris 1895). Mais pour être pratique ce procédé exigeait des tubes très courts. Or les tubes courts ont été condamnés par O'Dwyer.

par les médecins américains, par Bonain et autres, parce qu'ils ne préservent pas suffisamment le larynx.

Le procédé de l'énucléation du tube n'étant pas applicable aux tubes longs, nous avons cherché et nous croyons avoir trouvé un procédé pour extraire le tube du larynx plus facilement qu'avec le procédé d'O'Dwyer.

En effet cet auteur ainsi que ses disciples, ont toujours cherché à extraire le tube du larynx en faisant rentrer les mors de l'introducteur dans son orifice supérieur. Mais cet orifice est toujours difficile à trouver; par contre on sent toujours une partie du pourtour de la tête alors ne peut-on pas accrocher cette tête par la périphérie?

Tel fut notre point de départ. Nous en avons fait part à M. Mathieu qui a fait fabriquer des tubes en aluminium admirablement polis. Ces tubes absolument pareils à ceux d'O'Dwyer présentent cette particularité, que le point le plus culminant de leur tête se termine en boulette. Cette boulette, après l'introduction, va se loger très naturellement dans l'angle formé par les deux cartilages aryténoïdes.

Lorsqu'on introduit le doigt dans la gorge on pénètre dans le pharynx, on sent les cartilages aryténoïdes, et plus bas le chaton du cartilage cricoïde. En remontant un peu on sent la boulette terminale. Une simple anse suffit alors pour accrocher et retirer le tube.

L'instrument que M. Mathieu a fait fabriquer sur nos indications est constitué par un manche universel Schrœter : sur ce manche on peut monter par deux systèmes de vis soit un dilatateur s'écartant parallèlement et destiné à fixer et à introduire le tube, soit une deuxième pièce en forme de serre-nœud dont l'anse est destinée à extraire le tube en s'accrochant à la légère encoche située en dessous de la boulette.

Avantages de cet instrument :

1) *Introduction facile du tube.*

2) *Extraction sûre* et beaucoup plus facile qu'avec l'extracteur d'O'Dwyer.

3) Impossibilité de blesser le larynx.

4) Anse pouvant s'allonger à volonté pour s'adapter à tous les âges.

5) Anse formant avec le tube une articulation mobile et non une tige rigide comme l'extracteur ordinaire fixé au tube.

Avantages de nos tubes :

1) Les tubes en aluminium quoique très légers, ne sont jamais expulsés du larynx pendant les accès de toux.

2) Tous les enfants que nous avons intubés ont pu avaler les solides et les liquides très facilement.

5) Chez tous les enfants que nous avons intubés nous n'avons jamais observé l'obstruction de la lumière du tube par des fausses membranes.

Outre ces avantages ces tubes sont faciles à fabriquer et à polir; ils sont inoxydables, et gardent leur brillant si on évite de les plonger dans le sublimé ou dans l'eau bouillante boriquée ou non (qui les ternit), et si l'on prend le soin de les désinfecter non pas à l'autoclave, mais à l'étuve sèche, ou, en son absence, tout simplement dans l'acide phénique concentré, ou dans la teinture d'iode et l'alcool après nettoyage et brossage préalable à l'eau et au savon.

Pour notre compte, après avoir placé nos tubes dans un cylindre en verre, bouché à ses extrémités avec de la ouate, nous les stérilisons dans l'étuve sèche à 180 degrés.

DISCUSSION

M. Sevestre. — M. Tsakiris a dit que beaucoup de médecins, en France comme en Amérique, avaient renoncé à l'emploi des tubes courts, à cause des inconvénients qu'ils leur avaient reconnus. Je ferai remarquer tout d'abord que les tubes courts américains diffèrent totalement des tubes courts français et j'ajoute que ces derniers sont toujours employés, d'une façon presque générale, dans les deux hôpitaux d'enfants de Paris et que l'on ne paraît pas disposé à y renoncer.

M. Tsakiris a fait construire ses tubes en aluminium; c'est un métal très léger, ce qui dans l'espèce me paraît constituer un avantage, mais qui est aussi très altérable. Il y a cinq ans, j'ai fait usage dans mon service, chez plusieurs malades, des tubes fabriqués par M. Collin; malheureusement ces tubes étaient, au bout de 2 ou 3 jours, lorsqu'on en fit l'extraction, recouverts et comme incrustés de débris organiques et après un nettoyage qui ne réussit que difficilement à enlever ces débris, ils avaient perdu leur poli. M. Collin me dit qu'il n'était pas très surpris de cette circonstance, l'aluminium étant un métal poreux, facilement altérable; la dorure du tube permettrait de remédier à cet inconvénient, mais elle est elle-même difficile à obtenir

Quant à la forme des tubes de M. Tsakiris, j'avoue que je n'aime pas beaucoup la saillie postérieure qui se trouve en haut de ce tube et cela non pas seulement à cause de la pression qu'elle peut exercer sur le larynx, mais encore en raison des inconvénients qui pourraient en résulter si le tube était avalé par l'enfant: or c'est une circonstance qui n'est pas absolument rare avec les tubes ordinaires, longs ou courts, et qui se produirait tout aussi bien, je pense, avec les tubes de M. Tsakiris; généralement le séjour du tube dans les voies digestives est de 2 à 3 jours et je n'ai jamais vu qu'il en résultât d'inconvénients. Je ne serais pas aussi tranquille avec les tubes de M. Tsakiris.

Enfin il me semble que l'introducteur (nouveau modèle) est d'un mécanisme un peu compliqué et que la stérilisation en est peut-être assez difficile.

TUBAGE ET TRACHÉOTOMIE DANS LE CROUP COMPLIQUÉ

par M. Martinez VARGAS,

de Barcelone.

L'auteur rapporte deux observations, où le croup était compliqué de broncho-pneumonie et qui témoignent en faveur de la trachéotomie ; la trachéotomie favorise l'expectoration qu'on peut être parfois obligé de faciliter encore par l'introduction dans la canule d'une sonde de gomme molle aseptique. Par ce procédé, on abrège la durée de la maladie plus que par le tubage.

DISCUSSION

M. GUINON (de Paris) accorde que les cas de broncho-pneumonie secondaire, où on suppose que l'expectoration devrait être abondante, sont justiciables de la trachéotomie, mais ces cas sont très rares. Il a suffi fréquemment de pratiquer la respiration artificielle à plusieurs reprises dans la journée pour favoriser l'expulsion des mucosités. L'application du drap mouillé froid, préconisée par M. Sevestre, peut aussi réveiller des quintes de toux salutaires.

TRAITEMENT DE LA PARALYSIE DIPHTÉRIQUE

par M. le docteur Ramon Gomez FERREZ,

de Valencia.

Mon but est de faire connaître sommairement deux observations que j'ai recueillies et qui prouvent selon toute probabilité que :

1° Certaines paralysies diphtériques sont dues à la présence du bacille de Klebs-Loeffler dans les centres nerveux, comme le font prévoir les études de Barbier et Ulmann[1].

2° Que le meilleur traitement pour ces cas est le sérum antidiphtérique.

1re Observation. — Enfant Vincent, âgé de deux ans, de bonne constitution et de bonne santé habituelles. Sa mère le conduisit à ma clinique de la Faculté de Valencia le 24 octobre 1899. Il présentait des symptômes de paralysie du voile du palais (voile pendule avec

1. H. BARBIER et ULMANN. *La diphtérie*. Paris, 1899.

sensibilité faible), des muscles constricteurs laryngiens (chute du lait dans le larynx, toux en avalant), parésie des cordes vocales inférieures (voix rauque), parésie du diaphragme (cris faibles, aspiration faible) et peut-être même parésie des muscles de Reisessen (accumulation ou dépôt des mucosités dans les bronches, râles sous-crépitants, légère cyanose), paralysie des muscles trapèze et sterno-mastoïdien (tête pendante), paralysie flasque des muscles des extrémités (impossibilité de se tenir debout et de saisir les objets), pouls faible, battements cardiaques sourds.

La succion, ainsi que les mouvements des yeux, l'intelligence et les autres fonctions semblent normales, sauf un léger catarrhe de la conoactive de l'œil droit. L'affection de cet enfant commença, au dire de a mère, un mois environ après une éruption vésiculeuse généralisée (impétigo ?), plus marquée sur les extrémités, qui conservaient encore les taches rougeâtres couvertes d'un épiderme desséché et rugueux.

Un mois environ après cette éruption, l'enfant eut une suppuration de l'oreille droite qui disparut bientôt par de simples irrigations d'eau boriquée.

A peine cette suppuration eut-elle disparu, et cela sans fièvre apparente, que les symptômes de paralysie commencèrent, et ils ont environ un mois de date lors de mon observation.

La mère reconnut en premier lieu la paralysie des membres inférieurs, le nasonnement et la difficulté d'avaler.

Je n'ai pas pu faire l'exploration électrique et, d'autre part, les ensemencements faits avec le mucus du pharynx ne donnèrent aucun résultat positif quant au bacille diphtérique : malgré cela, je diagnostiquai une paralysie diphtérique en raison des régions premièrement envahies, — de leur manière de s'étendre et d'attaquer plus fortement les muscles du pharynx, du larynx et de la nuque, — du caractère de la paralysie flasque, et de l'absence d'atrophie, — de l'absence absolue de tares héréditaires syphilitiques ou autres.

Je considère que la suppuration de l'oreille ou les lésions cutanées ont pu être la porte d'entrée du bacille.

En me reportant aux études de Barbier et Ulmann déjà citées, je fis aire cinq injections de sérum antidiphtérique Roux de 20 centimètres cubes chacune, les 27, 29 octobre, les 1er, 6 et 10 novembre.

Le 6 novembre, c'est-à-dire quand l'enfant avait reçu déjà 60 centimètres cubes de sérum en trois injections, la voix prit un timbre moins nasal, l'enfant avalait mieux et la force augmentait dans les extrémités, surtout dans les membres inférieurs.

Le 10 novembre, quand on donna la dernière injection, l'enfant remuait bien la tête et pouvait la maintenir droite assez longtemps, le timbre nasal avait disparu presque complètement, et la force était revenue presque tout à fait aux membres.

L'enfant n'est plus revenue à ma clinique, mais j'ai su par le médecin de son village que la guérison a été rapide et complète.

2e Observation. — Mercédès Garcia, petite fille âgée de neuf mois, fut présentée à ma clinique particulière vers le 10 décembre dernier. Sa voix était faible, le lait tombait dans le larynx quand elle tétait et provoquait chaque fois une toux forte, la figure était boursouflée et pâle, les lèvres légèrement cyanotiques, les muscles de la nuque, du dos et des extrémités paralysés ou parétiques, la tête tombait dans tous les sens, et l'enfant ne pouvait pas se tenir assise. Il y avait aussi paralysie du muscle droit externe de l'œil gauche et parésie de l'orbiculaire, anémie, pouls faible et fréquent (140), température 56,°5.

Dans les régions mastoïdiennes, l'enfant présente des ulcères couverts d'une fausse membrane diphtéroïde.

Ayant ensemencé cet exsudat de fausse membrane dans du sérum solidifié, il se produisit des colonies semblables à celles du bacille de Klebs, et l'examen bactériologique fait par mon ancien élève, le docteur Campos Fillol, révéla un bacille court et gros, fortement cloisonné et analogue au bacille de Loeffler, autant dans la culture de l'exsudat des ulcères et dans le mucus pharyngien que dans les examens directs.

Toutefois, de nouveaux ensemencements de ce bacille dans le bouillon et dans le sérum ne prospérèrent pas.

Les antécédents pathologiques de cet enfant dans le mois d'octobre présentent une affection gastro-intestinale fébrile à marche lente, et des symptômes cérébraux à la fin (congestions suivant le médecin qui la soignait), qui motivèrent l'application de petits vésicatoires derrière les oreilles ; ce fut ce qui produisit les petits ulcères dont j'ai parlé plus haut.

Dans le mois de novembre, les bras et les jambes faiblirent, et la voix aussi, en même temps que sur le cou se présentait une éruption exsudative et une adénite, qui suppura abondamment, donnant un pus verdâtre et épais, avec une légère réaction fébrile.

Ayant diagnostiqué la paralysie diphtérique due probablement à l'infection des ulcères rétro-auriculaires, je décidai le traitement suivant :

Quatre injections de sérum Roux de 20 centimètres cubes chacune, qui furent faites les 15, 16, 17 et 18 décembre ; en outre, chaque jour, neuf gouttes de solution de perchlorure de fer (50 degrés Beaumé) et de petites doses d'hypophosphites de soude et de chaux avec quelques gouttes de teinture de noix vomique.

Le 21 décembre, l'enfant put s'asseoir, elle soutenait mieux sa tête et ne toussait plus toutes les fois qu'elle tétait : en un mot tous les symptômes cédèrent peu à peu.

Après cela, je n'ai plus suivi cette enfant, mais j'ai su que la guérison avait été rapide et complète, et qu'en ce moment, fin juillet 1900, elle se porte tout à fait bien, et a un développement normal.

Réflexions. — Deux cas sont sans doute peu pour formuler des conclusions : mais la rapidité avec laquelle la paralysie a disparu, sous l'action exclusive du sérum dans le premier cas, et presque exclusive dans le second, me fait croire qu'il ne s'agit pas d'autre chose que de la paralysie diphtérique, qui est seule attaquée avec succès par le sérum.

Je crois de même, que, par les deux cas, il est bien prouvé que certaines paralysies diphtériques sont dues à la présence du bacille diphtérique dans les centres nerveux bulbo-protubérantiels et peut être même médullaires.

Je crois aussi au grand avantage du traitement par le sérum antidiphtérique sur le traitement classique, qui donne des résultats si lents et si variables.

Je constate enfin, sur mes deux petits malades, l'inocuité et la parfaite tolérance de ces enfants pour le sérum Roux injecté à doses considérables.

DISCUSSION.

M. Guinon pense aussi que les injections répétées de sérum de Roux sont utiles dans ces cas : mais sa pratique ne lui permet pas de conclure d'une manière définitive. En tout cas il a constaté, lui aussi, la parfaite inocuité de cette médication.

VI

COQUELUCHE

LES COQUELUCHES FÉBRILES NON COMPLIQUÉES

par M. Gregorio ARAOZ ALFARO,

Professeur suppléant à la Faculté de médecine de Buenos-Ayres.
Chef du service d'enfants à l'Hôpital Saint-Roch.

La coqueluche est considérée, par la grande majorité des auteurs et praticiens modernes, comme une maladie absolument apyrétique, pendant la période spasmodique. On accepte volontiers que le stade catarrhal peut s'accompagner d'une fièvre plus ou moins légère, toujours de peu d'importance, mais une fois la période spasmodique survenue, la fièvre doit disparaître totalement.

C'est là, pour ne pas nous appesantir trop, l'opinion de Rilliet et Barthez, Jaccoud, Descroizilles, Cadet de Gassicourt, Baginsky, Unger, Uffelmann, West, Goodhart, Moncorvo, Henoch, Steffen, Eichhorst, Monti, Comby, Ausset, etc.

La presque totalité des médecins acceptent presque comme un aphorisme les assertions de Cadet de Gassicourt, lorsqu'il proclame, dans ses mémorables *Leçons*, que « *la coqueluche est une maladie absolument apyrétique, excepté parfois dans les premiers jours de la période catarrhale, et encore la fièvre, quand elle existe, est-elle toujours faible et de courte durée ; donc toute élévation quelque peu sérieuse de la température vous annoncera une complication pulmonaire, la seule qui s'accompagne de fièvre.... *»

Cependant, il est facile de trouver la relation d'anciennes épidémies de coqueluche où la fièvre a été observée fréquemment dans la période spasmodique. Aaskow constata le type intermittent quotidien à Copenhague (1766) et Ozanam l'observa de même à Milan, en 1815. Le type tierce fut décrit par Rosenstein (1775) en Suède, par Mellin (1769), Butter (1775), Stoll (1781), Hufeland (1786), Jahn (1805), et, plus récemment, par Winogradow, à Moscou (1825). Mellin décrit aussi un type double-tierce en quelques cas de 1769. Götz parle aussi d'une épidémie avec fièvre intermittente survenue dans la Russie méridionale, en 1866.

D'ailleurs, tous les auteurs modernes n'ont pas méconnu les formes fébriles de la coqueluche.

Trousseau dit qu'on peut voir la fièvre initiale persister sept, huit, douze, et même quelquefois quinze jours, bien qu'il ne parle pas du type qu'elle peut affecter.

Roger parle de l'état fébrile permanent quoique modéré (37°,5, 38 et même 39 degrés), qu'on peut observer lorsque la forme catarrhale est très accentuée. Et, en traitant de l'*hyper-coqueluche*, il ajoute qu'on peut voir des frissons plus ou moins accentués suivis de quelques accès fébriles à exacerbations et rémissions irrégulières.

D'après d'Espine et Picot, on observe exceptionnellement des accès éphémères de fièvre.

Filatow est bien explicite au sujet de la possibilité de voir la fièvre se maintenir à la période spasmodique en dehors de toute complication.

Guéneau de Mussy et Richardière signalent aussi dans la période convulsive des accès fébriles, périodiques ou non.

Enfin, Guérin, dans sa thèse inaugurale, faite sous l'inspiration du professeur Hutinel, insiste avec raison sur l'obscurité qu'on trouve généralement à ce sujet, et présente des observations très intéressantes d'accès fébriles intenses et éphémères, en pleine période spasmodique, sans complication appréciable. Il étudie aussi la fièvre plus ou moins prolongée pendant la période convulsive et incline, comme Roger, à la placer toujours sous la dépendance d'une bronchite catarrhale plus accentuée que d'ordinaire.

En présence de ces contradictions frappantes et du manque de détails qu'on trouve chez les auteurs sur ces mouvements fébriles, dont la connaissance est aussi délicate au point de vue du diagnostic et du pronostic, j'ai cru intéressant d'appeler l'attention de cette savante assemblée sur cette question, en lui soumettant les résultats des observations que j'ai été à même de faire jusqu'à présent.

Je crois pouvoir rattacher ces modalités fébriles à quelques types principaux.

I. — *Accès fébriles, brusques*, isolés ou répétés irrégulièrement, précédés ou non de frissons.

Ils ont déjà été signalés, comme nous l'avons dit plus haut, et il n'est pas juste de les rattacher toujours à une complication pulmonaire fugace (congestion pulmonaire, pneumonie abortive), comme l'ont prétendu quelques auteurs (Cadet de Gassicourt, Germain Sée, etc.).

Certainement, il y a des cas, et ils sont nombreux, où la fièvre, l'accélération du pouls et, quelquefois, un frisson initial, ne sont accom-

pagnés, ni suivis, d'aucun phénomène d'auscultation ou de percussion, ni de modification de la toux ou des crachats, ni même d'une dyspnée hors de proportion avec la température.

II. — *Fièvre prolongée* pendant toute, ou la plus grande partie de la période convulsive, de *type rémittent*, avec exacerbation vespérale et rémission matinale.

Cette forme a déjà été signalée par plusieurs observateurs et mise par la plupart d'entre eux en rapport étroit avec l'exagération du catarrhe bronchique, catarrhe considéré par eux comme une complication, bien qu'il soit ordinaire à un degré atténué.

Or, quoique nous ne puissions pas nier que la bronchite soit,

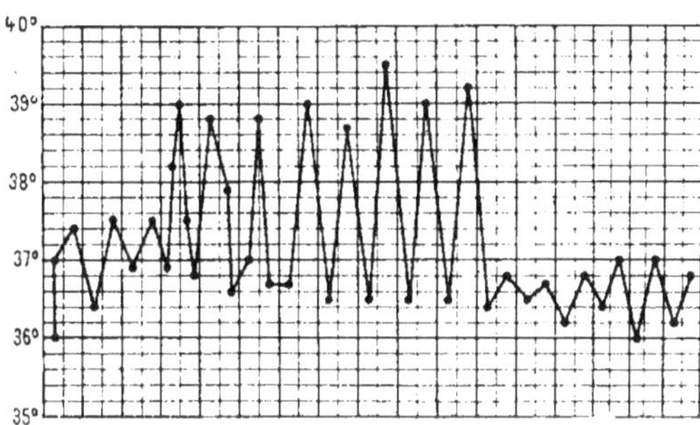

Fig. 1.

réellement, bien plus accentuée en quelques cas de coqueluche fébrile, *il est hors de doute pour nous que la même forme pyrétique peut être observée sans que le catarrhe soit plus appréciable que dans les cas communs, apyrétiques, et même en étant nul ou presque nul.*

III. — *Fièvre intermittente prolongée*, ordinairement quotidienne, quelquefois tierce ou irrégulière, avec ou sans frissons.

Nous avons déjà vu que Aaskow, Ozanam, Rosenstein, Mellin, Hufeland, Stoll, etc., l'avaient décrite il y a longtemps, et c'est la faute de la plupart des auteurs modernes de l'avoir oubliée.

Comme exemple de cette forme, très peu connue de nos jours, je peux présenter le graphique ci-dessous (fig. 1), qui se rapporte à un enfant de six ans, sans manifestations catarrhales d'aucune espèce, qui n'avait jamais été paludéen, avec un état général excellent, sans hypertrophie de la rate, et qui, d'ailleurs, guérit sans l'intervention de la quinine.

On peut voir que la température, sub-fébrile au commencement de la période spasmodique, s'élève au bout de quatre jours, en prenant le type nettement intermittent. Pendant trois jours, l'exacerbation se fait le matin ou à midi; puis, après, il y a apyrexie le matin, fièvre élevée le soir.

L'enfant se porte très bien aujourd'hui, deux ans après sa coqueluche.

IV. — J'appellerai, finalement, l'attention sur une *forme intervertie de fièvre*, qu'il m'a été donné d'observer deux fois.

Il s'agissait, dans l'un de ces cas, d'une coqueluche avec bronchite intense et même avec des foyers de congestion, et, probablement, de broncho-pneumonie. Dans l'autre observation, au contraire, le malade,

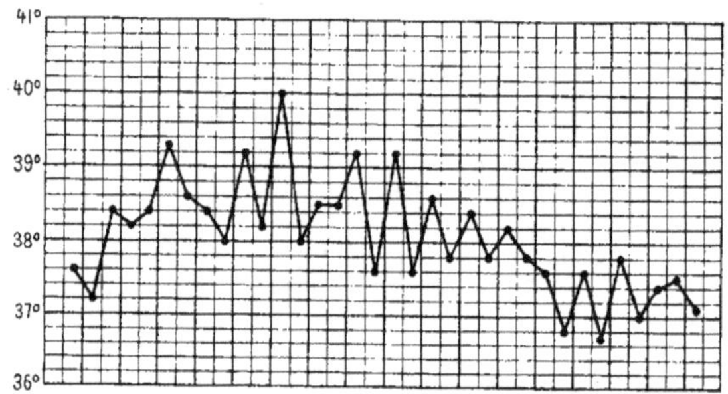

Fig. 2.

âgé de cinq ans, n'avait aucune manifestation catarrhale particulière.

Voilà un de ces graphiques, qui présente, comme vous pouvez le voir, l'exacerbation matinale et la rémission vespérale (fig. 2).

Vu l'importance qu'on a prétendu conférer au type interverti de la fièvre comme une manifestation tuberculeuse, il est doublement intéressant de savoir qu'on peut l'observer dans la coqueluche sans complication, ou avec bronchite intense, sans tuberculisation.

Nos deux observations, en effet, se rattachent à des enfants qui se portent tout à fait bien, deux et trois ans après leur coqueluche.

BELLADONE A TRÈS HAUTE DOSE DANS LA COQUELUCHE

par M. H. GILLET

Lorsqu'on est obligé de prolonger l'usage d'un médicament, il est bien rare qu'on ne soit pas contraint d'en augmenter progressivement la dose.

C'est ce qu'on est amené à faire dans la coqueluche en particulier.

Jusqu'ici, il faut bien l'avouer, nous n'avons pas de médication pathogénique réellement efficace, malgré des essais multiples. L'avenir, il faut l'espérer, nous en réserve une.

En attendant, il nous faut agir au mieux de l'intérêt des petits malades et nous adresser, faute d'autre, à une médication symptomatique : à la médication antispasmodique.

Nous ne manquons pas de médicaments qui répondent à l'indication, mais il s'en faut, surtout parmi les nouveaux venus, le bromoforme par exemple, pour n'en citer qu'un, qu'ils soient tous exempts de danger, dès qu'on veut un peu pousser la dose.

Or quoiqu'en général il faille être très sobre de médicaments chez les enfants, surtout très jeunes, ceci est d'une nécessité absolue. Il faut, dans la coqueluche, en augmenter les doses progressivement ou changer de médicament. C'est avec raison que le regretté Cadet de Gassicourt répétait, dans son enseignement, que dans la coqueluche un médicament avait épuisé son effet au bout de 8 jours.

Pour pouvoir employer des doses élevées, il faut s'adresser à des substances facilement tolérées sans accidents. De ce nombre paraît être la belladone entre autres.

Parmi les différents traitements, que j'ai mis en œuvre dans les services de consultation d'enfants dont je suis chargé, je me suis arrêté depuis un certain temps, après divers essais avec plusieurs médicaments, antipyrine, bromure, etc., à cette substance bien vieille en thérapeutique, à ce traitement nullement nouveau, mais en somme, quoique agent purement symptomatique, d'une certaine valeur, à la belladone. C'est l'ancien traitement de Guersant, de Trousseau.

Sous forme de solution titrée au millième de sulfate neutre d'atropine, je l'avais vu manier d'une façon très avantageuse, par mon estimé maître M. A. Sevestre, pendant mon internat à l'hospice des Enfants-Assistés.

J'ai pensé qu'en attendant le vrai spécifique, sous forme de sérum anticoquelucheux ou autre, il y avait peut-être intérêt à se limiter à peu de substances, à une seule même, à la belladone, au lieu de papillonner de l'une à l'autre, et à chercher à en bien définir les applications. On peut arriver à posséder ainsi une arme d'un maniement sûr, dans une main expérimentée, et savoir ce que peut donner le médicament et comment il peut le donner.

C'est l'expérience acquise par une pratique de plus de six années qui fera l'objet de cette note.

Je prescris exclusivement la teinture de belladone. Cette préparation est faite avec les feuilles de la plante dans cinq fois leur poids d'alcool à 60 degrés. On traite par déplacement 10 grammes de feuille de belladone par 50 grammes d'éther alcoolisé à 0,76 (éther 712 p. alcool à 90° 288 p.). Elle donne 55 gouttes au gramme, c'est une préparation au quart par rapport à l'atropine, 0 gr. 04 d'alcool répond à 0,01 d'atropine.

Le mode d'administration peu compliqué se résume à donner soit simplement la teinture de belladone, 5 à 10 grammes en provision, et à faire fractionner toutes les deux ou trois heures.

En potion, on incorpore la teinture de belladone dans une certaine quantité de julep, d'eau chloroformée, de sirop de tolu aux autres.

On peut aussi associer, dans la même formule, la teinture de belladone avec une faible dose d'eau de laurier cerise. Ce sont là les seules variantes du traitement. Il est inutile de faire des ordonnances longues d'une aune avec des formules polypharmaques.

La teinture de belladone a été ordonnée pendant les douze heures de jour, une dose toutes les deux ou plutôt trois heures, jamais plus rapprochée, et au besoin avec prises supplémentaires la nuit, mais toujours avec un intervalle minimum semblable. Parfois, lorsque les quintes prédominent beaucoup la nuit et s'espacent le jour, on retranche une ou deux prises diurnes, et l'on fait surtout l'administration nocturne, mais toujours avec espacement des doses de deux à trois heures au moins.

Les doses employées et absorbées ont toujours été fortes, graduellement et rapidement augmentées, jusqu'à atteindre des quantités qui semblent énormes.

Les premières doses, mais les premières doses seules, restent toujours très modérées pour tâter la susceptibilité du petit malade, puis l'on élève les doses rapidement et progressivement. À chaque nouvelle administration on augmente d'une fraction de la dose, par conséquent plusieurs fois dans une seule journée de façon à pouvoir arriver rapidement à des doses plus élevées.

Lorsqu'on arrive à une quantité forte, on ne néglige jamais d'expliquer et d'écrire les recommandations suivantes, pour éveiller l'attention sur les phénomènes de saturation voisine de l'intoxication : *surveiller la sécheresse réelle de la gorge et de la bouche, la dilatation des pupilles, les rougeurs de la face.*

Sur le nombre des enfants que j'ai soignés par cette méthode, j'ai pu recueillir 54 observations détaillées de sujets bien suivis et les utiliser ici.

Si je les range par âge, j'obtiens le résumé suivant :

Age.	Dose initiale.	Augmentation par dose	Dose extrême.
1 mois.	1/6 à 1/5 goutte.	1/12 à 1/6 goutte. 1/2	I. II.
5 mois.	1/5 à 1/2	1/4	V.
7 mois.	1	1/2	VI.
1 an. .	1	1/2	— IV. XII (?)
14 mois.	I. II.	1/2, 1.	III. VI. VIII.
1 an 1/2	1/2, III.	—	III, VIII.
1 an 3/4	II.	—	III, VII. XII.
2 ans. .	II, III.	—	VI. XIV, XVIII.
5 ans. .	1, II, IV.	I.	III, IV, V. VI. X. XII, XX, XXVIII.
4 ans. .	III, IV.	I, II.	V, XII. XVI, XX XXVI, XLII. XLV.
5 ans. .	III, IV.	—	X. XVI, XX, XLV.
6 ans. .	1, III, V.	I, V.	VI, XVI. XXII. XXX, LXV,
7 ans. .	—	—	XL.
8 ans. .	X.	IV.	LX.

Si l'on veut donner des chiffres ronds. on pourra adopter les suivants :

Chez les enfants au-dessous de six mois. 1/2 à 5 gouttes, soit 5 à 30 gouttes en vingt-quatre heures.

Chez les enfants au-dessus de six mois, jusqu'à un an, 5 à 10 gouttes (1 goutte par mois), soit 30 à 60 gouttes en vingt-quatre heures.

Chez les enfants entre un an et deux ans, 10 à 20 gouttes, soit 60 à 120 gouttes en vingt-quatre heures.

Chez les enfants de deux ans à trois ans, 20 à 30 gouttes. soit 120 à 180 gouttes en vingt-quatre heures.

Chez les enfants entre trois et cinq ans, de 30 à 50 gouttes, soit 180 à 508 gouttes en vingt-quatre heures.

Chez les enfants au-dessus de cinq ans, de 50 à 60 gouttes et plus. soit 308 à 360 gouttes en vingt-quatre heures.

Ces doses paraîtront en effet énormes, lorsqu'on les compare avec celles indiquées dans la posologie habituelle, d'après R. Noguès et Dauchez :

de 0 à 15 mois.	abstention.
à 1 an.	2 gouttes.
à 2 ans	4
à 5 ans	6
à 4 ans	8 à 10
à 5 ans	10 à 20
de 5 à 10 ans	20 à 40

La méthode consiste en somme à débuter toutes les trois heures, par une dose très modérée dans les premiers mois : 1 10, 1 6, 1/4 de goutte, 1 2 goutte jusqu'à plus d'un an, 1 goutte après, puis de 1 à 10, de deux à huit ans.

Comme DOSE EXTRÊME on voit que jusqu'alors on ne va guère qu'à 1 GOUTTE PAR MOIS D'AGE TOUTES LES TROIS HEURES, quatre au besoin ; qu'ensuite on pousse jusqu'à environ 10 GOUTTES dans le même intervalle, PAR ANNÉE D'AGE, toujours répétées toutes les 3 heures.

Il est évident que ces fortes doses ne représentent pas les doses initiales. On tâte d'abord le terrain avec une dose modérée, une demi-goutte, 4 gouttes, 10 gouttes toutes les deux ou trois heures, suivant qu'on a affaire à un nourrisson, à un enfant de cinq à six ans ou à un sujet déjà grand.

La dose du début toujours minime, 1 10, 1 6, 1/4 de goutte de teinture de belladone dans la 1ʳᵉ année, 1/5, 1 2, I, II, etc., après, toutes les 3 heures, ne se fixe pas d'une manière systématique ; mais, d'après diverses considérations prises en dehors de l'âge, par exemple sur l'état spasmodique plus ou moins accentué, sur la date plus ou moins éloignée du début de la maladie et dans ce cas sur la nécessité de regagner, s'il se peut, le temps perdu.

Ces mêmes raisons influent sur la marche à suivre dans l'augmentation des doses.

Chaque augmentation ne se chiffre que par une fraction modérée de la dose initiale, 1 6, 1 4, 1 5. La valeur plus ou moins grande de la fraction subit des oscillations qui obéissent aux mêmes raisons que celles qui ont présidé à la fixation de la dose initiale.

Il n'y a pas non plus nécessité à pousser jusqu'aux doses extrêmes, si les quintes cèdent rapidement. Ces doses servent seulement de témoins, pour nous montrer qu'on peut, sans danger, avec surveillance, aller jusque-là.

En somme, la méthode consiste à atteindre assez rapidement les hautes doses. Au lieu d'imiter la pratique de Trousseau, qui consistait à donner en une seule fois la forte dose, on répète l'ingestion du médicament, mais à intervalles suffisamment espacés, toutes les trois heures et plus au besoin, même lorsque les quintes s'éloignent.

On évite ainsi l'accumulation des doses.

Les doses extrêmes se maintiennent jusqu'à cessation de quintes typiques ; dès qu'elles s'amendent, on redescend graduellement.

Si nous entrons plus avant dans le détail de la médication belladonée, nous indiquerons la nécessité qu'a le médecin de surveiller de près ses petits malades, surtout au moment des fortes doses. A ce moment, je vois les enfants au moins tous les deux jours.

Les parents et les personnes destinées à soigner les coquelucheux doivent être stylés. Ils doivent donner le médicament toutes les trois heures, mais pas mathématiquement: le sommeil, les repas peuvent faire reculer l'heure d'administration. Il ne faut pas l'avancer. Pour faire manger les petits malades, on attendra qu'une quinte soit terminée pour faire prendre la belladone et, quelques minutes après, on donnera quelque nourriture.

La belladone n'empêche pas de prendre toutes les autres précautions, calme, silence, aération, atmosphère humide. Il en est de même du changement d'air. Elle n'interdit pas l'emploi simultané de toniques, de café, etc.

Qu'obtient-on avec ce traitement? Certainement, pas l'idéal, pas ce qu'on voudrait, pas la cessation rapide, absolue, mais tout au moins une grande atténuation de quintes. C'est tout ce qu'on peut demander à une médication purement symptomatique. Demander plus, c'est exiger plus que le possible.

La belladone compte avec le mercure parmi les médicaments les mieux supportés par les enfants, surtout lorsqu'on l'administre à dose graduellement progressive.

Pour observer des accidents, il faut donner d'un coup et sans accoutumance des quantités colossales. Deux fois j'ai été témoin d'une *intoxication belladonée* chez l'enfant. La première fois ce n'était ni chez un coquelucheux, ni à la suite d'une prescription régulière. Du reste, tout s'est terminé favorablement: on a été quitte pour une chaude alerte. C'était chez une enfant de deux ans à laquelle on avait administré par erreur des gouttes d'une solution au centième, préparée pour l'usage ophtalmologique, c'est-à-dire dix fois la dose prescrite. La sécheresse extrême de la gorge et de la bouche, la dilatation des pupilles avec injection et sécheresse conjonctivale, la rougeur de la face, le délire de paroles et d'actions, d'allures bruyantes avec tremblement, accès de rire, tous ces accidents finirent par cesser sous l'influence d'un vomitif, de l'administration large de café par la bouche et le rectum et par la sinapisation énergique. Les accidents avaient duré près de quatre heures. Aucune suite fâcheuse.

J'ai observé encore (fin octobre 1897) un accident survenu par la belladone; mais, dans ce cas, on ne peut incriminer la dose prescrite

L'enfant dont il s'agit, le jeune F...., âgé de quatre ans, traité depuis quelques jours pour la coqueluche, devait prendre 6 gouttes de teinture de belladone toutes les deux ou trois heures. La provision d'une journée, soit 36 gouttes incorporées dans six cuillers à café d'eau. était préparée à l'avance dans une bouteille. L'enfant, pendant que sa mère était occupée à autre chose, s'empara de la bouteille qu'il vida d'un trait.

La mère essaya bien de le faire vomir, sans administrer d'ipéca toutefois; mais l'enfant présenta de la rougeur sur la face et le corps, et pendant six heures resta endormi d'un sommeil dont on le tirait difficilement: pas de délire.

On sait, du reste, en particulier, depuis les travaux de Meuriot, que l'intoxication par la belladone, lorsqu'elle n'a pas été poussée trop loin, disparaît rapidement.

Mais ces faits d'empoisonnement à pronostic bénin, du reste, n'ont rien à voir avec le traitement belladoné à haute dose. C'est en dehors de celui-ci qu'ils se sont produits: ils ont même l'avantage de montrer, en somme, la grande tolérance qu'a l'organisme humain pour la belladone. Elle n'égale pas celle du lapin qui, dit-on pourrait impunément faire sa nourriture des feuilles de belladone, mais elle est cependant encore assez grande.

La médication belladonée à hautes doses ne comporte pas d'accidents, mais seulement quelques inconvénients. Dans les observations sur lesquelles je m'appuie, je n'ai noté que tout à fait exceptionnellement les signes de saturation.

De temps en temps, les petits malades accusent de l'amblyopie, les rougeurs de la face apparaissent, mais la cavité buccale reste humide. Deux fois le prurit a paru lié au traitement. Du côté du cœur, c'est à peine si l'on note un peu d'accélération. La diarrhée n'a rien de constant. Un enfant de six ans, qui prenait 65 gouttes par dose répétée toutes les 3 heures, fut tout le temps constipé.

Comme conclusion, on peut dire que, comme médication symptomatique, la belladone à fortes doses progressives représente une méthode d'une certaine valeur et d'une grande simplicité d'application. Quoique bien ancienne, elle mérite d'être conservée jusqu'à ce que les progrès de la science nous apportent la médication vraiment spécifique.

Mon intention n'est pas d'encourager à la témérité thérapeutique, mais d'indiquer jusqu'à quelles limites on peut, avec les précautions nécessaires, pousser les doses de belladone.

TRAITEMENT DE LA COQUELUCHE PAR LES BAINS D'AIR COMPRIMÉ

par **M**. le docteur ROCAZ.

Chef de clinique médicale des enfants à la Faculté de Bordeaux.

et par **M**. le docteur **J**. DELMAS.

Chargé du service hydrothérapique de l'Hôpital des enfants de Bordeaux.

Il est peu de maladies dont la thérapeutique soit aussi variée et paraisse aussi riche que celle de la coqueluche : richesse apparente faite pour nous illusionner sur notre réelle pauvreté, et notre triste impuissance devant une affection dont le remède spécifique reste encore à trouver. Chaque jour voit éclore une nouvelle médication qui a son moment de vogue plus ou moins durable, après lequel elle retombe dans l'oubli. Que de médicaments nous ont été ainsi présentés dans ces dernières années, nés la veille et morts le lendemain ! Et cependant la coqueluche est toujours sérieuse, souvent grave par elle-même, par les complications qui viennent s'y greffer et par les lésions qu'elle est capable de laisser à sa suite. Nous devons tout mettre en œuvre pour lutter contre elle, et, puisque nous n'avons que des palliatifs à lui opposer, devons-nous choisir parmi eux les moins inefficaces.

La médication dont nous allons vous entretenir et qui consiste dans l'emploi des bains d'air comprimé est déjà ancienne. Elle a déjà été mise en œuvre plusieurs fois, et en des pays divers, presque toujours avec succès. Nous n'avons ni l'intention ni le loisir de faire ici l'historique de cette question. Qu'il nous suffise donc de citer les noms de Shandhal (de Stockholm) qui nous a présenté une statistique aussi importante qu'encourageante (100 cas avec 85 succès évidents) ; de Moutard-Martin qui, en 1885, préconisait la méthode à la Société de Thérapeutique ; de Schliep, qui au Congrès de Wiesbaden tenu en 1887 nous apportait une observation des plus probantes, sur laquelle nous reviendrons.

Pourquoi cette thérapeutique, réellement efficace et connue depuis si longtemps, n'est-elle pas d'un usage plus courant ? C'est qu'elle nécessite un matériel qu'on ne rencontre pas partout, et que, d'autre part, elle exige plusieurs heures de traitement par jour, ce qui n'est pas à la portée de tous les parents. Cette première objection tombe d'elle-même dans les grandes villes pourvues d'un établissement aéro-thérapique, et le meilleur moyen de favoriser la création de ces établissements. aussi bien dans les hôpitaux qu'en ville, nous paraît consister dans la proclamation des résultats que donne la méthode. Quant à la seconde objection, elle ne saurait être de grand poids en face d'une coqueluche sévère, compromettant l'existence, et devant laquelle les familles n'ont rien à refuser. Aussi croyons-nous faire œuvre utile en tirant de l'oubli une médication qui a déjà fait ses preuves, et à laquelle nous n'avons pas hésité de soumettre les malades que nous avons eu l'occasion d'observer depuis un an environ.

Nous n'insisterons pas sur la partie technique de la méthode, dont la description se trouve un peu partout. Nos jeunes malades étaient placés, avec leurs parents, dans deux grandes cloches, réservoirs métalliques hermétiques éclairés par plusieurs hublots de verre épais. De chaque cloche partaient deux conduits, dont l'un communiquait avec un compresseur d'air actionné par un moteur à gaz, et l'autre avec l'extérieur. Ces deux conduits étaient commandés par deux robinets dont la manœuvre simultanée permettait de faire varier la pression à volonté: un manomètre très sensible nous donnait constamment la mesure de celle-ci. L'air envoyé dans la cloche était puisé à l'extérieur et filtré sur plusieurs couches d'ouate destinée à la stériliser.

La pression à laquelle étaient soumis nos coquelucheux a varié de 10 à 40 centimètres de mercure; ce minimum n'était guère dépassé dans la première séance; mais dans les séances suivantes une pression de 30 centimètres était la moyenne. La compression se faisait lentement (1 minute par centimètre de mercure); la période de pression stable variait entre une demi-heure et une heure; quant à la période de décompression, moment le plus délicat du bain, elle était environ d'une durée double de la période de compression : une telle prudence a eu pour effet de nous mettre à l'abri de tout accident. Ajoutons que grâce à la réfrigération du compresseur par un courant d'eau froide, et grâce au volume d'air considérable circulant constamment dans la cloche, la température de celle-ci restait à peu près constante, et que les malades n'en étaient nullement incommodés. Après chaque séance la cloche était soigneusement désinfectée.

Nous avons ainsi traité une cinquantaine de coqueluches.

Dans l'étude des résultats fournis par la méthode, il nous paraît nécessaire de ne faire entrer que les cas probants; il faut en effet éliminer tous ceux dans lesquels la coqueluche est déjà ancienne, c'est-à-dire capable d'une guérison spontanée rapide : un succès dans ces conditions n'est pas plus imputable à la thérapeutique qu'à l'évolution même de la maladie. Nous diviserons donc nos observations en deux groupes : le premier comprend toutes les coqueluches remontant à plus de 15 à 20 jours : constatons qu'elles ont toutes rapidement guéri : mais n'en tirons aucune conclusion, et occupons-nous exclusivement du second groupe formé par les coqueluches récentes, datant d'une quinzaine de jours, avec quintes caractéristiques survenues depuis huit ou dix jours seulement. C'est dans la lecture de ces dernières observations que nous puiserons les conclusions de ce travail.

Dès le début du traitement la quinte est modifiée dans son intensité, sa durée et sa fréquence. La diminution d'intensité et de durée est manifeste dès les premiers bains. Notons tout d'abord que la quinte est très rare dans le bain : exceptionnelle pendant la période de compression, elle ne survient généralement qu'à la fin de la décompression. Nous avons plusieurs fois observé que des quintes durant plusieurs minutes, et dans lesquelles on comptait de 10 à 20 reprises, étaient en quelques jours réduites à une durée deux ou trois fois moindre, le nombre des reprises diminuant dans les mêmes proportions.

Plus manifeste encore et plus facile à constater est la rareté relative des quintes chez les enfants traités par l'air comprimé. Nous ne saurions résister ici au désir de vous citer quelques chiffres. Voici tout d'abord une fillette de 11 ans qui nous est présentée avec une coqueluche de 15 jours caractérisée par plus de 20 quintes par jour (25 quintes la veille de l'examen) dont la violence se traduit par une bouffissure extrême de la face, et par la présence de deux grandes ecchymoses sous-conjonctivales recouvrant toute la sclérotique ; dix jours après le début du traitement, le nombre des quintes ne dépassait pas 8 en vingt-quatre heures. Un enfant de trois ans présentait 10 à 12 quintes par nuit, huit jours après l'apparition de sa coqueluche : cinq jours plus tard, c'est-à-dire après avoir pris cinq bains d'air comprimé, ce chiffre tombait à 2. Il serait fastidieux de vous communiquer toutes nos observations, qui concordent toutes, et qui sont toutes probantes à des degrés divers.

La durée totale de la coqueluche se trouve ainsi singulièrement abrégée. Dans la constatation de ce résultat deux causes d'erreur sont à éviter : qu'il s'agisse de coqueluches déjà vieilles, ou bien de formes très légères par elles-mêmes, presque abortives. Nous avons dit comment nous nous étions mis à l'abri de cette première erreur : et quant à la seconde, nous l'avons également évitée en ne comptant dans notre statistique que des coqueluches sévères, les seules qui nous parussent exiger un traitement énergique, auquel des raisons matérielles nous empêchaient de soumettre tous nos malades. Cette durée de l'affection chez les enfants traités par l'air comprimé est évidemment variable, mais elle est certainement bien moindre que chez les autres. Elle dépend de plusieurs facteurs dont les deux principaux sont l'intensité de la maladie, et l'époque à laquelle est appliqué le traitement. Nous avons noté en effet, — et cette constatation nous paraît avoir une grande valeur, — que le traitement devait durer d'autant moins qu'il était appliqué plus tôt. Une dizaine d'enfants soumis aux bains d'air comprimé dès l'apparition des quintes caractéristiques ont vu leur coqueluche terminée en trois semaines. Vingt bains constituent en effet la moyenne qu'on est rarement obligé de dépasser quand on intervient au début.

Le catarrhe bronchique qui accompagne presque toujours la coqueluche est heureusement modifié par l'air comprimé. Le fait ne doit pas nous étonner : car tous ceux qui ont quelque pratique de l'aérothérapie savent combien les sécrétions bronchiques sont diminuées par cette médication.

L'état général bénéficie également de cette thérapeutique. L'appétit, qui sombre si fréquemment dans les coqueluches graves, réapparaît à la suite des premiers bains. Il se passe donc chez les jeunes coquelucheux ce que Bertin, Hayem et Paul Delmas ont signalé chez les tuberculeux, les bronchiteux et les emphysémateux. La fièvre, quand elle n'est pas occasionnée par quelque infection secondaire, tombe rapidement ; et cette anémie spéciale, compagne de toute coqueluche sévère, trouve dans cette suroxygénation du sang son meilleur remède.

Les complications de la coqueluche qui relèvent directement de la quinte sont évidemment amoindries ou évitées par le bain d'air comprimé ; l'emphysème pulmonaire, les hémorragies disparaissent en même temps que les quintes diminuent de fréquence et de violence : l'emphysème, d'ailleurs, bénéficie largement de l'aérothérapie dont l'efficacité chez les vieux emphysémateux est démontrée depuis longtemps. Les vomissements deviennent également plus rares.

Dans l'étiologie des infections secondaires, il faut à la fois considérer le milieu dans lequel vit l'enfant et où il puise le germe morbide, d'une part, et, d'autre part, sa plus ou moins grande résistance en face de ce germe. Ce second facteur est, naturellement, le seul influencé par l'air comprimé. Mais nous savons combien cette question de terrain a d'importance, et ne sommes-nous pas étonnés en constatant qu'aucun de nos malades n'a été atteint de broncho-pneumonie, quoique la plupart aient été observés en hiver et que leur hygiène fût très défectueuse. L'heureuse action de l'aérothérapie sur la bronchite, point de départ de la broncho-pneumonie, doit également être prise en considération dans l'explication de ce phénomène.

Comment agissent les bains d'air comprimé dans la coqueluche? La question est complexe et difficile à résoudre. Tout d'abord le bain semble exercer une action antispasmodique spéciale sur la quinte, que nous devons rapprocher de « l'effet sédatif exercé sur le système nerveux » dont nous parle Hayem. Faut-il, avec Hayem, la rattacher à l'absorption de l'azote atmosphérique? Ne faut-il pas plutôt la considérer comme un simple réflexe dont la marche nous est encore inconnue?

Ce que nous savons mieux, depuis les beaux travaux de Paul Bert c'est que le séjour dans l'air comprimé augmente l'absorption de l'oxygène par le sang. Cette augmentation, manifeste à toutes les pressions, est proportionnellement considérable pour les pressions inférieures à une atmosphère au-dessus de la normale, c'est-à-dire pour les pressions employées en thérapeutique. Cette suroxygénation du sang joue dans la coqueluche un rôle incontestable, qu'ont récemment mis en lumière les tentatives de traitement de la coqueluche par les inhalations d'oxygène ou de vapeur d'eau oxygénée. Ajoutons enfin à ces deux facteurs l'action exercée par le bain sur l'état général et sur les sécrétions des voies respiratoires.

Nous n'avons jamais observé le moindre accident, soit pendant la durée du bain, soit après son application. Les mères qui accompagnaient leurs enfants dans la cloche ont quelquefois accusé un peu de douleurs d'oreilles, dues, à une obstruction plus ou moins complète de la trompe d'Eustache, s'opposant ainsi à l'équilibre de pression sur les deux faces du tympan : nos petits malades ne s'en sont jamais plaints.

La dilatation du cœur droit qu'on rencontre si fréquemment, à des degrés divers, dans les coqueluches sévères ne nous a pas paru constituer une contre-indication à la méthode. Nous savons en effet que cette dilatation cardiaque aiguë est le résultat de la gêne circulatoire produite par la longue durée, l'intensité et la fréquence des quintes, sur lesquelles le bain d'air comprimé a une action inhibitoire manifeste. Ce bain nous paraît donc constituer le meilleur traitement prophylactique de cette cardiopathie. Il nous paraît cependant prudent, en cas de fatigue cardiaque évidente dans une coqueluche grave, de recourir à l'emploi de la caféine avant l'administration des premiers bains. C'est la conduite que nous avons tenue dans un cas sévère, caractérisé par des quintes d'une fréquence et d'une violence extrêmes, et où les contractions cardiaques étaient si faibles que, pendant une semaine, nous redoutions la mort subite par arrêt du cœur. Cet enfant a d'ailleurs guéri en moins d'un mois de traitement.

Le très jeune âge des sujets n'est pas davantage un obstacle à l'usage des bains d'air comprimé. Nous avons traité plusieurs enfants âgés de moins d'un an. Ils ont tous admirablement supporté cette thérapeutique. Un enfant de six mois fut soumis pendant trois semaines à un bain quotidien dont la pression oscilla entre 50 et 55 centimètres de mercure; un bébé de quatre mois prit un bain quotidien, à la même pression pendant 16 jours, au bout desquels il était entièrement guéri. Ni l'un ni l'autre n'en éprouvèrent la moindre fatigue.

Pour être efficace l'application de l'air comprimé doit être poursuivie jusqu'à la disparition complète des quintes. Nous croyons même prudent de continuer le traitement un peu au-delà, en espaçant les séances. Plusieurs fois nous avons constaté la réapparition des quintes chez des malades qui avaient cessé les bains dès que celles-ci avaient disparu. Schliep nous cite une observation absolument semblable. Dans les nôtres, il suffit de suspendre le traitement pendant quelques jours pour obtenir une guérison définitive.

La guérison peut d'ailleurs être très retardée quand la coqueluche est compliquée d'adénopathie trachéo-bronchique très volumineuse ou de lésions pulmonaires de nature tuberculeuse.

En résumé, nous considérons le bain d'air comprimé comme un excellent traitement de la coqueluche, car il tempère la maladie, l'abrège et en écarte les principales complications. De tels titres nous paraissent suffisants pour rendre cette thérapeutique digne d'une plus grande notoriété et d'un emploi plus fréquent.

VII

FIÈVRES ÉRUPTIVES

DE L'ANGINE PULTACÉE COMME SIGNE PRÉCOCE, AVERTISSEUR, DE LA ROUGEOLE

RAPPORT

par M. le docteur R. SAINT-PHILIPPE,
de Bordeaux.

Dans une récente épidémie de rougeole, il m'a été donné d'observer un phénomène pathologique sur lequel l'attention n'a pas encore été attirée et qui peut avoir des conséquences prochaines et éloignées des plus intéressantes. Il s'agit d'une *angine pultacée* précédant de quelques jours l'invasion de la rougeole. J'ai observé cette angine une quinzaine de fois sur une centaine de rougeoleux, tant en ville qu'à l'hôpital.

Elle se caractérise cliniquement par de petits points isolés, à apparence bleuâtre plutôt que sale, rarement par une plaque véritable avec ou sans engorgement ganglionnaire, par de la dysphagie ordinairement légère, de la fièvre et quelques phénomènes réactionnel, sans gravité. Tantôt elle évolue huit ou dix jours avant la période d'invasion, tantôt elle précède cette période seulement de quelques jours, et il y a encore quelques taches blanches quand apparaissent le signe de Koplick, la stomatite érythémato-pultacée et le pointillé rouge du voile du palais.

L'analyse bactériologique a révélé dans quelques cas la présence dans d'autres cas, plus fréquents, l'absence du bacille de la diphtérie. Dans un cas où l'analyse avait été positive, l'enfant fut dirigé vers le pavillon de la diphtérie où il apporta la rougeole.

Ces faits pourraient expliquer ce qui se passe à la suite, et parfois au début même de la rougeole, on connaît la diphtérie secondaire. On sait moins que les phénomènes d'invasion de la rougeole peuvent prendre des proportions telles, une telle intensité que le tubage, la trachéotomie ou l'injection de sérum sont pratiqués d'urgence. Il y a vingt ans j'ai publié des faits de ce genre dans les Bulletins de la société de médecine et de chirurgie de Bordeaux.

A l'exemple de ce qui se passe trois fois sur quatre pour le croup dit « d'emblée » ou pour le croup fruste, c'est l'angine du début, qui a pu être assez légère pour passer inaperçue, qui est alors la cause du méfait. Ce sont les rougeoles précédées d'angine blanche qui s'accompagnent sans doute le plus fréquemment de croup secondaire.

Dans le numéro de juillet dernier des *Archives cliniques de médecine infantile*, M. Comby signale sans y insister d'ailleurs spécialement, dans les quatre cas de rougeole familiale qu'il rapporte, deux cas où il y a eu une angine à points blancs.

On ne peut donc pas dire absolument, comme Trousseau, que la rougeole n'aime pas le pharynx. Il faudra, au contraire, regarder avec soin la gorge des enfants en danger ou en passe d'avoir cette fièvre éruptive. La notion d'épidémie régnante aura ici une importance facile à saisir.

La constatation de cette angine pourra offrir en de certaines circonstances, la valeur d'un symptôme prémonitoire, véritablement avertisseur, et servira à prendre quelques mesures de prophylaxie générale.

D'autre part, il faudra éviter, si cette angine se présente en temps d'épidémie ou si elle s'accompagne déjà du catarrhe oculo-naso-laryngé, de diriger l'enfant vers un service de diphtérie et en tout cas de le réunir à d'autres enfants atteints de rougeole simple.

Enfin son apparition, suivie de près de l'apparition de la rougeole, devra éveiller l'attention du médecin, pour que l'enfant soit maintenu dans les meilleures conditions d'hygiène et d'antisepsie, au point de vue du greffage précoce ou tardif des accidents du croup.

Quel rapport faut-il voir entre cette angine et la rougeole? Y a-t-il relation de cause à effet ou simple coïncidence? Je ne suis pas en mesure de le dire aujourd'hui. Mais l'avenir nous l'apprendra sûrement.

PHOTOTHÉRAPIE DE LA ROUGEOLE
per M. CHATINIÈRE.

de Paris.

La méthode est la suivante : occlusion des orifices lumineux de la chambre du malade par des rideaux rouges.

Avec ce simple appareil, j'ai, dans vingt-deux cas, obtenu une évolution rapide de la rougeole, une guérison complète, et les symptômes qui m'ont paru les plus influencés sont : l'état général, la fièvre, l'éruption, l'absence de complications.

M. Comby et d'autres ont, je le sais, essayé ma méthode, avec des succès variables. J'ai cherché les causes de cette variabilité des résultats. Elle m'a paru résider dans la méthode d'application. J'ai moi-même, en effet, eu des résultats différents suivant la perfection de l'application.

La photothérapie demande, pour s'exercer efficacement, des rayons lumineux brillants, une coloration bien rouge de l'étoffe interposée : enfin l'exposition directe aux rayons rouges du corps du malade. En effet, les parties du corps des malades, découvertes, ont une éruption beaucoup plus fugace que les parties recouvertes.

En un mot, les insuccès de la photothérapie m'ont paru dus à des fautes d'application.

DISCUSSION.

M. Saint-Philippe (Bordeaux) se range à l'avis de M. Comby, et n'a pas constaté les bons effets de la photothérapie.

M. Guinon ne l'a appliquée que dans un cas, où la médication n'a apporté aucune modification.

DE LA LUMIÈRE ROUGE DANS LE TRAITEMENT DE LA ROUGEOLE
par M. le docteur PUJADOR.

de Barcelone.

Quoiqu'on ne puisse pas désigner la lumière rouge sous le nom de traitement curatif de la rougeole, comme quelques-uns le prétendent, cependant elle doit être considérée comme un moyen de traitement, qui, outre la facilité de son application, produit des résultats positifs pour les malades.

D'après le nombre d'observations que j'ai notées, nombre qui dépasse la centaine, j'ai pu constater dans tous les cas une diminution notable de la fièvre, et surtout si l'on soumet le malade à la lumière rouge, dès le commencement de la maladie, par exemple, dès l'apparition du signe de Flindt Koplik, dans le voile du palais, l'éruption se vérifie plus rapidement, mais le dessèchement ou dessiccation de l'exanthème résulte beaucoup plus lent.

La meilleure manière de pratiquer ce système consiste à mettre de petits rideaux rouges dans les ouvertures de l'habitation, et à veiller à ce que la lumière blanche ne pénètre d'aucun côté, car, dans le cas contraire, les qualités sédatives de la lumière se perdraient, et le petit malade serait plus exposé aux attaques convulsives.

On veillera autant que possible, lorsque la lumière rouge est très intense, à ce qu'elle n'aille pas directement sur les yeux du malade, et en tout cas, il vaut mieux que celui-ci tourne le dos à la lumière.

Ce petit supplément au traitement de la rougeole est intéressant pour le pédiatre qui l'emploie, à cause du caractère de bénignité qu'il inspire à la maladie.

DE L'ACTION DE L'ESSENCE DE TÉRÉBENTHINE DANS LA VARIOLE ET DANS L'ÉRYSIPÈLE

par M. le docteur PUJADOR,

de Barcelone.

Continuant mes observations cliniques sur l'essence de térébenthine dans le traitement de la rougeole (observations dont je rendis compte, Congrès international de Moscou), je dois ajouter ce qui suit, au sujet de la petite vérole et de l'érysipèle des enfants en particulier, et aussi des adultes.

Variole. — Si dès les premiers moments de la période éruptive, lorsque les papules commencent à se montrer sur le visage, on administre au malade l'essence de térébenthine à la dose de 1 gramme par jour (émulsionné dans une solution gommeuse) pour l'enfant, et de 5 grammes par jour, pour l'adulte (en perles, à raison de deux par heure, prises avec de l'eau bi-carbonée ou eau de Vichy), en arrivant à la période suppurative, nous trouvons que les papules se dessèchent, et les vésicules qui entrent en suppuration le font sans produire de réaction dans l'organisme, c'est-à-dire sans fièvre : dans les autres cas où l'on est arrivé tard pour l'application du remède, ou dans lesquels la dose a été insuffisante, la période de suppuration se manifeste, mais avec une fièvre si légère que je ne l'ai vue en aucun cas s'élever à plus de 38°5. En un mot, j'ai toujours observé une diminution dans la gravité, et par là-même, une diminution importante dans tous les symptômes.

Cette observation étant tirée de l'expérience de 118 cas cliniques, je sollicite à ce sujet, l'attention de mes confrères, leur manifestant que dans beaucoup de cas, ils observeront de meilleurs effets en augmentant lesdites doses.

Érysipèle. — Cette maladie étant d'une nature streptococcique, il n'est pas étonnant que l'essence de térébenthine agisse sur elle d'une manière importante.

Après avoir observé de très nombreux cas, je crois pouvoir conclure que si, en réalité, l'éruption ne disparaît pas tout de suite, dès le commencement du traitement, cependant le cycle d'évolution se vérifie avec une notable diminution : la plupart de mes observations se rapportent à des érysipèles à la tête, et en augmentant ou en diminuant les doses d'essence de térébenthine indiquées pour la petite vérole, j'ai vu avec surprise que la fièvre disparaissait même totalement et que l'éruption se désséchait.

Ce résultat serait-il dû à l'efficacité de l'essence de térébenthine, ou peut-être au peu de virulence ou de gravité de l'infection? Ce qu'il y a de certain, c'est que je n'ai noté aucun décès depuis que je pratique le traitement indiqué, soit pour les malades atteints d'érysipèle, soit pour ceux qui sont atteints de la petite vérole.

VIII

MALADIES INFECTIEUSES

UN SERVICE ANTISEPTIQUE DE MÉDECINE
STATISTIQUE DE DIX ANNÉES
par M. le professeur J. GRANCHER

« La prophylaxie des maladies contagieuses est une des questions les plus intéressantes de la médecine contemporaine. Dans l'hôpital, dans la maison, dans la famille, le problème se pose à peu près toujours de la même façon. Il s'agit de préserver les voisins du malade, ceux qui le soignent et l'entourent, contre la contagion; il s'agit aussi de préserver le malade contre ses voisins et contre lui-même, si on veut éviter les infections secondaires toujours si redoutables. Pour cela, nous avons deux moyens : l'*isolement* et l'*antisepsie*. »

J'écrivais ces lignes en 1890[1] pour justifier les réformes que je venais de réaliser dans mon service à l'hôpital des Enfants-Malades, et en même temps, je donnais les premiers résultats, très favorables, de ces réformes.

Dès 1880-1885, les médecins d'enfants avaient le souci de préserver leurs petits malades du sort que leur réservait l'hospitalisation alors très imparfaite de l'Assistance publique.

Les maîtres les plus autorisés, Parrot, Archambault, etc., avaient protesté contre la morbidité et la mortalité liées à la contagion et avaient, mais en vain, réclamé des mesures d'isolement.

A. Ollivier fut plus heureux: la science avait marché et sa tâche était plus facile, appuyée par une expérience médicale plus éclairée. Notre collègue put ainsi, dans de nombreux rapports au Comité de salubrité de la Seine, démontrer l'utilité, l'urgence de l'isolement pour la rougeole, la diphtérie, etc... et aussi la nécessité de préserver à la consultation les enfants sains de la contagion qu'apportent avec eux tant d'autres enfants.

Vers la même époque (1885), j'eus l'occasion d'étudier l'étuve à vapeur sous pression de Geneste et Herscher et d'en démontrer la su-

---

1. GRANCHER. Essai d'antisepsie médicale. *Revue d'hygiène*, 1900.

périorité sur toute autre étuve, et aussi l'insuffisance des étuves à air sec installées déjà dans plusieurs hôpitaux[1].

Enfin, les idées pastoriennes de pathogénie et de prophylaxie, si lumineuses, si bienfaisantes, supplantaient peu à peu, dans le domaine médical, les études moins fécondes de la physiologie et de l'anatomie pathologique. Ces dernières sciences, sous l'impulsion des Cl. Bernard et des Charcot, avaient épuisé leur sève première, et l'heure était venue des nouveaux horizons ouverts à la chirurgie, à l'obstétrique et à la médecine.

Après quelques tâtonnements inévitables, chirurgiens et accoucheurs trouvèrent assez vite la formule d'application des méthodes du laboratoire à la salle d'opération et à la maternité. Les médecins hésitèrent plus longtemps. En effet, il ne s'agit plus ici de la simple protection d'une plaie, chose relativement facile; le problème est beaucoup plus complexe, au moins en apparence, parce que les sources de la *contagion* semblent plus nombreuses et plus variées, et parce qu'elles sont moins connues.

Aussi l'*isolement* et la *désinfection* par l'étuve à vapeur sous pression parurent être les mesures idéales de protection contre la contagion *médicale* et furent réclamées de toutes parts : comités d'hygiène, sociétés savantes, etc. Mais si la *désinfection* ne peut se faire utilement que d'une seule façon, l'*isolement* peut s'entendre de bien des manières et il a plusieurs formules.

L'idéal serait l'application du plan de notre confrère du Val-de-Grâce, M. Richard, qui demandait en 1889, pour les rougeoleux, l'isolement individuel ou cellulaire afin de les préserver contre la broncho-pneumonie.

Je venais de démontrer, en effet[2], que l'isolement des rougeoleux dans des salles particulières et des diphtériques dans un pavillon spécial, à l'hôpital des Enfants, n'avait diminué ni la contagion ni la mortalité.

Aussi, la proposition de M. Richard, si elle parut impraticable alors, sembla-t-elle conforme aux vues scientifiques, et il arrive aujourd'hui qu'on tend à se rapprocher de ce desideratum, au moins pour les rougeoles et diphtéries, etc., compliquées. A celles-là, on réserve des chambres ou box d'isolement à un ou à deux lits.

C'est ce que M. Sevestre, sous cette formule : *Isolement* dans l'*isolement*, organisait par chambres de deux et quatre lits à l'hôpital des Enfants-Assistés. C'est ce que M. Hutinel a réalisé avec grand profit,

1. Recueil des travaux du Comité consultatif d'hygiène.
2. GRANCHER. *Revue d'hygiène* et *Bulletin médical*, 1889.

sous forme de box, au même hôpital. C'est ce que M. Roux vient de mettre en pratique avec toute la rigueur de la formule de M. Richard : *un box pour un enfant* au nouvel hôpital Pastorien, où chaque malade contagionnant aura sa chambre particulière, close jusqu'au plafond. Au contraire, les nouveaux box de l'hôpital des Enfants sont de simples loges sans plafond et sans porte, ouverts ainsi largement dans la salle commune. En fait, c'est la salle commune divisée en loges par des cloisons de verre de 2 mètres 70 de hauteur. Chaque enfant occupe une loge, ou box, pourvue d'un lit, d'une table de nuit lavabo, de deux chaises, et munie de tabliers, de serviettes et de cuvettes qui ne quittent pas le box et permettent un service commun, par des infirmières communes (voir fig. 1 et 2).

L'aération, la ventilation, la surveillance sont meilleures ou plus faciles dans cette salle commune divisée en box, plus clairs et plus gais qu'une chambre close ou qu'un box fermé.

Ce mode d'isolement que j'ai imaginé parce que la place est toujours insuffisante dans nos grands hôpitaux, rendra, je pense, les mêmes services que les box à deux et quatre lits de M. Hutinel, et que les chambres individuelles de l'hôpital Pastorien mais à la condition expresse que l'*antisepsie* y sera rigoureusement appliquée. Car, ou l'infirmière est « *antiseptique* » et la porte est inutile ; ou l'infirmière n'est pas « *antiseptique* » et la porte n'empêchera pas les contagions.

L'ANTISEPSIE ! *Avec elle*, L'ISOLEMENT *du malade, même imparfait, donne des résultats excellents ; sans elle*, L'ISOLEMENT, *fût-il individuel et cellulaire, n'arrêtera pas la contagion.*

L'antisepsie médicale est tout aussi simple à concevoir et facile à réaliser que l'antisepsie chirurgicale ou obstétricale. J'en ai fourni la preuve dans mon service, et la statistique des dix dernières années que je publie aujourd'hui après la statistique déjà publiée la première année (1889), démontre qu'on peut, avec elle, se mettre à l'abri de la contagion pour toutes les maladies, sauf la rougeole et la varicelle. Et encore, la contagion de la rougeole a-t-elle été réduite des deux tiers, dans la proportion de 5 à 1.

L'antisepsie procède de cette idée, que les germes morbides sont attachés au malade et couvrent son corps, ses mains, son visage, sa peau, ses muqueuses, ses vêtements et son lit, mais ne flottent pas autour de lui dans l'atmosphère et ne la souillent pas.

La contagion par l'air n'existe pas dans nos salles où les enfants ne crachent pas, et où la poussière est supprimée. Au contraire, la contagion par les objets, c'est-à-dire par le contact direct ou indirect, existe pour toutes les maladies.

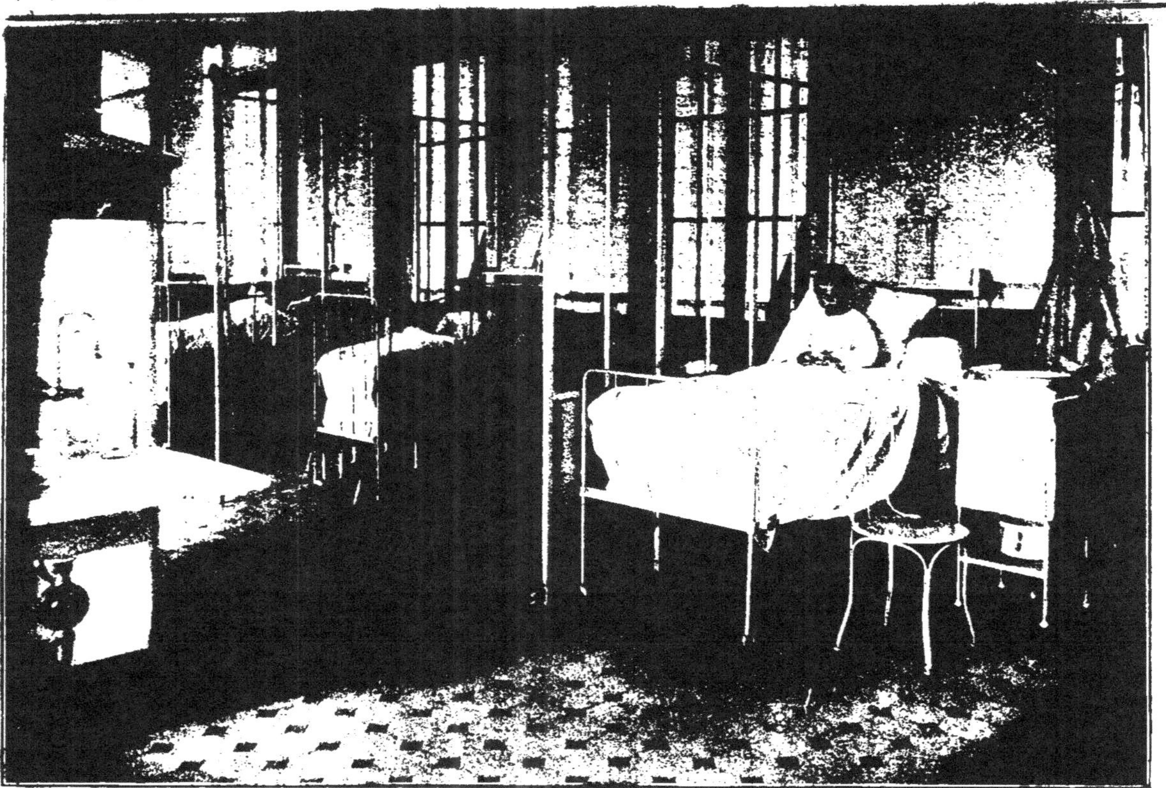

Fig. 1. — Vue du nouveau pavillon de la rougeole et de ses box ouverts, sans porte et sans plafond. Chaque enfant occupe ainsi une chambrette dans la salle commune.

Cette idée, prise au laboratoire de Pasteur, était la mienne en 1885, lorsque je fus appelé à remplacer Parrot dans la chaire de clinique infantile, mais elle était loin, à cette date, d'être l'idée commune des médecins. Ceux-ci pensaient, au contraire, que l'atmosphère est le véhicule ordinaire de la contagion, et pour ce motif préconisaient l'*isolement* avant tout et partout.

Sans combattre l'*isolement* comme moyen de prophylaxie, parce que c'est à mon sens, quand on peut s'en servir, la meilleure manière de supprimer les contacts, je pensais que dans maintes circonstances on ne pourrait isoler tous les malades contagionnants, et qu'il convenait d'apprendre à éviter les contagions, même dans une salle *commune* où tant de germes virulents vivent côte à côte, et où se font tant de contagions de rougeole, scarlatine, diphtérie, varicelle, oreillons, coqueluche, impétigo, etc…, avant qu'on ait isolé celles qui sont pourvues de pavillons spéciaux.

C'est là le côté original et personnel de ma méthode.

Partant de cet *a priori* que la contagion par l'atmosphère n'existe pas, je m'appliquai :

1° A purifier immédiatement les objets et les mains souillés par les contacts nécessaires à l'examen des malades et aux services hospitaliers :

2° A diminuer les contacts avec les enfants contagionnants ou supposés tels.

Ainsi l'ISOLEMENT *passait au second plan, et* l'ANTISEPSIE *au premier*. Car je m'occupais surtout et avant tout d'éviter le transport des germes morbides d'un enfant malade à un enfant sain *par le personnel hospitalier* ou *médical*. C'est lui, lui seul que j'incriminais quand un cas de contagion apparaissait dans le service. Bref, j'assimilais la *contagion médicale aux contagions chirurgicale et obstétricale*, et j'employais pour lutter contre elles les mêmes moyens.

Tout ce que j'ai vu depuis dix ans n'a fait que fortifier ma conviction et apporter des preuves nouvelles à la doctrine de la contagion par les mains ou les objets : contagion OBJECTIVE que j'oppose à la contagion ATMOSPHÉRIQUE.

Chemin faisant, mes opinions se sont modifiées sur des points secondaires, par exemple sur la fréquence relative de la contagion directe ou de la contagion indirecte dans la rougeole, sur sa durée d'incubation, etc…, mais l'idée fondamentale de l'innocuité de l'atmosphère non chargée de poussière et de la nocuité des contacts s'est imposée peu à peu à tous mes collaborateurs : chefs de clinique, etc…. Elle vient de recevoir la confirmation la plus éclatante d'une communication récente de M. Moizard, à la Société médicale

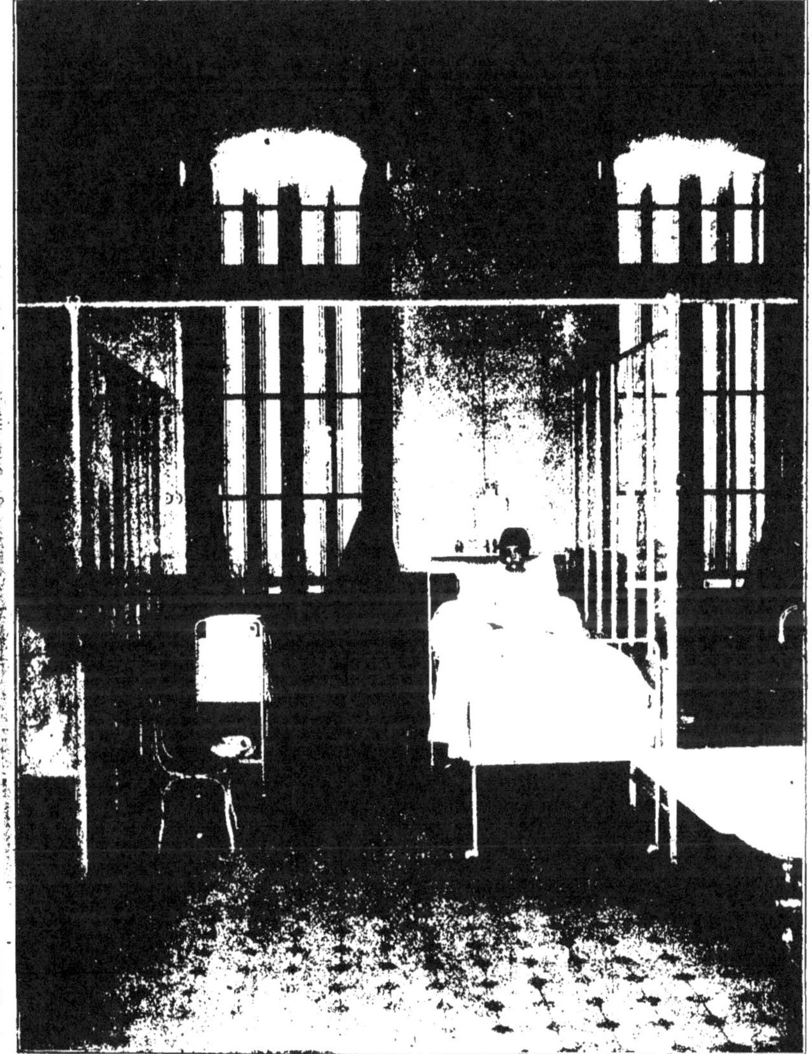

Fig. 2. — Pavillon de la rougeole. Un box ouvert de face. Deux cloisons de verre le séparent des box voisins.

des hôpitaux[1]. Mon collègue, chargé du service des « douteux » de-

1. *Bull. de la Soc. méd. des hôpitaux*, 7 juin 1900.

puis 1896, reçoit ses malades dans des salles divisées en box fermés,
mais sans plafonds, les cloisons de verre qui séparent les box ayant
2 m. 10 de hauteur. Chaque malade est donc isolé dans une chambrette qui n'a de commun avec les chambrettes voisines que l'air
atmosphérique. En outre, M. Moizard a veillé aux mesures les plus
rigoureuses d'antisepsie, c'est-à-dire que chaque box a sa ou ses
blouses, et que médecins ou infirmières n'abordent l'enfant qu'après
les avoir revêtues, et ne quittent le box en y laissant la blouse
qu'après un lavage soigneux des mains avec des liquides désinfectants, etc.

C'est exactement ce qui se fait dans mon service depuis 1888.

Dans ces conditions, M. Moizard a vu la contagion de la rougeole
se réduire à quelques unités, exactement à 7 cas de contagion, sur
5016 malades qui ont traversé son service en quatre années.

Quant au mode de contagion de la rougeole, M. Moizard se range
à mon opinion sans hésiter, et il accuse nettement les objets et les
personnes et non pas l'atmosphère.

L'idée a donc fait son chemin et ses preuves ailleurs que chez moi,
et j'en suis heureux: mais il me sera bien permis de dire que M. Moizard, en prenant, le 1ᵉʳ janvier 1896, le service des douteux organisé
sur les bases que M. Roux et moi avions indiquées à M. l'architecte
Belouet en 1894, et en y appliquant *terme pour terme* la méthode
d'antisepsie qui fonctionne dans mon service depuis avril 1888, avait
la tâche assez facile.

Loin de moi la pensée de diminuer le mérite de mon très distingué
collègue qui a supprimé à peu près la contagion dans son service.
Mais le pavillon qu'il dirige n'a pas trouvé de plus chaud partisan
que moi et j'ai beaucoup contribué à sa création; or, on pourrait
croire, à lire les dernières lignes de la page 685 des *Bulletins de la
Société médicale des Hôpitaux*[1] que j'ai pu songer, un moment à remplacer le pavillon des douteux par mon propre service, ou mieux, à
faire de mon service une salle de douteux. Telle n'a jamais été ma
pensée. Le service des « douteux » et mon service sont deux choses
tout à fait distinctes, et M. Moizard a bien raison de dire que la sélection des malades ne pouvait se faire que dans un service spécial.

L'organisation de ce service en 1896 a été l'un des progrès de l'hygiène prophylactique à l'hôpital des Enfants depuis vingt ans. L'étuve
à vapeur sous pression, installée dès 1886, avait ouvert l'ère nouvelle
avec la tentative de perfectionnement de la consultation à l'entrée,

____

1. 7 juin 1900.

tentative restée bien imparfaite. Enfin, tout récemment, les pavillons nouveaux de la diphtérie, de la scarlatine et de la coqueluche ont été inaugurés.

Entre temps (1888), l'organisation de mon service a marqué une date importante, je crois, dans l'amélioration de l'hygiène hospitalière à l'hôpital des Enfants. Cela autant peut-être par l'exemple donné de ce que peut l'antisepsie *dans une salle commune* que par les résultats obtenus. Ceux-ci sont excellents toutefois et méritent d'être connus. Si j'ai attendu dix ans pour les publier, c'est que je tenais à donner la statistique d'une longue période, et, par cela même, des chiffres incontestables et incontestés.

Les tableaux de la statistique de mon service démontrent, si on les compare à la statistique des services similaires voisins, tout ce que peut l'antisepsie contre la contagion *médicale*. Cependant ces services, au moins dans les dernières années, ont bénéficié de tous les progrès : étuve à vapeur désinfectant le linge de tout l'hôpital; sélection des malades à la consultation et au pavillon des « douteux »; création des pavillons spéciaux : diphtérie, scarlatine, etc.

La morbidité par contagion n'y reste pas moins très supérieure à celle de mon service.

ORGANISATION ET FONCTIONNEMENT DU SERVICE
DE LA CLINIQUE DEPUIS 1888.

Mon service se compose de quatre salles :

Salle *Bouchut* (garçons) : 24 lits;

Salle *Parrot* (filles) : 24 lits;

Salle *Husson* (nourrissons) : 8 lits;

Salle des chroniques (filles), *Husson* : 12 lits.

Pour des motifs budgétaires, je n'ai pu réaliser mon programme d'antisepsie que dans deux salles, Bouchut et Parrot, les plus actives du reste, celles où le succès ou l'insuccès devait être le plus éclatant : voici les réformes que j'ai fait appliquer.

1° *Suppression des poussières*. — Pour cet objet, le parquet a été refait, paraffiné et lavé deux fois par jour à la serpillière imbibée d'une solution de sublimé. Les murs ont été repeints et sont lavés au sublimé deux fois par semaine.

2° *Isolement des contagieux*. — Tout enfant atteint ou suspect d'une maladie contagieuse est mis en box. Cela veut dire que son lit est entouré d'un paravent métallique treillagé de 1 m. 25 de hauteur.

Isolement tout à fait relatif, puisque l'enfant reste dans la salle commune. Mais ce paravent, dont une feuille fixée au mur par un crochet
sert de porte pour le service, suffit à prévenir les contacts d'enfant à
enfant et à obliger les médecins ou infirmières qui pénètrent dans le

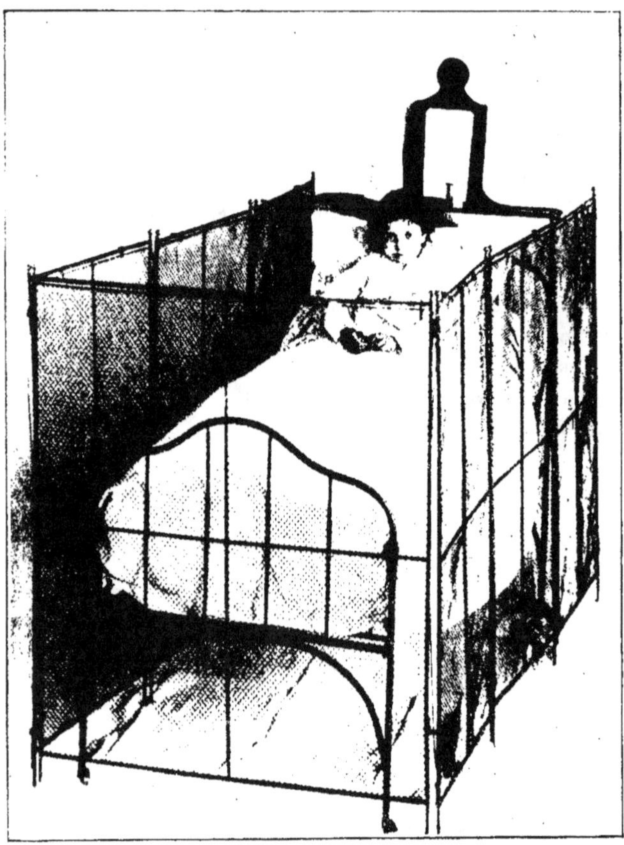

Fig. 3. — Box ou paravent métallique pour isoler le lit de l'enfant
contagieux, dans la salle commune.

box : a) à revêtir la blouse du box en y entrant, à l'y laisser en sortant; b) à se laver et désinfecter les mains à la sortie du box. (Voir
fig. 3 et 4.)

Ainsi, les contacts sont réduits au minimum, les vêtements protégés, les mains souillées purifiées.

Sans doute, ce box est imparfait, très inférieur aux chambres-box du pavillon des douteux ou de la rougeole; il est trop petit surtout et oblige à se laver les mains hors du box et à laisser la blouse sur le pied du lit. Tel quel, cependant, il nous a rendu les plus grands services, car le paravent est léger et mobile et permet d'isoler suffisam-

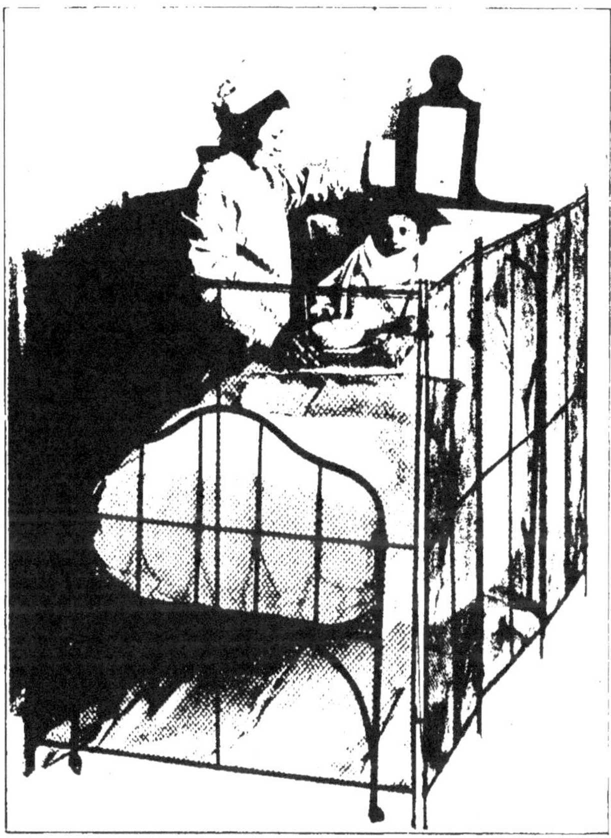

Fig. 4. — Box ou paravent métallique pour isoler le lit de l'enfant dans la salle commune. L'infirmière a pénétré dans le box, revêtu la blouse du box, et donne le repas de l'enfant.

ment autant de malades que l'on veut dans des salles toujours trop petites pour les besoins hospitaliers. En fait, il ne prend aucune place et se borne à transformer un lit *ouvert* en un lit *fermé*, où le petit malade peut voir et être vu, surveillé, sans aucun danger de contagion pour ses camarades.

Ce simple paravent ajouré réalise donc *pour la salle commune* un *isolement minimum* très précieux, et je crois qu'il sera nécessaire tant que nous n'aurons pas autant de pavillons distincts que de

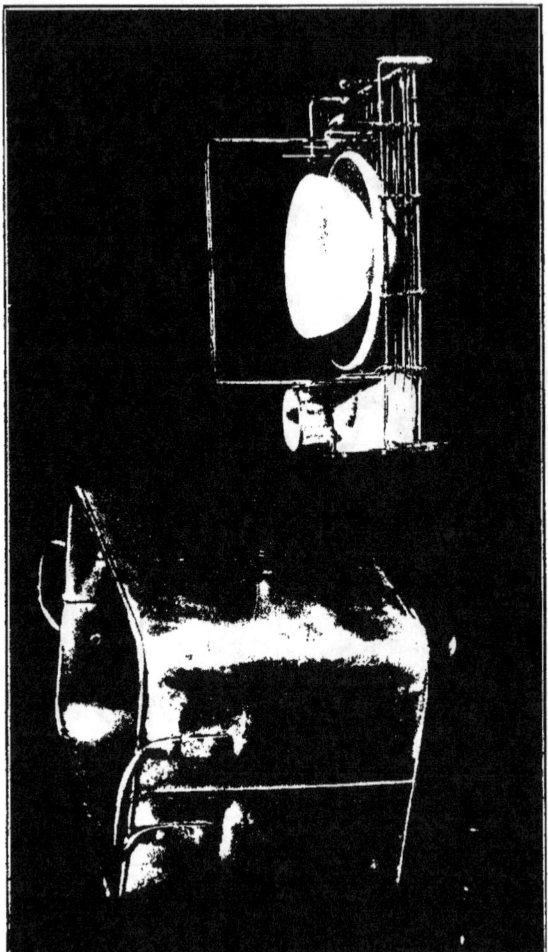

Fig. 5. — Petite cuve métallique et panier de laiton pour stériliser par l'eau bouillante carbonatée tout ce qui a servi au repas de l'enfant.

maladies transmissibles. Or, celles-ci, dans la pathologie infantile, sont si nombreuses, que nous sommes encore loin de cet idéal.

5° *Désinfection*. — Celle-ci consiste : 1° dans le lavage des mains à l'eau de savon et à la brosse, puis au sublimé au 1/1000°; 2° dans le passage à l'étuve des lits, sommiers, matelas, qu'un malade conta-

gieux vient de quitter : 3° dans la lessive des linges et l'ébouillante-
ment des objets qui viennent de servir aux repas.

Pour atteindre ce dernier but, j'ai fait faire des petits paniers en fil
de laiton et à compartiments pour la timbale, fourchette et couteaux,

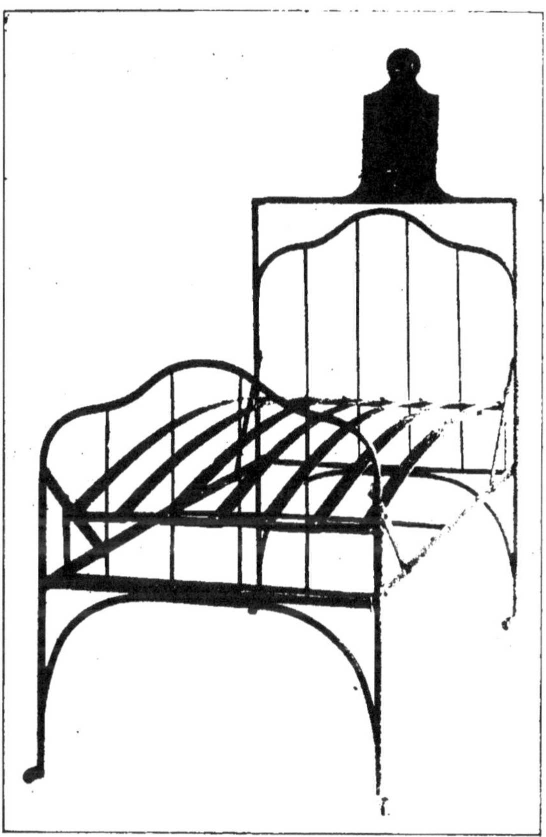

Fig. 6. — Lit en fer creux démontable dans toutes ses parties, pour la
stérilisation à l'étuve ou le lavage à la brosse.

assiette et bol, serviette. Le panier chargé du repas est porté dans le
box et déposé sur le lit recouvert d'une toile caoutchoutée. Après le
repas, l'infirmière le porte directement dans l'office et le met, avec
tout son contenu, dans une bouilloire ou marmite *ad hoc*, à demi
pleine d'eau chargée d'un peu de carbonate de soude. L'eau est ainsi

chauffée jusqu'à 105 degrés centigrades pendant cinq minutes et l'opération est finie. (Voir fig. 5.)

De même, les lits sont en fer creux, légers et démontables par compartiments; on peut ainsi ou les porter à l'étuve ou les laver sur place à la brosse et au sublimé acidifié. (Voir fig. 6.)

Ce dernier mode de désinfection a remplacé, depuis plusieurs années, l'étuvage, moins pratique: il suffit parfaitement.

Pour le bon fonctionnement de ce service, j'ai demandé et obtenu une infirmière supplémentaire — 4 par salle au lieu de 3 — mais pendant la nuit la veille est toujours confiée à une seule infirmière, et c'est, naturellement, la dernière venue, la plus jeune, la moins instruite, en conséquence, à qui incombe le fardeau. Beaucoup de nos contagions viennent, sans aucun doute, de l'insuffisance de cette partie du personnel hospitalier: mais sur ce point nous nous sommes heurté aux nécessités budgétaires de l'Assistance publique.

Il n'est que justice de dire ici, en revanche, que l'intelligence et le dévouement de nos deux surveillantes, Mmes Robin et Poux, nous ont beaucoup aidé à remplir notre programme. Sans elles, sans leur bonne volonté incessante et leur vigilance infatigable, nous aurions échoué. Le rôle de la surveillante et des infirmières, dans un service antiseptique de médecine, est, en effet, bien plus important que le rôle du même personnel hospitalier dans un service de chirurgie. Cela se conçoit de reste, et il me paraît superflu d'en donner les raisons. Qu'on veuille bien seulement remarquer ceci : en dehors de la présence du médecin, tous les contacts impurs, c'est-à-dire toutes les contagions dépendent du personnel hospitalier obligé de toucher dix fois par jour à chaque enfant, en passant de l'un à l'autre. Pour diminuer ces contacts dangereux, j'avais à l'origine chargé une infirmière, toujours la même, du service des box. Elle ne devait toucher à aucun autre enfant. Mais le petit nombre de nos infirmières nous a forcé à renoncer à ce système, car l'infirmière des box était ou surchargée ou presque inoccupée, selon que les box étaient plus ou moins nombreux.

En dehors des contagions inhérentes à quelques infirmières négligentes ou étourdies, qu'il a fallu renvoyer, d'autres, tout aussi inévitables, nous sont imposées par l'enseignement même et par le stage hospitalier. Une faute est vite commise par un élève encore ignorant de toutes les causes de contagion et des précautions simples, mais constantes, qu'exige l'antisepsie.

Ce fut la tâche de mes collaborateurs, MM. Hutinel et Marfan, et de mes chefs de clinique, de maintenir la discipline et de former la

SALLE BOUCHUT (année 1890).

Service de M. le professeur GRANCHER. — Chefs de Clinique : MM. DESCHAMPS et MARTIN DE GIMARD

MALADIES	MALADES entrés en incubation ou en évolution.	CONTAGIONS par importation.	CONTAGIONS DANS LE SERVICE				TOTAL des CONTAGIONS dans le service.	TOTAL GÉNÉRAL des CONTAGIONS
			CONTAGION d'enfant *isolé* par enfant *isolé*.	CONTAGION d'enfant *isolé* par enfant *libre*.	CONTAGION d'enfant *libre* par enfant *libre*.	CONTAGION d'enfant *libre* par enfant *isolé*.		
Rougeole	12		1	6	2		9	9
Diphtérie	7	2	1				1	5
Scarlatine.	5							
Coqueluche	14							
Broncho-pneumonie.	17							
Varicelle	5							
Oreillons								

COMMENTAIRES

Rougeole. — Parmi les 9 cas intérieurs, 8 se rapportent à des enfants contagionnés par d'autres enfants qui, pour des raisons diverses, n'étaient pas isolés au moment de leur éruption. Un seul cas a trait à la contagion par un enfant isolé.

Diphtérie. — Parmi les cas intérieurs de diphtérie, 1 cas, celui de Louis P... (5544), s'est produit 24 jours après l'entrée de l'enfant à l'hôpital, et 52 jours après le dernier cas de diphtérie dans la salle. Un mois après ce cas, un autre enfant, Édouard M... (5551), voisin du précédent et entré le même jour que lui, prenait la diphtérie. On a supposé que le contage avait été apporté par les médecins de la Clinique, chargés également à ce moment du service spécial des diphtériques.

SALLE BOUCHUT

Tableau des dix années (de 1890 à 1899).

MALADIES	MALADES entrés en incubation ou en évolution.	CONTAGIONS par importation.	CONTAGIONS dans le service.	TOTAL GÉNÉRAL DES CONTAGIONS
Rougeole	66	9	15	52
Diphtérie	26	5	1	6
Scarlatine.	15	5	2	.
Coqueluche	154		4	4
Broncho-pneumonie.	158			
Varicelle.	57	4	15	17
Oreillons	15		1	1

SALLE PARROT

Tableau des dix années (de 1890 à 1899).

MALADIES	MALADES entrés en incubation ou en évolution.	CONTAGIONS par importation.	CONTAGIONS dans le service.	TOTAL GÉNÉRAL DES CONTAGIONS
Rougeole	75	6	51	57
Diphtérie	17			
Scarlatine.	6	1		1
Coqueluche	205		5	5
Broncho-pneumonie.	102			
Varicelle	72		22	22
Oreillons	8			

conviction scientifique des élèves incessamment renouvelés. De ce chef, nous aurons, je l'espère, essaimé çà et là les bonnes doctrines.

Mais le service médical et le service hospitalier sont impuissants contre les imprudences du flot des visiteurs du dimanche et du jeudi. Que de fois, malgré l'avis, la prière des surveillantes, les box étaient ouverts, les enfants contagieux caressés, embrassés, et après ceux-ci les voisins! Comment empêcher une brave femme très tendre, mais très ignorante, de partager les gâteaux qu'elle apporte à son enfant avec le petit camarade qui, ce jour-là, n'a pas reçu de visites ni de gâteaux!

Il y a plus, et nous avons relevé, durant ces dix années, beaucoup de contagions dues à l'*importation*. Celle-ci se fait ou par les médecins ou par les visiteurs des dimanches et jeudis : c'est un élève en invasion de rougeole sans le savoir, et qui sème sa maladie; ou c'est une maman qui soigne chez elle un enfant atteint de diphtérie, de rou-

geole... et l'apporte à l'hôpital. étant elle-même indemne. Et c'est la
seule explication possible quand rougeole et diphtérie sont absentes
du service depuis des semaines et des mois.

Malgré tous ces dangers de contagion qui rôdent autour d'un service de médecine *antiseptique*, et l'empêcheront toujours d'être *aseptique*, nous n'avons pas à regretter nos efforts, et les tableaux que
nous publions (voir page 990 et 991) sont une récompense précieuse
pour nous, puisque nous avons conscience d'avoir fait quelque bien[1].

Commentaires généraux.

1° ROUGEOLE

Contagions de la rougeole en 1885, 1886 et 1887, dans mon **service** :
1885 : 57 cas ; 1886 : 59 cas ; 1887 : 54 cas.

En 1889, après un an de service antiseptique, nous avions encore
25 cas, et je concluais à un échec en ce qui concernait la rougeole[2].

Mais depuis 1890, notre statistique, même en ce qui concerne la
rougeole, s'est beaucoup améliorée, parce que j'ai fait mettre en
box d'abord pendant quatorze jours, puis sur l'initiative de M. Martin de Gimard, pendant vingt et un jours, tout enfant que les parents déclaraient n'avoir pas eu la rougeole. Ce seul fait de traiter
comme suspect d'incubation tout enfant non vacciné a beaucoup
amélioré nos résultats ; voici le tableau des contagions de 1890-
1899 :

```
1890. . . . . . . . . . . . . . . . . . . . . . . . . . .  16
1891. . . . . . . . . . . . . . . . . . . . . . . . . . .   8
1892. . . . . . . . . . . . . . . . . . . . . . . . . . .   8
1893. . . . . . . . . . . . . . . . . . . . . . . . . . .  12
1894. . . . . . . . . . . . . . . . . . . . . . . . . . .   7
1895. . . . . . . . . . . . . . . . . . . . . . . . . . .  11
1896. . . . . . . . . . . . . . . . . . . . . . . . . . .  23
1897. . . . . . . . . . . . . . . . . . . . . . . . . . .   9
1898. . . . . . . . . . . . . . . . . . . . . . . . . . .  14
1899. . . . . . . . . . . . . . . . . . . . . . . . . . .   2
                                         Total. . . .    110
```

Le total des contagions pour la rougeole en dix années est donc de
110 cas, soit 11 par an. au lieu de 56, moyenne des contagions, pendant les trois années 1885-1886-1887.

---

1. Nous ne pouvons publier ici les 20 tableaux (10 par salle) mais seulement
l'un d'entre eux à titre de spécimen et les deux tableaux récapitulatifs suivis de
commentaires généraux.
2. *Revue d'hygiène*. 1890.

Tel est le relevé de nos registres. Ceux du bureau de l'hôpital diffèrent d'une fraction et donnent 115 contagions en dix ans au lieu de 110. L'écart est peu de chose et il s'explique assez facilement. D'un « passage » à la rougeole exécuté aujourd'hui tardivement dans la soirée et inscrit seulement le lendemain au bureau, il résulte que le même malade peut être inscrit sur nos registres aux cas extérieurs et au bureau de l'hôpital aux cas intérieurs. 14 jours étant la date réglementaire qui sépare le contagionnant du contagionné. Aussi, les chiffres du bureau accusent-ils quelquefois un écart défavorable, ailleurs favorable, à notre statistique. Par exemple, la contagion de la scarlatine est comptée sur les registres de l'hôpital pour notre salle Bouchut à 3 cas, et à 5 cas sur nos registres. C'est l'inverse pour la salle Parrot. Et encore, nous comptons 6 cas de contagion de diphtérie, et l'hôpital 5 seulement. salle Bouchut.

Ces petits écarts, du reste, ne changent pas la physionomie d'une statistique qui porte sur un nombre si considérable de maladies et sur dix années. Mais nous avons, naturellement. pris les chiffres de nos propres registres pour les comparer à ceux. antérieurs, des mêmes registres.

Au contraire, pour la comparaison des diverses salles d'hôpital (salles de maladies aiguës similaires aux nôtres) et qui sont les salles Blache, Chaumont, Gillette et Baffos-Baudelocque. nous avons pris, de même que pour nos salles Bouchut et Parrot, les chiffres du bureau.

Ces chiffres ont été relevés par mon interne, M. Rosenthal, que je remercie bien pour ce travail délicat et fastidieux. Tels quels. ils permettent de voir que l'hygiène de nos deux salles Parrot et Bouchut. même en ce qui concerne la rougeole, est très supérieure aux autres salles de l'hôpital, puisque la contagion y est beaucoup moindre.

Nous donnons ici pour nos deux salles d'abord :

1° Le nombre total décennal et annuel des malades;

2° Le nombre total décennal et annuel des contagions de rougeole;

3° L'équation qui donne le coefficient des contagions.

Le même tableau. fait pour les salles voisines, permet de se rendre un compte exact de la supériorité de notre statistique.

Tableau des contagions de ROUGEOLE.

(Salles Bouchut et Parrot.)

Nombre décennal des malades (1890 à 1899 . . . . 6.541
Nombre annuel des malades. 654
Nombre décennal des contagions de rougeole. 115

Nombre annuel des contagions. 11

Équation et pourcentage. . . . . $x = \dfrac{11 \times 1}{654} = 0.01$

Le coefficient de la contagion de nos deux salles est de **0,01**.

Tableau des contagions de ROUGEOLE.

(Salle Blache).

Nombre décennal des malades (1890 à 1899). 6.555
Nombre annuel des malades. 655
Nombre décennal des contagions de rougeole. 195
Nombre annuel des contagions. 19

Équation et pourcentage . . . . $x = \dfrac{19 \times 1}{655} = 0.02$

Le coefficient de contagion de la salle Blache est de **0,02**.

Tableau des contagions de ROUGEOLE.

(Salle Chaumont).

Nombre décennal des malades (1890 à 1899). 4.527
Nombre annuel des malades. 452
Nombre décennal des contagions. 12

Équation et pourcentage. . . . . $x = \dfrac{12 \times 1}{452} = 0.02$

Le coefficient des contagions de la salle Chaumont est de **0,02**

Tableau des contagions de ROUGEOLE.

(Salle Gillette).

Nombre décennal des malades (1890 à 1899). 5.520
Nombre annuel des malades. 552
Nombre décennal des contagions de rougeole. 179
Nombre annuel des contagions. 17

Équation et pourcentage . . . . $x = \dfrac{17 \times 1}{552} = 0.03$

Le coefficient des contagions de la salle Gillette est de **0,03**.

Tableau des contagions de ROUGEOLE.

(Salle Baffos-Baudelocque).

Nombre décennal des malades (1890 à 1899). 3.786
Nombre annuel des malades. 578
Nombre décennal des contagions de rougeole. 157
Nombre annuel des contagions. 15

Équation et pourcentage . . . . $x = \dfrac{15 \times 1}{578} = 0.03$

Le coefficient des contagions de la salle Baffos-Baudelocque est de **0,03**.

Conclusions relatives à la rougeole.

Ces conclusions se dégagent toutes seules de la comparaison de nos deux statistiques personnelles, avant et après l'application des mesures d'antisepsie.

Nous avons réduit de 54 à 11 le chiffre de la contagion morbilleuse, soit de 5 à 1.

La comparaison de notre statistique avec celle des salles similaires de l'hôpital (tous les chiffres pour toutes les salles, y compris les nôtres, étant ceux de l'hôpital) donne en faveur de nos salles une diminution de contagion de moitié ou des deux tiers. Le coefficient de contagion de nos salles est de 0,01. Celui des salles de l'hôpital de 0,02 ou 0,05.

On peut ainsi calculer l'économie de morbidité et, en conséquence, de mortalité que nous avons obtenue en dix années.

2° DIPHTÉRIE

Sur les tableaux récapitulatifs de nos registres, on peut voir qu'en ce qui concerne la diphtérie, nous avons eu, salle Bouchut, 6 cas de contagion et 0 cas salle Parrot — en dix années. Mais il convient de faire une remarque. Sur les 6 cas relevés salle Bouchut à notre passif, 5 sont des cas d'importation. Ce serait donc, en bonne justice, un cas, un seul cas de contagion de diphtérie qu'il faudrait nous attribuer, pour nos deux salles et en dix ans!

La statistique *officielle*, qui ne distingue pas les contagions dans la salle d'avec les importations, ne nous attribue que 5 cas au lieu de 6 pour les deux salles et pour dix ans.

Comparons d'abord *nos* deux statistiques de contagion diphtérique avant et après l'antisepsie.

Pour une période de trente-deux mois, du 1ᵉʳ novembre 1885 au 14 juin 1888, nous avons eu, salle Parrot, 52 cas de contagion de diphtérie et, salle Bouchut, 54 cas, ce qui donne une moyenne de 12 *cas par an* pour chaque salle.

Or, nous avons eu 6 cas en dix ans pour les deux salles, soit 0,5 cas par an et par salle, 0,5 au lieu de 24! Et, je le répète à dessein, 5 de ces cas sur 6 sont dus à des importations et non à des contagions dont le service soit responsable.

On peut donc dire que nous avons supprimé la contagion diphtérique.

La comparaison de nos statistiques avec celles des autres salles

nous est également très favorable. Voici les chiffres recueillis pour
une période de dix ans sur les *registres de l'hôpital*, par M. Rosenthal.

Cas de contagion de diphtérie :

    Baffos-Baudelocque. . . . . 20 cas.
    Blache. . . . . 56 —
    De Chaumont   9
    Gillette. 51
    Bouchut . . . . 5 —
    Parrot . . . . 0 —

Je ferai ici deux remarques : la première, c'est que nos contagions
sont moins nombreuses, et de beaucoup, que partout ailleurs; la seconde, c'est que la contagion de la diphtérie a diminué dans toutes
les salles de l'hôpital dans une proportion considérable depuis 1889,
époque à laquelle le directeur d'alors, M. Magdelaine, fit étuver, *ad-
ministrativement*, toute la literie des enfants contagieux ou suspects.

Ce qui tend à prouver une fois de plus que le germe de la diphtérie est peut-être, plus que tout autre, justiciable de l'antisepsie qui
s'exerce utilement sur les objets et les linges souillés sur lesquels il
adhère et où il vit pendant des mois, si la lessive ou l'étuvage ne viennent le détruire.

Avant l'organisation de notre service antiseptique, notre mortalité
par cas de contagion égalait, selon les salles, le *quart*, le *tiers* ou
même la *moitié* de la mortalité totale. (Voir planche I.)

*Tout cela est changé, et, par exemple, lorsque autrefois, nous avions
en une année, salle Parrot, douze contagions et sept morts de diphtérie,
aujourd'hui, en dix années, nous n'avons pas un seul cas de contagion!*

5° SCARLATINE, COQUELUCHE, BRONCHO-PNEUMONIE, VARICELLE
ET OREILLONS

Ici, je serai plus bref, sous peine de redites, et aussi, parce que
les documents de comparaison me font défaut, car je n'ai pas de statistique personnelle antérieure à 1889 sur ces maladies. Mais je puis
donner le tableau comparé des contagions de scarlatine depuis dix
ans dans nos salles similaires de l'hôpital. Ces chiffres ont été recueillis sur les registres officiels, les voici :

Contagion de la scarlatine de 1890 à 1899.

    Salle Baffos-Baudelocque. . . . . 51 cas.
      —   Blache. 58 —
      —   de Chaumont . . . . 16 —
      —   Gillette . . . . 14 —
      —   Bouchut. 5 —
      —   Parrot . . . . 4 —

C'est, comme pour la diphtérie, la preuve évidente de la supériorité de nos salles Parrot-Bouchut et de l'action très efficace de l'antisepsie.

La lecture des tableaux récapitulatifs montre enfin que, dans notre service, la contagion de la coqueluche, de la broncho-pneumonie et des oreillons est à peu près supprimée.

CONCLUSION GÉNÉRALE

L'antisepsie médicale, comme l'antisepsie chirurgicale ou obstétricale, existe.

Elle donne, bien appliquée, des résultats tout aussi excellents, *même dans les salles communes consacrées à l'enseignement.*

Je termine donc par ce vœu :

Que tous les services de tous les hôpitaux d'enfants deviennent promptement des services antiseptiques.

C'est facile, peu coûteux, et cela épargnera beaucoup d'existences humaines.

Mortalité dans le service pendant une année : 1885-1886, d'avril en avril.

SALLE HUSSON

Total des décès. 15

Décès par cas intérieurs : 7. . . . {
Par rougeole. 5
» diphtérie. 5
» coqueluche. 1

D	Décès par diphtérie. .
R	» rougeole. .
C	» coqueluche.
V	» varicelle. . .	Cas intérieur
	» dus à toute autre cause.

Mortalité dans le service pendant une année : 1885 1886, d'avril en avril.

SALLE BOUCHUT	SALLE PARROT
Total des décès 71	Total des décès 58
Décès par cas inté-{ Par rougeole. 15	Décès par cas inté-) Par rougeole. 7
rieurs : 19. . . . . { » diphtérie. 5	rieurs : 15 . . . .) » diphtérie. 7
{ » varicelle. 1	

SALLE BOUCHUT

D	D	D	D	D
R	R	R	R	R
R	R	R	R	R
	V	R	R	R

SALLE PARROT

D	D	D	D	D
D	D	R	R	R
R	R	R	R	R

A 1889

ÉTAT DE LA SALLE BOUCHUT (15 ET 16 AVRIL)

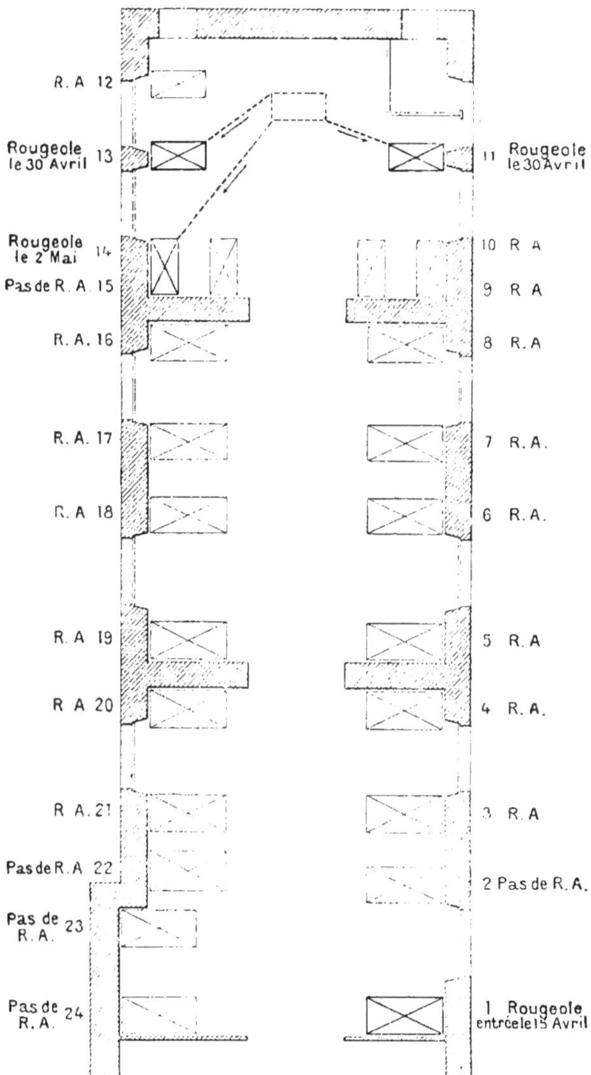

R. A. veut dire que l'enfant qui occupe ce lit a eu la rougeole.
Pas de R. A. veut dire que l'enfant n'a pas eu la rougeole

B (1889)

ÉTAT DE LA SALLE PARROT (10 FÉVRIER)

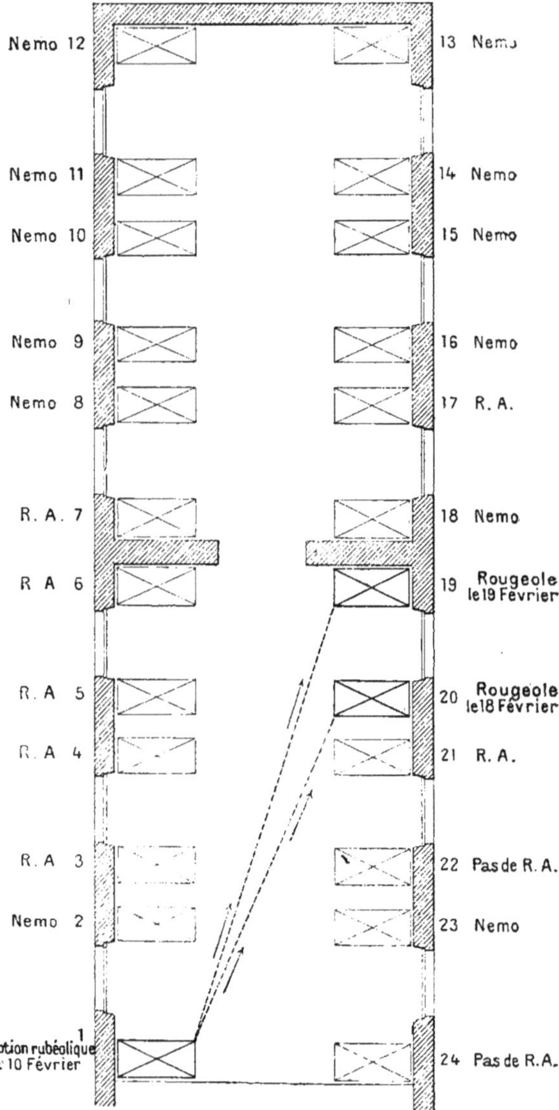

Même signification des lettres R. A. et *Pas de* R. A.
Nemo veut dire que le lit est inoccupé.

Légende du tableau A

Salle Bouchut, le 15 avril 1889, Lipowsky Joseph, qui venait de la consultation, attendit avec ses parents son tour d'interrogatoire. Un externe prenait quelques notes sommaires sur les nouveaux venus. Or, les parents du petit Lipowsky déposèrent sur le lit n° 11 une couverture qui enveloppait leur enfant et s'approchèrent des enfants couchés aux n°° 15 et 14. Du 30 avril au 2 mai, ces trois enfants étaient en éruption rubéolique. Quant à Lipowsky, suspecté dès son entrée, il fut placé dans un box (lit n° 1), à l'autre extrémité de la salle, où il resta vingt-quatre heures. Cependant aucun de ses voisins immédiats ne fut contaminé : ni les n°° 22, 25 et 24, placés en face, ni le n° 2, placé à ses côtés, qui n'avaient pas eu la rougeole antérieurement.

Depuis cette épidémie, l'interrogatoire des enfants ne se fait plus dans la salle, mais à la polyclinique. Mais cette seule faute nous a donné 6 rougeoles sur 24 dans notre statistique.

Le moins qu'on puisse conclure de ces faits, c'est que la rougeole, comme la diphtérie et tant d'autres maladies, se transmet sûrement par les mains ou les vêtements contaminés d'une tierce personne.

Légende du tableau B

Le 11 février 1889, deux fillettes atteintes de scarlatine occupèrent deux box dans la salle Parrot, aux n°° 1 et 19. Le n° 19 est dans la rangée opposée au n° 1 et placé, en ligne oblique, à 12 mètres de distance. Les deux enfants ne pouvaient quitter leur lit, et elles étaient soignées par la même infirmière, et par elle seule. Mais il arriva que la petite Jourdain Edwige, couchée au n° 1, avec la scarlatine, était en même temps en incubation de rougeole, qui fit son éruption le 10 février. Or, Chauffournier Angèle, couchée au n° 19, eut une éruption de rougeole le 19 février. Il est donc certain que les germes de la maladie sont partis du lit n° 1 au début de la période d'invasion de la rougeole, vers le 5 ou le 6 février, et ont été transportés au lit n° 19.

Comment? Par l'atmosphère ou par les mains de l'infirmière? Cette dernière hypothèse semble la plus probable, car l'infirmière, qui avait à soigner deux scarlatines et ne soupçonnait pas la rougeole du n° 1, passait de ce lit au lit 19 sans désinfection préalable.

Toutefois, la voisine immédiate du 19, le 20, fut prise aussi de rougeole le 20 février, et la contagion pour elle comme pour le lit 19 est venue du n° 1. Or, l'infirmière des box a déclaré qu'elle n'avait point touché Pauline Ledoledec, couchée au n° 20 (?). Elle passait devant son lit, voilà tout.

On pourrait donc ici incriminer l'atmosphère, si, beaucoup plus près du n° 1, les lits 22 et 24 n'avaient été occupés par deux enfants susceptibles de prendre la rougeole et restés indemnes.

DISCUSSION

M. Bézy (Toulouse). — Je désire, à propos de la remarquable communication de M. Grancher, insister sur deux points : 1° la formule de M. Grancher est très exacte : « réduire le contact au minimum ». C'est ce que j'ai toujours fait dans mon service de clinique infantile, à la Faculté de Toulouse. Les malades contagieux sont réunis par maladie (rougeole, scarlatine, diphtérie, etc.) chacun dans des chambres séparées, mais les diverses chambres sont voisines et une partie du personnel est commune. Je n'ai jamais eu de contagion, grâce à une antisepsie rigoureuse, pratiquée selon les principes indiqués. Au contraire, dans mon service de non contagieux. j'ai eu plusieurs fois des cas de contagion venus du dehors; 2° si les principes sont aujourd'hui adoptés partout, cela n'a pas été sans longues luttes et sans grandes difficultés. Nous avons la bonne fortune d'avoir dans cette salle les deux hommes qui ont le plus lutté, dans ce but depuis de longues années. MM. Grancher et Sevestre, sans oublier ceux qui ont combattu depuis le même combat. Je pense dire tout haut ce que pense tout bas chacun de vous en disant à MM. Grancher et Sevestre qu'ils appartiennent à cette catégorie de savants modestes et laborieux qui, sans faire de bruit, ont rendu d'immenses services à l'humanité.

LES MICROBES ANAÉROBIES EN PATHOLOGIE ET SPÉCIALEMENT EN PATHOLOGIE INFANTILE

par M. A. VEILLON

Vous avez entendu, il y a quelques jours, une communication de M. Tissier qui a paru vivement vous intéresser: ce n'était cependant qu'un point limité des recherches d'un ordre beaucoup plus général que je poursuis depuis plusieurs années dans le laboratoire de M. le Professeur Grancher avec l'aide de mes amis et dévoués collaborateurs : Zuber, Hallé, Guillemot, Cottet, Tissier, Rist et Morax.

Les faits apportés par M. Tissier, à propos de la gastro-entérite des enfants, ne sont point encore capables d'élucider complètement cette difficile question, mais je crois que, mieux que des théories, ils peuvent apporter un peu de lumière, et la bienveillante attention que vous avez prêtée à son exposé m'engage à vous parler de la méthode générale employée et des résultats qu'elle nous a permis d'acquérir, résultats importants, croyons-nous, pour beaucoup de maladies infantiles, et surtout importants parce qu'ils nous permettent d'avoir une conception pathogénique des processus gangreneux et putride.

Il y a déjà 7 à 8 ans[1], j'étudiais, soit pour mon instruction personnelle, soit à la prière de mes maîtres dans les hôpitaux, des produits pathologiques, pus, exsudats, tissus recueillis au cours d'opération.

Parmi ces pus ou exsudats, il y en avait qui n'avaient rien d'intéressant et dans lesquels on trouvait les microbes habituels et bien connus des suppurations; d'autres, au contraire, m'ont paru d'abord incompréhensibles à cause des résultats inattendus que me donnait leur analyse.

---

1. A. VEILLON. Sur un microcoque anaérobie trouvé dans les suppurations fétides. *Soc. de biol.*, 1895.

Ces pus, en effet, examinés au microscope, fourmillaient de bactéries, et cependant les cultures sur les milieux usuels restaient stériles. On disait alors que ces microbes étaient morts; cette explication ne me satisfaisait pas, car je ne pouvais comprendre que des lésions en pleine évolution ne fussent pas infectées par un virus encore vivant. Je croyais donc qu'il s'agissait là de microbes vivants, mais que je ne pouvais cultiver. Ayant remarqué que ces pus, si curieux bactériologiquement, appartenaient tous à un même type, le processus gangreneux ou putride, je me suis demandé s'ils n'étaient pas causés par des organismes anaérobies stricts, comme le vibrion septique qui provoque justement un processus gangreneux.

J'ai alors ensemencé ces pus non seulement sur des milieux aérés, mais encore dans des conditions d'anaérobiose rigoureuse.

J'ai alors obtenu des cultures extrêmement riches d'organismes anaérobies stricts. Ces premiers résultats ont été publiés à la Société de biologie en 1895. Mes études successives m'ont permis de constater que les affections causées par ces microbes n'étaient pas rares, et qu'elles étaient très diverses; mais les recherches devenaient de plus en plus compliquées et difficiles, car beaucoup d'espèces microbiennes étant associées, je n'arrivais pas à les isoler; j'avais la preuve que dans ces affections il y avait de nombreux microbes anaérobies, mais je n'arrivais que difficilement et exceptionnellement à obtenir des cultures pures et successives de ces microbes qui étaient très délicats. C'est alors que je me suis ingénié à trouver une méthode permettant un isolement sûr, pratique et relativement facile.

Je ne vous dirai pas ici, messieurs, pour quelles raisons multiples j'ai été obligé d'abandonner les procédés classiques, boîtes de Petri, cloches, tubes de Vignal, tubes et boîtes de Kitasato et les appareils de nombreux expérimentateurs; ceux que cette question intéresserait la trouveront discutée dans un mémoire que j'ai publié dans les *Archives de médecine expérimentale*[1]. Après bien des tâtonnements, j'ai trouvé que le plus simple était d'utiliser un dispositif que nous avons tous sous la main depuis longtemps: le tube de Liborius. Vous savez que ce savant expérimentateur, un des pères de la bactériologie des anaérobies, faisait des cultures dans des tubes à essais contenant de l'agar-agar en couche profonde, mais il ne s'en servait que pour des cultures de microbes déjà isolés. J'ai, au contraire, trouvé dans ce simple petit appareil un merveilleux procédé d'isolement, et, sans insister, permettez-moi en quelques mots de vous expliquer comment

---

1. VEILLON et ZUBER. Recherches sur quelques microbes strictement anaérobies et leur rôle en pathologie. *Arch. de méd. expérim.*, 1898.

je procède, car tout réside dans le *manuel opératoire*, et les résultats qu'on peut obtenir sont tellement importants que je voudrais voir vulgariser cette méthode. Tous les bactériologistes peu nombreux, qui ont écrit sur les anaérobies, laissent voir dans leurs mémoires les difficultés qu'ils ont pour l'isolement, à tel point qu'ils ont tous cherché un dispositif spécial, qui n'est malheureusement qu'une complication en général d'appareils déjà compliqués. Ceux de nos collègues étrangers à qui j'en ai parlé se plaignent tous de la difficulté de la technique. Vous m'excuserez donc de consacrer quelques minutes à vous montrer comment je procède.

Je prépare des tubes à essais que j'ai remplis sur une hauteur de 10 centimètres environ de gélose ordinaire, contenant seulement 12 grammes pour 1000 d'agar, et 15 grammes de glucose. Ces tubes, stérilisés, sont conservés en provision comme les milieux habituels. Quand je veux faire un ensemencement de pus contenant des anaérobies, je fais fondre au bain-marie une dizaine de ces tubes, et, quand ils sont fondus, je les refroidis à 39°-40° dans de l'eau tiède, puis, avec une pipette à longue effilure, je transporte une gouttelette de pus dans le 1er tube, puis je transporte une goutte du premier mélange dans un 2e tube, puis du 2e dans un 3e et ainsi de suite. J'ai soin d'agiter la pipette dans le milieu pour bien égaliser la distribution des microbes; j'ai ainsi des dilutions successives dans un milieu solidifiable, absolument comme on le fait pour des plaques ordinaires. Mais, au lieu de verser ces tubes dans des appareils compliqués où on fait le vide, dans des boîtes de Kitasato par exemple, je me contente des les laisser ainsi, de les faire refroidir pour que l'agar fasse prise, et de les mettre à l'étuve. Le milieu nutritif de ces tubes contenant un corps réducteur, la glucose, l'oxygène de l'air qui arrive librement dans le tube ne pénètre pas dans le milieu au delà d'un centimètre (je m'en suis assuré par l'analyse chimique). Les anaérobies peuvent donc s'y développer; et, en effet, on voit bientôt apparaître des colonies plus ou moins éloignées, selon le degré de dilution, et chaque colonie, correspondant à un seul microbe mis en suspension, est constituée par une culture pure. Voici un exemple de ce qu'on obtient. Il s'agit maintenant de prendre purement une de ces colonies soit pour en faire un examen microscopique, soit pour la réensemencer et avoir des cultures successives. Pour ce faire, il n'est nullement besoin de casser et de sacrifier le tube; on choisit la colonie qu'on veut obtenir, en la regardant soit à l'œil nu, soit au microscope, ce qu'on peut faire facilement sans rien déranger à la culture, puis avec une pipette à longue effilure munie d'un tube de caoutchouc, on va toucher la colonie choisie, et, en aspirant légèrement, on cueille cette colonie, purement, sans toucher aux voisines et sans compromettre ultérieurement le développement de ces dernières. Rien alors n'est plus facile que de transporter cette colonie dans un autre tube, ou de l'examiner au microscope après en avoir fait une préparation comme d'habitude. Voilà en quoi consiste ce procédé d'isolement; il est simple, relativement peu compliqué et donne d'excellents résultats, puisqu'il nous a permis d'isoler au moins 14 espèces de microbes anaérobies non décrites, espèces pour la plupart très fragiles, difficiles à cultiver, qu'on ne peut obtenir par les autres méthodes. Ces microbes, vous les trouverez décrits soit dans mes publications à la Société de biologie ou dans mon mémoire des *Archives de médecine expérimentale*, soit dans les thèses et travaux de mes collaborateurs. Je n'y insisterai donc pas, je veux seulement vous dire quelques mots sur le rôle qu'ils jouent.

Ces microbes sont les principaux agents de toute une série d'affections de nature gangreneuse ou putride, en particulier de celles qui prennent naissance au voisinage des cavités naturelles du corps humain, aériennes ou digestives. Agents fréquents de certaines otites, ces anaérobies pathogènes provoquent également des mastoïdites, si fréquentes chez les enfants, des thromboses septiques, des abcès intracraniens ou cérébraux, et forment les embolies septiques des complications métastatiques viscérales et articulaires d'origine otique; car nous voyons un pus gangreneux faire de la gangrène dans l'organe où l'embolie s'est arrêtée. Ils peuvent provoquer autour de l'œil, au niveau des glandes lacrymales ou dans l'orbite des phlegmons à caractère putride. Les sinusites de la face à pus fétide relèvent des mêmes germes. Ce sont là des cas qui intéressent la pédiatrie, car ils sont surtout fréquents chez les enfants. La carie dentaire et ses complications suppuratives, les phlegmons gangreneux et septiques du plancher de la bouche, certaines angines et certains phlegmons de l'amygdale, des adénophlegmons sous-maxillaires et cervicaux doivent leurs caractères spéciaux à la présence de ces microorganismes.

Dans l'appareil respiratoire, c'est la gangrène du poumon embolique ou aérienne, les pleurésies putrides qui ne sont pas rares chez les enfants.

Toutes les suppurations à point de départ intestinal leur doivent leur caractère de fétidité et leur allure gangreneuse: en particulier, les gangrènes et les abcès appendiculaires avec leurs complications immédiates de péritonite septique localisée ou diffuse, ou leurs complications à distance de suppurations hépatiques ou pleurales. Autour du tube digestif encore, les anaérobies pathogènes peuvent être les agents de la transformation purulente de certains kystes (kyste ovarique. kyste hydatique).

L'appareil génital de l'homme et de la femme offrent des portes d'entrée nombreuses à ces germes qui existent parfois sur leurs muqueuses saines ou malades.

Chez la femme, ce sont certaines complications puerpérales, — rétentions placentaires fétides. abcès péri-utérins. certaines formes de l'infection puerpérale, — ou bien certaines suppurations vulvaires, les bartholinites par exemple.

Chez l'homme, les anaérobies sont les agents actifs des infiltrations d'urine, d'un grand nombre d'abcès urineux et de leurs complications par continuité à la vessie, au rein et à son atmosphère. (Albarran et Cottet.)

Ainsi, dans tous les domaines de la pathologie humaine les anaérobies interviennent activement et les études ultérieures ne peuvent, croyons-nous, que montrer encore mieux l'étendue de leur rôle. Sans insister plus longtemps sur ce point, nous devons dire que cette énumération n'est pas théorique. que nous avons réuni un grand nombre de cas où l'analyse bactériologique a été faite complétement, et que toujours nous avons retrouvé nos espèces microbiennes lorsqu'il s'agissait d'un processus gangreneux et putride. Nous en sommes encore à trouver un cas de gangrène — je dis de gangrène vraie, et non pas de nécrose — où il n'y ait pas de microbes anaérobies. Certes, ces microbes sont souvent associés à des aérobies, ils sont souvent associés ensemble; mais la constance de certaines espèces semble les mettre au premier rang comme le *b. ramosus*, le *b. funduliformis*, le *c. fetidus*. Les preuves de leur rôle important ne sont pas seulement constituées par la constance avec laquelle on les trouve dans ces processus spéciaux. mais d'une part. par ce fait qu'ils existaient seuls dans nombre de cas, et qu'enfin. par l'expérimentation, nous avons reproduit le même processus : la gangrène pulmonaire par inoculation dans les veines. la gangrène d'un membre par inoculation dans le bout terminal d'une artère. Certains faits cliniques sont de véritables expériences : des foyers métastatiques sous-cutanés, formés par embolie loin du foyer primitif. étaient de la même nature que ce dernier et contenaient à l'état pur un de ces anaérobies. J'abrège, messieurs. il me faudrait plusieurs heures pour vous donner en détail l'histoire bactériologique de chacune des affections énumérées plus haut : résumons seulement les caractères généraux de ces organismes.

Ce sont des anaérobies stricts : on ne peut en obtenir de culture qu'à l'abri de l'oxygène libre, ils sont plus ou moins délicats, mais poussent sur les milieux de composition chimique habituelle. La plupart décomposent les sucres ; quelques-uns donnent des gaz abondants, presque tous dégagent une odeur plus ou moins fétide. Au point de vue pathologique, ils ont la propriété de nécroser les tissus, et, en même temps, de leur faire subir un processus de désintégration analogue à la putréfaction. Ce sont donc les agents des processus gangreneux et putrides. Ils produisent non seulement ces lésions importantes dans les tissus où ils ont été inoculés ou bien dans les organes où ils ont pénétré, mais encore, par embolie, ils peuvent aller former des foyers éloignés, où ils provoquent des lésions de nature gangreneuse et putride analogues à ce qu'on avait observé au foyer primitif. On peut même les rencontrer dans le sang de la circulation générale, où vraisemblablement ils n'ont pas pullulé, mais où ils ont pénétré par effraction du système circulatoire. Non seulement ils provoquent dans l'organe où ils se multiplient des lésions gangreneuses et putrides intenses, mais par les toxines qu'ils sécrètent, ils amènent une intoxication profonde de tout l'organisme, rappelant les grandes septicémies ; mais, en général, les accidents généraux d'intoxication causés par ces microbes ont des caractères un peu spéciaux. Ce sont de la fièvre, un état typhique, une prostration profonde, de la pâleur et une teinte plombée de la peau, des sueurs gluantes, une asthénie rapide du muscle cardiaque se terminant le plus souvent par le collapsus et la mort. Leur rôle en pathologie se résume donc par ces quelques mots : gangrène, suppuration fétide, toxi-infections. Des recherches encore en cours tendent à démontrer que, au moins dans quelques cas, ces organismes sont les hôtes habituels des cavités ouvertes, telles que le tube intestinal, ce qui expliquerait la nature spéciale fétide des suppurations autour de cet organe. Des recherches toutes récentes du docteur Tissier, que vous avez entendu, permettent de soupçonner le rôle important que la flore anaérobie joue dans l'état physiologique et pathologique de l'intestin de l'enfant. Les toxines, que nous commençons à isoler, nous laissent entrevoir la solution de bien des problèmes pathogéniques soulevés par la connaissance de ces organismes, et nous permettent d'espérer que la thérapeutique, grâce à la sérothérapie, ne sera plus désarmée devant les toxi-infections si graves qu'ils provoquent.

QUELQUES ÉTATS TOXIQUES POST-INFECTIEUX CHEZ LES ENFANTS
par M. le docteur ALVAREZ.

de Madrid.

Les toxines, qui empoisonnent l'organisme, comme un produit des agents infectieux qui y vivent, ont déjà été signalées, que ces toxines microbiennes agissent sur la crase sanguine, ou sur certains organes, en produisant des dégénérescences, ou encore sur le système nerveux.

Je n'aurai à m'occuper, dans cette communication, ni des infections secondaires, invasion de nouveaux hôtes dans l'habitat d'autres microbes pathogènes, ni des toxhémies infectieuses et post-infectieuses, ni des localisations de l'infection ou de ses agents : je me bornerai exclusivement à exposer *quelques états toxiques de nature nerveuse*, ou, pour parler plus exactement, produits par l'action des toxines sur le système nerveux; et encore, parmi ces derniers, non de ceux qui accompagnent l'infection, mais exclusivement de ceux qui la suivent, qui apparaissent après la disparition du tableau symptomatique par lesquels l'infection se manifestait.

Il est beaucoup plus fréquent d'observer des états toxiques post-infectieux chez les enfants que chez les adultes, pour deux raisons : 1° à cause d'une plus grande fréquence des infections pendant l'enfance et, partant, de leurs conséquences; 2° à cause de la plus grande susceptibilité de l'organisme des enfants, due à la loi de *rapide activité* dans toutes ses fonctions, par suite de laquelle cet organisme est plus facilement vulnérable et plus impressionnable, surtout dans le système nerveux et spécialement le cerveau. Plus qu'aucun autre viscère, le cerveau se trouve en effet avoir une activité de développement exagérée, d'où il résulte des conditions de moindre résistance contre les agents qui s'exercent sur lui.

On peut réduire à trois groupes principaux les états toxiques post-infectieux du système nerveux que j'ai observés :

I. Perturbations de la sensibilité et du mouvement.

II. Perturbations de l'intelligence et de la force psycho-motrice.

III. Perturbations neurotrophiques.

Je vais exposer succinctement quelques cas de chaque groupe; j'en donnerai l'interprétation théorique qui me semble leur convenir, et finalement je dirai quelques mots de leur traitement.

I. Perturbations de la sensibilité et du mouvement par l'effet des toxines post-infectieuses.

On comprend dans ce groupe les anesthésies, hyperesthésies, hétéro-esthésies sensorielles ou non, et les paralysies consécutives à des infections: c'est pourquoi il suffit de les énumérer :

Les névralgies post-grippales, les anesthésies sur diverses régions de la peau et sensorielles, les hétéro-esthésies olfactives et gustatives, fréquentes aussi comme conséquence de la toxine *pfeifféienne* ou grippale; la paralysie pharyngienne du voile du palais, très fréquente dans la diphtérie; celles plus rares des membres et du pneumo-gastrique, généralement observées dans les convalescences de ces infections.

Elles sont toutes plus ou moins transitoires; cependant, dans certains cas, elles ont une telle persistance ou une telle intensité qu'elles révèlent une importante lésion centrale annihilant la fonction par la destruction de l'organe ou de l'appareil.

Dans la convalescence de la grippe, nous avons observé, principalement chez les adultes, des perturbations dans la sensibilité spéciale : l'abolition dans certains cas et la perversion dans d'autres, du goût et de l'odorat. Dans certains cas, ces perversions se sont maintenues plus d'un an.

Luigi Concetti signale deux cas dans la convalescence d'une attaque d'influenza, où il observa de la myo-asthénie et dans un autre une névralgie de courte durée.

II. Perturbations de l'intelligence et de l'activité psycho-motrice, dues aux intoxications post-infectieuses.

Il est évident que, dans les cas que nous citerons, il faut sous-entendre que l'infection a disparu chez le sujet en question; autrement il ne s'agirait pas de post-infection, car de semblables manifestations ou perturbations peuvent se produire au cours de l'infection.

Les manifestations toxiques post-infectieuses de l'intelligence et de la force psycho-motrice peuvent se classer, comme le fait Manheimer en étudiant les perturbations mentales chez les enfants, en changements de l'émotivité, de l'intelligence, de l'activité psychique ou volition, et en d'autres plus complexes et plus généralisés, qui proviennent de l'altération primitive de la conscience.

Les effets des intoxications sur l'encéphale sont très variés. Nous avons vu souvent, principalement dans la convalescence des fièvres typhoïdes, deux degrés bien marqués de perturbations de l'émotivité: l'un léger, l'enfant est triste, pleure plus facilement qu'à l'ordinaire, se laisse conduire, repousse avec indifférence les jouets qui le passionnaient précédemment; l'autre degré est plus fort: le convalescent est indifférent à tout ce qui l'entoure, regarde quand on attire son attention d'un regard éteint et triste, et ferme bientôt les yeux: il y a souvent du mutisme: nous ignorons si cette aphasie est produite par amnésie de la parole ou par épuisement cérébral. Dans deux cas de convalescence de fièvre typhoïde d'enfants de 4 et 7 ans, le mutisme persista cinq et sept jours respectivement. Généralement la sensibilité de la peau est diminuée.

Peu à peu cet organisme réagit, et tout disparaît lentement.

C'est un état particulier de fatigue, d'épuisement du système nerveux, comme le démontre l'hypotension artérielle. Manheimer dit qu' « il s'agit dans ces cas de changements vaso-moteurs primitifs et généralisés »; « c'est un sentiment de diminution de l'innervation et de la tonalité musculaire », dit Lange et aussi de Fleury.

Les perturbations de l'intelligence que nous avons observées le plus fréquemment se rapportent, dans certains cas, à la faiblesse de toutes ses manifestations, à la lenteur de la perception du jugement et de la volonté, à une véritable psycho-asthénie, plus fréquentes après la fièvre typhoïde et la grippe qu'après d'autres infections.

D'autres fois, les perturbations intellectuelles se sont traduites par des hallucinations et du délire à marche plus ou moins rapide et à intervalles répétés.

En 1897, Kuhn a publié des cas de perturbations mentales post-diphtériques.

En 1896, Kalischer a publié une observation d'excitation maniaque alternant avec des phénomènes de stupeur consécutive à la grippe chez une petite fille de deux ans.

En 1898, Régis et Séglas se sont occupés des délires de l'infection et de l'auto-intoxication.

Voici trois cas très clairs de perturbation intellectuelle post-infectieuse parmi les divers que j'ai observés.

Le premier est celui d'un enfant guéri, par le sérum de Roux et le tubage, de diphtérie pharyngo-laryngienne intense: il fut affecté d'hallucinations visuelles: il voyait courir autour de lui, de-ci de-là, un rat, le suivant du doigt et suppliant la sœur de charité qui le soignait de le prendre et de le lui donner attaché à une corde pour jouer. Ce délire dura plusieurs minutes, se reproduisit vingt heures après et l'enfant mourut quatre heures plus tard de paralysie du pneumo-gastrique, trois jours après que tous les symptômes de l'infection diphtérique avaient disparu.

Le deuxième cas est celui d'un enfant de 8 ans, en pleine convalescence de la rougeole; il a de violents délires qui se répètent plusieurs fois, jour et nuit, à intervalles rapprochés; il en arrive à se jeter à bas du lit en fureur et comme fuyant, plein de terreur, de graves dangers, sans obéir aux personnes de sa famille qui le soignaient, ni les reconnaître. Ces délires étaient accompagnés d'hallucinations acoustiques et visuelles que l'enfant expliquait, une fois passées, en disant que des « hommes et des animaux criaient après lui et qu'il voyait des bêtes très laides qui se dirigeaient vers lui ». — Le délire et les hallucinations se répétèrent deux jours. Les hallucinations gustatives se prolongèrent encore trois jours; le malade éprouvait la sensation de cheveux sur la langue, ce qui l'obligeait à passer une serviette sur la langue; il repoussait le lait, le bouillon, l'eau et tous les aliments, car, disait-il, il y avait dans tout cela des cheveux qu'il cherchait et ne trouvait naturellement pas. Cinq jours après, tous ces phénomènes disparurent pour ne plus revenir.

Le troisième cas est celui d'une petite fille de neuf ans, sœur de ce dernier, qui tomba malade de la rougeole quelques jours après. Dans la convalescence se présentèrent les mêmes phénomènes que chez son frère, et les hallucinations durèrent le même temps. Après qu'elles eurent disparu, la peau de la malade présenta un phénomène *que je n'ai observé que cette fois-là* et dont nous nous occuperons plus tard dans l'étude des perturbations neurotrophiques.

L'activité psychique est fréquemment diminuée et pervertie par suite des intoxications post-infectieuses. Apathie pour tout mouvement, qui arrive parfois à l'immobilité de tout le corps, semblable aux états mélancoliques et à la confusion mentale; changement radical dans les goûts physiques et moraux habituels de l'enfant; obscurcissement de la conscience qui perd la notion du temps et de l'espace; véritable état de stupeur; voilà ce que l'on observe le plus fréquemment.

On voit généralement disparaître toutes ces perturbations en peu de jours à mesure que l'organisme élimine les toxines qui l'empoisonnent.

III. Perturbations toxiques post-infectieuses neurotrophiques.

C'est à cette catégorie que correspondent les dégénérations aiguës presque subites, que nous observons dans la convalescence de la scarlatine, l'hypertrophie graisseuse du cœur, la néphrite albuminurique, et une forme spéciale que j'ai eu l'occasion d'observer quatre fois : trois dans la convalescence de la scarlatine, et une dans celle de la fièvre typhoïde, chez des enfants de deux à six ans.

Voici le tableau : l'enfant, bien rétabli et levé, s'alite de nouveau au bout de 5 ou 4 jours avec une légère fièvre, provoquée par une inflammation polyarticulaire, principalement dans les petites articulations, symétriquement, aux pieds et aux mains, simulant une légère attaque de rhumatisme polyarticulaire aigu, quoique n'ayant de commun avec cette affection que la douleur et la tuméfaction articulaires très légères ; dans ce cas, le diagnostic différentiel devenait par conséquent très facile.

Cette lésion neurotrophique a duré de 4 à 8 jours, due sans aucun doute à l'action des toxines de ces infections sur le système nerveux, sans que l'on puisse dire la raison pour laquelle la perturbation vaso-motrice se localise dans les tissus *péri* ou *intra-articulaires*.

Le cas observé dans la convalescence de la fièvre typhoïde fut celui d'un enfant de trois ans. Son état était si bizarre que deux célèbres professeurs furent induits à diagnostiquer des tubercules cérébraux. Les pieds étaient en extension légèrement inclinés en dedans, les mains en flexion accentuée sur l'avant-bras et légèrement tournées en dedans, et les doigts en flexion forcée en complète symétrie ; on ne découvre pas de changement de coloration ni de tuméfaction articulaire ; le corps conserve constamment une attitude d'immobilité ; l'enfant pleure au moindre mouvement qu'on lui fait faire. Les docteurs jugèrent que cet état était des contractures provoquées par la lésion cérébrale, alors que ce n'était qu'une position instinctive motivée par la souffrance.

Cette forme d'intoxication post-infectieuse, que l'on appelle rhumatisme scarlatineux, est si peu fréquente que ces confrères ne l'avaient jamais observée et n'y crurent pas. Tous ces troubles avaient disparu le cinquième jour. Deux ans se sont écoulés, et l'enfant continue à jouir d'une santé parfaite et à se développer normalement.

Baginski a observé une névrite sciatique accompagnée d'une paralysie atrophique, consécutive à une infection grippale ; Kohts, une encéphalite hémorragique ; et Massalongo, une sclérose en plaques.

Chauffard a eu à l'hôpital Cochin un cas remarquable de polynévrite ériphérique post-grippale accompagnée de paralysie, dans lequel tous les accidents furent si rapides qu'ils disparurent avant un mois à compter du début de la maladie

Aux troubles névrotrophiques post-infectieux correspondent, à mon avis, les œdèmes et les anasarques, qui ont été principalement observés par les pédiatres, après la scarlatine, sans y trouver de signes de néphrite. C'est de cette anasarque que s'est occupé le docteur Cassel dans son rapport présenté à la Société de médecine de Berlin (séance du 7 février dernier) : il a observé ces œdèmes et anasarques dans la convalescence des éruptions, sans trouver d'albumine dans l'urine et sans lésion cardiaque, et après des entérites infectieuses observées aussi par Henoch qui les attribue à la diminution de l'énergie cardiaque et au thrombus (non démontré) des grosses veines, quand il n'y a pas de néphrite.

Ces œdèmes et anasarques ont aussi été décrits par Philippe, de Berlin, pendant une épidémie de scarlatine, et dans la plupart des cas sans albumine dans l'urine.

Rilliet, Barthez et Cadet de Gassicourt les ont observés après la fièvre typhoïde.

Stark, de Kiel, l'a observée après la rougeole et l'appelle anasarque essentielle. Filatow en a observé aussi divers cas après la scarlatine et d'autres exanthèmes aigus. Le distingué pédiatre moscovite est absolu, et avec raison à mon avis, dans son affirmation de l'indépendance des œdèmes et de la néphrite ; il assure qu'il n'y a pas le moindre rapport entre elles, car le terme en est heureux et rapide, et parce qu'on n'y observe jamais d'albuminurie ni d'urémie : il l'explique en établissant la théorie que « les principes toxiques dans le sang frappent les tubes capillaires de la peau et des membranes séreuses et altèrent les centres nerveux du cœur ».

Dans cette même séance de la Société de médecine de Berlin, le Dr Senator admet ces œdèmes en les expliquant par l'altération de la crase sanguine qui rend les vaisseaux cutanés perméables à l'albumine et au sérum.

Nous pensons que ces cas d'œdèmes plus ou moins généralisés sans albuminurie, sans lésion cardiaque, sans une anémie prononcée, que l'on observe quelquefois après des infections, ne sont autre chose que des effets toxiques post-infectieux dont nous croyons que le mécanisme est le suivant : action de la toxine sur le système nerveux, trouble consécutif dans les vaso-moteurs qui se traduit par de la parésie, faiblesse consécutive circulatoire périphérique qui, ajoutés à la diminution de plasticité du sang, facilite l'extravasion du sérum.

Pour terminer l'énumération des troubles toxiques post-infectieux, nous décrirons le cas remarquable dont j'ai parlé plus haut d'altérations neurotrophiques de la peau.

Quand la petite fille de neuf ans qui, après la rougeole, eut du délire et les hallucinations dont nous avons parlé plus haut, fut guérie et entra franchement en convalescence. il apparut, au bout de trois jours. de l'abattement. de la pâleur. et une démangeaison extraordinaire sur toute la surface de la peau ; la nuit fut agitée : en l'observant le matin, je trouve sur toute la surface du corps des ampoules confluentes de caractères spéciaux.

Leur dimension variait depuis celle d'un grain de millet jusqu'à celle d'un petit pois, de forme parfaitement ronde, excepté quelques-unes qui par leur union à quelque autre voisine présentent une forme allongée, sans changement de coloration en les regardant verticalement à la peau : il est dans ce cas difficile de les voir malgré leur volume, tant ces vésicules étaient transparentes, et normale la coloration de leur base. En regardant dans le sens du diamètre de la base sur la tangente de la partie examinée, se détachaient sur le fond de l'atmosphère autant de protubérances qu'il existait de vésicules sur la surface tangente, unique moyen pour bien les voir, transparentes et constituées par une couche extrêmement mince ressemblant à la peau d'oignon. A un toucher doux on sentait l'irrégularité de la surface de la peau.

En les piquant avec une épingle, il n'en sortait pas une goutte de liquide et la peau s'aplatissait et se ridait : il était indubitable que des gaz avaient soulevé la couche la plus externe de l'épiderme et avaient constitué cette ampoule.

Cette éruption était entièrement généralisée ; elle se présentait même à la paume des mains et à la plante des pieds.

Au bout de 48 heures environ, toutes les vésicules s'étaient affaissées et ridées ; et 24 heures plus tard, la couche de l'épiderme était éliminée et il ne restait pas la moindre trace de l'éruption, ni en coloration, ni en aspérité, ni en croûte, ni même en élimination furfuracée ; et l'enfant recouvrait la santé et les couleurs.

Nous croyons que ce phénomène remarquable fut la conséquence de l'action des toxines produites par la rougeole, lesquelles, en s'éliminant par la peau. donnèrent lieu à ce phénomène neurotrophique du mécanisme duquel je ne parviens pas à me rendre compte. Il se produit quelque chose de semblable dans l'herpès labialis et dans le pemphigus simple que nous observons fréquemment chez les nouveau-nés, quoique dans ces derniers cas le fond de l'ampoule ainsi que ses bords apparaissent colorés en rouge.

Généralement tous ces troubles toxiques post-infectieux sont fugaces et révèlent une rapide action de l'agent qui les produit et de son épuisement, sans laisser de lésion dans le tissu ou organe sur lequel il a agi (guérison), ou. s'il subsiste une lésion, elle tarde à disparaître. Dans d'autres cas, elle détruit l'organe (origines pneumo-gastriques. paralysie cardiaque).

Il est indubitable qu'une fois l'infection passée. et par conséquent le microbe qui la produisait étant mort, il reste dans l'organisme un poison, une toxine, un produit de ses agents qui ont une action toxique principalement sur le tissu nerveux ou sur sa fonction, quand il n'est pas rapidement éliminé. C'est de là que provient la courte durée de son action, parce que, une fois éliminés et une fois morts les êtres qui la produisaient, il n'y a plus de production de toxine. C'est pour cela que les phénomènes toxiques durant l'infection sont plus intenses et plus durables et plus à craindre que les phénomènes post-infectieux, dans la plupart des cas.

On ne peut répondre que par des hypothèses à la question encore insuffisamment élucidée de la manière d'agir de ces toxines sur le système nerveux pour troubler ses fonctions tantôt légèrement, tantôt profondément.

Il est raisonnable de demander s'il n'existe pas de lésions qui expliquent, par exemple, la paralysie du pneumo-gastrique, si la toxine a agi en produisant une annihilation de fonction dans l'élément cellulaire neuronique, empêchant la fonction indispensable à la vie de la même façon que cela se produit dans les syncopes émotionnelles, car dans quelques cas l'action toxique est si rapide et si intense que nous croyons qu'il n'y a pas eu de temps suffisant pour que puisse avoir lieu la phase de dégénérescence de Marinesco (destruction des prolongements protoplasmatiques et de la substance fondamentale achromatique, chargée de la transmission nerveuse): et la phase de réaction ne tue pas.

Dans d'autres manifestations plus fugitives. comme les troubles intellectuels déjà signalés, il vient à l'esprit, quand on cherche l'explication de ce mécanisme, l'idée de l'existence d'un fluide nerveux ou psychique dans les substances protoplasmiques chromatophyles et achromatiques: l'une transmettant. l'autre alimentant, peut-être au bénéfice de ce même fluide, quelque chose de semblable à ce qui a été étudié par Crookes sous le nom de force psychique; ce fluide équitablement réparti dans les neurones garantit l'intégrité de leur fonctionnement: mais quand une cause, comme l'émotion. l'hypnotisme. la suggestion et peut-être ces toxines, rompent la distribution harmonique de ce fluide, la fonction de la cellule cérébrale se trouble de telle façon que la fonction d'un groupe cellulaire cérébral diminue en même temps qu'un autre, proche ou éloigné. s'excite là où peut-être le fluide nerveux a afflué en plus grande quantité, et il se produit ainsi des troubles intellectuels post-infectieux qui durent jusqu'au recouvrement de l'équilibre de ce fluide qui efface le trouble cérébral, comme s'effacent les ondulations de la surface d'un lac quand la force qui a ébranlé sa tranquillité s'est épuisée.

Quant au *traitement* de ces accidents, nous devons avouer notre impuissance, qui ne nous permet que d'aider un peu l'organisme pour l'élimination des toxines.

Tonifier et exciter le système nerveux, et surveiller les émonctoires naturels, c'est ce qui est indiqué pendant l'infection et après l'infection.

Il nous a semblé avoir obtenu de bons résultats avec les préparations à base de quinine, de kola et de coca, avec de légères doses d'alcool, tâchant qu'elles ne dépassent pas la dose inoffensive : selon Joffroy et Serveaux, un centimètre cube par kilogramme : je puis en dire autant des préparations glycéro-phosphatées.

Dans tous ces états, la bonne alimentation et l'air de la campagne sont bienfaisants au plus haut point.

Conclusions.

I. — Il arrive souvent que les infections sont suivies d'états pathologiques déterminés par des toxines produites par ces infections.

II. — Ces états toxiques post-infectieux sont plus fréquents chez les enfants que chez les adultes, principalement ceux qui ont leur siège sur les centres nerveux.

III. — Ces états sont généralement de courte durée, transitoires. Cependant quelquefois les toxines ont un tel pouvoir toxique qu'elles tuent rapidement (paralysie du pneumo-gastrique).

IV. — Les troubles toxiques post-infectieux qui ont leur siège sur le système nerveux peuvent être groupés en trois catégories : 1° troubles toxiques post-infectieux de la sensibilité et du mouvement ; 2° troubles toxiques post-infectieux de l'intelligence et de la force psycho-motrice ; et 3° troubles toxiques post-infectieux neurotrophiques.

V. — Je trouve très remarquable le cas de troubles cutanés toxiques post-infectieux ; c'est la première fois que je les ai observés.

VI. — Jusqu'à ce jour le mécanisme de ces accidents demeure inexplicable : la relation entre la cause et l'effet nous est inconnue.

VII. — Il faut reconnaître dans le dynamisme cérébral un fluide nerveux ou force psychique dont la distribution harmonieuse dans les substances protoplasmatiques des neurones est peut-être troublée par les toxines, et cela pourrait donner une idée du mécanisme de ces accidents.

VIII. — Notre pouvoir thérapeutique se borne jusqu'à présent à aider l'organisme pour l'élimination des toxines.

INFLUENCE DU SALOL SUR LA DIAZORÉACTION D'ERLICH ET SON ACTION THÉRAPEUTIQUE DANS LA FIÈVRE TYPHOÏDE CHEZ LES ENFANTS

par M. le professeur N.-C. THOMESCO,

de Bucarest.

Pendant une petite épidémie de fièvre typhoïde à Bucarest, nous avons remarqué que la réaction d'Erlich apparaissait et disparaissait chez le même malade. En observant de plus près, nous avons constaté que toutes les fois que nous employions le benzonaphtol, le bétol, le salicylate de magnésie ou de bismuth, la réaction d'Erlich était très manifeste; pour disparaître d'une manière constante toutes les fois que nous administrions le salol.

Alors nous nous sommes dit : si le salol fait disparaître la diazoréaction, employons-le d'une manière systématique dans la fièvre typhoïde.

La dose du salol a été de 3-4 et 5 grammes, par jour, en petites doses de 20 jusqu'à 50 centigrammes, chaque heure ou chaque heure et demie, la diazoréaction étant négative pendant tout le temps que le malade se trouve sous l'influence du salol.

Abaissement thermique. — En dehors de la disparition de la diazoréaction nous avons constaté une diminution de température de 1° jusqu'à 2°.

Amélioration de l'état morbide. — Avec l'administration du salol, l'état des malades s'améliore d'une manière sensible, ils deviennent plus réveillés et plus attentifs, tandis qu'un jour plus tôt, sous l'influence d'autres antiseptiques, les malades se trouvaient en état de prostration et de délire.

La durée de la maladie devient en même temps plus courte et très souvent la défervescence se fait d'une manière brusque.

Zez, évaporant au bain-marie les urines des typhiques avec la diazoréaction et dissolvant le résidu dans l'eau stérilisée, a injecté 5 cc.

dans le péritoine d'une souris blanche qui est morte après quelques moments, tandis que les souris de contrôle de Zez, auxquelles il avait injecté 5 cc. d'une solution aqueuse du résidu des urines ne présentant pas de diazoréaction, ne sont pas mortes. Nous avons répété aussi ces expériences sur les cobayes. Le cobaye auquel nous avons injecté le résidu aqueux des urines avec diazoréaction est mort deux jours après, tandis que celui injecté avec les urines après le traitement au salol n'est pas mort. D'où il résulte que : 1° la cause de la diazoréaction d'Erlich serait une substance toxique détruite par la médication du salol, et 2° le traitement antiseptique de la fièvre typhoïde serait le salol qui aurait une action quasi spécifique sur l'infection typhique.

DE LA GRAVITÉ DU RHUMATISME CHEZ LES ENFANTS
DANS SES RAPPORTS AVEC LES COMPLICATIONS CARDIAQUES
GRAVITÉ DES CARDIOPATHIES

M. H. BARBIER,

Médecin des Hôpitaux de Paris.

Le rhumatisme articulaire chez les enfants est une affection grave en raison de la fréquence et de la gravité des lésions cardiaques qu'il provoque presque fatalement chez eux. On sait que Bouillaud disait que dans l'enfance le cœur se comporte vis-à-vis le rhumatisme comme une véritable articulation, et que H. Roger considérait les manifestations cardiaques comme à peu près fatales. Cadet de Gassicourt donne une proportion de 81 pour cent d'affections cardiaques et Billet, Barthez et Sanné, 87 pour cent.

Ce qui constitue le danger de ces rhumatismes, c'est que souvent ils sont peu accusés, subaigus, traînants, ne s'accompagnant pas de gonflement et de rougeur des jointures, mais se manifestant par des douleurs plus ou moins accusées durant des semaines, exaspérées par les mouvements et par la pression au niveau des interlignes articulaires, affectant principalement les membres inférieurs, mais souvent aussi se manifestant par un torticolis, dont on peut méconnaître la nature articulaire si l'on n'explore pas les vertèbres cervicales où l'on constate alors l'existence de points douloureux, indice de l'arthrite vertébrale rhumatismale.

Le début de ces rhumatismes est souvent marqué par des phénomènes généraux : fièvre, céphalée, vomissement, etc., qui montrent bien que chez les enfants le rhumatisme a plus l'allure d'une maladie infectieuse générale que d'une arthropathie multiple, et que les localisations viscérales, sur le cœur en particulier, ne sont pas en rapport avec l'intensité des manifestations articulaires. La loi de coïncidence de Bouillaud, si souvent vérifiée chez l'adulte, ne s'applique donc pas avec la même certitude chez l'enfant. La plupart des rhumatismes que j'ai observés et qui se sont accompagnés de complications plus ou moins graves du côté du cœur, rentrent dans cette catégorie et ont cédé à quelques jours de traitement par le salicylate de soude.

Je n'ai observé qu'un exemple de rhumatisme sans complications.

Obs. I. — Rhumatisme léger. — Pas de complications. — B. 15 ans et demi. Salle Barrier, 27. Hôpital Trousseau, 21 août 1899.

Paralysie infantile ancienne (?) Depuis quelques jours douleurs dans l'articulation coxo-fémorale droite, puis le lendemain dans le coude gauche, puis le droit.

A l'entrée on constate, en plus, une douleur de l'articulation tibio-tarsienne droite sans gonflement notable. Les manifestations rhumatismales cèdent à l'administration de 5 grammes de salicylate de soude pendant 5 jours. Rien au cœur.

Au contraire, dans toutes les observations que je rapporte, les complications cardiaques ont été constantes et quelques-unes très graves.

Obs. II. — Rhumatisme subaigu. — Endocardite. — Anémie consécutive. — Ernest B. 15 ans. — Entré le 18 septembre 1899. Salle Barrier, 25.

Première attaque de rhumatisme l'an dernier. Depuis 5 jours se plaint de douleurs dans les jambes, qui cessent au bout de 5 jours d'administration du salicylate de soude.

Cœur gros, la pointe est au niveau de la 6ᵉ côte. Souffle systolique de la pointe se propageant vers l'aisselle; sort, le 24, très anémié.

Obs. III. — Rhumatisme récent. — Endocardite. — (Consult. Hôp. Bichat). — Marguerite A. 4 ans. Venue le 15 mai 1900.

Douleurs de toutes les articulations et en particulier du genou droit avec fièvre, depuis 8 jours. — Bien qu'elle ne se plaigne ni d'essoufflement ni de palpitation, on constate un bruit de souffle systolique de la pointe avec piaulement se propageant vers l'aisselle.

Les complications cardiaques du rhumatisme chez les enfants ne méritent pas seulement d'attirer l'attention par leur *fréquence*, mais aussi et surtout par leur *gravité*. A ce point de vue l'observation montre qu'elles affectent volontiers pour l'endocarde à la fois l'orifice mitral et l'orifice aortique, très souvent le péricarde et probablement aussi l'aorte ou les tissus qui englobent le plexus cardiaque, peut-être le cœur lui-même. Enfin, en raison probablement de cette complexité de lésions, leur *évolution ultérieure* est très grave, soit que les malades présentent une asystolie précoce et difficilement maniable par les médicaments, soit qu'ils présentent plus ou moins atténués des signes d'*angor pectoris*, ou des menaces de syncope qui peuvent amener la mort subite.

La multiplicité des lésions se manifeste cliniquement par des modifications dans le timbre des bruits, ou par des bruits anormaux aux orifices de la mitrale et des valvules aortiques : le plus souvent, bruits de souffle doubles, indiquant des lésions complexes au niveau de ces orifices.

Lorsque l'orifice aortique est lésé, j'ai observé parfois l'existence de signes plus ou moins accusés d'*angor pectoris*. Sensation d'étau, douleur précordiale survenant par accès passagers qui peuvent faire penser à la participation de l'aorte au processus inflammatoire.

Dans tous ces cas la *péricardite* est conjointement observée, et quand on observe les malades quelque temps après la crise rhumatismale, alors qu'ils viennent consulter pour les accidents cardiaques dont ils souffrent, on trouve en général une voussure, une augmentation de la matité précordiale plus ou moins accusée, la pointe du cœur abaissée et déviée en dehors, mais presque toujours aussi une ondulation très marquée de la paroi thoracique, un choc étalé du cœur, et quelquefois une rétraction systolique de la pointe.

Obs. IV. — Rhumatisme articulaire aigu récent. — Endopéricardite, pleurésie, anémie profonde. — (Consultation hôpital Bichat.)

La nommée X. (fillette d'une dizaine d'années) se présente à la consultation le 6 novembre 1899, pour une première attaque de rhumatisme dont elle souffre depuis 15 jours, ayant porté sur un grand nombre d'articulations qui ont été atteintes à plusieurs reprises. Depuis 3 ou 4 jours crises d'oppression nocturne.

État actuel. — Enfant très pâle, très oppressée, présentant encore de la tuméfaction et de l'œdème des deux mains.

Cœur. — Soulèvement ondulatoire de la région précordiale. Pointe du cœur abaissée et déviée vers l'aisselle, battant dans le sixième espace. A la palpation, battements précipités, faibles, accompagnés d'un frémissement (frottement). Pouls petit (150 p.).

Pouls veineux, très appréciable au cou. Douleur sur le trajet du nerf phrénique gauche.

A l'auscultation. Assourdissement des bruits du cœur, en particulier du premier bruit qui présente un retentissement métallique.

Poumons. — Signes de pleurésie avec épanchement léger base gauche.

Signes généraux : Anémie, sueurs très marquées.

Obs. V. — Rhumatisme subaigu. — Endocardite mitrale. — Péricardite. — (Hôpital Trousseau.)

Marc L., 24 ans, Salle Barrier, 27. Le 11 septembre 1899.

Douleurs dans les jointures, subaiguës, traînantes depuis 2 mois. Gonflement des cou-de-pied depuis trois semaines.

A l'entrée douleurs articulaires peu marquées qui cèdent au bout de trois jours à l'emploi du salicylate de soude, supprimé complètement le 19. A l'entrée on constate un souffle systolique de la pointe qui, après avoir présenté quelques modifications pendant le séjour de l'enfant à l'hôpital (endocardite en évolution), persiste à la sortie de l'hôpital. Le cœur à ce moment est un peu gros, la pointe abaissée et déviée en dehors.

On a constaté également à l'entrée, à la région moyenne, un frottement péricardique.

Obs. VI. — Rhumatisme subaigu traînant. — Endocardite mitrale et aortique. — Asystolie légère. — (Hôpital Trousseau.)

Henri M., 12 ans, 51 juillet 1899, Salle Barrier. — Première attaque à l'âge de 9 ans. Douleurs vagues dans les membres inférieurs depuis 2 mois. Essoufflement, dyspnée d'effort.

A l'entrée : pas de rhumatisme.

Cœur. — Hypertrophié; la pointe bat à 5 travers de doigt au-dessous et en dehors du mamelon gauche. — Souffle prolongé de la pointe, avec piaulement (Insuffisance et rétrécissement mitral).

Souffle systolique et diastolique de la base (aortite avec insuffisance aortique).

Palpitations, dyspnée, pouls petit, irrégulier, intermittent à 96; pouls capillaires.

Foie tuméfié, déborde sensiblement les fausses côtes droites.

Sort amélioré le 20 août (repos, lait, digitale).

Obs. VII. — Affection cardiaque rhumatismale complexe; insuffisance aortique, symphyse cardiaque (?). — (Consultation de l'hôpital Bichat.)

Joseph J., âgé de 15 ans, se présente le 5 janvier 1900. — Première atteinte de rhumatisme à l'âge de 6 ans, sans troubles cardiaques apparents à la suite; ceux-ci se sont montrés pour la première fois il y a trois ans (oppressions, crises de palpitation).

Nouvelle atteinte de rhumatisme à 14 ans, il y a un an. Ce rhumatisme a duré tout l'hiver, et depuis ce moment les troubles cardiaques se sont accentués et n'ont pas cessé.

État actuel. — Enfant pâle, oppressé, présentant au niveau du cou des battements artériels énergiques, surtout dans le creux sus-sternal droit.

Cœur. — Voussure de la paroi thoracique. Pointe abaissée et déviée vers l'aisselle, à deux travers de doigt en dehors de la ligne mamelonnaire. Choc au doigt au moment de la rétraction.

A la palpation, battements de cœur énergiques et léger frémissement. A la percussion, matité transversale augmentée, débordant le bord droit du sternum. A l'auscultation, souffle diastolique à la base, se prolongeant le long du bord gauche du sternum. — Souffle très fort, accompagné d'un souffle systolique ayant son maximum dans les vaisseaux du cou et en particulier dans le creux sus-sternal. A la pointe, bruit de galop, bruits du cœur sourds et clangoreux.

Les vaisseaux du cou chez cet enfant présentaient l'aspect éréthique qu'ils ont dans certains cas de goître exophtalmique.

Foie et poumons : normaux.

Obs. VIII. — Rhumatisme subaigu, avec mouvements choréiformes. — Endopéricardite. — (Consultation. hôpital Bichat.) — Lésions multiples. — Aortite (?)

Jeanne G., âgée de 15 ans. venue à la consultation le 24 décembre 1899.

Bien portante jusqu'au mois de mai 1899. A ce moment elle est prise, la nuit. de douleur et de gonflement au niveau des articulations du genou, du cou-de-pied, de l'épaule, du coude et du poignet. Huit jours après, elle a eu pendant cinq jours des mouvements choréiformes.

Au bout de quinze jours de maladie, les accidents disparurent; la malade conserva seulement des douleurs vagues dans les articulations de la main et de l'oppression pendant la marche et la montée des escaliers.

Au mois de juin, un médecin constata pour la première fois des lésions cardiaques.

Au mois de juillet, la malade fut prise brusquement d'une douleur précordiale (sensation d'étau ou de griffe), accompagnée de dyspnée violente, surtout pendant la nuit.

Ces accidents cessèrent au bout de six jours.

Depuis cette époque la malade se réveille fréquemment la nuit avec de l'angoisse.

État actuel. — Enfant pâle, faible, peu développée, oppressée.

Cœur. — Voussure précordiale.

Soulèvement ondulatoire de la paroi thoracique. Rétraction systolique de la pointe qui bat dans le sixième espace, fortement déjetée en dehors.

Augmentation de la matité transversale. Souffle systolique très fort *à la pointe*. se propageant dans l'aisselle et dans le dos.

Souffle systolique et diastolique *à la base*. Le pouls est petit, rapide (125 p.) et présente un retard sensible sur le choc de la pointe du cœur.

Foie. — Le foie congestionné déborde de trois travers de doigt le rebord des fausses côtes.

Poumons. — Congestion des deux poumons. avec submatité dans le tiers inférieur.

Cette enfant a été suivie jusqu'au mois de novembre (21 novembre).

Sous l'influence du repos, de la digitale et du bromure de potassium. d'une part, et d'une révulsion persistante au-devant du cœur au moyen de vésicatoires répétés. les phénomènes asystoliques se sont améliorés; mais. le 21 novembre. on pouvait constater la persistance des bruits de souffle et l'existence d'un frottement péricardique fort appréciable à la main. Le foie était moins gros, mais débordait cependant encore d'un travers de doigt les fausses côtes.

En résumé, cette enfant. à la suite d'un rhumatisme peu violent et de durée relativement courte, avait fait des lésions graves de son endocarde, de son péricarde. et peut-être de l'aorte, et présentait les signes d'une asystolie permanente avec crises qui se rapprochent singulièrement de l'*angor pectoris*.

Obs. IX. — *Troisième attaque de rhumatisme. — Lésions multiples du cœur.*

Charles Del., 15 ans et demi. Légère angoisse de poitrine. (Hôpital Trousseau.) — Entré le 28 septembre 1899, salle Barrier, lit 25.

Mère rhumatisante, soignée en ce moment à l'hôpital Saint-Antoine. L'enfant a déjà eu deux attaques de rhumatisme : la première à l'âge de 10 ans, la seconde à 12 ans.

Il est atteint d'une troisième atteinte de rhumatisme depuis 16 jours, qui a débuté par les coudes et les hanches ; ces douleurs ont disparu au bout de 8 jours, et ont été remplacées par une douleur précordiale continue avec angoisse, qu'il a déjà ressentie d'ailleurs lors de sa deuxième attaque ; céphalalgie notable.

État à l'entrée. — Aucune tuméfaction, ni douleur articulaire.

Cœur. — Hypertrophié. La pointe bat dans le cinquième espace. A l'auscultation : frottements péricardiques à la pointe ; roulement présystolique et souffle systolique se propageant vers l'aisselle. A la base, souffle systolique et souffle diastolique se propageant le long du sternum. Lors de son entrée ces bruits n'étaient pas très nets et leur interprétation avait paru quelque temps douteuse ; mais au bout de quelques jours, il n'y avait plus de doute sur leur existence.

Foie gros, débordant les fausses côtes.

Sous l'influence du repos, de la révulsion précordiale, etc., les symptômes d'angoisse précordiale disparaissent pour se montrer de nouveau le 26 octobre, après que l'enfant se fut plaint d'une légère douleur de l'épaule gauche.

Il est sorti de l'hôpital le 26 octobre, avec les lésions cardiaques constatées à l'entrée.

Un dernier facteur de la gravité des manifestations cardiaques des rhumatismes, c'est la sévérité de leur évolution ultérieure.

Les accidents peuvent être rapides et précoces, et être provoqués par des accidents d'embolie cérébrale dus au morcellement des dépôts fibrineux formés au niveau d'une valvule malade.

Nous en avons étudié un cas avec M. Tollemer, chef de laboratoire de l'hôpital Trousseau. Cette observation devant être publiée en détail, je n'en donne ici qu'un résumé.

Obs. X. — *Rhumatisme articulaire. — Endocardite végétante. — Embolies cérébrales et périphériques multiples. — Mort. — Résumé.* (Sera publiée en détail ultérieurement. Hôpital Trousseau.)

Marguerite M., 11 ans, salle Blache, n° 8, 15 septembre 1899.

La malade se plaignait depuis 8 jours de douleurs dans les membres inférieurs, puis dans l'épaule droite et dans le pied gauche, lorsque dans la nuit du 14 au 15 elle cesse brusquement de parler sans paralysie et sans ictus. Au début, il y a eu de la fièvre, des vomissements, de la céphalée. On constate une aphasie motrice et sensorielle, avec intégrité du mouvement et de l'intelligence ; le 18, une légère paralysie faciale droite ; le 19 une monoplégie bronchiale droite progressive, en même temps que

le genou droit est devenu douloureux et s'est tuméfié. Hémiplégie droite à
peu près complète les jours suivants.

Le 21 escarre sacrée droite; la malade succombe le 28, après avoir
présenté un purpura terminal avec ecchymoses sous-cutanées et sous-
muqueuses.

L'autopsie montre *au cœur* une endocardite mitrale avec végétations
volumineuses; dans le *cerveau* des embolies multiples avec foyers de ramollissement multiples, très étendus, et probablement d'âges divers.

Mais c'est là un accident relativement rare. Ce qui l'est moins, c'est
1° une asystolie précoce, rebelle au traitement; 2° c'est la possibilité
de la mort subite ou rapide par syncope, dans le cours de cette
asystolie ou au contraire avec des symptômes d'asystolie peu accusés.
Dans le premier cas, au bout de quelques mois, quelquefois plus tôt,
les malades présentent le tableau de l'asystolie, avec une prédominance cependant à localiser leur asystolie dans le foie qui est toujours
gros, dur, douloureux; quand on percute chez ces malades le foie et
le cœur lui-même dilaté et hypertrophié, on limite à la région moyenne du corps une énorme zone de matité en forme de sablier oblique
de haut en bas et de gauche à droite, dont le renflement inférieur
remplit la partie supérieure et droite de l'abdomen, et correspond au
foie, et dont le renflement supérieur intra-thoracique correspond au
cœur.

Les œdèmes périphériques peuvent être peu accusés. La mort peut
survenir de 5 à 6 mois après le début du rhumatisme chez des enfants
antérieurement bien portants.

Obs. XI. — Rhumatisme en septembre 1899. — Endocardite et péricar-
dite. — Asystolie progressive.
Louise B., 9 ans. Venue à la consultation le 2 janvier 1900.
Douleurs articulaires au mois de septembre.
Depuis cette époque, palpitations, et dès le mois d'octobre, œdème des
jambes, de la face et probablement déjà ascite; oppression la nuit.
À l'entrée : anasarque, pâleur, oppression, pouls veineux cervical. —
Pouls petit (145 p.).
Cœur hypertrophié, pointe abaissée et déviée en dehors, matité trans-
versale augmentée. — Choc de la pointe étalé, ondulation manifeste de la
paroi. — rétraction systolique de la pointe.
Auscultation : Souffle prolongé et frémissement présystolique.
Foie. — Déborde de cinq travers de doigt les fausses côtes. — Ascite
assez considérable.
Poumons. — Congestion des deux poumons.
Par la suite, sous l'influence de la digitale, du calomel, du repos et du
régime lacté, il y eut une amélioration sensible, mais passagère. Pendant
ce temps on put constater, d'une façon très nette, une rétraction systo-

lique de la pointe dans le 7ᵉ espace, et, à plusieurs reprises, la malade eut des crachats hémoptoïques (apoplexie pulmonaire).

Vers le 50 janvier, des phénomènes d'insuffisance cardiaque réapparaissaient malgré le régime ; le foie se tuméfiait de nouveau, l'ascite réapparaissait. L'enfant ne s'est pas représentée à la consultation.

Obs. XII. — Le 25 août 1899, on me conduit chez moi un enfant de 7 ans, le jeune K., très bien développé, n'ayant jamais été malade jusqu'à un rhumatisme dont il a été atteint il y a deux mois et ayant duré six semaines. Depuis ce moment il est essoufflé, sa voix est faible, il est bouffi, très anémié, dyspeptique, avec des crises de toux après le repas et la marche.

A l'examen : *cœur* hypertrophié, frémissement présystolique, souffle systolique, pouls rapide 120, petit. *Foie* gros et douloureux.

Deux mois après, l'enfant succombait subitement dans une syncope (d'après les renseignements que j'ai pu avoir).

On peut voir également la marche rapide des accidents cardiaques dans l'observation que je relate plus loin, dans laquelle l'enfant Berthe L. succomba deux mois après le début du rhumatisme.

J'ai observé à la consultation de l'hôpital Bichat, en 1899, un enfant se présentant avec tous les caractères des deux observations précédentes.

A quoi tient la gravité de l'évolution des cardiopathies chez l'enfant ? Sans vouloir en discuter ici toutes les causes : aortite, myocardite, etc., je crois qu'il faut en attribuer une bonne part à *la péricardite*.

Dans la plupart des observations que nous avons relatées plus haut, on pourra relever un certain nombre de signes attribuables à la péricardite adhésive. Cette péricardite adhésive évolue parfois très vite et peut amener les accidents précoces d'asystolie que nous avons signalés. Dans une observation où la mort est survenue au bout de deux mois, nous avons pu constater à l'autopsie l'existence de cette péricardite qui avait été soupçonnée pendant la vie.

Obs. XIII. — Rhumatisme. — Endopéricardite. — Mort par syncope. — Autopsie. — Symphyse péricardique. (Obs. prise par M. Lefas.)

Berthe L., 8 ans et demi ; 28 août 1895. Salle de Chaumont, nᵒ 56. Enfants-Malades. Service de M. Descroizilles, que je remplaçais.

Le 14 juillet, attaque de rhumatisme articulaire frappant les membres inférieurs, ayant duré un mois. Depuis cette époque : palpitations, toux, œdème des membres inférieurs. Depuis deux jours : vomissements, tendances lipothymiques.

A l'entrée : enfant pâle, dyspnéique, cyanosée ; l'œdème des membres a disparu.

Cœur. — Ondulation de la paroi sterno-costale, surtout au niveau des 4ᵉ, 5ᵉ et 6ᵉ espaces gauches. Battements artériels très apparents dans les vaisseaux du cou. Cœur hypertrophié, la pointe bat à 9 centimètres de la ligne médio-sternale, et à 4 centimètres au-dessous du mamelon. Le choc est faible, *la pointe ne se déplace pas quand on fait changer de position la malade.* La percussion est douloureuse: matité verticale : 11 centimètres, transversale : 9 centimètres: elle déborde le bord droit du sternum.

A l'auscultation : souffle aux différents orifices du cœur avec un maximum net à la pointe se propageant vers l'aisselle. Bruit de frottement à la partie moyenne du cœur. Pouls faible, irrégulier, intermittent, 70.

Congestion des deux poumons, foie gros déborde les fausses côtes droites. Urines rares, troubles, 250, légèrement albumineuses.

Malgré le régime lacté et la digitale, le cœur ne se relève pas. Dès le 4 septembre : tendance au refroidissement périphérique et aux sueurs froides. Accélération du pouls depuis trois jours (de 120 à 140).

Le 7 septembre l'enfant succombe dans une syncope cardiaque après avoir vomi pendant deux jours.

A *l'autopsie* on trouve une symphyse du péricarde au niveau de la face antérieure du ventricule gauche sur une étendue de 5 centimètres en hauteur et de 2 centimètres en largeur. Adhérences fibreuses, peu vasculaires. Endocardite de la valvule mitrale.

Ces faits viennent à l'appui de ceux qui ont été publiés autrefois par Cadet de Gassicourt, et qu'il a résumés en disant que la péricardite est fréquente dans le rhumatisme chez l'enfant, et qu'elle amène dans un grand nombre de cas la terminaison fatale. (*Traité des maladies de l'enfance*, t. II.)

Les accidents peuvent être continus et progressifs, amenant la mort rapide dans les 2 ou 5 mois qui suivent le rhumatisme (Obs. II) (Cadet de Gassicourt a observé cette forme 6 fois sur 97 cas), ou bien être l'origine d'une asystolie plus tardive, mais non moins grave.

SUR UNE VARIÉTÉ D'ÉRYTHÈME INFECTIEUX CHEZ LES ENFANTS

par M. ESCHERICH,

de Graz.

Déjà, en 1890, j'ai eu l'occasion d'observer une éruption particulière que les médecins de Graz connaissent sous le nom de « rubéole localisée ». La maladie débute par le visage sous forme de plaques rougeâtres, confluentes, unies, et parfois atteint secondairement le dos, les extrémités, tandis que le tronc reste toujours indemne. La durée de cet exanthème est de huit à quinze jours, et pendant tout ce temps on n'observe aucun trouble morbide, aucun phénomène général. J'ai pu recevoir les enfants atteints de cette affection, dans mon service d'hôpital, sans voir aucun cas de contagion, et pendant tout le cours de la maladie, l'éruption a ressemblé à de l'érythème beaucoup plus qu'à de l'exanthème aigu. La différence très nette de cette sorte de rubéole avec la rougeole m'est apparue d'une façon indiscutable lors d'une épidémie de rougeole que nous avons eue à Graz l'an dernier. En effet, des enfants qui venaient d'avoir cet érythème gagnèrent, tout comme les autres, la rougeole.

Je propose de décrire cette affection particulière sous le nom « d'érythème infectieux ».

M. Escherich termine sa communication en présentant des dessins coloriés reproduisant l'éruption en question.

DISCUSSION.

M. Hutinel. — Je désire demander des renseignements à M. Escherich, au sujet de son intéressante communication. Je me suis beaucoup occupé des érythèmes infectieux depuis dix ans; je les ai rencontrés, au cours ou dans la convalescence de quelques maladies nettement caractérisées : fièvre typhoïde, diphtérie, rougeole compliquée de broncho-pneumonie, scarlatine avec infection maligne du naso-pharynx et des ganglions, entérocolites graves. Je les ai vus aussi dans des affections beaucoup plus bénignes : angines simples ou colites légères. Souvent il m'a semblé que ces érythèmes étaient sous la dépendance d'une infection streptococcique, démontrée par l'examen des muqueuses et quelquefois par celui du sang; mais, parfois, des infections staphylococciques nettement caractérisées, avec ostéomyélites, des infections pneumococciques, etc., ont déterminé des éruptions plus ou moins pareilles.

Quelques-uns de ces érythèmes s'accompagnent de symptômes généraux graves : vomissements verts, porracés, rétraction de l'abdomen, faciès grippé, albuminurie, et entraînent la mort dans un délai très court.

D'autres, au contraire, sont extrêmement légers, et cependant la localisation de l'éruption sur les coudes, sur les genoux, sur les fesses et la face, le tronc restant à peu près indemne, est toujours la même. Dans ces cas, j'ai presque toujours noté soit une angine, soit une colite, en un mot une infection locale à laquelle on pourrait attribuer l'apparition de l'érythème. J'ai pensé longtemps que l'infection streptococcique était la cause la plus habituelle de ces érythèmes. Cependant, dans une petite épidémie récente, M. Widal ne paraît pas avoir trouvé d'infection à streptocoques chez les typhiques qu'il observait. Je suis donc certain que des toxi-infections multiples peuvent causer les érythèmes. Je viens demander à M. Escherich si, dans les cas qu'il a étudiés, il a constaté dans la gorge ou dans l'intestin de ses malades les traces d'une inflammation qui aurait pu servir de porte d'entrée à une toxi-infection.

M. Chaumier (Tours). — J'ai observé une petite épidémie analogue à celle que décrit M. Escherich. Les enfants eurent pendant cinq ou six jours la face rouge, puis la guérison suivit sans que la cause de cet érythème ait pu être connue.

M. KOPLIK (New-York). — J'ai observé des cas d'érythème infectieux analogues à ceux décrits par M. le professeur Escherich. Je les ai toujours considérés comme une éruption toxi-infectieuse n'ayant pas de rapport avec les différentes formes d'érythèmes multiformes, avec la rubéole ou la rougeole. Ces cas ont été observés dans mon service d'hôpital. Ils ne présentaient ni fièvre, ni aucun autre symptôme général, ni localisation gastro-intestinale. Jamais je ne les ai vus apparaître épidémiquement.

M. WINSCOUROFF (Odessa). — Je demande à M. Escherich d'indiquer la marche habituelle de la maladie. Observe-t-on, par exemple, des périodes analogues à celles de toutes les maladies infectieuses? L'examen des urines a-t-il donné la réaction d'Ehrlich, constante dans la rougeole?

M. ESCHERICH. — Au sujet de l'érythème, je ne puis dire qu'une chose : c'est qu'il y avait absence de tous phénomènes généraux et que les enfants sont restés absolument bien portants. La maladie survient habituellement au printemps ou à l'automne, et se voit dans les familles ou à l'école. La cause en est inconnue.

LA PERLÈCHE ÉTUDE BACTÉRIOLOGIQUE

par M. le docteur Georges EYMERI.

Médecin-major de l'armée. Professeur suppléant à l'école de médecine de Limoges.

Depuis 1886, époque à laquelle M. J. Lemaistre[1] fit connaître le résultat de ses études sur la perlèche, la bactériologie de cette affection a fait l'objet de nombreuses recherches, sans qu'il soit possible jusqu'à présent d'attribuer à aucun microorganisme un rôle pathogène spécifique.

On sait que J. Lemaistre avait trouvé : A. *A l'examen direct*, dans l'épithélium des commissures labiales. 1° des diplococci et des sphérobactéries mobiles; 2° des streptocoques à chaînettes longues, enchevêtrées, intra ou extra-cellulaires.

B. *En cultures sur bouillon*, les mêmes microorganismes, avec prédominance des streptocoques agglomérés en longs chapelets et enchevêtrés, d'où le nom de plicatilis donné à ce streptocoque, que M. Lemaistre considéra comme l'agent spécifique de la perlèche.

Cette spécificité s'appuyait d'autre part sur la présence du streptococcus plicatilis dans les eaux qui alimentent les quartiers de la ville de Limoges où la perlèche est la plus fréquente.

1. La perlèche et le streptococcus plicatilis (*Journal de la Soc. méd. de la Haute-Vienne*, Limoges, 1886).

Les recherches entreprises par d'autres auteurs et, notamment par
M. Paul Raymond, sont moins exclusives en ce qui concerne l'unicité
de l'agent. C'est ainsi que M. P. Raymond, soulevant l'épiderme macéré, au niveau des fissures recueillit les produits épidermiques qu'il
ensemença sur gélose : il obtint des colonies de staphylococcus cereus
albus et plus rarement aureus. M. Raymond exprima dès lors l'opinion « que ces divers staphylocoques n'ont rien de spécifique, et jouent
dans la genèse de la perlèche le même rôle que dans l'impétigo qui
peut être produit par plusieurs microbes pyogènes ». Or, nous savons
aujourd'hui que l'impétigo est précisément le résultat d'un streptocoque spécial isolé et cultivé par Ch. Leroux (1892), et après lui par
Kurth (1895), Daum (1895), Franck Brocher (1896). Inoculé aux lapins
par Balzer et Griffon, ce streptocoque a déterminé des abcès, des
érysipèles de l'oreille et même des septicémies mortelles.

N'en est-il pas de même pour la perlèche? Et les staphylocoques
trouvés par M. P. Raymond ne représentent-ils que des microorganismes
surajoutés à un agent spécifique encore inconnu?

Les recherches ne permettent pas encore de résoudre ce problème
d'une façon décisive.

M. Tenneson[1], de même que M. Raymond, avait observé que la perlèche coïncide souvent avec d'autres lésions suppuratives de la face
ou du cuir chevelu (impétigo, ecthyma, furoncles). Ses recherches
l'amenèrent à penser que les organismes vulgaires, surtout les staphylocoques, en étaient la cause efficiente, et que rien n'autorisait à les
rattacher à un parasite spécial. Pour M. Tenneson, la perlèche serait
donc simplement un impétigo de la commissure auquel succède une
ulcération linéaire.

MM. Malherbe et Guibert[2], dans l'unique cas de perlèche étudié
par eux, ne retrouvèrent ni le streptococcus plicatilis de J. Lemaistre,
ni le staphylocoque aureus de P. Raymond. Ils ne trouvèrent que le
staphylocoque albus.

A son tour, M. René Planche[3] a procédé, sous la direction de M. P.
Raymond, à de nouvelles recherches, en s'entourant de toutes les précautions nécessaires pour éviter les microorganismes étrangers à la
perlèche. Il a trouvé constamment le staphylococcus aureus; et,
s'appuyant sur la coïncidence fréquente de la perlèche avec l'impétigo et la stomatite diphtéroïde, il fait de ces diverses affections des
manifestations variées d'une même infection polymicrobienne : opinion

1. TENNESSON. — Des stomatites in *Journal des Praticiens*, 15 décembre 1894.
2. Voir Thèse de René Planche, La perlèche (Paris, Jouve, 1897).
3. Voir Thèse de René Planche.

confirmée par les recherches de M. Leloir qui a vu des enfants atteints de perlèche communiquer soit l'impétigo, soit la perlèche elle-même, à des enfants de la même école, et qui considère ces affections comme des pyodermites sans caractère spécifique, survenant à la suite d'inoculation d'origine variable.

Telle est, sommairement résumée, l'histoire bactériologique de la perlèche. Malgré la concordance des résultats précités qui tendent à faire de cette affection une manifestation banale de la staphylococcie, il nous a semblé difficile, à M. J. Lemaistre et à moi, de les admettre sans contrôle. J'ai l'honneur de présenter aujourd'hui les résultats de recherches bactériologiques qui portent sur 58 nouveaux cas de perlèche, observés sur des enfants des écoles de la ville de Limoges.

Les ensemencements ont été faits sur les milieux ordinaires : bouillon-peptone, sérum humain, gélose, gélatine, lait, après asepsie rigoureuse de la surface cutanée immédiatement contiguë aux fissures des commissures labiales. Je portais le fil de platine, préalablement flambé dans la profondeur de ces fissures ou sous les croûtelles épidermiques.

Ces 50 examens m'ont donné les résultats suivants : le *staphylococcus aureus* a été rencontré 18 fois, l'albus 50 fois. Deux fois, les cultures ont montré un bacille court mobile, se décolorant par le Gram ; une fois, le leptothrix buccalis. En milieu anaérobie, les cultures sont toujours restées stériles.

Dans 4 cas d'eczéma concomitant de la face, du nez et des lèvres, les microorganismes (staphylococcus aureus et albus) étaient, soit à l'examen direct, soit en cultures, les mêmes qu'au niveau des lésions fissuraires de la perlèche. Fallait-il conclure de cette enquête que la perlèche est une affection de même ordre que les dermatoses banales des lèvres et de la face? Nous ne l'avons pas pensé. Nous avons essayé de chercher la solution du problème dans l'inoculation aux animaux des cultures pures de staphocoques fissuraires de la perlèche, d'autre part de l'eczéma concomitant : affections évoluant ensemble chez le même sujet. Six lapins furent donc inoculés avec des staphylocoques blancs de la perlèche : 2 par la voie intra-veineuse, 2 par injection sous-péritonéale; 6 autres lapins reçurent des inoculations semblables avec le staphylocoque albus provenant de lésions eczémateuses.

Les premiers lapins présentèrent les lésions suivantes :

1° Lapins inoculés avec 50 cc. de staphylococcus albus en culture pure dans bouillon, par voie sous-cutanée. Après 18 heures, abcès localisé au point d'inoculation; 2° lapins inoculés par la voie intra-veineuse : mort par septicémie au bout de 56 heures ; 5° lapins inoculés dans le péritoine : mort au bout de 50 heures par péritonite purulente généralisée.

Pour la seconde série de lapins en expérience, les accidents ont évolué avec moins de rapidité.

1° Lapins inoculés par la voie sous-cutanée : abcès sous-cutané localisé au point d'inoculations; 2° lapins inoculés par la voie intraveineuse : infection purulente avec abcès métastatiques et mort au bout de 8 jours; 5° lapins inoculés par la voie intra-péritonéale : suivie dans un cas. Dans l'autre, mort au bout de 8 jours, avec des symptômes de péritonite purulente.

Les expériences sur le cobaye m'ont donné sensiblement les mêmes résultats.

Il semble donc que le staphylocoque albus de la perlèche soit réellement doué d'une virulence supérieure à celle du même microorganisme récolté sous les croûtelles de l'eczéma concomitant de même âge et évoluant chez le même sujet.

Les conditions d'exaltation de cette virulence nous paraissent résider dans le siège même de la lésion : cutanéo-muqueuse dans un cas, exclusivement cutanée dans l'autre. La végétabilité du microorganisme est sensiblement différente dans l'un et l'autre cas. Rien de surprenant dès lors que, par suite de la malpropreté infantile, de l'humidité constante des commissures, etc., le même agent produise, dans un cas, des dermatoses banales, eczémateuses ou autres, dans l'autre, des lésions fissuraires aiguës, subaiguës ou chroniques, qui constituent la perlèche et ne se différencient des autres dermatoses que par leur siège, cause lui-même de l'exaltation de végétabilité et de virulence des germes.

DE LA PERLECHE

par **M.** le docteur Justin **LEMAISTRE**,

de Limoges.

Je tiens à dire quelques mots à propos de la communication que vient de faire mon excellent ami le docteur Eymeri, et à indiquer quelques faits nouveaux que j'ai observés à propos de la perlèche. — La contagiosité de cette maladie ne fait de doute pour personne, mais je crois que c'est surtout, et peut-être spécialement par l'intermédiaire des vases à boire, que se produit cette inoculation.

Voici deux faits assez curieux que j'ai observés depuis quelques années et qui semblent le prouver :

1° Dans une famille composée de huit personnes, adultes et enfants, sept avaient la perlèche. Toutes cependant buvaient l'eau du même seau, puisée avec le même godet.

Je cherchai la cause de cette immunité chez cette huitième personne — une femme de 24 ans — et j'en eus bien vite l'explication. Elle était gauchère : elle prenait donc, pour boire, le godet de la main gauche, et appliquait ses lèvres sur la partie de la circonférence de ce godet qui n'était jamais en contact avec la bouche des sept autres buveurs, tous droitiers.

C'était en somme comme si elle avait bu dans un autre vase. J'engageai cette femme à boire pendant quelque temps à l'aide de la main droite, c'est-à-dire à mettre ses lèvres en contact avec le bord du godet contaminé par les autres membres de la famille.

J'ai su, quelques jours après, qu'elle aussi était atteinte de la perlèche.

2° J'ai vu une nourrice — ne donnant pour toute nourriture que le sein à son enfant — avoir la perlèche, et son fils âgé de 6 mois, en être absolument indemne. Elle était cependant très bonne mère, aimait son enfant et ne se privait pas de l'embrasser.

Ces deux faits semblent bien prouver que c'est surtout par l'application de l'objet contaminé aux commissures des lèvres que se fait la contagion et que l'action de boire dans un vase favorise complètement ces conditions.

Le docteur Martinez, dans les écoles publiques de Buenos-Ayres, a vu disparaître la perlèche depuis que chaque enfant a un vase particulier pour son service.

Je ne nie pas les autres moyens de transmission de la perlèche qui ont été indiqués, mais je crois qu'ils sont rares.

Je me suis aussi occupé d'un autre point de la question, et cela depuis les travaux de MM. Raymond, Comby, Leloir, Planche, sur cette maladie.

M. Leloir a vu des enfants atteints de perlèche communiquer l'impétigo à des enfants de la même école, et la perlèche succéder à de l'impétigo, à du coryza, à des ophtalmies.

Je n'ai jamais observé pour ma part de faits semblables.

Dans les campagnes, dans les écoles, les enfants d'une bonne santé générale n'ont que la perlèche et ils la gardent pendant des mois et même des années sans qu'ils aient sur la figure le moindre bouton d'impétigo, la moindre croûte. Jamais ils n'ont communiqué à d'autres enfants autre chose que la perlèche.

Dans certains milieux et notamment dans les hôpitaux, il peut en être autrement. Là les enfants sont malades, ils entrent pour de l'impétigo ou autres affections suppurantes de la face ; rien ne les empêche d'avoir en outre la perlèche. Pour moi, ces deux affections évoluent côte à côte.

Dans mon service des enfants à l'hôpital de Limoges, où je fais une très grande attention aux cas de perlèche, j'affirme que jamais je n'ai observé un enfant atteint d'impétigo, donner la perlèche à un autre enfant, et cependant l'impétigo est très fréquent dans ce service. J'ai toujours vu la perlèche venir de la perlèche, jamais de l'impétigo, et jamais je n'ai vu l'impétigo produire la perlèche. M. le docteur Eymeri vient de faire des études très complètes sur la bactériologie de cette affection. Les résultats auxquels il est arrivé sont différents de ceux que j'avais obtenus en 1886 et concordent avec ceux indiqués par MM. Raymond, Leloir, Planche. Ils semblent donner tort à l'idée de spécificité de cette affection, que j'avais émise.

J'avoue que je ne puis me ranger à leur opinion. Les études que mes confrères ont faites semblent très complètes, mais celles que j'ai publiées en 1886, et les faits cliniques que j'ai indiqués plus haut et aussi à cette époque, m'empêchent d'accepter cette idée. Je ne puis croire que ce soient les microbes vulgaires de la bouche et de toutes les croûtes et suppurations de la face qui produisent la perlèche. On fait jouer, il me semble, à tous les staphylocoques, un rôle trop important. On les trouve partout, il est vrai, mais ils ne me paraissent pas être la cause du mal. Voyez d'ailleurs ce qui s'est passé pour l'impétigo. On a accusé pendant longtemps les staphylocoques d'être les coupables, actuellement il paraît prouvé que c'est un streptocoque qu'on a pu cultiver qui est l'agent de cette maladie. Je crois, pour ma part, que la question de bactériologie n'est pas encore élucidée. Est-ce le streptococcus plicatilis que j'ai trouvé et décrit, est-ce un autre agent pathogène qui est la cause du mal ? Je n'ose rien affirmer mais, je le répète, je ne puis croire à cette puissance des staphylocoques.

La perlèche, pour moi, est une maladie bien définie, ne ressemblant en rien à l'impétigo par exemple, et évoluant toujours en dehors de lui. L'impétigo d'ailleurs est long à guérir, la perlèche disparaît très vite dès qu'elle est soignée. — Au point de vue de la symptomatologie et des conséquences de la perlèche, tout a été dit dans les diverses publications parues sur ce sujet. J'ai cependant observé deux nouveaux faits intéressants.

1° J'ai vu, il y a quelques jours, dans une école, un enfant de 12 ans ayant des végétations, de véritables crêtes de coq, aux deux commissures des lèvres. Cet enfant a la perlèche depuis très longtemps. Je dois dire que c'est la seule fois où j'ai observé ce cas.

2° Un autre fait m'a frappé, c'est le mauvais état des dents, les caries dentaires nombreuses observées chez les enfants ayant la perlèche, caries atteignant de préférence les dents de la première dentition. Je n'ai pas poussé loin cette étude, et surtout je n'ai pas fait de recherches comparatives sur la dentition des enfants atteints de perlèche et sur celle des enfants indemnes, mais il m'a semblé que dans le premier cas, la dentition est toujours mauvaise.

CONTRIBUTION AUX SUPPURATIONS DE LA PLÈVRE CHEZ L'ENFANT

par MM. les docteurs BEZY et BAUBY,

de la Faculté de médecine de Toulouse.

Il a été publié, dans ces derniers temps, de très nombreux travaux sur les accidents pleuraux chez l'enfant. Presque tous tendent surtout à démontrer les difficultés du diagnostic, donnant lieu souvent à des erreurs, et l'utilité du traitement chirurgical.

Nous n'avons aucunement l'intention de reprendre cette grosse question, renvoyant ceux qui voudraient de plus amples détails au chapitre « Pleurésie » écrit par M. Netter dans le quatrième volume du *Traité des maladies de l'enfance*, à une revue générale sur la pleurésie interlobaire chez l'enfant, parue dans les *Archives de médecine des enfants* en mars 1900, à un article sur la même question traitée au point de vue surtout thérapeutique, publiée dans le même journal, en décembre 1899, par M. Baltus, à un travail sur 7 cas d'empyème de nécessité chez l'enfant, publiée par MM. Audion et Bourgeois dans la *Revue des maladies de l'enfance* en septembre 1899, enfin à toute une série d'articles parus dans les journaux de médecine générale et de maladies de l'enfance publiés depuis peu de temps. Cette simple contribution n'a d'autre but que d'apporter trois observations de notre pratique personnelle, et de les faire suivre de quelques remarques.

OBS. I. — Pleurésie gauche à pneumocoque: deux ponctions. Empyème de nécessité. Ouverture. Drainage. Guérison.

Henri F... est âgé de quatre ans quand nous le voyons en avril 1897. Nous avons à l'examiner parce qu'il est porteur d'un impétigo, en même temps que deux autres enfants de sa famille, et qu'il présente, au cours de cette affection, un œdème généralisé. Les urines sont albumineuses. L'enfant est mis au régime lacté pendant un mois ; le 20 mai, il allait très bien, quoique ayant eu pendant ce temps une pneumonie.

Le 28 mai, nous sommes appelé d'urgence auprès de l'enfant parce qu'il présente une dyspnée intense. L'examen fait immédiatement constater un œdème assez marqué de la paroi thoracique, et très intense du bas gauche, et tous les signes d'un vaste épanchement de la plèvre gauche avec refoulement de la pointe du cœur. M. le professeur Caubet, qui veut bien examiner le malade avec nous, pratique une ponction aspiratrice d'urgence, et retire environ 2 litres de pus que ses caractères physiques et l'examen bactériologique, pratiqué par M. Daunic, chef des travaux d'anatomie pathologique, révèlent être du pus à pneumocoque.

Huit jours après, empyème de nécessité ; nouvelle ponction aspiratrice qui donne un litre de pus analogue à celui de la première, mais la collection sous-cutanée ne se vide pas.

On procède alors le lendemain à l'ouverture de la collection qui est lavée et drainée. L'orifice est fermé au bout de sept ou huit jours. Depuis lors, l'enfant, qui a aujourd'hui 7 ans, se porte très bien.

Nous n'insisterons pas sur l'albuminurie impétigineuse qui a été signalée, ni sur les dangers possibles de l'impétigo, affection que les parents sont toujours portés à considérer comme une évacuation aussi salutaire que respectable. Nous insisterons seulement sur les points qui confirment les faits déjà énoncés : marche latente et utilité du traitement chirurgical.

OBS. II. — Pleurésie purulente post-typhoïdique (?) Pleurotomie. Guérison.

Joseph N..., 9 ans, habitant la campagne. Père et mère bien portants. Ils n'ont eu que cet enfant, qui a été mal nourri et n'a jamais été solide. Il est petit, maigre, nerveux, intelligent. Il n'a eu aucune maladie grave.

Le 8 août 1898, il va boire dans une rigole d'arrosage de l'eau croupissante et trouble qui s'échappe au moment où l'on ouvre la vanne. Il trouve cette eau mauvaise. Le soir même, à 9 heures, il s'éveille, se plaint de coliques et de douleurs de tête ; fièvre, agitation. Il aurait eu, à ce moment, des vomissements et de la diarrhée, et serait resté sérieusement malade pendant environ quinze jours, avec les allures d'une fièvre typhoïde (épistaxis, taches rosées, prostration, délire, convulsions).

Il y a eu aussi de la toux, mais on ne peut nous renseigner sur les résultats de l'examen stéthoscopique pratiqué à ce moment.

Dans les premiers jours de septembre, l'enfant, encore faible, mais convalescent et apyrétique, se plaint de nouveau de courbature, céphalalgie ; puis surviennent du frisson, de la fièvre, et un point de côté. Le Dr Jourda (de Muret), qui voit l'enfant à ce moment, assiste au développement rapide d'une pleuro-pneumonie. Bientôt signes d'un épanchement qui ne tarde pas à remplir la cavité gauche de la plèvre, refoulant le cœur à droite, et provoquant une violente dyspnée.

Le 28 septembre, l'enfant est amaigri, présente des sueurs, des yeux brillants, le faciès septicémique : la langue est un peu sèche, le pouls petit et fréquent, la peau chaude (39°,4), la respiration rapide. Le côté droit du thorax se dilate beaucoup plus largement que le gauche. Pas de déformation, thoracique ou vertébrale. Toux fréquente et pénible. Vibrations thoraciques à peu près nulles à gauche, très nettes à droite. Submatité à peu près uniforme dans tout le côté gauche, à la région postéro-latérale. Matité et résistance très marquées dans la pointe de l'omoplate. Le côlon est légèrement refoulé à droite.

Désinfection soigneuse de la peau; ponction aspiratrice à la seringue de Roux en pleine région suspecte : pas de pus, non plus à une seconde ponction. La troisième ayant amené du pus, la seringue est retirée et la canule laissée en place pour guider le bistouri. (La région avait été anesthésiée à la cocaïne). Dans le septième espace intercostal, au-dessous de la pointe de l'omoplate, est pratiquée une ouverture de 5 centimètres environ, dont le milieu répond au siège de l'aiguille enfoncée. Il s'écoule environ 120 centimètres de pus jaune crémeux, bien lié, d'assez mauvaise odeur. Il est recueilli dans un flacon lavé à l'alcool et à l'eau bouillie.

Le petit doigt pénètre assez difficilement dans l'espace intercostal et permet de reconnaître que la cavité est limitée par des parois lisses et régulières : elle paraît étalée en profondeur et s'engage dans l'espace interlobaire. Cette cavité est lavée à l'eau bouillie, puis au sublimé à 0.50 c. p. 100, puis de nouveau à l'eau bouillie. Drainage. Pansement.

L'examen bactériologique du pus, fait par le Dr Rispal, chef du laboratoire des cliniques, montre une association de streptocoques et de coli-bacilles.

La température baisse dès le lendemain (de 39° à 38°), l'état général s'améliore : mais peu après, l'état reste stationnaire à mi-chemin de la guérison.

Le 15 octobre, l'amélioration est réelle, mais légère : rien cependant ne révèle la présence du pus dans la cavité qui est du reste à peu près fermée. Un peu de submatité persistante fait penser à un foyer enkysté et presque impossible à atteindre.

Trois jours après, l'état s'aggrave, et dans un effort de toux, l'enfant rend environ un demi-verre de pus, à ce que l'on nous dit.

Dès lors l'amélioration se complète, et progresse très rapidement et en novembre l'enfant va très bien.

Cette observation est intéressante d'abord au point de vue pathogénique : le début de l'affection est marqué par un état typhoïdique, lequel semble avoir brusquement débuté après l'ingestion d'une eau malsaine. Pendant que les rigoles sont à sec, le bétail va y paître et y dépose ses excréments. N'y a-t-il pas une relation entre le fait et la présence du coli-bacille dans le pus de la plèvre ?

En second lieu, la présence du deuxième abcès aurait pu faire croire un moment à l'inutilité du traitement chirurgical et induire en erreur la famille et le praticien.

Enfin, cet enfant nous a présenté ce que M. Baltus a si bien appelé la vomique libératrice, événement des plus heureux qui n'est pas absolument rare, et dont on va voir un cas encore plus important dans l'observation suivante.

OBS. III. — *Pleurésie putride droite. Diagnostic longtemps douteux. Vomique. Longue convalescence. Guérison.*

Georges C..., 50 mois. Cet enfant est le fils d'un de nos confrères et amis que nous remercions d'avoir bien voulu prendre cette observation et nous autoriser à la publier. On va voir de quelle importance ont été les soins paternels dans la guérison de cette maladie aussi longue qu'insidieuse.

Du côté paternel, tendance à acquérir la fièvre typhoïde et à des crises de gastro-entérite; du côté maternel, plusieurs cas de coliques hépatiques.

Enfant nourri au sein par une nourrice mercenaire, constipée. Ictère pendant le premier mois. Tendance à la constipation quelquefois avec teinte subictérique des lèvres. Après le sevrage, la constipation s'accentue; on a toujours lutté contre elle.

L'été dernier, l'enfant étant en pleine campagne, avait été déconstipé par les raisins et se portait très bien en septembre, mais il trompait souvent la surveillance, mangeait des fruits souvent gâtés, et buvait dans des rigoles d'arrosage, de l'eau chargée de matières organiques.

C'est en octobre 1899, où il est souvent surpris dans ces conditions, qu'il est atteint d'une diarrhée glaireuse à 8 et 10 selles par jour, et que l'on peut admettre le début de la maladie. La diarrhée est traitée par l'antisepsie intestinale, s'arrête pendant huit jours, et voici alors ce qui se produit chaque jour pendant vingt jours du 7 au 30 octobre : matinée bonne, apyrétique. A midi légère poussée fébrile (38°); l'enfant cesse ses jeux et réclame son lit; de 3 à 5 heures 39°, puis crises profuses de sueurs; à 7 heures la gaieté revient, la fièvre cesse, l'enfant demande à se lever. La langue reste blanche tout le temps, la constipation est opiniâtre. Un peu de toux au début, quelques râles disséminés, mais éphémères. Régime lacté, œufs, entéroclyse. Quinine sans aucun résultat, antipyrine, avec une réussite relative.

Au bout de trois semaines la fièvre cesse; l'enfant a beaucoup maigri. La constipation et l'état de la langue persistent, malgré les modifications du régime alimentaire, le ventre est ballonné. Chaque quatre ou cinq jours, poussée subfébrile (38°,5).

En décembre, à la suite d'une promenade par un temps froid, l'enfant tombe et a presque une syncope qui disparaît par la position allongée. Un peu de fièvre dans la nuit. L'intestin ayant toujours appelé l'attention, on agit toujours de ce côté-là, tout en se demandant s'il ne s'agit pas d'une infection tuberculeuse latente. Les jours suivants, mêmes phénomènes avec fièvre.

Le 6 décembre, poussée de vésicules plates dans la bouche. Certaines forment, par leur réunion, un amas d'aspect pseudo-membraneux qui en impose pour une fausse membrane, et on injecte, en prévision, 10 centimètres cubes de sérum Roux. Le lendemain, la culture donne du streptocoque. Ces vésicules persistent deux mois, et sont constamment lavées avec des solutions antiseptiques.

Jusqu'au 12 décembre, fièvre (de 58°,5 à 59°,6), langue sale, constipation, toux sans aucun signe stéthoscopique, amygdales rouges, insomnie, congestion et pâleur successive de la face, inégalité pupillaire. On se demande si on ne va pas se trouver en présence d'une fièvre typhoïde ou d'une méningite : l'hypothèse d'une tuberculose est aussi envisagée. Pas de signe de Kernig. Le séro-diagnostic est négatif. On fait de l'enveloppement au drap mouillé.

Le 15 décembre apparaît une toux quinteuse quelquefois suivie de vomissements. Deux ou trois jours après, l'haleine devient fétide.

Le 17 décembre, apparaissent des signes importants : matité au sommet du poumon droit, et souffle intense de la même région. Vibrations thoraciques diminuées en ce point. En rapprochant ces faits de la toux quinteuse, de la fétidité de l'haleine, nous pensons à un abcès de la plèvre, comprimant le sommet du poumon droit.

Dès le lendemain matin nous nous préparons à faire une ponction exploratrice. Il est convenu que si elle permet de trouver la collection, on interviendra immédiatement, malgré l'affaissement du malade. Mais au moment où la ponction allait être pratiquée, l'enfant est pris d'une crise de suffocation, et rend un gros verre à bordeaux d'un liquide purulent, d'odeur infecte, rappelant celle qu'avait l'haleine les jours précédents. Cette vomique vient, malheureusement un peu trop tôt, confirmer notre diagnostic.

L'examen bactériologique du pus, pratiqué par M. le professeur agrégé Rispal, donne du streptocoque, du staphylocoque, du coli-bacille, et surtout des espèces très allongées que l'on rencontre ordinairement dans les pleurésies putrides.

Après les vomiques, les phénomènes stéthoscopiques disparaissent, et il devient impossible d'aller à la recherche du foyer. On continue l'antisepsie intestinale, et on désinfecte les voies respiratoires, soit avec des fumigations de créosote, soit en injectant par la trachée avec la seringue de Bayeux de l'huile avec de l'eucalyptus. La créosote est aussi donnée en lavement, à la dose de 50 à 50 gouttes, et amène deux fois des accidents d'intoxication.

Du 18 décembre 1899 au 5 janvier 1900, cet état persiste en s'aggravant. La toux augmente et donne quelquefois lieu à de petites vomiques. Le poumon droit fait entendre à l'auscultation de gros râles humides un peu partout. Œdème généralisé; pas d'albumine.

Du 5 au 7 janvier, cet état semble s'améliorer un peu : mais du 7 au 16, la température s'élève de nouveau. A ce moment, il y avait une épidémie de grippe dans la famille. Injections sous-cutanées de chlorhydrate de quinine (0,20 centigr. pour 1-2 cc. d'eau). Cette médication ne donne pas de résultat, et la fièvre semble surtout céder aux lavements créosotés.

Le 17, aggravation : oppression, cyanose, gargouillements dans la trachée, pouls presque incomptable. Enveloppement à la moutarde et à la térébenthine. Amélioration. Le soir, fièvre (59°,5). Rémission après enveloppement du thorax. A 7 heures du soir, nouvelle crise très grave; l'en-

fant semble près de mourir. Injection de caféine, enveloppement térében-
thiné. Amélioration.

Du 19 janvier au 4 février, aggravation, anurie, la sonde fait sortir de
la vessie un peu d'urine albumineuse. Lavements et bains froids. L'albuminurie disparaît, mais il y a de l'anasarque. Faiblesse extrême, injections d'eau salée caféinée pendant huit jours. Vers le 4 février, amélioration qui dure jusqu'au 19 malgré un amaigrissement considérable et une
grande faiblesse.

Pendant toute sa maladie, l'enfant a été autant que possible alimenté
(lait, œufs, etc.).

Le 19 février l'enfant est conduit à la campagne. Le voyage, qui dure
deux heures en voiture, est parfaitement supporté. Le temps étant très
beau, l'enfant est sorti tous les jours. Des lavements d'huile créosotée
sont donnés.

Au bout de quinze jours l'enfant engraisse légèrement. Cet état va toujours en s'améliorant, et à l'heure actuelle (juillet 1900) il est en parfaite
santé. Il reste seulement un peu de matité et d'obscurité respiratoire au
sommet droit.

Cette observation présente plusieurs points intéressants : 1º Son
début qui, comme dans le cas précédent, est marqué par des accidents
intestinaux, dus à l'ingestion d'eau malsaine. Y a-t-il relation de cause
à effet ; 2º cette éruption de vésicules buccales, dues sans doute au
pus qui sortait peu à peu des bronches et inoculait la muqueuse ; 3º les
énormes difficultés du diagnostic, les symptômes s'étant presque tout
le temps manifestés sur l'appareil digestif et n'ayant pas appelé l'attention vers les voies respiratoires qui étaient cependant soigneusement
explorées chaque jour ; 4º l'apparition d'un souffle de compression qui
finit par mettre le diagnostic sur sa véritable voie et fait espérer une
intervention utile ; 5º l'apparition opportune de la vomique, à l'instant
même où cette intervention allait être pratique et la rendant impossible pour le moment ; 6º la tolérance de l'enfant pour cet état et la
guérison après une situation des plus graves. Cette guérison est due
en grande partie aux soins du père de l'enfant qui, comme nous l'avons
dit, est un de nos confrères ; 7º la fétidité de l'haleine coïncidant avec
l'éruption buccale, et qui avait fait plutôt penser à une affection de la
bouche, erreur facile, sur laquelle nous insistons pour l'éviter à
d'autres. Imbu de cette idée, nous avons failli commettre naguère une
erreur en sens inverse, en présence d'une angine à bacille de Vincent,
l'odeur de la bouche étant, comme chacun sait, infectée dans ces
cas-là ; 8º l'espoir déçu de voir fermer la fistule, ce qui aurait de nouveau enfermé l'abcès, et aurait permis au chirurgien d'intervenir avec
plus de facilité.

Comme nous l'avons dit en commençant, nous n'avons d'autre but que d'apporter trois faits intéressants, et nous ne reviendrons pas sur les difficultés du diagnostic, ni sur les avantages du traitement chirurgical, ni sur la possibilité de la vomique libératrice. Nos observations viennent simplement corroborer ces notions déjà indiquées par d'autres, et ajouter trois faits cliniques qui nous ont paru intéressants à l'histoire, très étudiée de nos jours, des suppurations de la plèvre et des pleurésies putrides chez l'enfant.

DISCUSSION

M. Vargaz (Barcelone) demande à M. Bézy, à propos de la pleurésie purulente, s'il est partisan ou non de l'irrigation pleurale. Au Congrès de Bordeaux (1895), M. Vargaz a fait une communication tendant à montrer l'inutilité des irrigations pleurales. Depuis, il a opéré 52 cas de pleurésie purulente qui l'ont confirmé dans cette manière de voir.

A propos du diagnostic de ces épanchements, M. Vargaz croit qu'il y a, en effet, des cas obscurs, de véritables épanchements latents. Cependant, dans la majorité des cas, on peut arriver au diagnostic, soit par la percussion, par la percussion plus que par l'auscultation, soit par la ponction exploratrice.

M. Geffrier dit qu'il ne faut pas d'une manière générale presser l'intervention chirurgicale. Il recommande le procédé de Feréol, qui consiste à renverser la tête du malade de façon à provoquer et à faciliter les vomiques.

M. Bézy dit que ce procédé peut, en effet, rendre des services, mais qu'il est souvent difficile à employer.

Quant à ce qui est du diagnostic des pleurésies purulentes, il est bien certain qu'on y arrive le plus souvent; mais c'est justement à cause de l'absence de symptômes et de la difficulté du diagnostic qu'il a rapporté les cas en question. Reste le point de la meilleure technique chirurgicale ; ceci est affaire du chirurgien, et nous n'avons guère lieu ici de nous en préoccuper.

CURE DE QUINQUAUD (EMPLATRE AU CALOMEL A DEMEURE)
DANS LA SYPHILIS DE L'ENFANT

par M. H. GILLET

Parmi les procédés divers qui servent à appliquer le traitement mercuriel chez l'enfant, il en est un dont l'emploi n'a pas acquis la notoriété qu'il mériterait, c'est celui qui consiste en applications externes de préparations emplastiques au calomel.

Cette application purement externe d'un emplâtre à base mercurielle, principalement au calomel, à l'exclusion de tout autre traitement, en particulier de tout traitement interne ou autre, peut suffire à elle seule à la cure de la syphilis.

Dans un travail scientifique très documenté et très étudié, mon regretté maître, Ch. Quinquaud [1], a démontré, jusqu'à l'évidence, la réalité et le bien fondé des effets d'une telle thérapeutique.

Il ne s'agit nullement ici de l'emplâtre au calomel utilisé comme agent local, destiné à agir in situ sur telle ou telle manifestation cutanée, mais de l'emplâtre au calomel appliqué à demeure faisant seul tous les frais du traitement, comme peuvent le faire les frictions d'onguent mercuriel.

Le principe d'une telle méthode n'est pas nouveau absolument, il n'est que renouvelé.

Déjà, il y a 200 ans environ Martinus Rolandus préparait une espèce d'emplâtre mercuriel, appelé de son nom Cingulum Rolandi, qu'il faisait porter, cousu dans une gaine de toile, aux syphilitiques qu'il soignait.

C'est encore sur le même principe qu'est basé l'emploi de la flanelle mercurielle de Merget.

Il y a quelques années, M. Balzer a de même essayé des sachets remplis de mercure éteint dans la chaux (Hydrargyrum cum creta): M. Jullien a fait usage de la traumaticine mercurielle en badigeonnage plus ou moins étendus comme moyen de traitement spécifique.

Des sachets préparés avec l'onguent mercuriel double font partie de la pratique de M. le Professeur Welander (de Stockholm).

Dans ces différents procédés l'absorption du médicament mercuriel a lieu et par la peau, surtout pour les emplâtres par transformation insensible et continue, et aussi, en partie et dans certaines conditions, par les poumons pour les autres préparations par suite de la volatilisation partielle du produit.

Ce dernier point ne semble pas niable. M. Welander a cité le cas d'une femme dont les urines contenaient du mercure par le seul fait de vivre près de son mari qui portait des sachets à l'onguent mercuriel.

Dans son mémoire, Ch. Quinquaud fait voir l'efficacité réelle de l'emplâtre à base de calomel en application externe dans le traitement de la syphilis de l'adulte. La clinique par les résultats curatifs, la chimie par la recherche du mercure dans l'urine, prouvent l'action du médicament employé.

1. Ch. Quinquaud, Société française de dermatologie et de syphiligraphie Annales de dermatologie et de syphiligraphie, 11 avril 1890.

Ce mode de traitement, qu'on peut à juste raison, en vénération d'un grand travailleur, appeler la cure de Quinquaud convient parfaitement chez l'enfant, comme une expérience, vieille aujourd'hui de près de dix ans, nous l'a montré.

Mais dans la mise en œuvre du procédé, il y a quelques remarques importantes à faire au sujet des détails que comportent son adaptation au traitement de la syphilis de l'enfant.

L'emplâtre primitivement employé par Quinquaud se composait de :

Emplâtre diachylon des hôpitaux.	5000
Calomel à la vapeur.	1000
Huile de ricin.	500

Étendre sur des bandes de toile. Chaque décimètre carré de l'emplâtre obtenu doit contenir environ 1 gr. 20 de calomel.

Cet emplâtre s'applique aussi bien à l'enfant qu'à l'adulte, de même que les formules similaires avec l'emplâtre simple, sans litharge, l'emplâtre savonneux, même l'emplâtre caoutchouté, etc.

C'est surtout au point de vue du dosage que la question prend de l'importance.

Tandis que chez l'adulte on se contente, ou du moins Quinquaud semblait se contenter pour obtenir le résultat thérapeutique désiré, d'appliquer des *morceaux d'emplâtre* de 10 centimètres sur 12 chez l'homme, de 8 centimètres sur 10 chez la femme, il faut chez l'enfant des *surfaces non proportionnellement, mais absolument plus étendues que chez l'adulte*, soit 10 centimètres sur 15, 15 centimètres sur 20 et même 50, et dès les premiers mois, selon l'étendue des lésions, c'est-à-dire une bonne demi-ceinture.

Tous les 8 jours, sur la peau bien propre, on applique l'emplâtre, une fois en arrière, une fois en avant, ou bien alternativement sur un des côtés, sur la région hépatique, sur la région splénique et ainsi de suite, tant que doit durer le traitement. On profite du jour où l'on enlève l'emplâtre pour donner un grand bain à l'enfant.

Du reste l'emplâtre n'empêche pas de donner un bain rapide plus souvent.

Lorsqu'on retire l'emplâtre, au bout de la semaine, on trouve l'épiderme légèrement macéré, mais sans trace d'inflammation ni sous l'emplâtre, ni autour du point d'application.

Il est absolument rare, qu'il faille cesser le traitement par suite d'une irritation trop vive de la peau par susceptibilité individuelle.

Du reste, puisqu'on peut changer la région d'application chaque fois qu'on met un nouvel emplâtre, on peut ainsi donner à la peau le temps de revenir à son état normal.

D'après mon expérience personnelle, chez l'enfant le revêtement cutané supporte assez bien l'emplâtre laissé à demeure.

Une fois, une seule fois, sur nombre d'applications, chez un nourrisson de 2 mois 1/2, aujourd'hui âgé de 2 ans 1/2 et souvent revu, nous avons dû, mais tout à fait momentanément, suspendre l'emploi de l'emplâtre au calomel. Le premier emplâtre de 20 centimètres sur 50 placé à demi-ceinture postérieure, avait produit une dermite localisée avec phlycténisation partielle.

L'ablation de l'emplâtre, le poudrage de la peau altérée avec un mélange de talc et d'oxyde de zinc permit la guérison rapide de l'accident thérapeutique. Même, dans la suite, on put reprendre le traitement par l'emplâtre au calomel, sans qu'il y eut à nouveau rien de semblable.

Il faut ici faire la part de la prédisposition du sujet.

Dans une ordre d'idée analogue, l'emplâtre de Vigo, d'un emploi si répandu, cause exceptionnellement de dermite, même chez les enfants. Une seule fois, depuis que j'en ai vu appliquer ou appliqué moi-même dans ma pratique, j'ai observé une telle éventualité. C'était chez un jeune garçon de 7 à 8 ans, atteint d'une adénite au cou. L'emplâtre de Vigo fit naître, au-dessous et tout autour de lui sur une assez large surface, une dermite assez accentuée. Le placard érythémateux était parsemé de fines vésiculettes à contenu lactescent. L'emplâtre enlevé, la poudre de talc et d'oxyde de zinc en vint facilement à bout.

À l'hôpital Saint-Louis, l'emplâtre de Vidal, qui fut à un moment si couramment mis en usage, et par son auteur et par les autres médecins, a de même peu d'inconvénient de cette nature.

La cure de Quinquaud, comme nous l'avons déjà montré il y a plusieurs années[1], donne de bons résultats chez l'enfant.

Cependant je crois que bien peu de médecins l'emploient, faute de connaître la méthode, je suppose.

On ne voit guère les raisons qui l'empêcheraient d'être plus usuelle.

Depuis 1890-1894, époque à laquelle nous avions déjà réuni 11 cas de syphilis chez l'enfant ainsi traitée, nous avons continué jusqu'à ce jour à employer la cure de Quinquaud chez 7 nouveaux petits malades.

Ce sont donc les résultats d'une pratique, peut-être restreinte, mais déjà suffisamment ancienne que nous voulons présenter aujourd'hui.

Depuis le moment où nous avons commencé à mettre en pratique l'emploi de l'emplâtre au calomel comme traitement exclusif de la

[1] P. GILLET. Traitement de la syphilis de l'enfant par l'emplâtre au calomel de Quinquaud. *Annales de la Policlinique de Paris*, mars 1894.

syphilis chez l'enfant, nous avons pu suivre un certain nombre d'enfants, nous avons pu suivre un certain nombre d'enfants jusqu'à ce jour.

Nous pouvons ainsi donner un compte rendu assez fidèle non seulement immédiats de la méthode, mais aussi des résultats éloignés.

S'il est utile de connaître l'action du traitement sur les accidents spécifiques existant au début et qui ont nécessité l'emplâtre, il est non moins intéressant de savoir ce que l'avenir réserve aux sujets ainsi soignés, au double point de vue, d'une part des récidives possibles, de lésions spécifiques sur tel ou tel organe, peau, viscère, etc., et d'autre part, des lésions dystrophiques ou parasyphilitiques.

C'est ce que nous avons essayé de résumer dans la statistique détaillée ci-dessous, qui comprend l'ensemble de mes observations personnelles :

Nombre de cas traités :

	Vivants	Morts de syphilis	d'autres causes
18 { Syphilis héréditaire. 17	15	1 (le lendemain de la visite).	2 (grippe)
{ Syphilis acquise . . 1			

Nature des accidents traités :

Syphilides cutanées avec	{ Coryza { Syphilides anales { Syphilides labiales	5
Syphilides cutanées avec	{ Coryza { Syphilides anales { Pseudo-paralysie	1
Syphilides cutanées avec	{ Coryza { Pseudo-paralysie	1
Syphilides cutanées avec	{ Coryza { Testicule syphilitique	5
Syphilides cutanées avec	{ Coryza { Onyxis	1
Syphilides cutanées avec	{ Coryza { Hépatite { Coloboma irien	1
Syphilides cutanées		8

Durée du traitement :

5 mois (mais pas uniquement par l'emplâtre. Souvent Van Swieten	1
2 mois.	1
5 semaines	4
1 mois.	2
4 mois (emplâtre seul), friction dermite.	1
5 semaines	5
2 semaines (?) (non revus).	4
(non suivis, non revus).	2

ÉTAT DES ENFANTS REVUS :

Nombre	Âge à la dernière visite	
	9 ans	Développement physique intellectuel en retard. A 4 ans accidents méningitiques. Palais ogival. Encore en observation.
1	7 ans 1 2	Un peu chétif, mais plus rien. Encore en observation.
1	6 ans	Bon aspect général. dents cariées. 15 dents à 15 mois 1 2, marche à 15 mois. Poussée de kératite à 4 et 5 ans.
1	4 ans 1 2	Bon état. Premières dents à 10 mois. Marche à 16.
1	5 ans 1 2	Développement satisfaisant. A 2 ans 1/2 convulsions. Adénite cervicale chronique suppurée à 5 ans 1/2.
1	3 ans	Bon état. Premières dents à 6 mois 1 2. Marche à 16 mois 1 2. Toujours en observation.
1	2 ans	Bel enfant. 9 kilogrammes à 22 mois 1/2. Premières dents à 6 mois 1/2. Marche à 16 mois 1/2. Toujours en observation.
1	5 mois	En observation.
5	?	Non revus.

Les résultats semblent assez satisfaisants et tout à fait comparables à ce qu'on obtient avec tout autre mode d'administration de mercure, pour nous encourager à persister dans cette voie et pour recommander la méthode à tous points de vue.

Ce n'est certes pas un médicament nouveau, ni une médication nouvelle. C'est simplement un emploi particulier, parmi bien d'autres, du mercure. On ne peut lui demander ni plus ni moins que les autres préparations mercurielles.

Il présente un certain nombre d'avantages : 1° celui de respecter les voies digestives, parfois si fragiles dans le tout jeune âge.

2° L'application ne présente aucune difficulté.

3° L'absorption s'effectue d'une façon absolument continue et sans être à la merci d'un oubli ou d'une irrégularité d'administration.

4° On peut, à volonté, par l'ablation immédiate de l'emplâtre, faire cesser la médication. La peau n'en renferme plus qu'une minime proportion déjà emmagasinée.

5° C'est aussi un moyen de déguiser la médication mercurielle soit lorsqu'elle est systématiquement refusée par les parents, soit que des circonstances particulières nous obligent à ne pas dévoiler à l'entourage l'existence de la syphilis.

Il va s'en dire que l'emplâtre au calomel ne fait qu'office de traitement mercuriel, il cède la place en temps voulu au traitement ioduré : mais on le prolonge toujours un peu au delà du moment où les lésions visibles ont disparu.

IX

RACHITISME

RECHERCHES MICROSCOPIQUES ET NOUVELLES OBSERVATIONS SUR LE RACHITISME FŒTAL

par MM. F. FEDE et G. FINIZIO,

de Naples.

Les présentes recherches sont la continuation de celles déjà initiées par l'un de nous (Fede) et Cacace, et référées au Congrès pédiatrique de Turin en 1898, et après, plus en détail, à l'Académie de Médecine et de Chirurgie de Naples en 1898.

Personne n'ignore qu'il existe encore de grandes discussions sur la fréquence et même sur l'existence du rachitisme du fœtus. Nous ne rappelons pas ici la littérature au sujet, qui a été complétement exposée dans le travail cité ci-dessus. Nous répétons seulement que si Bednar, Kassowitz, Feyerahend, Cohn, Quisling, Lentz ont considéré le rachitisme fœtal comme très fréquent, d'autres au contraire l'ont déclaré fort rare. Parmi ces derniers, nous rappelons Eschistowitsch, Guérin, qui avait signalé 5 cas de rachitisme congénital sur 546 malades, et Chaussier 1 cas sur 25195 naissances. Grand nombre toutefois le nient positivement, et soutiennent qu'un nom semblable a été donné jusqu'à présent à plusieurs entités morbides, bien diverses de rachitisme. Parmi ceux qui appuient la dernière opinion, nous citerons les noms de Schidlowski, Porak, Scholtz, Kaufmann, Ballantyne, Urtel, Clivio Salvetti et Margarucci.

Fede et Cacace, après de minutieuses observations cliniques, faites sur 500 nouveau-nés à la *Maternità degli Incurabili*, sont arrivés à la conclusion que les nouveau-nés avec notes cliniques de rachitisme sont très rares, n'ayant rencontré qu'un seul cas offrant tous les caractères cliniques de rachitisme, et sur quatre la craniotabes d'Elsässer. Toutefois, dans plusieurs cas, ils ont trouvé les fontanelles plus ou moins larges et les sutures écartées.

Nous avons continué les observations cliniques sur 475 nouveau-nés de la même *Maternità degli Incurabili*. Sur chaque enfant, nous avons observé non seulement les notes possibles du développement irrégulier du squelette. mais même le poids et les principales dimensions du corps. Pour la mesure de la longueur du corps, nous nous sommes servis du bréphomacromètre inventé par Fede et Cacace, et pour les autres mesures d'un centimètre ordinaire.

Résumé des observations cliniques.

Nouveau-nés : 475

			Garçons	Filles
Nés à 9 mois	459	—	246	— 215
8	1 2	1	0	1
8		9	5	4
7		5	4	— 1
6		1	0	— 1

Poids du corps parmi les nés à 9 mois.
- Moyenne totale . . . . 2969 grammes
- — chez les garçons . . 2959 —
- — chez les filles . . . . 2982 —
- Maximum . . . . 4050 —
- Minimum . . . . 2100 —

N. B. — Dans cette moyenne ne sont compris ni deux nouveau-nés, un garçon et une fille du poids exceptionnel de 4850 grammes le premier et de 4700 la seconde, ni les enfants nés jumeaux : le poids que nous avons vérifié dans ces derniers a été de 2000 à 2650 grammes.

Longueur du corps parmi les nés à 9 mois.
- Moyenne totale . . . . 48 cm. 19
- — chez les garçons . . . . . 48 » 24
- — chez les filles . . . . . . 48 » 14
- Maximum 55
- Minimum 42

Circonférence de la tête parmi les nés à 9 mois.
- Moyenne totale . . . . 55 cm. 19
- — dans les garçons . . . . . 55 » 57
- — dans les filles . . . . . 52 » 99
- Maximum 57
- Minimum 27

Circonférence du thorax parmi les nés à 9 mois.
- Moyenne totale . . . . 51 cm. 11
- — dans les garçons . . . . . 51 » 56
- — dans les filles . . . . . 50 » 86
- Maximum 56
- Minimum 27

Fontanelles et sutures dans les nés à 9 mois.

1) Fontanelle antérieure régulière
Fontanelles postérieure et latérale fermées
Sutures régulières. } Nouveau-nés 220 sur 459

2) Fontanelle antérieure ample
Fontanelles postérieure et latérale non fermées
Sutures écartées. } Nouveau-nés 166 sur 459

Dans cette catégorie sont compris :

a) 28 cas dans lesquels un des diamètres de la fontanelle antérieure était entre 40 et 50 millimètres.

b) 10 cas dans lesquels un des diamètres de la fontanelle antérieure était de plus de 50 millimètres.

c) 9 cas dans lesquels la suture métopique était persistante.

3) Fontanelle antérieure très petite
Fontanelles postérieure et latérale fermées
Sutures régulières
\ Nouveau-nés / 40 sur 459

4) Fontanelle antérieure presque fermée
Fontanelles postérieure et latérale fermées
Suture sagittale avec bords superposés.
/ Nouveau nés \ 10 sur 459

5) Fontanelle antérieure ample
Fontanelles postérieure et latérale fermées
Sutures écartées.
/ Nouveau-nés \ 8 sur 459

6) Fontanelle antérieure ample
Fontanelles postérieure et latérale non fermées
Sutures régulières.
/ Nouveau-nés \ 7 sur 459

7) Fontanelle antérieure ample
Fontanelles postérieure et latérale non fermées
Sutures régulières.
/ Nouveau-nés \ 4 sur 459

8) Fontanelle antérieure régulière
Fontanelles postérieure et latérale non fermées
Sutures régulières.
/ Nouveau-nés \ 4 sur 459

Craniotabes.   Nouveau-nés 5 sur 459
Double *genu varu*.   6 sur 459
Épiphyses des os longs enflées.   —   5 sur 459

Ces trois derniers nouveau-nés présenteraient encore d'autres signes cliniques pour lesquels ils sont déjà compris dans certaines des catégories précédentes. Et ils offraient précisément la fontanelle antérieure plus ou moins large, les fontanelles postérieure et latérales non fermées, les sutures écartées, et deux d'entre eux aussi double *genu varum*. Par les observations cliniques précédentes, nous pouvons déduire les conclusions suivantes :

Sur 459 nouveau nés, nous avons notés parmi trois cas seuls quelques caractères cliniques du rachitisme. Également sur trois autres, nous avons trouvé la craniotabes et dans quatre le double *genu varum*. Pour ces derniers, nous faisons observer que la craniotabes peut exister aussi sans le rachitisme, comme dans l'hydrocéphalie (Fede), et même dans les limites du développement physiologique (Friedleben, Ritter); que le double *genu varum* peut devoir son origine au défaut de conformation ou aux lésions nerveuses; enfin que dans ces nouveau-nés, il n'y avait aucune note clinique évidente de rachitisme, et par conséquent il nous semble qu'on ne peut les déclarer avec sûreté, rachitiques. Toutefois, même en admettant que ces enfants soient certainement rachitiques, nous avons vu que le rachitisme fœtal ne se trouverait que chez les 2,1 pour 100 des nouveau-nés. Et ce chiffre est toujours inférieur au tant du cent donné par d'autres observateurs, c'est-à-dire du 10,5 pour 100 (Quisling), du 50 pour 100 (Cohn). du 68 pour 100 (Feyerabend), du 86 pour 100 (Schwarz).

Mais, selon nos observations, il résulte encore que chez les nouveau-nés on rencontre fréquemment, environ parmi les 52 pour 100, des irrégularités dans les os du crâne, comme la fontanelle antérieure plus ou moins large, la fontanelle postérieure et les latérales non fermées, les sutures écartées. La fréquence de ces lésions a été observée même par Fede et Cacace. Mais quelle est leur valeur clinique? Est-ce l'expression du rachitisme à son début ou de développement insuffisant?

Déjà Elsässer, Friedleben, Filatow, Bohn ont affirmé que la distance des os du crâne ne constitue pas un symptôme de rachitisme. Fede et Cacace se sont déclarés en faveur de cette opinion dans leur ouvrage. Selon eux, ces lésions doivent être interprétées comme arrêt de développement chez les nés des femmes mal nourries et obligées, pour cacher leur faute, de se serrer outre mesure. Pour définir la question, nous avons cru nécessaire de faire des recherches microscopiques sur les os du crâne des morts, ou morts peu après leur naissance, et qui présentaient les fontanelles très larges et les sutures écartées. Nous n'avons trouvé aucun enfant avec les épiphyses des os longs gonflées, ou avec une autre note évidente de rachitisme. Toutefois, parmi ces cas, l'examen microscopique n'aurait pas eu une grande importance, car nous ne nous proposions pas d'étudier les lésions du rachitisme fœtal, mais de nous assurer si ces lésions existaient ou non dans les cas en controverse ci-dessus.

Nous avons fait les recherches microscopiques sur six enfants, examinant de préférence les parties des os du crâne qui constituaient les sutures ou les fontanelles larges.

La décalcification a été exécutée par l'acide picrique en solution saturée, ou par une solution d'acide nitrique et d'alun, l'inclusion à la paraffine, et la coloration à l'hématoxyline.

Dans aucun des cas examinés nous n'avons trouvé des lésions qui autorisassent à reconnaître un rachitisme au début; au contraire, nous n'avons pas trouvé de lésions ou bien nous avons observé des signes de développement irrégulier ou insuffisant. Pour être brefs. nous indiquerons seulement ce que nous croyons le plus typique.

Premier fœtus (frontal, section qui correspond à la fontanelle antérieure). La couche osseuse n'arrive pas à la limite de la section, qui correspond à la fontanelle antérieure, mais elle s'arrête à une distance

remarquable. L'espace entre la couche osseuse et la limite de la section
est occupé par un tissu conjonctif très serré et abondant d'éléments
fixes, plutôt allongés. Dans ce connectif des îles de tissu osseux de forme
et de grandeur variées sont répandues çà et là. Vues en section elles sont
allongées, comme un S. rondes, représentées par un cercle mince, qui
entoure le tissu connectif. Les corpuscules osseux de ces îles sont un
peu plus nombreux et plus serrés que les corpuscules correspondants de
la couche osseuse.

Deuxième fœtus (pariétal). La plus grande partie de la section est faite
d'un connectif abondant d'éléments fixes. Seulement, à une importante
distance de la limite qui est vers la fontanelle, distance plus importante
que dans les autres cas, on observe une mince couche osseuse, qui à mesure qu'elle avance devient graduellement plus grosse. Une telle couche
n'est pas continuelle, mais présente des interruptions, dans lesquelles
l'introduit la couche interne du périoste. Entre la couche osseuse et celle
du périoste il y a un abondant tissu médullaire, qui manque toutefois
dans les endroits ou le périoste s'introduit dans les lamelles.

Donc, les observations cliniques nous confirment dans l'idée que
le rachitisme fœtal est rare, cette idée prend plus de consistance
d'après les observations microscopiques. Celles-ci nous autorisent à
soutenir que les fontanelles larges et les sutures écartées, chez les
nouveau-nés, ne sont pas toujours criterium de rachitisme, et que,
au moins dans la majorité des cas, ils sont le signe d'une ossification
retardée.

RACHITISME CONGÉNITAL

par M. ESCHERICH

M. Escherich présente la radiographie d'un cas de rachitisme congénital.

DISCUSSION

M. Marfan, au sujet de la radiographie présentée par M. Escherich,
dit que la photographie ne permet pas de se faire une idée exacte, parce
que les épiphyses sont invisibles. Sont-elles gonflées? Ce gonflement des
épiphyses est caractéristique du vrai rachitisme. Si je fais cette question,
c'est qu'à l'heure présente je n'ai pu me convaincre encore de l'existence
d'un vrai rachitisme congénital. Les faits décrits sous ce nom, ainsi que
je l'ai déjà dit, me paraissent rentrer, non dans le rachitisme vrai, mais :
1° dans l'achondroplasie de Parrot; 2° dans le myxœdème congénital;
3° dans les déformations consécutives à l'oligamnios. Mais je ne nie pas
l'existence d'un vrai rachitisme congénital.

LA CURE MARINE DU RACHITISME
AUX SANATORIUMS DE BANYULS-SUR-MER ET DE SAINT-TROJAN
par M. le docteur Charles LEROUX.

Je ne viens pas vous entretenir de nouveau des résultats excellents

Arrivée.   Départ.

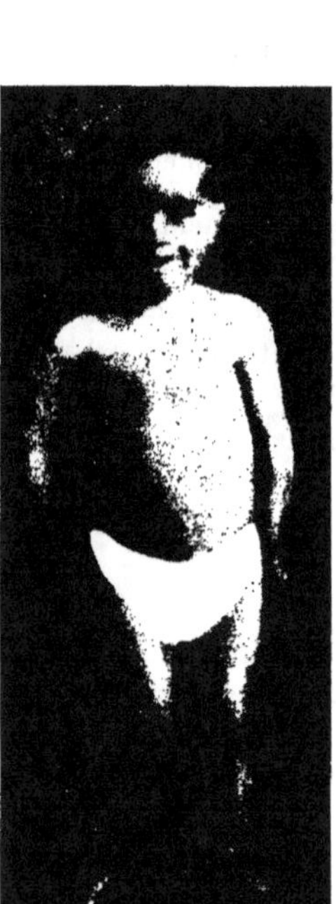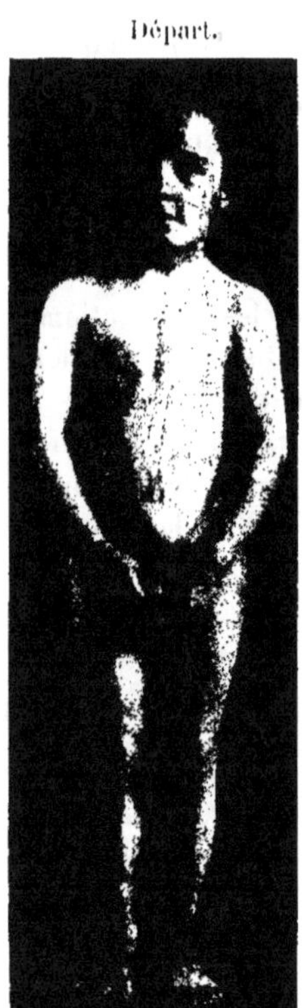

Fig. 1. — R. J., 5 ans. Rachitisme.

que donne la cure marine dans le traitement du rachitisme infantile,
la preuve en est faite aujourd'hui.

Je désire surtout vous présenter diverses photographies de rachitiques faites à l'entrée et à la sortie, qui, mieux que toute description,
entraînent la conviction.

Voici, par exemple, la photographie du jeune R. J... (fig. 1), entré

le 10 mai 1895, à l'âge de 5 ans, atteint de rachitisme avec double
genu valgum très accentué : l'écartement entre les talons est de
26 centimètres. Après un séjour de trois ans (sorti le 2 mai 1898), la
modification est considérable. Les jointures ont repris leur volume,
les genu valgum ont disparu, et les membres inférieurs sont complètement droits, sans la moindre intervention autre que la cure marine.

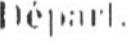

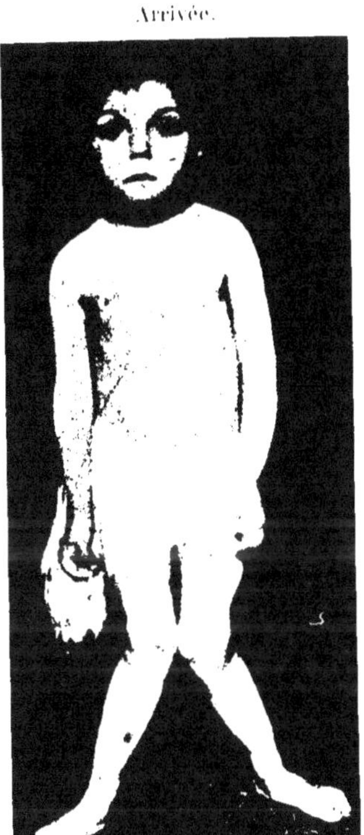
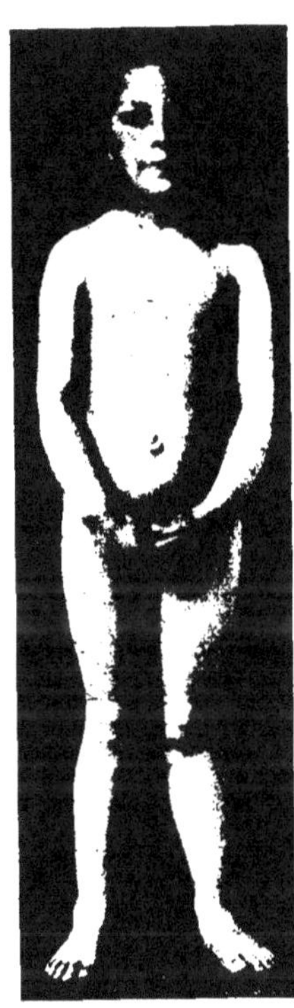

Fig. 2. — Genu valgum rachitique.

La seconde photographie est relative à une fillette de 4 ans,
Eulalie B.... Cette enfant est complètement déformée par le rachitisme ; les jambes sont arrondies en demi-cercles, les extrémités des
os sont gonflées, les côtes déformées ; le ventre est gros. L'enfant
marche très difficilement en raison de l'incurvation des membres.
Après un séjour de plusieurs années, la transformation est manifeste.
Les membres inférieurs sont parfaitement droits ; les os ont repris
leur volume normal ; la poitrine n'est plus déformée. L'enfant est

méconnaissable : le poids a passé de 12 kilogrammes à 20 kil. 500 ;
la taille a augmenté de 24 centimètres. La photographie faite à la
sortie montre bien cette transformation.

Le troisième exemple est également curieux. Il s'agit ici d'un petit
sujet de 2 ans et 10 mois qui est apporté au sanatorium dans un état
de déformation rachitique extrême. La planche que je vous présente

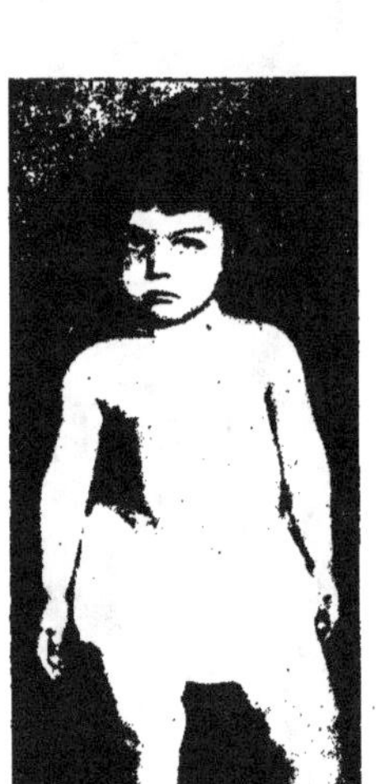
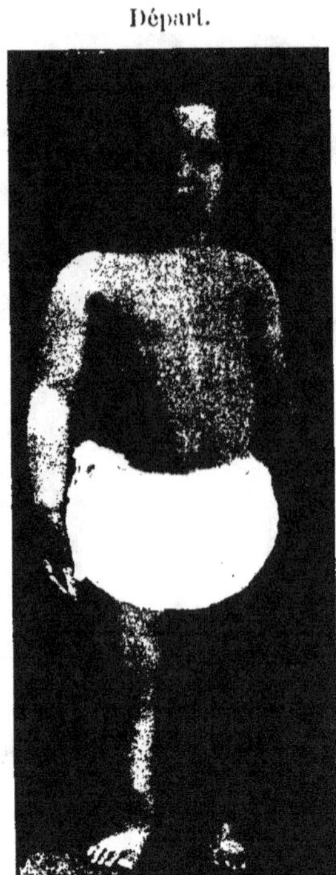

Fig. 5. — Rachitisme.

en dit plus que toute description : c'est un petit squelette qui n'a plus
forme humaine. Après un séjour de 1262 jours, la transformation est
considérable. Le redressement n'est pas complet, mais l'enfant marche facilement ; il est gros et gras et le résultat est relativement fort
intéressant.

Cette autre photographie représente une fillette de 6 ans (fig. 2),
Éloïse R.... atteinte d'un genu valgum rachitique très prononcé. Le
redressement est presque complet. Il est d'autant plus intéressant à

noter qu'à cet âge, on ne peut plus guère compter sur un redressement spontané, sans intervention chirurgicale.

La planche suivante, faite d'après les photographies, représente deux jumeaux âgés de 4 ans, d'une ressemblance extraordinaire et tous deux atteints de déformations rachitiques des membres inférieurs, des membres supérieurs, du thorax, etc. Soumis au même traitement, l'amélioration a été progressive et identique chez ces deux enfants. Ils sont sortis bien guéris ainsi que l'indique la deuxième figure, après un séjour de 5 ans et 8 mois. Ils pesaient tous les deux le même poids 16 kil. 200, et avaient la même taille : 1 mètre chez l'un, 1 m. 01 chez l'autre.

Je pourrais multiplier à l'infini les exemples, je me contente de vous faire passer sous les yeux encore quelques photographies (fig. 5) qui suffisent à donner une idée de l'influence favorable exercée sur les jeunes rachitiques par la cure marine.

Les résultats généraux ont été les suivants après 10 années d'exercice : sur 156 rachitiques traités, nous avons obtenu 108 guérisons, soit plus de 69 pour 100.

32 ont été améliorés; 11 sont sortis sans modification aucune; 5 sont morts de troubles digestifs, de maladies intercurrentes ou de tuberculose.

Tous ces rachitiques, transportés au bord de la mer, dans un milieu aussi aseptique que possible, soumis à une hygiène alimentaire convenable, soumis à la cure d'air marin et des bains de mer chauds ou froids suivant la saison et l'âge, modifient progressivement leur état.

La nutrition subit une accélération notable, ainsi que l'indiquent les pesées faites à l'entrée et à la sortie. Tous augmentent de poids pendant leur séjour[1] et quelques-uns, à la sortie, sont au-dessus de la moyenne correspondante à leur âge, d'après les tableaux de Quetelet.

La taille subit la même progression, mais avec moins de constance et moins de régularité. Les déformations rachitiques diminuent et disparaissent en totalité pour la plupart des enfants, partiellement pour la minorité.

Les résultats ne sont pas toujours parfaits, mais cela tient à deux causes.

La première est que beaucoup d'enfants sont trop âgés, quand on

---

1. Voir *Bulletins de l'œuvre des hôpitaux marins*; et 1er Congrès de Thalassothérapie à Boulogne-sur-Mer, 25-29 juillet 1894. *La médecine infantile*, 15 octobre 1894.

les soumet à la cure, 6, 8, 10 ans et même davantage, et que les déformations sont souvent à cet âge définitives.

La seconde cause est que leur séjour à la mer est beaucoup trop court. Certains enfants ne passent souvent que quelques mois au sanatorium alors que la moyenne de durée du séjour est environ de dix-huit mois à deux ans, pour les cas de guérison.

Il existe actuellement dans la plupart des sanatoriums maritimes, et particulièrement dans ceux que dirige l'Œuvre des hôpitaux marins à Banyuls-sur-Mer et à Saint-Trojan, des services spéciaux pour les jeunes rachitiques, qui y sont reçus à partir de 2 ans, en raison même de la constance et de la facilité de la guérison à cet âge.

C'est en m'appuyant sur ces courtes considérations que, dans l'intérêt des rachitiques et des hôpitaux et sanatoriums marins, je vous demande la permission de vous soumettre le vœu suivant :

Vœu :

Le Congrès, convaincu de l'efficacité de la cure marine dans le traitement du rachitisme, engage les médecins à envoyer dans les sanatoriums maritimes les jeunes rachitiques dès l'âge de 2 à 5 ans et à prévoir toujours un séjour prolongé, de deux années au moins.

DISCUSSION

M. Chaumier (Tours) fait remarquer que, sans nier l'influence de la cure marine, le rachitisme guérit très bien dans la famille.

M. Marfan. — Il est certain que des déformations rachitiques très accusées peuvent se redresser spontanément tant que l'enfant est âgé de moins de 3 ou 4 ans. Mais, après cet âge, un redressement complet de déviations très marquées devient fort rare. Ce qui me frappe dans les photographies de M. Leroux, c'est que quelques-uns de ces enfants étaient âgés de 4 ou 5 ans, qu'ils avaient des déviations très prononcées des membres inférieurs et que la cure marine les a presque complètement redressés. C'est un brillant résultat. Dans les conditions où étaient ces enfants, j'avoue que j'aurais eu la pensée de recourir à l'intervention chirurgicale.

RÉFUTATION DES DIVERSES THÉORIES
DE LA PATHOGÉNIE DU RACHITISME AYANT COURS ACTUELLEMENT
EXPOSÉ DE LA THÉORIE INFECTIEUSE

par M. le docteur Edmond CHAUMIER.

de Tours.

Dans une communication au Congrès de Rome, j'ai déjà prouvé que le rachitisme est une maladie infectieuse, contagieuse, épidémique et héréditaire.

J'ai rappelé que lorsqu'on l'a étudié pour la première fois en Angleterre, son épidémicité n'a fait de doute pour personne, et que sa contagion, qui à cause des théories régnantes, ne pouvait être admise, a été discutée.

J'ai dit que les crèches et les garderies d'enfants sont des endroits dangereux où parmi d'autres maladies on gagne le rachitisme; que les nourrices qui élèvent à la fois un certain nombre d'enfants ne sont pas moins nuisibles.

J'ai relaté des épidémies de rachitisme chez des jeunes porcs, tous les animaux d'une même portée étant pris à des degrés divers. J'ai présenté des préparations histologiques prouvant qu'il s'agissait bien du rachitisme. J'ai signalé, après bien d'autres, la fréquence du rachitisme dans les ménageries chez les jeunes animaux. Les jeunes lions y sont particulièrement sujets, et comme pour les porcelets, tous les animaux de la même portée sont pris à la fois.

Voilà bien des preuves, si je ne me trompe, de la nature épidémique, contagieuse, infectieuse en un mot du rachitisme.

Une maladie qui en même temps envahit tous les petits d'une même portée est bien épidémique et contagieuse; surtout, si comme je l'ai vu pour les porcs, tous les jeunes de la contrée sont pris à la même époque.

Malheureusement pour la thèse que je défends, les femmes sont moins fécondes que les animaux dont je viens de parler.

Cependant en fouillant mes notes, j'ai pu trouver six familles de jumeaux, que j'ai vues et dont je veux vous parler :

Voici d'abord Marguerite V. 2 ans 1/2; elle a marché à 25 mois. Elle a le thorax un peu bombé en haut avec les côtes déjetées en bas; un gros ventre; de très gros poignets; des articulations tibio-tarsiennes un peu grosses et du genu valgum. C'est bien une rachitique.

Son frère jumeau, un peu moins atteint, a marché à 18 mois : il a le front saillant et un genu valgum léger.

Voici maintenant deux jumelles : Marguerite et Suzanne G., âgées de 19 mois : elles ne marchent ni l'une ni l'autre. Marguerite ne se tient pas debout, Suzanne s'y tient un peu : Marguerite n'a que 5 dents, Suzanne en a 15, à peu près son compte. Marguerite a la fontanelle antérieure très largement ouverte et le front saillant ; Suzanne a la fontanelle fermée.

Suzanne a la poitrine un peu bombée de chaque côté ; Marguerite a un chapelet costal peu développé ; Suzanne a un chapelet plus marqué.

Marguerite a de gros poignets et des articulations tibio-tarsiennes grosses ; Suzanne a également de gros poignets et de grosses articulations tibio-tarsiennes, plus grosses que celles de Marguerite.

Marguerite a du genu valgum très prononcé, surtout à gauche ; Suzanne a moins de genu valgum.

Suzanne a un gros ventre.

Marguerite et Suzanne ont 5 frères : l'aîné, 16 ans, a marché à 18 mois ; le second, 7 ans, a marché à presque 5 ans ; le troisième, 4 ans, a marché à 15 mois.

Deux autres jumelles : Thérèse et Sidonie B. ont 28 mois ; Thérèse marche par la main ; Sidonie ne marche pas. Sidonie a du genu valgum, bien plus prononcé à gauche ; les clavicules sont difformes ; le thorax est bombé ; les poignets sont gros ; le chapelet costal peu marqué. 16 dents.

Thérèse n'a pas de genu valgum, mais le tibia droit est un peu courbé sur le plat, le chapelet costal existe ; les poignets sont gros. Les clavicules sont à peu près normales : 16 dents.

Le frère aîné, 15 ans, a marché à 22 mois ; il avait du genu valgum.

Le 2ᵉ enfant, une fille, 11 ans, a marché à 15 mois.

Le 3ᵉ, un garçon, 9 ans, a marché à 16 mois.

Le 4ᵉ, 7 ans, a marché également à 16 mois.

Le 5ᵉ, une fille, 5 ans 1/2, a marché à 4 ans et 3 mois. Je l'ai vue pour la première fois 2 mois après le début de la marche, et l'ai revue plusieurs fois. C'est un type très accentué de rachitisme, ayant touché à un haut degré la plupart des os.

Voici maintenant un jumeau et une jumelle. René et Yvonne C., que je vois à 17 et à 50 mois.

À 17 mois, René marchait le long des chaises ; mais il n'a marché réellement qu'à 19 mois. A 17 mois il a 6 dents, à 50 mois on note : des poignets un peu gros, une courbure à concavité interne assez marquée du tibia droit ; un gros ventre ; une poitrine un peu bombée ; du chapelet costal, mais peu développé ; les fémurs et les avant-bras un peu courbés, une tête un peu grosse ; de plus la démarche en canard des rachitiques ; il n'a que 16 dents.

Yvonne à 17 mois ne marche pas, ne se tient même pas debout ; elle n'a que 6 dents.

A 50 mois elle a 16 dents dont 2 viennent de pousser ; elle ne marche pas encore seule ; elle s'appuie aux meubles ; la figure est petite, le front gros ; la fontanelle est encore large ouverte. La taille est peu élevée. Les poignets sont un peu gros ; le chapelet costal existe, mais n'est pas très développé ; le ventre est un peu gros ; le thorax est bombé ; les côtes inférieures sont un peu déjetées : il y a un creux manifeste dans la ligne axillaire. Les 3ᵉ et 4ᵉ côtes droites semblent avoir été brisées : la clavicule du même côté est très irrégulière. Il y a du genu valgum, mais peu.

Auguste et Maria S., 2 ans et 10 mois. Je les ai vus à 21 mois pour la première fois. Ils ont un rachitisme très léger : Auguste a marché à 25 mois et Maria à 24 mois 1/2.

Leur frère, Camille, qui a 19 mois au moment de la note prise sur ses frères, n'a marché qu'à 25 mois, et n'a aussi lui qu'un rachitisme peu accentué.

La mère a marché à 2 ans.

Restent 2 jumelles que je n'ai pas vues, qui ont marché, l'une à 26 et l'autre à 52 mois, mais dont j'ai vu la sœur âgée de 4 ans 1/2 et qui présente encore des traces de rachitisme. Les jumelles sont placées entre cette sœur et 2 frères aînés âgés de 12 et 11 ans, qui ont marché, le premier à 20 mois, le second à 28.

La mère a marché à 18 mois.

J'ai tenu à transcrire ici les observations de ces six familles parce qu'elles sont très probantes et très instructives.

Elles montrent le rachitisme non seulement chez les enfants jumeaux, mais aussi dans quelques-unes chez des frères et chez les parents.

Si le rachitisme qui n'atteint que des enfants d'un âge déterminé était une maladie de courte durée, comme la rougeole, on pourrait ne le trouver que sur des sujets isolés.

Mais le rachitisme évolue lentement et sa période contagieuse doit être de longue durée. C'est ce qui explique l'existence du rachitisme chez un certain nombre de sujets d'une même famille. La conservation des germes dans les habitations, comme cela est bien prouvé pour la diphtérie et la pneumonie, doit également jouer ici un rôle.

L'hérédité existe puisque, dans certaines observations, l'un ou l'autre des parents, ou même les deux sont rachitiques.

Vous me permettrez de citer une observation très intéressante à ce sujet.

Il s'agit d'une famille de 19 enfants dont 15 sont morts.

Le père qui était noué n'a marché qu'à 4 ans. La mère qui n'a marché qu'à 2 ans est restée excessivement petite : elle a cependant les jambes droites et pas de genu valgum.

L'aîné est mort à 10 mois de convulsions.

Le 2ᵉ, mort en 1896 à 18 ans 1/2, a marché à 2 ans. Il avait 1 m. 57 de hauteur.

3ᵉ, 4ᵉ, 5ᵉ, grossesse triple : enfants morts à 2 jours.

6ᵉ, 7ᵉ, grossesse double : mort-nés.

8ᵉ, garçon, mort à 5 ans de convulsions, était resté 1 an au lit : était très difforme, avait les jambes et les bras courbés, ne pouvait porter les mains à sa bouche.

9°, garçon mort à 8 mois de convulsions.

10°, garçon mort à 1 an : ne marchait pas et avait les jambes de travers.

11°, fille, 19 ans 1/2 : très petite (1 m. 55 à 17 ans 1/2). Elle n'a marché qu'à 7 ans. Elle porte encore les traces d'un rachitisme intense. Elle a du genu valgum, les femurs sont très courbés à convexité antéro-interne. Les tibias sont excessivement courbés et en lame du sabre.

12°, garçon mort de convulsions à 2 ans 1/2 ; ne marchait pas ; il avait les jambes de travers.

13°, garçon, 16 ans. Il a marché à 2 ans ; puis a cessé de marcher de 4 à 5 ans : de 5 à 9 ans il a marché très mal. Comme sa sœur il a gardé des traces très marquées de rachitisme grave. Le front est très bombé, la tête un peu grosse, la face petite. Les courbures des clavicules sont exagérées ; la gauche semble avoir été brisée en deux endroits.

Le genu valgum est très prononcé : les tibias sont très cambrés et en lame de sabre. Les femurs sont très courbés. En marchant, ses genoux se cognent l'un l'autre.

14°, un garçon mort à 26 mois de bronchite et de convulsions ; ne marchait pas : ne se tenait pas debout ; avait les jambes de travers.

15°, garçon mort à 5 mois de convulsions.

16°, fille, 11 ans, a commencé à marcher à 2 ans, mais jusqu'à 5 ans elle marchait très mal. Elle a le front bombé, la face petite ; les clavicules difformes, très saillantes dans le quart interne, renfoncées dans les 3/4 externes. Le genu valgum est très prononcé ; les genoux se touchent et les pieds sont très écartés, les tibias sont courbés et en lame de sabre ; les femurs sont également courbés.

17°, mort-né.

18°, garçon mort à 2 jours.

Enfin 19, fille de 8 ans, qui a marché à 18 mois, et présente à peine quelques traces de rachitisme.

J'ai dit que cette observation était très intéressante : elle l'est à plusieurs points de vue : d'abord parce qu'elle montre bien l'hérédité du rachitisme : parce qu'elle montre l'hérédité grave, attaquant gravement tous les enfants qui ont vécu assez de temps pour cela, excepté la dernière fille qui a été légèrement touchée ; parce qu'elle montre enfin une polymortalité, qui n'a de comparable que celle de la syphilis ; polymortalité à laquelle il est impossible que le rachitisme soit étranger.

Est-ce qu'une maladie qui frappe ainsi une famille entière, après avoir frappé dans leur enfance le père et la mère, peut être autre chose qu'une maladie infectieuse ?

Jamais on ne me fera croire que c'est la diarrhée qui est la cause du mal et ni M. Comby ni M. Marfan ne me persuaderont que les toxines des microbes quelconques se trouvant dans l'intestin ont pu produire cela : mais je reviendrai sur cette question.

J'ai retrouvé dans mes notes, en plus des cas déjà cités, 85 observations de familles ayant plusieurs enfants rachitiques, ou bien dans lesquelles la contagion ou l'hérédité sont évidentes.

De ces 85 observations je n'en rapporterai qu'une en détail, donnant les autres sous forme de tableaux.

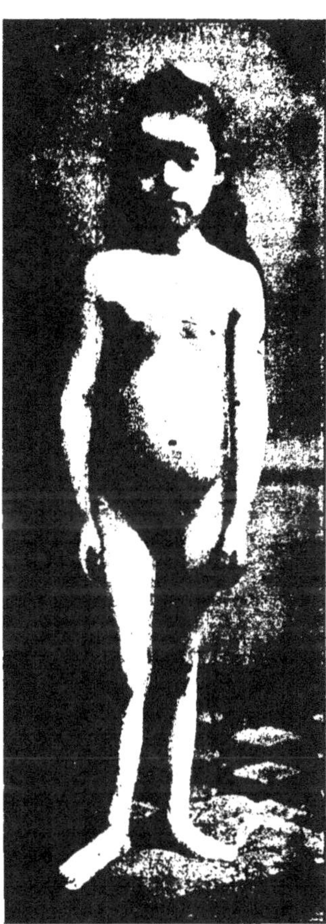
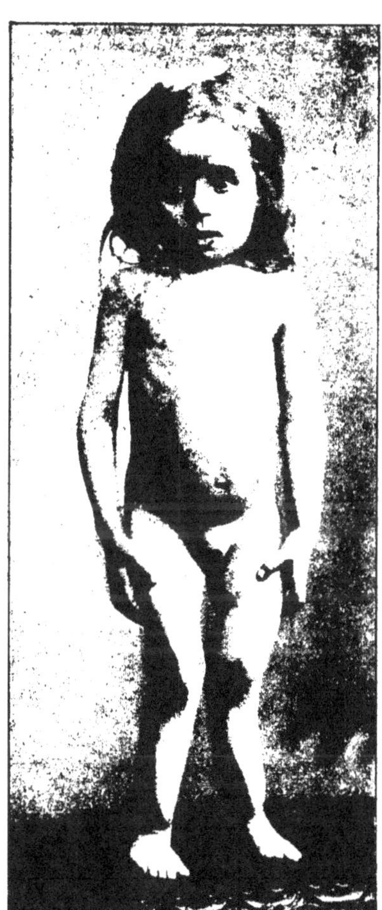

Celle que je rapporte est toute semblable aux autres, je l'ai choisie tout simplement parce que je puis vous présenter les photographies des enfants rachitiques.

Il s'agit de 5 sœurs que j'ai suivies d'assez près, mais dont je veux seulement résumer l'histoire.

Suzanne a actuellement 8 ans : elle a marché à 15 mois ; puis, après avoir marché pendant 1 mois, est restée 5 mois sans marcher. Je l'ai vue pour la première fois à 28 mois : elle avait du genu valgum droit, disparu aujourd'hui.

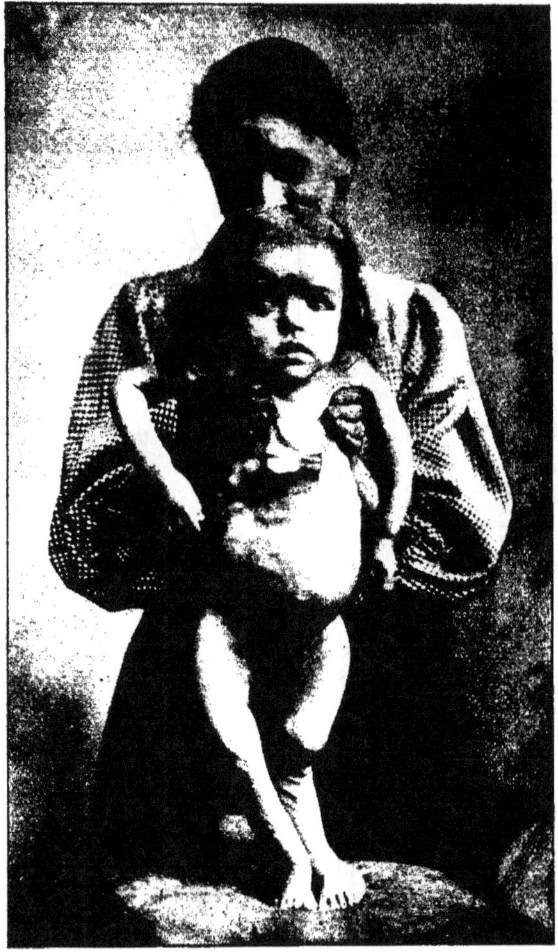

Cette fillette, atteinte de rachitisme léger, a aujourd'hui la taille des enfants de son âge.

Marguerite a eu 6 ans le 1er mars dernier. Je l'ai vue pour la première fois à 8 mois : elle a marché à 50 mois 1/2 ; à 55 mois elle a cessé de marcher pendant 5 mois ; 2 mois plus tard, elle s'est brisé une cuisse en tombant.

A 26 mois elle n'a que 6 dents et la fontanelle n'est pas fermée: le thorax est un peu bombé en haut, le chapelet costal est très prononcé, les poignets sont gros. Il y a du genu valgum, les tibias sont plats et courbés.

A 5 ans je note : encore genu valgum: les fémurs sont très courbés; les tibias présentent la courbure déjà signalée; il y a de l'ensellure avec renversement du bassin.

A 5 ans et 8 mois la hauteur est de 0 m. 97 1/2; elle a augmenté de 5 centimètres en 7 mois.

Madeleine a actuellement 5 ans. A 4 ans elle ne se tenait pas debout; à 4 ans 1/2 il faut la tenir des 2 mains pour la faire marcher; maintenant elle marche le long des meubles.

A 2 ans 1/2 elle n'avait que 11 dents; à 5 ans et 5 mois la fontanelle était encore largement ouverte; à 5 ans elle n'est pas complétement fermée.

Le thorax est très déformé, les côtes inférieures sont très déjetées. Le chapelet costal est très prononcé. Les poignets sont très gros. Les os des avant-bras et des bras sont courbés. Les fémurs et les tibias sont très difformes; le genu valgum est très prononcé, surtout à gauche. Le ventre est très gros; le bassin est renversé et semble déformé.

Voici maintenant sous forme de tableaux mes autres observations au nombre de 84. J'en ai fait 3 divisions : d'abord les familles dans lesquelles les enfants seuls sont notés comme rachitiques, n'ayant pas de renseignements sur les parents.

Ensuite les enfants ayant pu gagner le rachitisme en dehors de leur famille.

Enfin les cas dans lesquels l'hérédité a pu jouer un rôle.

I

Familles ayant plusieurs enfants rachitiques[1].

N°s	HISTOIRE DES MALADES	OBSERVATIONS
1	**FAMILLE V.** CHARLES, à 16 mois 1/2, ne marche pas : n'a que 5 dents ; rachitisme des jambes : gros ventre : côtes déjetées. — A marché à 18 mois. A 7 ans il a encore un peu de genu valgum, les poignets un peu gros. CÉLINE. A marché à 17 mois. A 5 ans je note : le front saillant ; le thorax aplati sur les côtés, dans la ligne axillaire. A 5 ans, tête encore grosse : 0m,52 de circonférence. Hauteur : 1m.06. PAUL. A 15 mois je note : front très bombé ; 2 dents ; très gros poignets : thorax un peu bombé ; chapelet très marqué ; gros ventre, genu valgum, fémurs courbés. Il a marché à 26 mois : il n'avait alors que 12 dents. HUBERT. Mort à 15 mois, ne marchait pas. SUZANNE. 1 an : pas de dents ; ventre un peu gros : ne marche pas, se tient un peu debout : pas de signes probants de rachitisme.	
2	**FAMILLE B.** CHARLES, 21 mois : a marché à 15 mois. Gros poignets : genu valgum double ; un peu de chapelet costal. CHARLOTTE, 5 ans : a marché à 17 mois.	Marcher à 17 mois n'est pas absolument une preuve de rachitisme. La fillette a été rachitique, mais je n'ai pas de note à son sujet.
3	**FAMILLE W.** PAUL, 5 ans. A 17 mois j'ai noté : chapelet costal : genu valgum gauche : grosses jointures : poitrine bombée : a marché à 15 mois. BERTHE, 5 ans. J'ai noté à 2 ans : a marché à 15 mois : se berce en marchant ; léger genu valgum gauche : gros poignets : grosses articulations tibio-tarsiennes : laxité de la hanche.	
4	**FAMILLE G.** MARGUERITE, vue à 22 mois : ne marche pas : ne se tient pas debout seule : lésions rachitiques des membres. EUGÈNE, a marché à 25 mois.	Il y a bien des chances qu'un enfant qui ne marche qu'à 25 mois soit rachitique : c'est pour cela que je cite ce cas.

1. Parmi les observations rapportées ici, il y en a assurément de très incomplètes, de trop incomplètes même : mais s'il peut y avoir doute pour quelques-unes, celles qui sont complètes sont en assez grand nombre pour fournir des preuves plus que suffisantes de la doctrine que je soutiens.

N°·	HISTOIRE DES MALADES	OBSERVATIONS
5	**FAMILLE V.** MARCELLE, 18 mois; ne marche pas; 7 dents. L'aîné a marché à 11 mois. Le second, mort à 50 mois, ne marchait pas. Le 5ᵉ a marché à 55 mois. La 4ᵉ (fille) a marché à 17 mois.	Mêmes réflexions que ci-dessus.
6	**FAMILLE L.** ANGÈLE, 18 ans; a marché à 19 ou 20 mois. OCTAVIE, 12 ans; a eu les jambes de travers; a marché à 19 ou 20 mois; est restée petite. MATHILDE, 2 ans; commence à marcher, tombe souvent; gros ventre; éventration; fontanelle ouverte; signes légers de rachitisme.	
7	**FAMILLE B.** GERMAINE, 3 ans; gros ventre; chapelet costal; genu valgum; ne marche pas; ne se tient pas debout; a marché à cinq ans et 5 mois. CONSTANT, 6 ans 1/2; a marché à 20 mois.	
8	**FAMILLE V.** Fille, 12 ans, a marché à 1 an. CAMILLE, 9 ans 1/2; a marché à 17 mois; étant petit, les genoux étaient écartés et ses pieds se touchaient; les jambes formaient un O. GABRIEL, 8 ans; a marché à 11 mois; était comme son frère, pire même; actuellement, lorsqu'il marche, il met les pieds en dedans et les jambes reprennent la forme en O. HENRIETTE, 5 ans 1/2; a marché à 14 mois. BERTHE, 4 ans; a marché à 15 mois; ses jambes ont un peu de tendance à faire un O.	
9	**FAMILLE B.** RENÉ, 22 mois, ne marche pas; 8 dents; front bombé; léger genu valgum; articulations de la hanche lâche; a marché à 5 ans. A 4 ans 1/2 je constate: front peu bombé; avant-bras courbés; poitrine très bombée; chapelet très marqué; fémurs très courbés; genu valgum peu prononcé. MAURICE, 5 ans 1/2; a marché à 5 ans moins 4 mois; genu valgum double, plus prononcé à gauche; fémurs cambrés; ventre assez gros; côtés très déjetés; chapelet costal; poitrine bombée, très aplatie sur les côtés; avant-bras courbés. BERTHE, 10 mois, pas de dents; fontanelle énorme; peut-être extrémités costales un peu grosses; rien autre encore.	

N°	HISTOIRE DES MALADES	OBSERVATIONS
10	**FAMILLE M.** JOSEPH, 21 ans, a marché à 15 mois. PIERRE, 15 ans, a marché à 19 mois. EUGÉNIE, 10 ans, a marché à 15 mois. FIRMIN, 9 ans, a marché à 15 mois. MARGUERITE, 7 ans, a marché à 19 mois : a encore du genu valgum droit. GEORGETTE, 5 ans, a marché à 15 mois : a encore du genu valgum. ANDRÉ, 20 mois, a marché à 17 mois.	
11	**FAMILLE S.** JULIE, 10 ans; a marché à 15 mois. JULES, 9 ans : a marché à 16 mois. EDMOND, 6 ans : a marché à 22 mois. ALFRED, 5 ans : a marché à 19 mois, il avait du genu valgum.	
12 13	**FAMILLE G.** PHILOMÈNE, 20 ans; a marché à 20 mois. JULIA, 19 ans : a marché à près de 5 ans : est restée très petite. LÉON, 10 ans; a marché à 19 mois; a encore un peu de genu valgum. LOUIS, 7 ans 1/2; genu valgum : gros genoux; grosses articulations tibio-tarsiennes : tibias à concavité interne. YVONNE, 26 mois, a marché à 19 mois 1/2, un peu de genu valgum : un peu de chapelet costal ; front bombé.	
14	**FAMILLE M.** MARGUERITE, 20 ans : a marché à 5 ans. Encore un peu de genu valgum : articulations tibio-tarsiennes un peu grosses. Le tibia droit est un peu cambré en avant et en dedans; le gauche l'est moins. ALICE, 8 ans : genu valgum très prononcé : les genoux se touchent. Elle a marché à 2 ans.	
15	**FAMILLE B.** JEANNE, 12 ans : a marché à 10 mois. ROBERT, 5 ans : a marché à 22 mois : encore traces de rachitisme. FÉLICIE, 5 ans 1/2 : a marché vers 16 mois ; se dandine en marchant : thorax un peu bombé : un peu de chapelet; très gros poignets : courbure des avant-bras : genu valgum très prononcé ; tibias un peu courbés, en lame de sabre : grosses jointures des pieds.	

N°	HISTOIRE DES MALADES	OBSERVATIONS
16	**FAMILLE F.** MARIE-LOUISE, 5 ans; a marché à 15 mois; avait la jambe gauche tournée. Front un peu bombé. ANDRÉE, 4 ans, a marché à 15 mois; puis a cessé pendant 2 mois; a marché à nouveau pendant 5 mois, puis a cessé. Elle a remarché à 59 mois; gros front; chapelet très prononcé; très gros poignets; genu valgum très prononcé surtout à gauche; très gros ventre.	
17	**FAMILLE E.** MARGUERITE, 15 ans; a marché à 14 mois. GEORGES, 9 ans; a marché à 20 mois. VICTOR, 4 ans, a marché à 18 mois. ROGER, 25 mois; ne marche pas; 10 dents; front un peu bombé; grosse tête; thorax très déformé; un peu de chapelet costal; poignets un peu gros; genu valgum très prononcé; parésie très marquée; gros ventre. 26 mois : ne marche pas, ne se tient pas debout.	
18	**FAMILLE A.** ALFRED, 4 ans; a marché à 19 mois. MARGUERITE, 19 mois, ne marche pas; front saillant; chapelet costal; gros poignets; un peu de genu valgum gauche.	
19	**FAMILLE R.** FILLE, 25 ans; a marché à 16 mois. GARÇON, 19 ans, a marché à 25 mois. MARTHE, 6 ans, a marché à 25 mois; a été nouée.	
20	**FAMILLE G.** MATHILDE, 15 ans; a marché à 16 mois; se berçait en marchant, cela a disparu. Vue à 12 ans, avec encore un peu de genu valgum gauche et des tibias un peu arqués, à concavité interne. MARIE, 15 ans 1/2, a marché à 18 mois. MAXIME, 12 ans, a marché à 20 mois. MARGUERITE, 5 ans; à 21 mois ne marchait pas; poitrine bombée; chapelet costal; a marché à 5 ans.	
21	**FAMILLE D.** EUGÉNIE a marché à 14 mois. ANTOINETTE, 1 ans; a marché à 2 ans 1/2; genu valgum très prononcé; poignets gros; gros ventre; poitrine très bombée. AUGUSTE, 18 mois; ne marche pas. Poitrine globuleuse, aplatie sur la ligne axillaire; gros poignets; laxité articulaire; genu valgum; gros ventre; éventration.	

Nᵒˢ	HISTOIRE DES MALADES	OBSERVATIONS
22	**FAMILLE L.** MAXIME, 28 mois, a marché à 19 mois : à 15 ans j'ai noté : genu valgum ; gros ventre ; éventration. CHARLES, 9 mois ; poitrine un peu bombée ; gros ventre ; un peu de genu valgum gauche : rien aux jointures.	
23	**FAMILLE A.** MARGUERITE, 11 ans 1/2, a marché à 27 mois. AUGUSTE, 7 ans, a marché à 2 ans. EMMANUEL, 18 mois, ne marche pas.	
24	**FAMILLE R.** LÉONCE, 26 mois ; ne marche pas ; ne se tient pas debout. Front saillant ; poitrine globuleuse ; clavicule gauche déformée, avec cal ; chapelet costal très accentué ; dernières côtes déjetées : creux considérable dans la ligne axillaire ; gros poignets ; genu valgum double ; grosses articulations tibio-tarsiennes ; très gros ventre. MARCEAU, 6 mois ; un peu de genu valgum gauche ; gros ventre ; chapelet ; dernières côtes déjetées ; poitrine bombée ; front un peu gros.	
25	**FAMILLE F.** ALPHONSINE, 6 ans : a marché tard ; poitrine en bréchet. FÉLICIE (morte), aurait 4 ans ; avait les jambes de travers. MARTHE, 2 ans 1/2 ; a marché à 2 ans : genu valgum.	
26	**FAMILLE L.** 1ᵉʳ mort à 14 jours. 2ᵉ mort à 10 jours. 3ᵉ mort à 14 mois. 4ᵉ fille, 9 ans ; a marché à 11 mois. 5ᵉ mort à 2 ans : aurait 5 ans : a marché à 21 mois. 6ᵉ SIMONE, 28 mois : a marché à 22 mois : se berce un peu en marchant ; un peu de genu valgum droit ; poignets gros.	Les 2 derniers nés d'un second mari.
27	**FAMILLE B.** HENRIETTE, 5 ans 1/2 : a marché à 15 mois : avait les jambes tordues à 9 mois : les avait encore de travers quand elle a marché. Un frère mort l'an dernier à 21 mois ne marchait pas.	

N°	HISTOIRE DES MALADES	OBSERVATIONS
28	**FAMILLE R.** 1. Fille, 13 ans, a marché à 15 mois. 2. — A marché à 20 mois ; mort à 5 ans. 3. — Mort à 9 mois. 4. — Mort à 2 ans 1/2, ne marchait pas. 5. — Mort à 22 mois, ne marchait pas. 6. FERNAND, mort à 2 ans 1/2, ne marchait pas. Vu à 2 ans. Thorax un peu bombé ; grosses jointures ; genu valgum double ; gros ventre. 7. LUCIEN, 4 ans, a marché à 18 mois ; gros poignets ; grosses articulations tibio-tarsiennes ; incurvation interne des tibias, surtout du gauche. 8. ROGER, à 2 ans et 3 mois, ne marchait pas. 9. Mort-né.	
29	**FAMILLE X.** 1. Garçon, 12 ans, a marché à 18 mois. 2. Fille, 9 ans, a marché à 16 mois. 3. Garçon, 6 ans, a marché à 16 mois. 4. GEORGES, 3 ans, a marché à 17 mois ; grosse tête, thorax un peu bombé ; un peu de genu valgum.	
30	**FAMILLE D.** ALBERTINE, 5 ans 1/2, a marché à 18 mois ; avait les jambes de travers. HENRI, 7 mois ; tibias un peu incurvés ; très peu de genu valgum ; extrémités des côtes inférieures un peu grosses ; poitrine bombée.	
31	**FAMILLE T.** MARIE-LOUISE, 16 mois ; ne marche pas ; ne se tient pas debout ; chapelet costal ; gros poignets ; genu valgum, surtout à gauche ; grosses articulations tibio-tarsiennes. Une sœur, morte l'an dernier d'angine, à 21 mois, ne marchait pas, commençait à se tenir sur les jambes.	
32	**FAMILLE P.** ALPHONSINE, 8 ans ; thorax bombé ; a marché à 18 mois. EUGÈNE, 6 ans ; a marché à 20 mois ; genu valgum double. ÉMILIENNE, 4 ans 1/2 ; a marché à 18 mois ; poitrine un peu bombée ; à 2 ans, se berçait en marchant. GEORGETTE, 2 ans, ne marche pas ; gros poignets ; grosses articulations tibio-tarsiennes. Déformation des tibias et des fémurs. Extrémité supérieure du tibia faisant saillie en dedans.	

N⁰ˢ	HISTOIRE DES MALADES	OBSERVATIONS
53	**FAMILLE V.** ALICE, 4 ans, a marché à 19 mois. ROBERT, 15 mois : ne marche pas : pas de dents : côtes déjetées : genu valgum double : gros ventre. A marché à 2 ans.	
54	**FAMILLE R.** ISABELLE, 4 ans : a marché à 30 mois : poitrine bombée : genu valgum double. MAURICE, 17 mois : ne marche pas : genu valgum double.	
55	**FAMILLE C.** JEANNE, 15 ans : a marché à 15 ans. ALBERT, 6 ans 1/2 : a marché à 2 ans : a les jambes de travers.	
56	**FAMILLE D.** MAURICE, 6 ans : a marché à 18 mois. SUZANNE, 4 ans : vue à 2 ans, avait 7 dents seulement et du genu valgum. RENÉE, 2 ans, a marché à 17 mois.	
57	**FAMILLE B.** MARIE, 14 ans ; a marché à 25 mois. HOMÈRE, a marché à 18 mois : a cessé au bout d'un mois, avait du genu valgum.	
58	**FAMILLE M.** 1. Fille, 16 ans : a marché à 2 ans. 2. Fille, 13 ans ; a marché à 16 mois. 3. Fille, 11 ans ; a marché à 14 mois. 4. MAURICE, 7 ans 1/2 : a marché à 3 ans : front saillant ; poitrine très bombée : genu valgum double, surtout à gauche : tibias en lame de sabre.	
59	**FAMILLE L.** FÉLIX, 6 ans : a marché à 17 mois. JEANNE, 5 ans : a marché à 14 mois. FERNAND, 3 ans : a marché à 18 mois : genu valgum.	
40	**FAMILLE A.** RENÉ, 2 ans : a marché à 20 mois ; chapelet : côtes déjetées : genu valgum droit très prononcé : gros ventre.	
41	HENRI, 1 an : ne marche pas : un peu de genu valgum : un peu de chapelet.	

N°˅	HISTOIRE DES MALADES	OBSERVATIONS
42	**FAMILLE A.** GARÇON, 7 ans: a marché à 2 ans. YVONNE, 2 ans; a marché à 16 ou 18 mois: encore un peu de genu valgum.	Un cousin du même âge que Yvonne a marché tard: ils étaient ensemble 2 ou 3 fois par semaine.
43	**FAMILLE M.** YVONNE, 15 mois: ne marche pas: chapelet léger: genu valgum gauche. Un frère a marché à 22 mois. Un autre à 28 mois.	
44	**FAMILLE L.** Fille, 9 ans: a marché à 14 mois. Fille, 4 ans, a marché à 28 mois. JEANNE, 2 ans et 5 mois: ne marche pas; poitrine difforme; poignets très gros: jambes très incurvées en dedans; gros ventre.	
45	**FAMILLE A.** 1. MARGUERITE, 13 ans: a marché à 26 mois: avait les jambes de travers: rachitique. 2. Fille morte à 5 semaines. 3. EMMANUEL, 9 ans: a marché à 2 ans. 4. Fausse couche.	
46	**FAMILLE D.** MARIE, 10 ans: a marché à 10 mois. EUGÈNE, 6 ans; a marché à 12 mois. FERNAND, 7 ans, a marché à 14 mois. ALPHONSE, 5 ans: a marché à 15 mois: gros front: gros ventre; genu valgum double. ROGER, 3 ans; a marché à 19 mois; poignets un peu gros: poitrine un peu bombée: à peine genu valgum. LUCIEN, 16 mois: ne marche pas: gros front: fontanelle large: gros ventre: genu valgum double: poitrine bombée; côtes inférieures déjetées: 4 dents. A marché à 2 ans.	En même temps que Roger, la mère a eu un nourrisson, qui a marché à 18 mois.
47	**FAMILLE L.** MARCELLE, 12 ans; a marché à 15 mois. GABRIELLE, 11 ans; a marché à 17 mois. ERNEST, 10 ans; a marché à 2 ans 1/2: au début il marchait sur le côté du pied. Il a encore une légère déformation des tibias, qui sont concaves en dedans.	
48	**FAMILLE G.** MARCELLE, 3 ans 1/2: a marché à 2 ans. RENÉ, 2 ans 1/2: a marché à 18 mois: gros ventre: gros poignets. MAURICE, 10 mois et 10 jours: gros ventre: fontanelle très large.	

N°°	HISTOIRE DES MALADES	OBSERVATIONS
49	**FAMILLE L.** CÉLESTIN, 8 ans : a marché à 17 mois. MAXIME, 5 ans 1/2 ; a marché à 21 mois : avait le ventre gros et une jambe de travers (la droite).	
50	**FAMILLE P.** ADRIENNE, 12 ans : a marché à 17 mois. MANUEL, 6 ans ; a marché à 2 ans : avait un gros ventre, une grosse tête, et quelque chose aux jambes. ISABELLE, 5 ans 1/2 : a marché à 17 mois. GEORGES, 17 mois : ne marche pas : gros front : figure petite : fontanelle énorme : genu valgum : gros poignets : thorax très déformé ; chapelet ; gros ventre. A marché à 29 mois.	
51	**FAMILLE B.** MAURICE, vu à 18 mois ; a marché à 15 mois : chapelet costal peu développé : un peu de genu valgum : grosses articulations tibio-tarsiennes ; fontanelle assez grande. MARGUERITE, 5 ans : a marché à 15 mois ; un peu de genu valgum ; un peu de laxité de la hanche.	
52	ROGER (1892), 14 mois : ne marche pas : genu valgum ; grosse tête. 1re dent à 21 mois : a marché à 21 mois. JEANNE (1896), 21 mois ; a marché à 17 mois : front bombé : 1re dent à 15 mois. LOUIS (1898), 10 ans : a marché à 15 mois : 1re dent à un an.	
53	**FAMILLE E.** MATHILDE (1892), 18 mois : ne marche pas : grosses jointures : chapelet, tibia gauche courbé. A marché à 20 mois. PAUL, 8 ans 1/2 : a marché à 19 mois.	
54	**FAMILLE P.** SUZANNE, 6 ans : a marché à 11 mois : jambes bien droites. ODETTE, 5 ans : a marché à 16 mois : poignets gros : articulations tibio-tarsiennes grosses : ensellure considérable : un peu de genu valgum : un peu de courbure à concavité interne des tibias : poitrine bombée. GERMAINE, 4 ans ; a marché à 16 mois : genu valgum : grosses articulations tibio-tarsiennes. C'était plus marqué étant plus jeune. FRÉDÉRIC, 5 ans : a marché à 26 mois : genu valgum droit : un peu de chapelet encore : poitrine bombée.	

N°*	HISTOIRE DES MALADES	OBSERVATIONS
55	**FAMILLE G.** PAULINE, 5 ans; a marché à 11 mois.	
56	LÉOPOLD, 21 mois: ne marche pas: un peu de genu valgum, surtout à gauche; poignets un peu gros; chapelet: côtes un peu déjetées: gros ventre: poitrine un peu bombée. A marché à 5 ans; à cet âge les lésions sont beaucoup plus accentuées. YVONNE, 7 mois, gros ventre: chapelet: genu valgum: gros front: fontanelle énorme: poignets gros; poitrine bombée. A 25 mois ne marche pas: les lésions sont très accentuées.	Léopold avait commencé à marcher par la main à 11 mois: a marché seul à 15 mois 1/2, une seule fois. On l'a mis à la crèche: a cessé de marcher: à la crèche il y avait un enfant de 2 ans 1/2 qui ne marchait pas.
57	**FAMILLE C.** LOUISE, 5 ans et 8 mois: a marché à 16 mois: vue à 2 ans, j'ai noté : léger genu valgum; ventre un peu gros; elle tombe souvent. ROGER, 2 ans et 5 mois: front gros: un peu de genu valgum; ventre un peu gros: peu de chapelet.	
58	**FAMILLE P.** FERNAND, 16 ans: a marché à 18 mois. GEORGES, 13 ans: a marché à 12 mois. Fille, 11 ans: a marché à 28 mois, était nouée. Fille, 6 ans; a marché à 14 mois.	
59	**FAMILLE J.** 1. Mort à 2 mois. 2. Mort à 2 jours. 3. Garçon, 7 ans ; a marché à 12 mois. 4. Garçon, 6 ans; a marché à 13 mois. 5. Fille, 4 ans: a marché à 20 mois. 6. Mort à 2 mois 1/2. 7. PIERRE, 25 mois ; a marché à 22 mois: ventre un peu gros: chapelet: un peu de genu valgum: un peu de laxité des hanches ; pas très gros front.	
60	**FAMILLE L.** MARIE-LOUISE, 7 ans : a marché à 9 mois 1/2. JEANNE, 6 ans: a marché à 21 mois. FERNANDE, 52 mois: a marché à 22 mois: rachitisme très peu marqué.	
61	**FAMILLE P.** GEORGES, 4 ans (1895): a marché à 18 mois. GEORGETTE, a marché à 18 mois. LUCIE, 9 mois (1897): poignets un peu gros: chapelet costal; un peu de genu valgum: gros front : grande fontanelle; gros ventre. RAOUL, 14 mois (1899): 2 dents, fontanelle énorme, gros front: chapelet: laxité de la hanche.	

N^{os}	HISTOIRE DES MALADES	OBSERVATIONS
62	**FAMILLE B.** 1er MARIAGE : 1. Fausse-couche. 2. Mort à 5 mois (variole). 3. Fille, morte à 6 ans; nouée: a marché à 2 ans.	
63	4. Garçon, a marché à 2 ans 1/2 : noué. 2e MARIAGE : 5. Garçon, a marché à 14 mois. 6. Fille, morte à 6 mois 7. Fille, a marché à 18 mois. 8-9. ÉMILIE, jumelle, a marché à 18 mois : l'autre jumelle, morte à 11 jours. 10. Fille, morte à 11 mois. 11. Fille morte à 6 mois; plus 5 mort-nés à terme.	
64	**FAMILLE V.** EUGÉNIE, 11 ans; a marché à 5 ans : était nouée. PAUL, 8 ans, a marché à 2 ans; petit genu valgum.	
65	**FAMILLE C.** LOUISE a marché à 10 mois. GEORGETTE a marché à 16 mois. JOSEPH a marché à 10 mois. YVONNE a marché à 28 mois; avait un très gros ventre. Lésions rachitiques notées à 2 ans: poitrine très bombée, lésions des clavicules. CÉLINE, morte à 15 mois; a marché à 15 mois. BASTILLE, a marché à 29 mois; front bombé: gros poignets; très gros ventre; genu valgum; poitrine bombée; côtes très déjetées : chapelet. RENÉE a marché à 15 mois: tête un peu grosse: genu valgum gauche; articulations un peu grosses; gros ventre; a toujours eu la fontanelle très grande: poitrine un peu bombée; laxité articulaire : marche en écartant les pieds et en se dandinant (21 mois).	
66	**FAMILLE B.** LOUIS, genu valgum assez prononcé. RENÉ, genu valgum. ÉDOUARD, genu valgum: ces trois frères ont été photographiés.	
67	**FAMILLE A.** JULIETTE, 5 ans: ne marche qu'avec une béquille: appuie le côté interne du pied: genu valgum double: déformation considérable de la poitrine; courbure des avant-bras. EUGÉNIE, 2 ans: ne marche pas: genu valgum: chapelet.	

II

Enfants ayant pu gagner le rachitisme en dehors de leur famille.

N°	HISTOIRE DES MALADES	OBSERVATIONS
68	**FAMILLE F.** Henri a marché à 26 mois; à 25 mois n'a que 12 dents; gros front; poitrine très saillante; côtes déjetées; gros ventre.	De 2 à 11 mois est resté dans une maison où était l'enfant d'un mois plus âgé que lui, et qui n'a marché qu'après 2 ans.
69	**FAMILLE P.** Gaston, 5 ans 1/2; a marché à 10 mois. Yvonne, 15 mois; ne marche pas; grosse tête; fontanelle largement ouverte; poitrine bombée; chapelet; poignets gros; gros ventre.	Yvonne a passé les 5 premiers mois dans une maison où était un enfant de 9 mois plus âgé et qui n'a marché qu'à 18 mois.
70	**FAMILLE G.** Auguste, 55 mois 1/2; a marché à 20 mois; chapelet rachitique.	Élevé par sa grand'mère, qui fait le métier de nourrice, et qui a élevé 2 frères dont l'un de 9 mois de plus que Auguste, et qui a marché à 29 mois; l'autre a marché à 24 mois.
71	**FAMILLE B.** Adolphe, 12 ans; a marché à 17 mois; poitrine un peu bombée; a encore un peu de genu valgum.	Un voisin du même âge à peu près, mort à 18 mois, ne marchait pas.
72	**FAMILLE B.** 1. Fille, 19 ans; a marché à 10 mois. 2. Fille, 17 ans; a marché à 11 mois. 3. Fille, 16 ans; a marché à 12 mois. 4. Garçon, 14 ans; a marché à 14 mois. 5. Marcel, 27 mois; ne marche pas seul; 12 dents; chapelet costal; grosses jointures; genu valgum; ventre énorme.	Marcel a été chez une nourrice dont les enfants ont marché à 5 ans.
73	**FAMILLE B.** Charles, 7 ans; a marché à 11 mois. Élevé par sa mère. Eugénie a marché à 17 mois; élevée en nourrice.	La nourrice d'Eugénie avait 5 enfants qui tous ont marché très tard. Celui du même âge qu'Eugénie a marché à 2 ans 1/2, ainsi qu'un qui avait un an de plus.
74	**FAMILLE M.** Marie, 25 mois; ne marche pas; symptômes rachitiques. Entrée à 9 mois en nourrice.	Chez la nourrice 2 enfants ont marché très tard.

N^{os}	HISTOIRE DES MALADES	OBSERVATIONS
75	**FAMILLE L.** ISABELLE, 5 ans : a marché à 16 ou 17 mois. Ses frères ont marché très tard ; l'aîné presque à 2 ans.	Un voisin du même âge que l'aîné, habitant la même cour, a marché très tard : il avait les jambes de travers.
76	**FAMILLE M.** SIMONE, 15 mois (a marché à 16 mois) ; ne marche pas : genu valgum ; grosses articulations ; chapelet costal : 8 dents.	Les parents habitent depuis 2 ans leur maison actuelle. Les personnes qui l'habitaient avant avaient 2 enfants : un âgé de 16 mois quand ils ont quitté la maison et qui ne marchait pas ; un de 3 ans qui avait les jambes de travers.
77	**FAMILLE M.** GERMAINE, 31 mois 1/2. — En nourrice dès la naissance. A marché à 20 mois. Le ventre n'est pas énorme, mais il l'a été : front bombé : côtes déjetées en bas : chapelet : genu valgum assez prononcé : fémurs très courbés. RENÉ, 16 mois. Chez la même nourrice dès la naissance : ne marche pas : se tient debout depuis 8 jours : 8 dents : gros poignets : très gros ventre : côtes déjetées en bas : chapelet ; genu valgum : gros front.	La nourrice a un nourrisson de 3 ans qui n'a marché qu'à 18 mois. Tous les enfants qu'elle a élevés ont marché tard ; entre autres 4 de la même famille. On avait prévenu la mère de GERMAINE et de RENÉ que chez cette nourrice les enfants marchaient tard.
78	**FAMILLE L.** DELPHINE, 11 ans, a marché à 9 mois. RACHELLE a marché à 24 mois. LUCIEN, mort à 1 an, a marché à 10 mois. ÉMILIENNE, morte à 17 mois (rougeole), a marché à 14 mois. YVONNE, 4 ans, a marché à 11 mois.	Un petit voisin de RACHELLE, plus âgé, a marché à 3 ans 1/2.
79	**FAMILLES P et M.** SUZANNE P. en nourrice, 16 mois : ne marche pas : chapelet : gros poignets : genu valgum. BLANCHE M., même nourrice : 15 mois : ne marche pas ; 3 dents.	

III

Cas dans lesquels l'hérédité a pu jouer un rôle.

Nᵒˢ	HISTOIRE DES MALADES	OBSERVATIONS
80	**FAMILLE J.** 1. 6 ans, a marché à 11 mois. 2. 4 ans 1/2, a marché à 11 mois. 3. Mort à 11 mois 1/2, ne marchait pas. 4. ALPHONSE, 20 mois ; a marché à 17 mois : actuellement marche en écartant les jambes ; genu valgum : la mère s'en est aperçue il y a 5 ou 6 mois.	Les 2 aînés ont un peu de *genu valgum, comme le père.* Lorsque la mère était enceinte de Alphonse, il y avait dans la même maison un enfant qui avait les jambes de travers, et qui n'a marché qu'à 5 ans. Alphonse avait 7 mois quand il a quitté le voisinage de l'autre.
81	**FAMILLE G.** ARMAND (nov. 1891), 27 mois ; a marché à 18 mois : 1ʳᵉ dent à 15 mois ; genu valgum. ALBERTINE (nov. 1895), 2 ans et demi. Genu valgum : 1 dent à 15 mois ; a marché à 18 mois. Frère, 14 mois, ne marche pas : pas de dents.	Le père a du genu valgum.
82	**FAMILLE J.** ROBERT, 2 ans 1/2 : a marché à 17 mois : genu valgum.	La mère a marché à 18 mois.
83	**FAMILLE P.** JOSÉPHINE, 14 ans, a marché à 2 ans ; avait de gros poignets. EUGÉNIE, 12 ans ; a marché à 18 mois. LOUIS a marché à 18 mois.	Le père a marché tard, à 18 mois ou 2 ans. la mère à 18 mois.
84	**FAMILLE V.** 1. Mort à 14 mois, ne marchait pas. 2. Fille, morte à 5 ans, a marché à 18 mois. 3. Garçon, 25 ans, a marché à 18 mois. 4. LÉOPOLD, 17 ans 1/2 : a marché à 2 ans : avait les jambes très de travers : cela a été en diminuant. Il a encore un peu de genu valgum. 5. Fille morte à 15 mois, ne marchait pas.	La mère a marché à 2 ans.
85	**FAMILLE T.** RENÉE, 6 ans 1/2 : a marché à 21 mois. GASTON, 4 ans : a marché à 21 mois.	La mère a marché à 20 mois ; le père à 17 mois.

N°	HISTOIRE DES MALADES	OBSERVATIONS
86	FAMILLE B. JULIETTE. 8 ans : a marché à 25 mois. ERNEST. 6 ans : a marché à 3 ans. Étant plus petit avait le gros ventre. Front saillant : un peu de genu valgum : tombe en marchant. ARMAND. 3 ans 1 2 : a marché à 26 mois : front un peu bombé : ventre un peu gros : avait les jambes de travers : cela s'est rectifié.	Le père a marché tard. Dans le même village, une fille de 9 mois de plus que Juliette a marché à 26 mois.
87	FAMILLE G. MAXIME. en nourrice chez Mme S., 27 mois : a marché à 2 ans. Front un peu gros : un peu de genu valgum.	Un autre nourrisson qui était en même temps que Maxime a marché à 22 mois. La nourrice a eu beaucoup de nourrissons, dont un grand nombre ont marché tard. Le fils de la nourrice a marché à 3 ans 1/2, et la fille de ce dernier, élevée par Mme S, morte à 3 ans, ne marchait pas.
88	FAMILLE R. ARMELLE. 2 ans : ne marche pas, ne se tient pas debout. A marché à 28 mois, très mal, en écartant les jambes. A 4 dents à 2 ans : gros front : poitrine bombée : peu de chapelet : très gros poignets : genu valgum gauche.	La mère a marché à 3 ans ; avait la tête grosse.

Je veux dire maintenant quelques mots des diverses théories ayant cours actuellement sur la nature du rachitisme. Je ne parlerai pas de la théorie syphilitique, tout le monde étant d'accord aujourd'hui pour la repousser.

La théorie inflammatoire de Kassowitz, en tant que théorie pathogénique, s'allie très bien avec l'infection. Kassowitz appelle inflammation la lésion osseuse du rachitisme. Pourquoi ne serait-ce pas de l'inflammation : nous sommes loin de la définition de l'inflammation : rougeur, chaleur, tumeur.

Pour Kassowitz cette inflammation est causée par un stimulus inconnu circulant dans le sang. Mais ce stimulus ne peut-il pas être spécifique, ne peut-il pas être un microbe ou sa toxine.

La théorie alimentaire et la théorie d'auto-intoxication par les produits de la fermentation gastro-intestinale, par les toxines secrétées par les nombreuses espèces microbiennes habitant le tube digestif, sont les théories en honneur en France où elles ont pour principaux défenseurs MM. Marfan et Comby.

Depuis que j'ai démontré au Congrès de Rome la nature infectieuse du rachitisme, un certain nombre de travaux, thèses ou articles d'encyclopédies, ont été écrits en faveur de ces deux théories que, si elles ne se confondent pas complétement, vous me permettrez de confondre dans ma discussion.

Or, dans presque tous ces travaux il y a cette petite phrase ou une autre analogue : « Il y a bien encore la théorie microbienne soutenue par Chaumier et par Mircoli, mais cette théorie n'a rien de sérieux. » Et c'est là toute la réfutation.

Moi je pourrais dire de même : « Il y a bien la théorie alimentaire, la théorie d'intoxication par les toxines intestinales, soutenues par *tel* et *tel*, mais cette théorie ne mérite pas qu'on s'y arrête. » Et je serais d'autant plus autorisé à dire cela que dans un certain nombre de thèses dont je parle on accumule comme observations de rachitisme des histoires de malades qui ne sont pas du tout rachitiques.

Je ferai remarquer que dans le présent travail j'apporte des observations inattaquables; j'expose les symptômes de mes malades afin que chacun puisse faire le diagnostic aussi bien que moi.

Or voici des modèles d'observations sur lesquelles on se fonde pour prouver que la diarrhée est la cause du rachitisme :

Enfant de trois mois, diarrhée, gros ventre. — rachitisme.

Enfant de six mois, diarrhée, gros ventre, grande fontanelle, — rachitisme.

Enfant de cinq mois, diarrhée, gros ventre, occiput mou, — rachitisme.

Or je tiens à le dire très haut, il ne suffit pas pour être *rachitique* qu'un enfant ait la diarrhée et le gros ventre; il ne faut pas davantage le dire rachitique parce qu'il a une fontanelle large ou un occiput mou.

Depuis bientôt trois ans je note l'état de la fontanelle et de l'occiput de tous les jeunes enfants que je vois. Je ferai un peu plus tard un travail à ce sujet; mais je puis dire dès aujourd'hui qu'il y a des enfants à fontanelle large qui marchent de bonne heure et ne présentent pas trace de rachitisme; j'en dirai autant du craniotabès, qui a été par erreur considéré comme une lésion du rachitisme.

Je ne nierai pas que la diarrhée soit fréquente chez les rachitiques; mais il n'est pas prouvé que la diarrhée ait précédé le rachitisme. Et puis. bien que j'aie des notes sur près de mille rachitiques, le rachitisme c'est l'exception, si on compare avec le nombre des jeunes enfants diarrhéiques. Mais ceci a déjà été dit maintes et maintes fois, et maintes et maintes fois encore on a dit que ce que la diarrhée prolongée produisait chez le jeune enfant ce n'était pas le rachitisme avec ses lésions spéciales, mais simplement de la faiblesse, de la maigreur, comme on observe après toutes les maladies sérieuses.

Aussi faut-il d'autres arguments : voici celui que j'apporterai.

Je soutiendrai, et cela avec des preuves aussi sérieuses, sinon plus, que celles apportées par les auteurs, que le rachitisme n'est pas d'origine gastro-intestinale, mais qu'il est lié à une lésion du système respiratoire.

En effet sur 100 rachitiques il y en a bien 95 qui ont des lésions de la cage thoracique, un thorax bombé, déformé.

Le gros thorax ne vaut-il pas le gros ventre.

Et pourquoi ces 95 rachitiques ont-ils ce thorax déformé? Apparemment parce que la fonction respiratoire ne se fait pas bien; parce que ces enfants ont des bronchites à répétitions, des broncho-pneumonies, du spasme de la glotte, du faux croup, de la sténose naso-pharyngée avec ou sans lésions auriculaires.

Et ceci est la réalité. On n'a qu'à examiner une série de rachitiques, de vrais rachitiques, à lésions bien nettes, et les moins clairvoyants verront que chez eux les troubles du côté de l'appareil respiratoire sont bien plus marqués que les troubles de l'appareil digestif.

Et pour appuyer ce raisonnement je dirai :

Qu'y a-t-il d'étonnant à ce que des troubles du côté de l'appareil respiratoire produisent du rachitisme : les neuro-pathologistes n'attribuent-ils pas certaines lésions osseuses à des affections pulmonaires (maladie de Marie). La maladie bleue, qui est une lésion autant pulmonaire que cardiaque, n'amène-t-elle pas des déformations des doigts?

La sténose naso-pharyngée causée par les végétations adénoïdes ne produit-elle pas une déformation de la poitrine absolument semblable à celle du rachitisme, au point qu'on a donné comme rachitiques des enfants qui avaient simplement des végétations du pharynx nasal.

Est-ce que beaucoup d'adénoïdiens n'ont pas le gros front et la face atrophiée du rachitisme? Est-ce que beaucoup d'adénoïdiens n'ont pas l'anémie des rachitiques, la faiblesse musculaire, l'atrophie même des rachitiques? Est-ce qu'un certain nombre ne marchent pas en retard comme les rachitiques: est-ce qu'il n'y en a pas, comme les rachitiques, qui sont en retard au point de vue intellectuel?

Est-ce que ce raisonnement ne prouve pas surabondamment que le rachitisme a son origine dans un vice de fonctionnement du système respiratoire?

En tout cas, est-ce qu'il n'est pas plus probant, aussi probant, si l'on veut, que le raisonnement qui attribue le rachitisme à des troubles gastro-intestinaux?

Je dirai, pour finir, que le rachitisme n'est point dû au poumon, n'est point dû à l'intestin; que, dans le rachitisme, il y a des troubles dans tous les organes; que le tube digestif est malade: que ses annexes le sont; que dans ces conditions la diarrhée s'explique, et le gros ventre qui tient en grande partie à de la parésie musculaire.

Ce que je dis du tube digestif s'applique au système respiratoire; s'applique au système nerveux, car le système nerveux aussi est malade? Est-ce que la grosse tête des rachitiques ne tient pas à un certain degré d'hydrocéphalie? Est-ce que ce ne sont pas des lésions du système nerveux qui produisent la parésie généralisée : parésie qui fait que les jambes se plient autant que dans une paraplégie, lorsqu'on veut mettre l'enfant debout; qui fait que dans les cas graves les enfants ne peuvent se servir de leurs membres supérieurs.

Il me sera donc permis de dire encore que le rachitisme est une maladie infectieuse, épidémique, contagieuse et héréditaire; je dirai de plus que c'est une maladie spécifique et que le rachitisme ne peut être produit que par le rachitisme.

Il reste à déterminer le microbe: à chercher son habitat dans le corps du rachitique; à déterminer les lésions produites par ce microbe, par sa toxine ou par les deux réunis; à déterminer l'influence des infections secondaires ou concomitantes (bronchites, diarrhée, etc.) sur la virulence du microbe et la toxicité de sa toxine, etc.

Un point que je tâcherai d'élucider dans un autre travail à l'aide des documents que je possède, c'est la durée de contagion de son microbe dans les habitations.

Pareille étude a été menée à bien par M. Netter pour la pneumonie, étude pour laquelle je lui ai fourni quelques documents.

J'ai déjà dit que dans les traités de pathologie, dans les thèses, etc., on avait l'habitude, à propos de la théorie microbienne du rachitisme, de rapprocher le nom de Mircoli du mien. Ma manière de voir diffère pourtant absolument de celle de Mircoli. Tandis que je regarde le rachitisme comme une maladie spécifique, naissant du rachitisme et produisant le rachitisme, Mircoli attribue le rachitisme aux microbes pyogènes, particulièrement au staphylocoque jaune. Il prétend même avoir reproduit le rachitisme en injectant des cultures de staphylocoques à de jeunes animaux. Il a certainement obtenu quelque chose ressemblant un peu aux lésions osseuses du rachitisme, mais ce qu'il a obtenu est tout simplement de l'ostéomyélite légère.

Du reste on peut obtenir par divers moyens chez les jeunes animaux des lésions osseuses ressemblant à s'y méprendre aux lésions osseuses du rachitisme, témoin les expériences de Delcourt avec le phosphate de soude et celles de Spillmann avec de l'extrait de matière fécale de rachitiques. M. Delcourt a bien voulu tout dernièrement, pour me montrer le résultat qu'il avait obtenu, m'envoyer des préparations histologiques d'os d'animaux ayant absorbé du phosphate de soude. Je l'en remercie ici très sincèrement.

Si M. Spillmann avait plusieurs observations au lieu d'une seule, je dirais que ses observations ne font que confirmer ma manière de voir, car il y a sans doute dans l'intestin des rachitiques les toxines du microbe du rachitisme et rien ne s'oppose à ce qu'on pense que ces toxines puissent produire les lésions osseuses.

DISCUSSION.

M. MARFAN. — J'hésite à prendre la parole pour répondre à M. Chaumier, parce que je crains que nous ne soyons pas bien d'accord sur ce qu'on doit entendre par rachitisme. Cependant, puisque M. Chaumier m'a directement mis en cause, je dirai quelques mots.

M. Chaumier paraît croire que le rachitisme n'existe pas chez les très jeunes enfants. Je le crois au contraire très fréquent à partir du troisième mois; dans le cours de la première année, il se manifeste d'abord par le chapelet costal, le gonflement de l'épiphyse du poignet et la cranio-malacie, qui est bien, dans certains cas, une lésion rachitique.

Je ne pense pas que M. Chaumier ait démontré que le rachitisme est une maladie infectieuse spécifique.

Pour qu'une maladie puisse être regardée comme infectieuse et spécifique, ou il faut prouver qu'elle est contagieuse, contagieuse d'une manière évidente, comme la rougeole et la syphilis; ou il faut que son microbe ait été isolé et que les cultures de ce microbe, inoculées aux animaux, reproduisent la maladie; ou, la connaissance du microbe faisant défaut, il faut tout au moins que la maladie puisse être reproduite par inoculation à l'animal. Or, M. Chaumier n'a fait aucune de ces démonstrations.

Le fait de trouver la maladie chez plusieurs enfants de la même famille prouve seulement, ou qu'il y existe une prédisposition héréditaire, ou que ces enfants ont été victimes des mêmes conditions d'existence et d'alimentation.

Enfin, si, vraiment, le rachitisme est contagieux, on ne s'explique pas pourquoi la contagion épargne les enfants nourris au sein, qui sont si rarement rachitiques, et frappe surtout les enfants soumis à l'alimentation artificielle, qui sont si souvent atteints par la maladie.

LE RACHITISME EN RUSSIE
par M. V. IOUKOVSKY

Le rachitisme est fréquent en Russie; c'est ce qui en fait l'intérêt pour le public médical russe; les nombreuses statistiques donnent il est vrai sur sa fréquence des résultats différents, mais elles n'ont sans doute pas été édifiées sur les mêmes bases.

Sur la fréquence, il y un nombre considérable de statistiques plus ou moins concordantes. Pour Zeleusky, 50 pour 100 des enfants de la classe pauvre de Saint-Pétersbourg seraient rachitiques; pour Woronickline et Reitz, 51 pour 100 des garçons et 25 pour 100 des filles, près de 50 pour 100 chez les enfants d'un an; pour Roussoff, 75 pour 100, pour van Puterem 65 pour 100.

Pour l'auteur lui-même, si on tient compte des manifestations légères, on pourrait compter 95 pour 100, mais 55 pour 100 seulement de formes graves.

L'étude histologique des os des nouveau-nés a été faite par Tchistowitch; il aurait constaté ainsi 8.5 pour 100 de rachitisme congénital (probablement Achondroplasie).

Dans la région de Saint-Pétersbourg, les auteurs s'accordent à reconnaître le rachitisme chez 60 à 80 pour 100 des enfants; en Crimée, au contraire, le rachitisme est très rare; à Tackkent, où l'on croyait qu'il n'existait pas, les travaux récents l'ont montré dans 47 pour 100 des cas.

Krussowski a étudié les déformations rachitiques du bassin: on ne les rencontrerait que dans 1/2 pour 100 des cas, sans doute parce que la mort frappe beaucoup de rachitiques pendant l'enfance.

Rauchfuss a préconisé le traitement de la maladie par l'huile phosphorée; Lemtscenko y est au contraire opposé, ainsi que Kissel, qui a montré expérimentalement sur les jeunes animaux l'action nocive du phosphore sur la croissance.

Une série de travaux a été faite sur la théorie hygrométrique du rachitisme, sur la carie des dents dans cette affection (Arkadieff), les modifications du tube digestif, les déformations et leur traitement orthopédique.

Korsakoff et Troïtsky ont essayé de reproduire expérimentalement cette affection; mais ils n'ont produit qu'une maladie analogue symptomatiquement et différente histologiquement. Philippoff a étudié la mortalité par rachitisme; elle serait de 0.65 pour 1000. Filatoff a étudié la parenté du rachitisme et de la scrofule, enfin une série de travaux d'anatomie pathologique est consacrée aux différents organes des rachitiques.

La deuxième partie du travail comporte une série de dessins et de photographies reproduisant un grand nombre de déformations rachitiques.

X

ALBUMINURIE INTERMITTENTE, URICÉMIE ET DIABÈTE

DES ALBUMINURIES CYCLIQUES DE L'ADOLESCENCE
PATHOGÉNIE ET CLASSIFICATION

par M. le docteur H. DAUCHEZ,

de Paris.

L'albuminurie cyclique est une affection rare, peu connue, et dont les origines sont généralement difficiles à déterminer, en raison des conditions pathogéniques qui président à son éclosion. Mais ce que la plupart des observateurs acceptent comme bien établi, c'est que l'albuminurie cyclique affecte un type à part, original, à évolution particulière.

Il importe donc tout d'abord de définir, ou mieux de rappeler ce qu'est l'albuminurie cyclique, pour ne pas la confondre avec les albuminuries intermittentes de la convalescence des néphrites banales.

On peut dire, croyons-nous, qu'un adolescent est atteint d'albuminurie cyclique (la seule que nous veuillons étudier ici) lorsque celle-ci est périodique, perceptible à heure fixe, lorsqu'elle disparaît en dehors de ces heures pathologiques quelle que soit l'attitude du sujet, alors surtout que celui-ci conserve un bon état de santé générale, n'a ni fièvre, ni cylindres rénaux dans ses urines, que le régime lacté ni le repos n'ont aucune influence sensible sur le syndrome qui nous occupe.

Cette définition, quelque peu schématique, serait incomplète si nous n'ajoutions à ces grands traits de l'albuminurie cyclique les conditions certainement prédisposantes que nous retrouvons dans nos observations et dans celles des autres auteurs :

1° Le terrain goutteux, arthritique des sujets si bien dénommés par Lécorché et Talamon sous le nom de prégoutteux, à tendance névropathique (Legendre).

2° Dans d'autres cas, l'état de convalescence de certaines maladies infectieuses (fièvre typhoïde, amygdalites, etc.).

L'albuminurie périodique diffère donc de l'albuminurie orthostatique, dont la cause est encore inconnue[1]. Nous n'en voulons pour preuve que l'observation citée plus loin, dans laquelle la jeune fille par nous observée se levait le matin sans que l'albumine paraisse, se couchait de midi à 7 heures du matin et chez laquelle l'albumine reparaissait invariablement de 4 heures à 10 heures du soir, quels que soient le régime, le traitement, en dépit de tous les traitements, classiques, sans que l'influence des repas se fasse sentir comme l'avait observé Tessier (de Lyon).

En regard des faits rares d'albuminurie cyclique, non orthostatique, il en existe d'autres où l'albuminurie apparaît tous les jours à la même heure, le matin par exemple, après la classe, après les exercices religieux notamment, dans lesquels l'attitude variable fait apparaître ou cesser l'albuminurie. Il existe donc des faits, comme celui de notre seconde observation, où un adolescent atteint d'hématurie, puis d'albuminurie permanente, devient nettement *cyclique sous l'influence de la station verticale*, et cesse dès que le malade reste assis.

Malgré leur point de contact, c'est-à-dire l'apparition passagère et périodique de l'albuminurie à heure fixe, ces deux affections nous paraissent essentiellement distinctes, en dépit de leur tendance commune à la guérison.

C'est ce qu'exprime très nettement notre collègue le Dr J. Renault (de Paris)[2], lorsqu'il propose de ranger en deux groupes les albuminuries cycliques, les unes dérivant, comme notre première malade, de la diathèse goutteuse marquant le début d'une néphrite goutteuse qui évoluera lentement, bien ou mal : les autres, indices d'une néphrite infectieuse susceptible ou non de guérir.

Nous n'entreprendrons pas ici de décrire l'albuminurie cyclique des adolescents déjà si bien étudiée par Pavy[3], par Teissier (de Lyon)[4], par Merley[5], nous contentant de poser la question de la nature des albuminuries cycliques.

S'agit-il dans ces cas de néphrite ou de pseudo-néphrite? Pour notre

---

1. Ce qui prouve que la station verticale n'a qu'une influence discutable dans l'albuminurie cyclique, c'est que les malades de Stirling et d'Arnozan (Congrès de médecine, 1896) continuaient à marcher l'après-midi. L'albuminurie reparaissait cependant avant que les sujets ne se remettent au lit.

2. Traité des maladies de l'enfance, par MM. GRANCHER, COMBY et MARFAN. — Album. et néphrites, par J. RENAUT, t. II. p. 287.

3. PAVY. Albuminuria in the apparent healty. Also *Med. Times* et *Gaz. London*, 1885 p. 529-551. Congr. Assoc. Britan. of Tardif. et *Lancet* London, 1885, p. 706 et 708. Cf. *Ind. medic.* 1885.

4. J. TEISSIER (de Lyon) in *Lyon médic.* 1887. p. 565.

5. MERLEY. Alb. intermitt. *Thèse de Lyon.* 1887.

excellent maître M. le D' Labadie-Lagrave, l'albuminurie cyclique, indépendante de toute maladie infectieuse, n'est pas une néphrite : c'est une maladie absolument à part, liée à l'évolution, à la croissance apyrétique, sans retentissement sur la santé, caractérisée par l'absence de cylindres rénaux, dans laquelle l'urotoxicité existe[1], qui guérit toujours, sans régime spécial, indépendante des néphrites cycliques infectieuses.

Pour tout dire en un mot, l'albuminurie cyclique de l'adolescence, suivant M. Labadie-Lagrave, est une pseudo-néphrite : notre maître est donc franchement dualiste et refuse toute comparaison entre cette pseudo-néphrite et les néphrites vraies.

Tout autre au contraire est l'opinion de MM. Lécorché et Talamon, qui en font une néphrite, et du D' Rendu, qui l'attribue à une néphrite partielle.

Enfin, plus éclectiques sont MM. Teissier (de Lyon), Arnozan (de Bordeaux) et Renault (de Paris), à l'opinion duquel nous croyons légitime de nous rallier.

Dans l'albuminurie cyclique proprement dite (obs. I), l'abondance des leucocytes renfermés dans l'urine semblerait plaider en faveur d'une fausse albuminurie dépendant plutôt d'une fluxion du rein, d'origine menstruelle, que d'une lésion rénale proprement dite.

OBS. I. — PERSONNELLE. — Albuminurie cyclique vespérale, d'abord quotidienne, plus tard intermittente, rappelée par les règles, par les marches forcées, par la fièvre typhoïde. — Amélioration progressive depuis deux ans.

La malade qui fait le sujet de cette observation, Mlle G. C.... avait douze ans lorsque nous fûmes appelé près d'elle pour la première fois en *décembre* 1898. Les antécédents héréditaires de Mlle G... sont très caractéristiques au point de vue arthritique et on peut à coup sûr la considérer comme atteinte d'albuminerie prégoutteuse. Son père est rhumatisant, souffre de coliques néphrétiques; sa grand'mère maternelle est franchement goutteuse. L'une de ses tantes est goutteuse; son jeune frère est atteint depuis son enfance d'une myélite dite rhumatismale avec déformations articulaires considérables des genoux et des doigts aujourd'hui complètement ankylosés.

Un seul de ses frères a succombé à des accidents urémiques consécutifs à une scarlatine méconnue.

Jusqu'à douze ans notre jeune malade n'a à son actif qu'une varicelle légère et une *céphalée frontale ou bipariétale continue* qui en 1897 et en 1898 s'accompagna de *troubles gastralgiques et dyspeptiques persistants.*

Les crises ayant plusieurs fois cédé au régime lacté, mais reparaissant

---

1. L'urotoxicité peut diminuer comme chez notre malade (Obs. I), mais cette diminution n'est pas toujours l'indice d'une néphrite. Elle peut aussi dépendre d'un défaut de production des toxines, lorsque l'alimentation (régime lacté par exemple) réduit celles-ci à leur minimum (D' Noël).

néanmoins, l'idée me vint d'examiner les urines moi-même le 9 *décembre* 1898 au soir. J'y trouvai des flots d'albumine.

Le lendemain matin 10 *décembre*, M. Desbruères, pharmacien de la famille C.... n'en trouvait pas.

Le soir du 10 *décembre*, nous en trouvions tous deux par tous les réactifs connus (acides picrique, acétique, nitrique, par la chaleur, par le réactif de Tanret, par l'acide trichloroacétique).

En versant dans un verre à expérience 15 grammes d'acide nitrique dans ces urines, il se précipitait un abondant dépôt de nitrate d'urée.

Pendant *dix jours* (du 9 au 15 *décembre*), la malade est maintenue au lit, au régime lacté strict, au traitement révulsif classique. — L'albumine paraît quand même de trois à sept heures du soir (0,20 à 0,50 centigrammes). — Elle cesse un jour, le 19 *décembre*. Pendant *quatre jours* (20 au 24 *décembre*), *époques des règles*, l'albumine reparaît l'après-midi *seulement*.

Les urines redeviennent abondantes (1000 gr.) aussitôt après la cessation des règles.

Du 25 *au* 31 *décembre* 1898, le régime lacté est repris intégralement, en raison de la réapparition de l'albumine pendant les règles.

Deux échantillons A et B d'urines sont adressés à M. Desbruères, pharmacien.

L'échantillon A a été recueilli *deux heures après le repas* (chocolat, œuf, biscuit, confitures).

L'échantillon B *trois heures après le lever*.

Ces deux échantillons renferment tous deux de l'albumine, mais en quantité sensible *élevée* dans l'échantillon B.

Au microscope, l'échantillon A ne renferme que des débris épithéliaux et très peu de leucocytes, enfin quelques cristaux d'oxalate de chaux.

L'échantillon B renferme des débris épithéliaux et *surtout des leucocytes en très grande quantité*. — Aucun cylindre ne peut être décelé dans l'échantillon B.

L'augmentation d'albumine dans l'échantillon B paraît due à la présence des leucocytes.

Les 26, 27, 28, 29 *décembre*, la malade se lève quand même à 5 heures de l'après-midi, tout en suivant le régime lacté. L'albumine ne reparaît plus le soir. Les urines sont même d'une extrême limpidité, ne se troublent pas à la chaleur, sont plutôt aqueuses et décolorées. Chose bizarre : le 30 *décembre*, sans changement de régime, l'urine redevient louche le matin, et le soir on constate 30 centigrammes d'albumine.

Année 1899. — *Du 1ᵉʳ au 9 janvier*, nous autorisons quelques aliments (œuf, biscottes, pain grillé, riz, farine d'orge, purées).

En même temps, nous laissons lever la malade jusqu'à midi.

L'après-midi, elle se remet au lit. Les urines du soir renferment presque tous les jours quelques flocons très nets d'albumine trois heures après le coucher.

Le 9 *janvier*, malgré le régime lacté, l'albumine reparaît le soir.

Du 9 *au* 15 *janvier*, Mlle Germaine C... est prise d'une telle intolérance gastrique qu'elle vomit le lait. Nous revenons au régime mixte (œufs cuits, bouillon de légume, biscotte).

Et pendant tout ce temps, elle reste au lit.

L'albumine cesse. Ce régime mitigé est bien toléré.

Le 15 *janvier*, elle se lève quelques heures. Le même jour les règles reparaissent.

Immédiatement l'*albumine vespérale* reparaît (0,50 centigr.).

Du 15 *au* 18 *janvier*, le régime des purées, œufs, chocolat, est repris le matin. Mlle G. se lève à deux heures. Elle n'a point d'albumine. De deux à sept heures, elle se lève; l'albumine (0,50 centigr.) reparaît quand elle se couche.

Du 19 *au* 24 *janvier*, nous ajoutons au régime alimentaire du bouillon, du fromage, de la crème, sans que l'albumine reparaisse.

Incidemment, je dois ajouter que la céphalée, la gastralgie ont disparu, et que nous n'avons jamais constaté de bruit de galop.

Le 24 *janvier*, sans aucune provocation, les urines de l'après-midi renferment 1 gramme d'albumine, avec débris épithéliaux et des cristaux d'oxalate d'urée.

Pour contrôler la perméabilité rénale, nous administrons à Mlle G. C... un cachet de bleu de méthylène (0,25 centigr.).

Pendant quatre jours la malade excrète des urines bleues, puis verdâtres, sans albumine. Le bleu a paru une demi-heure après l'ingestion.

Du 25 *au* 31 *janvier*, amélioration manifeste. L'albumine cesse, malgré un régime libéral (légumes, viandes blanches, bouillies), malgré des sorties.

Du 1er *au* 8 *février*, la malade sort, se lève, mange abondamment (viandes froides). Pas d'albumine, mais retour de la gastralgie et de la migraine que le régime lacté fait rapidement cesser.

9 *février*. Les règles reparaissent. L'albuminurie vespérale reparaît. Les urines sont très claires, non teintées de sang, recueillies après une toilette génitale.

Cette albuminurie *intermittente* n'a duré que vingt-quatre heures.

Du 9 *au* 20 *février*, l'albumine cesse malgré le régime animalisé, mais le 20 *février*, après une marche prolongée par un temps de brouillard, l'albuminurie reparaît le soir (1 gr. au moins).

Pendant trois jours, la malade persiste à sortir; l'albumine continue le soir (1 à 3 gr.).

Du 25 *au* 28 *février*, malgré des sorties quotidiennes, l'albumine cesse le soir.

Du 1er *au* 16 *mars*, pas d'albumine. Pour ralentir la fluxion menstruelle nous injectons cinq jours de suite une injection de chlorhydrate d'hydrastinine à 1/10e.

La dernière injection d'hydrastinine est pratiquée le 12 *mars*.

Néanmoins, du 18 *au* 20 *mars*, les règles reparaissent avec l'albuminurie vespérale (2, 3, 4 gr. dosés). Aucune trace d'albumine le matin.

L'analyse pratiquée à cette date (20 *mars*) par M. Desbruères signale l'existence de leucocytes, de cylindres hyalins et granuleux en petite quantité, et quelques débris épithéliaux dans l'échantillon présenté.

Le 24 *mars*, l'albumine disparaît *jusqu'au* 1er *avril* 1890

Ce jour-là, Germaine C... sort à midi. Rentre avec de l'albuminurie qui cesse le lendemain 2 *avril* jusqu'à six heures du soir et reparaît de huit à dix heures du soir.

Du 2 *au* 15 *avril*, notre jeune malade part en vacances à Villecresnes, s'y repose, s'y suralimente, sort l'après-midi, quelquefois le matin, reçoit même un jour une violente averse qui la transperce sans que l'albumine reparaisse.

Le 16 *avril*, Germaine C.... rentre à Paris : les règles reparaissent, l'albumine reparaît aussitôt.

Cette fois l'albumine (0.50 centigr. à 2 gr.) reparaît matin et soir, plus le soir (2 gr.) que le matin (1 gr.) du 16 *au* 25 *avril*, sans cause appréciable, sinon la date des époques menstruelles.

Du 16 *au* 30 *avril*, pas d'albumine.

Du 1ᵉʳ *au* 18 *mai*, l'albumine reparaît tous les soirs de quatre heures à dix heures du soir (0.50 à 1 gr.) et fait défaut tous les matins.

Elle cesse complètement *jusqu'au* 2 *juin*, alors que la malade s'alimente et prend même des douches froides pendant six jours, époque à laquelle les règles arrivent.

Le 5 *juin*, apparition des règles. Retour de l'albumine le matin (0.50 centigr.) et le soir (0.50 centigrammes à 2 grammes).

A dater de 15 *juin*, l'albumine devient de plus en plus rare. Elle reparaît une fois toutes les trois semaines (1 gr., 2 gr., 3 gr. ou 4 gr.). La céphalée a cessé. Seule la gastralgie reparaît assez souvent, au moindre excès de table. L'état général est bon. La jeune malade ne maigrit pas.

Du 6 *novembre au* 6 *décembre* 1899, on ne trouve que quelques centigrammes d'albumine tous les vingt jours.

Le 1ᵉʳ *janvier* 1900, traces passagères d'albumine, de loin en loin. L'enfant suit la vie commune.

Le 27 *janvier* 1900, brusquement, au cours d'une épidémie de grippe, Germaine C... est prise d'une violente céphalée, de douleurs intercostales et de fièvre (39°5, 40, 40°5), enfin de crises très aiguës d'entéro-côlite avec douleur, nausées, vomissements, diarrhée, adynamie, langue saburrale, rouge au bord, insomnies. — La température reste élevée matin et soir du 27 *au* 31 *janvier*.

Le séro-diagnostic est pratiqué le cinquième jour de la maladie par M. le Dʳ H. Jolly, chef de laboratoire à l'Hôtel-Dieu. L'épreuve du séro-diagnostic est négative, comme l'avait fait pressentir l'examen attentif du ventre, douleur localisée au côlon, ténesme et douleur rectale, selles glaireuses et sanguinolentes, absence de ballonnement du ventre). Le Dʳ H. Rendu, appelé en consultation, conseille chaque soir un suppositoire à l'extrait thébaïque (0.05), le matin l'entéroclyse, et le soir un grand bain tiède, la diète au lait glacé.

En quarante-huit heures, la fièvre tombe à 39°.

1ᵉʳ et 2 *février* 1900. — Mais en même temps, et *sous l'influence combinée des règles de l'hyperthermie et de l'entéro-côlite*, l'albumine reparaît (0.80 centigr., Desbruères).

Le 5 *février*, l'albumine disparaissait définitivement, la température restait cependant à 38° le matin et le soir, la diarrhée s'installait, le ventre se ballonnait, l'insomnie se prononçait.

Bref le séro-diagnostic, répété le 21 *février* par le Dʳ Jolly, affirmait cette fois l'existence d'une fièvre typhoïde avec agglutination des bacilles au contact du sang de la malade.

Le 5 *avril* 1900, nous revoyons Mlle G. C... guérie de sa fièvre typhoïde, sans retour d'albuminurie même à l'époque de ses dernières règles.

Pendant les mois d'*avril, mai, juin* 1900, l'analyse des urines est renouvelée deux fois par semaine, sans que l'albumine reparaisse, même pendant les époques menstruelles.

Mais la céphalée reparaît presque continuellement. Aussi la remettons-nous le 8 juillet au régime du lait.

Le 12 *juillet* 1900, l'urine de l'après-midi renferme encore un louche d'albumine.

Ce même jour, nous prions M. Labadie-Lagrave de vouloir bien nous permettre de rechercher à son laboratoire le pouvoir urotoxique de Mlle C....

L'expérience, pratiquée très gracieusement par M. le D' Noë, chef de laboratoire du D' Labadie-Lagrave, a fourni les résultats suivants qu'a bien voulu nous consigner M. le D' Noë dans la note ci-jointe :

Poids du lapin inoculé.	1750 grammes.	
Nombre de centimètres cubes d'urine injectée.	55 cent. cubes.	
Urotoxicité par kilogramme d'animal.	41	—
Quantité d'urine fournie par la malade en 24 h.	600	—
Poids intoxiqué en 24 heures.	14 kilogrammes.	
Poids de la malade.	65	—
Coefficient urotoxique.. . . . . = 0,222		

Donc diminution de la toxicité de ces urines d'environ de moitié, soit par défaut d'élimination des toxines, soit par défaut de production du fait du régime alimentaire insuffisant (Noë).

Le 1er *août* 1900, la malade a présenté dans l'après-midi un nuage d'albumine.

Sa santé se maintient assez bonne.

Elle continue à prendre sous notre surveillance son auto-observation.

Cette observation peut se résumer en quelques mots :

1° L'albuminurie toujours vespérale, sauf en avril 1899, a paru au début influencée par le régime lacté qui a en même temps modifié la céphalée et la gastralgie ; celles-ci, reparaissant en dehors de l'albuminurie, peuvent être considérées comme liées soit à l'arthritisme, soit aux toxines dues à la dyspepsie elle-même et incomplètement éliminées par le rein.

2° L'albuminurie a reparu très nettement et très périodiquement pendant six ou huit mois sous l'influence des règles.

3° Quelquefois elle a coïncidé avec des marches exagérées.

4° Elle nous a paru indépendante des influences atmosphériques. Ni le froid humide, ni les douches froides ne l'ont réveillée.

5° Le régime à partir du deuxième mois n'a plus eu aucune influence sur le syndrome, sauf sur les troubles dyspeptiques.

6° Les affections fébriles intermittentes ont rappelé très nettement, mais très passagèrement, l'albuminurie.

7° Celle-ci, non rétractile, paraît liée à la profusion des leucocytes trouvés dans les urines, celles-ci renfermant aussi des débris épithéliaux, des cristaux d'oxalate d'urée, mais pas de cylindres, et le rein resta perméable au bleu de méthylène.

8° L'arthritisme, la goutte comme causes prédisposantes, la fluxion menstruelle et l'âge adolescent sont les seuls facteurs appréciables de cette fluxion rénale qui manifestement évolue vers la guérison, mais qui est rappelée par les pyrexies aiguës, et pourrait plus tard se réveiller en cas de grossesse. — Sans une hygiène très sévère, très prolongée, absolument nécessaire pour la guérison, le mariage ne doit pas être conseillé.

OBS. II. — Albuminurie cyclique consécutive à une fièvre typhoïde.

L'observation suivante, que nous devons à l'obligeance de notre excellent confrère le D⁰ L. Bagot (de Saint-Pol-de-Léon), se rapproche de la précédente par sa périodicité, par l'influence absolument nulle du régime par sa tendance spontanée à la guérison.

Toutefois elle en diffère par son origine manifestement infectieuse, par l'influence nulle de la station à genoux, enfin par sa relation évidente avec le froid aux pieds.

Voici, résumée, cette très intéressante observation.

Au mois de juin 1897, le fils aîné de notre confrère est atteint, à l'âge de douze ans, d'une fièvre typhoïde grave, avec rechute durant deux mois et s'accompagnant d'hématuries permanentes pendant les deux premières semaines de chaque reprise de la fièvre typhoïde. La convalescence dure trois mois pendant lesquels l'albuminurie, parue après l'hématurie, va toujours en décroissant et devient imperceptible.

Novembre 1897. — Une angine commune avec hyperthermie (40°) s'accompagne d'une nouvelle hématurie. L'albuminurie reparaît, persiste quelques semaines, devient nettement intermittente.

Chaque matin l'albumine manque au réveil. En d'autres termes, les urines de la nuit sont normales. Malgré la vivacité de l'enfant, qui joue de sept à huit heures, l'albumine ne reparaît jamais qu'au retour de la classe, c'est-à-dire de dix à onze heures et demie du matin. Jamais elle n'apparaît après le repas du matin ou de midi, sauf après l'ingestion de blancs d'œufs.

L'albuminurie ne paraît de dix à onze heures et demie que de temps en temps, lorsque l'enfant a froid aux pieds. Jamais elle n'a reparu pendant une série de bains de mer pris pendant l'été de 1898.

En hiver, pendant la saison froide, en 1898, l'enfant a été repris d'albuminurie périodique le matin, à l'heure de la messe. Si l'enfant reste assis, l'albuminurie manque, s'il se met à genoux, elle apparaît. Elle cesse dans la station verticale.

Bien plus, l'exercice modéré semble la faire disparaître.

En résumé, le froid est le seul agent qui rappelle, avec certaines attitudes, l'albuminurie cyclique du malade de M. le Dr Bagot.

Le régime lacté strict n'a jamais modifié l'albuminurie. Aussi le jeune sujet a-t-il été mis au régime commun (potage, viande, légumes, œufs, farineux, etc.)

Nous avons, au début de ce travail, exposé les opinions en apparence contradictoires des auteurs sur l'albuminurie cyclique des adolescents. Ces divergences résultent de ce que certains auteurs ont mis en parallèle des faits dissemblables.

L'albuminurie cyclique de Pavy en effet, type rare à l'état de pureté, c'est-à-dire idiopathique, bénigne, sans fièvre primitive, n'est pas une néphrite pour M. Labadie-Lagrave. — Elle peut pourtant, croyons-nous, y aboutir, comme le prouve la réapparition de l'albuminurie au cours de la fièvre typhoïde, des amygdalites, des affections fébriles en général.

L'albuminurie permanente compliquant les maladies infectieuses peut à son tour devenir cyclique et, comme la maladie de Pavy, tendre à la guérison, éventualité fréquente dans les néphrites les plus banales : mais on n'est en droit d'affirmer la guérison que longtemps après.

En tout état de cause, la périodicité dans ces albuminuries infectieuses n'est qu'un trait de ressemblance avec la maladie cyclique de Pavy, spéciale et dont la survie est très prolongée. Pavy cite des cas où l'albuminurie resta périodique jusqu'à quarante-trois ans.

C'est alors vraisemblablement que la méconnaissance de cette variété clinique d'albuminurie peut aboutir à la néphrite partielle.

Mais, pour éviter une confusion regrettable, nous croyons nécessaire de réserver à ces troubles périodiques du rein le nom d'albuminurie cyclique, de préférence au terme impropre d'albuminurie intermittente, qui s'applique à toutes les néphrites en voie de guérison.

ALBUMINURIES INTERMITTENTES DES JEUNES SUJETS

par M. le docteur H. GILLET

Je ne me dissimule pas les difficultés que soulève à l'heure actuelle la question des albuminuries intermittentes.

Aussi n'aurai-je pas la témérité de prendre un tel sujet de communication et de le développer devant vous, sans demander au préalable toute votre bienveillante indulgence.

Faute de pièce anatomo-pathologique, que je ne puis fournir pas plus que tout autre, tout un chapitre reste forcément en suspens. Le champ est libre à toutes les hypothèses; aussi les théories ne manquent pas.

Ce serait, à mon avis, besogne stérile de nous évertuer à diriger nos efforts de ce côté, puisque nous ne pouvons pas discuter sur des faits palpables, mais seulement sur des déductions.

Dans l'espérance d'acquisitions attendues dans le domaine de l'anatomie pathologique, nous pouvons nous contenter de chercher par l'analyse et la critique des faits à nous faire une opinion basée sur la stricte observation. Mais en tout cas, il est possible dès aujourd'hui d'envisager les albuminuries intermittentes dans leur ensemble en ce qui concerne l'observation clinique et l'analyse urologique.

C'est ce que j'ai l'intention de faire devant vous.

Les matériaux sur lesquels je m'appuierai se composent d'une série de 16 observations, dont quelques-unes se rapportent à des sujets suivis depuis plusieurs années, 7 ans pour quelques-uns.

Dans 5 ou 6 cas, les analyses d'urine ont pu être fréquemment renouvelées et le plus souvent sans interruption, par périodes de 4 ou 5 jours et même 15 jours plusieurs mois de suite.

On en trouvera les détails complets dans une publication en cours dans les *Annales de la policlinique de Paris*[1].

C'est donc plutôt des documents qu'une théorie que je me permets de vous offrir.

Définition. — D'abord une définition : l'albuminurie est dite intermittente, par opposition à l'albuminurie continue, quand l'albumine n'existe dans l'urine qu'à certains moments de la journée et pas à d'autres.

Sous le nom d'*albuminurie intermittente*, on doit donc comprendre une albuminurie plus ou moins quotidienne, tout au moins par période, mais ne se produisant seulement que *pendant une fraction de temps de la journée*, au lieu de durer pendant tout le cours de la journée et même de la nuit comme dans l'*albuminurie continue*.

Dans cette dernière la quantité d'albumine peut varier dans de très larges limites durant la journée et la nuit, mais il y en a toujours dans l'urine à quelque moment qu'on l'examine.

Lorsque l'albuminurie ne se présente qu'à long intervalle, plusieurs jours, surtout des semaines, des mois, elle est alors dite passagère,

---

1. H. GILLET. Albuminuries intermittentes des jeunes sujets. *Annales de la Policlinique de Paris* (janvier, février, mars, mai, juin, juillet, août 1900 et à suivre), J.-B. BAILLIÈRE, édit., 1901.

transitoire. Elle peut être dans ces conditions ou continue, c'est-à-dire durer toute une journée, ce qui est rare, ou intermittente, mais elle n'est pas forcément intermittente.

Une albuminurie continue, mais qui manque à certains jours ne devrait pas être confondue avec l'albuminurie intermittente.

Enfin on réserve le nom d'*accidentelle* à toute albuminurie qui n'apparaît qu'une fois par hasard et qu'on ne peut plus retrouver ensuite.

Inutile d'ajouter d'autres signes distinctifs, comme l'absence de cylindres, quoique le plus souvent vraie, et surtout l'absence de lésions rénales, puisqu'on n'a aucune preuve de ce dernier fait sur lequel on discute, et que le contraire contient peut-être la vérité.

DIAGNOSTIC. — *Nécessité absolue de l'examen fractionné systématique de l'urine.*

La notion même d'intermittence entraîne avec elle l'obligation de l'*examen fractionné des urines*, c'est-à-dire la recherche de l'albumine effectuée non sur l'urine globale ou mélangée des 24 heures, mais l'analyse faite à part pendant un jour et une nuit de l'urine émise au cours des mictions échelonnées, pour la pratique sur les quantités émises pendant la matinée, la journée, la soirée, la nuit. En tout 4 échantillons, pour simplifier, si l'on veut, 3, matinée, journée et soirée, nuit.

Sans l'examen fractionné on passe forcément à côté des albuminuries intermittentes. On peut présumer à ce sujet qu'elles sont plus fréquentes qu'on ne le suppose.

On pourrait croire qu'on se fût mis dans de bonnes conditions d'examen et qu'il fût suffisant de recueillir les urines des 24 heures et de rechercher dans le mélange par l'examen global la présence de l'albumine, et au seul cas où l'on en trouverait, de procéder ensuite à l'examen fractionné.

Ce serait une erreur de pratique très préjudiciable à l'établissement d'un bon diagnostic.

Sans l'examen fractionné systématique, on ne peut être sûr de ne pas laisser inaperçue l'albuminurie intermittente.

Si l'on trouve de l'albumine dans l'urine mélangée des 24 heures, on ne sait si cette albumine est ou n'est pas intermittente. Il faut faire une recherche qu'on aurait évitée si l'on avait commencé par faire l'examen fractionné.

Si l'on n'en trouve pas, on ne peut même pas affirmer qu'il n'y en a pas à un moment donné. En effet, il peut y avoir une faible quantité d'albumine dans un temps très limité. Cette urine albumineuse est perdue au milieu de l'urine non albumineuse du reste des 24 heures. La limite de sensibilité des réactifs ne permet plus de la déceler. Nous avons vérifié à maintes reprise la possibilité de cette erreur et nous y avons insisté[1].

Il faut de plus *examiner plusieurs jours de suite et à plusieurs reprises*, pour éviter de tomber sur un moment où l'albuminurie s'arrête.

Quand on s'astreint à ces prescriptions on trouve que les albuminuries intermittentes sont très fréquentes chez les jeunes sujets.

Syndrome urologique dans les albuminuries intermittentes. — S'il règne encore une certaine obscurité sur l'état physiologique et surtout anatomique du rein chez les sujets atteints d'albuminurie intermittente, l'ensemble des constatations, tant cliniques qu'urologiques, semblent cependant dès maintenant permettre une vue d'ensemble sur ce syndrome.

En effet, bien que très diverses étiologiquement, bien que d'origines variées, les albuminuries intermittentes rentrent assez bien dans un cadre urologique commun.

Dans le syndrome urinaire l'albuminurie ne représente qu'un épisode d'un cycle, dont on retrouve au moins la trace, même dans les cas les moins typiques.

La majorité des albuminuries intermittentes semblent ainsi cycliques.

L'évolution complète de ce *cycle urologique* comprend une succession de phases ou *crises* qu'on peut ainsi résumer :

Cycle
- *crise minérale.* . . . { excès de carbonates } isolés ou / excès de phosphates } associés.
- *crise chromogène* . . { excès d'uroérythrine. / UROBILINE. / indican.
- *crise albuminurique.*
- *crise azotée.* . . . . . . { excès d'acide urique. / excès d'urée.

C'est, en somme, à quelques détails près, le cycle déjà si bien décrit par M. le professeur J. Teissier (de Lyon), qu'on retrouve assez net dans les cas typiques, plus fruste, seulement esquissé dans d'autres.

L'ordre de succession des crises ne subit pas d'interversion, mais elle admet des empiétements et des lacunes.

C'est ici un schéma général. De plus il ne faut pas croire à un excès

1. H. Gillet. Société médico-chirurgicale, janvier 1900.

vrai, mais seulement apparent par alcalinité (phosphates), par concentration (urée).

Remarque importante, ce n'est pas l'albuminurie qui se montre la plus constante, il semble que ce soit l'urobilinurie surtout, peut-être aussi l'excès d'uroérythrine. A certains jours la crise albuminurique peut manquer, la crise chromogène fait rarement défaut.

Autres caractères des albuminuries intermittentes : 1° *influence, positive très manifeste de la station debout et surtout de la marche* et de l'ascension sur la production de l'albuminurie au bout d'un temps ou très court ou un peu plus prolongé.

D'une façon générale, l'albuminurie intermittente n'est pas nocturne. L'urine de la nuit ne contient pas d'albumine.

Dans deux observations que nous avons publiées, cette règle semble infirmée. Il n'y a qu'apparence de contradiction. Il s'agit de deux cas absolument spéciaux. Dans l'un c'est une fillette de 7 ans 1/2 qui, dans la période de desquamation de la scarlatine, présente dans l'urine de la nuit une quantité infime d'albumine, probablement de la nucléo-albumine. L'autre cas montre une albuminurie tout accidentelle, d'un seul jour de durée, chez une fillette de 13 ans, au moment d'un érythème survenu 15 jours après une injection de sérum antidiphtérique.

Tout à fait exceptionnellement, on voit de l'albuminurie nocturne chez des sujets à albuminurie diurne habituelle, mais le nombre en est infime et en tout cas leur albuminurie est si régulièrement diurne, un nombre de fois si considérable qu'on peut tout au plus noter l'irrégularité qui parfois a sa raison particulière.

C'est après le lever, après la marche qu'on voit naître l'ALBUMINURIE INTERMITTENTE. Elle EST DONC DANS LA GRANDE MAJORITÉ DES CAS ORTHOSTATIQUE.

Il semble qu'il n'y ait pas nécessité absolue de décrire à part les albuminuries orthostatiques, dont la station debout serait la seule et unique raison efficiente nécessaire et suffisante.

Qu'il y ait quelques cas, rares, au dire même des auteurs, qui répondent à ces conditions et pour lesquels aucune autre cause ne puisse être invoquée, c'est possible ; cela ne veut pas dire, peut-être, qu'il n'y en ait pas une plus ou moins cachée.

Pour notre part, dans les faits que nous avons observés, nous n'avons pas vu d'albuminuries orthostatiques réellement pures ou du moins qui méritent ce nom.

Du reste, orthostatiques, on pourrait presque dire que les albuminuries intermittentes le sont toutes, par ce seul fait que même celles qui persistent le plus pendant le jour, s'interrompent, malgré tout, la nuit.

Comme moment d'apparition dans la journée, l'albuminurie intermittente affecte des heures un peu différentes selon les sujets. Chez les uns, c'est le type matinal qui prédomine, matinal précoce, très rapidement après le lever, matinal tardif après quelques heures. Chez d'autres, on observe un type diurne, très rarement vespéral.

Parfois, il y a deux périodes d'albuminurie, une matinale, une diurne ou vespérale, coupées par une période intermédiaire dans laquelle l'urine reste exempte d'albumine.

Il est probable que cette absence d'albumine intercalée entre deux crises albuminuriques coïncide avec la position assise prise pendant le repas, qui provoque la fin du cycle urinaire.

Dans certains cas, on remarque une certaine fixité dans l'heure d'apparition de l'albuminurie, d'où la dénomination de *cyclique*; mais cette heure se déplace. Ce n'est qu'une fixité relative, par périodes de temps plus ou moins longues.

Toutes les combinaisons paraissent du reste possibles. 2º *Influence négative encore plus manifeste de la position horizontale*, moindre de la position assise, par conséquent urine de la nuit, urine des malades au lit, et malgré la fièvre d'une maladie intercurrente sans albumine.

A titre d'exemple, voici un fait pris entre d'autres :

19 jours consécutifs une petite albuminurique intermittente est maintenue au lit avec de la fièvre à 40º passés pour une angine folliculaire, qui se complique d'otite externe suppurée. Pendant ces 19 jours consécutifs l'examen fractionné des urines est pratiqué, soit en tout sur 52 échantillons, 2 fois seulement et le même jour (25 février) il fut possible de déceler un peu d'albumine donnant un précipité et par la chaleur avec addition d'acide acétique et par l'acide azotique, 8 fois l'acide nitrique ne donnait lieu à aucun louche, tandis que la chaleur et l'acide acétique provoquaient un très léger trouble.

Si la station verticale, surtout avec marche, possède une puissance provocatrice indéniable, la position horizontale montre un pouvoir d'arrêt encore plus actif.

Malgré l'attitude debout et la déambulation, les malades peuvent ne pas avoir d'albumine dans leur urine. C'est ce qui arrive vers la soirée ; passé 5 à 6 heures ou plus tard, très rarement plus tôt, l'albuminurie non apparue n'apparaît plus ou cesse si elle a existé. Elle peut cependant réapparaître si on prolonge la veille avant dans la nuit, exception qui confirme la règle, car c'est recommencer une nouvelle journée, en faisant de la nuit le jour. L'albuminurie existante cesse donc, l'agent provocateur, la verticalité, persistant.

Un nombre assez grand de sujets n'ont pas d'albuminurie quotidienne, mais par séries de jours coupés de séries de jours sans albumine.

Par contre, il suffit de faire coucher, même parfois asseoir le sujet, pour qu'au bout d'un temps variable, mais cependant relativement court, l'urine ait cessé d'être albumineuse.

Par le cubitus, on est le maître absolu de commander à l'albumine de disparaître.

La force inhibitrice l'emporte manifestement sur la force provocatrice.

L'influence négative de la position horizontale ne semble même pas pouvoir être contre-balancée par les efforts musculaires, même par les mouvements des membres inférieurs, semblables à ceux de la marche.

D'autres influences peuvent exister, froid, règles, fatigues, émotions, mais il faut en plus la verticalité.

Déjà M. Pierre Marie[1] a signalé le fait. A celles de nos petites malades que nous avons soumises au repos forcé plus ou moins prolongé, nous avons toujours recommandé de faire de la gymnastique dans leur lit. L'urine excrétée au moment de ces exercices ne contenait pas d'albumine.

Il n'en serait pas de même pour les mouvements provoqués par la faradisation des muscles, d'après une observation publiée par MM. Ch. Achard et Lœper[2].

L'albuminurie contenue dans l'urine est de la sérine, parfois mélangée à la globuline, quelquefois c'est de la nucléo-albumine.

Il ne faut pas limiter les investigations à la seule constatation de l'albumine et de ses causes apparentes.

L'examen de l'urine peut encore nous fournir quelques données sur l'état fonctionnel du rein et sur l'état général du sujet.

1° Il y a dans la majorité des faits OLIGURIE manifeste. Cette oligurie coïncide chronologiquement avec le moment d'apparition de l'albuminurie, mais elle est encore en rapport plus intime avec la station verticale et la marche, car elle peut exister dans ces conditions avant que l'albumine n'apparaisse et même sans albuminurie aucune.

C'est donc un *phénomène plus constant que l'albuminurie*.

La *statistique urinaire* est *intervertie*; le sujet urine par heure moins le jour que la nuit.

1. PIERRE MARIE. De l'albuminurie cyclique (*Semaine médicale*, 5 février 1896).
2. CH. ACHARD et LŒPER. Albuminurie orthostatique (Société médicale des hôpitaux, Paris, 22 juin 1900).

Parfois, malgré cette oligurie diurne, il y a *polyurie paradoxale*, parce que les urines de la nuit et celles de la position horizontale compensent au delà le déficit des urines du jour et de la station debout.

2° Dans les mêmes conditions d'orthostatisme il y a *urobilinurie* et CETTE UROBILINURIE ORTHOSTATIQUE PEUT EXISTER AVEC L'OLIGURIE SANS ALBUMINURIE.

L'orthostatisme provoque donc d'abord l'oligurie et l'urobilinurie, avant de faire naître l'albuminurie, il peut même n'aboutir qu'à l'oligurie et qu'à l'urobilinurie sans albuminurie.

C'est pourquoi l'on pourrait peut-être, sans trop de paradoxe, dire des albuminuries intermittentes qu'elles devraient être considérées comme des *urobilinuries avec albuminurie*.

Cette mise à un second plan relatif de l'albuminurie semble légitimée par les résultats donnés par l'exploration de la perméabilité rénale.

J'ai signalé[1] les particularités présentées dans deux cas soumis à l'épreuve du bleu. La matière colorante se présenta bien en temps voulu dans l'urine à peu près comme à l'état normal, mais elle n'en disparut pas aussi vite que chez les sujets sains et cette prolongation avait lieu par poussées intermittentes.

Contre mes expériences, on pouvait soulever quelques objections : 1° la forte dose employée, 20 centigrammes au lieu de 5, dose habituellement usitée; 2° la nature de la matière colorante, bleu de méthyle, au lieu de bleu de méthylène.

Mais la question vient d'être reprise et l'expérience renouvelée dans toute sa rigueur avec le bleu de méthylène à dose convenable, par MM. Ch. Achard et Lœper[2].

Chez la jeune fille, sujet de l'observation et soumise à l'épreuve, le bleu se montrait au bout d'une demi-heure, mais son excrétion se prolongeait de 5 à 7 jours.

En plus de cette vérification, nous devons retenir la remarque importante signalée par les auteurs, que cet état de la perméabilité rénale restait le même et pendant les périodes où l'albuminurie existait et pendant celles où elle faisait défaut.

L'albuminurie à elle seule ne donne donc pas la note de l'état du fonctionnement rénal insuffisant.

A côté du passage intermittent de la matière bleue injectée expérimen-

---

1. H. GILLET. Albuminuries intermittentes des jeunes sujets. perméabilité rénale *Annales de la Policlinique de Paris*. mars 1898).

2. CH. ACHARD et LŒPER. Albuminurie orthostatique (Société médicale des hopitaux. 22 juin 1900).

talement, on peut noter la variabilité extrême dans la couleur de l'urine.

En dehors des variations de colorations habituelles on remarque parfois dans les albuminuries intermittentes une véritable intermittence dans la teinte de l'urine qui passe rapidement du jaune foncé au jaune pâle.

Il est arrivé une fois qu'on m'a présenté des urines tellement incolores, qu'on les aurait prises pour l'eau à peine blanchie par un peu d'orgeat. J'ai dû rechercher l'existence de l'urée pour me convaincre qu'on ne m'avait pas trompé.

Il s'agissait d'un jeune garçon de 11 ans, atteint de fièvre typhoïde grave en octobre 1891 et que j'ai vu pour une albuminurie intermittente irrégulière de mai 1892 jusqu'en août 1895.

A noter encore l'existence fréquente de mucus.

L'absence de cylindres ou tout au moins de cylindre granuleux se vérifie dans la plupart des examens.

De l'examen urologique nous pouvons de plus tirer des renseignements qui nous instruisent sur l'état de la nutrition.

Déjà, Pavy avait noté l'*oxalurie*: M. Alb. Robin a décrit une albuminurie avec *phosphaturie*.

Les urines donnent une réaction à peine acide, même alcaline à l'émission. La *toxicité urinaire*, d'après J. Teissier, est *augmentée*.

Comme lui j'ai noté l'*aspect graisseux* de ces urines. Parfois, en s'altérant, elles ont plutôt une *odeur de putréfaction* que d'ammoniaque; le fait semblait très net dans une de mes observations.

L'*urée baisse* de quantité.

Cette baisse peut être notable, aussi un de nos malades, adulte de 56 ans, voit en mars 1896 son urée à 21 gr. 50, en juin seulement 15 gr. 56. Ce sujet avait bien antérieurement 26 grammes et même 52 grammes par jour.

Le *coefficient azoturique abaissé* témoigne du trouble nutritif général. Dans les albuminuries digestives de M. Alb. Robin il y aura plutôt élévation du coefficient. Dans deux observations où nous avons fait l'analyse l'abaissement descendait à 79,97 chez une fillette de 11 ans, et chez un adulte de 56 ans même à 58,85 et remontait à 78 après une cure à Saint-Nectaire.

Clinique. — A ces constatations urologiques correspond une histoire clinique.

D'une façon générale on peut faire trois classes dans les observations.

Dans une première catégorie l'albuminurie intermittente constitue une surprise. Le sujet a les apparences de santé satisfaisante. C'est le type Pavy, Teissier, Heubner.

C'est, si l'on veut bien fouiller l'examen, une rareté.

On découvre le plus souvent quelque tare sous roche.

Un second groupe comprend toute une variété d'individus qui présentent quelques symptômes variables. C'est le plus grand nombre. Pour eux, on pense aux diagnostics d'anémie, de lymphatisme, de nervosisme, de neurasthénie vague, de dyspepsie légère et diverse, de troubles de croissance, de neuro-arthritisme, etc. En somme, troubles fonctionnels vagues, diagnostic vague.

En tout cas rien ne cadre avec une affection quelconque des reins.

Il n'en est pas de même de quelques sujets, qui forment la troisième série chez lesquels on constate quelques symptômes, qu'on rencontre dans les néphrites, céphalée, œdème léger, fugace, localisé surtout à la face, aux paupières, pas d'œdème tibial, douleurs lombaires, bouffées de chaleur, etc.

Il n'y a rien de plus, en général, pas de bruit de galop, même après course, parfois un peu d'irrégularité cardiaque.

Par contre on constate assez souvent un *pouls* un peu *ralenti*, mais surtout une *pression basse*, comme J. Teissier l'a déjà fait remarquer et comme je l'ai vérifié.

Mais en somme, manifestations morbides minimes.

ÉTIOLOGIE. — On note l'hérédité dans certains cas; dans une observation la mère avait eu de l'éclampsie à la naissance de l'enfant (observation 10): on relève aussi des antécédents nerveux et arthritiques des jeunes sujets, etc.

Dans nos observations, à côté de ces conditions étiologiques, nous avons trouvé d'une façon presque constante l'INFECTION OU L'INTOXICATION, COMME A L'ORIGINE DES NÉPHRITES. De sorte qu'on pourrait dresser la classification suivante des albuminuries intermittentes :

1° des néphrites
- initiale.
- résiduale, cicatricielle (1 obs. personnelle).

2° des infections
- scarlatineuse (4 obs. pers. dont 1 ? poitrine).
- diphtérique (1 obs. pers. ? nocturne).
- typhique (1 obs. pers.).
- rubéolique (1 obs. pers.).
- ourlienne (1 obs. pers.).
- choréique (1 obs. pers.).
- grippale (1 obs. pers.).
- syphilitique.
- tuberculeuse, prétuberculeuse (J. Teissier).
- blennorragique.
- impaludique.

N° D'ORDRE	ÉTIOLOGIE	CARACTÈRE			SEXE	DÉBUT PROBABLE	DURÉE	GUÉRISON	STATIONNAIRE	AGGRAVATION
		DIURNE	NOCTURNE	ORTHOSTATIQUE						
1	Néphrite	Diurne.		Orthostatique.	F	A 7 ans 1 2.	-		Amélioré après 4 ans.	
2	Scarlatine (desquamat.)		Nocturne.		F	Id.	8 jours?	Guérie.		
5	Post scarlatine . . .	Id.		Id.	H	A 15 ans.	?	?		
4	Id.	Id.		Id.	F	A 6 ans 1 2.	2 mois?	Guérie.		
5	Diphtérie éryth. séroth.		Id.		F	A 15 ans.	1 jour?	Guérie.		
6	F. typhoïde	Id.		Id.	H	A 12 ans.	?	?	Non revu.	
7	Rougeole	Id.		Id.	F	A 11 ans.	5 ans?	Guérie.		
8	Oreillons	Id.		Id.	F	A 7 ans 1 2.	"		Récidive après 7 ans.	
9	Chorée	Id.		Id.	F	A 10 ans 1 2.	"		Stationnaire après 5 ans 5 4	
10	Post grippal, etc. .	Id.		Id.	H	A 9 ans.	"	"	Vu récemment.	
11	Infections multiples.	Id.		Id.	F	A 11 ans.	"		Non revu.	
12	Id.	Id.		Id.	H	A 12 ans.	"		Stationnaire?	
15	Arthritique	Id.		Id.	H	A 44 ans.	4 mois?	Guéri.		
14	Dyspeptique	Id.		Id.	H	A 12 ans.	1 mois?	Guéri.		
15	Id.	Id.	Id.	Id.	F	A 15 ans 1 2.	1 jour?	Guéri.		
16	Dyspepsie, surmenage	Id.		Id.	H	A 56 ans.	"		Très amélioré après 5 ans.	

3° des diathèses \ arthritique } cyclique des jeunes sujets.
et dyscrasies / prégoutteuse (1 obs. pers.).
diabétique.

4° des auto-in-
toxications
{ dyspeptique (5 obs. pers.).
hépatique, cirrhotique.
chlorotique, chlorobrightisme (Dieulafoy).
nerveuse, surmenage \ physique { soldats. cyclistes.
intellectuel.

5° des intoxica-
tions.
{ saturnisme.
morphinisme. etc.

DURÉE. MARCHE. — Les albuminuries intermittentes peuvent se prolonger non seulement des mois, mais des années. Nous avons en observation des sujets depuis 5 et même 7 ans.

L'albuminurie intermittente peut persister sous forme quotidienne, mais souvent il y a accalmies, il y a des périodes avec albuminurie et des périodes sans albuminurie qu'il ne faut pas escompter comme guérison.

Il peut. rarement peut-être, se faire des récidives. Dans un cas d'albuminurie intermittente décelé à la suite des oreillons, j'ai vu une récidive 7 ans après avoir pensé pouvoir considérer la petite malade comme guérie.

PRONOSTIC. — Sauf la durée, parfois très longue, puisqu'on cite des albuminuries intermittentes remontant à 30 ou 40 ans, le pronostic, *quoad vitam* tout au moins, semble bénin.

Il ressort, du reste, de ce fait, qu'on n'a pas de pièces anatomiques à montrer. donc qu'il n'y a pas d'autopsie de ce chef, donc pas de mortalité.

Reste le point noir de l'avenir rénal du sujet.

Ici, il y a des pessimistes et des optimistes.

Il paraît difficile de faire un pronostic général tout d'un bloc. *Il y a des albuminuries intermittentes et non une albuminurie intermittente.* Toutes les circonstances particulières à chaque cas doivent être prises en considération.

On doit tenir en ligne de compte l'âge, la rapidité d'apparition de l'albumine. sa quantité, la durée de la crise albuminurique, le type quotidien ou plus éloigné de l'intermittence, la durée antérieure. la modalité de réaction chimique, la perméabilité rénale, l'état général, le coefficient azoturique. l'urobilisme, la nature étiologique.

On doit être réservé dans son diagnostic de guérison, et avant de le formuler il faut exiger la disparition de l'albuminurie depuis plusieurs mois constatée par des examens fractionnés répétés par périodes de 3 à 4 jours de suite, au besoin de toute une semaine.

Tant qu'il y aura de l'urobilinurie, un coefficient azoturique bas, il faudra se tenir sur ses gardes.

De ces 16 cas, 2 sont à mettre à part, le n° 2 et le n° 5. Le n° 2 appartient à une fillette qui n'eut que dans l'urine de la nuit une quantité infime d'albumine, probablement de la nucléo-albumine, pendant la desquamation de sa scarlatine.

Le n° 5 provient d'une autre fillette de 15 ans qui n'eut qu'une seule fois, la nuit, un peu d'albumine, au cours d'un érythème survenu 15 jours après une injection de sérum antidiphtérique.

Le tableau suivant résume le résultat de nos observations personnelles.

ÉTAT DU REIN. — Ici, il n'y a la place que pour l'hypothèse.

Toutefois, si l'on considère en dehors de l'albuminurie, les autres facteurs du fonctionnement rénal, l'oligurie avec renversement de la statique urinaire, la perméabilité rénale intermittente, en dehors même des légers symptômes rénaux présentés par quelques malades, l'urobilinurie même et l'indicanurie, on arrive à penser qu'il n'y a pas un simple trouble fonctionnel. Il y a lésion du rein, lésion infime, si l'on veut, curable aussi le plus souvent, mais lésion pas moins. Ce n'est pas, si l'on veut, une néphrite, mais il est à présumer que l'épithélium glomérulaire, tout au moins, peut-être aussi pour une petite part, celui des tubuli, n'a pas son intégrité absolue.

Si la fonction fait l'organe, à fonction troublée, organe altéré.

TRAITEMENT. — Cet état présumé du rein doit nous guider dans le traitement et crée une première indication, en dehors de la cause (dyspepsie, infection, arthritisme etc.).

Mais dans l'albuminurie intermittente, il faut voir au delà du symptôme rénal, au delà surtout du seul symptôme albuminurie.

Il faut voir du côté du trouble, parfois profond de la nutrition générale, du côté du foie, du tube digestif, du système nerveux et circulatoire.

Du côté du foie et du tube digestif, nous y invitent l'urobilinurie, l'indicanurie, la toxicité urinaire augmentée, l'abaissement du chiffre de l'urée, du coefficient azoturique. Du côté du système circulatoire et du système nerveux, le ralentissement du pouls, l'abaissement de la pression.

L'organisme de l'albuminurique intermittent est en état d'hyponutrition, de nutrition pervertie.

Le traitement sera surtout hygiénique.

1° *Hygiène alimentaire.* — Le régime lacté absolu semble ne pas convenir. On gardera le lait dans le régime mixte, mais on lui adjoindra les légumes, surtout farineux, les fruits cuits. On ne permettra qu'un usage excessivement modéré de viande, grillée, bien fraîche.

Suppression de toute boisson alcoolique.

2° *Hygiène générale.* — On mettra en œuvre tout ce qui peut activer la nutrition, hydrothérapie, selon les cas, cure d'air, cure hydrominérale, Saint-Nectaire, en particulier. Pas de fatigues intellectuelles, ni corporelles.

Frictions stimulantes, massage.

3° *Traitement proprement dit.* — L'action inhibitrice de la *position horizontale* la fait prescrire comme moyen curatif. Il y a quelques guérisons à son actif.

J'ai échoué après 6 mois chez une fillette de 10 ans, malgré un séjour au lit absolu.

En tout cas les albuminuriques intermittents doivent rester *debout le moins possible.*

Il faut veiller aux fonctions intestinales, restreindre les auto-intoxications.

On peut ajouter des révulsifs sur la région lombaire, comme médicaments, les tanniques, le perchlorure de fer, peut-être, quoique je n'aie pas eu de résultat, l'opothérapie, soit hépatique soit rénale, cette dernière surtout et avec des extraits tirés d'organes très jeunes. Pas de médicaments irritants pour le rein.

En résumé, on s'est trop attaché, dans l'étude des albuminuries intermittentes, au symptôme albuminurie; on a trop négligé l'état général du sujet.

L'albuminurie ne représente qu'un épiphénomène dont le déterminisme appartient aux conditions spéciales du moment dans le système nerveux et surtout circulatoire, mais le tout commandé par une susceptibilité spéciale du rein dérivée elle-même de l'infection ou de l'intoxication antérieure ou concomitante.

DISCUSSION

M. Daccmez objecte à M. le Dr Gillet que la situation horizontale n'interrompt pas forcément l'apparition de l'albuminurie cyclique, comme le prouve l'observation I de son mémoire. Les malades cités en 1896 au Congrès de médecine par Stirling et Arnozan étaient dans le même cas.

M. Gillet répond que l'on doit tenir compte de tous les faits, même ceux qui semblent en dehors de la généralité. Il y a une cause à la périodicité de l'albuminurie: le plus souvent c'est la station; mais il y en a probablement d'autres. Du reste, à moins d'une très grande quantité d'observations, on ne peut pas, en médecine et en biologie, dire *toujours*, ni *jamais*.

L'URICÉMIE CHEZ LES ENFANTS

par M. le docteur J. COMBY.

Médecin à l'Hôpital des Enfants malades.

I

L'insuffisance des combustions organiques, qui se traduit par l'excès d'acide urique et d'urates alcalins dans la circulation, a été peu étudiée chez les enfants. C'est dans la goutte de l'adulte surtout que, depuis Garrod, on a poursuivi la recherche de l'acide urique dans le sang, les humeurs et les tissus.

Mais la goutte, dans ses manifestations classiques, est exceptionnelle dans le jeune âge, et il ne faut pas attendre son apparition pour reconnaître l'uricémie, l'arthritisme et ses débuts.

Quand on étudie de près les descendants d'arthritiques, de goutteux, d'uricémiques, on saisit, dès les premières années de la vie, les germes d'une diathèse, d'une dyscrasie latente qui s'épanouira plus tard avec plus ou moins d'ampleur.

Les symptômes de l'uricémie infantile ne sont pas toujours d'une netteté absolue; ils veulent être cherchés avec soin, ils exigent une grande sagacité clinique. Les difficultés de la tâche expliquent le silence à peu près complet des écrivains médicaux sur l'uricémie, sur l'arthritisme embryonnaire des enfants.

II

Cependant je dois signaler des tentatives de synthèse plus ou moins heureuses dues à la plume du D' H. Cazalis (France), du D' Whitney, du D' Rachford (États-Unis). Ce dernier surtout, dans les *Archives of Pediatric* (*Symptomatology of lithæmia*, septembre 1897), s'est efforcé de décrire l'ensemble des états morbides que nous visons sous le nom d'*uricémie*.

Voici les grandes lignes de ce travail. Les nouveau-nés éliminent des *urates* en excès dès les premiers jours de la vie, et on peut trouver dans leurs langes des sables rouges en plus ou moins grande abondance.

Très acide, l'urine des nouveau-nés ne contient pas seulement des urates en excès. mais parfois aussi des oxalates. Les cristaux d'acide urique se précipitent dans les tubuli du rein. irritant parfois mécaniquement les voies urinaires. Les conséquences à prévoir. le professeur A. Jacobi y a insisté. sont l'albuminurie. l'hématurie. les calculs de la vessie.

Pour prévenir ces complications. pour prévenir encore la fièvre (*inanition fever* de Emmet Holt). la dysurie. l'incontinence d'urine, etc.. on cherchera à provoquer la diurèse par des boissons abondantes (lait ou eau); plus le nouveau-né boira, plus il sera en état de balayer, de chasser au dehors les poussières et graviers qui encombrent ses reins.

Parmi les accidents uricémiques. M. Rachford distingue des *troubles gastro-intestinaux* et des *troubles nerveux*.

1° Voici un enfant de souche arthritique (goutte du côté paternel et du côté maternel). frère de quatre ans, ayant des accès caractérisés par de la fièvre, des douleurs, des nausées et vomissements, de la constipation. accès d'ailleurs soudains. disparaissant aussi vite qu'ils sont apparus. L'intolérance gastrique du début a été remplacée plus tard par la somnolence. la céphalalgie, la migraine.

Le petit malade, dont nous venons d'indiquer les antécédents héréditaires et collatéraux. n'a que cinq mois : à partir de deux mois, toutes les quatre à six semaines. il a présenté des troubles intestinaux attribués à la mauvaise qualité du lait, mais persistant malgré le changement de lait, la stérilisation, la réglementation des repas.

Le 8 février. il refuse le lait et vomit : le 9, vomissements ; le 10, agitation. nausées et vomissements, algidité: le 11. même état, fièvre, dyspnée. le lait est refusé mais l'eau est acceptée : le 12, cris, état grave : le 13, calomel à doses fractionnées. un peu de lait est gardé : le 14, guérison.

L'uricémie des enfants peut donc se traduire par des troubles digestifs paroxystiques (nausées. vomissements. etc.), durant un. deux ou plusieurs jours. Rapidement l'enfant maigrit. s'affaisse. présente un état inquiétant. Il peut y avoir des convulsions. Un intervalle de plusieurs mois peut séparer les crises: la santé est bonne dans les périodes intercalaires. Cependant certains enfants restent pâles, tristes. languissants. Rachford insiste sur la diversité des accès, sur la dyspnée toxique, sans lésion pulmonaire. qui les accompagne parfois.

2° Les enfants uricémiques sont précoces intellectuellement, mais nerveux et irritables. Éclampsie fréquente dans les premières années. Développement physique satisfaisant.

Un enfant de dix-neuf mois a des convulsions suivies de trois à cinq jours de fièvre, de vomissements, puis tout cesse : de nouveaux accès identiques se déclarent périodiquement, à quelques semaines d'intervalle. Ainsi jusqu'à quatre ans ; alors les convulsions cessent, mais les troubles digestifs sont plus fréquents et plus graves.

Pour Rachford, les accidents nerveux, convulsifs, épileptiformes, seraient dus à l'action de la xanthine ou des leucomaïnes sur les centres nerveux. A côté de l'épilepsie essentielle, il décrit l'épilepsie uricémique (*lithæmic epilepsy*), qui serait associée à la migraine, aux troubles digestifs et autres manifestations de la diathèse urique. Parmi les poisons à incriminer, il distingue l'acide urique et ses composés, qui, étant peu ou pas solubles, agiraient surtout localement, et les poisons plus diffusibles (xanthine, para et hétéroxanthine, etc.).

Dans la migraine vraie, il a trouvé que les paroxysmes coïncidaient avec l'excrétion urinaire d'énormes quantités de xanthine.

Mais la chimie, sur ce point, est bien loin d'avoir dit son dernier mot.

L'esquisse du D' Whitney sur le vomissement périodique, *cyclic vomiting* (*Arch. of. Ped.* 1898), mérite aussi d'attirer l'attention.

Un garçon de huit ans et demi, après quelques malaises, de la fièvre, de l'anorexie, est pris le 25 juin 1898 de vomissements qui continuent pendant douze heures, malgré la diète : ces vomissements étaient muqueux, pituiteux, striés de sang. Le troisième jour, amélioration spontanée, et le lendemain, le lait n'est pas vomi. Cette attaque, assez légère, avait été précédée d'attaques semblables et à peu près périodiques (25 décembre 1896, 20 mars, 20 mai, 18 août et 18 novembre 1897).

Les accès, malgré un régime sévère, reviennent tous les trois mois à peu près. La première attaque date du 14 septembre 1896, à l'âge de six ans, elle fut très grave : pendant cinq jours, vomissements incoercibles avec collapsus, amaigrissement, pouls petit, faible, irrégulier. Antécédents héréditaires : goutte chez le grand-père maternel, tuberculose chez le père, folie chez une tante paternelle, suicide chez un oncle, folie chez une sœur, etc.

Enfant nerveux, pas de convulsions, pas de troubles digestifs dans l'intervalle des accès.

Tel est ce syndrome uricémique dont nous pouvons fixer les traits, d'après les observations concluantes que nous venons de résumer.

Un enfant, faible ou fort suivant les cas, est pris tout à coup ou après des malaises de courte durée, de vomissements répétés, incoercibles, alimentaires d'abord, puis muqueux, bilieux, sanguinolents. Toute ingestion est suivie d'un rejet immédiat. Pendant un jour, deux jours, parfois quatre ou cinq jours, les vomissements se répètent. Il y a de la fièvre le plus souvent, l'état général est très ébranlé, la prostration très accusée. Le ventre, loin d'être ballonné comme il arrive dans l'appendicite, la péritonite, l'occlusion intestinale, est affaissé, aplati, excavé.

Bientôt la crise cesse, les vomissements s'arrêtent, l'appétit revient, la digestion reprend son cours normal.

Tel est le vomissement cyclique dans sa forme habituelle et typique.

Autour des symptômes principaux peuvent se grouper d'autres manifestations plus ou moins insolites : céphalalgie, gastralgie, faiblesse et arythmie du cœur, refroidissement des extrémités, dyspnée, agitation et délire, convulsions. Constipation habituelle, d'où le terme de *choléra sec* (Hutinel) qui pourrait convenir à certains cas.

Les crises se reproduisent tous les deux, trois, six mois ; santé parfaite dans l'intervalle.

Comment expliquer ces paroxysmes? Ils rappellent d'une façon générale les intoxications, les empoisonnements (urémie, empoisonnement par les champignons, par les viandes gâtées, etc.). Ils sont évidemment dus à une auto-intoxication. Mais de quelle nature est-elle? Si l'on a égard aux antécédents héréditaires (arthritisme), aux antécédents personnels, au tempérament des sujets, à leurs appétits, à leur manière d'être, à leur hygiène alimentaire, on arrive à se convaincre de l'origine uricémique des accidents.

D'où la sagesse des conseils donnés par Whitney: soigner le régime alimentaire dans l'intervalle des crises, prescrire la diète quand elles surviennent et ne revenir que très graduellement à l'alimentation normale. Interdire la viande de boucherie, recommander le régime végétarien, faire prendre des alcalins (salicylate de soude, bicarbonate de potasse), combattre la constipation, voilà le traitement dans ses grandes lignes.

Outre ces deux syndromes, céphalalgies et vomissements périodiques, on peut décrire d'autres troubles d'ordre uricémique. Je les examinerai chemin faisant en exposant le résultat de mes observations personnelles.

III

J'ai vu un certain nombre d'accidents paroxystiques analogues à ceux de Rachford, de Whitney, et, avant d'aller plus loin, je vais en résumer les observations.

Obs. I. — Un garçon de douze ans accuse des douleurs de tête qui bientôt le font retirer du collège où il était. On lui donne des leçons particulières à domicile. Le moindre travail intellectuel provoque des crises céphaliques pénibles avec anorexie, insomnie, faiblesse générale. On note peu à peu un découragement absolu et une neurasthénie inquiétante. Nuits agitées, lassitude plus grande au réveil qu'avant le coucher. Un séjour prolongé à la campagne, deux cures à Bagnères-de-Bigorre améliorent l'enfant sans le guérir. Pendant plus de trois ans la céphalalgie paroxystique et la neurasthénie ont persisté.

Cependant un bon régime alimentaire, les alcalins, la noix vomique, les jeux et exercices au grand air ont assuré la guérison.

Accidents héréditaires et collatéraux. — Père rhumatisant, nerveux, ayant eu des attaques hystériformes; mère nerveuse, glycosurie; sœur nerveuse également, avec des craquements articulaires, des poussées d'hydarthrose aux genoux, neurasthénie après la puberté. En somme famille arthritico-nerveuse.

La céphalalgie du jeune garçon, qui n'était pas nettement périodique, qui n'avait pas les caractères de la migraine, se compliquait d'autres manifestations nerveuses (insomnie, inaptitude intellectuelle, neurasthénie) qui avaient fait craindre pour l'avenir cérébral de l'enfant. Car le traitement de l'uricémie a mis un terme à tous les accidents.

Obs. II. — Un médecin arthritique, goutteux et graveleux, père de quatre enfants, en a deux qui sont pris périodiquement, sans aucune provocation, en moyenne de quinze en quinze jours, de vomissements incoercibles qui durent deux à trois jours et s'accompagnent de fièvre. Pendant la crise, intolérance absolue de l'estomac. L'aîné des enfants a, de plus, des douleurs de tête atroces coïncidant avec les vomissements, et ayant fait craindre, au début, la méningite, d'autant plus que l'enfant a, pendant la crise, de la photophobie, etc.

Un 3ᵉ enfant a eu des convulsions éclamptiques répétées également, d'origine arthritique et uricémique.

Obs. III. — Garçon de huit ans, très nerveux, très grand pour son âge, de mère arthritique et eczémateuse, de père goutteux, est pris, il y a cinq mois, au début des vacances scolaires, de crises céphalalgiques très courtes, se montrant surtout le soir. Un séjour de trois semaines à la campagne les fait disparaître. Mais trois mois après, l'enfant est repris de douleurs de tête, à l'école, et se plaint également du ventre. La crise est soudaine : l'enfant, en train de jouer, s'arrête tout à coup, porte la main à la tête et crie. Au bout de quelques minutes, il reprend ses jeux. Ces accès se reproduisent plusieurs fois par jour et ne s'accompagnent pas de nausées ni de vomissements. Appétit excellent, l'enfant mange beaucoup, surtout des viandes rouges. De temps à autre on a noté des spasmes musculaires, des tics, des convulsions oculaires et au début une toux nerveuse, une sorte d'aboiement qui rappelle la toux hystérique. Retiré du collège, l'enfant est traité sans succès par les bromures et l'antipyrine.

L'analyse des urines donne :

Densité à 15°, 1028; urée, 55 grammes; acide urique (5 centigrammes, traces d'albumine, excès d'urates), etc. Donc azoturie et uricémie, augmentation de la densité, de l'acidité, albuminurie, phosphaturie. Un mois après, sous l'influence du régime végétarien et des alcalins, l'analyse des urines donne :

Densité 1025, urée 28, albumine 0.

Une troisième analyse faite plus tard montre que l'azoturie et l'uricémie ont disparu en même temps que la guérison est complète.

Voilà donc un cas très net de céphalalgie paroxystique qui semble bien lié à la dyscrasie urique, puisqu'elle disparaît le jour où les urines de l'enfant se rapprochent de la normale. Quant à l'albuminurie légère, signalée dans cette observation, elle s'est retrouvée chez d'autres malades.

Obs. IV. — Une fille de huit ans, grosse et forte, de souche arthritique, ayant eu de l'ictère catarrhal il y a un an, souffrant habituellement de constipation, a eu récemment plusieurs accès subits et peu durables de céphalalgie revenant de préférence le soir. Depuis longtemps elle a en outre une arythmie cardiaque très marquée (faux pas toutes les 5 à 6 pulsations), sans souffle, analogue à celle qu'on observe assez souvent chez les enfants arthritiques et nerveux.

Une analyse des urines, faite sur ma demande, donne : Acidité forte avec 1 gr. 10 d'acide oxalique par litre, densité 1024, excès de phosphates et de chlorures, urée 16 gr. 42, albumine 5 centigrammes. Cette albuminurie, très légère, a été constatée, il y a huit mois, dans une première analyse.

L'enfant a vu disparaître sa céphalalgie sous l'influence du traitement habituel : régime végétarien, alcalins, noix vomique, pain de Graham.

Obs. V. — Une fille de 10 ans, grande, élancée, de mère arthritique et dyspeptique, accuse dans la tête et dans les membres, depuis plusieurs mois, des douleurs qu'on a attribuées à la croissance. Elle mange beaucoup et presque exclusivement de la viande. L'analyse des urines a donné : Albumine 22 centigrammes par litre, urée 52 grammes, acide urique en excès, beaucoup de phosphates et de chlorures, densité 1052. Sous l'influence du traitement, l'albuminurie, l'azoturie ont disparu, et la densité s'est abaissée.

Dans un autre cas, j'ai relevé une glycosurie passagère.

Obs. VI. — Garçon de douze ans et demi ayant, tous les mois ou toutes les six semaines, des crises atroces de céphalalgie.

L'examen des urines a donné :

Densité 1027, glycose 2 grammes par litre, urée 20 grammes, acide urique 67 centigrammes. Il y avait donc à la fois glycosurie, azoturie, uricémie. Tout s'est modifié rapidement par le régime.

Dans quelques cas les douleurs peuvent occuper la continuité des membres ou les articulations et l'on peut, après la céphalalgie uricémique, décrire des arthralgies uricémiques.

Obs. VII. — On me conduit un jour une fille de quatorze ans, pesant 60 kilog., ayant un appétit exagéré (plusieurs obèses dans la famille). A neuf ans elle a eu ses règles ; à dix ans, nouvelle perte ; depuis cette époque, plus rien. Elle avait dix ans quand elle a accusé pendant deux mois, sans avoir ni fièvre, ni gonflement, ni fluxion, des douleurs articulaires vives. Outre ces arthralgies des membres, l'enfant a souvent du lombago.

Les urines sont très acides et contiennent de l'urée et de l'acide urique en excès.

Aux céphalalgies périodiques et paroxystiques de l'uricémie, on peut donc ajouter d'autres manifestations douloureuses: arthralgies, ostéalgies, myalgies, lombago, pseudo-névralgies. Toutes ces manifestations, observées dans certaines circonstances d'âge, de tempérament, d'hygiène générale, peuvent dénoter l'intoxication uricémique. Il y a encore d'autres manifestations d'ordre nerveux.

J'ai noté, chez un enfant uricémique, des crises hystéro-épileptiques qu'on ne pouvait attribuer à une autre cause que la diathèse urique, et qui se sont d'ailleurs terminées par la guérison.

Il n'est pas téméraire de ranger certaines convulsions éclamptiques du premier âge dans la classe des accidents uricémiques; peut-être faut-il y comprendre aussi l'excitation cérébrale, l'insomnie, les terreurs nocturnes, le spasme de la glotte, la tétanie, etc.

J'ai vu des enfants de goutteux de diabétiques, présenter à l'occasion d'une maladie infectieuse (grippe, pneumonie, angine) des accidents nerveux inquiétants et assez durables pour faire croire à la pseudo-méningite: délire, convulsions, strabisme, état comateux. L'étude des antécédents héréditaires et personnels m'a permis plusieurs fois de rassurer les familles.

Obs. VIII. — G... Marie, sept ans, de tempérament nerveux, est prise de raideur de la nuque avec torticolis; comme elle a en même temps un peu de fièvre, on pense au rhumatisme et on donne du salicylate de soude. Puis ce sont des douleurs de tête, de la somnolence, des spasmes musculaires, des convulsions épileptiformes, du strabisme. On parle de *méningite*. Pendant huit à dix jours, l'état est inquiétant. Cependant l'enfant a guéri complètement.

Elle appartient à une famille neuro-arthritique. Le père, gros et fort, a eu du diabète intermittent, de la goutte, et il porte nettement l'estampille de l'arthritisme. La mère a souffert de rhumatisme.

On pourrait donc décrire une *pseudo-méningite* mécanique, qui serait la plus haute expression et la plus effrayante de la localisation neuro-arthritique sur le cerveau, la céphalalgie, l'excitation cérébrale, etc., n'en étant que des expressions atténuées. Outre les décharges uricémiques sur le système nerveux, il peut s'en faire sur les autres appareils organiques: appareil respiratoire, estomac et intestin, cœur, voies urinaires, peau, etc.

Obs. IX. — Un garçon de huit ans, nerveux, excitable, de mère obèse et arthritique, a des hémorrhoïdes depuis l'âge de cinq ans. De temps à autre il présente des spasmes vésicaux, de la pollakiurie et rend une grande quantité de sable urique qui se dépose au fond du vase, quand on recueille ses urines. Cependant il n'a pas eu encore de véritables coliques hépatiques.

Parmi les manifestations uricémiques, il n'en est pas de plus saisissante que le vomissement périodique dont je vais rapporter brièvement trois observations inédites.

Obs. X. — Le 51 mars 1900, on me conduit un petit garçon de six ans. Le père est bien portant, la mère très migraineuse, la grand'mère maternelle a la gravelle. Pas d'autre enfant. Le petit malade est né à huit mois, avec une double cataracte congénitale (iridectomie d'un côté, énucléation de l'autre). Vue mauvaise, nystagmus. Nourri au sein, l'enfant a marché tard sans présenter de stigmates rachitiques. Il est excité, nerveux, toujours en mouvement, dort mal, grince des dents. Assez bien développé, intelligent et docile.

A l'âge de deux ans et demi, première crise de vomissements ayant duré quarante-huit heures, avec peu ou pas de fièvre. Ces vomissements revinrent d'abord tous les mois, puis s'éloignèrent au point de ne se reproduire que tous les huit ou dix mois. Les vomissements étaient précédés de crises nerveuses avec perte de connaissance durant 15 à 20 minutes. Santé parfaite dans l'intervalle des vomissements.

Rien à l'estomac qui ne paraît pas dilaté : à l'auscultation du cœur, souffle systolique de la pointe. L'analyse des urines donne : Densité 1052, cristaux d'acide urique en abondance.

Obs. XI. — Le 15 juin 1900, on me conduit une fille de dix ans que j'ai soignée déjà pour des troubles digestifs. Mère migraineuse, dyspeptique, asthmatique, ayant un rein mobile. Père migraineux et rhumatisant. Arthritisme des deux côtés.

L'enfant, dès l'âge de deux ans, a eu la migraine. Actuellement, elle n'a plus d'accès, mais elle se plaint de la tête (céphalalgie frontale) quand elle travaille. Depuis deux ans les migraines qu'elle avait autrefois ont été remplacées par des crises périodiques de vomissements incoercibles. Ces vomissements durent trois ou quatre jours et reviennent tous les six mois. Ils laissent l'enfant amaigrie et anémiée. La dernière crise date de trois jours seulement. L'enfant est très pâle et j'entends nettement un souffle continu avec redoublement dans les vaisseaux du cou.

Au moment des crises, clapotage gastrique. Sable urique dans le vase de nuit. Traces d'albumine dans les urines.

L'examen du ventre montre un rein flottant à droite : ce rein, très mobile, est porté en haut et en avant. Il n'est pas douloureux. La région de l'appendice (lors d'une crise on avait pensé à l'appendicite) est saine. Il n'y a pas de fièvre au moment des crises.

L'analyse des urines donne : Densité 1028, urée 24 grammes, acide urique 60 centigrammes, albumine traces.

Je conseille le régime végétarien, les affusions froides, les alcalins, le grand air, la vie à la campagne, l'eau d'Évian.

OBS. XII. — Le 6 août 1900, je suis appelé à voir un garçon de sept ans, dont j'ai soigné le frère aîné pour des troubles nerveux et de l'entérite muco-membraneuse. Cet enfant, très court de taille, bien musclé, ayant les côtes un peu évasées (stigmate de rachitisme), a été en retard pour la marche et la dentition. Nourri au biberon. Il a de la dilatation de l'estomac et le rein droit mobile. Il a toujours vomi facilement, par exemple sous l'influence d'une grippe, d'une angine, d'une indisposition quelconque. Mais il ne présente de *vomissements cycliques* que depuis huit mois. La première crise date du mois de décembre 1899. A cette époque il a été pris de vomissements incoercibles qui ont duré trois jours et se sont accompagnés de fièvre. Trois autres crises depuis cette époque.

Enfant gros mangeur de viande, refusant les légumes, constipé habituellement. Père asthmatique, mère goutteuse. L'arthritisme héréditaire est évident.

Prescription habituelle : régime végétarien, alcalins, frictions cutanées.

Aux crises de vomissements périodiques rappelées plus haut, il faut ajouter les douleurs de ventre, les coliques intestinales, les flux diarrhéiques soudains et passagers, sans cause occasionnelle appréciable.

On peut encore comprendre, dans cette liste déjà longue des accidents uricémiques : les sueurs profuses, les rhinites spasmodiques, les accès asthmatiformes, les palpitations de cœur, l'arythmie cardiaque, les bronchites sibilantes, certaines formes d'eczéma, etc.

OBS. XIII. — Le 28 juin 1899, on me conduit un garçon de neuf ans dont le père est goutteux, graveleux et obèse (poids 105 kilogrammes), la mère obèse, rhumatisante et nerveuse.

Un frère âgé de dix-sept ans, actuellement bien portant, a été diabétique de quatre à neuf ans, ayant eu jusqu'à 60 grammes de sucre par litre. Ce diabète, qui a fini par guérir d'une façon complète, s'était déclaré à la suite d'une frayeur.

Nourri au sein, notre petit malade a souffert, entre six semaines et quatre ans, d'un *eczéma* de la face et du tronc rebelle à tout traitement. Il persiste aujourd'hui, à la racine des cuisses, et sur le scrotum, un état lichénoïde de la peau avec démangeaisons. Recrudescences de temps à autre.

A cet eczéma arthritique, il faut ajouter des crises soudaines de céphalalgie, beaucoup plus tardives, puisqu'elles ne se sont déclarées que depuis six mois. Elles sont d'ailleurs de courte durée. Constipation habituelle, arthralgies sans fièvre.

Les urines, très acides, ont une densité élevée (1054); elles contiennent beaucoup d'urates.

Outre les manifestations localisées sur un organe ou un appareil, on trouve des manifestations générales sans localisation précise.

Telle la *fièvre uricémique*, dont je vais donner deux observations et qui simule la fièvre intermittente quotidienne. Cette fièvre, que je ne savais à quoi attribuer la première fois que je l'ai observée, que d'autres avant moi avaient également méconnue dans sa nature et ses origines, saturant en vain les enfants de quinine, d'arsenic, etc., a été éclairée d'une vive lumière quand, au cours d'un de ses accès, le premier malade a été pris d'un accès typique de goutte (*Obs. XIII*). La fièvre uricémique présente les caractères suivants :

Un enfant, qui peut être très jeune (première année, première enfance), ou âgé de plusieurs années (seconde enfance), est pris un jour d'un accès typique de fièvre, avec les stades de frisson ou d'algidité, de chaleur et de sueurs. Cet accès dure cinq, six heures ou davantage. Il apparaît le matin ou le soir, aucune règle ne préside à son évolution. Il se répète les jours suivants pendant deux, trois, cinq jours, une semaine, plusieurs semaines. La température atteint et dépasse 40 degrés pendant l'acmé pour retomber à 37 degrés ensuite, de sorte que la courbe thermique donne tout à fait l'idée d'une fièvre intermittente quotidienne.

Cependant l'enfant est pâle, abattu, amaigri, et sa convalescence est très pénible.

On ne trouve rien du côté du foie, de la rate, du cœur, etc.

Les paroxysmes sont souvent précédés de mal de gorge, il y a parfois même une véritable angine. Après quelques mois, parfois six mois ou un an de santé parfaite, les accès réapparaissent et ainsi pendant des années.

Obs. XIV. — N... âgé de huit ans, pâle, anémié, est atteint depuis plusieurs années de fièvres pseudo-intermittentes très intenses, revenant par séries d'accès tous les six mois. La température dépasse 40°, et les accès quotidiens se prolongent huit, quinze jours, trois semaines parfois, laissant l'enfant dans un état de faiblesse et d'anémie extrêmes. Des doses fortes de quinine par la bouche ou par la voie sous-cutanée n'ont rien produit. L'arsenic, l'hydrothérapie, la cure de la Bourboule sont restées inefficaces. La moelle osseuse de veau, que j'avais conseillée, a fortifié l'enfant sans prévenir les accès.

L'examen du sang n'a montré ni *hématozoaires* de Laveran, ni leucémie, ni filariose (Thiercelin).

Au printemps de 1900, je suis appelé à voir l'enfant dans un nouvel accès aussi grave que les précédents. Après sept ou huit jours, douleurs atroces au niveau des pieds avec gonflement œdémateux; c'est un accès de goutte très violent que nous traitons avec succès par le salicylate de soude.

D'ailleurs, au point de vue arthritique, l'enfant a de qui tenir. Nous trouvons chez ses ascendants la goutte, l'asthme, la migraine, etc.

Obs. XV. — Le 8 août 1900, je vois dans mon cabinet un grand garçon de neuf ans, pâle, amaigri, sortant d'un accès dont je parlerai plus tard. Nourri au sein par une bonne nourrice, l'enfant a marché de bonne heure, a eu une dentition précoce, n'a pas souffert de troubles digestifs graves. Depuis l'âge de six mois, il a, toutes les deux, trois, quatre semaines, des accès de fièvre, durant deux, trois, cinq jours. Ces accès, qui sont violents (plus de 40°), débutent par un frisson suivi de chaleur et de sueurs profuses. On a usé et abusé de la quinine sans succès; on a prescrit le changement d'air, la Bourboule, l'hydrothérapie, sans obtenir le moindre résultat.

L'enfant est très nerveux, très excitable. Il boit beaucoup et mange vite; je trouve son estomac dilaté. Mais la dyspepsie atone ne donne pas ces fièvres intermittentes que je viens de décrire. Il faut chercher ailleurs. Les urines sont acides, denses, chargées d'urée et d'acide urique, avec traces d'albumine.

Rien au foie, à la rate, au cœur, aux poumons.

Le père de l'enfant est arthritique, goutteux, eczémateux, migraineux. Du côté maternel, nous trouvons la migraine, le rhumatisme musculaire.

J'oubliais de dire que les accès, chez cet enfant, moins atteint que le précédent, commencent aussi par un mal de gorge, par une angine d'ailleurs bénigne.

J'ai prescrit un régime sévère, surtout végétarien, le rationnement des liquides. J'ai conseillé le drap mouillé, quoique l'enfant soit très sensible au froid, et j'ai donné des alcalins.

Les observations qui précèdent montrent presque toutes l'augmentation de densité, l'acidité exagérée des urines, l'azoturie, l'uricémie. Dans quelques analyses, on a pu noter l'albuminurie, la glycosurie, l'oxalurie, sans parler des bases xanthiques dont l'analyse offre de trop grandes difficultés pour être faite couramment.

Ces observations montrent encore la grande diversité des manifestations uricémiques chez les enfants. Mais, quelle que soit la diversité de ces accidents, n'est-il pas légitime de les rapprocher, de les grouper ensemble comme membres étroitement unis de la même famille? N'y a-t-il pas, dans les humeurs, dans le sang des malades, une altération identique qui serait le lien pathogénique de tous les désordres?

Pour ma part, j'en demeure convaincu, et les analyses d'urine qui ont été faites autorisent à incriminer la combustion incomplète des déchets de l'organisme, c'est-à-dire l'intoxication uricémique (*litharmia* des auteurs américains).

Il est vrai que cette conception, toute rationnelle qu'elle paraisse, ne concorde pas avec les recherches les plus récentes (*Traité de pathologie générale* de Ch. Bouchard, t. III, 1900, article de Lambling). D'après ces recherches, l'acide urique ne serait pas un produit de combustion incomplète, mais un produit de dédoublement des *nucléines*.

Ce dédoublement donnerait lieu, outre l'acide urique, aux bases xanthiques (xanthine, hypoxanthine, adénine, guanine), qui sont très voisines de l'acide urique. Quoi qu'il en soit, le dernier mot n'est pas dit sur l'interprétation chimique des accidents. Et, en attendant, je vais essayer de réunir, dans une courte synthèse, les documents cliniques que j'ai recueillis, pour aboutir à une thérapeutique rationnelle et autant que possible efficace.

IV

ESQUISSE DIDACTIQUE DE L'URICÉMIE INFANTILE.

ÉTIOLOGIE. — L'hérédité domine la pathogénie de l'uricémie. Quand on scrute les antécédents des enfants, on trouve presque toujours, chez les parents ou les grands-parents, une ou plusieurs des affections suivantes : goutte, obésité, diabète, gravelle, asthme, migraine, névroses et vésanies, dermatoses, etc.

Toutes les modalités de la diathèse neuro-arthritique sont susceptibles de se transmettre à la descendance sous une forme semblable ou dissemblable (hérédité homéomorphe ou hétéromorphe).

La prédisposition héréditaire ne s'accuse pas dès la naissance ; elle est d'abord cachée, latente, se dévoilant plus ou moins tard, dans la seconde enfance ou l'adolescence. A la prédisposition innée, à la tare héréditaire viennent d'ailleurs s'ajouter des influences accidentelles, et l'héritage peut s'enrichir d'acquisitions personnelles. Il semble même quelquefois que la maladie puisse s'acquérir de toutes pièces.

L'hygiène alimentaire figure au premier rang des causes de l'uricémie acquise. Si l'enfant a mangé trop tôt des substances trop azotées, trop fortes, trop abondantes : si ses capacités digestives, ses facultés d'assimilation, de combustion organique ont été dépassées : s'il n'a pu utiliser parfaitement ni éliminer suffisamment des aliments, ingérés sans mesure : s'il a ainsi fait de la surcharge graisseuse, s'il a encombré et irrité les cellules de son foie, de ses reins, de son cerveau ; s'il s'est empoisonné lui-même par les déchets de la suralimentation, alors il pourra présenter l'une ou l'autre des manifestations que j'ai décrites :

1° Céphalalgie périodique ; 2° vomissements cycliques ; 3° convulsions ; 4° albuminurie ; 5° troubles urinaires ; 6° dermatoses ; 7° fièvre uricémique, etc.

J'ai dit que l'uricémie était rare dans la première enfance ; toutefois elle devrait être considérée comme fréquente si l'on voulait y faire rentrer la lithiase rénale des nourrissons athrepsiés et déshydratés.

que j'ai étudiée dans un mémoire précédent (*Archives de médecine des enfants, octobre, 1899*).

Ordinairement, ce n'est que dans la seconde enfance, les observations en font foi, que l'uricémie se révèle.

Les garçons semblent être plus souvent atteints que les filles, mais ces dernières ne sont pas épargnées, il s'en faut.

On remarquera que certaines classes sociales paient un lourd tribut à la maladie : l'uricémie s'observe surtout chez les riches, chez les citadins, chez les intellectuels, chez les travailleurs de la pensée, chez tous ceux qui abusent de leur estomac et de leur cerveau.

La pathogénie est loin d'être élucidée complètement. On incrimine à bon droit, il me semble, l'acide urique ou lithique, élément quaternaire, azoté, dont les combinaisons avec la soude forment la base des dépôts urinaires. Mais on ne sait pas encore bien le mode d'action de ce produit de combustion incomplète ou de dédoublement, et surtout s'il agit seul dans les auto-intoxications révélées par la clinique. Malgré les travaux du Dr Gigot-Suart (*l'Uricémie*, 1 vol., Paris, 1875), il est probable que l'acide urique n'est pas seul en cause, et nous devons compter avec la xanthine et autres corps alloxiniques que les chimistes sont en train d'étudier. Quelques-uns soutiennent même que l'acide urique n'est pas toxique ; ce produit serait moins acteur que témoin de la diathèse urique.

SYMPTÔMES. — On a vu que les symptômes de l'uricémie sont très variables. Ils peuvent affecter presque tous les appareils organiques.

1° Les *symptômes nerveux* figurent parmi les plus communs et aussi les plus pénibles : céphalalgie périodique ou paroxystique, douleurs osseuses ou articulaires, excitation cérébrale, éclampsie, insomnie, terreurs nocturnes, neurasthénie, pseudo-méningite, etc. De tous ces symptômes, le mal de tête est le plus saillant.

2° Les *troubles digestifs* viennent ensuite : vomissements périodiques ou cycliques, coliques intestinales, flux diarrhéiques ou constipation, entérite muco-membraneuse et lithiase intestinale, etc. Parmi toutes ces manifestations, le vomissement périodique est à retenir.

3° Les *voies urinaires*, très souvent intéressées, nous donnent : lithiase rénale et vésicale, coliques néphrétiques, albuminurie, glycosurie, hématurie, dysurie et spasmes de la vessie, etc. Chez des enfants polyphagiques, mangeurs de viande, j'ai observé des envies incessantes d'uriner, des spasmes douloureux du col vésisal, de l'incontinence nocturne d'urine, qui cédaient à la suppression du régime carné et à son remplacement par le régime végétarien, par le lait, par la diète aqueuse.

Les urines trop azotées, trop concentrées, irritent la vessie, congestionnent le col ; il suffit de l'abstinence de certains aliments et d'une abondante dilution des urines par les boissons aqueuses pour faire cesser les désordres.

Le D⁾ Abt (*Ann. of. gyn. and ped.*, décembre, 1898) a vu, chez deux garçons de quinze à seize mois, une urétrite purulente avec rougeur du méat, douleurs à la miction, gonflement du prépuce, qui ne pouvait s'expliquer que par d'abondants dépôts uratiques dans les urines. A côté de l'urétrite gonococcique, il faut faire une place à l'urétrite uricémique.

4° L'*appareil respiratoire* participe, plus souvent qu'on ne le croit, aux manifestations de la dyscrasie urique : coryza spasmodique et éternuements, fièvre des foins, épistaxis, laryngites spasmodiques, bronchites sibilantes, accès asthmatiformes, congestion pulmonaire, etc.

Le D⁾ L.-H. Watson (*South. med. Record*, 1899) regarde l'acide urique comme une des causes de l'asthme et il se loue du traitement inspiré par cette conception étiologique.

5° L'*appareil circulatoire* est également touché par l'intoxication uricémique : palpitations, tachycardie, arythmie cardiaque, signes d'hypertrophie du cœur.

6° La *peau*, en sa qualité d'émonctoire, ne saurait manquer d'être fréquemment atteinte : sueurs abondantes, éruptions prurigineuses et lichénoïdes, poussées d'eczéma alternant parfois avec des crises d'asthme. L'eczéma tenace et récidivant des jeunes enfants est souvent d'origine arthritique et uricémique.

7° *Fièvre uricémique* : accès intermittents quotidiens revenant sans règle à longs intervalles.

Il peut y avoir sans doute d'autres manifestations de la dyscrasie urique : je me suis borné à énumérer les principales.

DIAGNOSTIC. — Le diagnostic se fait non pas tant d'après les symptômes pris en eux-mêmes que d'après les antécédents héréditaires et personnels. Par elles-mêmes, les manifestations cliniques ne sont pas toujours et absolument caractéristiques. Elles sont même parfois trompeuses et les premiers accès de vomissements cycliques de céphalalgie paroxystique peuvent faire penser à la méningite. Il y a des cas même où le tableau de la méningite est presque complet. Les vomissements incoercibles, quand ils coïncident avec des douleurs abdominales et de la fièvre, évoquent naturellement l'idée d'une péritonite appendiculaire. On peut encore songer à un empoisonnement accidentel. La fièvre uricémique est toujours confondue avec les fièvres palustres : mais on ne trouve pas l'hématozoaire de Laveran. Ce qui permet de classer le syndrome, de le catégoriser, c'est le terrain sur lequel il a poussé, ce sont les liens de parenté, les relations de famille qu'il affecte avec d'autres états morbides.

L'anamnèse pourra rendre, à ce point de vue, de très grands services, et les renseignements qu'elle donnera seront complétés par l'étude de l'enfant, de ses attributs physiques, de son tempérament, de ses appétits, etc. Enfin l'analyse détaillée des urines servira d'appoint au diagnostic clinique.

Pronostic. — Le pronostic n'est pas grave dans le présent, mais il comporte des réserves pour l'avenir. Les uricémiques sont marqués d'une tare constitutionnelle qui appelle la sollicitude de l'hygiéniste et du médecin.

Leur avenir sera bon, médiocre ou mauvais, suivant les soins dont ils auront été entourés, suivant la vie qu'ils auront menée. Il dépend d'eux et de leur entourage, que la diathèse aille en s'atténuant ou en s'aggravant, qu'elle reste stationnaire ou suive une marche ascendante, qu'elle devienne de plus en plus fruste avec les années, ou au contraire qu'elle se renforce et engendre des manifestations de plus en plus sévères.

Traitement. — Avant d'aborder le traitement, disons un mot de la prophylaxie. On est en présence d'enfants sur lesquels pèse un héritage fâcheux. Il ne faut pas attendre qu'ils aient présenté des accidents pour les soumettre à une hygiène convenable.

L'alimentation d'abord sera très surveillée. Après un allaitement naturel prolongé ou un allaitement artificiel bien réglé, on se gardera de commencer trop tôt l'alimentation carnée. Même si l'enfant, sevré depuis longtemps, témoigne d'un goût marqué pour les viandes de boucherie, le gibier, les mets épicés, on lui refusera ces aliments qui favorisent la production de l'acide urique en excès et des toxines. La viande doit être tardivement et parcimonieusement concédée aux uricémiques héréditaires. On recommandera la sobriété et on réglera strictement les repas pour éviter la suralimentation.

Repas réguliers, à heure fixe, et en petit nombre (trois ou quatre par vingt-quatre heures) : mets choisis et de facile digestion, régime végétarien mitigé : viandes blanches, poissons, œufs, laitage, légumes farineux, pâtes, macaroni, fruits cuits, etc. On pourra donner des légumes verts bien cuits, des salades cuites, en interdisant l'oseille et les tomates. Pas de charcuterie ni viandes faisandées. Pas de vin pur ni liquides alcooliques, usage très modéré du thé ou du café, boissons aqueuses ou lait.

Les fonctions intestinales seront surveillées de très près. On combattra la constipation par des remèdes, on cherchera à la prévenir par le régime des légumes verts et des fruits cuits. Le pain de Graham (pain complet) convient spécialement en pareil cas. On fera fonctionner la peau à l'aide des bains, des ablutions froides, du tub, du drap mouillé, des frictions sèches ou alcooliques.

On ne négligera pas les exercices physiques, on évitera la claustration prolongée, la sédentarité, le surmenage cérébral; on prescrira la vie au grand air, le séjour à la campagne.

Quand la maladie se sera déclarée sous l'une ou l'autre des formes cliniques étudiées plus haut, on ne manquera pas d'insister sur l'hygiène physique que je viens d'exposer, tout en agissant par quelques remèdes appropriés.

Les alcalins sont à essayer avant tout : bicarbonate de soude ou de potasse, citrate de potasse, magnésie calcinée, carbonate ou benzoate de lithine.

L'association de la noix vomique aux alcalins est très recommandable : je prescris au maximum un centigramme de poudre de noix vomique par jour et par année d'âge. Ce médicament a une action très efficace sur l'atonie gastro-intestinale. Voici la formule dont on peut se servir :

<pre>
Bicarbonate de soude. . . . . ⎫ āā 0ᵍʳ,20
Magnésie calcinée. . . . . ⎭
Poudre de noix vomique. 0ᵍʳ,01
</pre>

pour un paquet; en prendre deux ou trois semblables avant le repas, dans une cuillerée de lait ou d'eau sucrée, suspendre après huit ou dix jours d'usage. On peut remplacer, dans cette formule, le bicarbonate de soude par le bicarbonate de potasse ou par le citrate de potasse.

Quand on donne la lithine, on ne dépasse pas 10, 15, 20 centigrammes par jour.

Le traitement hydrominéral a une très grande importance. Voici les principales sources françaises qu'on peut conseiller suivant les diverses localisations de la diathèse :

Aux douleurs, craquements articulaires, névralgies uricémiques, conviennent les eaux chlorurées sodiques chaudes de Bourbonne, Bourbon-l'Archambault, Bourbon-Lancy, sans parler des boues de Dax, Saint-Amand, Reibacq. Plombières revendique les entérites, les flux intestinaux, les douleurs abdominales rhumatoïdes ; Châtel-Guyon s'adresse surtout aux enfants constipés, ayant des selles muco-membraneuses, du sable intestinal, etc. L'albuminurie des uricémiques est très favorablement traitée à Saint-Nectaire. La gravelle rénale relève de Contrexéville, Vittel, Martigny, Capvern, Évian. L'anémie uricémique peut être soignée à Royat, La Bourboule, Saint-Gervais. Les enfants lymphatiques, affaiblis, à nutrition languissante, seront soumis aux chlorurées sodiques fortes (Salies-de-Béarn, Briscous, La Mouillère, Salins, etc.).

Les dyspeptiques iront à Vichy ou à Pougues. Les uricémiques excitables, neurasthéniques, seront envoyés à Bagnères-de-Bigorre, Divonne. Les dermatoses uricémiques pourront être traités à La Bourboule, Uriage, Luchon.

Les paroxysmes aigus, les vomissements périodiques notamment seront traités par la diète absolue, la diète hydrique. Si l'estomac ne tolère rien, on soutiendra l'enfant par les lavements nutritifs et les injections de sérum artificiel. Les crises de céphalalgie commandent, le repos absolu, l'interruption des études, sans préjudice du traitement général indiqué plus haut.

Au demeurant, c'est sur l'hygiène qu'il faut surtout compter pour redresser dans la mesure du possible le vice de nutrition qu'est l'uricémie : hygiène de la digestion, de la peau, des muscles, du poumon, du cerveau. Des aliments bien choisis, en quantité convenable, des repas réguliers pris avec sobriété, des boissons aqueuses ; — des bains, des pratiques hydrothérapiques variées, voir le massage général et la gymnastique suédoise ; — des exercices physiques et jeux au grand air ; — pas de surmenage cérébral. Voilà l'hygiène qui convient aux uricémiques.

Avec cela et quelques remèdes prescrits opportunément et avec mesure, on obtient beaucoup pour le redressement d'un organisme mal équilibré.

CONCLUSIONS

L'uricémie est l'arthritisme en germe : c'est l'ensemble des désordres et des symptômes morbides déterminés dans la première ou la seconde enfance par la diathèse urique.

Parmi ces symptômes, les plus saillants sont : la céphalalgie périodique et le vomissement cyclique étudiés par Rachford et Whitney.

Ces paroxysmes douloureux, pénibles, inquiétants parfois, semblent révéler une auto-intoxication : et, dans cette intoxication, l'acide urique ou les corps qui s'en rapprochent joueraient le principal rôle. Quoi qu'il en soit, l'hérédité arthritique s'accuse dans la plupart des observations. A cette tare héréditaire peuvent s'ajouter des acquisitions personnelles. L'hygiène alimentaire joue un grand rôle dans l'uricémie acquise (abus de la viande, suralimentation).

En général, les accidents ne se montrent pas avant la seconde enfance, et sont plus fréquents chez les garçons que chez les filles, dans les classes riches et intellectuelles que dans la classe pauvre.

Les symptômes peuvent affecter la plupart des systèmes organiques.

1° *Système nerveux:* Céphalalgie paroxystique, ostéalgies et arthralgies, éclampsie, excitation cérébrale, insomnie, terreurs nocturnes, neurasthénie, pseudo-méningite.

2° *Tube digestif:* vomissement périodique ou cyclique, coliques, diarrhée et constipation, entérite muco-membraneuse et sable intestinal.

3° *Voies urinaires:* lithiase rénale et vésicale, albuminerie, glycosurie, hématurie, dysurie, spasmes du col vésical, incontinence d'urine, urétrite.

4° *Appareil respiratoire:* coryzas spasmodiques, épitaxis, laryngites, bronchites sibilantes, accès asthmatiformes.

5° *Appareil circulatoire:* tachycardie et arythmie cardiaque, hypertrophie du cœur.

6° *Peau:* sueurs, prurigo, lichen, eczéma à répétition.

7° *Fièvre* uricémique du type intermittent quotidien.

Pour faire le diagnostic, il faut remonter aux antécédents héréditaires et personnels, étudier le tempérament de l'enfant, faire analyser ses urines. On trouvera souvent un excès de densité, d'urée, d'acide urique, etc.

Le pronostic n'est pas grave, mais on peut craindre, pour plus tard, des manifestations arthritiques de plus en plus accentuées. Les soins hygiéniques et le traitement influent d'ailleurs beaucoup sur le pronostic.

La prophylaxie, comme le traitement, repose sur une bonne hygiène alimentaire, sur l'usage tardif et discret des viandes de boucherie. Sobriété, repas bien réglés, régime surtout végétarien, boissons aqueuses, voilà ce qui convient aux uricémiques.

Assurer un bon fonctionnement de la peau (frictions, hydrothérapie, exercices au grand air), éviter la sédentarité et le surmenage cérébral, sont de grande importance.

Parmi les médicaments, les meilleurs sont les alcalins (bicarbonate de soude ou de potasse, citrate de potasse), les amers (noix vomique), les laxatifs quand il y a de la constipation (magnésie, etc.). La lithine (carbonate ou benzoate) peut être également employée.

Les eaux minérales qui peuvent rendre service aux uricémiques sont très nombreuses : Bourbonne, Bourbon-l'Archambault, Bourbon-Lancy pour les uricémiques arthralgiques ; Plombières et Châtel-Guyon pour les uricémiques qui souffrent de l'intestin ; Saint-Nectaire pour les albuminuriques ; Contrexéville et similaires pour les graveleux ; Royat, la Bourboule pour les anémiques ; Salies-de-Béarn et autres du même genre pour les lymphatiques et débilités ; Vichy pour les dyspeptiques ; Divonne pour les nerveux ; Uriage, Louhan, La Bourboule pour les eczémateux.

Quant aux paroxysmes aigus (vomissement cyclique, céphalalgie), il faut les traiter par le repos absolu, la diète hydrique, et, dans les cas graves, par les injections de sérum artificiel.

DISCUSSION.

M. HUTINEL, tout en félicitant M. Comby de sa très intéressante communication, fait remarquer qu'en somme les enfants en question sont des neuro-arthritiques. Quant à l'uricémie, elle n'est pas démontrée dans tous les cas ; il y a souvent une dose normale ou même inférieure d'acide urique dans les urines. Aussi se demande-t-il jusqu'à quel point cette dénomination est exacte.

M. COMBY. — J'accepte la valeur des objections que vient de m'adresser M. Hutinel. Quand on examine les urines des petits malades on ne trouve pas toujours un excès d'acide urique. Le terme d'uricémie n'est donc pas irréprochable, mais il est adopté et permet de classer, sous un vocable connu, toute une catégorie de manifestations en apparence très divergentes. Ces enfants neuro-arthiliques ne sont peut-être pas intoxiqués par l'acide urique ; mais ils sont fils de goutteux, ils sont destinés à le devenir, et cliniquement ils relèvent de la diathèse urique. Et puis, quand on s'inspire, pour le traitement, de cette idée d'uricémie, on obtient des résultats remarquables.

Au point de vue doctrinal, M. Hutinel a raison peut-être. Mais sûrement, au point de vue pratique, il est d'accord avec moi.

LE DIABÉTE SUCRÉ OBSERVÉ CHEZ UNE ENFANT DE SIX MOIS — GUÉRISON

par M. L. BAUMEL,

Professeur de clinique des maladies des enfants à l'Université de Montpellier.

La connaissance de cette maladie, même chez l'adulte, est de date relativement récente. Ce n'est en effet que vers la fin du xviii° siècle que Pool et Dobson parvinrent à démontrer cliniquement, par l'évaporation et la fermentation, la présence du sucre dans l'urine. Cependant, pour être juste, il est bon de mentionner que, quelque cent ans plus tôt, Thomas Willis (1674) avait remarqué la saveur mielleuse de l'urine chez certains de ses malades ; mais ce n'était là qu'un fait d'observation clinique, ne reposant encore sur aucune base scientifique.

Chez l'enfant, ce n'est, on peut dire, que dans ce dernier siècle et plus particulièrement dans ces vingt-cinq dernières années que le diabète sucré a été sérieusement étudié.

Presque tous les auteurs reconnaissent au diabète infantile une gravité exceptionnelle et le rangent en général parmi les cas de diabète maigre. Les Allemands signalent toutefois une forme légère de la maladie[1].

Chez l'adulte on distingue un diabète nerveux, un diabète gras et un diabète maigre, ce dernier caractérisé par un amaigrissement considérable et une grande quantité de glycose dans les urines (Lancereaux). On voit des diabétiques éliminer 8 à 900 grammes de sucre dans les vingt-quatre heures.

Le diabète infantile a été surtout observé dans la seconde enfance.

J'ai eu l'occasion d'en voir deux cas : l'un, dans ma clientèle, chez un enfant de 15 ans qui finit par succomber ; l'autre, à l'hôpital. Dans ce dernier cas, le malade étant mort aussi, l'autopsie révéla l'existence d'une atrophie manifeste du pancréas.

Avant d'aller plus loin dans l'étude qui nous occupe, il serait intéressant de savoir si le diabète peut exister pendant la vie intra-utérine ou pendant les premiers mois après la naissance. En d'autres termes, existe-t-il un diabète fœtal ?

M. Ballantyne (d'Édimbourg) a signalé tout récemment, à cet égard, les observations de Ludmig, de Rossa, de Bell.

Ce qui frappe, à la lecture de ces trois observations, c'est qu'aucune n'est absolument probante au point de vue du diabète fœtal ; elles permettent toutefois d'en entrevoir la possibilité.

Ludwig, dans un cas de diabète chez la mère, trouva du glycose dans le liquide amniotique. Comme, en outre, ce liquide était en quantité énorme, il songea à la possibilité du diabète sucré du fœtus ; mais, ce dernier étant mort-né, la question ne put être résolue.

Rossa, également, observa un cas semblable ; mais, bien que l'enfant survécût assez longtemps, il ne trouva, à aucun moment, du glycose dans ses urines.

1. H. Leroux. *Diabète sucré*. — Granchér. *Traité des maladies de l'enfance*. Paris, Masson. 1897, t. II, p. 51.

Quant au cas de Bell, il a trait à un nourrisson chez lequel le diabète apparut dès l'âge de 5 mois[1].

C'est seulement sur ce dernier fait que l'on pouvait se baser pour avancer que, probablement, le diabète sucré peut survenir pendant la vie intra-utérine.

Cette probabilité devient presque une certitude si l'on en rapproche le fait de Kitselle, rapporté plus récemment encore par MM. d'Espine et Picot, qui en observa un cas sur son propre fils âgé de 14 jours[2].

Certains auteurs sont allés jusqu'à prétendre que le diabète observé pendant les premiers mois de la vie n'était pas le diabète sucré, mais le passage du lactose, sucre de lait, dans les urines, véritable lactosurie momentanée, due à certains troubles gastro-intestinaux. Resterait encore à démontrer la véritable nature de ces troubles.

Pour mon compte, je considère toute glycosurie, même passagère, comme un degré plus ou moins atténué du diabète sucré. Je me propose d'ailleurs d'y revenir un peu plus loin.

Dans ces formes de diabète sucré infantile, les uns veulent faire jouer un grand rôle à l'hérédité, les autres à l'infection.

Ni l'une ni l'autre de ces deux causes ne nous paraît avoir le rôle prépondérant qu'on est porté à leur accorder généralement.

Nous devons rappeler cependant que M. Charrin a expérimentalement produit le diabète chez les animaux en injectant des germes dans le canal de Wirsung[3].

Lancereaux veut que le diabète maigre soit le seul dans lequel le pancréas est lésé[4].

D'autres auteurs ne voient dans le diabète sucré, quelle que soit sa forme, qu'un *trouble de la nutrition*.

Pour moi, depuis longtemps déjà, aussi bien dans le diabète gras que dans le diabète maigre, que même dans le diabète nerveux, *le pancréas est toujours en cause*, soit directement, soit indirectement.

Seulement, tandis que les lésions pancréatiques, dans le diabète maigre, sont macroscopiques, elles sont généralement, dans le diabète gras, légères, peu profondes, microscopiques et passent facilement inaperçues. Elles sont purement *dynamiques*, dans le diabète

1. BALLANTYE. Maladies du fœtus (diabète fœtal) in Grancher: *loco citato*, Paris, Masson, 1898, t. V, p. 212.
2. D'ESPINE et PICOT. *Maladies de l'enfance*. Paris, J.-B Baillière et fils, 1899, p. 327.
3. CHARRIN *Diabète pancréatique expérimental d'origine infectieuse*. Congrès français de médecine. Lyon, 1894, p. 101.
4. LANCEREAUX. *Eodem loco*, p. 52 et suivantes.

nerveux[1], sans que nous sachions au juste le rôle dévolu dans chacune de ces formes à la sécrétion interne dont parle M. Lépine et dont le ferment, d'ailleurs, n'a pas été encore, que nous sachions, isolé.

L'observation qui nous est personnelle est relative à une fillette de 6 mois. La voici :

OBSERVATION. — A. B..., née le 4 juin 1898, entre à l'hôpital suburbain. (service de M. le professeur Baumel), salle des nourrissons, lit n° 2, le 20 décembre 1898.

Antécédents héréditaires. — Père bien portant, nous affirme la mère (fille mère).

Celle-ci a eu la *chorée* à 15 ans. Elle a avorté au quatrième mois de sa précédente grossesse, il y a trois ans.

Antécédents personnels. — Née à terme; *éruption généralisée* de nature inconnue, le *quatrième jour après la naissance.*

Histoire de la maladie actuelle. — Cette enfant nous fut présentée par sa mère, à la consultation externe, *quinze jours avant son entrée à l'hôpital.*

On nous raconta que la fillette avait, *depuis une vingtaine de jours environ, les paupières enflées* ainsi que les *mains* et les *jambes:* il fut facile de constater, à ce moment-là, qu'il en était encore ainsi.

On ajouta que la petite malade *urinait souvent et beaucoup plus* que ne le font, d'ordinaire, les enfants de cet âge; que les urines étaient totalement décolorées et semblables à de l'eau ; que la fillette *désirait constamment le sein et qu'elle n'était jamais rassasiée ;* qu'elle vomissait parfois; *qu'elle se démangeait.*

La mère avait déjà montré sa fille à deux médecins de la ville ; le premier lui avait dit qu'il s'agissait d'un refroidissement (néphrite); le second avait demandé à faire l'analyse des urines qui fut pour lui *négative.*

Ce dernier, comme les urines étaient absolument décolorées, demanda à la mère si elle ne lui avait pas apporté tout simplement de l'eau de fontaine.

Après ce récit, nous examinâmes, à notre tour, la petite malade.

Nous fûmes tout de suite frappé par l'*œdème* très accusé dont les paupières, les jambes, le dos, les mains, étaient le siège.

Nous ne trouvâmes rien au poumon, rien au cœur.

Le pouls était plutôt rare pour un enfant de 6 mois. Il ne donnait que 75 à 80 pulsations à la minute.

Le *ventre était volumineux, légèrement météorisé.*

Cet examen terminé, nous procédâmes à l'analyse des urines que la mère avait eu la bonne idée de nous apporter.

Comme coloration elles ressemblaient à de l'eau de fontaine.

---

1. BAUMEL. Pancréas et Diabète in *Montpellier médical,* 1881-1882.
Pour notre théorie pancréatique du diabète nerveux, voir le rapprochement établi par nous, dès 1881-82, entre la remarquable expérience de Cl. Bernard sur le pneumogastrique relative au diabète expérimental et celle, tout aussi intéressante et identique d'ailleurs, de Bernstein concernant la sécrétion pancréatique.

Nous en fîmes une analyse qualitative au point de vue albumine d'abord, elle fut négative.

Nous regardâmes ensuite au point de vue sucre. Sur-le-champ nous n'obtînes rien. Notre embarras était grand et nous avions conclu à l'existence d'une néphrite aiguë sans albumine (?).

La petite et sa mère étaient parties et déjà loin de nous, lorsque nous nous aperçûmes que le tube, dans lequel nous avions mis en présence e chauffé la liqueur de Fehling et l'urine, contenait un *précipité*, peu abondant il est vrai, mais *couleur rouge brique* caractéristique, qui s'était formé insensiblement et, pour ainsi dire, après coup.

Heureusement, cette femme et sa fille vinrent se présenter à la consultation une seconde fois, huit jours après, ce qui nous permit de procéder à un nouvel examen des urines au point de vue du sucre. Le *précipité rouge brique* ne se montra de *nouveau* que deux ou trois minutes après que l'urine et la liqueur de Fehling eurent été mélangées et chauffées.

Nous conseillâmes à la mère d'entrer à l'hôpital avec sa fille pour nous livrer à de nouvelles et plus précises recherches. Elle accepta, mais elle n'entra que huit jours plus tard.

Ce même jour, nous pûmes encore nous rendre compte que l'œdème des paupières, du dos, des mains, des jambes et des pieds était stationnaire.

La polyurie, la polydipsie, les démangeaisons cutanées, persistaient, d'après la mère, avec la même intensité qu'auparavant.

Le 20 décembre 1898, la mère et l'enfant entrent à l'hôpital.

Poids de la fillette, 4 kil., 210.

Paupières, dos, mains, jambes, toujours œdématiés; urines aqueuses, pas de diarrhée, ventre ballonné.

L'examen qualitatif des urines ne donne rien pour l'albumine, mais révèle, au moyen de la liqueur de Fehling, la présence du sucre.

Pas de dents. Signes d'évolution dentaire (salivation, mâchonnement, etc.).

Traitement. — Eau de lactophosphate de chaux à 5 pour 100, 20 grammes. Tétées toutes les trois heures.

Le 22, les œdèmes ont légèrement diminué; un peu de bronchite, quelques *vomissements*.

Looch blanc 120 grammes, benzoate 60 centigrammes.

Le 25, *vomissements, muguet, diarrhée verte*. OEdèmes diminuent.

Collutoire au borate de soude et miel rosat àà p. é. potion du muguet (à l'eau de chaux, 60 grammes pour 150).

Précipité rouge brique dans les urines chauffées avec la liqueur de Fehling.

Le 27, œdèmes à peu près disparus. Toujours *précipité rouge brique*. Poids : 4 k. 110. L'enfant a perdu 160 grammes. Cette diminution de poids, coïncidant avec la disparition des œdèmes, lui est attribuée.

2 janvier 1899, *toujours précipité rouge brique avec la liqueur de Fehling*.

5, poids : 4 k. 165. Augmentation sur la précédente pesée de 55 grammes, soit 8 grammes par jour.

5, envoi d'un échantillon d'urine à M. le docteur Moitessier, professeur agrégé de chimie, chef du laboratoire des cliniques, qui répond le lendé main : « L'urine envoyée jeudi, 5 janvier, du service de **M.** le professeur Baumel, contient 1 *gr.* 50 *de glycose par litre.* »

10, l'œdème des paupières reparaît. *Toujours réaction caractéristique du glycose avec la liqueur de Fehling.*

Poids : 4 k. 270. Augmentation sur la pesée précédente de 105 grammes, soit 15 grammes par jour. La polyurie et la polydipsie persistent.

12, œdème des paupières, des jambes et léger œdème du dos des mains.

M. Moitessier, à qui des urines ont été envoyées à nouveau, nous adresse une note ainsi conçue : « L'urine, envoyée le 11 janvier au laboratoire, contient 1 *gramme de glycose par litre.* »

13, œdèmes continuent; foie douloureux et augmenté de volume; gros ventre. La percussion de *l'estomac* est *tympanique.* Cet organe est dilaté. *La percussion profonde est douloureuse suivant une ligne transversale et pancréatique.*

15, œdèmes diminuent. Les deux incisives médianes inférieures sont sur le point de percer la gencive; elles se voient par transparence.

17, presque plus d'œdèmes aux paupières supérieures; encore un peu au dos, aux mains et aux jambes.

Poids : 4 k. 390. Augmentation de 120 grammes sur la pesée précédente malgré la diminution des œdèmes, soit 17 grammes environ par jour.

La liqueur de Fehling est légèrement *réduite.*

21, disparition à peu près complète des œdèmes. Des urines sont envoyées ce jour-là au laboratoire des cliniques.

24, note de M. Moitessier ainsi conçue : « L'urine qui a été envoyée au laboratoire, samedi 21 janvier, avec l'indication : Crèche : n° 3, A.... *réduit très légèrement la liqueur de Fehling et la liqueur d'Almen* (sous-nitrate de bismuth en solution alcaline). Les essais en vue d'obtenir des cristaux de glucosozone, pour l'identification de la substance réductrice avec le glycose, n'ont pas donné de résultat positif. »

26, œdèmes complètement disparus. *Plus de précipité rouge brique des urines traitées par la liqueur cupro-potassique.*

30, *plus de sucre dans les urines. Les démangeaisons continuent,* tandis qu'il se fait sur tout le corps une *desquamation furfuracée.*

La mère de notre petite malade demande qu'on lui signe son billet. Elle sort ce jour-là de l'hôpital.

Depuis lors, nous avons eu l'occasion de revoir la petite A. B... et de la soigner à plusieurs reprises, d'abord pour une broncho-pneumonie, puis pour une varicelle, enfin tout récemment pour une rougeole dont elle est complètement guérie depuis fin juin 1900. Elle a en ce moment la coqueluche.

La guérison de son diabète est restée définitive jusqu'à ce jour (23 juillet 1900).

RÉFLEXIONS. — Maintenant que nous connaissons l'observation ci-dessus dans tous ses détails. nous pouvons nous poser tout de suite la question de savoir si. chez cette fillette, le pancréas était en cause dans la production de son diabète et comment.

M. Lancereaux, dans un article paru, il n'y a pas bien longtemps, dans le *Journal de clinique et de thérapeutique infantiles*, a décrit une forme particulière de diabète sucré chez l'adolescent tenant à une *aplasie pancréatique*[1].

Il insiste tout spécialement sur cette cause : *l'arrêt de développement du pancréas*, donnant lieu à une forme grave du diabète ; mais, du même coup, il reconnaît *implicitement* à cette glande digestive un rôle prépondérant dans la production du diabète chez l'enfant.

Comme cet auteur, je suis intimement convaincu que certains cas de diabète de la seconde enfance peuvent tenir à un arrêt de développement du pancréas.

Ce n'est pas une simple hypothèse que j'émets, mon opinion est basée sur l'observation. J'en ai vu moi-même un cas chez un enfant de 15 ans.

Dans notre observation actuelle, nous sommes en présence d'une enfant de 6 mois que nous considérons comme ayant été atteinte de diabète et non de glycosurie, qui n'est, après tout, qu'un diabète atténué. Chez l'enfant, comme chez l'adulte, il y a des degrés divers dans le diabète sucré.

La glycosurie est au pancréas (je l'ai dit dès 1881-1882) ce que l'ictère est au foie. Le pancréas présente deux conduits, le foie un seul. Un de ces deux conduits peut être obstrué partiellement ou bouché complètement et l'autre être encore perméable.

Rörig n'a-t-il pas vu, dans un canal collatéral, une pierre qui comprimait le canal principal dilaté et formant un kyste rempli de suc pancréatique ?

Ce que je viens de dire et l'exemple que je viens de citer peuvent expliquer ces divers degrés dans la glycosurie, selon que les deux canaux ou un seul sont obstrués, ou qu'après l'avoir été un certain temps, ils recouvrent leur perméabilité.

Quoi qu'il en soit, c'est la première fois que j'observe le diabète chez un enfant de 6 mois. J'ai voulu, à cette occasion, attirer l'attention sur ce point de pathologie infantile, qui m'a suggéré certaines idées et certaines réflexions que j'ai cru bon de faire connaître.

Nous avons vu qu'il a été noté dans les antécédents personnels de notre malade une *éruption* survenue vers le *quatrième jour après la naissance*, éruption qu'il ne nous a pas été possible de déterminer, n'ayant pas assisté à son évolution.

---

1. LANCEREAUX. *D'une forme de diabète sucré des adolescents, liée à l'aplasie pancréatique.* Juin 1898.

Cette éruption n'était-elle pas déjà liée à l'existence du diabète? Celui-ci n'était-il pas congénital?

Peut-on invoquer, dans l'étiologie de ce cas de diabète sucré, l'existence de la chorée chez la mère à l'âge de 16 ans? Ceci pourrait satisfaire les partisans de l'*hérédité nerveuse* du diabète.

On note encore, chez la mère, un avortement au quatrième mois. Cet accident nous a fait tout de suite penser à l'existence possible de la syphilis, d'autant plus qu'il s'agit d'une fille mère. Toutefois, nous n'en avons pas trouvé la moindre trace, ni par l'interrogatoire, ni par l'examen direct. Ce que nous pouvons affirmer, c'est que cette fille mère n'était pas elle-même diabétique. A aucun moment, nous n'avons trouvé du sucre dans ses urines.

Loin de moi la pensée de nier l'*hérédité diabétique*; mais je suis d'avis qu'on ne doit l'incriminer que lorsqu'on n'a pas autre chose à invoquer.

Ne peut-il pas y avoir *contagion* quelquefois dans le diabète? Certains auteurs, M. Teissier, de Lyon, entr'autres[1], l'admettent.

Pour mon compte, je crois que dans certains cas une semblable étiologie peut être invoquée, surtout quand le diabète lui-même a été observé à la suite d'une maladie infectieuse.

Demandons-nous maintenant quelle est l'étiologie, quelle est la pathogénie relative à notre cas particulier, et, à ce sujet, faisons un peu de pathologie générale.

Ne voyons-nous pas journellement, chez l'enfant nouveau-né, une tuméfaction de l'une des glandes salivaires, tout simplement parce que, la sécrétion se produisant, l'excrétion n'a pas lieu?

Dans un autre ordre d'idées, ne voyons-nous pas également des nourrices primipares déclarées insuffisantes parce que la sécrétion lactée a une certaine difficulté à s'établir, chez elles, pendant les premiers mois qui suivent l'accouchement, alors qu'un peu plus tard cette sécrétion devient, chez ces mêmes nourrices, très abondante?

Pourquoi, ce qui se passe pour les glandes salivaires et pour les glandes mammaires n'aurait-il pas lieu pour le pancréas, soit par lenteur de développement, soit par imperméabilité momentanée ou définitive des conduits, d'où chimie biologique et digestive anormales par nullité ou insuffisance de la fonction pancréatique?

D'après moi et depuis longtemps déjà, le diabète ne serait qu'un syndrome pancréatique, au même titre que l'ictère est un syndrome hépatique. Il y aurait donc à rapprocher le diabète sucré des nouveau-nés de l'ictère du même âge.

1. TEISSIER. *La contagion du diabète.* Congrès de Lyon, 1894. p. 99.

De plus, le pancréas, après avoir acquis son développement normal, peut s'atrophier pour des raisons diverses, ainsi que j'en ai moi-même rapporté ailleurs plusieurs exemples (gastro-entérite. péritonite, etc.[1]).

Dans notre cas, l'alimentation ne saurait être incriminée. l'enfant ne prenait que le sein de sa mère.

Mais. si la cause, que nous venons de signaler et qui nous paraît avoir un *rôle prépondérant chez le nouveau-né et dans la première enfance*, ne peut être invoquée dans tous les cas de diabète passager. ne pourrait-on pas faire intervenir dans une certaine mesure l'évolution dentaire, exerçant une influence nerveuse analogue à celle qui est produite dans l'expérience de Cl. Bernard et de Bernstein?

Ne peut-il pas y avoir excitation du bulbe, de la protubérance. du cerveau même, par l'intermédiaire du trijumeau irrité?

On comprendrait alors que les terminaisons périphériques dentaires de ce nerf, excitées. puissent exciter à leur tour le centre glycosurique, comme dans la chorée de Sydenham elles vont produire l'excitation motrice du bulbe, de la protubérance et de la moelle.

Dans notre cas, c'est l'évolution dentaire *intra-maxillaire,* la plus pénible par conséquent, qui est en cause.

Notre petite malade, à 7 mois, n'avait pas encore ses premières dents, mais, bien qu'elles ne fussent pas encore sorties. elles évoluaient sûrement dans leurs alvéoles.

Il y a toute une pathologie bulbo-protubérantielle, disons mieux *nervoso-réflexe*, de dentition, dont le cadre ira sans contredit s'élargissant de jour en jour.

Il n'est, par conséquent, pas impossible que l'évolution dentaire elle-même joue un rôle dans la pathogénie de certains cas de diabète sucré.

De bonne heure, grâce à l'idée que je me fis dès les premiers temps de ce cas de diabète survenu dans les circonstances signalées, je le déclarai *curable* devant les élèves de mon service. La suite m'a donné raison.

Cette étiologie une fois admise. il est facile de prévoir quelle sera. en général, la thérapeutique du diabète chez le nourrisson.

Au point de vue du pancréas et dans le but de favoriser ses fonctions et sa sécrétion. les alcalins pourront être sagement et habilement administrés (v. plus loin).

On facilitera l'évolution dentaire par l'emploi des phosphates calcaires (lacto. chlorhydro ou glycérophosphate de chaux).

1. L. BAUMEL. *Loco citato.*

Comme l'évolution dentaire chez le nourrisson s'accompagne presque toujours de muguet, il sera bon de rechercher systématiquement cette complication et de la traiter par des badigeonnages à l'aide d'un collutoire composé en parties égales de borate de soude et de miel rosat et par la potion suivante, administrée toutes les trois heures à raison de 2 cuillerées à café dans l'intervalle des tétées :

Eau de chaux. . . . . ⎫ āā 60 gr.
Eau de laitue. . . . . ⎭
Sirop simple. . . . . 50 gr.
Teinture de musc . . . . IV gouttes.

On s'abstiendra, contrairement à la pratique de bien des médecins, de donner de l'eau de Vichy : car, à cause de l'acide carbonique libre qu'elle contient, elle engendre facilement la dilatation de l'estomac, si elle n'existe pas, et l'augmente, lorsqu'elle existe déjà.

Si l'on tient, malgré tout, à donner une eau alcaline, on prescrira de préférence l'eau de Vittel (grande source) ou, tout simplement, l'eau de chaux comme nous l'avons fait dans le cas qui nous est personnel.

L'état nerveux résultat de l'évolution dentaire pourra exiger l'emploi de quelques nervins, du bromure entr'autres.

Quant aux cas de diabète infantile qui résisteraient à ces divers traitements, on pourra les traiter par la pancréatine.

On se rappellera toutefois que cette substance est digérée par l'estomac. Aussi donnera-t-on peut-être un jour la préférence aux injections hypodermiques d'extrait pancréatique, tout en reconnaissant les inconvénients de toute piqûre chez l'enfant, en général, et les dangers qu'elles peuvent faire courir aux diabétiques, en particulier.

XI

SUJETS DIVERS

TROIS CAS DE MENSTRUATION CHEZ LES NOUVEAU-NÉS

par Mme le docteur KOUINDJY.

de Paris.

L'hémorragie génitale des nouveau-nés du sexe féminin pour quelques auteurs et la menstruation précoce pour d'autres, présente un certain intérêt vu sa rareté relative et nous croyons utile de signaler les trois observations que nous avons eu l'occasion de voir dans notre clientèle.

En faisant des recherches sur la fréquence de cet accident, nous avons trouvé que Naegelé considérait les cas d'hémorragie vulvaire comme autant des fables inventées à plaisir. Mais d'autres auteurs ont incontestablement vu ce phénomène se produire et nous voyons qu'Intervood en parle, ainsi que Billard, Olivier (d'Anger), Boivin, Barier, Banchut, etc.

En 1876, le Dr Cullingwort a présenté à la Société obstétricale de Manchester un travail où il a réuni 52 cas, parmi lesquels il a signalé deux cas personnels (un en novembre 1871, l'autre en mai 1875) et actuellement personne ne viendra contester la réalité de cet accident.

Le travail du Dr Cullingwort sert de base dans l'étude de cette question et de temps en temps un auteur vient ajouter un cas personnel à ce tableau fondamental.

Ainsi avons-nous eu l'occasion d'observer pendant les trois dernières années de notre exercice médical trois cas d'hémorragie vulvaire dont nous donnons les observations plus ou moins détaillées.

Obs. I. — Mme D..., âgée de 21 ans, primipare, n'a jamais été éprouvée par une maladie grave, mais elle est anémique et d'une santé plutôt délicate.

Réglée à 15 ans, mariée à 20 ans, elle a accouché le 18 octobre 1897 d'une petite fille bien constituée, pesant 3500 grammes.

Elle a eu une assez bonne grossesse. Les urines présentaient des traces d'albumine pendant les deux derniers mois de la grossesse. Le bassin était normal, mais la tête de l'enfant se maintenait à une certaine hau-leur dans le petit bassin jusqu'au commencement du travail, grâce à une particulière résistance de la paroi abdominale.

La rupture de la poche des eaux a eu lieu le 17 octobre, à minuit. Le travail a duré quinze heures. Présentation O. I. G. A. La petite fille bien vivante a crié aussitôt. J'ai fait la ligature du cordon au bout de quatre minutes. La délivrance naturelle a eu lieu au bout d'une demi-heure. Placenta et membranes complètes. Pas d'hémorragie anormale.

L'enfant bien portante, nourrie par sa mère, présentait des fonctions urinaires et digestives normales.

Le 4e jour après sa naissance on m'a signalé un écoulement génital muqueux. Le 5e jour l'écoulement est devenu sanguinolent. J'ai examiné attentivement l'enfant. Tout l'appareil vulvaire était rouge et turgescent et de l'orifice vaginal s'écoulait un sang rouge noirâtre peu abondant. Cet écoulement a duré jusqu'au 9e jour et n'a plus reparu. Comme traitement j'ai institué des lavages à l'eau boriquée et une garniture avec du coton hydrophile. L'enfant tout en criant pendant ces cinq jours plus qu'à l'ordinaire, a continué de téter et de bien se porter. Du côté des seins j'ai exprimé une certaine quantité d'un liquide lactescent, comme on en trouve chez tant d'autres nouveau-nés des deux sexes. La seule particularité à noter c'est que le cordon ombilical est tombé au bout de vingt et un jours.

Obs. II. — Le 28 février 1899, c'est-à-dire seize mois plus tard, la même Mme D... est accouchée d'une petite fille bien portante, qui pesait 5750 grammes.

A partir du 4e jour l'enfant présentait un écoulement sanguin vaginal qui a duré deux jours. Il n'y avait rien d'anormal à noter chez la mère ni pendant les couches, ni après.

L'enfant se porte bien. Nourrie par sa mère, son appareil digestif et urinaire fonctionnait bien. Le cordon ombilical est tombé au bout de seize jours.

Obs. III. — Mme R.... âgée de 35 ans, multipare, a été réglée à 14 ans. Mariée à 18 ans, elle a eu un garçon à 20 ans, un autre garçon à 25 ans et une fausse couche de 4 mois à 31 ans. Le 31 janvier 1900 elle est accouchée à terme d'une petite fille bien constituée.

Épuisée et anémique, cette malade a beaucoup souffert pendant toute la durée de sa grossesse. Pas d'albumine dans les urines.

Présentation O. I. G. A. Durée du travail trois heures. La délivrance naturelle a eu lieu au bout d'une demi-heure. Le cordon était très grêle; les membranes friables étaient comme tranchées sur le pourtour du gâteau placentaire. Une partie de ces membranes était retenue. Une forte hémorragie a suivi cette délivrance. Suites des couches fébriles. Injections intra-utérines 2 fois par jour avec 18 ou 20 litres d'eau bouillie antiseptique. Guérison et levée au bout de vingt-deux jours.

L'enfant née dans ces conditions, nourrie par sa mère, était très énervée, criait tout le temps et présentait le 4e jour après la naissance un écoulement sanguin vaginal, qui a duré deux jours. Les veines de cet enfant ne présentaient rien de particulier. L'appareil vulvaire était rouge et turgescent. Comme traitement j'ai employé des lotions boriquées et une garniture avec du coton hydrophile. Le cordon ombilical est tombé au bout de six jours. L'enfant se portait bien et ses fonctions digestives et urinaires s'accomplissaient avec régularité.

L'hémorragie génitale apparaît le plus souvent vers le 4ᵉ ou 5ᵉ jour après la naissance et, comme on voit, son pronostic est bénin et n'empêche en rien le développement ultérieur des enfants qui présentaient cette anomalie quelques jours après leur naissance.

Les opinions sur l'étiologie de ces hémorragies sont différentes. Ainsi le Dᵣ V. Gauthier (*Revue méd. de la Suisse romande*, 1884) pense que ces hémorragies dépendent uniquement d'un état catarrhal des organes génitaux comme on en voit chez les nouveau-nés de catarrhe oculaire nasal suivi ou précédé parfois par un écoulement sanguin.

Une autre théorie, celle de Camerer, explique ce phénomène par un trouble de la circulation pelvienne à la suite d'une ligature hâtive du cordon, alors que les battements funiculaires existent encore.

M. Ribemont-Dessaignes attribue ces hémorragies aux troubles circulatoires qui sont sous la dépendance d'une gêne de la respiration ou d'une disposition anormale du cœur ou des gros vaisseaux.

Le Dᵣ Cullingwort ainsi que beaucoup d'autres auteurs adoptent la théorie de Camerer. Même Billard qui a eu l'occasion de voir à l'autopsie de deux petites filles mortes peu de jours après la naissance du sang épanché et pris en caillot dans la cavité de l'utérus, accepta cette théorie.

Une autre théorie considère ces hémorragies comme un écoulement menstruel précoce. Ainsi Ollivier (d'Angers), dans une note ajoutée au chapitre des maladies des organes de la génération du Traité de Billard voit dans cet écoulement un « prélude de la nature ». M. Pinard a eu l'occasion de faire l'autopsie de trois petites filles ayant présenté cet écoulement sanguin précoce par la vulve et il a trouvé au niveau d'un ovaire un follicule de Graaf volumineux venant de se rompre.

En nous basant sur les observations de M. Pinard, il nous semble plus rationnel de considérer cet écoulement génital comme une menstruation précoce.

DISCUSSION

M. Perier demande à Mme Kouindjy si les phénomènes en question se sont reproduits. Il a observé des cas semblables avec répétition.

Mme Kouindjy dit qu'il n'y a pas eu répétition, bien qu'elle ait pu suivre ces enfants.

DE L'APROSEXIE CHEZ LES ENFANTS

par M. BROSIUS.

de Sayn-sur-Rhin.

L'aprosexie des enfants est : 1° au point de vue psychologique un trouble de l'esprit, une faiblesse intellectuelle dont le symptôme fondamental est l'inaptitude de fixer la pensée sur un objet quelconque, par conséquent le manque de conception, de reproduction, l'insuffisance de la mémoire, le retard du développement intellectuel.

2° Au point de vue anatomique une obstruction des fosses nasales et de la cavité nasopharyngienne, due surtout aux végétations adénoïdes.

3° L'embarras de la circulation pulmonaire qui en résulte a pour conséquence une altération nutritive de l'encéphale, une sorte d'auto-intoxication par les produits de déchets de la substance cérébrale.

4° M. le professeur Guy, d'Amsterdam, a proposé, en 1887, le terme d'aprosexie pour désigner cet état.

5° Le cancre scolaire est le type clinique de l'aprosexie. C'est un malade curable qu'il faut savoir soigner: aussi la connaissance de l'aprosexie est-elle importante au point de vue de l'hygiène scolaire et de la pédagogie.

DISCUSSION

M. Chaumier répond que les enfants atteints de végétations adénoïdiennes peuvent être rangés en deux groupes :

a) Ceux qui entendent bien et sont intelligents:

b) Ceux qui sont sourds et qui, par suite, peuvent présenter des troubles intellectuels.

ALCOOLISME DES ENFANTS EN NORMANDIE

par M. le docteur Raoul BRUNON,

de Rouen.

1° Nos documents ont été recueillis à la consultation de l'Hospice Général de Rouen, depuis 1892, dans une enquête faite auprès des instituteurs du département de la Seine-Inférieure, et dans la clientèle.

2° Il faut distinguer l'alcoolisme des enfants pauvres et celui des riches. Chez les premiers, le café noir donné le matin a remplacé le lait et la soupe. Or, en Normandie *le café ne se prend pas sans eau-de-vie*. Il en résulte que l'alcoolisme est la conséquence d'un caféisme primitif.

3° Tous les enfants, sans exception. sont élevés avec du café. Parmi les enfants de dix à quinze ans 75 pour 100 prennent de l'eau-de-vie en plus ou moins grande quantité.

4° La principale cause de cet usage de l'alcool est l'extension progressive de l'alcoolisme chez la femme. celui de l'enfant s'explique alors naturellement.

5° A la campagne, le privilège des bouilleurs de cru facilite l'empoisonnement de la famille entière.

6° Le caféisme et l'alcoolisme engendrent chez l'enfant une dyspepsie spéciale avec manifestations cutanées. Ils enlèvent aux enfants toute résistance aux maladies. Ils sont les promoteurs les plus actifs de la tuberculose. Ils expliquent l'effrayante mortalité infantile, qui est de 55 pour 100 à Rouen.

7° Les adolescents font un usage plus franc de l'alcool (absinthe et apéritifs). Les cas d'ivresse manifeste et publique sont extrêmement fréquents. On ne les remarque même plus dans la rue du samedi soir au mardi matin.

8° *Chez les riches*. La dyspepsie infantile existe par usage des vins généreux et médicamenteux. L'usage prématuré et l'abus de la viande remplacent le caféisme des pauvres.

Les adolescents tendent au contraire à être sobres. L'abstinence fait parmi eux de nombreux prosélytes.

9° Un très grand danger menace les populations normandes : elles sont attaquées dans leur descendance.

10° L'Université a le devoir d'organiser la lutte contre l'alcool dans toutes les écoles de la France. Actuellement cette lutte est conduite mollement.

SUR LE RÔLE DU THYMUS

par M. le docteur SVEHLA.

de Prague

On remarque souvent chez les enfants et même chez les adultes. mais plus rarement. que dans un état de parfaite santé, il arrive des accès de suffocation qui disparaissent ou amènent la mort, avec les symptômes d'accélération de la respiration. de cyanose, de dilatation des pupilles, engorgement des veines, asphyxie et de convulsions générales. On trouve, dans ces cas, à l'autopsie, de l'hyperhémie des méninges; le cœur est rempli de sang liquide rouge foncé; sur les poumons, la plèvre, le péricarde et la glande thymus, on constate des ecchymoses et quelquefois l'œdème du poumon; *l'hypertrophie du thymus est constatée dans tous les cas.*

Dans la littérature, nous rencontrons ce phénomène pathologique décrit sous diverses appellations : asthma thymicum, asthma de Kopp, asthma Millari, spasme de la glotte (laryngo-spasmus), mors thymica.

Les auteurs sont presque unanimes à constater une connexion entre cet état morbide et la mors thymica et l'hypertrophie de la glande thymique.

Prater est le premier qui en 1617 ait démontré cette relation de l'état morbide décrit ci-dessus et l'hypertrophie du thymus.

Mais si les auteurs sont d'accord à reconnaître que le thymus et son hypertrophie sont en connexion directe avec l'asthma thymicum et la mors thymica; il n'en est pas de même pour l'explication de l'action du thymus hypertrophié et de la manière dont se produit l'état morbide et même la mort.

On distingue deux opinions principales : l'une d'elles explique la mort par étouffement; l'autre par paralysie du cœur (Herztov).

Une série d'auteurs (Hirsch, Graf, Hauff, Montgomery, Scharlan, Meissner, Strassmann, Virchow, Klessin) sont d'avis que, dans les cas qu'ils ont observés, le thymus a produit les accès d'étouffement et la mort par la pression mécanique sur l'appareil respiratoire (trachée et poumons); mais ces auteurs ne fournissent pas de preuves directes qui puissent confirmer ce fait.

Pallauf se prononce contre ces auteurs en affirmant que, dans aucun cas de mort subite par étouffement, accompagné d'hypertrophie du thymus, il n'a constaté de modification quelconque de la trachée, produite par compression qui eût été certainement manifeste si elle avait atteint un tel degré que la mort eût pu s'ensuivre.

Schelle et Iamassia ont prouvé par des expériences qu'il faut une plus grande pression pour la compression de la trachée que celle que produit le thymus hypertrophié.

Iamassia dit que pour la compression de la trachée jusqu'à obstruction chez les enfants nés à terme, il faut un poids de 218 grammes et pour la production de la dyspnée, un poids de 125 grammes. D'après Schelle, il faut, chez les enfants d'un an, pour la compression totale de la trachée un poids de 2000 grammes.

Contre cette opinion de la compression de la trachée par la glande thymus, on trouve des cas dans lesquels, malgré la trachéotomie et le cathétérisme de la trachée, la mort a suivi.

Une autre série d'auteurs parmi lesquels Kopp, Hood. Velsen. Masse, Piédecocq, etc., affirme que le thymus hypertrophié comprime l'appareil circulatoire (cœur et grands vaisseaux) d'où résulte un engorgement de sang dans le cerveau produisant des accès d'étouffement.

Schelle prétend, au contraire, que le thymus hypertrophié ne suffit pas à comprimer la veine cave supérieure.

Roth, Palk, Reitel, Hauff, Münchmeyer sont d'avis que le thymus hypertrophié provoque des accès d'étouffement soit par effet réflexe, soit directement, d'une façon mécanique par excitation des nerfs moto-respiratoires.

Pott parle de la compression de la trachée ou des nerfs situés près de la trachée (recurrentes n. vagi) par tuméfaction subite du thymus. et conclut : le thymus hyperplastique exerce une influence lente ou subite sur la respiration et même sur la circulation et peut être, sous l'apparence de pleine santé, et au moins indirectement, la cause d'une mort subite.

Leydl résume son opinion ainsi : dans le cas de mort subite chez les enfants ayant le thymus hypertrophié, la mort est amenée par paralysie du cœur, par suite de compression du nerf cardiaque.

Une autre théorie a été émise par Paltauf et Recklingshausen qui ne voient dans le thymus hypertrophié qu'un simple symptôme d'état morbide général, désigné par eux sous le nom de constitution lympho-chlorotique, et non une cause directe de la mort qui, dans ces cas. est amenée par insuffisance cardiaque, provenant de dégénération du muscle cardiaque. Dans quelques cas, Pala a contaté cette dégénération; Dvornitschenka partage l'avis de Paltauf.

Friedleben estime être autorisé à affirmer que le thymus, même à l'état hypertrophié, ne peut produire le laryngospasmus, et que par conséquent l'asthma thymicum n'existe pas.

Nombre d'auteurs qui décrivent la mort subite accompagnée d'hypertrophie du thymus. faute d'explications suffisantes, laissent la question pendante de savoir s'il y a relation entre le thymus hypertrophié, les accès asthmatiques et la mort.

On voit donc par toutes les théories indiquées ci-dessus qu'il est impossible d'expliquer, par l'action mécanique du thymus, l'asthma thymicum et la mors thymica.

Me basant sur mes expériences faites sur des chiens. au moyen d'extrait aqueux de thymus de provenance humaine ou animale (de bœuf, de porc, de chien), expériences publiées dans mes travaux de l'année 1896, j'ai émis l'opinion que l'asthma thymicum et la mors thymica chez les enfants ayant l'hypertrophie du thymus, sont amenés probablement par hyperthymisation du sang.

Par l'injection de l'extrait aqueux du thymus dans les veines, j'ai démontré que cet extrait agit comme toxique sur les chiens, soit qu'on emploie un extrait de thymus de chien, de bœuf, de porc ou de thymus humain. Après l'injection de cet extrait, on constate de la dyspnée, l'accélération du pouls, du nystagmus, des convulsions partielles des extrémités, de la tête et des convulsions générales, une forte somnolence, et même la perte des réflexes, salivation, nausées, miction et défécation involontaires.

L'autopsie présente soit un résultat négatif ou bien de l'hyperémie des vaisseaux cérébraux; le cœur est rempli d'un liquide sanguin rouge foncé, avec ecchymoses sur le péricarde, la plèvre et les poumons.

J'ai pu confirmer ces constatations par des essais faits ultérieurement à l'aide d'extrait de glande sèche. mais, dans ces cas, la concentration a dû être plus grande.

L'extrait aqueux du thymus agit comme toxique, et même à petites doses, amène la mort chez les individus jeunes; chez les chiens âgés il ne produit pas une si grande intoxication.

La propriété toxique de cet extrait est plus en rapport avec l'âge qu'avec le poids de l'individu. c'est-à-dire qu'un chien âgé et de petite taille supporte une dose d'extrait de 100 centigrammes, sans grande difficulté: tandis qu'un *jeune* chien plus fort que le premier succombe après une injection de 10 centigrammes du même extrait.

L'injection de l'extrait de la glande surrénale provoquant une grande augmentation de la tension du sang, ainsi qu'une accélération du pouls, n'empêche pas la mort après injection d'une dose toxique léthale d'extrait de thymus. L'effet reste le même soit que l'injection de l'extrait de la glande surrénale ait été faite avant, pendant ou après l'injection toxique léthale de l'extrait de thymus.

De quelle manière l'extrait de thymus agit-il?

Les essais suivants ont été faits sur des chiens ; après une injection de curare avec ventilation artificielle des poumons ou après une narcose d'opium, une canule fut introduite dans l'artère carotide et reliée à un sphygmographe ; ensuite une injection d'extrait de thymus fut faite dans la veine fémorale.

J'ai démontré que l'injection d'extrait de thymus produit l'accélération du pouls et une dépression de la tension du sang.

J'ai démontré dans des essais ultérieurs faits dès l'année 1896 que l'accélération du pouls a lieu : 1° après la section du nerf vagus et une injection antérieure d'atropine ; 2° même après l'extirpation des ganglions stilata, la section simultanée du nerf vagus et la paralysie du vagus par l'atropine.

L'accélération du pouls après l'injection de l'extrait de thymus a lieu même après la section de la moelle opérée à la hauteur de la septième vertèbre cervicale.

Il résulte de ces expériences que l'injection dans la circulation du sang de l'extrait aqueux de thymus produit l'amélioration du pouls, par action directe sur le cœur.

J'ai tâché de rechercher au moyen des expériences suivantes la cause de l'abaissement de la tension du sang par suite de l'injection de l'extrait de thymus.

Après la narcose des chiens dont l'artère carotide est en communication avec un cymugraphe, je lie l'aorte thoracique et injecte l'extrait de thymus dans la veine jugulaire. J'obtiens ainsi un abaissement de la tension du sang ; le même fait se produit lorsque avant l'injection de l'extrait de thymus, je lie l'aorte sur le diaphragme, la radio-mésentérite et l'artère rénale, même quand je lie l'aorte et fais en même temps l'éventration totale.

Au cours de cette dernière expérience, j'ai introduit dans la seconde veine jugulaire une canule ouverte et j'ai observé l'écoulement du sang veineux. J'ai constaté que l'écoulement du sang diminue lorsque la tension du sang s'abaisse et augmente avec accroissement de la tension.

L'expérience de contrôle se fait de la façon suivante : après la ligature de l'aorte, j'ai injecté, au lieu d'extrait de thymus, une solution physiologique de chlorure de sodium, et j'ai démontré qu'aucun changement de tension du sang n'a lieu.

On voit, d'après ces expériences, que même l'abaissement de la tension du sang, après l'injection de l'extrait de thymus, est provoqué, en première ligne, par action directe de l'extrait sur le cœur et non sur les vaso-moteurs.

Il faut donc considérer l'extrait de thymus comme un poison spécial du cœur.

J'ai publié, en 1899, des expériences faites à l'aide de l'extrait de thymus provenant d'embryons humains d'enfants et d'adultes.

En même temps, j'ai fait des expériences à l'aide d'embryons de bœuf et j'ai fait usage de l'extrait de glande thyroïdea et de glande surrénale. J'ai démontré ainsi que chez l'homme les glandes thymus.

thyroïde et surrénale ne produisent pas en elles, à l'état embryonnaire, la matière active qu'on extrait par l'eau et qu'elle commencent à se manifester chez les enfants nés à terme, sans disparaître même avec l'âge. D'après mes propres recherches, Hyrst n'a pas raison d'écrire : « Le thymus n'existe en pleine évolution que dans la vie embryonnaire et dans la première enfance », de même Seyd qui écrit : « Le thymus, cet organe fœtal ».

Au cours de ces essais, j'ai observé que le degré d'activité relative de l'extrait des glandes thymus, thyroïdea, et surrénale varie selon l'âge de l'individu d'où elles proviennent. Le thymus est relativement le plus actif dans l'enfance ; ensuite la thyroïde ; enfin la glande surrénale est la moins active.

Pour apprécier plus nettement cette relation d'activité de l'extrait des glandes, j'ai pris dans de nouvelles expériences les organes entiers, le thymus, la thyroïde et la surrénale d'un individu et j'ai injecté l'extrait de cette mixture à des chiens.

J'ai constaté, après l'injection de l'extrait mixte, provenant d'un enfant venu à terme, une courbe cymographique semblable à celle du thymus ou de la thyroïde, c'est-à-dire une dépression de tension du sang, une accélération du pouls et non l'effet de l'extrait surrénal, c'est-à-dire augmentation de tension et accélération du pouls, ou excitation des nerfs vagus quand ceux-ci subsistent.

Dans un âge plus avancé, l'action de la glande surrénale est manifeste et même, ensuite, prédominante.

Quant à la constitution chimique de la matière active du thymus, j'ai pu jusqu'ici constater l'effet suivant : on peut l'extraire par l'eau, par l'alcool ; elle ne coagule pas à la cuisson par l'eau additionnée d'acide acétique et de chlorure de sodium ; on ne peut l'extraire de la solution aqueuse par l'éther sulfurique et elle ne se précipite pas par l'acétate de plomb.

J'ai fait usage de la méthode d'injection de l'extrait aqueux du thymus par la veine dans l'organisme, parce que cette manière s'approche le mieux du passage de la sécrétion du thymus, dans la vie réelle, dans l'organisme. Car Restelli et, après lui, Friedleben, ont observé que chez le veau, les éléments formés de la sécrétion du thymus passent dans la veine thymique : Friedleben n'a pas rencontré ces éléments dans la carotide.

En résumé, la glande thymus contient dans sa sécrétion une matière qui, amenée dans l'organisme d'une manière s'approchant le mieux de la voie naturelle, produit chez les chiens un état morbide cliniquement semblable aux symptômes observés dans l'asthma thymicum des enfants. Cette matière, même à petite dose, cause la mort, chez les jeunes individus, avec les mêmes symptômes que ceux observés dans la mors thymica des enfants.

L'autopsie des animaux d'expérience, présente après l'injection de l'extrait de thymus, le même résultat que celui observé à l'autopsie des enfants morts à la suite d'hypertrophie du thymus.

La matière active du thymus est un poison pour le cœur. On peut donc dire, en résumé, que très probablement chez les enfants ayant le thymus hypertrophié, et conséquemment une augmentation de sécrétion, sous l'influence de diverses causes (compression de glande par rejet brusque de la tête en arrière (Seydl), il se produit des accès d'asthme et même la mort par suite du passage d'une grande quantité de sécrétion du thymus dans la circulation ; c'est-à-dire par hyperthymisation du sang.

DISCUSSION

M. MARTINEZ-VARGAS. — Je viens d'entendre que le D' Svehla attache une influence exclusive à l'hyperthymisation du sang, dans la production des morts soudaines consécutives à l'hypertrophie du thymus. Nous ne pouvons laisser sans réplique cette manière de penser, puisqu'elle jette par terre plusieurs autres mécanismes qui ont été signalés par les cliniciens et démontrés par les autopsies. Je ne nie pas certaine valeur à l'intoxication, mais cependant ce n'est pas la cause principale ni la plus fréquente. Il faut rappeler les conditions anatomiques et physiologiques du thymus et des organes avec lesquels il est en rapport, les principales de ses relations étant avec la trachée, les nerfs et vaisseaux du cou, le cœur et les gros vaisseaux, comme l'artère pulmonaire et le tronc brachio-céphalique, etc.

Quelle que soit la cause, hypertrophie, néoplasmes ou syphilis, ou autres troubles, le thymus augmente son volume et ne peut pas vaincre dans le cou le cercle osseux que forment la colonne vertébrale, le sternum et les clavicules, et par conséquent il doit produire certaine compression dans la trachée, surtout si l'enfant pendant le sommeil redresse son cou : c'est la cause qui expliquerait les morts survenues pendant la nuit et qu'anciennement on attribuait à l'étouffement déterminé par la mamelle de la nourrice fermant la bouche du nourrisson. C'est un des mécanismes de mort, c'est-à-dire celui de la compression de la trachée ; cette compression a été démontrée par les autopsies ; en effet, on a vu des cadavres d'enfants avec un enfoncement de la trachée et avec aplatissement ou ulcération. Dans ce cas la mort est tout à fait rapide.

On doit accepter un second mécanisme. Quand l'agrandissement du thymus se produit dans sa partie inférieure, soit par l'hypertrophie, soit par les néoplasmes, il peut déterminer la compression directe du cœur, mais surtout de l'oreillette droite ou de l'artère pulmonaire. Donc si la pression est capable d'interrompre la circulation du sang et de produire la mort, l'accident n'est pas si rapide que dans le cas antérieur et en outre il s'accompagne de symptômes de cyanose, d'asystolie, etc. La clinique nous a montré des cas semblables.

Troisième cause. Quand il y a des accès préalables de spasme de la glotte et d'autres troubles nerveux, il faut penser à l'excitation produite par le thymus sur le nerf laryngien inférieur ou le vagus.

Enfin il y a un autre mécanisme de mort à invoquer, celui qui se rapporte aux belles expériences de mon confrère Svehla avec les chiens, c'est-à-dire l'intoxication par la substance thymique. Cette théorie a besoin de quelques confirmations dans la clinique humaine. De toutes manières, en acceptant l'intoxication, elle ne pourrait pas expliquer tous les cas de mort il y a contre un argument irréfutable : si toujours la mort fut produite par l'hyperthymisation du sang et seulement par elle, comment pourrait-on expliquer la mort soudaine par un thymus agrandi par une néoplasie qui a détruit tout le tissu de la glande? Alors il y a une grande augmentation de l'organe, mais il est impossible de produire du suc thymique et par conséquent d'intoxiquer le sang. Dans la littérature clinique on trouvera des preuves à cet appui.

M. SVEHLA dit qu'il n'a pas voulu expliquer tous les cas. Ce qui est certain c'est que la compression mécanique admise à l'exclusion de tout autre mécanisme par certains auteurs, n'est certainement pas vraie pour bon nombre d'entre eux.

DES DANGERS DE L'ÉTROITESSE PRÉPUTIALE CHEZ LES NOURRISSONS ET DES AVANTAGES DE LA DILATATION COMME MOYEN D'Y OBVIER

par M. le docteur R. SAINT PHILIPPE,

Médecin de l'Hôpital des Enfants malades, de Bordeaux.

Chez l'enfant naissant, le phimosis est presque de règle. Les cas où le gland passe à frottement entre les lèvres du prépuce constituent l'infinie exception. Mais il faut distinguer, comme l'a fait depuis longtemps Vidal de Cassis, entre le phimosis atrophique dans lequel le prépuce s'applique au gland sans le déborder, et le phimosis hypertrophique dans lequel le prépuce exubérant le dépasse parfois de 2 à 5 centimètres.

Je veux retenir l'attention sur la première variété, dont les inconvénients ne me paraissent pas avoir été tous mis en lumière.

On sait, en effet, que le phimosis banal est capable de produire des effets divers, bien étudiés et bien indiqués en France : des troubles fonctionnels du côté de la vessie et de l'urètre, des hernies, des prolapsus, du rectum, de l'hydrocèle et aussi des troubles réflexes à distance, étudiés par les Américains et frappant surtout, de façon bien inattendue, tout le système nerveux, tels que l'irritation cérébrale, l'insomnie, les convulsions, les attaques épileptiformes, la chorée, les palpitations, du strabisme. des parésies. des paralysies et même des contractions.

Ce que l'on sait moins, c'est que l'étroitesse de l'orifice préputial peut être un danger pour la vie même de l'enfant. Voici comment :

Le parallélisme n'est pas toujours exact entre l'orifice préputial et l'orifice du méat urinaire. L'urine commence par être retenue en petite quantité, après la miction : puis l'accumulation des sécrétions épithéliales et glandulaires, irritantes, la présence d'une urine épaisse et sédimenteuse, comme on l'observe parfois chez les enfants d'arthritiques et pendant les grosses chaleurs, amène l'inflammation du gland et du prépuce, et tout doucement l'orifice d'excrétion se ferme. L'infiltration d'urine s'opère et. peu à peu, la rétention elle-même s'établit.

L'enfant, si on n'intervient pas chirurgicalement sans hésitation. par de larges débridements, peut succomber alors, soit au progrès de l'infiltration rapidement suivie de sphacèle, soit à l'urémie aiguë.

Huit observations servent de base à mon articulation. On pourrait en relater bien d'autres.

L'une d'elle est très curieuse. Édifié par l'expérience sur les accidents promptement mortels qui peuvent survenir en pareil cas, je fis une fois prier un de mes collègues chirurgiens, au moment où je cédais mon service pendant les vacances, de surveiller de près un nourrisson qui présentait un prépuce serré. de la balano-posthite avec rareté des urines.

Ce chirurgien temporisa et fit appliquer des compresses résolutives. L'enfant mourait 24 heures après. J'ai donc raison de dire que ces faits ne sont pas assez connus.

Quand les événements revêtent une allure moins dramatique, c'est l'avenir qui est menacé. Ces enfants restent exposés aux conséquences fâcheuses du phimosis, et il faut intervenir pour les y soustraire. par une opération sanglante. dont les résultats ne sont pas toujours parfaits.

Mieux vaudrait intervenir de bonne heure. et de façon beaucoup plus douce.

Rien n'est plus facile que de rompre les adhérences balano-préputiales lorsque l'orifice du prépuce le permet. Il suffit de ramener cet organe en arrière du gland. et il serait à désirer. dit mon collègue. M. Pousson. que cette petite manœuvre s'introduisît dans toutes les maternités et que tous les nouveau-nés y fussent soumis là ou ailleurs.

Lorsque au contraire le prépuce ne peut pas découvrir le gland, lorsqu'on a affaire à un phimosis par excès de brièveté du prépuce, à une adhérence très étroite du prépuce et du gland, à plus forte raison à un tout petit pertuis, presque imperceptible, il faut avec une sonde cannelée ou un stylet, séparer les deux surfaces épithéliales fusionnées et rétablir la béance normale de l'orifice d'excrétion. Un jet d'eau boriquée lancée entre le prépuce et le gland aseptise ensuite le sac préputial et entraîne le smegma et tous les produits de sécrétion.

Enfin, lorsqu'on n'arrive pas au résultat désiré, il est de toute nécessité de recourir à la petite opération de la *dilatation* à l'aide d'une pince à forcipressure, par le procédé doux et instantané, préférable par sa rapidité à la dilatation méthodique et progressive. Si cette méthode préconisée par des hommes comme Verneuil, Lannelongue, de Saint-Germain et Chalot peut être contestée comme mode opératoire chez les enfants plus âgés et pour le phimosis ordinaire, elle ne peut plus soulever de discussion dans les cas dont il s'agit et pour des nourrissons dont il faut ménager les forces et le sang. Ce moyen est simple, à la portée de tous: il n'expose, quoi qu'on ait dit, ni aux rétractions, ni à la récidive. Un de nos élèves de Bordeaux vient de l'établir d'une façon très nette dans sa thèse inaugurale (Carrère, 1899), à l'instigation de mon collègue et ami M. Piéchaud qui donne lui aussi, dans la majorité des cas, la préférence à la dilatation de la STRICTURE préputiale.

DISCUSSION

M. AUDEOUD (de Genève) confirme l'opinion de M. Saint-Philippe et a vu des accidents graves dus à l'atrésie du phimosis, guérir par la dilatation.

TRAITEMENT DE LA PELADE INFANTILE

PAR LES PULVÉRISATIONS DE CHLORURE DE MÉTHYLE

par M. le docteur HÉRON.

de Tours.

M. HÉRON (Tours) signale les sérieux résultats obtenus dans son service d'enfants à l'hôpital de Tours par l'application des pulvérisations de chlorure de méthyle au traitement de la pelade. Ces pulvérisations précédées de lavages des plaques au sublimé étaient répétées tous les deux ou trois jours et chaque fois suivies d'enveloppement de coton hydrophile.

Les enfants traités avaient de 2 à 5 ans : les plaques de pelade de 2 à 6 millimètres. Toutes ont guéri au bout de deux à trois mois.

M. Héron demande à ses confrères s'ils ont fait des expériences semblables et, dans la négative, les prie d'expérimenter à leur tour ce moyen dans l'intérêt de leurs petits malades.

DISCUSSION

M. Jacquet répond à M. Héron que, tout en le félicitant de sa très intéressante communication, il y a beaucoup à dire sur certaines des ses affirmations.

Sur le premier point, la contagiosité de la pelade à laquelle il a fait allusion, M. Jacquet fait remarquer qu'à l'heure actuelle les dermatologistes sont très partagés, mais que l'hypothèse de la contagiosité perd de plus en plus de terrain. Pour sa part, M. Jacquet ne l'admet plus et donne à toute pelade une origine névrotrophique sur la nature intime de laquelle il est en train de faire des recherches.

Pour ce qui est du traitement proposé par M. Héron, M. Jacquet observe que l'auteur a mis d'instinct la main sur un très bon traitement. Mais ici, il faut s'entendre, et M. Héron est-il bien sûr d'avoir eu toujours affaire à la pelade vraie, quand il parle de ces guérisons rapides. En tout cas sa communication manque de précision sur ce point. Il ne faut pas oublier que chez les enfants, très fréquemment, on observe des plaques d'alopécie disséminées, sans gravité, contre lesquelles tout traitement réussit, et en particulier contre lesquelles doit particulièrement bien réussir le traitement proposé par M. Héron.

Mais à côté de ces alopécies, trop souvent qualifiées de pelade, il y a la pelade vraie, celle qui se caractérise par le découronnement de la nuque, par une alopécie qui, débutant au niveau de l'occiput, remonte derrière les oreilles, et où la peau présente cet aspect très spécial de l'aire péladique. A ce niveau, en effet, la peau a perdu son élasticité, elle est molle, si on la prend entre les doigts, elle vient comme un morceau d'étoffe, et ce fait montre bien que dans la pelade vraie il y a une sorte d'hypotonie des tissus. Cette hypotonie se retrouve sur d'autres organes, en particulier du côté du système veineux, ce qui montre bien que la pelade n'est qu'un phénomène localisé d'une altération nutritive généralisée, que M. Jacquet croit très profonde, et dont il est en train d'étudier la nature.

Quoi qu'il en soit, dans la pelade le traitement qui réussit le mieux est l'irritation légère et permanente du cuir chevelu ; aussi comprend-on que le traitement préconisé par M. Héron puisse rendre des services.

M. Héron trouve dans les observations de son savant confrère l'utilité de la communication qu'il a faite. Il sait bien que de petites plaques alopéciques se produisent au cours de maladies aiguës chez les enfants, et il les a observées aussi bien dans la clientèle de ville qu'à l'hôpital ; mais il ne s'en préoccupait pas outre mesure, car elles guérissaient presque sans traitement. Il n'en était pas de même des véritables plaques dont il a rapporté la relation et qui n'ont été améliorées et guéries que par le traitement en question. C'est le seul point qu'il a voulu signaler, pensant être utile à la cause qu'il sert.

Personne ne demandant plus la parole, M. Héron croit de son devoir de dernier inscrit de se faire l'interprète de ses confrères de la section de pédiatrie en remerciant les éminents maîtres et professeurs qui constituent le bureau pour les précieux enseignements qu'ils leur ont donnés, soit pendant les séances du Congrès, soit au cours des intéressantes visites dans les hôpitaux, ainsi que pour la constante courtoisie qu'ils ont mise à montrer leur science aimable et bienveillante.

ALLOCUTION

de M. le professeur GRANCHER

Messieurs, avant de prononcer la clôture de notre section, je tiens à vous rappeler qu'au début de nos travaux nous avons eu la douleur de perdre deux hommes qui, depuis vingt ans, ont été des maîtres incontestés en pédiatrie. Je veux parler de MM. Cadet de Gassicourt et Jules Simon. Ces deux hommes, par leur haute valeur scientifique, par leurs qualités, ont succédé dignement à des maîtres qu'il semblait impossible de remplacer, les Bouchut, les Roger, les Parrot.

Sans vouloir ici prononcer leur éloge, — ce ne serait pas le lieu, — je désire m'étendre un peu sur chacun de ces deux hommes.

Cadet de Gassicourt était tout de finesse et d'élégance. Il portait en lui une sorte d'aristocratie intellectuelle qui se retrouvait dans tous ses écrits, dans toute sa personne. D'un abord facile et charmant, il possédait un remarquable don d'observation, et, à cet égard, ses « cliniques » sont restées un modèle de science et de conscience. Elles me servent presque quotidiennement. Il n'est presque pas de sujet, pas de point qu'il n'ait abordé, et partout il y a apporté cette qualité maîtresse : l'exactitude de l'observation.

Quant à Jules Simon il était, bien que possédant lui aussi un esprit très fin, très délicat, d'un abord, d'un aspect tout différent. C'était un homme rond, d'allures très simples, adorant les enfants qui l'adoraient, sachant mieux qu'aucun autre comment les prendre, à cet âge surtout où le médecin d'enfants rencontre de si grosses difficultés. Il les captivait; aucun ne lui résistait, et, en même temps, Jules Simon savait plaire aux mères par le côté utile de la pratique médicale, par ces mille petites ressources qu'il savait leur indiquer, et, grâce à ces dons, il était arrivé à gagner une situation enviée et respectée.

Il ne faut pas oublier enfin que Jules Simon était également un homme d'avant-garde. C'est lui qui, le premier avec Roux, fit le diagnostic bactériologique de l'angine diphtérique, et c'est ainsi que cet homme, tout en gardant l'aspect, les apparences du vieux médecin, savait se montrer un médecin moderne dans toute l'acception du mot.

Jules Simon a rendu de grands services à l'enseignement, non pas par des leçons *ex cathedra* auxquelles sa modestie ne le conviait pas, mais par le soin avec lequel il instruisait à la consultation tant de jeunes générations médicales. Aussi a-t-il laissé un grand vide.

Je tenais à rapprocher ces deux hommes et à mêler leur nom à nos travaux pour qu'il ne soit pas dit que nous les oublions.

Le Congrès de pédiatrie, qui clôt ses séances, a fait en somme une très bonne besogne. Des rapports excellents, des discussions vigoureuses, utiles, un grand nombre de communications, voilà ce que nous avons entendu. Tous les membres de notre section ont compris l'utilité de cette mise en commun d'efforts et de bonne volonté, et ce ne sont pas seulement nos travaux, mais nos personnes qui ont pu ainsi mieux cimenter le travail de collaboration dans l'étude de cette branche de la médecine.

En terminant, je tiens tout particulièrement à remercier nos confrères étrangers et à leur dire combien nous leur sommes reconnaissants de leur empressement. A notre tour, nous irons chez eux leur porter le résultat de nos efforts, de notre travail, afin de resserrer encore les liens affectueux qui nous unissent.

TABLE ANALYTIQUE

DES COMPTES RENDUS DE LA SECTION DE MÉDECINE DE L'ENFANCE

I

ALLAITEMENT, ALIMENTATION ET HYGIÈNE DES ENFANTS

II

AFFECTIONS GASTRO-INTESTINALES

III

TUBERCULOSE INFANTILE

IV

MALADIES DES MÉNINGES ET DU SYSTÈME NERVEUX

V

DIPHTÉRIE

VI

COQUELUCHE

X

ALBUMINURIE INTERMITTENTE, URICÉMIE, DIABÈTE

XI

SUJETS DIVERS

SECTION DE CHIRURGIE DE L'ENFANCE

COMPTES RENDUS

publiés par M. VILLEMIN

Secrétaire de la Section.

CHIRURGIE DE L'ENFANCE

COMITÉ D'ORGANISATION DE LA SECTION

Président : M. LANNELONGUE.
Vice-Présidents : MM. KIRMISSON et PIÉCHAUD (de Bordeaux).
Secrétaires : MM. BROCA et VILLEMIN.
Membres : MM. BRUN, FÉLIZET, JALAGUIER, MAUCLAIRE, NOVÉ-JOSSERAND (de Lyon), VINCENT (de Lyon), PHOCAS (de Lille) et MÉNARD (de Berck).

Présidents d'honneur :

MM. BRADFORD (Boston), HOFFA (Würtzbourg), LORENZ (Vienne).

VENDREDI 3 AOUT

Séance de l'après-midi.

DISCOURS D'OUVERTURE

de M. LANNELONGUE, président.

MESSIEURS,

Permettez-moi tout d'abord de souhaiter la bienvenue à tous les étrangers à la France, en particulier à ceux venus de loin, d'autres continents que le nôtre, qui n'ont pas craint d'affronter de grandes distances pour assister à ce Congrès. J'y joins en suite nos amis de France qui eux aussi ont abandonné leurs affaires, et je me plais à croire que tous vous n'aurez pas de regret d'avoir consenti à venir prendre part à nos travaux pour y exposer vos recherches ou le fruit de votre expérience.

Il suffit de lire le nom des rapporteurs des questions qui vous ont été soumises, les Hoffa, les Lorenz, les Soubotine, les Bradford, les Trèves, les Roux, pour être fixés à l'avance sur la valeur des questions qui sont soumises à votre libre discussion. Ce sont les représentants les plus éminents dans les branches diverses de la pédiatrie qui ont été choisis pour mettre au point les questions pendantes, après en avoir fait l'objet d'un examen approfondi. De même que le nombre des communications inscrites témoigne non seulement d'un empressement justifié par l'importance des sujets, mais aussi du vaste champ de la pédiatrie qu'on ne fait en réalité que commencer à défricher.

Il était à peu près resté la propriété de la pathologie interne ou de la pathologie externe, malgré qu'il y eût depuis longtemps des hôpitaux spéciaux de maladies des enfants.

C'était le temps où les spécialités n'étaient pas très en honneur et où les hommes sérieux n'osaient s'y aventurer qu'après avoir acquis déjà une certaine notoriété par une culture générale étendue et un savoir apprécié.

C'est alors seulement qu'ils consentaient à se confiner dans un domaine plus étroit et comme rétréci, et ils y apportaient souvent des qualités vraiment peu communes d'observation et de tact.

Mais les temps allaient changer avec l'introduction de branches nouvelles dans la médecine. La science microscopique la première allait sortir d'une longue enfance et avec elle toute une série de vues nouvelles sur les diathèses, sur les métastases, sur l'évolution des maladies des organes que la pathologie cellulaire synthétisait admirablement.

Puis la bactériologie apparaissait à son tour et allait imprimer un essor nouveau à la pathologie proprement dite, en même temps que l'antisepsie allait donner toute carrière à toutes les hardiesses opératoires.

Il n'en fallait pas davantage pour donner aux spécialités une poussée vigoureuse et d'un caractère scientifique. De fait, les spécialisations se sont beaucoup étendues, trop peut-être, et un grand nombre de chercheurs y ont introduit les méthodes d'études nouvelles. Grâce à cette introduction, on peut dire que l'ère des spécialisations a amené un progrès très grand et très rapide et fourni des résultats plus nombreux et plus précis. La technique y a atteint un perfectionnement des plus importants et, en somme, on peut dire que les spécialités ont contribué grandement à l'avancement des sciences.

La pédiatrie dont la chirurgie infantile est certainement le plus grand héritier, le fils aîné par l'âge et pour les droits à l'héritage, n'est pas seulement une spécialité. Elle ne se borne plus aux maladies d'un organe ou d'un appareil, elle accapare la vie entière de l'homme presque durant sa première moitié au point de vue pathologique. Et comme tout adulte émane d'un âge antérieur, il en résulte que tous les hommes ont dû passer par elle ou peu s'en faut.

Vouloir dire alors de quoi elle s'occupe, ce serait passer en revue à peu près toute la pathologie, car elle a son chapitre urinaire comme celle du vieillard, de chirurgie d'urgence comme l'adulte, et elle a de plus en propre tout le groupe des maladies congénitales de développement.

Le nouveau-né, l'enfant et l'adolescent présentent, à quelques exceptions près, tout le cadre pathologique de l'adulte, seulement il prend chez eux une modalité spéciale inhérente à la composition des humeurs, à la jeunesse des cellules organiques et à l'active poussée de ces dernières.

Tout le groupe des maladies congénitales, embryonnaires et fœtales nous appartient en propre; il comprend l'orthopédie, cette branche si chirurgicale de notre art. Il soulève les problèmes les plus élevés de l'hérédité, qui ne borne pas ses effets à des manifestations aussi éclatantes que celles des anomalies ou des vices de conformation. La puissance de l'hérédité se montre sous de nombreux aspects dans le jeune âge, depuis l'influence tangible comme dans la syphilis, la tuberculose, l'hystérie, jusqu'aux manifestations occultes d'états morbides divers.

Et je ne puis qu'indiquer la part qui revient dans toutes les manifestations morbides à un développement qui n'est pas livré au hasard, s'accomplissant au contraire suivant des lois dont la régularité permet de prévoir les écueils de l'évolution, et par suite de la surveiller, de la protéger.

Le développement ne saurait par lui-même faire naître la maladie, il ne la crée pas, mais il peut, sous l'influence de certaines circonstances comme le surmenage, la fatigue, le traumatisme, préparer un terrain favorable aux manifestations morbides, à l'infection en particulier, en diminuant les défenses contre certains microbes, ou encore en rendant les microbes plus virulents.

Je m'arrête, Messieurs, me bornant à dire en terminant qu'il n'y a pas seulement qu'à glaner dans le champ où nous travaillons. Il s'y trouve des mines d'une grande richesse qu'il nous appartient d'exploiter avec plus ou moins de fruit.

L'OPÉRATION SANGLANTE DE LA LUXATION CONGÉNITALE DE LA HANCHE

RAPPORT

par le professeur A. HOFFA,

de Würtzbourg.

C'est avec bien du plaisir, que je réponds aujourd'hui à l'honorable invitation de donner une communication sur l'opération sanglante de la luxation congénitale de la hanche. Je voudrais traiter cette question très objectivement et vous prie de m'excuser, si je n'ai recours qu'aux observations faites par moi-même pendant quatorze ans. D'abord j'ai voulu donner un bref aperçu historique.

Le premier qui ait décrit la manière sanglante d'opérer la luxation congénitale de la hanche est *Guérin*. D'après sa théorie de la rétraction primaire des muscles, il pratiquait la ténotomie de tous les muscles autour du trochanter majeur, en même temps il faisait attention au développement insuffisant de la cavité cotyloïde, en voulant fixer par des scarifications sous-cutanées la tête du fémur bien directement à l'os iliaque. Les résultats qu'il obtenait de cette manière ne furent pas de longue durée. *Bouvier*, *Pravaz* le jeune, *Corridge* et particulièrement *Brodhurst* reprirent la ténotomie de *Guérin* et c'est bien *Brodhurst*, qui prétend avoir eu de bons résultats les dernières années qu'il pratiquait cette méthode. *Hueter* avait alors un plan rationnel. Il voulait, après avoir dénudé la tête atrophiée du fémur, détacher des lambeaux périostiques du fémur et de l'os iliaque et les suturer l'un à l'autre.

Il n'a jamais mis en pratique cette opération. *De Paoli* et *Israël* clouaient ou bien suturaient la tête du fémur à l'os iliaque pour lui donner un appui manifeste, mais n'obtenaient aucun bon résultat.

Koenig cherchait à donner une nouvelle loge osseuse ou un relief osseux contre la réascension de la tête en détachant de l'os iliaque un lambeau ostéo-périostique, qu'il rabattait et suturait avec la capsule, après avoir pratiqué une extension préparatoire pour abaisser le plus possible la tête du fémur.

Cette méthode suivie par *Koenig* et d'autres chirurgiens comme *Gussenbauer*, *Schoenborn*, a donné sur divers points une véritable amélioration. Elle fut cependant plus tard abandonnée par *Koenig* même. Une autre opération qui fut pratiquée pour la luxation congénitale de la hanche est la résection de la tête du fémur. Après qu'elle eut été premièrement faite par *Rose* et *Reyer*, elle fut vulgarisée par *Margary*, qui seul l'a pratiquée six fois. Plus tard, elle fut reprise en Italie par *Lumpagnani, Motta, Raffo, de Paoli, Postempski* et encore d'autres, en Allemagne par *Heusner, Schüssler* et *Läcke*, en Angleterre par *Ogston*, en France par *Vincent* et *Molière*.

Le résultat de la résection de la tête fémorale laisse encore beaucoup à désirer. La cause de la mauvaise marche après l'opération unilatérale est bien sans exception le raccourcissement absolu atteint par la résection, qui devient d'autant plus grand que le raccourcissement nutritif des parties molles autour de l'articulation de la hanche, acquis par la maladie elle-même, donne plus de résistance à la traction pendant l'extension. De plus, le glissement de l'extrémité supérieure du fémur contre le bassin n'est pas certainement enlevé par la résection.

En outre, il existe encore la lordose de la colonne vertébrale, au moins c'est le cas avec la luxation unilatérale.

Au contraire, il en résulte régulièrement une scoliose statique de la colonne vertébrale lombaire.

Ces observations nous indiquent que la résection n'atteint pas le but que nous pourrions exiger d'une opération de la luxation congénitale de la hanche.

Veut-on l'opérer, alors on doit la faire selon mon idée, dans les cas où on est assuré qu'on peut améliorer, d'un côté, la claudication et de l'autre, la lordose de la colonne vertébrale lombaire.

Si la résection est capable de faire disparaître la lordose, elle n'améliore pas au même degré la marche, le raccourcissement de la jambe et le déplacement de l'extrémité supérieure du fémur.

Ainsi, en général, je ne puis défendre la résection de la tête fémorale, et je la pratiquerais seulement quand il y a des symptômes arthritiques, comme souvent chez les personnes âgées.

L'opération qui à cette époque est à préférer, comme opération sanglante, est la reposition sanglante de la tête fémorale dans une cavité assez creusée.

Si cette opération réussit et si nous sommes capables de tenir la tête fémorale dans un contact continu avec la cavité maintenant bien creusée, la tête formera, chose certaine, une néarthrose.

Au courant de l'année, il serait donc obtenu, à la suite de l'usage de la jambe dans sa position normale et avec la réhabilitation des conditions statiques, que le pouvoir transformateur des os rétablisse l'architecture interne et la bonne conformation de l'os : ainsi on obtiendrait une véritable guérison dans le sens anatomique.

Telle était mon idée, quand je commençais, en 1887, au mois de juillet, ma première opération sanglante de la luxation congénitale de la hanche.

Je voulais faire la reposition sanglante et donner à la tête reposée un contact manifeste dans sa cavité ancienne.

A cette époque, c'était *Poggi*, je l'appris plus tard, qui avait déjà proposé une reposition sanglante, mais il ne l'avait pas continuée. Quand je faisais ma première opération j'avais encore l'idée que l'obstacle principal était le raccourcissement de tous les muscles autour de l'articulation luxée de la hanche. Ainsi j'ouvrais l'articulation au moyen de l'incision postérieure de *Langenbeck*, je détachais tous les muscles du trochanter, je creusais la cavité cotyloïde et je faisais la reposition.

Les résultats fonctionnels ne furent pas si favorables que j'avais cru, malgré la réussite de la reposition.

Lorenz en donnait bientôt la cause.

Il démontrait que les muscles pelvitrochantériens n'étaient pas raccourcis, mais au contraire allongés. Je modifiai ainsi ma méthode d'opérer, de sorte que j'ouvris l'articulation du côté antérieur et les muscles pelvitrochantériens restèrent intacts. Au contraire, il recommandait de faire d'abord la ténotomie des adducteurs et des muscles tubériens, afin d'éviter le raccourcissement de ces muscles.

Plus tard il se démontrait que toutes ces ténotomies n'étaient pas tout à fait innocentes et qu'il pouvait survenir un raccourcissement des muscles par une extension vigoureuse de la jambe pendant l'opération.

Quand après *Trendelenburg* nous montrait l'avantage des muscles glutæi pour la bonne fonction de l'articulation opérée, j'abandonnais mon incision postérieure et j'ouvrais l'articulation davantage en faisant une incision latérale, afin d'opérer ainsi comme *Lorenz* en évitant absolument les muscles.

Ma méthode d'opérer ne différait encore de celle de *Lorenz* que de la manière de faire l'incision.

L'incision antérieure de *Lorenz* est souvent la cause d'une contracture des muscles fléchisseurs, qu'on évite absolument avec ma manière de faire l'incision.

Je décris ainsi la technique de l'opération la meilleure comme étant la méthode *Hoffa-Lorenz*, ainsi qu'elle fut alors pratiquée.

Après tous les soins aseptiques, le malade est endormi et couché de côté sur la table opératoire.

Une contre-extension aseptique part du périnée. Pour les jeunes enfants, un assistant fait l'extension en tirant la jambe. Chez des personnes plus âgées on fait l'extension à l'aide d'une vis de *Lorenz*, qu'on applique aux malléoles de la jambe.

Pendant qu'on tire lentement et graduellement la jambe, on fait une incision qui part du bord supérieur antérieur du grand trochanter, à environ un demi-centimètre plus haut et finit à environ 6 centimètres en descendant. Après l'incision de la peau, on fait en droite ligne l'incision du fascialata, à laquelle, chez des enfants plus âgés, on ajoute encore une incision transversale. — Après le fascia on voit immédiatement les muscles glutaeus medius et minimus. A l'aide d'un crochet à pointe mousse, on tire les deux muscles fortement en haut, afin que la capsule de l'articulation de la hanche sorte entièrement et qu'on puisse facilement la sectionner.

Maintenant suit l'exarticulation.

La capsule est incisée, pendant qu'on maintient la jambe en abduction. Ainsi la capsule s'étend bien sur la tête. On la prend à son attache antérieure au trochanter avec une pince, on l'élève, on fait une petite ouverture pour voir la surface cartilagineuse de la tête, on introduit dans l'ouverture un bistouri boutonné et on sectionne la face antérieure de la capsule entièrement dans la direction de la tête fémorale jusqu'à son insertion au bassin.

En ouvrant la capsule, il s'en écoule souvent une petite quantité de synovie.

En général, cette incision suffit pour luxer la tête fémorale de la capsule. Si elle ne réussit pas, on sectionne la capsule aussi en haut. On procède en faisant une incision perpendiculaire à la première. Ainsi on fait l'incision en forme d'un T. Il peut arriver qu'on soit obligé de faire encore une incision, de manière à la transformer en une incision cruciale. Si la capsule est suffisamment ouverte, la tête pend encore au ligament teres, quand il existe. On détache alors de la tête le ligament à l'aide de ciseaux, on le prend avec une pince, on tire vigoureusement et on sectionne son insertion au bord inférieur de la cavité. Maintenant la tête fémorale est entièrement dénudée, on peut facilement la pousser de côté, l'examiner et la creuser.

La formation de la nouvelle cavité est le troisième acte de l'opération.

Pour l'évidement de la cavité, je fais usage de gouges courbées en baïonnette. C'est ici surtout que l'emploi de cet instrument est une question d'habitude.

J'ai essayé tous les instruments recommandés par des collègues, mais je suis toujours retourné aux miens : la question principale est de savoir que la cavité dans la luxation congénitale, même chez les enfants jeunes, est si épaisse, qu'on peut assez profondément l'excaver sans risque d'une perforation du bassin. A l'aide de la gouge et en se guidant avec l'index gauche, on excise le cartilage de l'ancienne cavité. On éloigne le tissu cartilagineux, afin qu'il ne puisse empêcher plus tard la guérison.

La cavité nouvelle doit être non seulement profonde, mais aussi bien élargie.

On doit aussi faire attention que les bords soient bien saillants ; ainsi on donnera à la tête vers le haut un bon appui. Ceci est plus facile, car les os sont surtout très épais en ce point.

Si on juge que la cavité nouvelle est bien conformée à la tête fémorale, on fait la reposition et on examine si elle a vraiment, dans toutes les positions de la jambe, un appui solide dans la cavité. On verra très souvent, qu'on est obligé d'approfondir un peu la cavité d'un côté ou de l'autre. C'est de la sculpture, qui sera le mieux faite par celui qui a du talent. Je dois encore remémorer en peu de mots les cas où la cavité est très rudimentaire. C'est ici que je dois exprimer ma conviction, que plusieurs collègues, qui n'auraient pas trouvé la cavité, l'ont cherchée à un faux endroit.

Moi-même, malgré ma grande habitude, j'ai souvent eu des difficultés à trouver la cavité. C'est la règle, que la partie antérieure de la capsule couvre la cavité, et il peut arriver qu'elle aboutisse à une ossification partielle avec l'os iliaque au bord supérieur de la cavité. Elle est alors entièrement couverte. On sent bien un bord supérieur, mais ce n'est que du tissu conjonctif qui descend. Si on découvre une pareille conformation de la capsule, on sectionne le tissu conjonctif au bord supérieur de la cavité, on l'enlève des deux côtés avec une rugine, et on est souvent étonné de trouver une cavité assez bien conformée. Les cas où on ne trouve pas une cavité et où elle est très rudimentaire sont très rares. Dans tous mes cas, je n'ai trouvé qu'une fois une écuelle au lieu d'une véritable cavité. Ainsi je n'avais jamais de difficultés pour bien élargir la cavité, et le résultat était favorable. Quand la cavité est creusée, je la nettoie avec de la charpie stérilisée pour éloigner toutes les parcelles cartilagineuses et osseuses. Suit maintenant la dernière et la plus importante action de l'opération : **la reposition de la tête fémorale**. La reposition de la tête fémorale dans la cavité nouvelle est généralement très facile chez les jeunes enfants ; chez des personnes âgées, au contraire, elle est souvent difficile. Les obstacles qui s'opposent dans ces cas sont formés surtout par les parties molles ; il est bien rare que la conformation de la tête même s'oppose à la reposition dans la cavité. Le raccourcissement des parties molles est évité par une vigoureuse extension et une ample incision de la capsule antérieure. Rarement il peut être nécessaire de faire une ténotomie partielle des adducteurs ou des tendons dans le creux poplité. La forme de la tête même donne très rarement un obstacle à la reposition. Je n'ai observé que deux fois au lieu d'une tête fémorale une masse osseuse sans forme et presque quadrangulaire. Dans les deux cas, j'ai essayé de donner une forme qui ressemblât le plus à la tête fémorale normale ; l'un, hélas ! s'est terminé par la mort à la suite de la longue durée de l'opération ; dans le second cas, j'ai très bien réussi. En tout cas, cette déformation est très rare. Chose remarquable : j'observai les deux cas chez de très jeunes garçons. Deux autres cas sont fournis par deux jeunes filles, l'une de quinze et l'autre de quatorze ans. La reposition ne réussissait qu'après une grande ablation de la tête fémorale déformée. Je formai alors le reste du col fémoral comme appui pour la cavité, et les résultats définitifs ont été bons. Le modelage de la tête se fait rarement. Quand la forme de la tête est très pointue, on fait bien de l'arrondir autant que possible. De même on doit enlever de la tête les exostoses, puisqu'elles forment un obstacle statique aux mouvements.

Il reste quelquefois un autre obstacle. On fait la reposition jusqu'au bord de la cavité, il manque encore quelques centimètres pour l'élever sur le bord de la cavité, mais la tête reste immobile, elle n'entre pas dans la cavité. Dans ces cas, on tâte encore les parties molles et la capsule antérieure, pour s'assurer s'il n'y a pas une bride, qu'on n'ait pas encore sectionnée. Souvent on la trouvera, on la coupera et la reposition se fera. Ou bien on remarque que la partie postérieure de la capsule se plie entre le bord de la tête et la cavité, de sorte qu'un relief de la capsule fixe la tête. On repousse alors la tête vers le haut, on sectionne la capsule en arrière et au milieu jusqu'à l'os iliaque, on la retire des deux côtés et on donne ainsi à la tête une situation grâce à laquelle elle glisse facilement dans la cavité. Quand un tel obstacle n'existe pas et qu'on ne trouve rien aux parties molles qui tienne la tête si immobile, on tâche d'élargir la cavité vers la partie postérieure et supérieure, ou bien on abrase les parties superficielles cartilagineuses et osseuses de la tête. Quelquefois on fait les deux et la reposition réussit. En ce qui concerne l'acte de reposition, on le fait différemment selon le cas qui se présente. On doit essayer comment il réussit le mieux. Quelquefois suffit, surtout chez des enfants, une simple extension à la jambe et la tête passe avec un bruit perceptible. D'autres fois on est obligé de faire une vigoureuse abduction et rotation en dedans. D'autres fois la reposition se fait le mieux quand on fléchit la jambe dans l'articulation de la hanche et du genou ; on fait ensuite une vigoureuse extension et rotation en dedans ou en dehors, pendant qu'on exerce une forte pression sur le trochanter. Plus la reposition est difficile, plus la joie est grande, quand au dernier moment la tête glisse avec un bruit dans la cavité. Je crois que la plupart des repositions, qui autrefois ne réussissaient pas, avaient pour cause qu'on ne faisait pas assez attention à la tension de la partie antérieure de la capsule. Dans l'avenir, nous procéderons, puisque nous le savons, avec beaucoup d'énergie contre cet obstacle et, à l'aide de la vis de *Lorenz*, la non-réussite de la reposition deviendra de plus en plus rare. Je veux encore faire mention d'un obstacle qui peut se présenter : c'est la narcose incomplète. Quand le malade n'est pas bien endormi, les muscles sont si contractés, qu'on a la plus grande difficulté pour finir la reposition. Une profonde narcose est alors absolument nécessaire pour une reposition facile. Si la tête est passée, on examine si elle se manifeste dans toutes les positions. Il faut qu'elle reste dans sa cavité même dans une forte abduction et rotation en dehors ; alors on sera assuré que le résultat de l'opération est favorable. Après la reposition, je tamponne la plaie avec de la gaze stérilisée, j'applique un pansement aseptique de gaze et au-dessus un pansement plâtré. L'assistant qui faisait l'extension tient la jambe dans la bonne position, c'est-à-dire dans l'abduction et la rotation en dedans.

Avec l'autre main il applique une contre-extension au bassin, afin que l'extension de la contre-extension soient correctes. Lorsque le plâtre est appliqué, je fais coucher les enfants dans un lit incliné de *Phelps*. Ceci est très avantageux, puisqu'on évite l'élèvement des enfants pendant les selles, on peut facilement les transporter dans un autre lit, et quand il fait beau, dans le jardin sans grande difficulté. Afin d'éviter l'infection du pansement, on applique aux jambes, à la partie inguinale, de la batiste imperméable de *Billroth*

Le premier pansement reste de quatre à huit jours. J'éloigne le tampon et je serre la plaie à l'aide d'une compresse roulée. Après huit jours, je change encore ce pansement ; quinze jours après le premier changement, la plaie est guérie. S'il existe encore une granulation superficielle, on la touche au nitrate d'argent et on la recouvre avec du taffetas. Si la plaie est guérie, nous arrivons au traitement consécutif comme chose principale. On doit avoir soin d'éviter, les contractures et faire attention que les muscles de toute la jambe et les muscles fessiers restent en bon état. En outre d'un massage énergique et de l'application de l'électricité, tous les jours on fait des exercices de gymnastique. Après on apprend aux enfants à rester debout seulement sur la jambe opérée. Au commencement ils ont besoin d'un appui, plus tard ils l'abandonnent. Ensuite on fait des exercices de marche, et on apprend aux enfants à abandonner l'habitude de vaciller. Plus tard viennent les exercices d'abduction. Les enfants sont couchés sur un côté et pendant qu'on applique une pression sur le bassin, ils doivent lever la jambe latéralement. Au commencement ceci leur est difficile; ensuite on lève la jambe si haut que possible latéralement et on oblige les enfants à la garder dans cette position; immédiatement la jambe tombe, mais peu à peu ils arrivent à le faire. Ensuite ils font des exercices d'abduction étant couchés sur le dos et ils écartent la jambe opérée si loin que possible sur commande. A la fin viennent les exercices qui ont pour but d'abaisser autant que possible le bassin du côté opéré. Si bien étant couchés sur le dos que placés avec la bonne jambe sur une planchette les enfants doivent apprendre à abaisser activement la jambe opérée sans fléchir l'autre, de sorte que la malléole interne de la jambe opérée descend le plus possible au-dessous de la malléole interne de la bonne jambe. Les muscles abducteurs seront assez vigoureux, quand le malade étant debout sur la jambe opérée aura le pouvoir de lever le bassin si haut, que le pli fessier du bon côté vienne aboutir plus haut que celui du côté opéré. En dehors de ces exercices d'abduction, on exerce aussi les autres muscles de la jambe. Surtout il est nécessaire de bien étendre le genou. Je ne touche pas aux articulations. Je n'ai vu que des inconvénients des mouvements forcés. Quand il arrive qu'une articulation est dans une position fléchie, on la corrige en faisant coucher le malade à plat ventre, avec un coussin sous le fémur au-dessus du genou, en appliquant des sacs de sable sur les fesses afin de provoquer une hyperextension.

Ensuite les hyperextensions passives seront nécessaires. Il est désirable que les malades eux-mêmes tâchent de mobiliser la nouvelle articulation. Excellents sont les appareils de *Krukenberg*, également la bicyclette, qui est aussi recommandée par *Lorenz*. Les enfants apprennent très vite le tricycle et exercent très facilement leurs articulations dans le sens de flexion et d'extension. S'il arrive le malheur qu'une articulation ait tendance à s'ankyloser, on doit éviter tous les mouvements brusques et appliquer des appareils d'extension. Il est très remarquable que la raideur des articulations s'améliore quand l'extension est appliquée pendant quelques semaines. On s'aperçoit bien que le traitement consécutif est une chose principale pour la réussite de l'opération.

C'est ici comme dans toutes les opérations orthopédiques. Nous recommandons spécialement de faire la plus grande attention au traitement consécutif dans le sens indiqué : on sera récompensé par les résultats définitifs.

J'insiste sur ce que le traitement consécutif n'a jamais duré longtemps. Les enfants ne restèrent jamais en traitement plus de quatre mois : j'insiste surtout, puisqu'avec notre méthode par l'opération sanglante, on atteint plus vite le but cherché qu'avec l'opération non sanglante de *Lorenz*.

La grande question qui est posée pour la méthode sanglante est le danger de l'opération.

Je puis vous assurer que l'opération n'est pas dangereuse, quand on suit la méthode indiquée. J'ai pratiqué 248 fois l'opération sanglante et sur ce nombre j'ai eu 10 décès ; 2 sont survenus à la suite d'une diphtérie et d'une scarlatine, après que les malades eurent quitté la clinique. 8 décès sont survenus à la suite de l'opération ; 7, hélas ! en payement cher d'apprentissage, afin d'arriver à la technique complète d'aujourd'hui ; le 8ᵉ à la suite de la narcose. De mes malades opérés en laissant intacts les muscles, c'est-à-dire de mes 152 dernières opérations consécutives, je n'en ai perdu aucun. — Une asepsie sévère est nécessaire pour la bonne réussite de l'opération. Ainsi on évitera de suturer la plaie, mais on la tamponnera les premiers jours après l'opération. En ce qui concerne les résultats, je vais vous communiquer ce qui suit : si l'opération est faite, nous pouvons immédiatement juger le résultat qu'elle donnera. Le pronostic est plus ou moins favorable selon la déformation de l'extrémité supérieure du fémur. On n'obtiendra jamais un état normal, ni par la meilleure opération sanglante ni par la non-sanglante. Ce que nous pouvons obtenir, on peut facilement le préciser. L'extrémité supérieure du fémur est dans toute luxation congénitale de la hanche déformée, même avec une opération précoce : elle diffère dans sa forme et dans sa direction beaucoup d'une extrémité normale.

La nouvelle cavité se laisse rarement conformer à la tête anomale, et la place où on fait la nouvelle cavité ne correspond pas complètement à celle où se trouve la cavité cotyloïde normale. On creuse à la suite de la déformation du bassin la nouvelle cavité beaucoup plus en avant et en haut qu'elle l'est à l'état normal.

Le tout résumé, nous ne pourrions obtenir même avec une néarthrose complète une restitutio ad integrum.

On aura toujours, même dans les cas les mieux réussis, des anomalies dans la position et dans la mobilité de la jambe. Prenons le cas où la nouvelle cavité se conforme bien à l'extrémité reposée, nous pouvons avec la déformation typique de la tête et du col du fémur obtenir les résultats suivants. Nous savons que l'angle du col fémoral n'existe plus et que la pointe du trochanter majeur est au même niveau que la plus haute pointe de la tête fémorale, quelquefois même plus élevée ; nous savons aussi que le col fémoral présente relativement souvent une déformation antéro-postérieure, de sorte qu'on est obligé de faire une très ample rotation en dedans pour obtenir une rétention de la tête dans la cavité. Ainsi nous avons ici la même situation à l'extrémité supérieure du fémur que chez les coxa vara, et on pourrait attendre qu'il se forme après la reposition une forme plus ou moins complète de coxa vara.

Nous avons provoqué une certaine forme de coxa vara artificielle. Nous trouvons ainsi, après l'opération, le trochanter majeur un peu plus élevé que la ligne de *Roser-Nélaton* et quelquefois une adduction et rotation en dehors de la jambe qui a pour cause la situation plus élevée de la nouvelle cavité, la petitesse de la tête fémorale, le peu de longueur du col fémoral, et aussi le raccourcissement comme suite de l'inactivité du fémur entier. Le raccourcissement, selon l'âge des malades, variera de 1 à 5 centimètres.

Un raccourcissement existera toujours, même dans l'opération la mieux réussie. Aussi nous ne pouvons obtenir une mobilité absolument normale de l'articulation nouvelle. On doit faire bien attention de donner un grand rebord à la nouvelle cavité pour que la tête ait un bon appui. Ainsi on donne un très grand arrêt mécanique, comme il existe dans l'articulation normale de la hanche. Les mouvements de l'articulation normale, comme ceux de la nouvelle, sont limités, parce que le col fémoral se pousse contre le bord de la cavité ; et il est naturel que le col raccourci, qui a une direction horizontale, trouve plutôt un arrêt à un rebord bien pointu de la cavité que le col normal, qui est long et plus raide. Nous ne pouvons donc obtenir une ample et libre excursion de la jambe.

Une flexion un peu plus grande que l'angle droit sera en général la mesure. Aussi l'adduction de la jambe sera un peu moins que la normale ; nous avons ici, comme je l'ai déjà mémoré, la même forme de l'extrémité supérieure du fémur que chez la coxa vara statica. Jusqu'à présent nous n'avons parlé que des rapports mécaniques de l'articulation opérée. Ceci ne suffit pas pour juger. La bonne fonction dépend aussi de la musculature. D'autant plus forts sont les muscles de la jambe et surtout les muscles fessiers par le traitement consécutif, d'autant meilleur sera le résultat fonctionnel. Si nous ne pouvons obtenir par l'opération une articulation absolument normale, les avantages pour le malade seront néanmoins suffisants. Dans la luxation unilatérale nous compensons le raccourcissement de la jambe, qui a pour cause l'élévation de la tête fémorale, et il ne reste que le raccourcissement, qui dépend de la formation du fémur. Nous donnons au fémur un bon appui au bassin, et nous rétablissons la traction correcte des muscles glutaei. En fortifiant la musculature par le massage et la gymnastique nous obtenons des résultats fonctionnels, et ce sont surtout ceux-ci qui sont irréprochables. Les enfants compensent le moindre raccourcissement par abaissement du bassin et marchent définitivement si bien, que le simple spectateur a souvent des difficultés pour juger quelle est la bonne ou la mauvaise jambe.

Dans la luxation bilatérale l'opération corrige la lordose, elle améliore la marche vacillante, elle rend aux jambes la bonne position et donne une meilleure abduction. Les résultats définitifs sont d'autant meilleurs que l'opération a été précoce. Selon mon idée, l'âge le plus favorable est de 5 jusqu'à 8 ans. Mais aussi dans un âge plus avancé les résultats peuvent encore avoir un succès complet. Mais puisque la déformation de l'extrémité supérieure du fémur augmente avec l'âge, on ne peut jamais garantir un succès complet. En outre, la reposition devient plus difficile et avec elle la difficulté de l'asepsie. Chaque faute dans l'asepsie augmente, car les microorganismes trouvent dans les tissus tirés et meurtris des circonstances particulières, qui prédisposent à la septicémie. Le risque d'une ankylose ou d'un exitus léthal est aussi plus grand chez les personnes âgées. Maintenant je voudrais vous expliquer les résultats que j'ai obtenus dans les 152 dernières repositions sanglantes que j'ai pratiquées en épargnant les muscles par la méthode déjà indiquée. Je vous ai déjà dit que je n'ai pas eu parmi ceux-ci un cas mortel. Les plaies ont presque toutes bien guéri et les malades ont quitté la clinique en moyenne après 4 mois. Dans les 152 opérations sanglantes, il y avait 82 luxations unilatérales et 25 bilatérales. Quand nous jugeons les 82 luxations unilatérales, 55 fois le résultat définitif était idéal dans le sens déjà mémoré. On peut dire que les malades sont guéris dans le sens anatomique et fonctionnel. 27 fois le résultat était bon dans le sens fonctionnel. La position de la tête n'était pas irréprochable; aussi la mobilité de la nouvelle articulation n'était pas absolument libre, l'adduction surtout n'était pas tout à fait normale.

La marche des enfants était très bonne, de sorte qu'on n'apercevait pas la moindre claudication. 6 fois nous avons obtenu une entière ankylose en bonne position moyenne de la jambe.

Ces cas ont rapport à des malades qui ont passé leur 8me année. Chez ces malades la tête fémorale est généralement très déformée, et il se forme, après la reposition, très facilement des obstacles mécaniques qui tendent à l'ankylose. Chez aucun de mes malades d'un âge inférieur à 8 ans il ne s'est formé d'ankylose. J'insiste ici particulièrement que, dans aucun des cas où l'articulation était mobile quand le malade a quitté la clinique, il ne s'est produit plus tard d'ankylose. Lorsque l'ankylose est survenue, c'était alors chez des malades non guéris ou chez des personnes âgées. 10 fois j'ai trouvé, après un examen consécutif, des contractures : ce furent des contractures de flexion-adduction qui furent seulement dans 5 cas si intensives, qu'elles influençaient vraiment la marche. J'ai amélioré plus tard la position de la jambe par une ostéotomie sous-trochantérienne, et en définitive j'ai obtenu une position parallèle des jambes et en outre une bonne fonction. Je n'ai jamais observé des reluxations en arrière ; au contraire, j'ai remarqué dans 4 cas une transposition de la tête. Dans ces cas il existe un grand raccourcissement de la jambe qui mesure jusqu'à 5 centimètres. Puisque les têtes fémorales sont immobiles, on peut très bien compenser le raccourcissement par une semelle élevée. Résumant les résultats, que j'ai obtenus par la reposition sanglante de la luxation unilatérale, je ne puis être que très content. Les résultats sont, aussi bien dans le sens anatomique que fonctionnel, plus favorables que ceux du même chiffre obtenus par l'opération non sanglante, malgré les plus grands soins. Les résultats chez les 25 luxations bilatérales sont moins favorables ; dans 14 cas j'ai obtenu seulement un résultat irréprochable ; dans 4 le résultat était bon d'un côté, de l'autre la jambe était raccourcie puisque la tête fémorale s'était élevée. Ces malades marchent encore assez bien avec une semelle élevée ; dans 5 autres une des jambes n'est pas seulement raccourcie, mais il existe encore une contracture en légère flexion-adduction ; chez 5 de ces enfants j'ai encore pu améliorer le résultat par une ostéotomie sous-trochantérienne. Dans un autre cas j'ai recommencé l'opération et par cette seconde opération j'ai obtenu une bonne position. Deux fois j'ai observé chez des enfants très jeunes, qui furent opérés dans leur 2me année, une reluxation antérieure bilatérale. La lordose est dans ces cas vraiment améliorée, la marche vacillante n'est pas entièrement corrigée. Ces cas m'ont prouvé qu'il n'est pas raisonnable de faire l'opération avant la troisième année. Des reluxations en arrière n'ont pas été observées. De même heureusement aucune ankylose bilatérale, comme je l'ai eu deux fois parmi mes premières opérations. — Les résultats dans la luxation bilatérale, comme vous le voyez, ne sont pas si favorables; en tout cas ils ne sont pas plus mauvais que ceux qu'on constate dans la luxation bilatérale traitée par la reposition non sanglante. 14 cas bien guéris pour les 25 opérations représentent un résultat satisfaisant. Nous devons aussi nous rendre compte que, pendant les dernières années, nous avons essayé d'abord la reposition non sanglante et que nous n'avons fait l'opération sanglante qu'après la non-réussite de l'autre.

Ainsi dans les cas opérés par la méthode sanglante il est toujours question de cas graves et inaccessibles à l'autre méthode. Ceci, messieurs, par rapport à mes résultats.

Je me permets de vous présenter maintenant un cas de luxation unilatérale. J'ai opéré les deux cas il y a 5 ans. Je vous prie de vous convaincre en examinant que ces cas sont vraiment à considérer comme entièrement guéris. Ils vous prouveront qu'il est vraiment possible d'obtenir par l'opération indiquée une guérison de la luxation congénitale de la hanche aussi bien dans le sens anatomique que fonctionnel.

Je me permets de vous montrer un grand nombre d'images de *Röntgen* qui vous montrent l'articulation avant, et plusieurs années après l'opération. Vous pourrez juger par ces images que la tête fémorale est irréprochablement restée dans la nouvelle cavité après plusieurs années et à la même hauteur que la tête fémorale de l'autre côté. Vous voyez que le col fémoral se présente après l'opération entièrement dans la position frontale et qu'il est dans la luxation unilatérale toujours un peu plus court que du côté sain; aussi vous pouvez remarquer qu'avec la croissance la nouvelle cavité se développe au même degré. Je n'ai jamais pu constater la supposition de *Lorenz*, que par la lésion de l'Y cartilagineux la croissance de la cavité pourrait s'arrêter. En tout cas je n'ai jamais aperçu le moindre trouble de développement de la cavité. Une des malades, que j'ai opérée il y a 7 ans pour une luxation unilatérale, s'est mariée, il y a un an et demi, et est accouchée, il y a quelques mois, d'un beau garçon. L'accouchement était très facile. Selon mes expériences on peut creuser la cavité sans crainte d'un arrêt du développement de l'anneau osseux du bassin. L'approfondissement même augmente le danger d'une infection, et celui qui n'est pas assuré de son asepsie fait mieux de laisser la cavité intacte, comme *Lorenz* le répétait encore récemment, et de reposer simplement la tête fémorale au niveau de la cavité. Pour ma part, je ne trouve pas que l'approfondissement au degré indiqué soit un tel obstacle, qu'il soit préférable de l'éviter. Je veux vous montrer une préparation intéressante d'un enfant de 4 ans qui est mort d'une diphtérie un an et demi après l'opération bilatérale, après avoir marché correctement. Vous voyez qu'il existe des deux côtés une néarthrose complète et que les deux têtes fémorales sont mobiles dans leur nouvelle cavité dans toute direction. Il résulte de cette description que je ne puis recommander cette opération chez les enfants que jusqu'à leur 10me année. Plus les enfants sont jeunes, plus l'opération sera facile. La limite sera en général la 10me année. Comment faut-il agir avec des personnes plus âgées? Avec le grand matériel, dont je dispose, j'ai posé souvent cette question, et, à la fin, l'étude de la pathologie anatomique m'a montré une méthode d'opérer les anciennes luxations bilatérales, qui, n'étant que palliative, est quand même très avantageuse.

Cette méthode est basée sur le fait que la tête ne trouve pas un appui suffisant sur l'os iliaque parce que la capsule s'est posée entre les deux os. Si l'on corrige cet obstacle, on peut donner un meilleur appui à la tête fémorale. Dans un cas très grave d'une luxation bilatérale chez une jeune fille de 15 ans, j'essayai cette opération, c'est-à-dire l'extirpation de la capsule interposée. Pendant l'opération je trouvai que la tête déformée avait trop peu d'appui sur l'os iliaque. Dans les cas suivants je pratiquai la résection de la tête même. Ainsi j'obtins le large contact de la plaie du fémur directement avec l'os iliaque, de sorte qu'il pouvait se former entre ces os une forte pseudarthrose. J'ai déjà pratiqué 22 fois cette opération, dont les résultats fonctionnels sont excellents, car elle corrige la lordose et la marche vacillante. La technique suivante s'est montrée la meilleure :

Par une incision latérale on ouvre l'articulation. Alors on détache les parties molles sous-périostalement du trochanter majeur et les insertions de la capsule du col fémoral, de sorte que la tête puisse être luxée librement hors de la plaie. A l'aide d'une sonde pointue on abrase la tête fémoral près de la ligne intertrochantérienne; on incise la partie postérieure de la capsule jusqu'à l'os iliaque, on sectionne les insertions au bord de la cavité, on détache toutes les adhérences, qu'on trouve toujours entre la capsule et le périoste de l'os iliaque et on extirpe les deux lambeaux de la capsule. Ainsi on donne à l'os iliaque un libre niveau périostal, contre lequel est posée la plaie de l'extrémité supérieure du fémur pendant que la jambe est en extension et en abduction.

Traitement consécutif : tamponnement avec de la gaze iodoformée, extension et appareil plâtré. Quand les malades se lèvent après 4 ou 6 semaines, ils reçoivent un corset qui rend la marche plus légère. Quand la plaie est guérie, on applique le massage et la gymnastique.

La durée du traitement est en moyenne de 5 mois. Je recommande spécialement cette méthode, que je nomme **opération de pseudarthrose**, puisque je tâche de provoquer une cicatrisation fibreuse. Pour vous donner un exemple de la valeur de cette méthode, je me permets de vous présenter une patiente que j'ai opérée il y a 4 ans par la méthode indiquée. Vous voyez qu'il n'existe chez la personne, qui, actuellement, est âgée de 20 ans, aucune trace de la maladie d'autrefois. Elle peut marcher pendant des heures sans douleur et sans fatigue. Les autres opérations ont donné les mêmes résultats. Tandis que cette opération de pseudarthrose ne s'applique qu'à une luxation bilatérale, nous avons aussi pour des luxations anciennes unilatérales une méthode très praticable.

C'est **l'ostéotomie sous-trochantérienne** qui fut recommandée et pratiquée premièrement avec succès par *Kirmisson*.

Comme j'ai mémoré plusieurs fois, la reposition sanglante donne chez les malades qui ont passé leur 10me année souvent un mauvais résultat, puisqu'il se forme très facilement comme suite de l'opération une ankylose. J'ai donc renoncé à l'opération typique dans ces cas. Quand il existe, comme suite de la luxation, une grande déformation, c'est-à-dire une grande adduction et raccourcissement de la jambe, l'opération de *Kirmisson* est très recommandable. J'ai préféré, non seulement pour corriger la difformité, mais en même temps le raccourcissement de la jambe, **l'ostéotomie oblique**.

L'ostéotomie oblique corrige non seulement la fausse position de la jambe, mais peut donner un allongement de 5 centimètres et de plus une bonne fonction, ce qui est la chose principale. Je pratique l'opération de la manière suivante :

D'abord incision sous-cutanée et percutanée des adducteurs tendus, des muscles qui s'insèrent au tuber ischii, et des fascias et des muscles qui descendent de l'épine iliaque antérieure. Puis une incision longitudinale à la partie extérieure du fémur. On sectionne le fascia qui est souvent très tendu transversalement, afin qu'il soit totalement relâché. Après, on incise à l'extérieur du vaste externe jusqu'à l'os. A l'aide de la rugine l'os est dénudé dans toute sa largeur. On écarte avec un crochet mousse les parties molles, pour qu'on puisse placer les ciseaux larges de *Konig* obliquement sur l'os. On coupe l'os à l'aide de coups forts frappés sur les ciseaux, pendant qu'on leur donne la direction vers le trochanter mineur. Si on veut que l'os soit presque coupé, on retire les ciseaux et on casse les dernières lamelles, pendant qu'on porte le fémur en position d'ample adduction.

Lorsque les fragments sont devenus entièrement mobiles, qu'ils peuvent se déplacer parallèlement en tirant la jambe. on tamponne la plaie avec de la gaze stérilisée et on applique dans la position d'abduction voulue un appareil d'extension. qui est chargé avec des poids de plus en plus lourds, jusqu'à 50 livres.

On enlève le tampon après 5 à 8 jours et on ferme la plaie. L'appareil d'extension est remplacé par un pansement plâtré. avec lequel les malades peuvent se lever et marcher. Après 6 semaines tout pansement est abandonné afin de faire maintenant énergiquement un traitement de massage et de gymnastique.

J'ai fait 10 fois l'opération avec la méthode indiquée jusqu'ici : j'ai été, ainsi que les malades et leurs parents. satisfait sous tous les rapports du résultat obtenu.

J'arrive à la fin! Encore dois-je m'excuser de n'avoir fait mention que de mes propres observations. J'ai voulu vous montrer ce que l'opération sanglante de la luxation congénitale de la hanche peut donner dans la main d'un chirurgien exercé dans cette opération.

Il a été fait des observations du même genre par d'autres collègues. Avec *Lorenz*, des chirurgiens comme *Broca*, *Kirmisson*, *Denucé*, *Doyen*, *Calot*, *Bradfort*, *Whitman* et encore d'autres ont fait cette opération avec bon résultat. J'espère que la discussion de cette partie donnera encore plus de clarté dans cette question. En tout cas la reposition sanglante du fémur luxé dans une nouvelle cavité ne mérite pas d'être mise ad acta, comme ont fait les enthousiastes pour l'opération non sanglante. et bien parce qu'ils ne sont pas capables de faire la reposition sanglante.

Je résume mes observations sur l'opération sanglante de la luxation congénitale de la hanche dans les conclusions suivantes :

1° Dans chaque cas de luxation congénitale de la hanche on essayera d'abord la reposition non sanglante. Si la non sanglante ne réussit pas à cause d'une raison quelconque, l'opération sanglante est indiquée.

2° Comme opération sanglante pour les enfants de la 5ᵐᵉ jusqu'à la 8ᵐᵉ année vient le choix de la reposition sanglante de la tête fémorale luxée dans une cavité nouvellement formée de *Hoffa-Lorenz*.

3° L'opération typique de *Hoffa-Lorenz* ne sera pas faite trop tôt ni trop tard. L'âge le plus avantageux est de la 5ᵐᵉ jusqu'à la 8ᵐᵉ année.

4° L'opération typique de *Hoffa-Lorenz* sera toujours accompagnée d'une réfection d'une cavité.

5° L'opération typique sanglante ne sera faite que par des chirurgiens, qui sont maîtres d'une asepsie complète.

6° Le danger de l'opération se trouve surtout dans l'infection septique de la plaie. Ce danger augmente avec l'âge du patient, auquel correspond aussi une plus grande difficulté de la reposition de la tête dans la cavité.

7° Avec une asepsie sévère et l'opération étant faite entre la 5me et la 8me année, très correctement selon les indications de *Hoffa-Lorenz*, la reposition sanglante n'est pas dangereuse.

8° Les plaies ne seront pas suturées.

9° Le traitement consécutif est d'une très grande importance, parce qu'il fortifie les muscles avec le massage et la gymnastique.

On doit éviter des mouvements passifs trop forts.

10° Des contractures de flexion-adduction s'évitent dans toutes les circonstances par des précautions spéciales pendant le traitement consécutif. Une contracture en flexion-adduction survenue peut être traitée avec bon résultat par une ostéotomie sous-trochantérienne.

11° Des ankyloses ne surviennent qu'après une suppuration de la plaie et quand on fait l'opération à un âge avancé. Comme limite extrême pour la reposition sanglante nous prenons la 10me année dans les cas unilatéraux, la 7me année dans les luxations bilatérales.

12° Une ankylose des articulations qui furent d'abord mobiles n'est pas à craindre. Une raideur postérieure ne survient que chez des personnes âgées et pour les articulations qui tendaient déjà dès le commencement à une mobilité incomplète.

13° Par l'opération sanglante de *Hoffa-Lorenz* une guérison de la luxation congénitale dans le sens anatomique et fonctionnel est possible.

14° La guérison complète est obtenue plus souvent dans la luxation unilatérale que dans la luxation bilatérale. Il est inexact qu'avec un traitement correct et un bon choix des cas, la situation après l'opération soit plus mauvaise qu'avant l'opération.

15° La durée en moyenne du traitement est environ de 4 mois; à partir du moment où le patient commence à marcher, il va de mieux en mieux. Après un an on peut considérer le résultat comme définitif.

16° Un obstacle de croissance pour l'anneau du bassin n'est nullement à craindre par la reformation de la cavité. Le bassin se développe plus normalement sous le bon chargement statique. Les accouchements se passent éventuellement sans difficulté.

17 Dans la luxation unilatérale des malades qui ont passé leur 8me jusqu'à la 10me année, l'ostéomie sous-trochantérienne **transversale** (*Kirmisson*) ou **l'ostéotomie oblique** (*Hoffa*) est recommandable. Dans ces cas-ci l'ostéotomie sous-trochantérienne est à préférer à la reposi

tion sanglante de la tête fémorale sans formation de la cavité (*Lorenz*).

18° Dans la luxation bilatérale chez des personnes âgées l'opération **de pseudarthrose de Hoffa** donne des résultats fonctionnels excellents.

RAPPORT SUR LE TRAITEMENT NON SANGLANT DE LA LUXATION CONGÉNITALE DE LA HANCHE

RAPPORT

par M. A. LORENZ
de Vienne.

Messieurs, pour me faire mieux comprendre par mes collègues français, je préfère lire mon rapport en français ; mais veuillez bien m'excuser si je vous expose à entendre écorcher votre belle langue que j'aime plus que je ne la possède.

Avant d'aborder mon sujet qui est le traitement non sanglant de la luxation congénitale de la hanche, je suis bien aise d'appeler votre attention sur ce fait, que c'est à des Français que nous devons les premières tentatives pour obtenir la réduction non sanglante de la hanche luxée ; c'est surtout à Pravaz que revient l'honneur d'avoir atteint le premier ce but par une méthode d'extension lente et continue, c'est-à-dire par une méthode qui, dans les derniers temps, sans doute modifiée, a été employée par M. Mikulicz et par M. Kirmisson, qui l'a appelée justement la méthode française.

Il paraît que Pravaz par cette méthode originale n'a obtenu que des insuccès ou du moins des succès transitoires, pour ainsi dire ; à cet égard, on ne doit peut-être pas accuser la technique comme imparfaite, elle était, au contraire, minutieusement perfectionnée ; la vraie cause en était l'âge trop avancé des enfants que Pravaz a soumis à son traitement.

De même a échoué la méthode de la réduction extemporanée — inaugurée par des chirurgiens français — par Jalade Lafont, Humbert de Morley et Jacquier, à cause de l'âge trop avancé des enfants soumis aux tentatives de la réduction extemporanée de la tête luxée.

C'est ainsi que toutes les tentatives d'une réduction non sanglante ayant échoué, on se borna à un traitement conservateur, c'est-à-dire à l'application d'appareils portatifs, jusqu'au moment où la réduction sanglante, inaugurée par M. Hoffa et perfectionnée par moi-même, commença à devenir la méthode dominante.

Je n'ai pas à parler de la réduction sanglante combinée à un approfondissement artificiel de la cavité cotyloïde; qu'il me soit seulement permis d'ajouter, qu'ayant opéré deux cent soixante cas par la méthode sanglante, j'en ai connu aussi bien les résultats parfaits que les échecs déplorables et c'est sur ces derniers que je veux m'arrêter.

Sur deux cent soixante cas que j'ai opérés, j'en ai perdu quatre par septicémie ; certainement ce n'est pas beaucoup, mais une opération orthopédique doit être tout à fait exempte de dangers.

Cinq fois j'ai eu à déplorer des ankyloses bilatérales dans les luxations doubles, certainement un malheur horrible ; je laisse à part les ankyloses unilatérales comme un accident de moindre importance. *Le danger de mort et l'ankylose absolue ou relative*, ce sont les deux désavantages qui sont à craindre immédiatement après l'opération sanglante.

Mais il y a encore à signaler un désavantage redoutable qui menace l'avenir des fillettes opérées. En creusant l'acetabulum par la gouge, on diminue ou amincit, on enlève même les zones du cartilage épiphysaire en forme d'Y, dont dépendent la croissance et le développement du bassin. N'est-il pas à craindre que le bassin ne se rétrécisse plus tard et que, la luxation guérie, ce rétrécissement n'entraîne de grands dangers dans le cas d'un accouchement?

Voilà les causes pour lesquelles je ne pratique plus le creusement de l'acetabulum rudimentaire.

D'autres chirurgiens ont aussi commencé à craindre la réduction sanglante et c'est M. Mikulicz et plus tard M. Kirmisson qui ont recommandé la réduction non sanglante par un procédé semblable à celui de Pravaz.

Quant à moi, j'ai recommandé la réduction non sanglante d'emblée, au contraire des autres chirurgiens et orthopédistes qui n'ont jamais cessé d'employer des appareils portatifs.

Disons tout de suite que, durant l'époque de l'unique emploi des appareils portatifs, tout le monde était d'accord pour reconnaître la luxation congénitale comme une affection inguérissable.

A mon avis, les résultats qu'on peut obtenir par des appareils quels qu'ils soient, et employés pendant beaucoup d'années ne sont pas le moins du monde comparables aux résultats que nous offre la réduction manuelle.

Avant l'époque de la réduction sanglante ou non sanglante, notre très honoré président, M. Lannelongue, a recommandé le traitement par des injections de chlorure de zinc, la méthode dite sclérogène.

Naturellement, ce n'est pas une méthode radicale, mais par elle on a pu obtenir des améliorations appréciables. Aussi pourrait-on combiner la réduction manuelle avec la méthode sclérogène, comme l'a proposé M. Lange (Munich).

En somme, il n'y a que deux méthodes non sanglantes qui rivalisent entre elles : ce sont la réduction lente et la réduction d'emblée sous chloroforme.

Tâchons d'apprécier sans préjugé les avantages et les désavantages de l'une et de l'autre méthode.

A mon avis, il y a *un seul avantage* du côté de la réduction lente, c'est que l'on peut se passer de la narcose : excepté cet avantage, je n'y vois que des inconvénients :

I. — La réduction lente ne se fait que chez des enfants tout petits ; au delà de la troisième ou quatrième année, la méthode ne laissera pas que d'être une œuvre de patience.

II. — La méthode de la réduction lente est complexe et demande une détention de longue durée dans la gouttière à extension, exposant les malades à tous les inconvénients de la position horizontale et à toutes les difficultés de la traction continue.

III. — Il ne sera jamais possible d'atteindre par la traction seule l'engagement intime entre la cavité cotyloïde et la tête du fémur, engagement qu'on obtient par les manœuvres de la pression et du percement de la réduction manuelle.

Quant à moi, je suis partisan absolu de la réduction d'emblée, en une seule séance, sous chloroforme.

Nous disposons de plusieurs méthodes de réduction en une seule séance ou d'emblée. La plus ancienne est celle de M. Paci. En général, chez des enfants un peu plus âgés, on n'obtient par cette méthode qu'un rapprochement de la tête du fémur et de la cavité cotyloïde. Chez des enfants tout petits, la réduction de la tête fémorale peut se faire par diverses manœuvres et certainement aussi par celles de M. Paci. Mais il sera *toujours* impossible de retenir la tête fémorale à sa place par l'abduction peu considérable, prescrite par la méthode italienne, qui ne peut pas se ranger parmi les méthodes radicales. On peut s'en servir dans des cas irréductibles, à cause de l'âge trop avancé des enfants pour obtenir une amélioration.

La méthode à traction horizontale de M. Schede, la méthode de la réduction au-dessus du rebord *supérieur* de l'acetabulum, est applicable à tous les cas. Elle permet de soumettre à la réduction même des enfants plus âgés : mais cet avantage devient probléma-

tique à cause de paralysies sciatiques produites par des tractions trop
forcées.

Quant à moi, je préfère en général la méthode de la réduction au-
dessus du rebord *postérieur* de l'acetabulum. c'est-à-dire la méthode à
traction *verticale*, combinée à une abduction forcée. admettant qu'il
n'y a pas de préférence *absolue* de l'une des méthodes sur l'autre ;
mais il y a des préférences relatives en faveur de la réduction au-dessus du rebord postérieur de l'acetabulum. Cette préférence relève du
fait. que le rebord postérieur de la cavité cotyloïde étant beaucoup
plus développé que le rebord supérieur. fait naître, au moment du
passage de la tête fémorale. des phénomènes physiques infaillibles,
qui indiquent *ainsi nettement* la réussite de la réduction, de sorte
qu'on n'est jamais dans le doute si la tête a pris ou non sa place sur
le fond de l'acetabulum.

Un deuxième avantage de la méthode d'extension verticale et d'abduction forcée consiste en ce que le grand appareil coûteux nommé
par M. Schede « table à extension » est tout à fait inutile. *Au contraire*, ma méthode de la réduction se fait *à main libre* et de la manière suivante qui est typique.

On commence par le déchirement sous-cutané des muscles adducteurs (myorhexis adductorum). au moyen du pétrissage des muscles
fortement tendus par une abduction forcée. Au cas d'un raccourcissement considérable on peut faire aussi une extension horizontale
manuelle et rythmique. pour abaisser la tête fémorale, mais ordinairement ce préparatif n'est pas nécessaire.

Ensuite. on exerce sur le fémur fléchi à angle droit une extension
verticale avec abduction jusque à peu près à 90 degrés, combinée à
la pression directe sur le grand trochanter.

La réussite de la réduction est accompagnée de symptômes physiques et cliniques infaillibles et peut être vérifiée par la radiographie.

C'est le principe du traitement post-opératoire de soumettre le fond
de la cavité cotyloïde à la pression du poids du corps au moyen de la
tête fémorale réintégrée; sous l'influence de cette fonction physiologique. la cavité cotyloïde s'élargit et s'approfondit. grâce surtout au
rehaussement de son rebord supérieur.

Pour retenir la tête fémorale dans la cavité cotyloïde, le fémur est
fixé dans une position d'abduction exagérée selon les circonstances
jusqu'à 90 degrés. combinée à l'hyperextension avec légère rotation
en dedans.

Ce n'est qu'au bout de quatre à cinq mois que l'on corrige cette
position extrême du fémur par une position moyenne (flexion et

abduction légères). et que l'on fixe *de nouveau* cette position moyenne durant quatre à cinq mois.

Il faut que pendant la durée de cette fixation le malade marche ou se tienne debout sur ses jambes le plus longtemps possible.

Le traitement finit par du massage et de la gymnastique des muscles pelvi-trochantériens (fessiers). les enfants restant libres sans porter des appareils quelconques.

Il faut ajouter que la méthode de réduction non sanglante est *sans aucun danger*, pourvu que l'on se borne à des cas qui n'ont pas dépassé la dixième année pour la luxation unilatérale. et la septième ou la huitième année pour la luxation double.

Quant aux résultats obtenus, il faut d'abord reconnaître que jusqu'à présent dans beaucoup de cas on n'a pas réussi à retenir la tête fémorale sur le fond de l'acetabulum et qu'à la fin il s'est produit une reluxation en avant et en haut.

Parlons d'abord de ces insuccès au point de vue anatomique.

A cela il y a sans doute des raisons diverses.

D'abord, on a fait beaucoup de fautes sous le rapport de la méthode de rétention qu'il faudra éviter dans l'avenir. On a aussi manqué de patience à l'égard de la durée de la fixation de la cuisse. Et, plus souvent encore, les causes de la non-réussite résultent des altérations anatomiques de l'articulation, la cavité cotyloïde n'étant pas assez développée et la tête fémorale présentant des déformations considérables : c'est *surtout* l'antéversion ou la torsion de la tête fémorale ou plutôt la torsion en avant de la partie supérieure du fémur qui est défavorable à la rétention. Dans de telles circonstances, le contact normal de l'acetabulum et de la tête fémorale ne peut s'obtenir qu'à la condition d'une rotation exagérée du fémur en dedans.

Pour remédier à cette position incompatible avec la démarche normale, M. Schede a recommandé de fixer le fémur d'après la réduction non sanglante quelques mois dans une rotation *en dedans* accentuée. La cuisse s'étant fixée dans cette position. M. Schede obtient la rotation *en dehors* de la partie inférieure du fémur au moyen d'une ostéotomie linéaire *sus*-condyloïdienne, après avoir fixé la partie supérieure de cet os dans sa position au moyen d'un clou d'acier, revêtu d'or, qu'il a fait pénétrer à travers le col et la tête fémorale dans le fond de l'acetabulum.

Certainement on ne saurait rien objecter à ce procédé opératoire, et sans doute il est possible d'en obtenir de meilleurs résultats anatomiques, *mais il ne faut pas oublier* que ces reluxations en avant et en haut. — malgré leur infériorité au point de vue anatomique, — ne laissent pas que d'être de très bons résultats fonctionnels, de sorte que je n'ai jamais jugé nécessaire d'achever *et de compromettre* en même temps la méthode non sanglante par une opération sanglante.

Les bons résultats fonctionnels de ces reluxations sont dus au fait que le rebord antérieur de l'os ilium chevauche sur la tête ou sur le col du fémur luxé, de sorte que le bassin prend un point d'appui osseux.

Il faut ajouter que, d'après mes expériences, ces bons résultats fonctionnels sont persistants et qu'ils s'améliorent au fur et à mesure que les muscles se fortifient par un traitement post-opératoire approprié.

Jusqu'ici, d'après la statistique qui m'est personnelle, à peu près dans la moitié des cas les résultats anatomiques sont mauvais, quoique très satisfaisants au point de vue de la fonction, comme j'ai déjà fait remarquer.

Dans l'autre moitié des cas, les résultats sont tout à fait satisfaisants aussi au point de vue anatomique, c'est-à-dire que la *tête fémorale réintégrée reste* à sa place et va être fixée par la cavité cotyloïde s'élargissant et s'approfondissant sous l'influence de la mise en fonction de l'articulation.

Dans beaucoup de cas, la cavité cotyloïde s'élargit et s'approfondit concentriquement, de sorte qu'on peut parler dans ces cas d'une restitution anatomique de l'articulation de la hanche ; mais, dans la majorité des cas, la cavité cotyloïde s'élargit excentriquement par la néoformation d'un rebord supérieur osseux, au-dessous duquel la tête fémorale reste appuyée. Cette néo-formation osseuse se présente sur les radiographies sous la forme de crêtes opaques et de faisceaux opaques rayonnés.

Dans les luxations doubles, les résultats anatomiques parfaits n'ont été obtenus jusqu'ici qu'à peu près *dans un quart des cas* sur les deux côtés ; dans le reste des cas les résultats anatomiques n'ont été obtenus que d'un côté, ou bien la reluxation en avant et en haut s'est produite des deux côtés.

Néanmoins, même dans ces derniers cas, on peut parler d'une guérison fonctionnelle, ou au moins d'une amélioration très considérable de la fonction, car la lordose lombaire disparaît complètement et la marche se fait presque sans claudication et sans fatigue.

Il faut mettre en lumière ce fait, que le moindre des résultats qu'on puisse obtenir et qui ne fait jamais défaut, c'est la marche sans fatigue.

La disparition complète de la claudication dépend moins de la perfection *absolue* du résultat anatomique que de la restitution de la force musculaire, ce qui constitue la *tâche* la plus importante du traitement post-opératoire.

Au cas où l'on ne pourrait réussir par la méthode non sanglante, on peut faire la réduction sanglante par l'arthrotomie en laissant intacte la cavité cotyloïde et en dirigeant le traitement post-opératoire d'après les principes de la réduction non sanglante.

Chez les adolescents, atteints d'une luxation congénitale unilatérale, où la réduction devient impossible à cause de l'âge, il faut se contenter d'une amélioration de la position de la tête fémorale en poussant celle-ci en avant par surextension et en forçant la jambe dans une abduction extrême et en maintenant cette position pendant quelques mois.

Par ce moyen on obtient tous les avantages de l'ostéotomie sous-trochantérienne d'une manière non sanglante, évitant en même temps le raccourcissement du fémur, qui en résulterait.

Tout en admettant que pour l'instant la méthode de la réduction non sanglante sous chloroforme ne soit pas irréprochable et en reconnaissant qu'elle nous a causé beaucoup de déceptions au point de vue anatomique par les reluxations antérieures en haut, il faut néanmoins lui concéder le nom de *méthode radicale*, puisqu'elle peut donner et a donné à tous les chirurgiens qui s'en sont servis un assez grand nombre de guérisons anatomiques.

Aussi appelons-nous la méthode sanglante de la réduction *méthode radicale*, malgré les mêmes reluxations qui surviennent.

Mais ce sont là des querelles théoriques qui ne sauraient diminuer la valeur pratique de la réduction non sanglante et je tiens à affirmer qu'il n'y a pas d'autre méthode, dont les résultats *pratiques* s'obtiennent d'une manière aussi rapide et aussi sûre sans exposer les malades à des dangers quelconques soit pour le présent, soit pour l'avenir.

TRAITEMENT DES LUXATIONS CONGÉNITALES DE LA HANCHE

RAPPORT

par M. E. KIRMISSON.

Les notions cliniques générales sur la luxation congénitale de la hanche datent surtout du mémoire de Dupuytren, publié en 1826 dans le *Répertoire général d'anatomie* de Breschet [1]. Son but, nous dit-il, est moins d'ajouter une infirmité nouvelle au catalogue déjà trop nombreux des infirmités humaines, que le désir d'éviter aux gens de l'art de graves erreurs de jugement, et aux malades des traitements aussi inutiles qu'ils sont rigoureux; ainsi donc, au dire de Dupuytren, il s'agirait là d'une difformité incurable, et le grand nom de l'auteur fit considérer pendant longtemps cette décision comme sans appel.

Il a fallu l'intervention de l'antisepsie pour révolutionner complètement cette question, comme, du reste, presque tous les chapitres de la chirurgie. Ce sont surtout les communications de Hoffa, soit devant la *Société allemande de Chirurgie* [2], soit au *Congrès international de Berlin*, en 1890 [3], qui ont donné le signal de cette révolution. L'idée directrice de Hoffa est la suivante : 1° sectionner les muscles trochantériens et, en particulier, les fessiers dont la rétraction s'oppose à l'abaissement de la tête fémorale; 2° creuser sur l'os iliaque une cavité cotyloïde nouvelle; 3° abaisser la tête fémorale et la replacer dans la cavité cotyloïde ainsi reconstituée.

L'idée première qui avait donné naissance à la méthode de Hoffa ne tarda pas à subir une importante modification; bientôt, en effet, Lorenz s'appliqua à démontrer que les muscles fessiers ne jouent pas, comme obstacle à la réduction, le rôle qui leur avait été attribué; il insistait d'ailleurs sur le grave inconvénient que présente, au point de vue de la marche ultérieure, la désinsertion de ces muscles, et les travaux de Trendelenburg n'ont fait que confirmer son opinion à cet égard. Pour ménager les fessiers, Lorenz porta donc l'incision en

---

1. DUPUYTREN. Mémoire sur un déplacement originel ou congénital de la tête des fémurs. *Répertoire général d'anat. et de phys. pathol.*, t. II, 1re partie, p. 82, 1826.

2. *Beilage zum Centralbl. für Chir.*, 1890, n° 25, p. 87.

3. *Verhandlungen der X Internationalen Medic. Congresses*. Band III, abtheilung VII a, p. 22.

avant, entre le couturier et le fascia lata. Le désavantage de cette
dernière incision est de ne permettre que difficilement l'accès jusque
sur la tête fémorale dans les cas où celle-ci est située très haut dans
la fosse iliaque externe; aussi, d'un commun accord, presque tous
les opérateurs placèrent-ils leur incision au côté externe de la hanche,
entre le fascia lata et le moyen fessier, ménageant, autant que possible, ces deux muscles, mais attaquant quelques-uns de leurs faisceaux dans les cas où la chose devient nécessaire pour se donner du
jour.

Quels ont été les résultats fournis par cette méthode? — Tout
d'abord, il est à noter qu'elle n'est pas absolument bénigne; tous les
opérateurs qui y ont eu recours ont perdu des malades. Si les accidents s'étaient produits entre les mains d'un seul, ou du moins d'un
petit nombre, on pourrait accuser l'impéritie du chirurgien. Du
moment, au contraire, où toutes les statistiques comptent des morts,
force est bien d'incriminer l'opération, et non l'opérateur. Et, point
plus particulièrement à mettre en relief, la cause de la mort ne varie
pas suivant le hasard des cas : elle est toujours la même, savoir la
septicémie et ses diverses modalités cliniques. Quand on réfléchit à
l'étendue de cette vaste plaie, à ses anfractuosités; quand on songe
à l'ouverture de la synoviale qui va verser dans la profondeur des
tissus un liquide prêt à s'infecter, on comprend la gravité du pronostic opératoire. Joignez-y l'abondance de l'hémorragie, la nécessité
de pratiquer des manœuvres de réduction parfois longues et difficiles,
au cours desquelles l'infection a chance de se produire; joignez-y,
enfin, la participation du tissu osseux lui-même au traumatisme,
source nouvelle d'infection chez les enfants toujours guettés par
l'ostéomyélite; de là, la recommandation qui s'impose de drainer
largement la plaie, ou même de la laisser complètement ouverte,
comme le conseille Hoffa.

Cette opération, avec les facteurs de gravité qu'elle comporte,
donne-t-elle du moins des résultats satisfaisants au point de vue
orthopédique? C'est là la question principale que nous devons envisager ici. Sans doute, dans un certain nombre de cas, les résultats
orthopédiques ont été des plus satisfaisants. Mais parfois, il faut bien
le dire, le malade n'a guéri qu'au prix d'une ankylose, ce qui est déjà
fâcheux dans les luxations unilatérales, et ce qui, dans les luxations
doubles, constitue un véritable désastre. Dans d'autres cas, au contraire, l'articulation a conservé toute sa mobilité, mais il en est résulté
un autre inconvénient, la reproduction plus ou moins rapide et plus
ou moins complète de la luxation. Joignez à cela la possibilité de voir

le membre se placer dans une attitude vicieuse où la flexion se combine à l'adduction, ce qui constitue pour la marche et la station une position singulièrement désavantageuse. Notons enfin que, même dans les cas les plus favorables, il n'est pas possible de faire disparaître complètement l'inégalité de longueur des membres. Il reste un raccourcissement qui, suivant les cas, mesure 1, 2, ou même 5 centimètres. On comprend donc que, dans ces conditions, on ait songé à trouver une méthode qui, avec de moindres dangers, permette d'obtenir des résultats égaux, ou même supérieurs, au point de vue orthopédique. De là l'intervention de la méthode non sanglante.

Déjà, en 1888, le professeur Paci, de Pise [1], émettait l'idée de traiter les luxations congénitales de la hanche d'après les mêmes principes qui guident le chirurgien dans le traitement des luxations traumatiques, c'est-à-dire par l'emploi de la méthode de douceur. Se servant du chloroforme, il imprime au membre une série de mouvements qui, commençant par la flexion complète, passent ensuite par l'abduction combinée à la rotation en dehors pour revenir à l'extension complète. En 1894, Paci présentait au *Congrès international de Rome* une pièce anatomique provenant du service de Nota (de Turin), sur laquelle on pouvait constater les heureux résultats fournis par sa méthode ; on y voyait, en effet, une cavité cotyloïde normale. Du reste, il ne faut pas l'oublier, jamais Paci n'a présenté sa méthode comme un moyen de guérison radicale des luxations congénitales; il l'a donnée seulement comme un moyen palliatif, capable d'améliorer la situation des malades.

A ce même Congrès de 1894, Mikulicz présentait l'appareil dont il se sert pour le traitement de la luxation congénitale, appareil dans lequel l'extension continue est associée à l'abduction. Déjà, du reste, Schede avait insisté sur la nécessité de placer le membre dans l'abduction, et avait construit un appareil réalisant cette position pendant la marche; aujourd'hui tous les chirurgiens sont d'accord sur la nécessité de l'abduction dans le traitement de la luxation congénitale.

C'est surtout Lorenz qui, après s'être fait l'ardent défenseur de la méthode sanglante, se constitua, en 1896, le champion de la méthode non sanglante. Il présenta sa méthode comme complètement différente de celle de Paci. En effet, aux moyens de douceur il substitue l'extension continue poussée très loin sous le chloroforme. S'il reconnaît, comme Paci, la nécessité des mouvements de flexion et d'abduc-

[1]. AGOSTINO PACI. *Studio ed osservazioni sulla lussazione iliaca comune congenital del femore et sua cura razionale.* Gènes, 1888.

tion, à la rotation en dehors il substitue, au contraire, la rotation en dedans. Enfin, différence essentielle, tandis que Paci terminait la série des manœuvres en replaçant le membre dans l'extension, Lorenz, au contraire, le laisse dans l'abduction complète.

Si les manœuvres diffèrent sur quelques points, les prétentions des deux auteurs étaient surtout complètement opposées. Paci, en effet, comme nous l'avons dit, n'avait d'autre prétention que d'améliorer le sort des malades en modifiant la situation de la tête fémorale ; Lorenz, au contraire, présentait sa méthode comme une méthode de guérison radicale : « En aucun cas, disait-il, ma méthode ne consiste à améliorer la position de la tête fémorale et à la fixer dans cette position. La reposition non sanglante est, comme la sanglante, une opération radicale, et non un moyen palliatif. »

Pour notre part, prenant en considération ce que l'anatomie pathologique et la pratique des réductions sanglantes nous avaient appris, savoir les déformations de la tête et du col fémoral, l'aplatissement ou même l'effacement complet du cotyle, la rétraction et l'étroitesse de la capsule, nous crûmes devoir faire des réserves formelles. « Sans doute, disions-nous, dans un grand nombre de cas on pourra réussir à améliorer la situation de la tête fémorale ; quant aux réductions vraies, elles nous semblent devoir constituer toujours une rare exception. » L'intervention de la radiographie est venue démontrer le bien fondé de mes réserves. En effet, dans une communication à l'*Académie impériale de médecine de Vienne*, à la fin de 1898, où il se propose de réfuter les objections que nous avions faites à sa méthode, M. Lorenz[1] reconnaît que la radiographie est venue détruire en partie ses illusions. « Le plus souvent, nous dit-il, il n'y a pas réduction vraie ; mais seulement transposition de la tête en avant. Cela, du reste, ajoute-t-il, n'a aucune importance, puisque le résultat fonctionnel est excellent. » Nous ne contestons nullement l'excellence des résultats obtenus ; mais, au point de vue scientifique, force est bien de reconnaître qu'on ne peut appeler radicale une méthode qui ne procure qu'exceptionnellement la réduction vraie.

Reprenant l'argumentation que nous faisions tout à l'heure au sujet de la méthode sanglante, nous dirons : « Si la méthode ne donne pas toujours des résultats orthopédiques excellents, est-elle du moins sans dangers ? » Il est intéressant de chercher dans les *Comptes rendus du Congrès allemand de Chirurgie* pour 1899 la réponse à cette question. Lorenz dit avoir observé une gangrène de la cuisse, conséquence

1. Verhandlungen ärztlicher Gesellschaften, in *Wiener klinische Wochens.*, 4e décembre 1898, n° 48, p. 1107.

de l'oblitération des vaisseaux fémoraux par la tête déplacée au pli de l'aine chez une jeune fille de 15 ans. Viennent ensuite 10 fractures du col fémoral chez des malades de 9 à 16 ans; une fracture de la branche horizontale du pubis, et un enfoncement de l'aile de l'os iliaque. Deux fois, il y a eu paralysie du sciatique poplité externe, 4 fois paralysie du triceps; toutes ces paralysies ont guéri spontanément. On a eu, en outre, à déplorer 5 morts par le chloroforme.

De son côté, Hoffa parle de déchirures des parties molles, de la vulve, de l'urètre; de fractures et de décollements épiphysaires, et surtout de paralysies du sciatique et du crural; d'hématomes suppurés dans la région des adducteurs. Il a même perdu un malade, enfant de 6 ans, très nerveux, qui, après la réduction d'une luxation unilatérale, a été pris de convulsions ayant entraîné la mort.

Narath (d'Utrecht) signale de volumineuses hernies crurales, ou plutôt de larges éventrations se produisant par déchirures de toutes les parties molles au-dessous de l'arcade de Fallope.

Ces accidents sont une grave objection contre la méthode non sanglante dont le principal avantage sur sa rivale devrait être de ne pas offrir de dangers. Ils démontrent tout au moins la nécessité de ne pas employer dans les manœuvres une force trop considérable.

Quant aux résultats fonctionnels, ils sont les suivants : sur 560 cas, Lorenz a échoué 22 fois; 15 fois, la luxation en arrière, dans la fosse iliaque, s'est reproduite et a pu être réduite. Ce qu'on observe le plus souvent, comme le montre la radiographie, c'est la reproduction de la luxation en haut et en avant. Sur 135 cas où la radiographie a été faite, il y a 56 cas douteux, et 79 résultats anatomiques satisfaisants.

Hoffa a employé 64 fois la méthode de Lorenz : 42 fois, la luxation était simple, et 22 fois, double. Dans tous les cas, la réduction a réussi. Sur les 42 luxations unilatérales, la réduction a persisté 4 fois seulement. Dans 1 cas, il y a eu luxation complète; 1 enfant est mort : 25 fois, il y a eu transposition en avant et en haut; 11 fois, transposition en avant et au voisinage de l'épine iliaque antérieure et inférieure.

Dans les luxations bilatérales, les résultats ont été moins bons. Jamais il n'y a eu réduction des deux côtés; 4 fois, il y a eu réduction d'un seul côté, et transposition du côté opposé; 5 fois, il y a eu récidive complète des deux côtés; 15 fois, transposition des deux côtés avec un bon résultat.

Dix-neuf fois, Hoffa a eu recours à la méthode de Schede, caractérisée surtout par la pression sur le grand trochanter jointe à l'extension. Sur 15 luxations unilatérales, il a obtenu une reluxation en arrière, 7 transpositions en avant et 5 au voisinage de l'épine iliaque. Sur 6 luxations doubles, il y a eu également 1 reluxation et 5 transpositions.

La méthode de Mikulicz, appliquée 7 fois chez de jeunes enfants de 5 ans et au-dessous, a donné 4 guérisons complètes et 3 améliorations. Enfin, Hoffa lui-même a adopté une modification consistant à maintenir le membre dans une position moyenne d'abduction jointe à la rotation en dedans. Il a traité par sa méthode 17 luxations unilatérales et 5 doubles. Sur 17 luxations unilatérales, il y a eu 9 guérisons et 8 transpositions ; sur les 5 doubles, une guérison obtenue sur 1 enfant de 5 ans et 2 transpositions.

Pétersen (de Bonn) rend compte des résultats obtenus à la Clinique de Schede. Comme les auteurs précédents, il considère la réduction vraie comme exceptionnelle. Sur 161 luxations, dont 70 doubles, elle n'a été obtenue que 10 fois, 8 fois sur des luxations unilatérales, et 2 fois sur des luxations doubles. En somme, Schede et Pétersen se contentent de transpositions, et ils en sont revenus au point de départ de Paci ; ils n'adoptent pas l'abduction forcée avec rotation en dehors préconisée par Lorenz.

Mikulicz exprime cette idée que toutes les méthodes de réduction non sanglante ont à peu près la même valeur ; Heusner (de Barmen) constate qu'on est obligé d'en rabattre beaucoup de l'enthousiasme qu'avait suscité d'abord la réduction extemporanée ; Lange (de Munich) et Kummell (de Hambourg) parlent dans le même sens.

On voit, par cette rapide analyse du Congrès allemand de 1899, combien l'avenir nous a donné raison, et combien les réserves *a priori* que nous faisions dès le début au sujet de la méthode de Lorenz étaient justifiées.

A côté des méthodes de traitement radical, il nous faut signaler les méthodes de traitement palliatif applicables dans les cas où les malades sont trop âgés, et les déplacements trop prononcés pour qu'on puisse songer à obtenir une vraie guérison. Hoffa a préconisé l'établissement d'une pseudarthrose dans la fosse iliaque externe. De mon côté dans les cas d'inversion complète du membre inférieur, c'est-à-dire dans les cas où la cuisse est placée dans la flexion marquée avec adduction et rotation en dedans, au point que les genoux s'entre-croisent pendant la marche et que la peau de la face interne du membre s'excorie par le frottement ; dans ces cas, dis-je, j'ai préconisé l'ostéotomie sous-trochantérienne oblique qui m'a fourni les meilleurs résultats. Elle permet de détruire l'ensellure, de placer le membre dans une position moyenne d'abduction et de lui fournir un point d'appui solide pendant la marche et la station.

Je me suis efforcé dans cette étude de porter un jugement aussi impartial que possible sur la méthode de réduction extemporanée des luxations congénitales de la hanche, soit par l'opération sanglante, soit par les procédés non sanglants. Il en résulte que rarement on peut compter sur une guérison radicale, absolue. Ce serait toutefois une très grande exagération que de nier les heureux résultats qu'on peut obtenir par une application judicieuse de ces méthodes. Il est assez difficile de dire dans quelles limites d'âge leur emploi doit être circonscrit. M. Lorenz (*Congrès allemand de chirurgie*, 1899) pense qu'on peut tenter la méthode de réduction non sanglante jusqu'à dix ans pour les luxations doubles, jusqu'à sept ou huit ans pour les luxations simples. J'ai pu obtenir un résultat satisfaisant, chez une jeune fille de 15 ans atteinte d'une luxation congénitale double. Mais je pense qu'en général on ne peut guère espérer réussir après 10 ans. Si la méthode de réduction extemporanée, non sanglante, n'a rien permis d'obtenir, on aura recours à l'opération sanglante. Il me semble qu'à l'heure actuelle, par un revirement dont l'histoire de la chirurgie nous offre plus d'un exemple, on tend trop à abandonner cette dernière méthode. Sans doute elle compte à son passif des accidents mortels, mais la méthode non sanglante elle-même, nous l'avons dit, n'est pas exempte d'accidents. Du reste, il se passe ici ce que l'on constate à l'avènement de toutes les méthodes opératoires nouvelles, les accidents, plus nombreux au début vu l'inexpérience des opérateurs, deviennent de plus en plus rares, au fur et à mesure que les chirurgiens se familiarisent avec la technique de l'opération. Quant au reproche que je trouve formulé contre la réduction sanglante dans le dernier congrès allemand de chirurgie, reproche d'après lequel l'opération exposerait aux arrêts de croissance ultérieurs du bassin, je n'ai rien vu dans ma pratique personnelle qui permette d'y ajouter foi.

En résumé, nous pouvons conclure que malgré les progrès considérables réalisés dans le traitement des luxations congénitales de la hanche dans ces dernières années, la question n'est pas encore complètement résolue. Dans ces conditions, il nous paraît indispensable de nous demander si tous les efforts qui ont été tentés jusqu'ici ont été faits dans une bonne direction. En somme, que fait-on? On assimile plus ou moins complètement les luxations congénitales aux luxations traumatiques, et l'on s'efforce en un seul temps d'en obtenir la réduction. Or, cette assimilation est-elle fondée? En aucune façon. Et je ne parle pas ici seulement de l'arrêt de développement de la cavité cotyloïde qui établit une différence essentielle entre les luxations congénitales et les luxations, soit traumatiques, soit pathologiques de la hanche. Mais je fais allusion surtout à l'évolution de la maladie.

Le tableau que nous a laissé Dupuytren de la luxation congénitale est celui de la luxation parachevée, avec passage de la tête dans la fosse iliaque externe, claudication manifeste, raccourcissement prononcé, ensellure considérable. On comprend que d'un pareil ensemble de lésions Dupuytren ait conclu à l'incurabilité de l'affection. Cela tient à ce que l'éminent chirurgien de l'Hôtel-Dieu avait observé surtout des adultes. Mais, quand on examine la maladie à son début, c'est-à-dire chez de très jeunes enfants, l'ensemble symptomatique est tout autre. Si Dupuytren nous a donné de la luxation confirmée un tableau qui ne laisse rien à désirer, il est un homme qui a parfaitement décrit l'évolution du mal à ses débuts : cet homme, c'est Palletta, le précurseur de Dupuytren dans l'étude de la luxation congénitale. C'est merveille de voir avec quelle exactitude il en décrit l'évolution et les symptômes. Je m'efforcerai de traduire aussi fidèlement que possible le style latin de Palletta, si pittoresque, et en même temps si plein de précision.

« Chez les enfants nouveau-nés, nous dit-il, la malformation ne saute pas aux yeux, soit parce qu'elle est tout à fait à ses débuts, soit parce que, sous l'influence de la traction de la main, les membres se laissent aisément ramener à la même longueur. Plus tard, quand les enfants font leurs premiers pas, le diagnostic n'est pas plus aisé, parce que les enfants vacillent, tombant tantôt à droite, tantôt à gauche et semblant boiter alternativement des deux côtés. Plus tard, quand ils marchent d'un pas plus sûr, c'est-à-dire entre 17 et 18 mois, la claudication devient manifeste.

« C'est seulement quand l'enfant leur est rendu par la nourrice que les parents la constatent. Ils entrent en fureur et rejettent toute la faute sur la nourrice, l'accusant d'avoir laissé tomber l'enfant, ou de lui avoir tordu les membres en le portant sur ses bras. »

C'est bien ainsi que les choses se passent : l'examen d'un nombre considérable de luxations congénitales nous permet d'affirmer que jamais la malformation n'est soupçonnée au moment même de la naissance. Et cela non seulement chez les malades pauvres de l'hôpital, mais aussi dans les classes riches de la société, où l'enfant est soigneusement examiné par les parents, par la garde et par la nourrice chargées d'en prendre soin, par l'accoucheur et le médecin de la famille. Force est bien d'admettre que si, dans ce nombreux entourage, personne ne découvre une imperfection quelconque, c'est qu'il n'y a rien d'appréciable.

S'il existait en effet une luxation vraie dans la fosse iliaque externe, l'attitude vicieuse du membre, le raccourcissement, la présence même de la tête dans la fosse iliaque ne sauraient passer inaperçus. Mais il n'y a qu'une laxité anormale de l'articulation, une tendance à la luxation plutôt qu'un déplacement véritable.

L'enfant sur lequel il m'a été donné de faire le diagnostic le plus précoce est une petite fille de 4 mois, atteinte d'une luxation congénitale de la hanche droite, avec un raccourcissement d'un centimètre. Encore le père de cette enfant était-il un vétérinaire, possédant par conséquent des notions exactes d'anatomie, et plus apte par là même à reconnaître et à apprécier l'importance des symptômes observés. Plus tard même, quand la malformation devient évidente pour tous les yeux, et que nous sommes appelés à examiner les petits malades, c'est-à-dire vers l'âge de 18 mois à 2 ans, il est tout à fait exceptionnel que nous rencontrions des déplacements considérables. Pour ma part, une seule fois, j'ai constaté une luxation iliaque droite chez un jeune enfant. Le plus souvent le raccourcissement atteint à peine 1 centimètre ou 1 centimètre et demi. Dans l'immense majorité des cas, sinon toujours, la tête est encore facilement appréciable par la palpation au pli de l'aine. Elle est seulement située plus en dehors, parfois plus en dehors et plus en haut qu'à l'état normal, se rapprochant de l'épine iliaque antérieure et inférieure; elle est en même temps plus superficielle, plus facile à sentir sous le doigt pendant les mouvements de rotation imprimés à la cuisse; ce qui démontre qu'elle n'est pas, comme à l'état normal, solidement encastrée dans la cavité de réception.

Plus tard, au fur et à mesure que l'enfant avance en âge, le raccourcissement augmente, en même temps que la claudication et l'attitude vicieuse du membre se caractérisent; en d'autres termes, sous la double influence de l'augmentation du poids du corps, et d'exercices de plus en plus violents, de plus en plus prolongés, la luxation se complète et s'exagère. Franchissant la ligne ilio-ischiatique ou de Nélaton, cette ligne que, dans mon enseignement journalier, j'appelle familièrement le *Rubicon*, la tête devient libre dans la fosse iliaque externe, en un mot, la luxation arrive à son dernier terme.

Au lieu d'abandonner les choses à elles-mêmes, et d'intervenir seulement quand le déplacement est parachevé, il importe, croyons-nous, de commencer le traitement dès l'âge le plus tendre, dès que le diagnostic est établi, soit vers l'âge de 18 mois à 2 ans. Tout nous permet d'établir une comparaison entre la luxation congénitale et le pied bot. Or, dans cette dernière affection, que faisons-nous? Abandonnons-nous les choses à elles-mêmes jusqu'à ce que des déformations osseuses plus ou moins considérables, une véritable subluxation dans l'articulation médio-tarsienne, nous obligent à recourir à des ténoto mies à ciel ouvert, à de larges arthrotomies médio-tarsiennes, ou même à des résections osseuses plus ou moins étendues? Nullement : nous agissons, au contraire, dès les premières semaines qui suivent la naissance; et par des moyens très simples, massage aidé au besoin de la ténotomie du tendon d'Achille, et suivi de l'application de petits appareils contentifs, nous arrivons à obtenir la guérison.

Ce sont ces principes qu'il nous semble indispensable de suivre dans le traitement de la luxation congénitale de la hanche. Pour ce faire, il n'est pas besoin d'avoir recours à la réduction extemporanée sous le chloroforme par la méthode non sanglante ou par la méthode à ciel ouvert. Le déplacement, en effet, est, avons-nous dit, le plus souvent insignifiant. Il suffit, pour rendre au membre sa longueur normale, d'une traction légère, en un mot, il suffit d'avoir recours à l'extension continue par la méthode qu'on peut appeler véritablement la méthode française. C'est elle en effet qu'ont employée autrefois Jalade-Lafont et Duval, dont les résultats encourageants sont consignés dans la thèse de Caillard-Billionnière et ont pu être vérifiés par Dupuytren lui-même; c'est elle encore qu'ont mise en usage Humbert (de Morley), et Jacquier, et, plus tard encore, Pravaz (de Lyon).

Si l'on a pu contester que ces auteurs aient obtenu des réductions vraies, tout le monde a été d'accord pour reconnaître qu'ils ont réalisé dans certains cas de remarquables améliorations. Malgaigne admet même la possibilité de la réduction : « Je crois pour mon compte, dit-il, qu'Humbert et Pravaz ont pu obtenir des réductions; mais je sais qu'une des guérisons les plus belles et les plus durables de Pravaz n'a point persisté[1]. »

Il est, du reste, indispensable de faire remarquer ici que tous les auteurs que nous venons de nommer ont tenté la réduction chez les adultes, ou, du moins, chez des enfants déjà avancés en âge. Il n'est pas étonnant dès lors qu'ils aient rencontré de sérieuses difficultés, ou même qu'ils aient échoué complètement. Chez les très jeunes enfants, il en va tout autrement : chez eux, l'extension continue amène rapidement la réduction et l'égalité de longueur des membres, mais le difficile est de maintenir la réduction.

Pour cela, le port d'un appareil contentif est indispensable. Mais ici

---

1. MALGAIGNE. *Fractures et luxations, luxations congénitales de la hanche.* t. II. p. 897.

encore il importe de modifier complètement les principes d'après lesquels ces appareils ont été construits jusqu'à ces dernières années. On s'est contenté d'ordonner le port de ceintures orthopédiques dites ceintures de Dupuytren, qui ont pour but d'exercer une pression sur la tête fémorale et de s'opposer à son ascension. En réalité, comme chacun a pu s'en assurer, ces appareils ne donnent aucun résultat utile. Ils laissent libre, en effet le membre inférieur qui se place dans une position de plus en plus marquée d'adduction, en même temps que la tête fémorale, par un mouvement inverse, se portant en dehors, abandonne de plus en plus la cavité cotyloïde et se luxe complètement dans la fosse iliaque externe. Ce qu'il faut, c'est immobiliser l'articulation coxo-fémorale au moyen d'un appareil qui embrasse à la fois la cuisse et le bassin : il faut, en un mot, appliquer à la luxation congénitale les principes qui nous guident dans le traitement de la coxalgie. Déjà nous avons noté la nécessité de placer le membre dans une position modérée d'abduction, de façon à ce que la tête appuie sur le rebord antérieur du bassin et qu'elle ait chance de se fixer solidement dans ce point. C'est là un principe du traitement sur lequel tous les chirurgiens sont aujourd'hui d'accord. J'insiste également sur la nécessité de faire un appareil qui immobilise complètement la hanche, sans permettre les mouvements de flexion. En effet, la flexion se lie à l'adduction, de même que l'extension est en rapport avec l'abduction ; or, permettre les mouvements d'adduction, c'est favoriser le déplacement de la tête dans la fosse iliaque externe. D'autre part si, à l'état normal, les mouvements de la tête fémorale dans la cavité cotyloïde peuvent être comparés à ceux d'une sphère accomplissant des mouvements de rotation autour de son point central, dans la luxation congénitale, au contraire, la tête fémorale subit un mouvement de translation ; elle décrit un arc de cercle autour de la cavité cotyloïde déshabitée, et, dans ce mouvement, elle tend à se porter de plus en plus dans la fosse iliaque. Immobiliser complètement la hanche, c'est donc s'opposer autant que possible aux déplacements de la tête fémorale, et favoriser l'établissement d'une articulation solide. Plus tard seulement, et au fur et à mesure qu'on avancera dans le traitement, on pourra permettre l'établissement d'une articulation.

Ces principes sont les mêmes que ceux que nous avons formulés déjà dans les études que nous avons publiées sur le traitement de la luxation congénitale, c'est-à-dire dans notre communication au *Congrès de Rome* en 1894, dans la discussion de 1897 à la *Société de chirurgie* et dans notre *Traité des maladies chirurgicales d'origine congénitale*. Nous les avons mis en œuvre dans bon nombre de cas et nous avons pu en tirer les résultats les plus avantageux. Nous sommes arrivés ainsi à maintenir la tête dans une position très voisine de l'état normal, c'est-à-dire qu'elle est située au pli de l'aine, en avant de la ligne de Nélaton, et que le raccourcissement est nul, ou, du moins, extrêmement modéré, ne dépassant pas, par exemple, un demi ou un centimètre. Nous sommes persuadé que là est l'avenir du traitement de la luxation congénitale. Il se résume à dépister le plus tôt possible les traces de la malformation, et à la traiter immédiatement par le repos joint à l'extension continue, suivi du port d'appareils contentifs, immobilisant rigoureusement l'articulation, jusqu'à ce qu'on soit assuré qu'il n'y a plus tendance au déplacement. Ce traitement employé avec persévérance pendant plusieurs années donnera une proportion considérable de succès. C'est seulement dans les cas où, pour une raison ou une autre, il n'aura pas pu être suivi, ou n'aura pas donné de résultat, que la réduction extemporanée sous le chloroforme, avec ou sans opération sanglante, restera comme une dernière ressource, capable de reculer les limites de l'action chirurgicale et de fournir encore des résultats avantageux. Les méthodes de traitement palliatif ne devront plus constituer qu'une rare exception.

TRAITEMENT DE LA LUXATION CONGÉNITALE DE LA HANCHE PAR LA MÉTHODE NON SANGLANTE

COMMUNICATION

de M. P. REDARD,

de Paris.

Nous désirons indiquer les résultats que nous a donnés la méthode de la réduction non sanglante dans le traitement des luxations congénitales de la hanche.

Après avoir employé avec quelques avantages sérieux le procédé de Paci (de Pise) qui nous a souvent donné un changement de position plus favorable de la tête fémorale luxée, nous cherchons, depuis plus de quatre ans, à obtenir chez tous nos jeunes sujets une véritable réduction des luxations congénitales de la hanche.

Notre statistique, qui porte sur 52 cas de réductions de luxations congénitales de la hanche, démontre d'abord que dans certaines limites d'âge et dans quelques cas à disposition anatomique favorable une véritable réduction de la luxation peut être obtenue.

Dans 12 de nos cas, chez de jeunes enfants de 2 à 7 ans, ainsi que le prouvent les radiographies et les résultats fonctionnels, la réduction anatomique a été obtenue. Les radiographies que nous présentons, et principalement nos radiographies stéréoscopiques, ne permettent pas de nier la réalité de cette réduction. Nous obtenons actuellement plus fréquemment des réductions véritables, persistantes, depuis que nous avons perfectionné notre technique opératoire.

La reproduction de la luxation en arrière, quelque temps après l'opération, sous l'appareil de contention, est assez rare, d'après nos observations. Cet accident, qui est la conséquence de l'application défectueuse de l'appareil contentif, peut facilement être évité.

Les transpositions antérieures sont assez fréquentes (4 fois sur nos 52 cas). Elles s'observent surtout chez les sujets âgés, à la suite de manœuvres trop violentes de réduction, à la suite de la position vicieuse du membre inférieur en rotation externe trop accentuée et surtout du maintien imparfait de la réduction par l'appareil plâtré.

Si on a souci d'observer par la radiographie la nouvelle position donnée à l'extrémité supérieure fémorale par les manœuvres de réduction, on peut éviter les transpositions et placer très exactement la tête du fémur dans la cavité cotyloïde. C'est ainsi que, d'accord avec Hoffa et Schede, nous recommandons dans quelques cas, après la réduction, la position en abduction de la cuisse, mais avec rotation en dedans de tout le membre inférieur. Chez quelques sujets, en effet, ce n'est que dans la rotation en dedans que la tête fémorale, le col et le grand trochanter peuvent se diriger directement sur la cavité cotyloïde.

Nous n'avons jamais eu aucun accident sérieux à déplorer dans nos nombreuses réductions de luxations de la hanche. Chez les jeunes sujets, la réduction se fait, en général, très facilement et l'on n'observe aucun accident primitif ou consécutif. Assez souvent, nous avons observé de volumineux hématomes dans la région génitale et des adducteurs qui se sont toujours graduellement résorbés. Nous avons quelquefois noté des rétractions douloureuses des muscles postérieurs de la cuisse dans les premiers jours qui suivent l'opération ou, plus tard, de la persistance de la rotation en dehors du pied et du membre inférieur.

Les accidents graves signalés par quelques auteurs (fractures, paralysies, etc.) tiennent certainement à la violence des manœuvres et

à la puissance des tractions qu'exige la réduction des luxations chez
des sujets âgés de plus de 10 ans.

Chez nos opérés âgés de plus de 10 ans, chez lesquels les manœuvres
de réduction ont été particulièrement pénibles, nous avons toujours
agi avec une grande prudence. Nous croyons qu'il est sage de ne pas
continuer l'opération si les manœuvres de réduction doivent être trop
prolongées et exigent le déploiement d'une grande force.

Les résultats fonctionnels ont été très satisfaisants chez 17 de nos
opérés. Chez 6 jeunes sujets, la marche se fait sans aucune claudication, d'une façon tout à fait normale. Chez les autres, on note un peu
de laxité articulaire, de la fatigue après la marche; dans deux cas, un
très léger raccourcissement du membre inférieur.

Dans nos cas de transposition antérieure ou d'antéversion du col et
de la tête fémorale, bien que la tête ne soit pas exactement placée
dans la cavité cotyloïde, les résultats fonctionnels sont néanmoins
très satisfaisants : la marche s'effectue sans claudication, avec une
certaine raideur.

Dans un de nos cas de réduction de luxation bilatérale, chez une
fillette de quatre ans et demi, la réduction des deux luxations a été
facilement obtenue, le résultat fonctionnel est excellent, l'enfant
marche sans aucune claudication.

Dans notre technique opératoire, nous cherchons d'abord à placer
la cuisse en forte abduction, mobilisant la tête fémorale, agissant par
des massages sur les muscles rétractés, principalement sur le groupe
des adducteurs.

Nous sommes peu partisans des tractions instrumentales, exécutées
avec la vis de Lorenz ou l'appareil de Schede, dans le but de faire
descendre la tête du fémur au niveau du cotyle. Ces tractions, indispensables chez les sujets âgés, sont la cause de sérieux accidents tels
que fractures, paralysies, surtout si elles sont brutales et violentes.
Dans tous les cas où nous employons ces tractions, nous mesurons la
force développée au moyen du dynamomètre.

Dans le cas de luxation sus-cotyloïdienne, nous transformons
d'abord la luxation en luxation iliaque que nous réduisons par le procédé ordinaire.

Les photographies que nous présentons représentent les divers
temps de la réduction d'après notre technique.

Dans les cas faciles, chez les jeunes sujets, après flexion à angle
droit de la cuisse sur le bassin et très forte traction, nous ramenons le
membre en abduction, nous contentant, pendant ce temps, de presser
avec notre main, dans la bonne direction, au niveau du grand tro-

chanter. Dans les réductions difficiles, pendant l'abduction forcée et les tentatives de propulsion de la tête fémorale du côté du cotyle, nous plaçons notre poing fermé en arrière du trochanter, de façon à donner un point d'appui au levier constitué par le fémur.

Ces manœuvres de levier, qui sont malheureusement indispensables pour obtenir la réduction des luxations chez des sujets âgés, exposent à des accidents et particulièrement à des fractures. Elles doivent être exécutées avec une grande prudence, en exerçant une forte traction sur le fémur et en évitant surtout de l'appuyer sur le bassin.

Dans toutes nos observations, nous avons obtenu une réduction ou une transposition. Dans trois de nos observations, chez des sujets âgés, les manœuvres de réduction ont duré plus de deux heures.

Si, chez des sujets âgés, des manœuvres répétées de réduction ne donnent aucun résultat, si la force à déployer doit être trop grande, nous conseillons d'interrompre l'opération, pour la renvoyer à plus tard ou pour s'adresser à d'autres méthodes. L'opération, dans ces cas, doit être considérée comme dangereuse et d'assez nombreux accidents ont été signalés.

La contention, après la réduction, doit être l'objet de tous nos soins. Il faut d'abord placer le membre en bonne position, de telle sorte que la tête fémorale repose très exactement dans la cavité cotyloïde, éviter ensuite le déplacement ultérieur de l'extrémité supérieure fémorale.

Nous aidant surtout des renseignements donnés par la radiographie, nous mettons le membre inférieur, après abduction, soit en rotation externe ou interne, suivant les cas.

L'appareil plâtré doit s'appliquer très exactement sur la peau, de façon à éviter tout vide et, par conséquent, tout déplacement du membre inférieur. Nous enroulons, depuis longtemps, nos bandes plâtrées sur un simple maillot en tissu des Pyrénées, dont nous revêtons notre opéré après la réduction et sans interposition de ouate.

Une très petite quantité de ouate est seulement placée au niveau de l'abdomen, des épines iliaques et de la région lombaire.

A l'exemple de Lorenz, nous ne faisons pas descendre l'appareil au-dessous du genou, excepté dans les cas où le membre inférieur doit être placé en rotation interne.

Nous modifions ensuite graduellement l'attitude en abduction, jusqu'à la position verticale, par une série d'appareils que nous changeons tous les trois mois.

Nous permettons à nos opérés pour luxation unilatérale de marcher en s'appuyant sur leur membre inférieur en abduction. La marche a dans ces cas une influence favorable pour la consolidation de la réduction ; elle n'expose pas à des récidives si l'appareil plâtré est correctement appliqué ; elle a le grand avantage de permettre d'éviter les inconvénients incontestables de l'immobilité prolongée, d'ailleurs si difficilement acceptée par les parents.

Dans les luxations doubles, nous faisons la réduction des deux côtés à la fois, afin d'éviter la trop longue durée du traitement consécutif. Chez les sujets âgés et chez lesquels la réduction d'un côté présente des difficultés, il est prudent de renvoyer à plus tard la réduction de la luxation du côté opposé.

Nous insisterons surtout enfin sur la question d'âge qui domine la thérapeutique des luxations congénitales de la hanche. Chez les jeunes sujets, de 2 à 6 ans, l'opération est simple, facile ; la réduction est presque toujours obtenue ; les résultats fonctionnels sont excellents. Chez les sujets plus âgés, à mesure que l'on s'éloigne de l'âge de 10 ans, les résultats sont plus incertains et l'on peut dire que la difficulté, la gravité de l'opération et l'imperfection des résultats définitifs sont en rapport avec l'âge des sujets. De là l'indication formelle de recommander la réduction des luxations congénitales de la hanche lorsque les sujets sont âgés de 2 à 7 ans.

Généralement, la réduction chez les sujets âgés de plus de 10 ans est dangereuse et donne de mauvais résultats. Il n'y a pas cependant de règle absolue et nous avons réduit récemment avec une très grande facilité une luxation congénitale double très prononcée chez une fillette âgée de 11 ans et pour laquelle nous nous attendions à de très graves difficultés opératoires.

En résumé, la réduction non sanglante exécutée chez de jeunes sujets et avec une technique régulière est une opération simple, exempte de dangers et qui donne, dans la généralité des cas, une réduction anatomique parfaite et surtout d'excellents résultats fonctionnels.

Nous rappellerons, en terminant, que nous avons insisté depuis longtemps sur l'importance de la radiographie pour l'étude et le traitement des luxations congénitales de la hanche. La radiographie permet, en effet, de se rendre compte sur le vivant, d'une façon assez précise, des détails de la configuration et du degré de malformation de l'articulation de la hanche, d'obtenir des indications pour la bonne direction du traitement et d'apprécier enfin les résultats thérapeutiques obtenus. A notre avis, la radiographie est le guide le plus sûr pour nos opérations curatives de luxations congénitales de la hanche.

Dans toutes nos réductions par la méthode non sanglante, nous faisons exécuter des radiographies de la hanche avant l'intervention et après chaque étape du traitement. Après l'opération de la réduction, les radiographies nous indiquent si la réduction est bien réellement obtenue, si la tête fémorale correspond bien au centre de la **cavité cotyloïde** : elles nous renseignent sur la meilleure position à donner au membre inférieur pour le maintien de la réduction de la luxation ; elles nous montrent si la rotation en dedans du membre inférieur doit être préférée à la rotation en dehors : elles nous démontrent enfin que la luxation est bien réduite ou qu'elle s'est reproduite. Un grand nombre de nos radiographies démontrent que la réduction véritable des luxations congénitales peut être obtenue chez de jeunes sujets. Les derniers perfectionnements apportés à l'opération de la luxation congénitale de la hanche ont pour base les précieuses indications fournies par la radiographie.

Depuis longtemps, nous nous servons de la radiographie comme guide pour le traitement des luxations congénitales de la hanche. Depuis quelque temps, nous avons adopté la **radiographie stéréoscopique** qui, mieux que les radiographies ordinaires, nous donne des images plus nettes, semblables en tant que forme et rapport de dimensions à l'objet réel radiographié et surtout des images en relief, avec plans superposés et des différences de profondeur qui donnent la position, la direction exacte des os et des surfaces articulaires. Cette méthode, croyons-nous, constitue un perfectionnement important qui mérite de fixer l'attention des orthopédistes.

Sur nos positifs radiographiques sur papier, examinés au stéréoscope, on obtient des images réelles, très nettes, en relief, de la luxation. La position des os, la superposition des plans et les différences de profondeur, leurs rapports sont très exactement représentés. La cavité cotyloïde peut être étudiée dans toutes ses particularités. La direction de l'extrémité supérieure du fémur peut être connue. Sur nos épreuves, on voit distinctement la différence de plan des deux fémurs, la direction du col et de la tête, variable suivant les cas, l'antéversion du col, la position de la tête fémorale dans la fosse iliaque ou au-dessus du bourrelet cotyloïdien.

Nos radiographies stéréoscopiques indiquent enfin très nettement les résultats du traitement et représentent avec exactitude les réductions obtenues.

DE LA RÉDUCTION NON SANGLANTE DES LUXATIONS CONGÉNITALES
DE LA HANCHE

COMMUNICATION

de MM. A. BROCA et A. MOUCHET.

Depuis plus de 5 ans, à l'hôpital Trousseau, nous avons traité par la méthode non sanglante de Lorenz : 58 sujets atteints de luxation unilatérale dont 55 filles et 5 garçons, et 24 sujets atteints de luxation bilatérale dont 21 filles et 5 garçons. Nous omettons volontairement 4 filles atteintes de luxation unilatérale chez lesquelles le résultat semble devoir être très favorable, mais qui sont trop récemment traitées pour pouvoir figurer dans notre statistique. En somme, nous avons traité 62 sujets (soit 86 articulations de la hanche), chez lesquels le résultat thérapeutique date d'un temps assez long pour pouvoir être définitivement apprécié. Nous avons suivi à la lettre la méthode de Lorenz.

Les enfants chez lesquels nous sommes intervenus avaient de 20 *mois à* 14 *ans*. Rares sont ceux que nous avons traités au-dessus de 10 ans : 2 à 12 ans, et 1 à 14 ans. Moins heureux que Lorenz qui a réussi à 12, 13 et 15 ans, nous n'avons eu dans les cas au-dessus de 10 ans que des échecs.

Nous pensons avec Lorenz et la plupart des auteurs qui se sont occupés de la question que le succès est assez aléatoire au-dessus de 10 ans et que plus l'enfant est traité de bonne heure, plus il a de chances de guérir favorablement. Nous avons eu cependant plusieurs fois des difficultés à réduire des luxations chez des sujets très jeunes à 3, 4 ans, alors que la tête rentrait dans le cotyle dès la première tentative chez des enfants de 8 et 9 ans. Dernièrement même, en ville, l'un de nous a réduit avec une extrême facilité une luxation bilatérale très accusée, vierge de tout traitement préalable chez un garçon de 10 ans : or, la luxation bilatérale est d'une façon générale plus difficile à réduire que l'unilatérale et la limite d'âge doit être en principe abaissée en vue de la réduction dans cette variété de luxation.

Il y a donc à tenir compte dans l'emploi de la méthode de Lorenz d'autres facteurs que de l'âge : l'état de la capsule fibreuse, l'état du cotyle, la situation élevée de la tête et plus accessoirement sa conformation sont des éléments avec lesquels il faut compter. Nous ne faisons point entrer dans notre statistique un certain nombre (10 environ) de luxations *antérieures* dans lesquelles la position de la tête fémorale bien fixée et la démarche satisfaisante du sujet nous ont paru contre-indiquer toute espèce d'intervention.

Nous n'avons réduit que des luxations *postérieures* ou *postéro-supérieures*.

Comme nous venons de le dire, les luxations unilatérales nous ont paru d'une reposition plus facile que les *bilatérales*.

Ces dernières ont été réduites le plus souvent des *deux côtés à la fois* dans la même séance (chez 16 sujets). Nous avons dans 4 cas seulement, et au début de notre pratique, réduit la deuxième luxation après guérison de la première et nous ne voyons aucun avantage à cette façon de faire qui allonge, au contraire, du double, la durée du traitement.

Enfin dans 5 cas nous n'avons pu reposer la tête fémorale que d'un côté. l'autre a été réduit chez deux de ces sujets par l'opération sanglante.

Une fois, chez une fillette de 14 ans. nous avons éprouvé un échec complet.

Nous n'avons employé avant l'intervention l'*extension continue* que chez les sujets ayant dépassé l'âge de 5 ou 6 ans ou dans les cas où nos premières tentatives ayant été infructueuses, nous voulions les renouveler. Cette extension était pratiquée avec des poids ne dépassant pas 6 à 7 kilogrammes au maximum et sa durée n'excédait pas 10 à 15 jours.

Malgré l'avantage que Lorenz assigne aux sections tendineuses sous-cutanées des muscles couturier, tenseur du fascia, demi-tendineux, demi-membraneux, biceps, adducteurs « pour abaisser la tête fémorale et forcer l'isthme de la capsule ». nous n'avons jamais cru devoir recourir à ces ténotomies.

Au cours de la réduction, lorsque nous éprouvions trop de difficultés à rentrer la tête. nous nous servions de la **vis** de Lorenz, mais nous devons reconnaître qu'elle ne nous a point, employée ainsi extemporanément, rendu de grands services, et nous avons dû le plus souvent dans les cas qui nous avaient paru exiger l'emploi de la **vis**, remettre à une autre séance de nouvelles tentatives de réduction ; en attendant. nous avons soumis le membre à l'*extension continue* qui a toujours eu le plus heureux résultat.

Nous n'avons jamais pratiqué la réduction qu'à *main libre*, selon l'expression de Lorenz: jamais nous ne nous sommes servis du coin que Lorenz a parfois utilisé.

Le *degré d'abduction* dans lequel nous avons laissé le membre pour assurer le maintien de la reposition est évidemment variable suivant les cas ; il dépend surtout du degré de saillie du rebord cotyloïdien postérieur : lorsque ce dernier est à peine marqué, il faut presque toujours une abduction très prononcée à angle droit, si l'on veut éviter la reluxation.

Quant au *sens de la rotation* dans laquelle il faut placer la tête fémorale, notre tendance primitive était favorable surtout à la rotation en dedans : c'est la position que recommande principalement Hoffa. Mais nous avons remarqué que cette attitude favorisait dans beaucoup de cas la reluxation, et nous préférons actuellement avec Lorenz une rotation indifférente, en avouant que, dans beaucoup de cas, la rotation externe est seule capable de maintenir la tête réduite.

Nous avons appliqué l'*appareil plâtré* après réduction comme Lorenz, et, amis de la simplicité, nous n'avons pas cru utile de recourir à la modification complexe prônée par Ducroquet.

Le *premier appareil* est laissé de 2 à 4 mois au maximum dans les luxations unilatérales ; plutôt 2 que 4. Dans les bilatérales qui sont réduites toutes les deux à la fois, le premier appareil n'est généralement laissé qu'un mois pendant lequel l'enfant, vu l'abduction exagérée des deux cuisses, ne peut évidemment pas marcher.

Dans les luxations unilatérales, nous faisons marcher l'enfant dans les jours qui suivent l'application de l'appareil plâtré, et cette marche est toujours possible, quel que soit le degré d'abduction, mais dès maintenant nous devons avouer qu'après la communication toute récente de Brun à la Société de chirurgie, nous nous demandons s'il ne serait pas préférable en vue d'obtenir un résultat ultérieur parfait de laisser pendant 2 ou 3 mois l'enfant absolument immobile, et de ne permettre la station debout et la marche qu'au bout de ce temps.

En tout, la durée d'application de l'appareil plâtré chez les malades que nous avons traités n'a guère dépassé 6 mois.

Une fois l'appareil supprimé, nos enfants ont été soumis à un *massage* méthodique fréquemment répété et à des exercices de *reluxation* ; ce traitement consécutif présente une importance considérable pour le bon fonctionnement ultérieur de la jointure.

Nous n'avons pas eu d'accident sérieux à déplorer par l'emploi de la reposition non sanglante des luxations congénitales de la hanche ; à l'exception de deux *fractures* sous-trochantériennes du fémur, qui n'ont eu du reste aucune influence fâcheuse sur le résultat définitif du traitement, nous n'avons vu survenir, après la réduction sous chloroforme, ni paralysie du nerf sciatique, ni paralysie partielle du nerf crural (paralysie du quadriceps), ni paralysie avec anesthésie et incontinence d'urine et des matières fécales, tous accidents signalés par Lorenz, sauf le dernier vu dans un cas seulement par Schlesinger.

Nous ne rangeons pas dans les accidents les *eschares* que nous avons observées, très exceptionnellement d'ailleurs, sur les apophyses épineuses des vertèbres lombaires et sacrées. Ces eschares, dont la présence nous était décelée par la douleur et par la mauvaise odeur communiquée à l'appareil, ne nous ont jamais obligés à supprimer ce dernier, nous nous sommes contentés de l'échancrer pour panser la plaie, en même temps que nous interdisions la marche pendant toute la durée du pansement. Une fois l'eschare guérie, nous appliquions un nouvel appareil.

Nos résultats se décomposent de la manière suivante :

15 *excellents* sur lesquels il y a 8 luxations bilatérales (2 de ces bilatérales ont dû être opérées d'un côté par la méthode sanglante). Ce ne sont pas les bilatérales qui ont fourni le moins bon résultat, loin de là, et, quand nous parlons d'excellent résultat, nous avons en vue autant la forme, l'esthétique de la hanche que son fonctionnement.

25 *résultats satisfaisants*, ce qui signifie que les enfants ont conservé une légère boiterie par raccourcissement ou une atrophie assez visible de la région fessière et crurale; mais il n'y a pas de dandinement, pas de fatigue après la marche, et en somme, le fonctionnement de la jointure est bon, parce que la suspension du tronc sur le fémur est bonne, parce que la surface d'appui présentée par le bassin à la tête fémorale est satisfaisante.

7 *résultats passables*.

5 *résultats mauvais* dont 3 chez des fillettes âgées de 12 et 14 ans : la reposition n'a pu être obtenue dans ces 3 cas et maintenue dans les 2 autres.

9 *résultats inconnus* (enfants non ramenés par leurs parents, enfants partis au loin dont on n'a pu avoir de nouvelles).

Enfin, 1 fillette, atteinte de luxation bilatérale, morte des suites de la *rougeole* en cours de traitement.

Telle est l'appréciation clinique des résultats que nous avons obtenus par la méthode de Lorenz. Il nous reste un dernier point à discuter : celui de la *situation anatomique* des têtes fémorales ainsi replacées. Y a-t-il reposition vraie ou seulement transposition?

Nous avons, pour trancher la question, eu recours à la *radiographie*. Employée dès le début, elle nous fournissait, concurremment avec l'examen clinique quelques renseignements utiles sur le degré de profondeur du cotyle, sur la situation de la tête par rapport à cette cavité, et nous pouvions ainsi prévoir jusqu'à un certain point la facilité plus ou moins grande que nous aurions à replacer la tête fémorale. Il ne faut cependant pas vouloir tirer de la radiographie plus qu'elle ne peut donner; il reste, après elle, bien des inconnus, quand ce ne serait que sur l'état de la capsule.

Une fois le traitement terminé, les sujets étaient de nouveau radiographiés et nous pouvions comparer à la situation ancienne de la tête, la situation nouvelle créée par la méthode de Lorenz.

Nous devons reconnaître que, sur nos 62 cas, nous n'avons obtenu la reposition *anatomique* vraie que 2 fois — chiffre absolument conforme à celui d'Hoffa dans son mémoire de 1898 (5 fois sur 90 réductions non sanglantes dont 20 bilatérales). Ce que nous avons obtenu presque toujours, c'est donc la transposition de la tête en avant, contre l'épine iliaque antéro-inférieure. Il est certain que la transposition est très souvent obtenue par la méthode de Lorenz; d'après la majorité des auteurs, elle serait la règle, et la reposition vraie l'exception. Il n'en est pas moins vrai que la reposition est l'idéal que l'on doit s'efforcer d'atteindre, car si la transposition est compatible avec un excellent fonctionnement de l'articulation, elle ne peut permettre de par le raccourcissement qu'elle entraîne, — dans les luxations unilatérales, — une marche absolument parfaite. Peut-être conviendrait-il afin d'obtenir sûrement la reposition — toutes les fois qu'elle est possible, s'entend — elle ne l'est certainement pas toujours — d'immobiliser les enfants pendant les premiers mois du traitement.

CONTRIBUTIONS AU TRAITEMENT ET A L'ANATOMIE PATHOLOGIQUE RADIOGRAPHIQUE DE LA LUXATION CONGÉNITALE DE LA HANCHE

COMMUNICATION

de M. le docteur FROELICH,

de Nancy.

Nous avons eu l'occasion dans ces quatre dernières années de traiter à la clinique de chirurgie orthopédique de l'Université 21 malades atteints de luxation congénitale de la hanche. De leur étude il s'est dégagé pour nous un certain nombre de faits et de conclusions que nous croyons utile de rapporter. Nous pensons ainsi, pour notre modeste part, faire progresser vers une thérapeutique définitive le traitement de ces malformations qui, malgré les innombrables travaux de ces derniers temps, n'est pas encore assis sur des bases solides et indiscutées.

Nos 21 observations ont porté sur 17 filles et 4 garçons.

13 luxations étaient doubles, 8 unilatérales dont 3 à droite et 5 à gauche.

Parmi les antécédents personnels de nos malades, nous notons 5 accouchements par le siège dont 2 laborieux. 7 de ces enfants étaient franchement scrofuleux.

Parmi les antécédents héréditaires nous devons signaler 5 fois la mère atteinte de la même lésion; 2 fois soit la tante soit un oncle; une fois la grand' mère.

Dans une observation assez curieuse nous voyons le père de l'enfant porteur d'un pied-bot varus équin double congénital, une sœur un pied bot de même espèce, une tante, un pied bot unilatéral, et enfin une autre tante une luxation congénitale de la hanche.

Dans une autre observation, une tante de l'enfant avait la même lésion, et une petite sœur, un pied bot varus congénital.

Les enfants étaient atteints 5 fois d'autres malformations : une fois d'ectopie pupillaire, une fois de graves hernies inguinales, une fois de hernie crurale.

Dans une de ces observations, celle d'un petit garçon, les deux hernies inguinales étaient d'un volume et d'une incoercibilité tels que je dus faire 4 fois la cure radicale pour enfin l'en débarrasser. Cette difficulté du traitement était due, comme le raconte un auteur déjà ancien (Vrolik), à la luxation en dehors du psoas iliaque qui ouvre toute grande à l'intestin la porte de l'abdomen.

Étiologie. — Nous avons l'impression que l'étiologie de la luxation n'est pas la même dans tous nos cas. Si dans l'immense majorité des cas nous la croyons due à une malformation congénitale, 5 fois elle nous a semblé attribuable à une autre cause. Deux fois elle nous a paru une conséquence de la paralysie infantile; la lésion était survenue à la suite d'une maladie fébrile, et la réaction électrique des muscles péri-articulaires était très diminuée. Une fois enfin elle fut une suite d'un épanchement intra-articulaire. Chez un petit garçon de 55 mois, était survenu depuis trois mois de la claudication; nous pûmes nous assurer grâce à l'amaigrissement que la capsule en arrière était distendue par du liquide, et que la tête avait franchi le sourcil cotyloïdien, sans qu'il y ait eu la plus légère douleur. S'agit-il du rhumatisme articulaire qui dans certains cas serait unique chez les enfants? (Marfan.)

Dans tous les autres cas, 18 sur 21, c'est à une malformation congénitale que nous avons eu affaire.

L'*anatomie radiographique*, que nous avons étudiée sur 15 de nos cas, nous a d'ailleurs permis de confirmer ce fait.

Nous avons procédé de la façon suivante pour étudier l'anatomie pathologique radiographique.

Si l'on examine un cliché de luxation congénitale on remarque que la cavité cotyloïde est représentée par un triangle dont le sommet se confond avec le vide qui indique le cartilage en Y.

Ce triangle a un bord supérieur qui est le toit osseux de la cavité, il a un bord inférieur, et enfin un bord externe opposé au sommet de la cavité.

Nous avons, dans la luxation unilatérale, mesuré ces côtés du triangle, noté la direction du bord supérieur, et nous les avons comparés au côté sain; et celui-ci à une hanche normale.

Dans les luxations bilatérales, nous avons également comparé ces mêmes mensurations à celles fournies par un enfant du même âge sain, et établi leur rapport réciproque.

Pour la tête fémorale nous avons noté son volume en mesurant son diamètre et nous avons comparé entre eux les angles que fait le col avec la diaphyse du fémur chez les différents sujets.

Pour le bassin dans sa totalité nous avons noté son volume et sa densité osseuse.

En agissant ainsi nous avons établi des moyennes pour des enfants de moins de 2 ans, des enfants de 3 ans, et enfin des enfants de 5 à 6 ans.

Dans les mensurations de la cavité le premier chiffre indiquera en centimètres la profondeur de la cavité cotyloïde; le deuxième chiffre marquera la longueur du toit osseux de la cavité; le troisième, enfin, le côté opposé au sommet de la cavité.

Il est évident que ces chiffres sont très approximatifs, qu'il ne peut être question de profondeurs réelles, puisque la radiographie ne permet pas de tenir compte des parties cartilagineuses.

Enfants de moins de 2 ans :

```
            0,5                 1,5                  2 et 2,5
Cavité luxée 1 à 2 côté sain 2,5 enfant normal 2,5
             2                   5                    5
```

Le toit est en pente douce se rapprochant de la verticale du côté luxé, tandis que, chez l'enfant sain, il tend vers la direction horizontale.

Tête du fémur. — Le noyau d'ossification est moins prononcé du côté luxé ; l'angle d'inclinaison du col et du corps du fémur est plus obtus que du côté normal et que chez l'enfant sain.

Os iliaques. — Ils sont plus grêles chez l'enfant luxé ; et de plus le bassin a l'apparence oblique ovalaire.

Enfants de 5 ans :

	1	2	5 et 4
Cavité luxée	2	côté non luxé 2.7 enfant normal 4	
	2.8	4	5.

Même remarque que précédemment pour le toit de la cavité.

Têtes du fémur. — Elles sont fortes, leur diamètre est de 2.6 ; l'angle d'inclinaison moins obtus.

Os iliaques. — Même remarque que précédemment.

Enfants de 5 ans :

	1	2	5 et 4
Cavité luxée	1	côté non luxé 2.5 enfant normal 5	
	1.5	5	4.

Le toit semble plus vertical ici ; les dimensions de la cavité luxée sont, fait curieux, proportionnellement plus petits que chez l'enfant plus jeune.

Têtes et cols. — Les têtes sont volumineuses débordant le col ; l'angle d'inclinaison du col avec le corps est plus prononcé avec tendance à l'angle droit.

S'il est permis de tirer des conclusions de ces mensurations fatalement soumises à de nombreuses causes d'erreur, nous dirons qu'il en résulte :

Que le côté luxé est toujours notablement plus grêle, bassin et fémur, que le côté non luxé, et que dans son ensemble un enfant ayant une luxation simple ou double a le bassin et les fémurs moins développés qu'un enfant normal du même âge.

La cavité est moins profonde du côté luxé et ses bords plus fuyants.

La différence est surtout remarquable chez l'enfant de moins de 2 ans, et chez celui de 5 ans.

Le toit des cavités luxées est presque toujours en pente douce c'est-à-dire se rapprochant de la verticale, tandis que chez l'enfant sain cette direction se rapproche de l'horizontale.

L'ossification du fémur est plus précoce du côté sain et chez le sujet normal.

L'angle d'inclinaison du col avec la diaphyse est plus ouvert chez le tout jeune enfant luxé et il semble que le col et le corps sont dans le prolongement l'un de l'autre.

Cette différence semble disparaître à 3 ans, mais vers 5 ans les rapports deviennent inverses, c'est-à-dire que le col luxé fait un angle plus fermé avec la diaphyse que chez un enfant normal du même âge. L'angle d'inclinaison du col luxé se rapproche de l'angle droit.

Enfin le col semble plus court que normalement, et la tête plus évasée.

Le bassin est toujours plus grêle du côté luxé que chez le sujet normal.

Dans la luxation simple ou double le bassin paraît le plus souvent asymétrique.

Évolution naturelle de la luxation congénitale. — En interrogeant les parents de nos malades atteints eux-mêmes de luxations, et nos malades âgés de 15 et 35 ans, nous avons pu nous convaincre que l'évolution spontanée de la lésion se faisait dans deux directions diamétralement opposées, tantôt l'âge améliore les troubles fonctionnels et tantôt il les aggrave.

Exceptionnellement la claudication, après avoir augmenté jusqu'à 10 ou 15 ans, semble disparaître, et la marche devient presque normale, ou même complètement parfaite.

Dans le plus grand nombre de cas, au contraire, la boiterie subit une diminution vers 10 ans, une aggravation après 15 ans, et de nouveau une sensible accentuation à la suite de couches ou de maladies.

Chez la plupart des malades, une marche un peu longue, une station debout prolongée sont pénibles et occasionnent même des douleurs.

Certains sujets en se forçant, comme ils disent, peuvent faire disparaître totalement la claudication, mais la contraction musculaire qui les améliore leur est très pénible et ne peut être continuée longtemps.

Traitement. — Avant d'aborder l'étude du traitement, nous signalerons une catégorie de luxés qu'il ne faut pas opérer. La radiographie est indispensable aux diverses phases du traitement : on rencontrera des cas comme dans une de nos observations concernant un petit garçon de 7 ans, atteint de luxation double dans lesquels la radiographie indiquera qu'une nouvelle cavité est en voie de formation, que cette cavité est déjà bordée par des productions osseuses. Dans ce cas l'intervention serait nuisible, elle détruirait le travail de guérison spontanée entrepris par la nature.

Dans notre observation, d'ailleurs très instructive, ce qui nous confirme dans cette opinion c'est l'histoire de la mère. Celle-ci actuellement âgée de 58 ans a boité jusqu'à l'âge de 12 ans, et maintenant elle marche à la perfection; ses articulations coxo-fémorales sont solides, et sauf l'ensellure rien ne ferait soupçonner sa lésion.

Chez cet enfant un corset moulé pour appliquer les fémurs dans les cavités cotyloïdes, et un talon surélevé d'un côté pour compenser l'inégalité de longueur des membres ont été le seul traitement.

Age où il faut intervenir. — L'âge le plus favorable à l'intervention nous a paru s'étendre entre la fin de la 2ᵉ année et la fin de la 3ᵉ année. On peut alors sans trop d'efforts, et sans extension préalable ni avec des poids ni avec la vis de Lorenz, remettre les fémurs en bonne position.

Dans le cours de la 4ᵉ et de la 5ᵉ année, les obstacles sont plus considérables. On parvient cependant presque toujours à les ramener avec de l'extension préalable ou extemporanée; jamais nous n'avons dû sectionner les adducteurs.

Après 6 ans les échecs sont nombreux, et les dangers assez grands.

Intervention. — Nous avons toujours pratiqué la réduction par l'opération de Paci-Lorenz, et employé le traitement post-opératoire de Lorenz quelque peu écourté : immobilisation en abduction de 70° à 90° pendant une première période de six semaines, une deuxième période de six semaines en diminuant l'abduction, et quelquefois une dernière période d'égale longueur.

Il nous a paru indispensable, même pour les luxations unilatérales de prendre les deux cuisses dans le plâtre, et de les maintenir écartées par une baguette en bois résistant, dont les deux extrémités étaient incorporées dans le plâtre.

Après l'ablation du plâtre que je ne laisse que trois mois en tout, et pendant le port duquel les enfants sont massés et électrisés au niveau des parties à jour des fesses et des mollets, nous faisons porter un corset moulé pendant 1 an ou 2, avec ou sans béquillons.

Pendant la nuit nous maintenons l'abduction de la jambe avec ou sans traction; quelquefois avec une couchette, sorte de gouttière en plâtre ou simplement avec un écarte-cuisse.

Le massage et l'électrisation des muscles péri-articulaires sont longtemps continués.

Résultats. — Les résultats que l'on obtient au bout d'un an ne sont jamais parfaits chez les petits enfants de 2 à 5 ans.

Il faut une période de deux à trois ans encore pour que la musculature se soit suffisamment développée dans sa nouvelle position pour bien fixer la tête fémorale, et permettre une marche assurée et sans balancement. Cette longue attente d'un résultat très bon fait quelquefois perdre patience aux parents des malades.

Les résultats anatomiques ont été huit fois parfaits dans nos observations. Mais, comme nous l'avons déjà fait remarquer dans une communication à la Société de pédiatrie de Paris, le contrôle du résultat anatomique par la radiographie n'est efficace et réel que si l'on prend une photographie oblique de la hanche en plus de la photographie directe.

La photographie directe, c'est-à-dire perpendiculaire au corps couché horizontalement, montre la tête parfaitement encadrée par la cavité, alors que cette tête en réalité peut être placée en avant de la cavité.

Il est difficile par la radiographie d'arriver à prouver que la tête n'est pas dans la cavité, mais au devant d'elle. Nous croyons y être arrivé avec l'aide de notre collègue et ami M. le D\u1d63 Guilloz (Nancy).

Si l'on place, dans un cas où la tête n'est pas dans le rudiment de cavité, mais bien en avant de cette dernière, l'enfant obliquement sur la table radioscopique, la plaque sur la partie antérieure du bassin et le tube obliquement en dehors et en haut, dans le plan de clivage supposé entre la tête et la cavité et que l'on fasse varier le tube dans ce plan, on voit la tête fémorale se déplacer et même sembler pénétrer dans le bassin tandis que, si la réduction est réelle, l'aspect et la position de la tête ne se modifient pas sensiblement.

Soumis à cette épreuve, qui nous paraît indispensable et sur laquelle, croyons-nous, personne n'a encore attiré l'attention, nos huit cas de résultats anatomiques en apparence parfaits se réduisent à quatre.

Accidents du traitement. — Les accidents, que nous avons eus à déplorer dans vingt-deux interventions différentes, n'ont pas été bien sérieux.

La plus grave fut une fracture du fémur à l'union du tiers supérieur avec les deux tiers inférieurs chez une petite fille de cinq ans et demi.

Puis vient une rétraction des tendons du creux poplité (donc les pelvi-cruraux) qui amena une flexion de la jambe très longue à vaincre.

Ces muscles, dès que l'ascension du trochanter est notable et que les enfants ont quatre à cinq ans, ne se prêtent pas immédiatement à l'allongement de la cuisse provoquée par la réduction ; mais, petit à petit, cet allongement se fait grâce à des mouvements provoqués toujours un peu douloureux et à du massage. Une seule fois cette rétraction persista pendant trois mois et nous causa beaucoup d'inquiétude. Elle disparut enfin.

De larges ecchymoses au niveau du pli génito-crural et fémoro-fessier dans deux cas. Chez les autres enfants, il apparaît presque toujours une petite ecchymose en demi-lune dans le pli cruro-génital à la suite de la réduction, mais elle n'a d'importance que quand elle a de fortes dimensions.

Dans quelques cas, la peau est légèrement fendillée, très superficiellement d'ailleurs, tout de suite après l'opération, quand l'extension à la vis avait été pratiquée.

Trois fois, nous avons eu de la rétention d'urine pendant trente-six à quarante-huit heures.

La constipation est presque toujours opiniâtre tant que les malades portent l'appareil plâtré.

Chez la plupart des opérés, il s'ensuit, pendant six à huit jours au plus, une élévation de température qui n'a jamais dépassé 59°.

Si, maintenant, nous portons un jugement sans parti pris sur les résultats que nous avons obtenus par l'opération de Paci-Lorenz, nous dirons que cette intervention ne mérite ni l'enthousiasme des uns, ni le dédain des autres.

Elle est excellente chez les petits enfants jusqu'à quatre ans ; sans grand traumatisme, on arrive à réintégrer la tête fémorale dans le rudiment de cavité cotyloïde ou au moins à la placer en avant de cette dernière.

On a ainsi donné au fémur un point d'appui solide. Le bassin repose sur un pilier osseux, tandis que, avant l'intervention, il était simplement suspendu par des sangles entre les deux fémurs.

Quant au résultat fonctionnel immédiat, il est beaucoup moins bon chez les petits enfants jusqu'à trois ans. Chez eux le système musculaire s'atrophie vite pendant le traitement, et les petits enfants ont de la peine à adapter leurs muscles péri-articulaires à la nouvelle position des surfaces osseuses. Mais plus on fortifie les muscles et plus on soigne la marche par une éducation rationnelle, et plus le résultat devient bon.

Chez les enfants qui ont dépassé quatre ans, la réduction est plus difficile, les résultats anatomiques généralement moins bons, mais le résultat fonctionnel immédiat est meilleur à cause du développement déjà plus grand du système musculaire et de l'intelligence plus grande des enfants à contracter, pendant la marche, les muscles péri-articulaires de façon à fixer solidement le fémur dans la cavité.

Pour les enfants qui ont dépassé six ans, je m'abstiens de conclure, nos résultats étant trop peu nombreux pour me permettre de le faire.

La conclusion pratique est que les enfants atteints de luxation congénitale doivent être traités le plus tôt possible par l'opération de Paci-Lorenz ; mais il faut bien savoir que ce n'est qu'après deux ou trois ans d'efforts que les résultats fonctionnels viendront récompenser la patience des parents et des chirurgiens.

APRÈS RÉDUCTION DE LA LUXATION CONGÉNITALE DE LA HANCHE
ON DOIT OBTENIR
UNE GUÉRISON ANATOMIQUE ET FONCTIONNELLE COMPLETE.
CAUSES DES ÉCHECS

COMMUNICATION

de M. DUCROQUET.

Me basant sur l'anatomie pathologique de la luxation congénitale et cherchant à interpréter ce que l'on faisait lors de la réduction, je fus amené à modifier sur bien des points la méthode du professeur Lorenz. J'ai déjà eu l'occasion du reste d'exposer ma technique dans diverses communications[1].

Plus je vais et plus je suis convaincu, si cela est possible, des conclusions que je déposais à la tribune de l'Académie en mai dernier, à savoir : *Que tout enfant atteint de luxation congénitale doit être, lorsque la réduction est obtenue, amené à la guérison complète anatomique et fonctionnelle.* Je ne dirai pas que cela soit chose simple et facile, il s'en faut, il arrive souvent quelque anicroche durant la route. Il faut s'armer d'une persévérance à toute épreuve.

Je ne parlerai pas de la réduction proprement dite, difficile dans les luxations postérieures : elle est facile, au contraire, dans les luxa-

---

1. Académie de Médecine, mai 1898 et avril 1899.
Société anatomique, février 1897.
Congrès de Marseille, octobre 1898.
Congrès français de chirurgie.

tions antérieures ou les sus-cotyloïdiennes. Jamais je ne me sers plus d'extension préalable, c'est chose tout à fait superflue.

Je ne touche plus que rarement aux muscles, c'est un massacre souvent inutile. Le pétrissage énergique des adducteurs facilite sans aucun doute la réduction. Mais, à cela, il y a deux grands inconvénients : 1° Lorsque la réduction est obtenue et surtout si la cavité est petite, on perd un aide précieux pour le maintien de la réduction. En effet, les adducteurs qui toujours plus courts qu'à l'état normal et par suite très tendus lorsque la réduction est obtenue sont, si je puis m'exprimer ainsi, comparables à des cordages pressant vigoureusement la tête fémorale contre le cotyle rudimentaire ; sont-ils détruits, la tête est ballante dans la fosse iliaque et, après réduction, elle se déplace sous le moindre effort, elle est comme folle dans cette fosse iliaque : 2° lorsque, à la fin du traitement, l'appareil est enlevé, on s'aperçoit souvent si la désinsertion a été tant soit peu énergique que les adducteurs ont mal refait leur insertion supérieure. La cuisse paraît cylindrique, ayant le même volume à ses parties supérieures et inférieures, et cela n'est pas sans nuire considérablement à l'esthétique de la marche. Malgré la réduction et la tête dans le cotyle, l'enfant boite encore beaucoup du fait de cette insuffisance musculaire. Le meilleur signe qui, en dehors de la radiographie, ainsi que je l'ai dit dans une de mes communications à l'Académie, prouve la réalité de la réduction, consiste dans la période douloureuse durant de trois jours à un mois qui accompagne la réduction.

Immobilisation.

1ᵉʳ *Temps.* — Comme Lorenz, je conserve avec soin la position que prend la jambe après réduction, mais mon appareil prend la jambe et presse sur la partie postérieure du grand trochanter. Je laisse les malades marcher avec une chaussure surélevée. La marche n'a du reste aucune influence sur le résultat final.

2ᵉ *Temps.* — Au bout de deux à six mois, je ramène la jambe à sa position normale. C'est dans cette dernière position que se trouve l'écueil de tout le traitement. La réduction conservée dans le premier appareil, une faute même légère amènera une transposition dans ce dernier temps.

Reconstitution du cotyle.

La formation d'une cavité solide dépend :
1° De la valeur du cotyle existant ;
2° De la rétraction de la capsule.

I.   Il est en général impossible, étant donné l'âge du malade de dire quel est l'état du cotyle. Avant trois mois, il est le plus souvent fort petit et plat à tel point que les auteurs ont coutume de le comparer à une assiette. On trouve rarement de belles cavités à cet âge. Vers quatre ans, au contraire, il arrive souvent que l'on a des surprises agréables. Le cotyle présente des déformations plus ou moins accentuées ; bien que déshabité, il se développe néanmoins. Une cavité présentant une mauvaise conformation à quatre ans est mauvaise encore à sept. Mais une cavité belle à quatre ans l'est beaucoup plus encore à sept et il n'est pas rare de rencontrer vers cet âge des cavités presque normales. Si l'on pouvait attendre, ce serait assurément l'âge de prédilection. Mais, et cela surtout lorsqu'il s'agit de luxations doubles ou de luxations postérieurement placées, il faut se hâter, parce que, toujours réductibles à 4 ans, il arrive parfois que, vers sept ans, on se heurte, quoi que l'on fasse, à des luxations irréductibles.

Il est évident que plus on aura affaire à une cavité grande, plus les conditions seront favorables et la durée du traitement moindre.

II. — *Rétraction capsulaire.* — La rétraction de la capsule est l'objectif capital, c'est le principal point de mire du traitement. Elle se fait de façon très différente et à des degrés très divers suivant les malades. Mais il est cependant un fait constant, c'est qu'elle est d'autant plus forte et plus rapide que le malade est plus âgé, et ce fait heureux est d'une grande importance, il permet de s'attaquer à des sujets déjà âgés et je suis arrivé à penser que vers dix et douze ans, si la réduction est obtenue, on obtient toujours un résultat plus favorable et plus rapide, aussi peut-on conclure qu'à cavité égale le résultat est d'autant meilleur que l'enfant est plus âgé. Chez le petit enfant de trois à quatre ans même, la rétraction capsulaire est toujours fort lente à se produire ; aussi, comme cela arrive souvent à cet âge, si la cavité est avec cela petite, la durée du traitement devient fort longue.

Dès que la réduction est obtenue, la jambe se trouve placée en abduction extrême et plutôt en hyperextension ; veut-on essayer de ramener la jambe vers l'axe du corps, tout aussitôt on voit la tête franchir le bord postérieur du cotyle en s'accompagnant d'un ressaut souvent très perceptible. De même, en appuyant sur la tête qui fait saillie au niveau du triangle de Scarpa, on la fait immédiatement filer en arrière. Cette reluxation est rendue possible par la très grande laxité de la capsule à sa partie postérieure et supérieure. Or, dans cette première position, cette partie de la capsule est au maximum de relâchement et plissée sur elle-même. Toute cette partie capsulaire va se rétracter considérablement durant le premier temps.

Pour que l'épiphyse reste dans le cotyle, il faut, lorsque l'on ramène la jambe vers la ligne médiane, imprimer à celle-ci une forte rotation interne, sinon ce serait la partie postérieure de la tête qui viendrait en contact avec le cotyle. La rotation interne tend au maximum la partie capsulaire postérieure et cela contribue par contre à presser vigoureusement l'épiphyse fémorale contre le cotyle. L'appareil immobilisant la jambe en rotation interne, la partie interne de la capsule qui avait été en surextension dans le premier temps est devenue trop lâche, elle se plisse sur elle-même et se rétracte sous l'influence d'une bonne immobilisation, à tel point qu'à la fin du traitement la tête fémorale, l'épiphyse particulièrement, est maintenue d'une façon extrêmement solide contre le cotyle par deux bandes très serrées qui la tirent l'une d'arrière, l'autre de devant.

La rétraction de la capsule se fait donc en deux temps : dans le premier, c'est la partie postérieure qui se rétracte, dans le second la partie antérieure.

Comment se fait la transposition.

Le mécanisme en est fort simple. Supposez que l'on ramène la jambe du premier temps à sa position normale, mais sans lui imprimer de rotation interne et avec un appareil s'arrêtant au-dessus du genou, par exemple, par conséquent n'empêchant pas la rotation externe de se produire, que va-t-il arriver? La partie postérieure de la capsule fortement rétractée va tirer le col du fémur en arrière et faire tourner le membre en rotation externe. L'épiphyse du fémur regardera directement en avant et quittera le cotyle, et ce sera la partie postérieure de la tête fémorale qui se trouvera en contact avec le cotyle peu profond et plus ou moins plan. On comprend alors facilement ce qui va se produire. Deux surfaces planes ne pouvant pas rester en présence, elles glisseront nécessairement l'une sur l'autre, la tête fémorale remontera progressivement au-dessus du cotyle et cela de plus en plus avec le temps.

On ne fait jamais assez de rotation interne dans le dernier temps et si parfois on est obligé de rattraper une transposition commençante, cela tient uniquement à la rotation interne insuffisante que l'on a faite[1].

Peut-on rattraper une transposition?

Oui cela est toujours possible, mais c'est chose délicate. Il faut être bien secondé et connaître soi-même très bien ce que l'on fait. Je l'ai

1. Voir Société anatomique 1897.

fait personnellement quatre fois. Une de mes malades n'a plus de plâtre depuis dix mois et se maintient néanmoins très bien depuis cette époque, une autre depuis deux mois.

Lorsque la radiographie montre que la tête est éloignée du cotyle un peu trop haute, bref qu'elle a perdu ses rapports normaux avec le cotyle par rapport au cartilage en Y, il ne faut pas hésiter à rendormir le malade et à faire une nouvelle réduction. Mais cette réduction que l'on va opérer est différente de la première, les conditions sont changées. Il s'agit de faire franchir à la tête fémorale non le bord postérieur du cotyle, mais son bord antérieur. Pour effectuer cette réduction le mieux est de placer la jambe à 45 ou 50 d'abduction et de lui imprimer de la rotation interne, l'une des mains maintenant le fémur au-dessus du genou et l'autre main, prenant le grand trochanter avec les quatre derniers doigts, essaie de le ramener en avant. On pousse, en outre, la tête avec le pouce vers le cotyle.

On s'aperçoit alors que la tête rentre dans le cotyle et ce, en s'accompagnant d'un léger ressaut, parce que le bord antérieur du cotyle qu'elle est obligée de franchir est beaucoup moins accentué que le postérieur. C'est une manœuvre très délicate, je le répète, qui demande une très grande attention. La réduction opérée, la jambe est prise dans un appareil plâtré qui la maintient en rotation interne, à tel point que parfois le talon, au lieu de regarder directement en arrière, regarde directement en avant. L'appareil est laissé de deux à trois mois. Ce qu'il y a de très curieux, c'est qu'après cette nouvelle réduction le malade souffre quelque jours comme s'il s'était agi d'une réduction première.

Lors de ma dernière communication à l'Académie, j'ai présenté huit malades dans le dernier temps. J'ai actuellement quinze malades dont le traitement est terminé, je vous présente leur radiographie. Vous pouvez juger que, chez tous, la tête se trouve dans le cotyle et non en transposition. Une de mes malades marche depuis douze mois et sept autres depuis huit mois et, chez tous, la réduction s'est maintenue. On ne doit jamais se contenter d'une transposition, on ne sait jamais ce qu'en sera le résultat final, c'est une amélioration et non une guérison. Le résultat orthopédique est bon au début, peu à peu la boiterie redevient visible au bout de quelques années pour l'œil le moins exercé. Mon excellent maître et ami, M. le Dr Brun, a bien voulu me permettre d'appliquer avec lui mon procédé dans son service. Je ne saurais trop le remercier et nous avons publié, il y a quelques jours, les observations de dix malades chez lesquelles nous avons obtenu un résultat anatomique complet.

Chez deux malades offrant une luxation postérieure très haut placée je n'ai pu obtenir une réduction. l'une était double et âgée de 10 ans et l'autre simple avait 11 ans.

Sur les quinze malades que j'ai opérés seul, j'ai obtenu quinze résultats anatomiques parfaits. Aussi je crois être en droit de conclure que, lorsque la réduction est obtenue. on doit, *d'une façon certaine, arriver à la guérison complète anatomique et fonctionnelle.*

Si j'ai de bons résultats, cela tient à l'usage de la radiographie que j'ai mise depuis trois ans à contribution à tout changement d'appareil.

TRAITEMENT OPÉRATOIRE DE LA LUXATION CONGÉNITALE DE LA HANCHE

COMMUNICATION

de M. DOYEN.

La cure radicale de la luxation congénitale de la hanche ne peut être obtenue que par l'opération.

Le temps principal est la réfection de la cavité cotyloïde.

On obtient une cavité cotyloïde parfaite et convenablement orientée en la creusant avec un tube tranchant cylindro-sphérique de diamètre approprié.

La réduction peut exiger l'emploi de l'appareil spécial que j'ai construit à cet effet. La tête, saisie par une cuiller métallique, est conduite par une puissante vis de rappel jusque dans le cotyle.

Dès que la réduction est faite. il est en général nécessaire de placer la jambe dans l'abduction avec rotation en dedans. Les insertions supérieures du premier et du second adducteur sont sectionnées si elles sont trop tendues et l'appareil plâtré est appliqué sur le brancard démontable que je présente au Congrès.

La direction défectueuse du col du fémur peut exiger pour la réduction une rotation en dedans de 50° à 60°.

Dans ces cas. le genou et le pied. qui occuperaient pour toujours une situation vicieuse. sont redressés par une ostéotomie supracondylienne du fémur suivie de rotation du fragment inférieur de dedans en dehors. Cette opération complémentaire est pratiquée au bout de trois à quatre semaines.

J'étudie en ce moment les avantages de l'interposition entre la tête fémorale et le nouveau cotyle, d'un fragment d'aponévrose frais et stérilisé, pour assurer la mobilité de la néarthrose.

***

LE TRAITEMENT DE LA LUXATION BI-LATÉRALE ET CONGÉNITALE DE LA HANCHE PAR LA MÉTHODE DE LORENZ DOIT-IL ÊTRE SIMULTANÉ OU ALTERNATIF?

COMMUNICATION

de M. le docteur MAUCLAIRE,

de Paris.

Je n'ai pas eu l'occasion de pratiquer l'opération de Hoffa, étant donné le refus des parents. J'ai suivi plusieurs fois la méthode de Lorenz. Tantôt la luxation a été irréductible et j'ai renoncé au traitement, tantôt l'abaissement était très grand et la réduction pour ainsi dire tangente mais non possible. J'ai alors proposé une intervention pour favoriser simplement la transposition antérieure en abrasant les surfaces osseuses iliaques ou une ténotomie des tendons trochantériens; mais les parents ont encore refusé cette simple opération.

Parmi les cas où la réduction fut possible, en voici un intéressant.

En février 1898 je réduisis sous chloroforme et très facilement la luxation droite. Je suivis très régulièrement la méthode de Lorenz. En juillet 1899, la transposition était parfaite. J'entrepris alors la réduction du côté opposé (côté gauche) et actuellement celle-ci est bien transposée en avant. Mais la tête fémorale du côté droit s'est légèrement déviée en arrière et la luxation est devenue un peu sus et rétrocotyloïdienne. J'attribue ce déplacement consécutif aux efforts que fit l'enfant pendant la marche au cours du traitement de la deuxième luxation. Aussi je pense que dans ces cas de luxation bilatérale il vaut mieux traiter les deux articulations en même temps. Dans tous les cas chez mon petit malade la lordose est très diminuée l'abduction et la flexion est presque complète des deux côtés. L'amélioration fonctionnelle est donc des plus grandes.

***

TRAITEMENT DE LA LUXATION CONGÉNITALE DE LA HANCHE

COMMUNICATION

de M. CALOT,

de Berck.

La luxation congénitale de la hanche, regardée comme incurable autrefois est entrée dans une phase nouvelle depuis une dizaine d'années.

Nous savons aujourd'hui obtenir la rentrée de la tête dans la cavité cotyloïde, c'est-à-dire réduire cette luxation congénitale.

On y peut arriver par deux méthodes : l'une sanglante, l'autre non sanglante.

La méthode sanglante assure une réduction bien solide, mais ce n'est qu'au prix d'une ankylose, non pas qu'on ne puisse obtenir une certaine mobilité de la nouvelle articulation, mais elle ne s'obtient guère qu'aux dépens de l'attitude.

Et une attitude vicieuse compromet bien davantage la marche qu'une raideur de la hanche.

Il faut même ajouter que cette raideur n'est presque jamais assez complète pour empêcher une déviation de se produire, et que l'on a souvent après l'opération sanglante, à la fois une hanche raide et une mauvaise attitude.

C'est pour cette raison que l'on doit préférer l'opération non sanglante lorsqu'elle peut nous donner la réduction. Elle peut nous donner cette réduction jusque vers 8 ans et dans quelques cas exceptionnels jusqu'à 10 ou 12 ans.

La réalité de la réduction nous sera démontrée par les rayons X.

Dans ce traitement, la contention est plus difficile à faire que la réduction.

Six à douze mois de traitement suffisent. Après ce temps, l'enfant est débarrassé de tout appareil et doit être massé, et on doit faire l'éducation de sa marche. Il est des cas où la guérison est obtenue sans boiterie.

Pour les cas irréductibles, reste la méthode sanglante après laquelle on recherchera l'ankylose complète, si la lésion est unilatérale.

Pour les luxations doubles, l'on n'arrive plus à la réduction par la méthode non sanglante après l'âge de 7 ans généralement.

Il n'y a pas à recourir ici à l'opération sanglante qui, nous donnant deux ankyloses de la hanche, ne fait qu'aggraver la situation de l'enfant.

Pour les luxations irréductibles, reste le massage longtemps continué et l'éducation de la marche. Même pour ces cas extrêmes on arrive ainsi à des améliorations fonctionnelles notables.

LUXATION CONGÉNITALE DE LA HANCHE

COMMUNICATION

de M. PAUL COUDRAY,

de Paris.

Dans ma communication en octobre 1899, au Congrès français de chirurgie, j'ai relaté dix observations relatives au traitement non sanglant de la luxation congénitale de la hanche; depuis cette époque, j'ai appliqué ce traitement dans quelques cas, mais ces cas ne sont ni assez nombreux, ni assez âgés pour qu'il y ait matière à une communication nouvelle.

Je me bornerai donc à quelques remarques visant surtout l'état des malades anciens. J'avais surtout obtenu en employant le procédé de réduction, soit de Paci, soit celui de Lorenz, des transpositions antérieures, la tête fémorale étant placée généralement un peu au-dessus et en dehors de l'épine iliaque antérieure et inférieure. La marche des malades était bonne, presque parfaite pour quelques-uns. J'ai pu revoir trois de ces malades atteints de luxation unilatérale et qui marchent sans appareil depuis 26 mois, 16 mois et un an, et j'ai constaté que la marche est excellente et que la tête fémorale est restée dans sa position.

Je ne nie pas du tout les réductions qu'on a obtenues ou cru obtenir dans bon nombre de cas, mais ces réductions, subordonnées à certaines conditions anatomiques plus qu'aux procédés de réduction eux-mêmes, doivent être vérifiées longtemps après que les malades marchent sans appareil. Il est utile aussi de publier les observations qui entraînent la conviction plus que les chiffres.

La réduction elle-même est préparée très utilement par l'extension continue; j'ai insisté sur ce point au Congrès de Bordeaux en 1895 et tout le monde est d'accord aujourd'hui.

Il est très difficile de fixer une limite à la réduction. Sans doute jusqu'à 8 et 10 ans on a les plus grandes chances de succès. Ultérieurement on obtiendra assez souvent des transpositions antérieures qui améliorent la marche sans doute, mais qui chez les enfants âgés, comme je l'ai vu chez une grande et forte fille de 15 ans, prennent l'aspect de luxations antérieures avec forte rotation externe et abduction. Encore ne peut-on rien fixer à cet égard. Récemment, en effet, j'ai vu M. Kirmisson réduire, selon toute apparence, une luxation chez une fille d'environ 15 ans.

Mais il ne faut pas oublier que ces réductions chez les enfants âgés nécessitent parfois des violences réelles.

Chez la grande fille chez laquelle j'ai fait une transposition, deux séances ont dû être pratiquées avec manœuvres très fortes. Un certain nombre d'accidents ont été signalés dans les cas de ce genre. Aussi, malgré tout ce que la méthode non sanglante a de séduisant, peut-on envisager comme préférable la méthode sanglante pour quelques cas de cette catégorie.

D'ailleurs Hoffa donne dans son rapport une conclusion, la première, que j'accepte complètement : « Dans chaque cas de luxation « congénitale de la hanche, on essaiera d'abord la reposition non « sanglante. Si la non sanglante ne réussit pas à cause d'une raison « quelconque, l'opération sanglante est indiquée. »

Il est cependant à noter que chez les enfants relativement âgés, après 8 ans, l'ankylose à la suite de l'opération sanglante se montre parfois puisque Hoffa en cite 6 cas.

Relativement aux luxations bilatérales, il est bon je crois, du moins chez les enfants d'un certain âge, de ne traiter qu'un côté dans une séance. Récemment sur une fille de 8 ans chez laquelle je crois avoir obtenu une bonne réduction, j'ai observé des douleurs assez vives pendant deux jours dans la hanche opérée. Il est certain que si les deux hanches avaient été opérées en même temps, il en fût résulté un traumatisme excessif. Au résumé, les travaux de Paci et de Lorenz en particulier ont marqué une étape importante dans cette question. Je crois qu'on pourra rendre les résultats très bons que nous obtenons aujourd'hui, plus constants encore en augmentant la durée de l'immobilisation en première position, c'est-à-dire en abduction à angle droit, en la portant par exemple à cinq ou six mois et en rendant cette immobilisation plus parfaite.

CONTRIBUTO ALLA TECNICA DELLA CURA CRUENTA RADICALE DELLA LUSSAZIONE CONGENITA DELL' ANCA.

COMMUNICATION

de **M. CODIVILLA**.

de Bologne.

Nel periodo di un anno e quattro mesi, cioè da quando io tengo la direzione dell' Istituto Ortopedico Rizzoli, sopra 62 atti operativi compiuti per curare individui affetti da lussazione congenita dell'anca, n 10 casi ho ricorso ad un'operazione cruenta. Non prendo in considerazione 5 di questi, nei quali l'atto operativo non ha avuto che uno scopo palliativo. In essi si trattava di individui in età piuttosto avanzata, nei quali il notevole accorciamento dell'arto, le alterazioni dell'estremità femorale, le complicazioni insorte nell'articolazione, e cioè, l'artrite cronica, la rigidità dolorosa ecc, non permettevano l'esecuzione di un atto operativo, che lasciasse sperare in un risultato che potesse dirsi radicale, e cioè seguito da condizioni normali dell'articolazione, sotto l'aspetto sia anatomico, sia funzionale.

In questi casi lo scopo dell'operazione fu quello di portare un miglioramento nella posizione dell'estremità femorale sul bacino, e di procurare a questo un appoggio sufficientemente stabile sopra il femore. Si comprende che in questi casi l'atto operativo ha variato a seconda delle circostanze: peraltro in tutti si è tentato di formare una neoartrosi solida sopra un piano frontale anteriore a quello tenuto dalla testa femorale, che trovavasi prima a contatto con una regione della metà posteriore della fossa iliaca esterna. La testa femorale è stata resecata in totalità od in parte in un punto adatto della sua porzione anteriore. l'osso iliaco è stato denudato dal periostio e scavato per formare una cavità atta a ricevere l'estremità del femore. la capsula è stata suturata al periostio ed alle parti molli che la circondavano. Dopo un periodo che ha variato dai 2 ai 4 mesi, nel quale l'articolazione dell'anca è stata tenuta immobilizzata. dapprima in posizione di abduzione notevole. che poi si è diminuita. è stato tolto l'apparecchio gessato e si è tentato di muovere la neoartrosi. In tutt'i casi si è ottenuta una mobilità articolare limitata. ma la deambulazione ha potuto compiersi in modo più facile. senza il rapido senso di stanchezza e senza il dolore. che insorgeva prima. Come pure il zoppicamento è notevolmente migliorato ed ha perduto la forte oscillazione, per trasformarsi nell'andatura rigida, che si nota negli esiti di coxite, coll'arto in buona posizione.

Sopra questi ammalati, nei quali, tutto sommato, la tecnica non si è scostata che in dettagli di poca importanza da quella comunemente usata, non desidero insistere. Ho intenzione invece di richiamare in modo speciale l'attenzione dei membri del Congresso sopra la tecnica da me tenuta nel praticare l'atto operativo negli altri 7 infermi, e ciò perché questa si allontana in parte dalla comune. Le storie dettagliate dei malati saranno presentate fra qualche tempo, quando sarà trascorso dall'operazione un periodo sufficiente a portare un giudizio sul risultato ultimo. In questo momento non è possibile, trattandosi di casi piuttosto recenti.

Lo scopo della presente comunicazione, fatta a modo di nota preventiva, è quello di poter avere un giudizio dal Congresso sulla razionalità o meno dei metodi operatori da me posti alla prova.

Debbo prima di tutto porre in evidenza che in alcuni casi i criteri, che mi hanno stimolato a sostituire un'operazione cruenta alla solita riduzione incruenta, sono alquanto diversi da quelli comunemate seguiti dagli ortopedici. Non parlo qui naturalmente dei casi, nei quali, dopo varî tentativi di riduzione, questa non è avvenuta. In essa gli ostacoli opposti alla ripresa per parte del femore de'suoi rapporti col cotile, non erano superabili colle manovre consigliate per la riposizione incruenta ed era giocoforza, se si voleva tentare la correzione della deformità, aprire l'articolazione e togliere tali ostacoli. Questa è la via tenuta da tutti, quando le condizioni locali e l'età parlano per la possibilità e la convenienza di una riduzione coll'intervento cruento.

Ma in 4 casi io ho eseguito l'operazione cruenta, quando pure la riduzione era riuscita colle semplici manovre esterne.

Non ostante questa riduzione ho giudicato necessario completare l'atto operativo con un intervento diretto sull'articolazione.

Il primo caso, che mi ha stimolato ad agire in tal modo, mi è stato fornito da un bambino di 6 anni (C. R.) nel quale fu eseguita la riduzione alla Lorenz il giorno 7 marzo 1900.

Di questo presento la radiografia praticata innanzi l'atto operativo. La riduzione riuscì molto facilmente col far passare la coscia dalla posizione di flessione sul bacino, nell'iperestensione, dall'abduzione negativa a quella ad angolo retto, dalla rotazione interna all'esterna ed aiutandomi colla mano a pugno, a guisa di cuneo, spinta posteriormente sul trocantere. La riduzione avvenne collo scatto e col rumore caratteristico, la coscia abdotta a circa 90° rimase fissata per l'azione delle resistenze muscolari. Ma al più piccolo tentativo di diminuzione dell'abduzione, la testa femorale si rilussava e si avvertiva che il bordo superiore del cotile non presentava che una lieve resistenza alla rilussazione.

La radiografia mostra infatti che la porzione ossea del cotile trapassa quasi senza tetto nella fossa primitivamente occupata dalla testa spostata. Peraltro la radiografia è meno propria della prova diretta a far giudicare della capacità di contenzione per parte del cotile, poichè la radiografia non può dare segno del rivestimento cartilagineo e dei bordi cotiloidei, i quali nella prima infanzia sono diafani per i raggi X. Ad ogni modo, nel caso cui ho accennato, questa capacità di contenzione era minima e fui obbligato ad immobilizzare l'arto nel massimo grado di abduzione (90°). La testa si rilussò durante l'esecuzione dell'apparecchio cosiche si fu costretti a ridurla nuovamente. 15 giorni dopo dall'esame dell'infermo fu giudicata una nuova rilussazione, non ostante l'immobilizzazione prodotta dalla gessatura.

Fu tolto l'apparecchio e si osservò che, anche semplicemente col portare in abduzione la coscia, mantenendola nel piano frontale, a patto di esercitare una pressione sul gran trocantere, allorchè la coscia era ad angolo retto sul tronco, la testa femorale entrava nella tasca cotiloidea, ma ne tornava subito fuori, quando si faceva percorrere alla coscia la via inversa. Ciò avveniva con un piccolo scatto. Dal modo col quale il capo del femore si spostava nel compiere questi movimenti, sembrava che il femore funzionasse come una leva di primo genere, il cui fulcro risiedesse circa in vicinanza del gran trocantere : il polo della testa femorale percorreva così una circonferenza il cui centro trovavasi circa in questa regione. Si applicò la vite di Lorenz per abbassare la testa, ma non si riesci che a spostarla di pochi millimetri. La causa della rilussazione, più che in una mancanza assoluta di contenzione per parte del bordo cotiloideo superiore, fu ammessa nelle trazioni che il segmento superoesterno della capsula esercitava sul collo femorale allorchè l'abduzione veniva diminuita.

A ciò faceva pensare la constatazione nella negativa radiografica di una striscia più chiara che dall'estremità del tetto della cavità, scavata dalla testa spostata, si abbassava fino a raggiungere la base del collo. Evidentemente quest'ombra, che non risalta più ora nella prova positiva, corrispondeva alla capsula ispessita. Mi era accaduto spesso di osservarla in radiografie di casi, nei quali al passaggio dalla prima posizione dopo la riduzione, nella seconda coll'arto meno abdotto, la testa fuoriusciva dal cotile per spostarsi verso l'alto e l'esterno. Il gioco delle trazioni esercitate sul collo in questi movimenti dalla capsula ispessita e fissata nella località anormale occupata dalla testa, può guidicarsi dalle figure schematiche che presento.

Nella posizione di forte abduzione la riduzione è possibile, poichè il punto d'attacco della capsula sul collo femorale trovasi vicino a quello sul quale la capsula si è fissata sulla fossa iliaca esterna. Diminuendo l'abduzione il polo femorale puo restare a contatto del punto d'unione delle cartilagini di coniugazione a patto che il collo sia libero d'allontanarsi in proporzione dalla fossa iliaca esterna. Se a questa è legato dalla capsula, questa trasforma, come ho detto, il femore in una leva di primo genere e fa salire il capo femorale rilussandolo verso l'alto. Le figure riescono completamente [di]mostrative di un tale concetto. In un altro caso di lussazione bilaterale, nel quale da un lato lo spostamento verso l'alto della testa avveniva, secondo il mio parere, collo stesso meccanismo, forti trazioni fatte colla vite di Lorenz ed un apparecchio gessato, praticato in modo da esercitare una pressione sul trocantere, bastarono a vincere la resistenza opposta dalla capsula.

Certamente questo non è il solo fattore, e, molto probabilmente, neppure il principale degli spostamenti del capo femorale verso l'alto e l'avanti, che avvengono con notevole frequenza, durante la cura incruenta della lussazione. Anzi dagli autori si suole dare ad esso poca o nessuna importanza.

Per solito la figura che nei trattati riproduce schematicamente i rapporti presi dal femore e dalla capsula coll'osso iliaco, non mostra alcun legame di questa colla fossa iliaca-esterna: il bacino figura come sospeso, non appoggiato al femore, e la capsula che si distacca dal bordo cotiloideo, va a ricoprire come di un cappuccio la testa femorale, ma si mantiene a distanza dall'osso.

Nei gradi più avanzati della lussazione posteriore iliaca può infatti ammettersi che il bacino sia sospeso, non appoggiato al femore, ma noi ben di rado abbiamo occasione di curare radicalmente lussazioni inveterate. In ogni modo, siccome lo spostamento è avvenuto a gradi, e le ricerche di Kölliker e di Hoffa provano che la lussazione è prima anterosuperiore, e cioè sopracotiloidea, poi gradatamente diviene posteriore, nel primo periodo i rapporti statici del bacino col femore saranno stati essenzialmente diversi, ed il bacino si sarà realmente appoggiato sull'estremità femorale, non sarà rimasto semplicemente sospeso ad essa.

Le radiografie mostrano, in quasi tutti i casi, nella fossa iliaco-esterna località, nelle quali la testa femorale si è scavato un giaciglio abbastanza profondo. Ora, in questi punti, la capsula ha certamente aderito al periostio iliaco. La prova si ha nei casi che si operano cruentemente.

Tutti accennano al grave ostacolo opposto all'abbassamento della testa dalla capsula ipertrofica, fissata in alto sull'ileo. Per vincere quest'ostacolo è necessario tagliare trasversalmente il tubo capsulare nella sua porzione anteriore ed esterna. Nei miei casi queste condizioni della capsula sono state riscontrate costantemente.

Gli altri fattori, che diminuiscono la stabilità della contenzione e che rendono facile lo spostamento verso l'alto e l'avanti della testa femorale, nel periodo che segue la riduzione, sono da ricercarsi nelle alterazioni che hanno colpito l'estremità femorale e le parti che concorrono a formare la cavità cotiloidea. Quest'ultima, oltre la deficienza di profondità, trovasi più anteriormente ed in un piano maggiormente inclinato verso il piano frontale, che in condizioni normali. Riesce facile quindi alla testa femorale lo sfuggire verso l'alto e l'innanzi, tanto più poi che questa è impiantata sopra un collo per solito valgo ed antiverso.

In queste condizioni le leggi meccaniche, che regolano la fissazione del bacino sulla testa del femore, sono notevolmente modificate da quelle di un caso normale.

In questo, nella stazione eretta, è la parte alta e mediale del fondo del cotile, che si appoggia sul capo femorale, mentre in un caso, nel quale il collo ha subìto le alterazioni accennate, il punto di appoggio dovrebbe trovarsi nella porzione laterale del segmento supero-anteriore del cotile.

Ora è appunto questa la parte più deficiente della regione cotiloidea, nessuna meraviglia adunque che la testa sfugga per questa via Sono molti perciò i fatti a cui si dovrebbe provvedere, se si volessero dare all'articolazione le condizioni anatomiche normali. Se ciò non può raggiungersi in modo completo, poco importa, purchè l'alterazione della funzione scompaja.

È necessario tuttavia dire subito che la riduzione incruenta ed il trattamento consecutivo per mezzo della funzione coll'arto immobilizzato in posizioni speciali (metodo di Lorenz) portano in alcuni casi. come a me pure gli studi radiografici hanno mostrato, modificazioni nell'articolazione, che, a trattamento finito, di poco la fanno restare dissimile da un'articolazione normale. Ciò peraltro accade soltanto in un numero limitato di casi. Nella maggior parte degli altri tuttavia, benchè il capo femorale si sposti più o meno dal centro del cotile, seguendo la via antero-superiore indicata, l'estremità femorale si fissa sull'ileo in posizione da rendere possibile una funzione o del tutto normale, o molto migliorata da quella antecedente all'atto operativo. I punti, nei quali il bacino può trovare un buon appoggio sul femore, sono situati lungo la linea segnata dal piano frontale determinato dal fondo del cotile. Si comprende pure come, a parità delle altre condizioni, la funzione sarà tanto più buona, quanto più il punto, nel quale la testa femorale resterà definitivamente fissata, si troverà in vicinanza del cotile stesso.

A contenere la testa nella cavità cotiloidea mira il trattamento che segue la riduzione incruenta. Questo compito, appare molto difficile, se, come io ho fatto sommariamente, si passano in rassegna tutte le condizioni che si oppongono a questa contenzione. Lorenz perciò ha dovuto modificare già le leggi che egli dettava dietro le sue prime esperienze. La durata della posizione primaria raggiunge ora i 4 od i 5 mesi: quella della immobilizzazione nell'apparecchio gessato oscilla dai 10 ai 12 mesi. Nel passaggio dalla prima alla seconda posizione Lorenz mette ora in accordo colla diminuzione dell'abduzione la flessione della coscia allo scopo di appoggiare la testa femorale contro il bordo cotiloideo posteriore e di allontanarne così l'appoggio dalla pericolosa regione supero-anteriore.

A giudicare spassionatamente i risultati, a cui egli stesso giunge pure con tali mezzi, si conclude, che, se essi appaiono soddisfacenti sotto l'aspetto funzionale, lasciano tuttavia a desiderare sotto quello anatomico, poichè in un gran numero di casi il capo femorale trova il suo giaciglio nella linea detta, ma più o meno lontano dal **punto** d'unione delle cartilagini di coniugazione cotiloidee. Questo **fatto, di** poca importanza, nei casi nei quali lo spostamento è lieve, è grave quando la distanza della testa dal centro cotiloideo è notevole, poichè le condizioni si avvicinano così a quelle di una vera e propria recidiva.

La stabilità della riduzione, e quindi la facilità della contenzione, possono riconoscersi all'esame dell'articolazione lussata, dopo che questa è stata ridotta. Quanto maggiore è l'angolo d'abduzione, che è necessario dare alla coscia, perchè la testa femorale resti a contatto del cotile, quanto più lieve è la forza che è necessario impiegare per determinare la rilussazione, tanto più imminente sarà la possibilità che la testa femorale abbandoni la regione cotiloidea, per venire ad appoggiarsi in un punto in alto ed in avanti di questa. Nel mio caso questi segni parlarono già all'atto della riduzione per questa possibilità e gli avvenimenti confermarono le cattive previsioni che si erano fatte sulla stabilità della articolazione ridotta.

Nel caso in questione si poteva in qualche modo impedire il ripetersi della rilussazione, togliendo alcune delle cagioni, che la rendevano facile? I rapporti delle superfici articolari erano tutt'altro che adatti a rendere sufficientemente stabile la riduzione. Il cotile piatto,

col bordo superiore poco sviluppato, il collo femorale corto ed antiverso, la testa piccola erano condizioni favorevoli alla recidiva, ma a
queste non si poteva provvedere. Nel caso speciale nulla poteva farsi
per modificare in modo conveniente l'estremità femorale, e l'esperienza
fatta eccezione di rari casi, ha già condannato quei metodi operativi,
nei quali lo scavare il cotile era uno dei tempi dell'intervento. Per
fortuna nel caso speciale una delle condizioni precipue della rilussazione, e cioè la trazione fatta sul collo dalla porzione laterale superiore della capsula, al diminuire dell'abduzione della coscia, poteva
essere vinta. Se per mezzo di un atto operativo, si fosse tolto l'anormale attacco capsulare sull'ildeo e se si avesse potuto dare un appoggio
più stabile alla testa femorale, nel punto verso il quale era diretta
nella posizione indifferente dell'arto, si fosse giunto cioè a formare
artificialmente il tetto normale dell'anca, si sarebbe impedita la rilussazione. Alle altre condizioni anormali del cotile e dell'estremità
femorale avrebbe, per quanto sarebbe stato possibile, provveduto
l'esercizio dell'articolazione.

Lo scopo a cui mira il trattamento della lussazione congenita col
metodo incruento alla Lorenz, è appunto la ricostituzione di un tetto.
e le radiografie mostrano che dopo un lungo periodo di cura ciò può
avvenire. È egli possibile, ricorrendo ad un intervento cruento, rendere
più rapida la formazione di questo valido ostacolo al risalire della
testa femorale? Guidato da questi criteri mi accinsi ad operare il caso
in questione.

L'atto operativo è eseguito il giorno 24 marzo 1900. L'incisione
della pelle è tracciata in linea retta, della lunghezza di 12 centimetri
circa, discendendo, a partire della S. J. A. S., lungo il bordo anteriore
del muscolo tensore fascialata. Attraversato l'interstizio, fra il gruppo
anteriore dei muscoli dell'anca ed il gruppo laterale, giungo sulla
regione articolare. La testa femorale è a contatto di un punto anteriore della fossa iliaca esterna, poco sotto il piano orizzontale determinato dalla S. J. A. S. In questo punto la testa del femore si è
scavata una nicchia. Liberazione della capsula dalle intime aderenze
che essa ha contratto col piccolo gluteo.

Un assistente riduce la lussazione colle solite manovre, mentre la
mano dell'operatore guida la testa femorale verso il cotile. La coscia è
mantenuta in abduzione.

La porzione capsulare, che incappucciava il capo, è strettamente
aderente all'ileo. Sul limite della porzione aderente è inciso il periostio, e collo staccaperiostio, questo, insieme alla capsula, viene tolto
dall'osso per tutto quel tratto, che la testa femorale ha percorso dal

cotile fino alla regione ultimamente da essa occupata. La specie di borsa ottenuta così dalla liberazione della capsula esuberante è ripiegata a formare una duplicatura verso l'esterno ed in tale disposizione è fissata con tre punti di sutura dati con seta numero due.

La figura schematica che presento mostra in che modo si sia formata questa duplicatura. Sutura dell'incisione cutanea. Immobilizzazione dell'arto in abduzione di 80°.

Un mese dopo si tolgono l'apparecchio ed i punti di sutura cutanei. Guarigione di prima intenzione. La testa è tuttora nel cotile, ma non sembra ancora stabilmente fissata. Si ripone l'apparecchio, diminuendo l'abduzione (60°).

Il bambino viene dimesso dall'Istituto e vi ritorna due mesi dopo. La riduzione si è mantenuta e l'articolazione sembra fissa. È facile a compiersi, tanto attivamente che passivamente, un'esagerazione dell'abduzione. Si avverte invece una resistenza ed il bambino mostra di sentire dolore nel tentativo di adduzione dell'arto. Il trattamento consecutivo mira ad una diminuzione lenta dell'abduzione mercè l'applicazione di un apparecchio estensivo nella notte e correggendo con adatti movimenti l'attitudine viziata.

La radiografia mostra le condizioni dell'articolazione nel momento attuale. La testa del femore si trova nella regione cotiloidea, piuttosto sotto la posizione abituale del capo nell'articolazione normale, che sopra. Il femore è ancora qualche poco abdotto.

Ciò che interessa è la constatazione che la riduzione, in un caso così poco favorevole, si è mantenuta in un modo completo. Più distinti all'esame della lastra radiografica, ma pure a quello della positiva che presento, si riscontrano segni di neoformazione ossea nella regione in cui è stata eseguita la duplicatura capsulare. L'atto operativo porta dunque realmente ad un miglioramento delle condizioni della contenzione per l'estremità femorale ridotta, e ad un'irritazione formativa atta a produrre una buona superficie d'appoggio dell'ileo sulla testa del femore. Era razionale il pensare alla possibilità di questo avvenimento, tenendo conto della facilità, colla quale il periostio iliaco riforma anche estese porzioni d'osso, quando si trovi in istato d'irritazione. Infatti Bergmann (di Riga) in un caso di osteomielite ha veduto riprodursi dal periostio tutta l'ala dell'ileo.

La quasi nessuna gravità dell'atto operativo (è rapido, poco traumatizzante, non apre l'articolazione) permette di porlo allo stesso livello di un'operazione radicale di ernia, e mi ha stimolato a metterlo alla prova in altri casi, variando le condizioni dell'esperienza. Ho scelto tre soggetti, che presentassero rispetto alla capacità di ritenzione condizioni, consimili a quelle del caso ora illustrato, ed ho preferito bambini in età avanzata, nei quali il trattamento incruento presenta lo svantaggio di facili rigidità consecutive alla lunga immobilizzazione. Potendosi col mezzo da me proposto diminuire il periodo di immobilizzazione dell'articolazione, ho avuto speranza si diminuisce pure il pericolo della rigidità. I soggetti hanno rispettivamente 10, 11, 12 anni.

In uno di questi l'atto operativo è stato eseguito in 2 tempi. Dapprima si è compiuta la riduzione colle solite manovre, e si è immobilizzato l'arto, poi, 15 giorni dopo, è stata praticata la duplicatura capsulo-periostea. Negli altri casi le manovre di riduzione si sono compiute immediatamente prima dell'atto operativo cruento. Mi è sembrato di constatare che in questi l'azione debilitante del trauma sia stata maggiormente sentita. È consigliabile perciò, nei casi meno facili e negli individui più deboli, di eseguire in un primo tempo la riduzione, ed in un secondo, alla distanza di circa due settimane, l'operazione cruenta.

In tutti tre i casi guarigione senza segno d'infezione. In uno (R. Z. di anni 10) dopo l'atto operativo l'arto è staro tenuto nella 1ª posizione per 15 giorni e per altri 12 è stato immobilizzato in attitudine meno abdotta.

Dopo si è lasciata camminare la bambina senza apparecchio. Il periodo di cura coll'apparecchio immobilizzante non ha durato che 27 giorni, meno di un mese quindi dall'atto operativo. In questo momento la bambina è ancora sottoposta a massaggio e ad esercizi. La funzione della deambulazione si compie con lievissima oscillazione e va sempre migliorando. I movimenti articolari sono ampi, facili e per nulla dolorosi.

La prova radiografica e la fotografica che presento sono prese a d 2 mesi dall'atto operativo. La prima mostra che la testa trovasi qualche poco più in alto della linea delle cartilagini del cotile. L'arto è infatti più corto di mezzo centimetro rispetto all'altro, ma il bacino è ben sostenuto sulla testa femorale da neoproduzioni prodottesi sulla regione del tetto. La fotografia dà un'idea dell'attitudine dell'arto, quando questo è tenuto in posizione indifferente.

Degli altri due casi, non posso dare alcun giudizio su uno (S. A. di anni 12), poiché porta ancora l'apparecchio immobilizzante che dovrà tenere per due mesi. Nell'altro (P. G. di anni 11) questo è stato tolto da pochi giorni, dopo averlo mantenuto per un mese e mezzo. Di questo caso presento le radiografie, l'una che mostra lo stato precedente all'atto operativo, l'altra al momento attuale. Da questa si può rilevare che la riduzione è perfetta, si constatano pure segni che parlano per la costituzione di un tetto dell'anca.

In questi tre casi l'atto operativo cruento è stato compiuto con lievi modificazioni da quello del C. R. È stato modificato soltanto il taglio cutaneo. Infatti l'incisione, limitata allo spazio sotto la S. I. A. S. rende difficili la liberazione della capsula, il distacco del periostio, e la formazione della duplicatura capsulo-periostea, poichè il cappuccio capsulare, che copre la testa del femore, trovasi annidato profondamente fra i muscoli e la fossa iliaca esterna, Percio in un caso ho tagliato l'attacco del tensore fascialata a livello della S. I. A. S. e negli altri, prolungando l'incisione cutanea lungo la cresta iliaca, sollevando il periostio dalla superficie esterna dell'ileo, ho staccato così le inserzioni anteriori del piccolo e medio gluteo. Compiuta la sutura della duplicatura capsulo-periostea, con alcuni punti ho ridato ai muscoli i rapporti normali.

Tale intervento, come ho potuto assicurarmi sulla R. Z., non ha disturbato l'importante funzione di questi muscoli. Ho preferito fare l'incisione fra il gruppo muscolare anteriore ed il laterale, staccando, in caso di bisogno, per rendere più ampio il campo operativo, le inserzioni del tensore e del piccolo e medio gluteo, insieme al periostio, perchè fra questi due gruppi muscolari sembrami sia segnata la via normale per l'attacco della regione antero-laterale dell'articolazione dell'anca. Lorenz. Sprengel preferiscono incidere fra il tensore fascia lata ed il piccolo gluteo, ma questa incisione porta lo svantaggio di cadere sopra un interstizio muscolare, meno libero e meno ampio di quello del lato interno del tensore, ed il danno, il più delle volte inevitabile, della lesione dei rami nervosi che partendo dai glutei vanno ad innervare il muscolo tensore, i quali traversano appunto tale interstizio. Se negli atti operativi sopra l'articolazione dell'anca, nei casi di lussazione congenita, si deve fare il massimo risparmio dei muscoli, la cui funzione è così importante per l'esito, l'incisione fra il fascialata ed i glutei, per la ragione detta, sembrami debba essere rigettata. Un'idea della linea d'incisione puo aversi dalla fotografia della R. Z.

È certamente precoce formulare delle conclusioni sopra l'importanza dell'operazione, che io ho posta alla prova nel trattamento della lussazione congenita dell'anca, poichè queste, basate su dei fatti recenti sarebbero premature. Parrebbe tuttavia che nei casi, nei quali la stabilità della riduzione del femore lussato è molto labile l'allontanamento dell'attacco anormale della capsula sopra la fossa iliaca esterna, la formazione di una duplicatura capsulo-periostea, che tolga il cul di sacco capsulare, nel quale può ad ogni momento trovare ricetto la testa del femore, quando abbandoni la regione cotiloidea, aumentino le condizioni che favoriscono la ritenzione. Io ho infatti trovato ridotta la lussazione e tale si è mantenuta anche quando, dopo un tempo relativamente breve (2 mesi e mezzo), ho liberato l'articolazione dall'apparecchio immobilizzante ed ho rapidamente diminuita l'abduzione, in individui, nei quali tutto parlava per la possibilità di una rilussazione. Anzi in uno dei casi questa era già avvenuta durante il trattamento consecutivo della riduzione incruenta.

L'aumento della stabilità articolare ed i segni presentati dalle prove radiografiche fanno pensare che l'atto operativo irriti formativamente la superficie esterna dell'ileo ed il periostio, e così avvii alla neoformazione del tetto dell'anca. Dall'esperienza fatta finora sembra pure che l'atto operativo abbrevî singolarmente la cura. Forse un mese solo di immobilizzazione è troppo poca cosa per assicurare un giaciglio stabile alla testa femorale nella regione cotiloidea, perchè infatti nella R. Z. si osserva che il femore si è qualche poco spostato verso l'alto, ma probabilmente 1 mese e mezzo o 2 mesi sono sufficienti. Su cio sarà l'esperienza ulteriore che permetterà di decidere. Lo stesso deve dirsi riguardo allo funzionalità dell'articolazione, dopo l'operazione cruenta.

Quale sarà il contegno della capsula raggrinzata, dei tessuti incisi. quale la funzione dei muscoli, di cui si sono staccate le inserzioni sull'osso iliaco e le aderenze anormali colla capsula? Non sarà che l'osservazione degli operati, dopo che l'articolazione si sarà esercitata per un tempo sufficiente, che darà la possibilità di giudicare. Sarà poi in seguito alle risposte che verranno date a queste questioni, che si potrà stabilire se l'intervento che io ho esperimentato, dovrà limitarsi, come eccezione, a pochi casi, oppure estendersi a molti che ora vengono sottoposti, con molto vantaggio, non è da porre in dubbio, alla sola cura incruenta.

Non aggiungo che due parole sul metodo operativo che io seguo nei casi, nei quali la riduzione non è possibile. che a patto di aprire l'articolazione. Mi è accaduto soltanto in 5 casi, rispettivamente dell'età di 13, 13 e 16 anni, di giudicare necessario ricorrere ad un intervento cruento dopo fallite le solite prove di riduzione incruenta. Gli ostacoli in tutt'i casi risiedevano nel tubo capsulare che. fissato sulla fossa iliaca ed ipertrofico. opponeva una forte resistenza ed era troppo ristretto nell'istmo. Coll'atto operativo ho innanzi tutto cercato di rimuovere questi ostacoli incidendo trasversalmente la capsula nella sua porzione laterale ed anteriore per favorire l'abbassamento del capo femorale ed allargando l'istmo per rendere libero l'accesso alla testa del femore nella tasca cotiloidea. Nè il fondo del cotile, nè l'estremità del femore sono state intaccate.

Nell'ultimo caso, dopo l'esperienza fatta sull'importanza della liberazione della capsula e del periostio dalle loro aderenze colla fossa iliaca e sull'irritazione neo-produttiva che questo distacco porta nella superficie esterna dell'ileo e nel periostio ho modificato l'operazione in questo senso. Dopo eseguita la riduzione ho resecato la porzione esuberante antero-laterale della tasca femorale, ho distaccato il lembo capsulo-periosteo dall'ileo e l'ho abbassato a chiudere la breccia fatta nel tubo capsulare, riunendone i bordi con un'accurata sutura. Chiusura immediata della ferita ed immobilizzazione con apparecchio gessato sull'arto in abduzione. L'atto operativo non varierebbe quindi da quello precedentemente esposto che pel fatto che la riduzione si compie ad articolazione aperta e dopo allontanati gli ostacoli capsulari.

Anche l'incisione, per mezzo della quale si giunge sull'articolazione è eseguita nello stesso modo. La tecnica da me tenuta diversifica tuttavia da quella comune anche durante il tempo intra-articolare dell'operazione. A dilatare l'istmo non pratico incisioni, nè asportazioni nella capsula, ma mi servo di un divulsore che agisce come l'apribocca di König.

La riduzione poi, che costituisce il tempo più difficile dell'operazione, mi è notevolmente agevolata dallo strumento che presento. Anche Doyen ha fatto costruire un apparecchio allo scopo di ridurre ad articolazione aperta la testa femorale nel cotile. Il mio ha su quello di Doyen il pregio della semplicità senza che certamente abbia minore l'efficacia. Consiste in una leva a doccia a lungo manico, che può essere fortemente impugnato dall'operatore. La leva ha il punto d'appoggio fisso sulla S. I. A. I. passando sotto il tendine del retto anteriore e gli attacchi ligamentosi della capsula. La spina è abbrancata da un uncino di forma acconcia col quale termina il bordo, che chiamerò anteriore della leva. Il bordo posteriore si foggia alla sua estremità pure ad uncino, ma molto meno sporgente del primo. Questo uncino posteriore non ha altro ufficio che di impedire la rotazione esterna alla leva quando è in funzione e si appoggia lievemente sul bordo cotiloideo posteriore o sull'osso iliaco in un punto immediatamente vicino a questo.

Il funzionamento dell'apparecchio è dei più facili. Dopo aperta l'articolazione e dilatato convenientemente l'istmo, è preparata la tasca cotiloidea. Allora la leva passata fra la testa femorale e l'ileo va ad abbrancare coll'uncino anteriore la S. I. A. I. ad appoggiarsi coll'uncino posteriore nella località detta. La testa. femorale è adagiata sulla doccia ponendo l'arto in rotazione esterna. L'operatore allora impugna con una mano il manico dello strumento e coll'altra abbranca la coscia sopra ai condili femorali. Le due mani agiscono ora simultaneamente tentando l'una d'allontanare la leva dalla fossa iliaca facendola ruotare nel suo fulcro, rappresentato dall'uncino che si fissa attorno alla S. I. A. I., mentre l'altra porta la coscia in abduzione. Lo strumento agisce così da leva di secondo genere, il femore da leva di primo genere (ipomoclio costituito dai punti d'attacco dei muscoli, della capsula, ecc.) ed ambedue portano la testa verso il cotile. Un assistente, se ciò si giudica necessario, può eseguire pressioni direttamente sopra il capo del femore, che deve scorrere sulla doccia. Andando con lentezza la testa discende nella cavità cotiloidea, senza soffrire contusioni.

Questo gioco di leve è capace di vincere le più forti resistenze e per mezzo suo la riduzione diventa di una facilità maravigliosa. L'apparecchio è stato adoperato in quattro casi, in tre di lussazione congenita, ed in uno (ragazza dell'età di 19 anni), di lussazione paralitica, ed in tutti ha mirabilmente corrisposto.

Nell'ultimo operato, un ragazzo di 16 anni, con lussazione iliaca posteriore, rigida con accorciamento di 6 cm la riduzione è avvenuta immediatamente, senza che antecedentemente si fosse fatta pratica alcuna per mobilizzare ed abbassare il capo femorale, per mezzo di trazioni continue o coll'applicazione della vite di Lorenz e dell'apparecchio di Schede-Eschbaum.

È tuttavia consigliabile di ricorrere, in questi casi di grave accorciamento, prima dell'atto operativo a trazioni continuate per qualche tempo, poiché nella distensione rapida fatta dall'apparecchio possono soffrire i tronchi nervosi.

In questo caso infatti, alla riduzione praticata colla leva ha seguito una paralisi del n. crurale, la quale ha obbligato a togliere l'apparecchio gessato ed a diminuire l'abduzione ed a porre la coscia in flessione. Questo fatto può far perdere alla testa femorale i rapporti col cotile, che l'atto operativo le ha dato.

L'arto operato da un mese e mezzo è ancora sottoposto all'immobilizzazione e non si può dire nulla sul risultato ultimo del caso. Nei due casi operati nell'anno decorso, nei quali non si è seguito, riguardo al trattamento della capsula e del periostio iliaco, lo stesso metodo che ora consiglio, l'atto operativo ha portato sullo stato antecedente, un notevole miglioramento funzionale. ma l'articolazione possiede mobilità limitata, e la testa femorale si è fissata sopra la regione cotiloidea.

E forse col metodo ora proposto che il trattamento cruento della lussazione congenita. nei casi, nei quali la riduzione non puo avvenire che aprendo l'articolazione ed intervenendo entro di essa, potrà dare risultati funzionali, che reggano il confronto con quelli buoni, forniti ogni giorno dalla cura incruenta.

<hr>

COMMUNICATION

de M. T. PIÉCHAUD,

de Bordeaux.
Professeur de clinique chirurgicale infantile.

Messieurs, après les communications que nous venons d'entendre, je veux ajouter seulement quelques réflexions.

Certaines populations, en particulier dans le sud-ouest de la France se montrent très hostiles à l'opération sanglante, dans la luxation congénitale.

Les parents s'informent des résultats possibles de l'intervention et n'acceptent pas un traitement qui peut faire courir des dangers alors que la lésion ne menace pas la vie. C'est donc à la réduction non sanglante où nous conduit le conseil actuel que nous aimons à nous adresser. Si nous félicitons M. Hoffa des brillants résultats qu'il a obtenus par l'opération sanglante nous sommes heureux de remercier M. Lorenz de nous avoir donné une action chirurgicale si simple et si féconde.

Je ne saisis pas très bien sur quels motifs s'appuient ceux qui parlent constamment de réduction intégrale. Je vais dans un instant rapporter ma statistique personnelle. C'est sur l'expérience qu'elle m'a donnée que je m'appuie pour penser que nous ne savons pas ce que nous pourrons obtenir en pratiquant la réduction non sanglante. Cette opération consiste à fixer la tête contre un obstacle où elle pourra créer un cotyle. Si d'aventure on fait une réduction véritable, tout est pour le mieux : mais c'est bien l'exception.

Pour assurer le résultat de créer un cotyle en fixant la tête fémorale il faut cependant ménager à cette dernière un certain degré de mobilité : aussi faisons-nous de suite et autant que possible marcher nos petites malades. C'est pour cela que je ne comprends plus la pratique de certains chirurgiens qui opèrent à la fois les deux côtés dans la luxation double. Les opérés ne marchent pas et ils ne guériront pas.

Messieurs, j'ai, depuis la lecture des remarquables publications de Lorenz, donné toute ma faveur à la réduction non sanglante et j'ai opéré cinquante enfants avec les résultats suivants.

Vingt-neuf sujets étaient atteints de luxation unilatérale.

11 d'entre eux sont encore en traitement. Restent donc pour le moment 18 résultats que je dois diviser de la manière suivante :

8 médiocres (amélioration simple).

2 bons (claudication très diminuée).

2 très bons (claudication légère).

6 excellents (boiterie supprimée).

Vingt et un enfants avaient une luxation double. 14 sont encore en traitement. Restaient donc 7 cas qui nous donnent 1 ankylose fibreuse un peu serrée mais en voie d'amélioration. Il s'agit d'une enfant arthritique, issue de parents rhumatisants et âgée de quatorze ans.

2 raideurs articulaires.

2 résultats médiocres.

2 résultats très bons, presque excellents.

Si j'ajoute que presque tous les enfants en traitement sont jeunes, nous ont par conséquent donné des réductions faciles, je vous ferai pressentir des résultats au moins égaux aux précédents surtout pour les luxations unilatérales. Des chiffres que je viens de placer sous vos yeux il ressort, en effet, que la luxation bilatérale ne promet pas de fournir à nos statistiques un appoint bien sérieux.

Je me crois, avec les résultats fort encourageants que m'ont donné 50 opérations, Messieurs, tout à fait en droit de conclure que l'opération non sanglante doit être désormais l'intervention de choix, car elle est bien, avec son innocuité, le traitement réservé à une malformation qui ne compromet ni la santé ni la vie.

PROCÉDÉ DE LA ROTATION INTERNE IMMÉDIATE

COMMUNICATION

de M. le docteur PIERRE

de Berck-sur-Mer.

Le docteur Pierre (de Berck) propose de passer, dès la première séance opératoire, de la première position de l'opération de Lorenz (abduction et rotation externe, jambe fléchie) à la deuxième position (abduction et rotation interne, jambe allongée). Il a réussi, par cette manœuvre, dans un cas qui avait résisté à 21 mois d'essais dans les mains du chirurgien qui avait traité l'enfant avant lui. Ce procédé aurait pour avantage : 1° de gagner beaucoup de temps, presque la moitié de la durée du traitement ; 2° d'éviter les risques de reluxation, de transpositions ou de fractures qui sont les écueils à craindre dans le passage si délicat de la première à la deuxième position de l'opération de Lorenz.

SAMEDI 4 AOUT

Séance du matin.

CONTRIBUTION A L'ÉTUDE DU REDRESSEMENT FORCÉ SUCCESSIF
DANS LA SCOLIOSE

Photographies et radiographies avant et après le traitement.

MÉCANISME SUIVANT LEQUEL S'OPÈRE LE REDRESSEMENT DU RACHIS.
MOYEN DE MESURER PAR DES CHIFFRES LE DEGRÉ DE CE REDRESSEMENT.

COMMUNICATION

de M. le docteur LOUIS MENCIÈRE, [1]

de Reims.

Les examens radiographiques montrent, à côté de vertèbres demeurant longtemps à peu près normales, des disques intervertébraux présentant des différences de forme variables.

Je vous soumets des dessins demi-schématiques de colonnes verté-

1. D'après nos observations, voici comment un chirurgien doit se comporter en présence d'une scoliose :

Avant toute chose, il faut être persuadé que les corsets orthopédiques journellement construits par les mécaniciens ne peuvent pas, employés seuls, enrayer une scoliose, même au début :

Ce mode facile de traitement, encore trop en honneur, ne donnera au praticien que déboires et lui laissera la responsabilité d'un traitement illusoire et sans efficacité. Tous les malades qui nous arrivent ont porté corsets sur corsets, le résultat a toujours été négatif.

Guidé par nos observations, voici notre façon habituelle de procéder :

1° Scoliose tout à fait au début, sans déformation des disques, sans déformation thoracique.

Tuteur amovible variant suivant le genre de déviation. Le tuteur n'est pas seul employé, nous avons largement recours aux mouvements, à l'électrothérapie, à la mécanothérapie, aux *appareils de détorsion.*

2° Scoliose encore au début mais un peu plus avancée, avec déformation des disques et légère déformation thoracique.

Le tuteur amovible, la mécanothérapie ne donneront aucun résultat dans cette scoliose, que beaucoup considèrent comme encore légère.

Les modifications subies dans les disques souvent dès le début de la scoliose, comme l'indique la présente communication, guideront notre manière de faire.

Notre tuteur *inamovible*, placé après avoir mis le rachis en hypercorrection permettra à la colonne et aux disques de récupérer leur forme.

Des trous sont ménagés dans l'appareil pour l'électrisation des muscles vertébraux. L'atrophie est ainsi combattue.

Plus tard, au tuteur inamovible succédera un tuteur amovible. La mécanothérapie et les massages referont la musculature vertébrale, mais seulement quand on aura obtenu la correction des disques et du rachis.

brales, représentant rigoureusement les radiographies obtenues dans notre laboratoire radiographique.

Remarquons tout d'abord que deux choses sont à considérer dans une colonne vertébrale déviée :

1° Le degré de déviation de chaque courbure soit dorsale, soit lombaire, considérée isolément ;

2° Le degré de déviation du sujet au point de vue de l'attitude, attitude qui dépend de la direction de la colonne vertébrale, considérée dans son ensemble, abstraction faite de chaque courbure particulière.

Je m'explique :

Il se passe pour la colonne vertébrale ce qui se passe pour un membre, quand nous pratiquons certaines ostéotomies; si les deux extrémités du squelette sont une même ligne droite, le membre paraît droit, bien que les fragments ne soient pas toujours anatomiquement dans une rectitude parfaite au niveau de leur point de jonction.

Voici la méthode que nous suivons pour juger mathématiquement du degré de redressement d'une colonne vertébrale. Nous prenons un fil-à-plomb que nous plaçons sur la radiographie au centre de la première vertèbre dorsale: la distance d séparant le fil-à-plomb du milieu de la vertèbre, qui occupe le sommet de chaque courbure particulière, mesure le degré de déviation de cette courbure.

Deux mensurations, prises l'une avant le redressement, l'autre après, donnent, par une simple soustraction, le degré de redressement obtenu pour chaque courbure prise isolément.

Mais, esthétiquement, le redressement d'un sujet ne dépend pas

L'échec de la mécanothérapie et des massages par la méthode suédoise vient précisément de ce que les praticiens ne tiennent aucun compte des modifications de formes que présentent les disques dès cette période de début. Corrigez d'abord les disques, faites ensuite des muscles!

3° Scoliose grave avec déformation thoracique et ankylose plus ou moins prononcée, mais cependant encore opérable.

1° Mécanothérapie pour assouplir le rachis et préparer le redressement, pendant un temps variable;

2° Redressements successifs, progressifs et périodiques (tous les trois ou quatre mois). On gagne de plus en plus à chaque séance.

Le redressement ainsi pratiqué ne ressemble en rien au redressement brusque, en une séance unique encore parfois employé et qui, lui, est dangereux.

Les redressements successifs, progressifs et périodiques ne présentent absolument aucun danger s'ils sont pratiqués par un chirurgien rompu aux difficultés de la chirurgie orthopédique.

Nous avons longuement décrit notre appareil muni de dynamomètres qui nous permettent de nous rendre compte de la force déployée.

La colonne vertébrale est ensuite maintenue dans notre appareil permettant l'électrisation des muscles.

Plus tard, un tuteur léger suffira pour soutenir le rachis redressé, pendant que la mécanothérapie, les massages, l'électrothérapie rendront à la colonne vertébrale la souplesse et permettront de refaire une musculature solide.

tant du redressement d'une courbure que de la correction de l'attitude générale de la colonne vertébrale. Le sujet sera droit, si le milieu de la colonne dorsale dans sa région supérieure se trouve sur une même ligne droite que le milieu de la colonne lombaire, pourvu toutefois que les courbures dorsale et lombaire ne présentent pas une déformation exagérée et que les gibbosités soient très peu accentuées.

Or, les redressements forcés successifs corrigent d'abord en partie la déviation de chaque courbure prise séparément; ils amènent une diminution considérable des gibbosités et ensuite et surtout ils corrigent, au delà de tout ce qu'il était permis d'espérer, l'attitude générale de la colonne vertébrale.

Ils font récupérer aux disques déformés une partie de leur forme. Au-dessus et au-dessous des disques ankylosés, trop solides pour céder, ils provoquent une correction en sens inverse des disques sus et sous-jacents non encore ankylosés.

Cette correction se fait insensiblement sur les disques, dans toute la hauteur de la colonne vertébrale, sans amener de fortes inflexions de cette colonne. C'est grâce à ce mécanisme que l'attitude générale de la colonne vertébrale se trouve corrigée. La ligne *d* mesurant, ainsi qu'on peut le voir sur les dessins que je vous présente, la distance du fil-à-plomb au centre de la colonne lombaire dans sa région inférieure, indique le degré de déviation de l'attitude générale de la colonne vertébrale. Or, la difformité du sujet dépend, abstraction faite de la rotation des corps vertébraux et des déformations costales, du degré de déviation de l'attitude générale de la colonne vertébrale.

Le degré de correction de l'attitude du sujet et de sa colonne vertébrale est mathématiquement donné par deux mensurations, faites l'une avant, l'autre après le redressement.

En mesurant, avant et après le redressement, la distance qui sépare du fil-à-plomb les apophyses épineuses de la région lombaire, on se rend compte du degré de correction de l'attitude de la colonne vertébrale considérée dans son ensemble.

Or, si la correction de cette attitude est obtenue, le sujet paraîtra droit, alors même qu'il présenterait anatomiquement des courbures légères dans la hauteur de sa colonne vertébrale.

Le redressement provoque la correction de l'attitude en atténuant chaque courbure particulière, et en obtenant le reste sur l'ensemble des disques intervertébraux au niveau desquels se produisent des corrections de compensation; de sorte que des sujets sont esthétiquement droits, alors que la radiographie nous décèle encore une courbure dorsale et lombaire, diminuée il est vrai, mais non totalement disparue. Tel est le mécanisme par lequel on opère le redressement forcé, dans les cas de scoliose assez avancée. Les pressions sur les gibbosités agissent d'autre part sur le degré de rotation des corps vertébraux.

Correction de l'attitude du sujet par le mécanisme énoncé plus haut, laquelle correction peut se mesurer, comme vous le voyez sur les figures que je vous présente, diminution des gibbosités obtenue par le redressement lui-même de la colonne vertébrale, et par les pressions qui diminuent la rotation des corps vertébraux : voilà ce que procurent les redressements.

J'ai insisté sur le mécanisme de ces redressements et sur la façon de les mesurer, pour que l'on ne soit pas surpris à l'avenir de voir le dos de certains sujets plus droit que l'examen radiographique n'aurait pu nous le faire soupçonner, en comparant chaque courbure prise séparément et sans avoir égard à l'attitude de la colonne vertébrale dans son ensemble. Si une courbure dorsale, par exemple, n'est pas anatomiquement disparue, il n'en est pas moins vrai que l'attitude générale du sujet, elle, peut être corrigée, c'est-à-dire que le milieu de la colonne dorsale dans sa région supérieure se trouvera alors sur la même ligne que le milieu de le colonne lombaire dans sa région inférieure.

Enfin il faut tenir compte que, dans tout examen radiographique, les déformations sont exagérées, par ce fait que la colonne vertébrale ne peut pas être appliquée immédiatement sur la plaque et que l'ombre projetée en est agrandie. C'est ce qui nous est arrivé, alors surtout que nous avons pris nos colonnes vertébrales après redressement. La plupart des sujets, dans leur grand désir d'être droits, contractaient leurs muscles vertébraux et malgré nos soins, se mettaient en ensellure pendant que nous prenions nos radiographies. La plaque était donc éloignée du dos: l'image a été agrandie et les déformations exagérées. Ceci devra s'ajouter à tout ce que nous venons de dire plus haut, et vous expliquera la légère dissemblance qui existe, en apparence, entre la photographie et la radiographie d'un même sujet.

Néanmoins vous constaterez sur les images prises après le redressement, que la radiographie elle-même accuse une correction anatomique considérable bien que les déformations s'y trouvent plutôt exagérées, ainsi qu'il nous a été facile de nous en rendre compte en suivant avec le doigt la ligne des apophyses épineuses.

Les mensurations montrent deux choses :

1° Les courbures considérées isolément sont toujours fortement diminuées

2° L'attitude générale de la colonne vertébrale est corrigée, parfois en hypercorrection : d'où la correction esthétique du sujet obtenue.

Vous me permettrez de vous présenter le résultat de l'examen radiographique et clinique de quelques malades, sous forme de tableau. Cet exposé sera peut-être aride, mais seul il peut nous permettre une vue d'ensemble.

I° Scoliose dorsale à convexité droite, datant de deux ou trois mois, consécutive à une pleurésie purulente, chez un enfant de sept ans. Gibbosité dorsale droite accentuée (fig. 1).

Vertèbres et disques très visibles par la radiographie et normaux. La courbure porte, en effet, sur l'ensemble des disques, de telle sorte

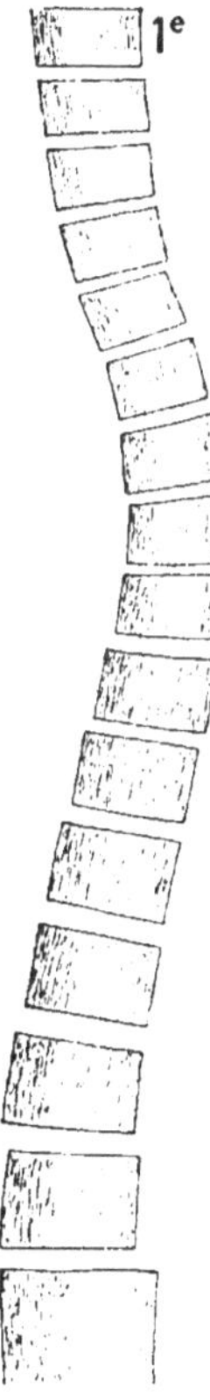

Fig. 1.

qu'aucun d'eux ne présente une diminution sensible de hauteur si l'on compare leurs côtés droit et gauche. Or, nous allons voir qu'il en est tout autrement pour les scolioses essentielles et de date plus ancienne, où certains disques, diminuant de hauteur du côté de la concavité et augmentant d'épaisseur du côté de la convexité, donnent à la colonne vertébrale sa direction définitive et déviée.

2° **Scoliose dorsale à convexité droite, datant d'au moins quatre ans, chez une jeune fille de quinze ans. Gibbosité dorsale droite accentuée** (fig. 2 et 3).

En comparant les figures 4 et 5 qui représentent les radiographies

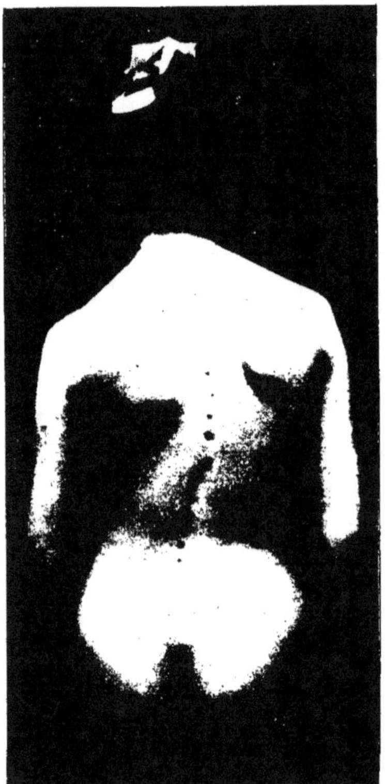

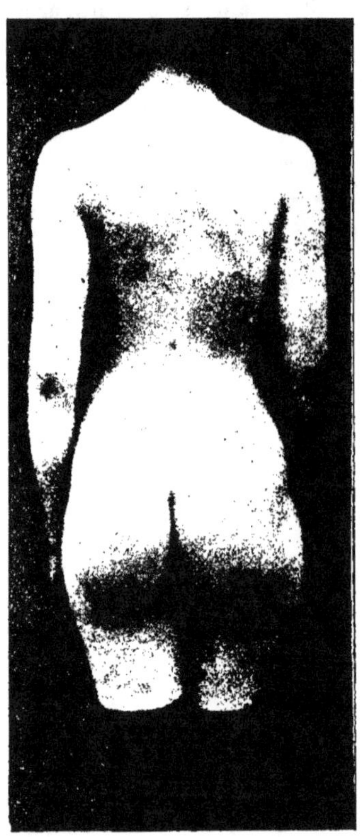

<table>
<tr><td>Fig. 2. — Avant l'opération
(28 novembre 1898).</td><td>Fig. 3. — Après l'opération
et le traitement (juin 1900).</td></tr>
</table>

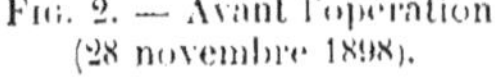

Scoliose dorsale à convexité droite, datant d'au moins quatre ans, chez une jeune fille de quinze ans. Gibbosité dorsale droite accentuée.

La malade est droite et la gibbosité qui était très apparente à droite, a presque totalement disparu. Le coup de hache à gauche, primitivement très accentué, est corrigé. L'épaule gauche qui était beaucoup plus basse que la droite est soulevée et mise au même niveau que celle-ci, qui elle-même a été abaissée. De novembre 1898 à juillet 1900, la taille s'est élevée de 4 cm. 1/2.

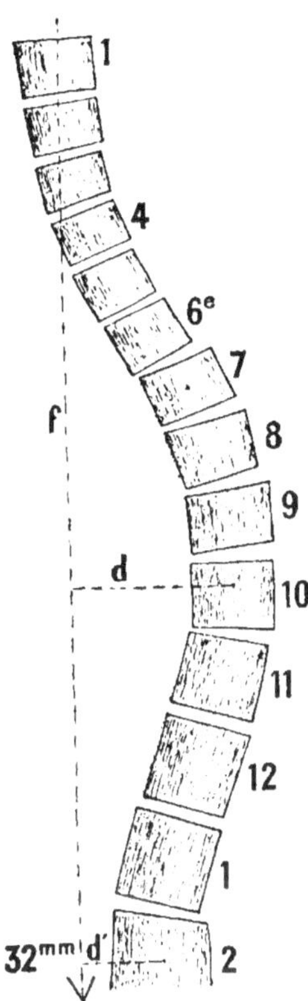

Fig. 4. — Radiographie
prise le 28 novembre 1898.

Le sommet de l'arc est constitué
par le milieu de la dixième dorsale,
et la distance du sommet de cet arc
à la corde sous-jacente *f*, indiquée
par la flèche *d*, mesure le degré de
déviation de la courbure dorsale prise
isolément. Cette distance est de
6 cm. 1/2.

La ligne *d'* distance du milieu de la
colonne lombaire au fil-à-plomb *f*, mesure la déviation de l'attitude de la
colonne vertébrale envisagée dans son
ensemble, le fil-à-plomb passe à 32 millimètres à gauche du milieu de la colonne lombaire.

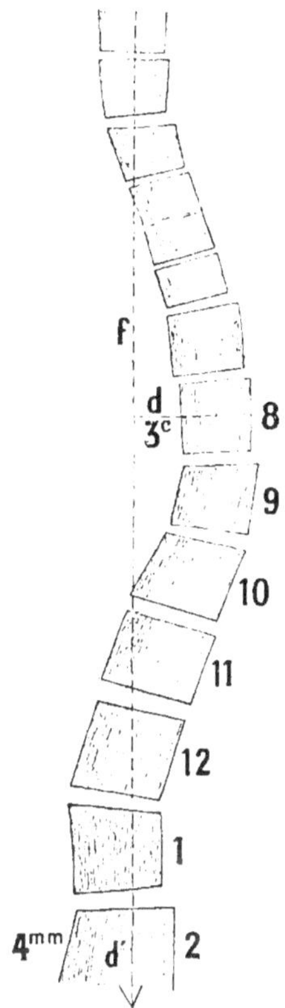

Fig. 5. — Radiographie
prise en juin 1900.

Le sommet de l'arc est situé sur la
huitième dorsale. La distance *d* du sommet de cet arc à la corde sous-jacente
est de 5 centimètres. La différence entre
6 1 2 et 5 représente le degré de redressement de la courbure dorsale en particulier. Le fil-à-plomb passe à 4 millimètres à droite du milieu de la colonne
lombaire. Il y a donc eu correction de
5 cm. 1 2 de la courbure dorsale et hypercorrection de l'attitude générale de
la colonne vertébrale, hypercorrection
indiquée par la ligne *d'* sur la seconde
radiographie

Ceci explique le redressement parfait
de la malade donné par la photographie,
bien qu'anatomiquement il existe encore
un certain degré de courbure dans la
région dorsale.

de la colonne vertébrale avant et après le traitement, vous constaterez que la colonne vertébrale a été anatomiquement très notablement redressée. Entre la septième et la onzième dorsale, les disques, qui avant le redressement, étaient deux fois plus épais à droite, côté convexe (fig. 4), ont récupéré leur forme normale (fig. 5).

Si l'on considère l'arc formé par la concavité de la colonne vertébrale et la corde de cet arc représentée par la ligne *f*, qui n'est autre qu'un fil-à-plomb dont le point d'attache serait fixé directement sur la radiographie, au centre de la première dorsale, on est amené à faire plusieurs remarques.

Sur la première radiographie (fig. 4) prise avant redressement, le sommet de l'arc est constitué par le milieu de la dixième dorsale, et la distance du sommet de cet arc à la corde sous-jacente, indiquée par la flèche *d*, mesure le degré de déviation de la courbure dorsale prise isolément. Cette distance est de six centimètres et demi.

Sur la deuxième radiographie (fig. 5) obtenue après redressement, le sommet de l'arc est situé sur la huitième dorsale. La distance *d* du sommet de cet arc à la corde sous-jacente est de trois centimètres. La différence entre six et demi et trois représente le degré de redressement de la courbure dorsale en particulier.

Sur la première radiographie, la ligne *d'*, distance du milieu de la colonne lombaire au fil-à-plomb, mesure la déviation de l'attitude de la colonne vertébrale envisagée dans son ensemble. Le fil-à-plomb passe à trente-deux millimètres à gauche du milieu de la colonne lombaire. Sur la deuxième radiographie il passe à quatre millimètres à droite du milieu de la colonne lombaire. Il y a donc eu correction de trois centimètres et demi de la courbure dorsale et hypercorrection de l'attitude générale de la colonne vertébrale, hypercorrection indiquée par la ligne *d'* sur la seconde radiographie.

Ceci explique le redressement parfait de la malade donné par la photographie, bien qu'anatomiquement il existe encore un certain degré de courbure dans la région dorsale.

Les figures 2 et 3 sont des photographies de la malade avant et après le traitement.

La première a été prise le 28 novembre 1898, époque à laquelle cette malade est amenée à notre Clinique de Chirurgie infantile et orthopédique de Reims. La seconde a été prise en juin 1900.

Les redressements forcés progressifs, périodiques et successifs, suivis de maintien dans notre appareil et à l'aide de notre minerve spéciale décrite antérieurement dans la *Médecine moderne*, numéro du 20 mai 1899, ont donné les résultats suivants :

La malade est droite et la gibbosité, très apparente à droite, est à peu près totalement disparue. Le coup de hache à gauche, très accentué, est corrigé. L'épaule gauche qui était beaucoup plus basse que la droite est soulevée et mise au même niveau que la droite, qui elle-même, a été abaissée. De novembre 1898 à juillet 1900, la taille s'est élevé de quatre centimètres et demi.

5° **Scoliose dorsale principale à convexité droite et courbure secondaire à convexité gauche datant de trois ans, chez un garçon de quinze ans. La gibbosité dorsale est très accentuée** (fig. 6).

Les disques entre la cinquième et la dixième dorsale, sont du double plus hauts à droite, côté de la convexité. Les vertèbres sont légèrement moins élevées à gauche, côté de la convexité.

Les disques entre la onzième dorsale et la troisième lombaire sont plus hauts à gauche, c'est-à-dire du côté de la convexité lombaire. Les vertèbres paraissent normales. En résumé, les disques sont plus épais du côté des convexités dorsale et lombaire. Il y a là un espace dépourvu d'éléments osseux. On peut donc espérer comprimer les disques de ce côté et non seulement leur donner leur forme normale, mais encore récupérer sur eux la déformation des vertèbres, qui d'ailleurs est légère.

Comparez les figures 8 et 9, vous constaterez le résultat anatomique du redressement.

1re radiographie (fig. 8). Flèche *d*. . . . . 5 centimètres
   Distance *d'*. . . . . 5 centimètres
2me radiographie (fig. 9). Flèche *d*. . . . . 4 centimètres 1/2
   Distance *d'*. . . . . 1 centimètre

C'est donc l'attitude générale surtout qui a été corrigée. La courbure dorsale l'a été beaucoup moins. Néanmoins le résultat esthétique est bon, comme on va le voir.

Les photographies (fig. 6 et 7), la première prise le 1er avril 1899, avant le redressement, et la seconde le 4 juillet 1900, indiquent que l'enfant, qui semblait tassé sur lui-même, est aujourd'hui élancé. Le malade paraît être droit; les gibbosités dorsales et lombaires, qui cependant étaient volumineuses et qui ont présenté assez de dureté à la réduction, sont diminuées dans des proportions considérables. Le coup de hache au-dessous de l'épaule gauche et le coup de hache au-dessus de la hanche droite sont corrigés; en un mot le résultat obtenu est très satisfaisant.

Le sujet, avant le traitement, mesurait 155 centimètres : il mesure aujourd'hui 169 centimètres. Il a grandi de 14 centimètres. La taille s'est donc rapidement accrue. Or c'est un fait constant d'observation, les enfants grandissent beaucoup après les redressements

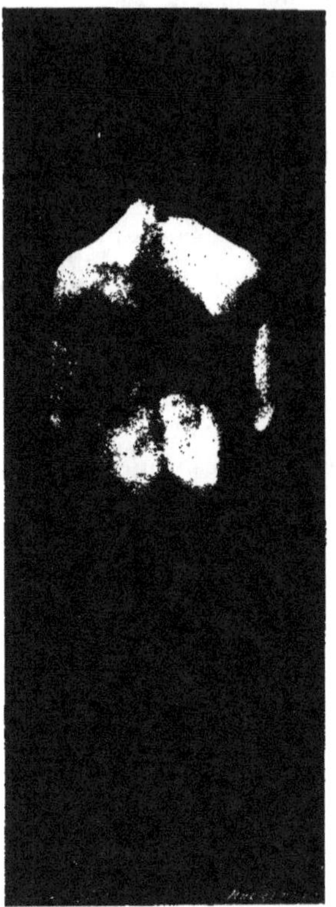

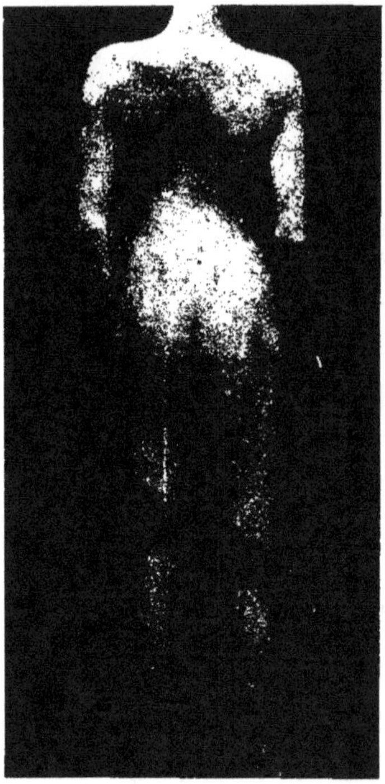

Fig. 6. — Avant l'opération.
1er avril 1899.

Fig. 7. — Après l'opération et le traitement.
4 juillet 1900.

*Scoliose dorsale principale à convexité droite et courbure secondaire
à convexité gauche datant de trois ans, chez un garçon de quinze ans.
La gibbosité dorsale est très accentuée.*

L'enfant, qui semblait tassé sur lui-même, est aujourd'hui élancé. Le malade parait droit, les gibbosités dorsales et lombaires, qui cependant étaient volumineuses et qui ont présenté assez de dureté à la réduction, sont diminuées dans des proportions considérables. Le coup de hache au-dessous de l'épaule gauche et le coup de hache au-dessus de la hanche droite sont corrigés, en un mot le résultat obtenu est très satisfaisant.

Le sujet, avant le traitement, mesurait 155 centimètres; il mesure aujourd'hui 169 centimètres. Il a grandi de 14 centimètres. La taille s'est donc rapidement accrue. Or, c'est un fait constant d'observation, les enfants grandissent beaucoup après les redressements.

forcés, nous le constaterons surtout dans l'observation 6, où un enfant ne grandissant plus, noué, suivant l'expression des parents, a vu sa taille s'accroître rapidement après le redressement. Cet accroissement

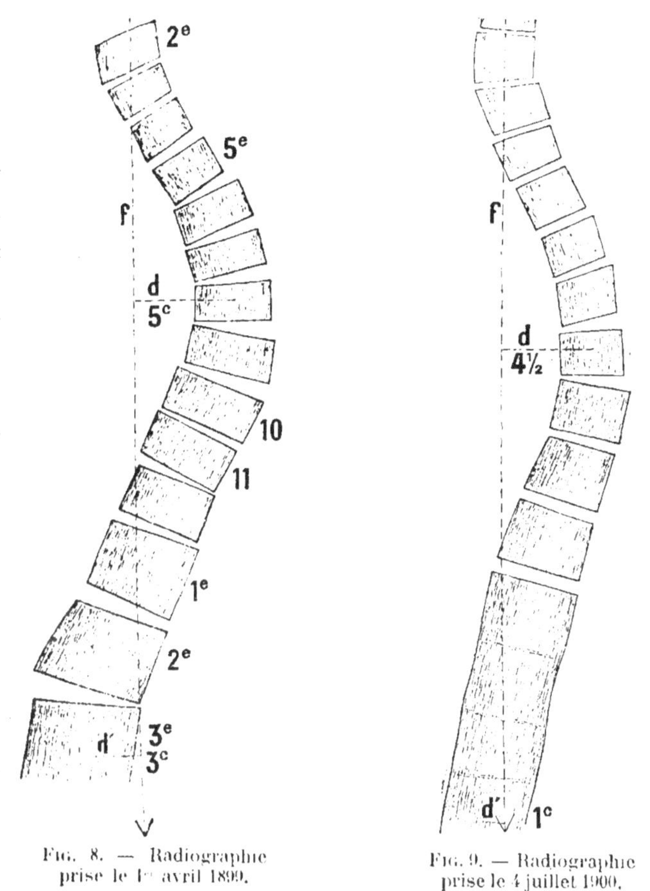

Fig. 8. — Radiographie
prise le 1er avril 1899.

Fig. 9. — Radiographie
prise le 4 juillet 1900.

Flèche d .... 5 cm.   Flèche d .... 4 cm. 1,2
Distance d' .... 5 cm.   Distance d' .... 1 cm.

C'est donc l'attitude générale surtout qui a été corrigée. La courbure dorsale l'a été beaucoup moins. Néanmoins le résultat esthétique est bon, comme le montrent les photographies.

de la taille en bonne attitude ajoute encore au redressement et augmente celui-ci.

4° **Scoliose principale dorsale à convexité droite, avec gibbosité accentuée à peu près irréductible, et scoliose secondaire lombaire gauche, datant de 4 ou 5 ans au moins, chez une jeune fille de 16 ans.**

Entre la septième et la onzième dorsale, les disques sont peu visibles et peu déformés, autant qu'on en peut juger (fig. 12).

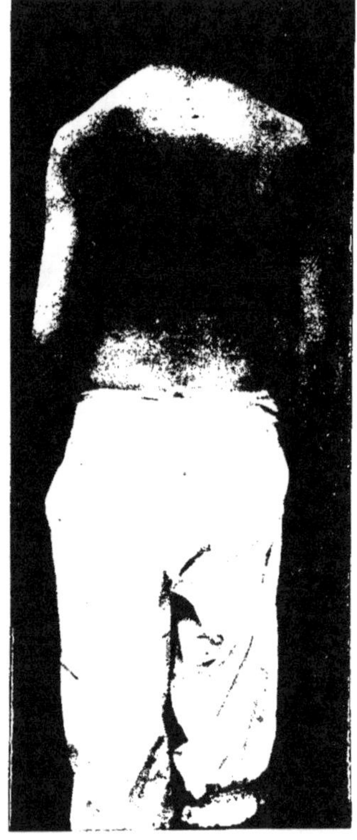

Fig. 10. — Avant l'opération
(22 juin 1899).

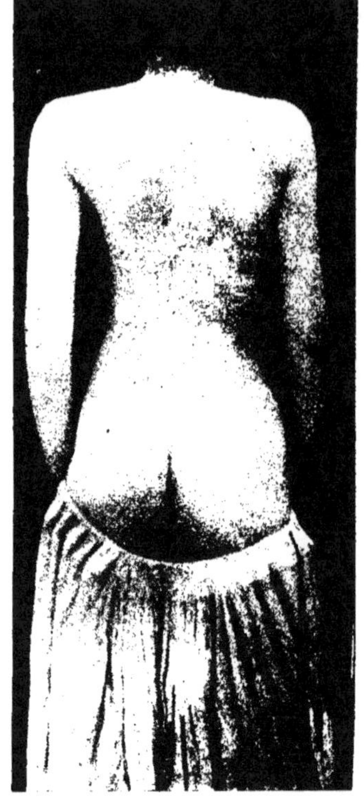

Fig. 11. —Après l'opération et le traitement
(9 juillet 1900).

Scoliose principale dorsale à convexité droite avec gibbosité accentuée à peu près irréductible et scoliose lombaire gauche datant de quatre ou cinq ans au moins chez une jeune fille de seize ans.

La gibbosité dorsale droite accentuée, qui était à peu près irréductible, a cependant cédé aux redressements successifs : aujourd'hui elle est presque totalement disparue, le thorax est à peine un peu plus gros de ce côté. Le côté gauche, qui était creux, a récupéré en grande partie sa forme.

La malade, qui était déjetée dans son ensemble à droite, est d'aplomb.

Le bénéfice procuré par le traitement est considérable et surpasse ce que pouvaient faire espérer l'état de la malade et la rigidité de la colonne vertébrale et des gibbosités.

Les disques entre la onzième dorsale et la troisième lombaire sont le double plus hauts à gauche.

La comparaison des radiographies 12 et 15 nous montre pour la

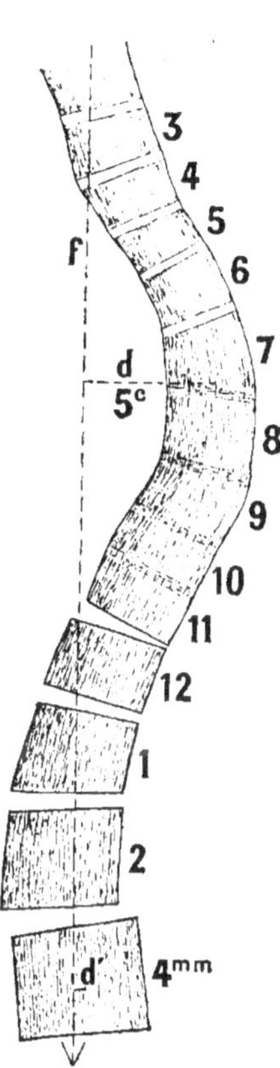

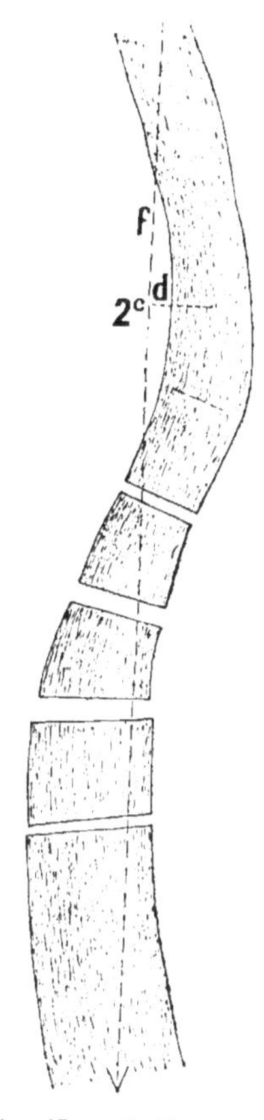

Fig. 12. — Radiographie
prise le 22 juin 1899.

Fig. 15. — Radiographie
prise le 9 juillet 1900.

Flèche *d* .... 5 cent.   Flèche *d* .... 2 cent.
Distance *d'* .... 4 mill.   Distance *d'* .... 0 cent.

Il y a donc eu une forte correction de la courbure dorsale et une correction totale de l'attitude.

Ce qui explique l'excellent résultat esthétique obtenu, comme il est facile d'en juger par les photographies 10 et 11.

première une flèche *d* de 5 centimètres : le fil à plomb tombe à 4 millimètres à gauche du milieu de la colonne lombaire. Sur la seconde radiographie, la flèche *d* est de 2 centimètres, le fil à plomb tombe exactement sur le milieu de la colonne lombaire.

Il y a donc eu une forte correction de la courbure dorsale et une correction totale de l'attitude.

Ce qui explique, comme on va le voir par les photographies, l'excellent résultat esthétique obtenu.

1° Photographie prise le 22 juin 1899 (fig. 10).

2° Photographie prise le 9 juillet 1900).

La gibbosité dorsale droite accentuée, qui était à peu près irréductible, a cependant cédé aux redressements successifs ; aujourd'hui elle a presque totalement disparu. le thorax est à peine un peu plus gros de ce côté. Le côté gauche, qui était creux, a récupéré en grande partie sa forme.

La malade, qui était déjetée dans son ensemble à droite, est d'aplomb.

Le bénéfice procuré par le traitement est, ainsi que vous pouvez vous en rendre compte par les figures 10 et 11, considérable et surpasse ce que pouvaient faire espérer l'état de la malade et la rigidité de la colonne vertébrale et des gibbosités.

Scoliose dorso-lombaire droite, datant de neuf années, chez une jeune fille de 15 ans. Gibbosité droite très notable. Coup de hache très accentué à gauche (fig. 14, 15, 16, 17).

Entre la première lombaire et la douzième dorsale, le disque est beaucoup plus haut à droite, côté de la convexité.

La première lombaire est moins haute à gauche, côté de la concavité.

Entre la première et la troisième lombaire, les disques sont libres, mais plus épais à droite.

Sur la première radiographie, la flèche *d*, distance du sommet de l'arc à la corde sous-jacente. mesure six centimètres et demi.

Sur la deuxième radiographie. cette distance est de trois centimètres et demi.

La différence de six centimètres et demi à trois centimètres et demi représente le degré de redressement de la courbure dorso-lombaire. La ligne *d'* mesurant l'attitude tombe à gauche du milieu de la colonne lombaire et mesure dix-huit millimètres sur la première radiographie. Sur la seconde le fil à plomb passe à droite du milieu de la colonne lombaire et à une distance de dix millimètres. Cette ligne s'est donc déplacée de vingt-huit millimètres donnant une hypercorrection de l'attitude, ce qui explique le bon résultat obtenu au point de vue esthétique. résultat constaté par les photographies 14 et 15.

En résumé, on a obtenu une forte correction de la courbure dorso-lombaire, et une hypercorrection de l'attitude.

Première photographie, le 17 août 1899 (fig. 14).

Deuxième photographie le 4 juillet 1900 (fig. 15).

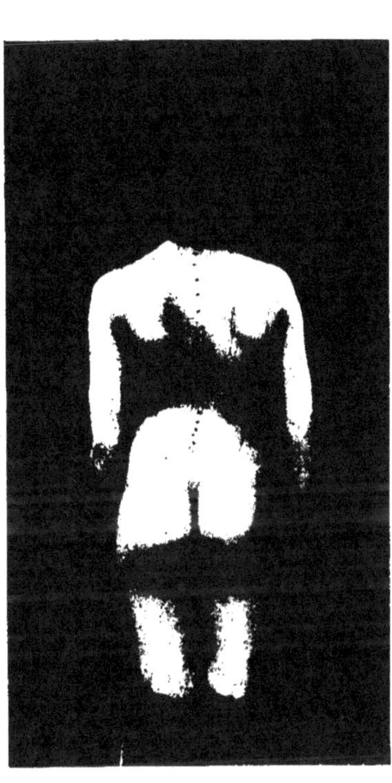

Fig. 14. — Avant l'opération
(17 août 1899).

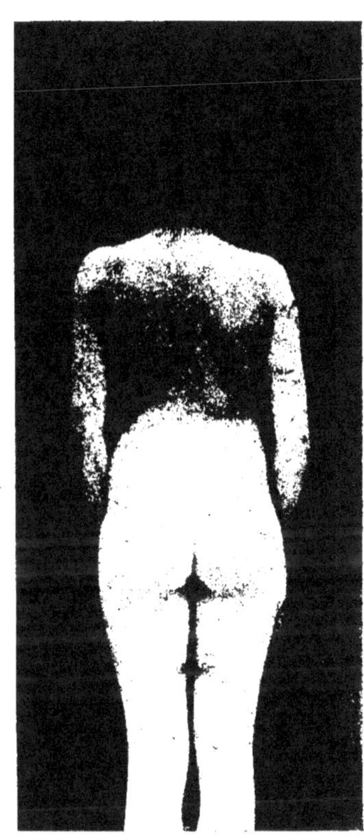

Fig. 15. — Après l'opération
et le traitement (4 juillet 1900).

Scoliose dorso-lombaire droite datant de neuf années, chez une jeune fille de quinze ans. Gibbosité dorsale droite très notable. Coup de hache très accentué à gauche.

L'enfant s'est déviée depuis l'âge de sept ans, elle a porté un corset orthopédique dès le début de sa maladie, elle s'est donc déformée sous le corset lui-même, ce qui indique le peu de valeur thérapeutique de ce moyen encore trop en honneur.

Le premier redressement a eu lieu le 17 août 1899. Actuellement, comme en fait foi la photographie, la malade est redressée, la gibbosité disparue et le coup de hache corrigé. Taille avant le traitement, 150 centimètres; taille après le traitement, 154 centimètres.

L'enfant s'est déviée depuis l'âge de sept ans, elle a porté un corset orthopédique dès le début de sa maladie, elle s'est donc déformée sous le corset lui-même, ce qui indique le peu de valeur thérapeutique de ce moyen encore trop en honneur.

Le premier redressement a eu lieu le 17 août 1899. Actuellement, comme en fait foi la photographie, la malade est redressée, la gibbo-

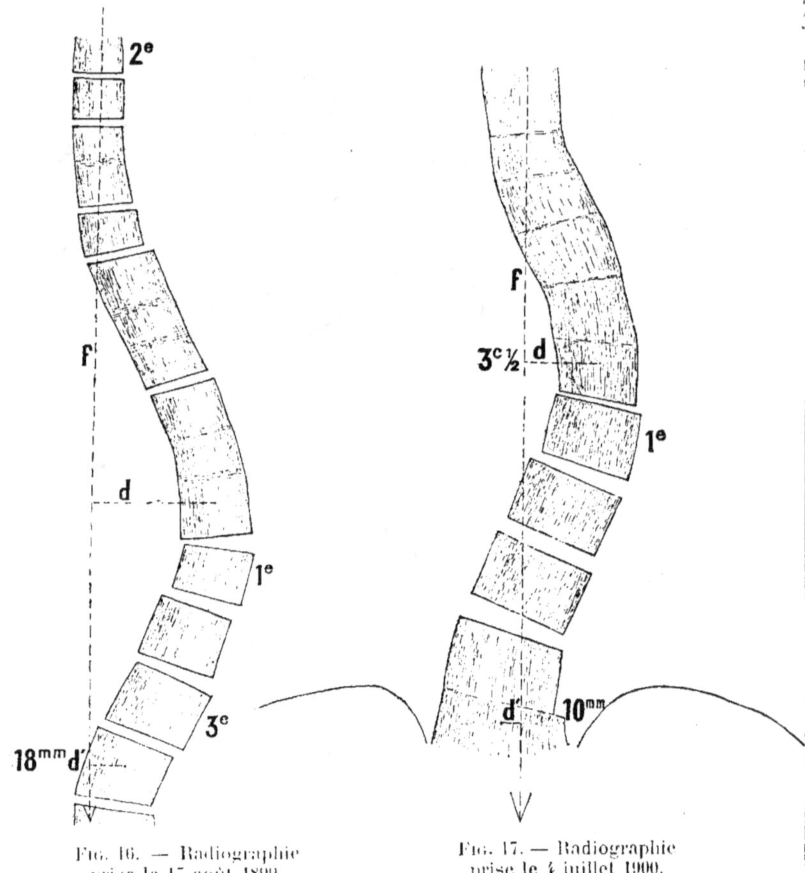

Fig. 16. — Radiographie
prise le 17 août 1899.

Fig. 17. — Radiographie
prise le 4 juillet 1900.

Flèche *d* .... 6 cent. 1/2   Flèche *d* .... 5 cent. 1/2
Distance *d'* .... 18 mill. à g.   Distance *d'* .... 10 mill. à dr.

. On a obtenu une forte correction de la courbure dorso-lombaire, et une hyper-correction de l'attitude.

La différence de 6 cent. 1/2 à 5 cent. 1/2 représente le redressement de la courbure dorso-lombaire. La ligne *d'* mesurant l'attitude tombe à gauche du milieu de la colonne lombaire et mesure 18 millimètres sur la première photographie. Sur la seconde le fil à plomb passe à droite du milieu de la colonne lombaire et à une distance de 10 millimètres. Cette ligne s'est donc déplacée de 28 millimètres donnant une hypercorrection de l'attitude, ce qui explique le bon résultat obtenu au point de vue esthétique. résultat constaté par les photographies 14 et 15.

sité disparue et le coup de hache corrigé. Taille avant le traitement
150 centimètres, taille après le traitement 154 centimètres.

**6° Scolio-cyphose principale dorsale gauche et scoliose secondaire
lombaire droite chez un garçon de quinze ans** (fig. 18, 19, 20, 21).

Gibbosité accentuée à gauche et à peu près irréductible.

Les clichés sont défectueux, néanmoins on perçoit des disques non

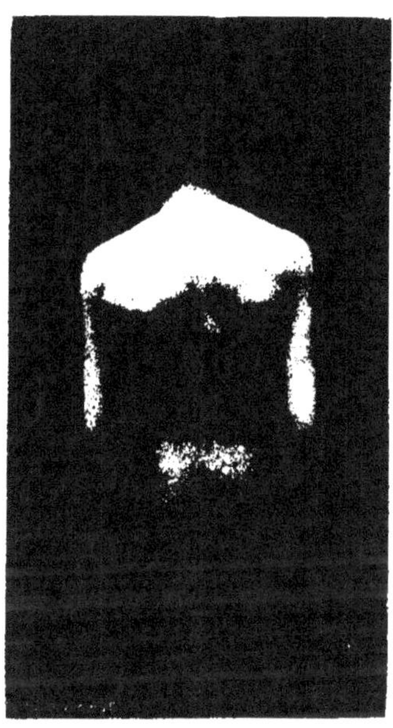

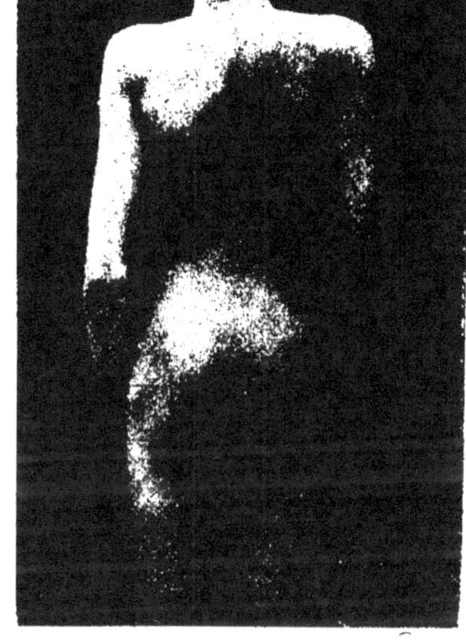

<table>
<tr><td>Fig. 18. — Avant l'opération
(mars 1899).</td><td>Fig. 19. — Après l'opération
et le traitement (2 juillet 1900).</td></tr>
</table>

*Scolio-cyphose principale dorsale gauche et scoliose secondaire lombaire droite
chez un garçon de quinze ans.*
Gibbosité accentuée à gauche et à peu près irréductible.

Le premier redressement a eu lieu le 12 juin 1899, après plusieurs mois d'assouplissement et de préparation. Malgré une ankylose à peu près totale, la scolio-
cyphose a pu être corrigée : la gibbosité gauche est diminuée dans des proportions considérables. Depuis plusieurs années, l'enfant ne grandissait plus. Avant
l'opération la taille était de 139 centimètres, aujourd'hui elle est de 156 cent. 1 2,
elle s'est donc accrue de 17 cent. 1 2. Un des résultats du redressement a été
d'amener une croissance très rapide chez un enfant chétif subissant un arrêt de
développement. L'enfant se plaignait fréquemment de douleurs dans la région
du thorax; celles-ci ont cessé dès le premier redressement. Dans la plupart de
nos observations nous avons noté le même fait.

soudés dans toute la hauteur de la colonne vertébrale à côté d'autres
moins visibles et paraissant ankylosés. Les disques sont plus nettement indiqués dans la région lombaire. On a néanmoins une image

donnant la direction de la colonne vertébrale. laquelle est fortement
déviée, surtout à gauche.

Sur la première radiographie, la ligne qui représente un fil à plomb
passe à trois centimètres et demi du milieu de la colonne vertébrale

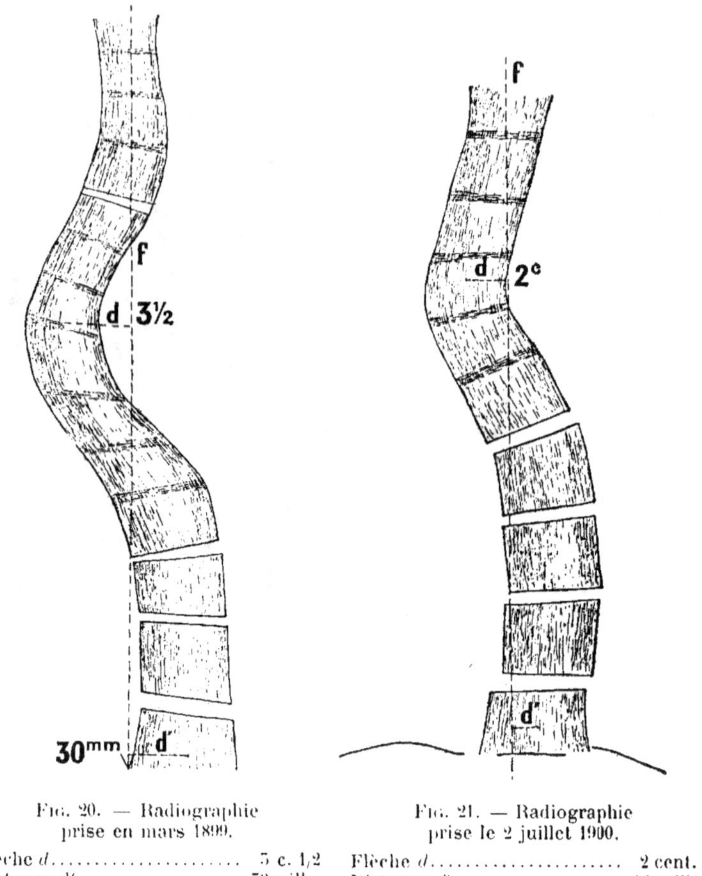

<table>
<tr><td>Fig. 20. — Radiographie
prise en mars 1899.</td><td>Fig. 21. — Radiographie
prise le 2 juillet 1900.</td></tr>
<tr><td>Flèche d...................... 5 c. 1/2
Distance d'................... 50 mill.</td><td>Flèche d...................... 2 cent.
Distance d'................... 12 mill.</td></tr>
</table>

Le résultat du redressement a donc été de mettre sensiblement sur la même
ligne les deux extrémités de la colonne vertébrale. tout en diminuant très notablement la courbure supérieure.

au niveau de la courbure supérieure. Sur la deuxième radiographie.
elle ne passe plus qu'à une distance de deux centimètres.

Plus bas. la ligne *f* passe à trente millimètres à gauche du milieu de
la colonne lombaire. Sur la deuxième radiographie elle tombe sur la

colonne lombaire à douze millimètres seulement du milieu de la vertèbre.

Le résultat du redressement a donc été de mettre sensiblement sur la même ligne les deux extrémités de la colonne vertébrale, tout en diminuant très notablement la courbure supérieure.

Première photographie prise en mars 1899, avant le redressement.

Deuxième photographie, le 2 juillet 1900.

Le premier redressement a eu lieu le 12 juin 1899, après plusieurs mois d'assouplissement et de préparation. Malgré une ankylose à peu près totale, la scolio-cyphose a pu être corrigée : la gibbosité gauche

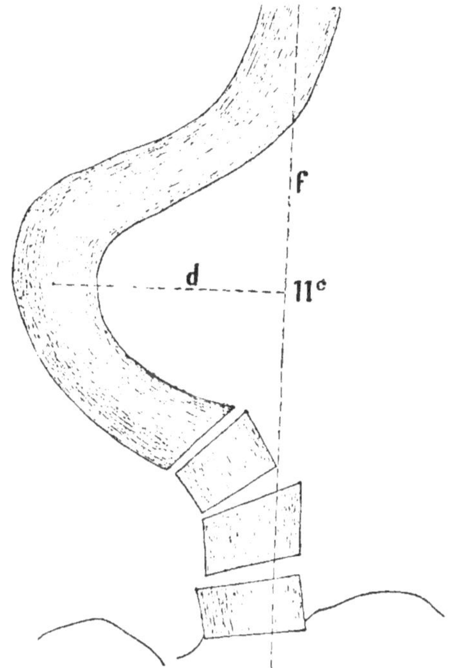

FIG. 22. — Radiographie d'une scoliose considérable totalement ankylosée et inopérable. Scoliose datant de dix ans, chez une jeune fille de seize ans. La colonne vertébrale paraît être d'une seule pièce, les vertèbres sont soudées entre elles et les disques ont disparu. Dans la région lombaire, les disques sont visibles et plus élevés à droite. Néanmoins, la dureté de la colonne vertébrale, jointe à l'examen radiographique, ne nous a pas permis de tenter un redressement.

est diminuée dans des proportions considérables. Depuis plusieurs années, l'enfant ne grandissait plus. Avant l'opération, la taille était de cent trente-neuf centimètres, aujourd'hui elle est de cent cinquante-six centimètres et demi, elle s'est donc accrue de dix-sept centimètres et demi. Un des résultats du redressement a été d'amener une croissance très rapide chez un enfant chétif subissant un arrêt de développement. L'enfant se plaignait fréquemment de douleurs dans la région du thorax; celles-ci ont cessé dès le premier redressement. Dans la plupart de nos observations nous avons noté le même fait.

7° Enfin je vous présente (fig. 22) la radiographie d'une scoliose considérable, totalement ankylosée et inopérable, scoliose datant de dix ans chez une jeune fille de seize ans.

La colonne vertébrale paraît être d'une seule pièce, les vertèbres sont soudées entre elles et les disques ont disparu. Dans la région lombaire, les disques sont visibles et plus élevés à droite. Néanmoins, la dureté de la colonne vertébrale, jointe à l'examen radiographique, ne nous a pas permis de tenter un redressement.

Conclusions.

I. — L'examen radiographique indique le siège des lésions anatomiques des disques et des vertèbres.

II. — Il montre que le maximum de la lésion siège et persiste fort longtemps dans les disques seuls, qui sont plus hauts du côté convexe et atrophiés du côté concave.

Ce fait, à lui seul, indique suffisamment l'utilité et la possibilité du redressement forcé, qui fait en partie récupérer aux disques leur forme normale, ainsi que l'indiquent les radiographies prises avant et après le traitement.

III. — Les redressements forcés, progressifs et successifs (tous les trois ou quatre mois), outre qu'ils sont sans danger dans la scoliose, pourvu que l'on veuille s'abstenir dans les cas trop anciens et trop ankylosés, pour lesquels la radiographie donnera de précieuses indications, fourniront des résultats que jusqu'ici aucun des moyens classiquement connus n'a pu donner.

Les photographies et les radiographies que je viens de vous montrer, prises avant et après le traitement, indiquent le mécanisme suivant lequel s'opère le redressement, redressement qui consiste dans la diminution de chaque courbure en particulier et la correction et souvent l'hypercorrection de l'attitude.

IV. — Il est possible de mesurer ces corrections par des chiffres, en suivant notre méthode.

V. — Dès qu'il y a des déformations anatomiques au niveau des disques ou des vertèbres, il faut les corriger, que ces déformations soient primitives ou secondaires, peu importe.

D'ailleurs, l'attitude corrigée est encore ce qui permet le mieux aux ligaments et aux muscles de récupérer leur longueur normale.

VI. — Il faut s'abstenir systématiquement, sous peine de discréditer la méthode, dans les cas trop défavorables où le bénéfice qu'on pourrait obtenir ne justifierait pas la longueur du traitement.

Dans les cas moins défavorables, mais présentant cependant un degré notable d'ankylose, à l'exemple de Redard, nous assouplissons et mobilisons le rachis avant le redressement.

VII. — La correction anatomiquement complète des courbures de la colonne vertébrale ne peut être réalisée que dans les cas relativement récents.

Dans les cas plus accentués, mais encore justiciables du redressement, on obtient une correction anatomique très notable de chaque courbure considérée isolément, et dans la plupart des cas, on obtient non seulement une correction, mais une hypercorrection de l'attitude générale de la colonne vertébrale.

Ces corrections se font aux dépens des disques, qui augmentent d'un côté et diminuent de l'autre. Elles se font également aux dépens des disques situés au-dessus et au-dessous d'une lésion déjà en partie ankylosée. Il se produit alors, au niveau de ces disques, des corrections de compensation qui dans leur ensemble amènent les colonnes dorsale et lombaire à se trouver sensiblement sur la même ligne, ce que l'on peut constater par le fil à plomb.

Il s'ensuit qu'en examinant le dos d'un sujet soumis au redressement, le résultat esthétique obtenu dépasse le résultat anatomique, si l'on considère chaque courbure prise isolément. Au contraire le résultat esthétique est directement proportionnel au degré de redressement de l'attitude générale de la colonne vertébrale.

VIII. — Les documents que je viens de vous soumettre montrent l'incontestable utilité du redressement dans la scoliose. Si les corsets orthopédiques et les mouvements méthodiques sont incapables de redresser un rachis, dont les divers éléments sont anatomiquement déformés, il n'en est plus de même pour le redressement forcé. Néanmoins les corsets et les mouvements méthodiques devront, après le redressement, longtemps servir pour le maintien du résultat laborieusement obtenu.

IX. — Sous l'influence de causes diverses, attitude, muscles, états morbides siégeant dans les disques, ceux-ci s'atrophient d'un côté et prennent une direction oblique; la colonne suit et se courbe plus haut et plus bas en sens inverse.

La raison d'être du redressement forcé est précisément de s'adresser non à une tige *rigide*, composée d'une seule pièce, mais à une tige formée d'une série d'anneaux séparés par des disques qui, bien que déformés, sont encore susceptibles d'une certaine élasticité.

En corrigeant les courbures, on dégage ou allonge le disque du côté atrophié. En maintenant longtemps la position, on permet au disque de récupérer une partie de sa forme. Le côté subissant une pression tendra plutôt à s'atrophier et l'autre à s'hypertrophier, c'est là une loi de physiologie générale.

Bien que quelques-uns des sujets, dont je viens de vous tracer succinctement l'histoire, aient encore besoin de nos soins, car nous évaluons à dix-huit mois environ la durée du traitement actif, les résultats acquis et que j'aurais voulu vous montrer à plus longue échéance, nous ont paru suffisamment beaux et instructifs pour être apportés devant le Congrès, comme contribution à la recherche des moyens de guérison d'une affection, qui trop longtemps a été systématiquement et classiquement considérée comme incurable.

Les travaux que quelques chercheurs ont publiés dans ces dernières années, et qu'ils n'ont cessé de poursuivre malgré le scepticisme des uns et le dédain des autres, les documents que je vous apporte aujourd'hui sont des bases suffisantes pour que chacun puisse établir sa conviction et être assuré qu'il y a mieux à faire que de suivre la plupart des observateurs actuels qui, se trouvant en face d'une scoliose, se contentent de la constater.

LES OPÉRATIONS DU PRÉPUCE

COMMUNICATION

de M. le docteur SAMUEL BERNHEIM,

de Paris.

L'auteur déclare avoir eu à intervenir plus de 5600 fois chez des sujets de tout âge et avoir encore examiné le prépuce d'un plus grand nombre d'individus. D'une pratique de 17 années, il tire les conclusions suivantes :

1° Le prépuce est un organe offrant souvent des malformations congénitales ou acquises : il est très irrégulier de forme. Ces malformations, gênantes pendant l'enfance, peuvent être le point de départ de mauvaises habitudes (masturbation) ou d'infirmités (rétention ou incontinence de l'urine). A l'âge adulte, elles constituent un empêchement aux rapports sexuels et favorisent toute espèce d'inoculations infectieuses (chancres simples, ou syphilitiques, blennorragie, épithélioma, végétations, tuberculose). Quelquefois même, elles sont la cause de la stérilité. Il est donc utile d'examiner chez tous les nouveau-nés cet organe anatomique ;

2° Quand il existe une de ces difformités rencontrées chez les nombreux enfants que l'auteur a examinés, on pratique : soit la rupture des adhérences préputiales, quand cette simple intervention suffit, soit une opération irrégulière ou régulière. Souvent, on est forcé de se contenter d'une opération irrégulière par suite de complications accidentelles. On opère alors suivant les circonstances et aucune règle chirurgicale ne peut être imposée. Les opérations régulières consistent à dilater le prépuce ou à en faire l'ablation. La dilatation ou l'excision partielle du prépuce sont de mauvaises opérations, puisqu'il se produit à la suite des phimosis cicatriciels. Au surplus, le prépuce est un organe absolument inutile et sa présence ou son absence n'influe en rien sur le sens génital ;

3° De toutes les interventions préputiales, la circoncision est donc la plus salutaire. Exécutée d'après un procédé simple, que l'auteur a pratiqué un très grand nombre de fois, cette opération n'entraîne que très exceptionnellement des accidents peu graves. Des statistiques nombreuses entre circoncis et non circoncis, on peut conclure que cette opération hygiénique est utile à différents points de vue moraux et matériels.

THÉRAPEUTIQUE DE LA SCOLIOSE : SCOLIOSE INFANTILE ET SCOLIOSE DES ADOLESCENTS

COMMUNICATION

de M. le docteur A. CHIPAULT.

Depuis que je m'occupe de la scoliose, je me suis efforcé de réagir contre deux tendances aussi fâcheuses l'une que l'autre :

1° La tendance à négliger complétement le traitement de cette affection, tendance qui n'est que trop répandue, non seulement chez les parents, naturellement timorés, des malades, mais encore chez les médecins qui préfèrent l'abstention à la responsabilité qu'entraîne la surveillance d'une affection laborieuse et longue à soigner. Au début, c'est l'insignifiance de la difformité qu'on invoque et l'éventualité, si rare, de la voir disparaître spontanément; plus tard, c'est la médiocrité de l'état général, avec cette formule toute faite : le malade est hors d'état de supporter un traitement sévère. Considérations aussi fausses l'une que l'autre.

2° La tendance, non moins fâcheuse, de beaucoup de spécialistes, à traiter toute scoliose, quels qu'en soient la nature, le degré et l'ancienneté, par un traitement toujours le même. Celui-ci, c'est un corset orthopédique qu'il ordonne, à prendre toujours chez le même fabricant: celui-là, ce sont des mouvements, gymnastiques ou autres, qu'il s'agisse d'une scoliose infantile ou d'une scoliose de l'adolescence, qu'il s'agisse d'une scoliose récente ou d'une scoliose ankylosée, avec les difformités secondaires les plus énormes.

Heureux lorsque ces prescriptions ne tombent que dans le ridicule : comme celle que j'ai vue, sur l'ordonnance d'un orthopédiste cependant bien connu, de se tenir debout, levant la jambe pendant un quart d'heure, matin et soir, du côté de la convexité, dans les cas de scoliose ancienne et irréductible.

Or, contrairement à cette indifférence et à ces prescriptions systématiques qui n'en sont au fond qu'une forme dissimulée, je crois que l'on peut toujours beaucoup dans la scoliose, mais à condition de mettre dans le choix et la direction de la thérapeutique à suivre, de l'expérience et du doigté.

C'est ce que je vais essayer de démontrer en passant successivement en revue les deux grandes formes de la scoliose, la scoliose des adolescents et la scoliose infantile, à leurs différentes phases.

I

SCOLIOSE DES ADOLESCENTS.

La scoliose des adolescents, scoliose de beaucoup la plus commune, scoliose type, doit être envisagée, pour plus de commodité, à trois étapes successives de son évolution, étapes qui comportent nécessairement entre elles toutes sortes d'intermédiaires, auxquelles seront applicables des traitements d'une gravité et d'une durée également intermédiaires.

1re étape. Cas sans difformité thoracique. — Une première série de

cas est présentée au chirurgien alors qu'il existe seulement une déviation vertébrale plus ou moins accentuée. A cette période, l'affection
passe parfois inaperçue des parents inattentifs, qui remarquent seulement que leur enfant se tient mal, qu'il a une épaule plus basse que
l'autre. Comme il s'agit presque toujours de fillettes, c'est à la corsetière à leur donner l'éveil. En leur disant que les corsets ne peuvent
rien contre l'affection qui se développe et qu'au contraire un traitement approprié remettra rapidement les choses en l'état, elle leur
rendra un réel service, car la scoliose est très loin de s'arrêter à cette
phase aussi souvent qu'on le croit, et on peut au contraire la faire
disparaître, entièrement, à l'aide d'un traitement nullement laborieux,
et qui durera quelques mois à peine.

Voici celui que je suis dans la circonstance :

1° J'applique, dans la suspension par les pieds, un corset plâtré
bien modelé.

Je demande tout d'abord que l'on ne s'effraie pas de cette suspension
par les pieds. Son emploi, innové par mon ami Levassort, qui l'a
décrit dans mes *Travaux de neurologie chirurgicale* (1898, p. 556) et
qu'il a bien à tort abandonné, est de tout point satisfaisant. Elle est
bien supérieure à la suspension par la tête, si pénible pour certains, ou même à la station debout prolongée, qui fatigue plus qu'on
ne saurait croire les sujets de grande taille. Au contraire, je n'ai
jamais vu aucun enfant se plaindre de la suspension par les pieds :
avertis, et doucement suspendus ils ne s'étonnent même pas, et
causent au chirurgien tout le temps que demande la confection de
l'appareil.

Je suis tellement convaincu que la suspension par les pieds, qui
n'est au fond qu'un degré de plus que la position de Trendelenburg,
est supérieure à la suspension par la tête que je ne saurais trop engager mes confrères à en faire l'essai, avant de s'en inquiéter.

Quoi qu'il en soit, la suspension par les pieds réalise, dans les cas
que nous étudions, le moyen de sustentation non seulement le moins
pénible, mais aussi le plus satisfaisant ; en effet :

a) Elle suffit à elle seule pour permettre à la colonne vertébrale,
par le simple poids de la tête, de reprendre sa rectitude ;

b) Elle permet de faire un corset plâtré parfait, très léger, ce qui
n'est pas à négliger, mais encore efficace et élégant : l'efficacité tenant à ce qu'on peut le faire remonter très haut sous les aisselles, et
descendre très bas sur les hanches où, s'appliquant par une large
surface, il ne détermine ni gêne, ni eschares, contrairement à un
corset qui y appuierait par ses bords : l'élégance à ce que, dans cette

attitude, on le fait, presque involontairement, cambré des reins, bien bombé en avant du thorax et bien appliqué en haut du dos. Son seul inconvénient esthétique est de tenir les épaules hautes : mais c'est une des conditions essentielles de son efficacité, et les mères, qui s'inquiètent d'un rien dans ces cas dont elles ne soupçonnent pas la gravité possible, doivent être assurées que le cou se dégagera à nouveau dès que l'appareil ne sera plus porté.

Quoi qu'il en soit, ce corset dont on vérifie et rectifie au besoin les proportions, lorsqu'il est sec, sur l'enfant mis debout, est fendu en avant sur la ligne médiane, puis recouvert d'une toile fine à laquelle sont adaptées de chaque côté de la fente, des rangées de crochets; on le termine en entourant le rebord qui portera dans l'aisselle d'une couche de molleton épais.

2° Une fois par jour, le matin au lever de préférence, ce corset est retiré: on procède au lavage complet du corps de l'enfant; on fait une séance de massage et d'exercices vertébraux, et l'on termine en passant le long de la colonne vertébrale une éponge imbibée d'eau froide alcoolisée.

Les massages et exercices seront les suivants :

a) L'enfant debout, on la fera se cambrer, soit en avant, soit en arrière, soit latéralement, en l'appuyant par sa colonne vertébrale sur le poing ou le genou.

b) L'enfant couchée sur le ventre on appuiera sur la colonne vertébrale et on la fera se redresser, à l'aide de ses mains; on la saisira ensuite à bras le corps, mains appuyées du côté de la convexité, et on la fera résister à ce mouvement.

c) On terminera par des manipulations le long de la colonne vertébrale, du côté de sa convexité.

La séance terminée, on replacera de suite le corset, en soulevant l'enfant par les aisselles pour augmenter l'intervalle entre celles-ci et les hanches et redresser la colonne vertébrale.

Ce traitement mixte, contention par le corset, exercices, devra durer de trois à six mois.

On le fera suivre d'une seconde période de six mois environ, pendant laquelle on habituera l'enfant à se passer de l'un et des autres. On fera faire par une corsetière, sur le modèle du corset plâtré, un corset bien haut et bien baleiné: ce corset sera tout d'abord porté quelques heures, puis toute la journée; le corset plâtré ne sera plus porté que la nuit, et enfin abandonné. Les massages et exercices seront également laissés de côté, et l'on se contentera des lotions froides vertébrales.

Le résultat devra être et rester parfait.

2e étape. Cas avec difformité thoracique légère. — Une seconde série de cas de scoliose des adolescents est constituée par ceux plus accentués que les précédents, où, à la déviation vertébrale, s'ajoute une déformation de la cage thoracique, qui tend à faire saillie d'un côté, sans se déprimer encore de l'autre, d'une façon appréciable.

Dans ces cas, on placera, dans la suspension par les pieds, un corset plâtré, fait avec les mêmes précautions que nous avons indiquées tout à l'heure : mais ce corset ne sera pas fendu : il restera inamovible, et l'enfant devra le porter nuit et jour pendant un laps de temps de trois mois environ.

C'est alors, mais alors seulement qu'on remplacera ce traitement immobilisateur par un traitement mixte, analogue à celui que nous avons décrit tout à l'heure et comprenant :

1° Le port d'un corset plâtré amovible :

2° L'ablation de ce corset, tous les matins, pour faire des séances de manipulations locales, des mouvements et des lotions.

Dans le cas particulier, on devra insister d'une façon toute spéciale sur les manipulations de la saillie thoracique et sur les mouvements de flexion latéro-postérieure du rachis.

Enfin l'on terminera par le port d'un corset de corsetière fait sur le modèle du corset plâtré, corset de corsetière porté d'abord concurremment avec lui, puis seul.

Ici encore, on pourra, avec de la patience, obtenir un résultat absolument complet.

3e étape. Cas avec difformité thoracique très accentuée. — C'est du reste seulement dans une troisième catégorie de cas, dans ceux avec difformité thoracique très accentuée, que le traitement deviendra véritablement laborieux.

Il comprendra alors quatre périodes :

a) Une première période, période d'assouplissement, comportera l'exécution de séances sur ma planche à plaques obliques.

Cette planche, que m'a construite M. Collin, permet d'exercer sur le sommet et les extrémités de l'arc scoliotique des pressions à l'aide de plaques à vis mobiles sur des rails parallèles au grand axe de la planche. Ces plaques sont susceptibles d'agir les unes horizontalement au-dessus du niveau de la planche, les autres obliquement de bas en haut et de dehors en dedans. Ces dernières ont l'avantage de joindre à la pression directe une détorsion qui n'est pas à dédaigner. Enfin, on pourra adjoindre aux pressions ainsi exercées, des tractions suivant l'axe, à l'aide de simples bandes de toile fixées, d'une part à la circonférence occipito-mentonnière, d'autre part aux genoux ou au bassin, et serrées par des vis adaptées aux extrémités de la planche.

Les séances pourront être nocturnes, d'une durée de huit à neuf heures, avec simple pression latérale, ou diurnes, d'une durée d'un quart d'heure environ, avec pression plus énergique et tractions surveillées par le chirurgien.

Cette période d'assouplissement doit être d'une sévérité et d'une durée variables suivant le cas: il en est de nombreux où cinq ou six séances diurnes, pendant une semaine suffisent; il en est d'autres, où séances diurnes et séances nocturnes doivent se compléter et s'associer pendant un ou même deux mois.

b) Une seconde période, période de redressement, succède à cette première: elle est essentiellement caractérisée par l'application de corsets plâtrés réducteurs, renouvelés et améliorés jusqu'à ce qu'on ait obtenu tout le redressement que l'on croit possible d'obtenir.

Pour les exécuter, j'ai fait construire par Chazal un appareil que je désigne sous le nom d'appareil vertical de détorsion à plaques. Cet appareil se compose d'un solide trapèze qui supporte en haut, à l'aide d'un crochet et d'une poulie, une tringle de fer en forme de T horizontal, avec une annexe verticale, à la jonction de ses trois branches; en outre le long de ses montants se fixent deux demi-cercles en cuivre, l'un antérieur, l'autre postérieur, sur chacun desquels on adapte, au point voulu, la tige d'une plaque de pression, que la disposition du cercle permet de diriger en porte à faux vers le centre de l'appareil; enfin ces mêmes montants supportent plus bas deux demi-anneaux d'emboîtement transversaux.

Cet appareil, aisément transportable et d'un placement très simple, est employé comme suit :

Le sujet, dont le rachis a été assoupli pendant la période précédente du traitement, est suspendu à la tringle supérieure à l'aide d'une mentonnière, et des poids sont suspendus à ses pieds préalablement munis de bottes plâtrées. Les demi-anneaux transversaux fixent de chaque côté le bassin. Les mains sont placées, celle correspondant à la saillie thoracique sur la branche postéro-antérieure de la tringle passant en dehors; l'autre sur la branche verticale, le bras passé en arrière de la branche transversale. Enfin, sur les demi-cercles sont adaptées : en arrière une plaque de pression allant porter à faux sur la saillie thoracique; en avant une autre plaque faisant, également à faux, de la contre-pression. On réalise ainsi, on le voit, des tractions, des pressions et de la détorsion, c'est-à-dire les trois éléments du redressement rationnel de toute difformité scoliotique.

Ces précautions prises, le chirurgien entoure le corps du sujet d'une mince couche de coton hydrophile, recouvrant les plaques de pression, puis construit le corset à l'aide de bandes étroites de tarlatane trempées extemporanément dans du plâtre de modeleur un peu épais. Le corset doit, comme je l'ai déjà dit, remonter très haut sous les aisselles et descendre très bas sur les hanches. Lorsqu'il est terminé, on retire les tiges des plaques de pression, qui restent ainsi englobées dans l'appareil, on enlève les poids des pieds et on met le sujet horizontalement sur le dos, jusqu'à ce que, d'ordinaire une demi-heure après, on puisse le faire se tenir debout, abraser économiquement les bords supérieur et inférieur du corset, en un mot lui donner sa forme définitive.

J'ai proposé de désigner le corset ainsi construit, du nom de corset plâtré de détorsion à plaques.

Ce premier corset sera changé au bout de quinze ou vingt jours et remplacé par un autre, changé à son tour au bout du même laps de temps et ainsi de suite, jusqu'à ce que le redressement obtenu soit ou parfait, ou tout au moins satisfaisant et correspondant à ce qu'on croit pouvoir obtenir. Cela demande de trois à cinq mois.

La seconde période de traitement, la période de réduction, est alors terminée.

c) La troisième période, période de contention permanente, est moins laborieuse.

Elle consiste à mettre au sujet, dont l'attitude est devenue satisfaisante, un corset plâtré ordinaire, dans la suspension tête en bas, suivant la technique que nous avons déjà indiquée. Ce corset simplement contenteur devra avoir les qualités que nous avons signalées pour les corsets de cette sorte, et, en plus, dans le cas particulier, une grande solidité ; il devra être changé tous les six mois environ.

Cette troisième période durera de un an et demi à deux ans.

d) Une quatrième période, période de contention intermittente, commencera alors.

A ce moment je recommande d'ordinaire :

Pendant la nuit, le repos dans une gouttière plâtrée, modelée sur le sujet placé dans le décubitus horizontal et légèrement rembourrée. Je n'insiste pas sur les détails de construction de cette gouttière analogue à celles de Hebel et de Vulpian. On suivra donc, pour sa fabrication, les conseils de ces auteurs sans y annexer les tiges d'acier et les bandes réductrices dont ils parlent et qui n'auraient rien à faire ici, puisque l'appareil, dans les conditions où nous l'employons, est destiné à jouer un rôle purement contenteur.

Pendant le jour, le port d'un corset plâtré léger, amovible, placé le matin après une heure de massage, d'exercices méthodiques et de lotions.

Avec le temps ce traitement deviendra de moins en moins sévère : en particulier on remplacera le corset plâtré par un corset de corsetière fait sur son modèle ; ce dernier devra être porté des années, sinon indéfiniment.

En résumé, dans les cas de ce genre, le traitement a pour but de substituer à l'ankylose pathologique en mauvaise attitude une ankylose thérapeutique en bonne attitude. La 1re période a pour but d'assouplir l'ankylose pathologique. La 2e période la détruit dans la mesure du possible. La 3e période permet au rachis de reconstituer la nouvelle ankylose. La 4e période, enfin, surveille cette ankylose, constate comment elle se comporte vis-à-vis d'une sustentation de moins en moins sévère du rachis, enfin redonne à celle-ci une certaine souplesse.

En effet, et cela on ne saurait trop le répéter, on doit, pour être sûr d'un bon résultat durable, avoir à la fin de la 3e période une colonne vertébrale plutôt trop droite et trop rigide et devoir ensuite défaire en partie ce qu'on a fait.

Il y a du reste des cas où malgré la durée de la contention, l'ankylose thérapeutique ne se fait pas : c'est alors que l'on recourra à la fixation apophysaire par les ligatures ou les griffes, moyen bien moins fréquemment indiqué que dans les cyphoses pottiques ou autres, mais qu'il est cependant bon de n'y point négliger, car il y donne, dans les cas où il est indiqué, des résultats qu'il est véritablement seul à pouvoir donner.

II

SCOLIOSE INFANTILE.

La scoliose infantile, trop souvent confondue avec la scoliose des adolescents, malgré l'âge différent des malades, l'évolution plus rapide, la gravité plus grande encore, demande, elle aussi, à être envisagée thérapeutiquement à plusieurs étapes de son évolution.

1re étape. Cas à la phase aiguë. — Dans les cas à la phase aiguë, caractérisée par de la fièvre, des douleurs rachidiennes, tous les symptômes des affections rachitiques à la période d'évolution, on appliquera dans la suspension par les pieds un corset plâtré inamovible qui, en deux jours, calmera les douleurs, et, en trois ou quatre mois, permettra l'ankylose en bonne attitude. Quelques séances de massage et d'exercices suffiront pour compléter le traitement.

On aura ainsi évité l'évolution d'une difformité déplorable, dont la seule trace subsistante sera un arrêt de développement du rachis qui donnera au tronc, par rapport aux membres, une longueur relativement moindre.

2ᵉ étape. Cas à la phase de déviation constituée. — Les cas à la phase de déviation constituée montrent quelle intensité peut, dans la scoliose infantile, atteindre la difformité. Le tronc effondré ne représente plus que 1/6 ou même 1/7 de la hauteur totale du corps; les fausses côtes plongent dans le bassin; l'abdomen bombe, énorme, au-devant du pubis et des cuisses; le thorax est porté en presque totalité d'un côté de la ligne verticale passant par l'entrejambe, le plus souvent à gauche et son axe coïncide avec l'axe du membre inférieur correspondant; la colonne vertébrale, déviée à l'extrême, se cache sous l'omoplate. Il existe des déformations secondaires souvent très accentuées, en haut du côté du cou et de la tête, en bas du côté du bassin et des membres inférieurs.

Le traitement doit être calqué sur celui que nous avons décrit à propos des cas graves de scoliose des adolescents.

Il comprendra donc quatre périodes :

a) Une période d'assouplissement;

b) Une période de redressement;

c) Une période de contention permanente;

d) Une période de contention intermittente avec massage.

Mais on doit savoir que, dans le cas actuel, les corsets de redressement ont besoin d'être surveillés avec une sévérité toute spéciale, tant qu'une attitude réellement satisfaisante n'est pas obtenue; on ne saurait en effet se faire une idée de la rapidité avec laquelle, dans la scoliose rachitique, l'ankylose se forme : c'est une difficulté, mais c'est aussi un grand avantage, car elle ne manque pour ainsi dire jamais, et l'on peut, sans crainte d'être déçu, compter sur elle pour maintenir le résultat obtenu.

C'est dire que la fixation apophysaire ne sera ici jamais utile.

En somme, on le voit d'après l'étude qui précède, et qui est bien loin d'avoir la prétention de répondre à toutes les données du problème, le traitement de la scoliose est loin d'être, ainsi qu'on le dit et l'écrit d'ordinaire, toujours le même; certes ses principes généraux ne peuvent que peu changer, mais leur application doit varier d'un cas à l'autre, au point qu'il n'y a vraiment, entre certains des traitements que nous avons eu à décrire, rien de commun, au moins en apparence.

Je crois toutefois devoir terminer par deux remarques générales, qui répondront à deux questions que soulève la thérapeutique de plus d'un cas de scoliose.

1° Quelle que soit la gravité des cas, le chloroforme n'est pour ainsi dire jamais utile : il n'y a pas dans la scoliose de contraction musculaire à vaincre. L'anesthésie y sera donc réservée aux malades peu raisonnables, et aussi à ceux chez qui l'on sera obligé de recourir à la fixation apophysaire directe.

2° Quelle que soit la durée et la sévérité du traitement, il n'a jamais d'influence fâcheuse sur l'état général du sujet. Au contraire, celui-ci, dont le rachis ne se fatigue pas, dont les organes ne sont plus comprimés et déplacés par les os déviés, reprend rapidement la bonne apparence et l'activité qu'il avait d'ordinaire perdues : c'est là une conséquence tellement constante du traitement régulièrement et méthodiquement suivie qu'on peut affirmer, si elle fait défaut, qu'il y a, dans son exécution, quelque erreur. Un bon état général est à proprement parler le critérium de son application rationnelle.

On ne devra point pour cela négliger d'associer au traitement orthopédique les précautions d'ordre général : les phosphates et glycérophosphates, le séjour, pendant l'été, dans les montagnes ou au bord de la mer, aideront, à n'en pas douter, utilement l'organisme à suffire à la réparation du squelette.

PATHOGÉNIE DE LA SCOLIOSE DORSALE GAUCHE CHEZ LES ADOLESCENTS

COMMUNICATION

de M. le docteur PIERRE,

de Berck-sur-Mer.

D'après la statistique de Drachmann, la scoliose dorsale gauche ne représente que 7.9 pour 100 de toutes les formes observées.

Cela explique qu'on la traite un peu sans façon dans les auteurs classiques ; qu'on passe légèrement sur sa pathogénie : qu'on en résume par un *vice versa* le traitement déjà décrit pour la scoliose dorsale droite. Même ceux qui mettent sur le compte de la prépondérance du bras droit la plus grande fréquence de la scoliose dorsale droite n'ont pas l'air de s'embarrasser outre mesure de l'objection qui coule à pic leur pathogénie quand la scoliose dorsale gauche est portée par un droitier.

C'est ce point de pathogénie que nous allons tenter d'éclaircir.

Avant d'être une maladie localisée à la colonne vertébrale, la scoliose est une maladie générale de la croissance, d'origine encore inconnue, coïncidant à peu près toujours avec des troubles dyspeptiques. Comme le rachitisme avec lequel elle a beaucoup d'analogies cliniques, la scoliose au début frappe tous les tissus, mais plus particulièrement le tissu osseux et, dans ce dernier, plutôt certaines parties du squelette que d'autres. C'est un fait d'observation courante que la plupart des scoliotiques sont atteints en même temps de genu valgum, ou de pied plat, ou de déformations rachitiques des cartilages chondro-sternaux. Parmi ces anomalies de développement, il en est une dont la fréquence est telle que beaucoup d'orthopédistes ont voulu lui attribuer la genèse de l'inflexion rachidienne dans la plupart des cas. Je veux parler du raccourcissement du membre inférieur gauche. On peut le constater dès la première heure, dès le premier soupçon de scoliose, lorsque les troubles dyspeptiques attirent encore davantage l'attention que la légère élévation de l'une des deux épaules. Ce raccourcissement est réel et non pas seulement apparent. On le constate, que le sujet soit mesuré debout ou couché : il s'aggrave parfois d'un pied plat du même côté. On s'explique cette localisation par une *inversion* de la loi de suractivité fonctionnelle, plus grande, comme l'a démontré M. P. Godin devant l'Académie des sciences, dans la séance du 15 février 1900, sur le membre inférieur gauche que sur le droit. Voici les conclusions de ce travail de M. Godin :

« 1° Le membre supérieur droit est plus gros que le gauche de 0 cent. 5 ;

« 2° Pour les membres pelviens, c'est au contraire le gauche qui l'emporte sur le droit ; la différence est de 0 cent. 5 et elle s'affirme au niveau du mollet ;

« 3° La suractivité fonctionnelle est donc croisée. La nutrition plus active qu'elle entraîne doit avoir autant d'influence sur l'allongement des membres qui en sont le siège que sur leur augmentation de volume. C'est, en effet, ce qui a lieu.

« Le membre supérieur droit moins la main (humérus et radius) est plus long que le gauche de 1 cent. Le membre inférieur gauche moins la hauteur du pied (fémur et tibia) est plus long que le droit de 1 cent.

Ces différences de longueur se retrouvent pour une part proportionnelle dans les segments des membres :

« 4° Les gauchers observés constituent un contrôle de valeur : chez un grand nombre, la supériorité de largeur et de longueur reste croisée, mais en sens inverse ;

« 5° La plus grande longueur du membre inférieur gauche, chez les droitiers, relève tout le côté correspondant du tronc ; l'épine iliaque gauche, plus haute de 1 cent., relève l'inclinaison du bassin. Il en est de même de la ceinture thoracique, dont l'extrémité scapulaire gauche domine la droite de 1 cent. en moyenne ;

« 6° Le mollet gauche, qui est le plus volumineux, est aussi plus bas que le droit de près de 1 cent. ;

« 7° Les oreilles offrent également une notable et presque constante asymétrie : en mesurant leur hauteur, on trouve 0 cent. 5 de plus en faveur de l'oreille gauche. »

Or, chacun sait qu'un organe est d'autant plus exposé aux processus morbides que la suractivité fonctionnelle en est plus grande. Le membre inférieur gauche, l'emportant normalement sur le droit, devait être atteint de préférence par la maladie scoliotique. Il l'est dans tous ses segments (pied, jambe, cuisse) qui sont à la fois plus courts et plus minces. La différence des pieds saute à l'œil ; celle des jambes est à peine mesurable ; celle des cuisses est très nette ; la différence de longueur, le sujet debout, porte presque entièrement sur le segment fémoral.

Qu'en conclure ? que ce raccourcissement entraînera une inflexion lombaire que compensera une inflexion dorsale et que toute la genèse de la scoliose est dans ce fait primordial ? Nous n'allons pas jusque-là : nous croyons que la colonne vertébrale peut être malade pour son propre compte, indépendamment du contre-coup que peut avoir sur elle le raccourcissement du membre inférieur, mais que ce dernier doit, dans la majorité des cas, jouer le rôle d'amorce en latéralisant l'axe des pressions vertébrales et attirant sur les corps vertébraux, par le fait amoindris dans leur résistance, le poison inconnu des déformations osseuses.

Si l'on admet ces prémisses, la plus grande fréquence de la scoliose primitivement lombaire se comprend de soi, ainsi que la production à droite de la courbure dorsale compensatrice. Si l'usage habituel du bras droit agit uniquement à titre de cause aggravante, par le même mécanisme, le raccourcissement du membre inférieur droit entraînera l'inflexion à droite du segment lombaire de la colonne vertébrale, et comme compensation, l'inflexion à gauche du segment dorsal.

On comprend qu'une paralysie infantile, qu'une tumeur blanche frappant le membre inférieur droit puissent, par contre-coup, produire une gibbosité costale gauche. Mais ce n'est là qu'une des deux causes, et peut-être pas la plus fréquente, de cette forme de gibbosité.

Au lieu d'alterner avec le membre le plus court, la courbure dorsale peut se trouver du côté homonyme. On peut avoir une gibbosité gauche avec un membre gauche plus court et *vice versa*.

J'ai rencontré pour la première fois cette disposition chez une fillette de 12 ans et demi, Marguerite D..., dont la scoliose remontait à l'âge de 6 ans et qui n'avait eu pour tout traitement jusque-là qu'un corset orthopédique, d'ailleurs porté peu de temps. La forte inclinaison à gauche frappait l'œil, sitôt qu'on la voyait. Le raccourcissement à la fois apparent et réel du membre inférieur gauche était de 1 cent., presque tout entier localisé à la cuisse. Le pied était de 1/2 cent. plus court et plus étroit que le droit. L'examen du dos, dessiné, révélait une triple courbure.

La première, de 5 millimètres de flèche, s'étendait de la cinquième vertèbre lombaire à la quatrième.

La seconde, de 1 cent. et demi de flèche, s'étendait de la quatrième vertèbre lombaire à la cinquième dorsale. Elle compensait la première : elle refoulait donc le flanc droit.

La troisième, courbure principale, s'étendait de la sixième dorsale à la deuxième cervicale. Elle mesurait 2 cent. et demi de flèche.

La gibbosité, considérable, beaucoup plus que ne semble l'indiquer la hauteur de la flèche, occupait toute la hauteur des côtes. Elle finissait en coup de hache, presque au niveau de la crête iliaque.

La jeune fille était *droitière*. Chose assez curieuse, la partie antérieure de la poitrine était à peine déformée. La bosse antérieure n'existait presque pas. Les seins étaient à peu de chose près au même niveau : ce qui tenait à ce que les côtes du côté droit avaient presque entièrement conservé leur place normale.

Voilà donc une bosse costale gauche pour la production de laquelle je n'ai trouvé d'autre facteur que le raccourcissement du membre inférieur gauche. Pour être complet, je dois ajouter que les organes du cou et de la face étaient parfaitement symétriques.

On m'objectera peut-être que la simple inflexion de la colonne vertébrale, compensatrice du raccourcissement de l'un des deux membres, ne suffit pas à créer une scoliose, qu'il y faut quelque chose de plus, un mouvement de torsion, la déformation angulaire des côtes, un ensemble de lésions trophiques. C'est de toute évidence. Aussi ai-je seulement dit que le raccourcissement amorçait la scoliose, qu'il en était la cause occasionnelle, qu'il en déterminait le sens. Si cela n'était pas, comment s'expliquer la si grande fréquence de la scoliose primitivement lombaire gauche ?

Pour résumer cette communication sous forme de conclusion, nous dirons :

1° Que toute scoliose droite ou gauche a son origine première dans la maladie générale qui atteint le tissu osseux de l'adolescent ;

2° Que la position de la gibbosité à droite ou à gauche de l'axe médian du corps est directement influencée par le raccourcissement de l'un des deux membres inférieurs, ordinairement le gauche ;

3° Que presque toujours la gibbosité se trouve du côté opposé au membre le plus court ;

4° Qu'il est des cas cependant où elle se trouve du même côté : ce sont ceux où les deux premières courbures se compensent dans les lombes et sont suivies d'une troisième qui occupe la région du dos ;

5° Qu'il en est ainsi dans une partie des cas de gibbosité dorsale gauche.

Cette pathogénie nous semble rationnelle et d'accord avec les faits observés.

PATHOGÉNIE DE LA SCOLIOSE DORSALE GAUCHE CHEZ LES ADOLESCENTS

COMMUNICATION

de M. le docteur PIERRE,

de Berck-sur-Mer.

Bien que la scoliose dorsale gauche ne représente, d'après Drachmann, que les 7,9 0/0 de toutes les formes observées, elle n'en est pas moins digne d'intérêt, ne serait-ce que pour sa pathogénie, laissée trop dans l'ombre par les auteurs classiques.

Normalement, la suractivité fonctionnelle des membres étant croisée, le membre supérieur droit l'emporte sur le gauche et le membre inférieur gauche sur le droit, en longueur et en grosseur.

Dans la scoliose, c'est justement l'inverse. Le premier effet de cette maladie, c'est justement l'arrêt momentané de la croissance du membre inférieur gauche qui devient plus court et plus mince que le droit. Étant donné le rôle joué par l'inégalité statique sur la production des courbures rachidiennes, ce raccourcissement entraînera l'inflexion à gauche du segment lombaire de la colonne vertébrale et, par compensation, l'inflexion à droite de la région dorsale. La gibbosité costale droite se trouvera du côté opposé au membre le plus court.

Par un mécanisme analogue, le raccourcissement du membre inférieur droit pourra produire une scoliose dorsale gauche.

Au lieu de se trouver du côté opposé au membre le plus court, la gibbosité costale peut se rencontrer aussi du même côté. Le raccourcissement du membre inférieur gauche peut déterminer une scoliose dorsale gauche : c'est toutes les fois que les deux courbures primaire et secondaire, au lieu de se faire équilibre, l'une au dos, l'autre aux reins, comme c'est la règle, se compensent sur un très court rayon dans la région lombo-dorsale, laissant place à une courbure tertiaire, la principale, qui occupe presque toute la hauteur du dos, du côté gauche, déterminant ainsi la gibbosité costale gauche.

CONSIDÉRATIONS AU SUJET DE DEUX CAS DE TUMEURS MALIGNES
DE L'ABDOMEN CHEZ LES ENFANTS

COMMUNICATION

de M. le docteur ALBERT MILLS,

Adjoint de la clinique de chirurgie infantile de M. le professeur CHARON, à l'hôpital St Pierre à Bruxelles.

Messieurs,

Permettez-moi de vous entretenir pendant quelques instants de deux cas de tumeurs abdominales malignes qui se sont présentées à notre observation dans le service, et sur l'histoire desquels des considérations intéressantes peuvent être émises. Il s'agit d'un cas de tuberculome du grand épiploon chez une fillette de onze ans et d'un cas de sarcome du mésentère chez un garçon de cinq ans. Ces cas présentaient des caractères propres à chacun d'eux et d'autres qui leur étaient communs.

Parmi les caractères communs nous trouvons la similitude des symptômes, au palper et à la percussion, l'absence de troubles généraux soit dans le fonctionnement du tube digestif, soit dans les fonctions des glandes dépendant du tractus intestinal, de plus l'absence d'amaigrissement des sujets dans les deux cas. Au nombre des caractères différentiels nous devons mettre l'évolution lente du tuberculome, comparée à la progression ultra-rapide du sarcome (trois semaines). L'intervention dans les deux cas a été opératoire, à savoir :

Laparatomie exploratrice simple suivie d'amélioration sinon de guérison pour le tuberculome, suivie de mort dans le cas du sarcome.

Vous voyez, Messieurs, combien dans le genre du cas qui nous occupe le problème se pose redoutable et combien sa solution est difficile, combien aussi le pronostic doit être réservé. Nous voyons la laparotomie exploratrice avec décollement partiel de la tumeur apparaître comme l'intervention de choix et curative dans le cas de tuberculome de l'épiploon et cette même intervention devenir un simple moyen de constatation dans le deuxième et ne pas empêcher la mort du sujet.

Un point sur lequel nous désirons encore attirer votre attention est la rareté de ces cas. En effet, Messieurs, sans vouloir faire ici un historique bibliographique complet de ces affections, nous donnerons néanmoins quelques renseignements à propos de chacun d'eux.

Les cas de péritonite tuberculeuse ne sont pas rares ; cependant, il n'est pas fréquent de trouver que des masses tuberculeuses de différents âges forment un ensemble tel qu'elles aient l'aspect d'une grosse tumeur caparaçonnant toute la région de l'estomac. Lucas-Championnière[1] cite un cas qui se rapproche du nôtre. Chez son malade le point de départ était une hernie qui avait déterminé une inflammation de l'épiploon, d'où épiploïte formant une grosse masse indurée, couvrant comme d'une cuirasse toute la paroi antérieure de l'estomac. Quoique le point de départ soit différent nous estimons qu'il y a entre ces cas des points d'analogie et que, sous la forme que nous citons, ces tumeurs sont rares.

En ce qui concerne le *sarcome du mésentère*, si nous recherchons les cas publiés en 1898, nous ne trouvons que les quelques observations suivantes : Vinogradow[2] a observé un sarcome globo-cellulaire qui, à la naissance gros comme une noisette, est devenu à six semaines gros comme une tête d'enfant ; l'auteur qui a fait à l'hospice des Enfants-Assistés de Saint-Pétersbourg plus de 5000 autopsies de nouveau-nés n'a trouvé de tumeurs semblables que quatre fois. Henoch pense que les sarcomes du mésentère chez les nouveau-nés ont, comme point de départ, l'hyperplasie embryonnaire des ganglions

1. Société de Chirurgie, Paris.
2. *Meditzinié Obozrinskoe*, mars 1898.

péritonéaux ou des reins. Doukanof[1] cite un cas de sarcome du mésentère : l'auteur a fait la laparotomie et l'excision, l'opération a été suivie de succès. Lejars[2] a observé un myxo-lipome du mésentère et du mésocôlon. Heinricius[3] considère comme des cas très rares les tumeurs abdominales constituées par des sarcomes primaires du mésentère ou de l'épiploon ; il a extirpé un sarcome primaire de l'épiploon constitué par des petites cellules rondes et par des éléments fusiformes ; la tumeur avait le volume d'une petite tête d'homme. La petite fille âgée de 5 ans a survécu à l'opération, mais est morte de récidive quatre mois et demi plus tard. Dans le cas qui nous occupe, la survie a été très courte, quelques heures seulement : le shock opératoire en est la seule cause. Il survenait chez un organisme débilité par un sarcome, occupant tout le mésentère, remplissant le bassin et enclavant dans sa masse le tube digestif presque tout entier, transformant les anses intestinales en véritable tuyau traversant une masse dure. Nous arrêtons ici cet aperçu historique, croyant bien que vous estimerez comme nous que la rareté des cas les rendait d'un intérêt puissant.

L'anatomie pathologique de ces deux cas nous a paru bien intéressante.

Le *tuberculome de l'épiploon* présentait des tubercules de tout âge, attestation évidente d'une formation lentement progressive. On rencontrait à la surface de la tumeur et tout près l'un de l'autre, des tubercules crus, roses et tout petits, à côté d'autres granulomes jaunâtres ou blancs, beaucoup plus gros, ayant déjà subi l'infiltration calcaire, la transformation colloïde ou la dégénérescence graisseuse, d'autres également durs et déjà scléreux. Nous n'avons pu pousser plus loin l'investigation de la tumeur à cause de l'issue favorable du cas.

Le sarcome du mésentère a été l'objet d'une étude beaucoup plus approfondie, nous avons fait des coupes nombreuses, épaisses de 30 à 40 μ en différents points de la tumeur, aussi bien dans la périphérie que dans la profondeur de la tumeur. Elles ont été colorées par les divers procédés de coloration (différents carmins, hématoxyline, bleu de méthylène) et ont démontré que la tumeur était constituée par des petites cellules rondes, sans substance intercellulaire, embryonnaires, d'un diamètre d'environ 15 à 20 μ, à gros noyaux centraux. Les cellules dans la constitution de leurs noyaux témoignaient d'une croissance ultra-rapide (noyaux indivis, protoplasme très

1. DOUKANOF. *Chirurgien*, t. III. p. 417.
2. LEJARS. Société de Chirurgie. Paris, 1898.
3. Finska läkarisälk, 1898.

hyalin, etc.), nous avions donc bien affaire à un sarcome à petites cellules rondes, la forme la plus rapide et la plus maligne de ce genre de tumeurs.

Une coupe sur laquelle notre attention a été particulièrement attirée est celle que nous avons faite en y comprenant la partie du sarcome enveloppant l'intestin et la paroi intestinale elle-même. Cette coupe nous montrait la paroi intestinale absolument saine (épithélium, membrane basale et tissu conjonctif sous-épithélial) et graduellement en s'enfonçant dans la profondeur de la tumeur, c'est-à-dire en s'éloignant de la paroi intestinale, les cellules sarcomateuses apparaissaient pour, finalement, remplir d'une façon intégrale et pure tout le champ du microscope. Ceci prouve à l'évidence et une fois de plus, l'origine mésodermique du sarcome aussi bien que sa parfaite innocuité, au point de vue de la malignité envers les tissus épiblastiques comme par exemple ici, l'épithélium de la paroi intestinale.

Nous croyons avec Henoch que l'origine de ces tumeurs existe dans une croissance embryonnaire mésodermique des cellules des ganglions lymphatiques du mésentère. Nos coupes nous ont semblé appuyer cette manière de voir par l'aspect des condensations cellulaires que l'on trouvait dans certaines coupes, la persistance de quelques fibres conjonctives et surtout par le fait de l'origine profonde de la tumeur et non péri-intestinale. Nous espérons, Messieurs, avoir, par les différents ordres d'observations que nous avons eu l'honneur d'exposer devant vous, justifié et de l'intérêt et de la raison de notre communication. Nous croyons que la conclusion scientifique à en déduire est une démonstration en plus de l'origine mésodermique et embryonnaire du sarcome et que le résultat pratique à en tirer est que, dans les cas de tumeurs malignes de l'abdomen chez les enfants, la laparotomie exploratrice est indiquée d'urgence. Elle doit être suivie si possible du diagnostic de la tumeur et, dans les cas de tuberculose épiploïque ou péritonéale abondante, suivie également de décollement étendu des feuillets péritonéaux; en agissant ainsi elle peut être curative.

DISCUSSION.

M. Villemin. — Dans les très intéressantes communications que vous venez d'entendre, comme dans ce qui a été écrit sur ce si difficile sujet de la scoliose, certaines contradictions m'ont toujours frappé. On nous parle d'une part, d'ankylose des corps vertébraux, d'arthrite ankylosante du rachis et, de l'autre, d'immobilisation prolongée pendant des mois et des mois dans des corsets plâtrés. Pourquoi dans le cas particulier de la scoliose mettre en œuvre des moyens thérapeutiques tout à fait opposés à ceux qui nous réussissent d'ordinaire? Pourquoi murer dans du plâtre pendant des mois, parfois des années, une ankylose vertébrale alors que tout le monde s'accorde à reconnaître la mobilisation et le massage comme constituant le traitement rationnel d'une ankylose du coude ou du genou par exemple?

C'est ce qui nous a engagés, mon ami le D' Mayet et moi, à chercher dans une voie tout à fait différente, celle de la mobilisation répétée, quotidienne, pendant toute la durée du traitement. Dans le service de M. le professeur Lannelongue, depuis cinq mois, 40 malades ont été mis en traitement de la manière suivante : le sujet est couché dans la position abdominale sur une table, la tête et les bras dépassant l'extrémité de cette table, la poitrine légèrement soulevée par un coussin dur; dans cette situation la gibbosité costale devient très saillante. Sur cette gibbosité avec la paume de la main on produit une série de refoulements vigoureux sous l'influence desquels au bout d'une dizaine de minutes on reconnaît d'une manière constante : 1° une diminution de la saillie de la gibbosité ; 2° une détorsion du rachis; 3° une diminution de la flèche vertébrale. Les séances ont lieu tous les jours ou tous les deux jours. Limité à ces séances de redressement le traitement a toujours produit une amélioration ; dans certains cas spéciaux il comprend en outre le port d'un corset agissant par refoulement à l'aide d'une série de plaques métalliques et maintenant les résultats obtenus. D'ailleurs peu importe le manuel opératoire employé : la mobilisation est à notre avis le traitement de choix de la scoliose. Depuis cinq mois que le D' Mayet poursuit ses recherches à l'hôpital des Enfants-Malades, il a toujours obtenu une amélioration considérable même dans les scolioses les plus graves et a enregistré nombre de guérisons dans les formes bénignes.

M. FROELICH (de Nancy). — Je m'associe volontiers à la remarque de M. Villemin, et je suis heureux de protester avec lui contre l'immobilisation prolongée dans un appareil plâtré des scoliotiques. Ce traitement est illogique et illusoire.

Illogique, car ce sont les muscles seuls qui redressent la déviation vertébrale et la maintiennent redressée.

Illusoire, car j'ai eu l'occasion plusieurs fois de déplâtrer des malheureux scoliotiques traités par cette méthode ; sans parler de leur amaigrissement et de leur saleté, je puis dire que les enfants flottaient dans leur cuirasse qui était inutile.

Hoffa, Vulpian et d'autres, après avoir essayé le redressement forcé et l'immobilisation plâtrée l'ont abandonné.

Depuis six ans, à la clinique de Nancy, je mobilise la colonne vertébrale, et je fortifie les muscles, et mes résultats sont très encourageants.

Quant au corset, qui doit toujours être amovible, il y a trois catégories de malades qui entrent en ligne de compte :

1° Les uns n'ont pas besoin de corset, leur système musculaire, mû intelligemment, les maintient redressés ;

2° Les autres portent un corset qui leur rappelle sans cesse qu'ils doivent se redresser et peut-être aider cet effort ;

3° Les troisièmes enfin portent un corset pour le même motif que les deuxièmes, mais en plus pour cacher leur difformité.

SAMEDI 4 AOUT

Séance du soir.

TRAITEMENT DU MAL DE POTT APRÈS LE DÉVELOPPEMENT
DE LA DIFFORMITÉ

RAPPORT

de M. le docteur BRADFORD,

de Boston.

Le traitement du mal de Pott, après le développement de la difformité, se présente à l'examen sous deux aspects : 1° le traitement de la maladie elle-même pour son arrêt et la guérison de la condition pathologique; 2° le traitement de la difformité pour la corriger ou pour empêcher son aggravation.

Premièrement, le traitement de la maladie elle-même.

C'est un sujet qui a été bien discuté, mais sur lequel le monde chirurgical est aujourd'hui d'accord. Il est bien entendu que la colonne vertébrale doit être placée dans une position qui fera diminuer ou disparaître la pression intervertébrale à l'endroit de la maladie jusqu'à ce que la cicatrisation soit complète. Cette fixation doit être aussi complète que le permettent l'exercice et l'air pur qui sont si favorables pour avancer les changements métaboliques salutaires et enrayer l'invasion de la tuberculose. Cet exercice, néanmoins, doit être réglé d'après les prescriptions chirurgicales pour éviter les lésions traumatiques des parties malades de la colonne vertébrale. En un mot, le traitement se borne à la fixation propre de la colonne vertébrale, soit dans une position couchée pour les cas les plus aigus, soit dans une fixation complète qui laisse la faculté de marcher dans les cas moins aigus ou pendant la convalescence, cela veut dire aussitôt que la plus petite secousse inévitable en marchant ne produit pas des effets nuisibles.

Correction de la difformité.

En examinant un nombre de colonnes vertébrales atteintes du mal de Pott, on constate qu'elles varient beaucoup dans leurs états et dans leurs courbures. Dans quelques cas. les corps ne sont que peu affectés : dans d'autres, les ravages sont grands. Dans certains cas, la courbure ne peut pas être grande grâce à la résistance des tissus osseux intacts qui sont assez forts pour supporter le poids qui est placé dessus. Mais si la maladie continue sans obstacle, la destruction de la vertèbre sera complète et nous aurons une inclinaison en avant de la colonne et une projection croissante de l'épine dorsale. Si une ostéite ossifiante se déclare, elle est suivie d'une guérison avec difformité. La difformité, comme Ménard l'a démontré, ne dépend pas seulement de la quantité du tissu osseux détruit mais aussi de la partie de la colonne affectée, la difformité étant bien plus grande, pour raisons statiques, dans la région dorsale.

Quoique les essais pour corriger la difformité soient aussi vieux que la chirurgie, le sujet n'a jamais été envisagé avec autant d'activité que de nos jours, grâce aux efforts des chirurgiens français. Autrefois, la courbure était regardée, non seulement comme une condition qu'on ne pouvait pas changer, mais aussi, comme le résultat nécessaire indiquant une guérison : aujourd'hui que la gibbosité est mieux connue on la regarde comme un mal, qui doit être évité ou corrigé quand c'est possible.

Depuis la publication des ouvrages chirurgicaux français sur ce sujet, des corrections forcées ont été entreprises par tout le monde chirurgical, et les résultats obtenus demandent à être considérés avec soin.

Le tableau suivant montre les statistiques d'une correction absolue qui ont servi à la rédaction de cet écrit.

659 cas par 54 opérateurs.
Temps écoulé : de quelques jours à trois ans et plus.

Des cas racontés séparément. 7 ont plus d'un an, 55 plus de six mois.

Morts constatées de tous les cas. 25
Maladies diverses. 5
Tuberculose générale. 4
Lésions traumatiques. suite de l'opération et chloroforme 5
Maladies intercurrentes. 7

Résultats immédiats :

Embarras des voies respiratoires. 7
Douleurs. 6
Choc grave. 5

Abcès présents avant l'opération. 19
    —   rompus 4
    —   soulagés ou absorbés 6
    —   ayant paru. 2
Paralysie constatée avant l'opération. 25
    —   améliorée 17
    —   non améliorée 2
    —   plus mal. 1
La paralysie s'est montrée après dans. . . .   4 cas.

Effet direct sur la difformité dans 240 cas.

Correction complète . . . . 130 —
Correction incomplète. . . . . 94 —
Aucune douleur. . . . . 16 —

Résultat sur 77 cas.

Aucune rechute. . . . . 20 cas.
Rechute légère . . . . 50 —
Rechute totale . . . .   7 —

Ces tableaux ont été relevés, par les Dᵣˢ Vose et Cotton, des publications citées à la fin de cet article.

Quoiqu'il ne faille pas attacher trop d'importance aux statistiques, néanmoins les tableaux que nous venons de voir nous montrent que l'on peut user, avec sécurité, plus de force pour essayer de corriger une gibbosité que cela semblait possible autrefois, 630 cas avec seulement 5 morts, pour l'opération seule.

La quantité de force qui doit être employée avec sécurité doit dépendre de la résistance et de la solidité des os affectés. Il est évidemment antichirurgical de produire des lésions traumatiques aiguës sur un os atteint de tuberculose dans le cours d'une cicatrisation conservatrice. La rectification d'une courbure est bienfaisante si, en diminuant la pression intervertébrale, on emploie peu de force qui puisse blesser. La rectification doit être entreprise d'autant plus promptement que la correction demande moins de force. Si la force est nécessaire pour produire une correction entraînant la fracture des tissus solidifiés, la méthode est inapplicable. L'ostéotomie ne se recommande pas. Si un large trou doit être laissé, demandant un pouvoir réparatif trop grand pour que les tissus malades puissent développer une ostéite ankylosante, on ne doit pas désirer une rectification complète.

Si une masse considérable de détritus caséeux est retenue dans la cavité de la cyphose et si la rectification fait dangereusement augmenter la pression de la masse tuberculeuse retenue sous une plèvre ou sous une paroi péritonéale, on ne doit pas employer de force pour corriger la gibbosité sans le faire avec beaucoup de soin et de jugement. La paralysie provenant du mal de Pott est quelquefois guérie par la correction. D'un autre côté, la paralysie peut avoir pour cause une correction par la force.

Il y a trois cas à examiner.

I. Quand le progrès est actif et lorsque la courbure flexible permet la rectification;

II. Quand la fusion de la partie postérieure de la colonne s'est produite, mais avec une cavité qui n'est pas guérie;

III. Quand la solidification et la fusion sont complètes et on a pour résultat la cure avec difformité.

Le traitement de correction n'est possible que dans le premier cas. Lorsque le traitement par force est entrepris, plusieurs méthodes sont employées : 1° la suspension verticale par la tête; 2° la suspension verticale par la tête et les bras; 3° la traction horizontale du patient couché, avec la force tirant sur la tête, les bras et les jambes; 4° la même chose, mais avec pression de haut en bas sur la gibbosité, le cou et les hanches fixés, le malade étant couché à plat-ventre; 5° traction de la même manière avec le patient couché sur le dos; 6° pression de haut en bas sur le bassin et la partie supérieure du tronc avec résistance remontant sur le dos au point maximum de la projection, le patient étant couché sur le dos, avec la traction de la tête et des pieds ou sans la traction; 7° le patient couché sur le dos avec une pression de bas en haut par le moyen d'une courroie, jointe avec une corde et une poulie, passée sous le patient au point de la projection; 8° correction avec le patient assis, la partie supérieure du tronc étant retenue en arrière pendant que la courbure est poussée en avant au point de la projection, pendant que le bassin est retenu par une courroie. Ces différentes méthodes entraînent deux manières d'appliquer la force, l'une par la pression, l'autre par la traction.

Les expériences sur les cadavres montrent que l'on doit préférer la pression plutôt que celle de la traction, pour une force corrective. La pression a des effets plus précis sur les tissus malades qu'une force de traction qui se perd, en partie, sur les courbes secondaires. Une force de traction entraîne un effort inutile sur le cou et dans la région lombaire, qui, quand un anesthésique n'est pas employé, cause des douleurs qui ne sont pas nécessaires à la correction. Une force de pression agit plus directement avec moins de force inutile.

On peut dire que la manière d'appliquer les forces correctives qui est désirable varie nécessairement selon les cas, mais la méthode qui doit être regardée comme la meilleure est celle qui peut être facilement contrôlée par le chirurgien et qui peut être employée avec le moins de désagréments pour le malade. On doit aussi préférer celle où la camisole de plâtre peut être appliquée facilement par le chirurgien et avec le moins de gêne pour le malade pendant que la colonne vertébrale est tenue dans une position correcte. Si l'on n'a pas besoin d'employer des forces sur les courbes secondaires ou sur le cou, souvent un anesthésique n'est pas nécessaire pour permettre au chirurgien d'user autant de force de correction qu'il est désirable.

La différence, produite sur une colonne vertébrale déformée, soit par les effets d'une force de traction, soit par une force de pression corrective, est démontrée par les expériences suivantes :

Expérience 1. — Le cadavre était celui d'un enfant de 5 ans, dont la mort avait été la suite du mal de Pott. Maladie d'une durée de plusieurs années avec abcès et amyloïdes. Il y avait dans la partie inférieure de la colonne dorsale une courbure enfermant deux vertèbres et une accumulation de pus sous le quadratus lumborum des deux côtés, mais plus marquée du côté gauche. La courbure était large et arrondie. L'abdomen étant ouvert et tous les organes enlevés, la traction fut appliquée à la tête et aux cuisses. Des épingles furent plantées à angle droit dans les vertèbres voisines du point de la maladie. Avant la traction la distance entre les têtes de ces épingles fut mesurée. Sous une traction très forte on obtint une séparation d'un demi-pouce. Le tronc étant couché et la traction se faisant dans le même plan que la table sur laquelle le tronc était placé, la face étant tournée en haut. Si un support était placé sous la projection, le soutenant, et une légère pression appliquée sur les épaules et sur les cuisses de haut en bas (sans traction) une séparation d'un pouce était facilement obtenue.

Expérience 2. — Spécimen au Musée de l'École de Médecine de l'Université Harvard. Une colonne vertébrale d'adulte avec maladie destructive de la troisième vertèbre lombaire; gibbosité d'une grosseur moyenne mais avec peu de déviation dans l'axe des vertèbres. L'épine placée le dos en dessus, une traction d'une force d'environ cent cinquante livres dans l'axe de la colonne vertébrale ne put pas corriger la difformité ou faire plus que tendre quelques adhérences. Mais en couchant l'épine avec le dos en dessous et attachant à la table la partie de l'épine sous la gibbosité, une pression sur la partie supérieure de l'épine de haut en bas commença à être effective avec une force de trente livres, et l'enlèvement complet de la cyphose fut possible en ajoutant là-dessus très peu de force. Après que l'adhérence fut rompue, une traction directe dans l'axe de la colonne fut de nouveau essayée; même, avec beaucoup de force, la meilleure correction obtenue fut celle qui est montrée dans le tracé N° 2. Mais quand une pression de haut en bas fut appliquée à la partie supérieure de l'épine (l'épine étant supportée avec le dos en dessous), très peu de poids suffisait pour faire une correction complète, ou même reverser de la difformité.

Expérience 5. — Spécimen dans le Musée de l'École de Médecine de l'Université d'Harvard. Celle-ci, comme la précédente, était une colonne vertébrale d'adulte avec une maladie destructive non guérie de la troisième vertèbre lombaire, mais dans ce cas-ci la gibbosité était petite. La traction dans l'axe de la colonne n'eut réellement aucun effet sur la difformité, même quand on usa beaucoup de force. Cependant, en soutenant la gibbosité de dessous, seulement le poids de la partie supérieure de la colonne suffisait pour séparer les épines, beaucoup au point de la maladie, et une très légère pression de haut en bas vers la région cervicale plaçait la colonne dans une correction presque normale.

Expérience 4. — La même colonne fut prise pour produire une cyphose artificielle. Une partie de l'os des huitième et neuvième vertèbres fut enlevée au ciseau et la colonne courbée dans une cyphose prononcée. Des crampons de fer furent alors insérés de la même manière que les épingles dans l'expérience N° 1; et entre ces crampons, on tendit des bandes de caoutchouc. En mesurant la longueur de ces bandes pendant les différentes manipulations et en vérifiant la force nécessaire pour les tendre de la même longueur lorsqu'elles étaient hors des crampons, il fut possible d'obtenir une estimation approximative de la force employée dans les différents modes de correction, On trouva que la réduction de la difformité correspondait à un effort d'extension à ce point de neuf livres. Pour arriver à une force de rupture en employant la traction, il fallait une force de vingt et une livres. Un effort de traction de seize livres corrigeait seulement la colonne dans une position assez bonne. Avec la colonne tenue par de légères tractions (le dos toujours en haut), une pression de quatre livres à la gibbosité était suffisante pour faire un semblant de correction. Avec le dos en dessous, autrement dit avec la difformité supportée et la partie inférieure de la colonne fixée, une pression de haut en bas à la partie supérieure de l'épine seulement d'une demi-livre ou d'une livre suffisait pour la correction complète.

Expérience 5. — Les conditions de la dernière expérience furent à peu près, reproduites sur un modèle en bois semblablement arrangé avec des crampons de fer et des bandes de caoutchouc : dans ce cas, une correction complète correspondait à une force de rupture de douze livres, comme elle fut mesurée par l'extention des bandes de caoutchouc. Pour accomplir cela par une traction directe d'un bout à l'autre, il fallait une force de traction de vingt livres. Avec les extrémités supportées, le dos en dessus, la pression demandée de haut en bas était de trois livres à l'angle. Avec la gibbosité et la partie inférieure supportée le dos en dessous, un peu moins d'une livre suffisait pour un redressement complet.

Une force de pression corrective antéro-postérieure du type de l'appareil Metzger-Goldthwait semble remplir les conditions nécessaires pour la correction et l'application du bandage, plus précis que la méthode de Calot parce que les forces de correction peuvent être exactement calculées par le chirurgien et parce qu'il y a moins de pertes dans les courbes secondaires.

Dans toutes les méthodes il se présente une difficulté qui est de prévenir une exagération de la courbure lombaire. La traction est la voie la plus efficace pour la prévenir, mais la flexion des cuisses (si l'appareil Metzger-Goldthwait est employé) peut aussi servir avantageusement.

On trouvera un avantage dans la position couchée sur le dos, sur la position couchée à plat ventre par une plus grande facilité pour l'application des bandages sur le devant, et parce que c'est la position où on a le plus besoin de l'application ferme de l'appareil.

Les plaques de pression (plaques d'aluminium ouatées) peuvent être laissées dans la camisole de plâtre, où des tiges d'acier aplaties peuvent être usées et enlevées après que le plâtre est sec.

Méthodes de contention après la correction. — Après la correction, il est nécessaire de maintenir l'épine dorsale dans une position correcte jusqu'à ce que l'intervalle fait pendant la correction soit réparé ou supporté par des ankyloses.

La réparation des os peut, dans des circonstances favorables, être rapide et considérable. Par exemple dans le cas de Nichols de Boston où un tiers de l'os huméral avait été enlevé au-dessous du périoste après une ostéomyélite étendue, un os nouveau, solide, fut refait en neuf mois. Un cas rapporté par le Dr H.-W. Cushing de Boston montre la néoformation de l'os tibial (après excision pour ostéomyélite) en neuf mois.

La formation de nouveaux os dans l'épine peut de même être rapide après fractures. Wagner et Stolper rapportent les autopsies (avec gravures) montrant des cals durs unissant les vertèbres brisées après dix, huit et quatre mois, huit semaines et même six semaines après la blessure.

Il ne s'ensuit pas, néanmoins, que de telles néoformations se produisent après la séparation par force des vertèbres malades. Il n'y a réellement aucune preuve que de tels intervalles aient jamais été fermés par un tissu osseux.

Les recherches de Ménard tendent à démontrer que la formation de nouveaux os par le périoste (reconnue essentielle pour une réparation solide en cas de fracture) est dans beaucoup de cas pauvre et tardive. Drehmann a étudié 47 spécimens et arrive aux mêmes conclusions.

Une étude de 21 spécimens, au Musée de Warren, à Boston, montre dans les cas les plus récents (au nombre de 10) une apparence de réparation seulement. L'enclavement des vertèbres est généralement causé par la difformité croissante et, dans certains cas, il y a fusion partielle des surfaces des vertèbres quand elles sont en contact, mais il n'y a pas formation de nouveaux os en masse. Les plus vieux spécimens montrent une fusion plus grande, dans certains cas ankylose de la partie postérieure de la colonne avec ou sans nouvelle formation considérable d'os dans cette région, mais seulement six sur onze offrent un nouvel os périostéal au siège de la maladie elle-même.

Des six cas, l'un est une cyphose, depuis longtemps guérie, datant de 45 ans avant la mort. Il fut guéri par la fusion des vertèbres et la masse considérable d'os périostal appartient évidemment à une ostéo-arthrite ankylosante qui n'est pas limitée au siège du vieux mal tuberculeux. Un second spécimen semblable est évidemment la suite d'une guérison ancienne. Les quatre autres présentent une formation d'os périostal en petite quantité ajoutée à une fusion solide. Dans ces quatre cas, le mal tuberculeux datait de 19, 14, 10 et 6 ans avant la mort.

Les spécimens présentés comme arguments par Calot, Krause d'Altona, Gayet et d'autres proviennent de sujets dont, selon toute apparence, la tuberculose a été guérie comme les spécimens du Musée de Warren. La conclusion inévitable est que la formation de nouveaux os en masse des vertèbres n'est pas la méthode ordinaire de réparation dans le mal de Pott et qu'une telle formation arrive seulement après des années, si elle arrive.

Comme preuve directe de cas après correction par force, des autopsies rapportées par Malherbe, Murray (2), Sherman, Braun, Krause, Anders (4), pas une ne peut démontrer trace de nouvelle formation d'os.

Les illustrations skiagraphiques ne semblent pas avoir prouvé aucune nouvelle formation; les dessins de Calot, d'après semblables radiographies, ne sont certainement pas convaincants.

Contention après la correction. — Il est évident qu'un moyen de contention est aussi important que la correction elle-même, et il est nécessaire qu'une fixation soigneuse, dans une position correcte, soit supportée pendant une longue période. Combien cette période doit-elle durer? C'est une question qui n'est pas encore définitivement déterminée, mais il est évident que le temps pour la cure accordé par quelques chirurgiens est beaucoup trop court.

Il est évident que chez les petits enfants avec courtes épines dorsales et aussi dans les cas de courbures en haut, une contention **suffisante** est impossible, et un certain relâchement de la courbure corrigée est inévitable dans bien des cas.

Des ceintures fixes de plâtre offrent la forme la plus pratique de fixation immédiate suivie d'abord de la position couchée qui enlève le poids superposé: mais, comme le repos est incompatible avec les conditions d'hygiène nécessaires à la réparation, la marche devrait être, aussitôt que possible, permise au malade[1].

Arrêt du développement de la courbure. — Quand la correction n'est pas possible pour plusieurs raisons, soit à cause de la place de la courbure, ou soit à cause des conditions pathologiques, le traitement par fixation du tronc avec accessoires doit être employé avec espoir d'arrêter le développement de la courbure. La contention de l'épine dorsale en la meilleure position possible est toujours importante, même si on a essayé la correction. Le traitement de fixation négligé, même si on a obtenu une correction satisfaisante, a pour suite un relâchement de la courbure.

Pour prévenir de l'augmentation de la courbure par des procédés mécaniques il faut beaucoup plus de soins et d'attention dans les détails, qu'il n'est ordinairement possible d'en donner dans les grands hôpitaux ou dans les grandes cliniques. L'augmentation de la courbure peut être arrêtée par un traitement de rectification en utilisant à plusieurs reprises les méthodes d'application employées dans la correction par la force, mais avec l'aide de moins de force. Cela constitue, avec les mesures propres de contention, un moyen rationnel de traitement dans le mal de Pott applicable à un grand nombre

---

1. Une description des différents appareils efficaces et amovibles, qui ont été et qui sont employés comme expédients pour les convalescents, prendrait beaucoup plus d'espace que celui que permet cette discussion. Pour cela on se reportera aux différents manuels de chirurgie orthopédique.

de cas, mais ce traitement demande une longue période de temps.

Les résultats suivants, obtenus grâce à la courtoisie du D' H. L. Taylor, de New-York, montrent un succès inusité dans sa pratique. L'auteur a eu l'occasion d'examiner personnellement les cas et de vérifier l'authenticité des rapports et, plus tard, des tracés.

Le traitement était entièrement ambulatoire dans la période de convalescence et consistait surtout en supports mécaniques antéro-postérieurs portés continuellement pendant des années.

Dans quelques cas une amélioration présente dans la courbure fut observée après des années de traitement, comme il l'a aussi été démontré par le D' H.-L. Taylor dans The Transactions of the American Orthopedic Association. Dans quelques cas, on trouvait une augmentation de la courbure; dans beaucoup, enfin, les progrès de la courbure étaient relativement petits, souvent nuls.

Arrêt de l'accroissement de la courbure. — Après que les progrès de la tuberculose dans l'épine dorsale ont été arrêtés, qu'une ankylose complète a suivi et que la cure est établie chez un enfant grandissant, on trouve, quelquefois, une augmentation de la courbure qui peut se produire pendant la croissance de l'enfant et qu'il faut attribuer, non à la condition des progrès de la tuberculose, mais à un changement dans la forme des vertèbres causé par la direction anormale des pressions superposées: comme une courbure rachitique peut augmenter chez un enfant grandissant dans les os longs, même après que les progrès du rachitisme lui-même sont arrêtés. L'extension de ces courbes secondaires et leur développement dépendent du degré de croissance de l'enfant et de la quantité de poids superposé plutôt que d'une condition d'ostéite. Pour arrêter cette croissance tordue il est nécessaire d'user des appareils de support plus longtemps que les conditions pathologiques ne sembleraient le demander. Dans des cas de cette sorte, il n'est possible d'arrêter la croissance de la courbe que par l'usage de tels appareils qui maintiennent, comme on le désire, la position propre.

Méthodes opératoires. — Il a été démontré que le support principal pour une épine dorsale malade résidait dans l'ankylose des articulations. Quand elles sont soudées, en connexion avec une ankylose des apophyses transverses et des épines, la nature a fourni le support le plus désirable pour une colonne vertébrale avec des vertèbres malades. Des essais pour avancer la solidification de ces tissus sont venus naturellement d'eux-mêmes à la pensée, mais on ne peut pas encore sûrement aujourd'hui présenter une méthode établie de traitement.

La question de laminectomie pour paralysie de même que le traitement opératoire pour abcès, ou séquestre vertébral, ne sont pas considérés comme devant prendre place dans ce rapport.

Il faut dire, comme conclusion, que la correction ou la rectification de la courbure du mal de Pott doivent être considérées dans tous les cas de maladie active avec une difformité. L'emploi de la force devrait dépendre des conditions pathologiques et non de la grosseur de la courbure. La force devrait être employée avec grande réserve. L'amélioration de la courbure doit être considérée dans tous les cas ; on peut essayer partout où la colonne vertébrale peut être redressée avec peu de force. La principale condition, cependant, pour un succès final, dépend des soins assidus et prolongés du chirurgien et de l'emploi de mesures de contention qui supportent l'épine dans la position la plus droite possible pendant un temps assez long pour permettre la consolidation des parties osseuses malades. Le succès est obtenu plus par une attention pleine de soins dans les moindres détails que par une opération.

DE LA RÉDUCTION DES GIBBOSITÉS DU MAL DE POTT

COMMUNICATION

de MM. P. REDARD et PAUL BEZANÇON.

Nous avons observé tant au dispensaire Furtado-Heine qu'en ville un grand nombre de maux de Pott. Depuis le mois de mars 1897, nous les avons traités non pas systématiquement ce qui serait dangereux et inutile, mais pour le plus grand nombre des cas par le redressement des gibbosités et l'immobilisation en bonne position ; nous n'avons eu qu'à nous louer de ce procédé et nous désirons présenter au Congrès international le résultat de notre pratique.

L'un de nous a déjà décrit l'appareil[1] dont nous nous servons ; nous ne l'avons pas sensiblement modifié depuis trois ans, en étant pleinement satisfaits.

Au début nous entourions l'enfant d'ouate ; depuis le mois de septembre 1897, l'un de nous a repris le maillot sur lequel Sayre appli-

1. P. REDARD Du traitement de la gibbosité du mal de Pott. — XI° Congrès français de chirurg., et XII° Congrès internat. Moscou, août 1897.

quait son corset plâtré : à l'essai, nous avons reconnu qu'une étoffe plus épaisse que le tricot était utile, et nous avons adopté le maillot en tissu des Pyrénées, taillé de façon à être collant, couvrant les épaules et assez long pour qu'on puisse, par une épingle à maillot ou deux cordons noués ensemble sous le périnée, tirer en bas l'étoffe de façon qu'elle ne plisse pas. On met à l'enfant une mentonnière de cuir si l'on ne doit mettre qu'un corset, une mentonnière faite d'une bande de toile, prenant le menton et la nuque, si l'on doit comprendre la tête dans l'appareil. L'enfant garde ses bas et on entoure ses malléoles d'une guêtre à deux ou trois boucles avec une cordelette en anse formant étrier. L'enfant est alors étendu sur la table où est fixé l'appareil de traction : aux deux extrémités une vis d'acier horizontale avec un crochet dans lequel on accroche un dynamomètre de Collin. L'enfant est mis sur le ventre, la partie antérieure des épaules reposant sur des béquillons qu'on peut à son gré éloigner l'un de l'autre ou élever au-dessus du plan de la table, la partie inférieure de l'abdomen appuyant sur un coussin dur. Une barre de fer transversale réunit les deux côtés de la mentonnière au dynamomètre ; une autre semblable réunit les deux pieds au dynamomètre placé de ce côté. Tout est ainsi prêt pour la traction. Celle-ci se fait en tournant les manivelles lentement et en surveillant le dynamomètre ; quand celui-ci marque 25 à 30 kilogs, exceptionnellement 35, il convient de s'arrêter ; encore ne faut-il arriver à ces chiffres qu'au bout de plusieurs minutes (10 à 15). L'enfant se plaint rarement d'une façon vive ; l'étrangeté de la position qu'on lui fait prendre l'effraie plus que la traction progressive ne le fait souffrir. On voit sous son influence la gibbosité diminuer notablement, souvent même, quand elle n'a que quelques mois de date, *disparaître* tout à fait. Il est *inutile*, comme on l'a fait au début, *de faire des pressions manuelles* dessus ; il est également *inutile d'endormir l'enfant*, car la traction triomphe aisément des contractures et la surveillance de la respiration serait bien difficile.

Aussitôt la gibbosité disparue ou diminuée, on met un peu d'ouate à son niveau (si l'on craint une eschare, de l'ouate hydrophile stérilisée qu'on glisse sous le maillot) ; on en met également un plastron sur l'abdomen et les épines iliaques et l'on commence le corset suivant le mode ordinaire en évitant soigneusement les plis des premiers tours de bande : nous nous servons d'ordinaire de *tarlatane* (jaconas) *non* apprêtée, saupoudrée par avance de plâtre et mouillée au moment de s'en servir. Quatre bandes de 8 mètres suffisent pour un adolescent ; trois bandes pour un petit enfant. Nous n'interposons rien pour renforcer le plâtre : notre technique vient du reste d'être décrite par notre élève M. Franck-Michel, dans sa thèse[1].

Si le mal de Pott siège au-dessus de la région dorsale moyenne, au corset il convient d'ajouter une minerve plâtrée. Pour cela, on laisse le corset durcir, puis l'enfant muni de sa mentonnière de toile est suspendu verticalement, le bout des pieds touchant terre. Il faut prendre bien soin que le plâtre ne vienne serrer l'angle des mâchoires et le devant du cou ; pour cela, nous recommandons de protéger la mâchoire et la nuque avec deux croissants de feutre épais doublés de tarlatane qu'on aura soin de maintenir en bonne place. La tête étant couverte d'ouate, on l'enveloppe de bandes plâtrées qu'on marie à celles du corset, les renforçant à la partie postérieure du cou par une solide attelle plâtrée verticale recouverte par les circulaires.

La minerve une fois sèche, on réséque toute la partie supérieure, de manière que l'appareil affleure sous le menton, à l'angle des mâchoires et à la nuque. Cette demi-minerve est *bien moins* gênante que le casque complet : elle suffit à maintenir la tête en rectitude.

L'appareil ainsi terminé, que faire de l'enfant ? Va-t-on le remettre sur ses jambes ? Notre opinion est formelle sur ce point : à part les maux de Pott lombaires ou des deux dernières dorsales (et encore), c'est dans la *position couchée* que doivent guérir les malades. Il est bien évident que le redressement de la gibbosité ne peut abréger les délais de consolidation de la carie vertébrale ; la gibbosité qu'on a fait disparaître ou diminuer tend à se reproduire, l'angle dont on a redressé les deux côtés tend à se fermer et, si le sujet est laissé debout, il faut craindre les *eschares* ; or l'eschare est le reproche principal qu'on a fait à la méthode de redressement : c'est l'inconvénient qu'il faut éviter avant tout et le meilleur procédé est le décubitus horizontal et en particulier le *décubitus abdominal*. C'est depuis des années que nous invitons les parents à tenir les enfants sur le ventre pendant la moitié du temps, si possible, et nous n'avons qu'à nous louer de cette pratique. Ajoutons qu'il faut les faire porter chaque jour dehors et leur faire respirer le meilleur air possible.

Un autre écueil du corset après redressement, ce sont les corps étrangers que les enfants laissent glisser dans leur corset, surtout dans les familles pauvres où ils sont peu surveillés ; c'est ainsi que nous avons maintes fois retrouvé dans les corsets des miettes de pain, des perles de verre, des épingles à cheveux, etc., tous objets qui avaient ulcéré la peau, fait des plaies et obligé à remplacer trop tôt le

---

1. Fr. Michel. Technique des appareils plâtrés, spécialement en orthopédie. Paris, juillet 1900.

corset. Il faut donc veiller à ce que le bord supérieur du corset ne soit pas béant et que les épaules soient toujours couvertes par la chemise et celle-ci bien fermée au cou.

A quels enfants s'applique la méthode de redressement?

Nous avons, au début, encouragés par la facilité du procédé, redressé des gibbosités datant de 4, 5, 7 ans et très accusées ; ces redressements se sont faits sans presque de douleur et avec peu de craquements ; nous sommes persuadés que si les parents de ces enfants avaient consenti à les maintenir étendus pendant 12 à 18 mois ils auraient guéri en bonne position ; mais il est certain qu'après 4 ou 5 ans de maladie, si les douleurs ont cessé, la patience des malades et de leurs parents est à bout et que le repos horizontal leur paraît inutile, et c'est dans les cas où les malades ont été presque aussitôt remis sur leurs jambes que nous avons observé des eschares, toujours ennuyeuses parce qu'elles retardent le traitement et affaiblissent le malade.

D'après une cinquantaine de cas pris au hasard dans notre statistique, c'est *en moyenne* à 18 mois après le début de la maladie que nous avons réduit la gibbosité ; ce chiffre ne résulte que du hasard des observations et n'est pas l'époque de choix ; car nous estimons que c'est bien avant 18 mois qu'il faut immobiliser le rachis pottique. Après 2 ans de date, nous pensons qu'il ne faut plus guère toucher aux gibbosités, à moins de se préparer à un repos encore long après la réduction.

Quels inconvénients peut présenter le redressement par la traction?

Nous avons parlé des eschares : on peut les éviter par le décubitus sur le ventre et en soignant bien les premiers tours de bande. Quelques chirurgiens font des fenêtres à l'endroit où siégeait la gibbosité ; ce moyen n'est qu'un pis aller ; la gibbosité s'y reforme, s'y loge à l'aise ; mieux vaut enlever le corset pour quelques jours, le temps que la peau se cicatrise.

Certains enfants trop anémiés ou tuberculeux pulmonaires supporteraient mal le corset et la traction ; à ceux-là nous réservons, si le mal de Pott siège aux premières dorsales, la gouttière avec appareil extenseur de la tête ; s'il siège plus bas, le lit plâtré, excellent appareil trop abandonné.

Comme accident *immédiat*, nous n'avons, sur 120 malades environ et après 500 ou 600 applications de la traction aux pottiques, constaté qu'une seule fois un certain degré de paraplégie avec incontinence des matières ; ce cas s'est produit au troisième corset, et sans presque de traction, dans un mal de Pott des 4e, 5e, 6e dorsales. Nous répétons que ce cas est unique dans notre série.

Nous ne parlons pas des incidents que peut donner le chloroforme, car nous sommes d'avis de ne pas anesthésier les sujets. Les accidents plus *tardifs* ne nous ont pas paru plus nombreux.

Les abcès froids ne sont pas influencés en mal, nous n'avons pas constaté de rupture d'abcès et leur évolution nous a semblé plus favorable.

La coexistence avec le mal de Pott d'autres tuberculoses (coxalgie, sacro-coxalgie, tumeur blanche du poignet) s'est rencontrée dans trois ou quatre cas où le mal vertébral était secondaire; elle constitue un élément de pronostic défavorable; mais nous ne l'avons pas vue suivre le redressement, non plus que la méningite. Chez un de nos patients, la maladie s'est terminée par des hématuries et de l'urémie; chez deux autres par la tuberculose pulmonaire. Cette terminaison se voit dans le mal de Pott, quelque traitement que l'on emploie.

Par contre les *résultats* de la méthode sont palpables et évidents : réduction complète, indolente des gibbosités récentes, grande diminution des saillies plus anciennes, redressement du thorax en avant, allongement de la taille, consolidation en bonne position.

Dans plusieurs cas, nous l'avons dit, les abcès froids préexistants nous ont paru diminuer. Dans trois cas, nous avons vu, chez des enfants tout à fait paraplégiques, quelques mouvements volontaires des membres inférieurs se produire le jour même de la réduction et persister dans la suite.

La *consolidation* du rachis dans la nouvelle position où on l'a mis s'obtient, quoi qu'on ait pu dire. Après la longue étape passée dans le décubitus, le malade redressé se lève et marche, parfois un peu en lordose; il peut reprendre ses occupations; la radiographie faite à cette période peut témoigner qu'il s'est reformé de l'os et que le rachis a repris son assiette. Certes les résultats ne sont pas comparables suivant la région qu'occupent les vertèbres malades : plus la lésion siège haut, plus le résultat est aléatoire, et la facilité avec laquelle se reproduit une saillie cervico-dorsale est parfois désespérante; nous avons dit que dans ces cas nous mettions le sujet sur un plan déclive avec de l'extension continue de la tête. Dans les maux de Pott dorsaux et lombaires, les résultats sont excellents.

Si, parmi nos observations, nous voulons ne tenir compte que de celles qui ont été longtemps suivies et des malades revus récemment, il en reste environ soixante. Sur ces 60 enfants, nous pouvons dire que :

14 vont bien.

29 vont assez bien ou passablement.

11 vont médiocrement soit par paraplégie, abcès ou tuberculose d'autres parties.

3 ou 4 sont morts, sans qu'on puisse imputer la mort au redressement, mais bien à la généralisation tardive de la tuberculose.

Cette statistique absolument sincère et comprenant des cas de tout genre nous paraît satisfaisante et démontre la grande valeur de la méthode du redressement des gibbosités pottiques.

SUR LE TRAITEMENT DU MAL DE POTT

COMMUNICATION

de MM. A. BROCA et A. MOUCHET.

Depuis 5 ans, à l'hôpital Trousseau, nous avons observé avec attention tous les maux de Pott qui se présentaient à notre consultation, et nous avons expérimenté au début, sur un grand nombre d'entre eux, le traitement local préconisé par Calot.

Ce traitement a subi de la part de son auteur des fluctuations diverses que nous n'avons pas jugé bon d'essayer successivement et nous nous sommes contentés du redressement brusque ; nous n'avons pas pratiqué d'opération osseuse préliminaire ; nous n'avons eu recours ni aux ligatures des apophyses épineuses, ni à l'ablation (sous-périostée ou non) de ces mêmes apophyses.

Le nombre des maux de Pott traités par nous depuis 5 ans s'élève au chiffre de 85, dont il faut défalquer 28 malades traités seulement depuis un an, c'est-à-dire depuis un temps trop court pour qu'on puisse apprécier sainement les résultats du traitement.

C'est donc seulement d'après 55 cas de maux de Pott bien suivis depuis au moins 2 ans, la plupart depuis 5, que nous formulons ici notre opinion sur le traitement du mal de Pott.

Sur ce chiffre 46 malades seulement (28 filles et 18 garçons) ont été soumis au redressement brusque de la gibbosité par la méthode de Calot.

Les autres malades, à gibbosité nulle ou toute récente, ont été mis seulement dans un grand appareil plâtré sous l'anesthésie chloroformique.

On ne trouvera sur nos 55 malades aucun mal de Pott cervical, parce que notre recherche presque exclusive des cas de Pott justiciables du redressement brusque, nous faisait éliminer dans les premières années le mal cervical.

Nous avons eu affaire surtout au mal de Pott dorsal (56 cas, dont 19 à la région dorsale moyenne), au lombaire (11 cas), au dorso-lombaire (8).

L'abcès par congestion constituait pour nous une contre-indication au redressement brusque, il en était de même d'un état cachectique trop accentué ou d'une tuberculose pulmonaire trop avancée. La paraplégie nous a paru, comme à la majorité des auteurs, constituer au contraire une indication nette, et nous devons reconnaître qu'elle nous a semblé dans plusieurs cas favorablement influencée par le redressement brusque de la gibbosité. Autant que possible, les gibbosités que nous avons tenté de redresser étaient choisies parmi les récentes, parmi celles dont le début ne remontait pas à plus d'un an, mais chacun sait quelle peine on a à obtenir des parents des renseignements exacts sur ce point et, d'autre part, quelle difficulté on éprouve à reconnaître l'âge d'une gibbosité.

La forme, les dimensions de la gibbosité nous importaient moins que leur âge: et le nombre des vertèbres intéressées, le rayon de courbure de la gibbosité, pourvu qu'elle ne fût pas trop ancienne, ne constituaient pas pour nous des contre-indications aux tentatives de redressement.

Nos redressements brusques ont tous été pratiqués suivant la technique primitive de Calot: nous l'avons trouvée simple, et nous devons avouer tout de suite que nous ne lui avons dû aucun accident; nous avons atténué, il est vrai, la brutalité des manœuvres de pression sur la gibbosité.

L'enfant était soumis à l'anesthésie chloroformique; une fois la résolution obtenue, l'enfant était maintenu par les aides au-dessus de la table, le dos en l'air, et nous faisions pratiquer sans appareil spécial la traction horizontale selon la première manière de Calot.

Cette seule traction arrivait parfois à faire disparaître la gibbosité dans les cas tout récents où celle-ci était à peine marquée.

Dans la plupart des cas, 9 fois sur 10, nous pressions sur la gibbosité avec nos deux mains superposées, et nous entendions les craquements caractéristiques. Une seule fois, où les craquements furent très bruyants, l'enfant eut un arrêt brusque de la respiration. Quelques mouvements de respiration artificielle, et tout rentra dans l'ordre.

Le redressement effectué, nous faisions endormir à fond le malade et, sans perdre de temps, nous le suspendions debout dans la position de Sayre, en ayant soin de supprimer les brassières axillaires et de remplacer le collier de tête en cuir par deux bandes de toile solidaires soulevant le menton et la nuque.

Nous n'avons jamais observé d'accidents au cours de cette chloroformisation dans la position de Sayre, et nous y avons eu recours plus de 100 fois chez des enfants de 2 à 16 ans. Dernièrement même, nous l'avons vue admirablement supportée en ville par un homme de 40 ans. La tâche du chloroformisateur est peut-être un peu plus délicate, parce que le bruit de la respiration est moins facile à entendre, mais ce n'est qu'une question de surveillance à laquelle nous avons vu successivement se plier les divers externes chargés de la chloroformisation. D'ailleurs si le malade a été endormi à fond avant d'être suspendu et si l'on ne met pas trop de temps à confectionner l'appareil plâtré, il suffit de quelques gouttes de chloroforme pour maintenir la résolution musculaire. Nous n'avons jamais eu d'alerte; une fois seulement nous avons vu asphyxier une enfant que nous avons dû dépendre en toute hâte; mais cette asphyxie était certainement due à la constriction trop forte de l'appareil plâtré, car elle a cessé par l'ablation de celui-ci.

L'utilité de la chloroformisation pendant la suspension dans le traitement du mal de Pott n'est pas contestable; c'est le seul moyen d'obtenir un relâchement musculaire complet comme n'en fournit jamais la suspension simple longtemps prolongée, à tel point que sans avoir subi aucune tentative de redressement brusque, les gibbosités récentes peuvent arriver à disparaître presque complètement.

Au début, nous avons essayé l'application de l'appareil plâtré dans la suspension tête en bas, à la façon de Levassort, mais nous avons vite constaté qu'il était difficile d'appliquer correctement l'appareil dans cette position.

Nous devons savoir gré à Calot de nous avoir vanté l'innocuité de la chloroformisation dans la suspension de Sayre, car l'efficacité de ce procédé dans la thérapeutique du mal de Pott nous paraît considérable.

Nous n'insistons point sur la confection du corset plâtré : un jersey, peu d'ouate, sauf sur la partie antérieure du thorax pour la respiration et de l'abdomen pour la digestion; nous employons des bandes de tarlatane humide que nous plâtrons au fur et à mesure avec une bouillie plâtrée un peu épaisse.

Nous avons réservé le grand appareil plâtré entourant la tête et le tronc tel que le recommandait Calot aux enfants atteints de mal de Pott dorsal supérieur et de mal cervical. Pour les maux de Pott de la

région dorsale moyenne (cas les plus fréquents) et de la région dorso
lombaire et lombaire, nous avons fait le corset plâtré entourant les
épaules, enserrant le cou dans une sorte de collier, et descendant au-
dessous des épines iliaques antéro-supérieures.

Le soir ou le lendemain de son application, le corset plâtré est
échancré : on dégage le cou, les aisselles, et on pratique une fenêtre
abdominale pour faciliter la digestion et la respiration.

Nous laissons le premier appareil 2 ou 3 mois autant que possible,
en condamnant les malades au décubitus dorsal absolu.

Mais que ces prescriptions fussent ou non observées, chez les trois
quarts des malades, des eschares survenaient au niveau de la gibbosité, qui nous obligeaient à enlever un carré de l'appareil plâtré.
Nous les reconnaissions moins à la douleur éprouvée par le malade
qu'à l'odeur sphacélique exhalée par le corset plâtré. Nous n'avons
jamais vu que des eschares très superficielles, et dont le diamètre
le plus considérable n'a pas excédé une pièce de 1 franc : la durée de
leur cicatrisation n'a pas dépassé trois à quatre semaines. Une fois
cette cicatrisation achevée, nous appliquions presque toujours un
nouveau corset plâtré. Ce dernier était renouvelé aussitôt qu'il nous
semblait un peu lâche ou un peu mou.

Nous soumettons les malades à l'immobilisation absolue pendant
une année au moins, et nous ne permettons au bout de ce temps la
station debout et la marche modérée que si nous constatons une évolution du mal assez favorable. Le corset est porté encore pendant
de longs mois.

*La correction obtenue par le redressement brusque de Calot se main-
tient-elle ?* Voilà la question importante à laquelle nous devions chercher à répondre d'une façon précise. D'abord cette correction n'est
pas toujours possible et nous avons échoué dans une dizaine de cas où
les gibbosités étaient peu accentuées, mais probablement déjà anciennes et ankylosées. Pour ces dernières, l'accord est fait, le redressement brusque doit être proscrit : il présente des dangers de l'aveu
d'un grand nombre de chirurgiens, et il est sans effet.

Des dangers, nous n'en avons point observé : sur les 5 morts que
nous avons relevées, 4 ont été dues à des fièvres éruptives, une seule,
par méningite tuberculeuse, ne saurait être imputable à la méthode,
puisqu'elle est survenue plusieurs mois après le traitement.

La correction, même si elle semble complète après le redressement
brusque, ne l'est plus au bout d'un temps assez rapide, bien que l'enfant ait été maintenu rigoureusement dans le décubitus dorsal. Quand
il survient une eschare au niveau de la gibbosité, — et c'est presque

la règle en pareil cas. — L'ouverture creusée dans le plâtre pour permettre le pansement nous montre la bosse tendant à faire hernie au dehors. C'est pourquoi nous n'avons pas cru devoir, comme Lorenz, Wolff, ménager un orifice au niveau de la saillie osseuse, dès l'application de l'appareil plâtré, en vue d'éviter les eschares.

Nous avons systématiquement reporté sur le papier la courbe de toutes les gibbosités, obtenue à l'aide d'un ruban de plomb flexible, et cela avant le redressement, comme à chaque renouvellement d'appareil. Or nous avons eu le regret de constater qu'au bout de quelques mois, la difformité se reproduisait presque aussi accentuée qu'auparavant.

Nous savons qu'on a parlé de consolidation par soudure des arcs postérieurs des vertèbres, de tassement postérieur, capable ainsi de remédier à l'énorme hiatus créé en avant du rachis par le redressement forcé; mais ces considérations nous ont toujours paru un peu théoriques et, — même prises comme telles, — insuffisantes à expliquer les faits. Il est vrai qu'on a prétendu trouver la preuve de cette consolidation dans des radiographies: mais notre expérience nous a toujours fait douter de la netteté de celles-ci, et nous craignons qu'une indulgente paternité n'ait donné à leurs auteurs une netteté de coup d'œil qui nous fait défaut.

En ce qui concerne les gibbosités récentes, le redressement brusque a-t-il de réels avantages? Nous ne le croyons pas. Dans les 10 cas où la méthode de Calot nous a fourni une diminution réelle et durable de la gibbosité, il s'agissait de maux de Pott tout au début pour lesquels il n'a pas été nécessaire d'appuyer sur la gibbosité: la simple traction horizontale exercée par les aides a suffi, — sous l'anesthésie chloroformique, bien entendu, — à rendre à la colonne vertébrale sa rectitude. Ce n'est donc point sur le compte du redressement brusque que ces succès doivent être mis, c'est à l'emploi de l'anesthésie chloroformique, c'est à la suspension de Sayre sous cette anesthésie qu'il faut les rapporter. La confection soignée d'un grand appareil plâtré maintenant bien les épaules et le bassin contribue ensuite pour une grande part à rendre le succès définitif.

On a dit que la paraplégie devait être considérée comme une indication du redressement forcé, et beaucoup d'auteurs ont signalé des améliorations de la paraplégie imputables à cette méthode. Pour notre part, nous avons constaté pareille amélioration chez 5 malades, mais il n'est pas bien certain que ce soit autre chose qu'une coïncidence : on connaît la tendance des paraplégies pottiques à guérir spontanément, et on sait comme il est exceptionnel qu'elles soient imputables à une compression osseuse. En tout cas, nos paraplégies auraient-elles dû leur amélioration à notre traitement que nous en attribuerions le mérite moins au redressement forcé lui-même qu'à la suspension sous l'anesthésie chloroformique.

Sur ce point spécial encore, nous proscrivons donc le redressement forcé, d'accord avec la majorité des auteurs.

Ce qu'il faut garder de la méthode de Calot, c'est la chloroformisation dans la suspension de Sayre, et l'application d'un appareil plâtré englobant les épaules et les hanches.

Par la chloroformisation, on obtient le redressement spontané des gibbosités récentes, de celles qui ne doivent leur accentuation qu'aux contractures des muscles des gouttières vertébrales.

Par l'application du grand appareil plâtré, on assure au rachis une sérieuse immobilisation qui tend à maintenir le résultat acquis et à imprimer au mal de Pott une évolution désormais favorable.

C'est dès le début qu'il faut soigner le mal de Pott; lorsque la bosse est constituée, il est trop tard, et le temps n'est pas encore venu où il n'y aura plus de bossus.

La tuberculose vertébrale est soumise dans son évolution à l'influence de trop de facteurs divers ; elle est, — particulièrement dans la clientèle hospitalière, — d'une chronicité trop désespérante chez les uns, d'une progression trop rapide chez les autres, pour qu'on s'illusionne sur les effets d'un traitement local, si bien dirigé soit-il.

Nous pensons, en tout cas, que ce dernier ne doit jamais être négligé par le chirurgien : il doit être longtemps prolongé pour être efficace, c'est par années que se chiffre sa durée.

Nous croyons enfin que c'est dans la voie que nous venons d'indiquer qu'on obtiendra les meilleurs résultats.

COMMUNICATION

de M. D. DUCROQUET.

J'ai assisté au début de la méthode de Calot et Chipault, j'ai fait et vu faire de nombreux redressements; je crois en avoir beaucoup simplifié la méthode, en ce sens que je fais la réduction en suspension et sans chloroforme; l'application de l'appareil est beaucoup plus facile.

Le redressement fait avec méthode est pour ainsi dire sans danger.

Quant aux résultats, les réserves que je faisais il y a 2 ans dans ma thèse se sont malheureusement confirmées. Dans le redressement des maux de Pott cervicaux et cervico-dorsaux la consolidation ne se fait pas. J'ai revu 20 malades opérés il y a 2, 3 et 4 ans et maintenus cependant jusque maintenant dans les appareils plâtrés bien faits : chez tous la gibbosité s'est reproduite.

Un des malades que j'avais redressé pour une assez forte gibbosité, A. P..., âgé de 4 ans, est mort. 7 mois après l'opération, de broncho-pneumonie. L'opération s'était faite très facilement. L'enfant était à la campagne et se portait à merveille avant d'avoir cette broncho-pneumonie. Depuis son redressement il avait beaucoup grossi. Lorsqu'après la mort j'ai fait l'autopsie, bien que son dos fût dans une rectitude parfaite, je trouvai à la partie antérieure du rachis une destruction complète des V⁰ et VI⁰ vertèbres dorsales; les IV⁰ et VII⁰ étaient en outre à moitié détruites et entre ces deux vertèbres extrêmes se trouvait un écart de 5 centimètres. Au niveau des lames vertébrales et des apophyses articulaires il n'y avait aucune trace de consolidation sauf l'articulation droite de l'apophyse articulaire de la V⁰ et VI⁰ dorsales. Dès que je mis l'enfant en position verticale la gibbosité se reproduisit immédiatement.

Mais ce que je trouvai de très intéressant dans ce cas, c'est l'absence totale de fongosités autour du foyer malade et les IV⁰ et V⁰ vertèbres dorsales, qui avaient été détruites en partie, semblaient avoir été nettoyées avec une éponge tant leur surface était nette, et dans ce cas si, après le redressement, le rachis ne s'était pas consolidé, il avait, je pense, par la décompression des surfaces malades amené une guérison bien rapide ou tout au moins une grande évolution vers la guérison du processus tuberculeux.

Dans le mal de Pott des régions inférieures le problème est un peu différent.

Considérons les conditions nouvelles du mal de Pott redressé. Le redressement qui a remis le rachis dans la rectitude va favoriser, grâce à des conditions particulières que je vais indiquer, la consolidation de la colonne vertébrale au niveau du rachis postérieur (arc, lames, tout ce qui est en arrière du corps vertébral); et cette consolidation de la gibbosité elle-même se fera d'autant mieux qu'elle siégera dans une position plus voisine du sacrum.

Avant d'examiner la genèse de cette consolidation et les divers cas qu'il faut envisager, voyons les conditions dans lesquelles va se trouver une gibbosité réduite.

Prenons, pour la facilité de la description, un mal de Pott dorsal inférieur ou lombaire. Je suppose qu'il y ait destruction totale de la II° lombaire, par exemple.

La gibbosité est assez prononcée, et si nous remettons le rachis dans la rectitude, il va se produire à sa partie antérieure une cavité dont la grandeur correspondra précisément au volume de la vertèbre disparue, 5 ou 4 centimètres par exemple, en hauteur.

Le rachis dans son état normal est maintenu dans la rectitude par l'empilement des divers disques vertébraux. Supprimez un corps vertébral et la gibbosité va immédiatement se reproduire.

Si nous replaçons ce rachis en sa position normale, et qu'au moyen d'un appareil de fixation nous le maintenions dans cette position, que va-t-il devenir ? A la partie antérieure, plus de corps vertébral, mais en arrière la continuité correspondante du rachis n'a pas disparu.

Il se maintient, grâce à l'articulation des apophyses articulaires. Mais celles-ci, dans la région qui nous occupe, sont à peu près verticales. Ces petites articulations ont des ligaments peu résistants, incapables en tout cas de supporter le poids de toute la partie du corps sus-jacente à cette vertèbre : il va en résulter fatalement les luxations des apophyses articulaires de la vertèbre disparue sur celles des vertèbres sus et sous-jacentes. Les lames vertébrales elles-mêmes sont à peu près verticales. Il va y avoir emboîtement réciproque des arcs postérieurs et la luxation ne cessera que lorsque les lames vertébrales seront arrêtées par leur contact réciproque. Si plusieurs vertèbres voisines ont été détruites par la carie tuberculeuse, le même phénomène se produira sur chacune d'elles, et la cavité que l'on aura artificiellement produite se trouvera réduite dans la proportion des 2/5 et même des 4/5.

J'ai envisagé, pour la facilité de la démonstration, le cas où une vertèbre entière était totalement disparue. Il arrive fréquemment que 2 vertèbres voisines ont disparu de moitié dans leurs parties adjacentes. Il est bien facile de prévoir que, là encore, la luxation va se produire, mais elle ne pourra pas être aussi complète que dans le cas précédent ; son évolution sera arrêtée au moment où les restes des vertèbres incomplètement détruites arriveront au contact, le rachis n'en conservera pas moins la rectitude. La consolidation de ces vertèbres peut alors se faire par soudure corps à corps comme cela a lieu dans le mal de Pott non réduit. Fort souvent la partie antérieure des corps vertébraux est détruite beaucoup plus que ne l'est leur partie postérieure et, dans ce cas, il n'y aura que les parties postérieures du corps de la vertèbre qui seront en contact : il restera en avant un petit hiatus.

La nature est capricieuse, et parfois il n'y a que la moitié latérale d'un corps vertébral de détruit, et celui-ci a la forme d'un coin dont l'axe serait transversal, la luxation va encore tenter de se faire : d'un côté elle est bientôt arrêtée par le contact du tissu restant, mais de l'autre côté le vide existant, la luxation des apophyses se fait davantage, elle est donc dans ce cas particulier surtout unilatérale. Il en résulte une déviation de la colonne vertébrale de ce côté ; le rachis est infléchi latéralement, cette courbure latérale n'a d'ailleurs que fort peu d'importance au point de vue de l'esthétique du dos, elle est corrigée en très peu de temps par des courbures de compensation ; un examen très attentif est nécessaire pour se rendre compte de ce fait que nous montre si clairement la radiographie.

Si plusieurs vertèbres sont détruites, ce cas peut se compliquer des précédents, il est facile en combinant les deux de se rendre compte de ce qui se passe.

Lorsque plusieurs vertèbres sont incomplètement cariées, cas fréquent, il reste souvent une partie plus ou moins considérable de la partie postérieure du corps vertébral attaché au rachis postérieur, le tassement produit par la luxation se fait suivant le mode ci-dessus décrit, et l'évolution de ce tassement se trouve limité par le contact des restes de tous ces corps vertébraux.

Toutes les lames vertébrales fortement pressées les unes contre les autres vont se dénuder réciproquement et se souder les unes aux autres, tel est le mode habituel de consolidation du rachis après redressement. La soudure pourra se faire sur toute l'étendue de l'arc postérieur : lame, apophyses épineuses, etc., et c'est pourquoi il faut, à l'encontre de Calot, respecter les apophyses épineuses dont l'ablation ne sert à rien et peut enlever un précieux moyen d'obtenir la solidité rachidienne.

L'intérieur des arcs postérieurs, surtout dans la région lombaire, est inégal et recouvert d'aspérités et l'on conçoit que le frottement des lames les unes sur les autres amène leur dénudation réciproque et leur soudure, soit par l'intermédiaire du périoste, soit d'os à os.

Ce qui se fait dans le cas de mal de Pott inférieur quelquefois à un degré extrême comme vous pouvez le voir sur cette radiographie, est de beaucoup moins prononcé dans les régions supérieures, et de plus, comme les maux de Pott lombaires n'offrent que rarement de grosses gibbosités, le traitement le plus élémentaire en entravant assez souvent l'évolution rend, par suite, la part du redressement forcé du mal de Pott très restreinte. Une des seules indications qui en restent est de pouvoir remédier à la paralysie dans grand nombre de cas.

On peut dire de cette intéressante période thérapeutique que la bosse n'était pas chose sacrée et qu'on pouvait la redresser à peu près sans danger, — mais, hélas! les espérances qu'elle promettait ne se sont point réalisées.

Efforçons-nous d'empêcher l'évolution du mal de Pott et cela nous le pouvons dans de grandes proportions.

Le redressement des bossus a été néamoins une tentative du plus haut intérêt. MM. Calot et Chipault auront fait bénéficier la science d'une étude fort intéressante.

DE LA RÉDUCTION DU MAL DE POTT

COMMUNICATION

de M. le docteur PHOCAS,

de Lille.

J'ai pratiqué 20 fois le redressement du mal de Pott. Dans une première série de 7 cas nous relevons 2 mauvais résultats et 5 bons au point de vue de l'état général.

Au point de vue local une gibbosité est restée réduite. Une autre s'est améliorée.

Dans un cas la paralysie préexistante a disparu.

Dans une seconde série comprenant 13 sujets traités par le redressement simple nous relevons un résultat nul chez 8 enfants sur 12. Une mort par compression de la moelle (Mal de Pott cervical). Six fois la réduction n'a pu être obtenue et 2 fois la réduction ne s'est pas maintenue.

Les résultats consécutifs sont les suivants :

Un seul cas réellement satisfaisant, trois autres assez bons. Deux morts consécutives par méningite (5 mois et 7 mois).

Deux abcès (l'un 4 mois, l'autre 7 mois après l'intervention).

En réalité il y a eu 5 bons résultats sur 20 et 5 morts dont l'une immédiate.

Avec ces résultats on peut juger la méthode.

Le redressement sous le chloroforme, même sans exercer la moindre violence, est une méthode dangereuse.

Elle n'est pas souvent efficace. Elle n'a réussi que dans 1 4 des cas choisis.

Faut-il la condamner absolument? Faut-il la réserver pour quelques cas particuliers?

En ce qui me concerne je crois qu'il y a lieu de la bannir comme méthode générale de traitement du mal de Pott, mais j'estime que dans certains cas exceptionnels cette méthode de traitement peut être appliquée.

Dans ces cas exceptionnels je citerai les gibbosités dorsales pas trop volumineuses, angulaires ou dorso-lombaires se redressant et se déroulant pour ainsi dire à la traction quand il n'y a pas d'abcès apparent et que l'état général est assez satisfaisant.

La paralysie est une indication à redressement.

Mais il faut se méfier du mal de Pott cervical.

Je dois ajouter que les gibbosités lombaires peu considérables se dissimulent si bien sous les vêtements qu'il est absolument inutile de les redresser.

En résumé, le traitement habituel du mal de Pott chez l'enfant est encore l'immobilisation pure et simple et ce n'est que dans certains cas exceptionnels que l'on peut avoir recours au redressement de la gibbosité en prévenant les parents du danger inhérent à cette opération, et de ses résultats aléatoires.

TRAITEMENT DE LA DÉFORMATION DANS LE MAL VERTÉBRAL

COMMUNICATION

de M. E. KIRMISSON.

Les résultats orthopédiques obtenus dans la cure du mal de Pott peuvent dépendre de trois éléments : 1° le siège même de l'affection; 2° l'étendue du mal à un plus ou moins grand nombre de vertèbres; 3° le mode de traitement employé.

Plus le mal de Pott siège à un niveau élevé, plus les circonstances sont défavorables au point de vue de la déformation. En effet, plus on s'approche de son extrémité supérieure, plus la colonne vertébrale devient mince, et moins elle est efficacement soutenue. Il n'est pas étonnant dès lors, que, si la lésion porte sur ces points élevés du rachis, elle aboutisse parfois à des déformations considérables.

Quant au second point, l'étendue des lésions, il tombe sous le bon sens que, plus la colonne de soutien sera interrompue dans une étendue notable, plus l'affaissement qui en résulte sera prononcé. Si la destruction osseuse est limitée à un seul corps vertébral, elle aboutit à la déformation angulaire et médiane classique, à sommet très court. Au contraire, si la perte de substance est étendue à un grand nombre de corps vertébraux, il en résulte une brèche énorme, et, pour la combler, le rachis s'infléchit en produisant une gibbosité angulaire considérable.

Le troisième élément qui intervient pour modifier le résultat obtenu, c'est le mode de traitement employé. Trop souvent il nous arrive de voir venir vers nous des enfants porteurs de gibbosités énormes, et qui n'ont jamais été soumis à aucun traitement. D'autres, dès le début de leur maladie, ont été affublés de corsets lourds et n'immobilisant que très incomplètement le rachis. Pourvus de ces corsets, ils n'ont jamais cessé d'aller et venir. Chez eux, l'action de la pesanteur se faisant sentir sur les points malades de la colonne vertébrale est doublement nuisible : elle entretient et aggrave le processus tuberculeux, et, au point de vue mécanique, elle exagère le tassement des éléments osseux, et, par suite, la difformité.

Alors même que les corsets employés remplissent bien le but, c'est-à-dire réalisent une immobilisation suffisante, ils ne suppriment pas l'action de la pesanteur. Au contraire, si les malades continuent à rester debout, au poids des parties supérieures du corps s'ajoute le poids de l'appareil lui-même, qui se fait sentir sur le foyer osseux. A cet égard, nous avons à nous demander si le corset plâtré dont la vulgarisation a été considérée comme un immense progrès dans le traitement du mal de Pott, n'a pas été quelquefois un mal.

Il est certain que, pour la population pauvre de nos hôpitaux, le corset plâtré qui n'est que d'un prix de revient très peu considérable, qui peut à chaque instant être renouvelé par le chirurgien, constitue un immense bienfait.

Mais, sous sa forme habituelle, le corset plâtré est passible de graves reproches. Il commence, en bas, à la région lombaire et laisse libres les articulations coxo-fémorales ; en haut, il se termine au-dessous des bras, au sommet de l'aisselle, et, par suite, il ne saurait immobiliser la partie supérieure de la région dorsale. Pourvus de ces appareils, les enfants sont laissés au lit : mais souvent, en dépit des recommandations faites aux parents, les petits malades sont assis pendant la plus grande partie du jour. Dès lors, on ne supprime pas l'action de la pesanteur sur le foyer pathologique. Depuis longtemps déjà, frappé de cet inconvénient grave, j'ai modifié la construction des appareils plâtrés destinés au mal de Pott. Au lieu de les arrêter au niveau de la région lombo-sacrée, je les prolonge jusqu'à la partie supérieure des cuisses au moyen d'un double spica de l'aine, de manière à immobiliser les articulations coxo-fémorales et à empêcher le petit malade de s'asseoir, absolument comme s'il était immobilisé dans une gouttière de Bonnet. De plus, pour peu que le mal de Pott dépasse la partie inférieure de la région dorsale, s'il occupe, par exemple, les 7° et 8° vertèbres dorsales, j'embrasse dans les bandes plâtrées les épaules et je fais remonter l'appareil jusqu'à la base du cou.

Il est un autre moyen dont on ne fait pas, suivant moi, dans le mal de Pott, un usage suffisant : je veux parler de l'extension continue. Sans doute, dans le mal cervical, tous les chirurgiens sont d'accord pour y recourir. Mais, dans le mal dorsal supérieur, celui qui siège au niveau des cinq premières vertèbres dorsales, qui s'accompagne assez fréquemment de paraplégie, et qui donne naissance à des déformations considérables, l'extension continue faite au moyen de l'appareil de Sayre, qui prend point d'appui à la fois sous les bras et sur l'extrémité céphalique, me rend chaque jour les meilleurs services. Pour cela, le malade est immobilisé dans une gouttière de Bonnet. Ceci m'amène à parler des modifications que j'ai fait subir à cette gouttière qui peut, dans le mal de Pott, donner les meilleurs résultats, si son usage est bien surveillé.

La gouttière de Bonnet, telle qu'elle existe chez nos fabricants, et telle qu'elle est généralement employée, a des rebords élevés qui prennent point d'appui au-dessous des bras; mais elle laisse complètement libre la région cervicale et la partie supérieure du thorax. Placé dans cette gouttière, l'enfant peut soulever incessamment la tête et la partie supérieure du tronc; et, dans le cas d'un mal de Pott dorsal supérieur, il n'est rien d'étonnant à ce qu'une immobilisation aussi insuffisante aboutisse à des déformations énormes. Je me suis préoccupé dès longtemps de parer à cet inconvénient grave, et, pour cela, j'ai ajouté à la gouttière des épaulières croisées au-devant du thorax, qui immobilisent rigoureusement les épaules et la région du cou. Un autre point qui, celui-là, a trait à l'hygiène générale, c'est la nécessité d'articuler l'un des membres inférieurs, de façon à pouvoir lui imprimer des mouvements d'abduction. On arrive ainsi facilement à laver toute la région périnéale, tandis que, dans les gouttières de l'ancien modèle, les deux membres inférieurs sont accolés l'un à l'autre, et il est très difficile de donner à l'enfant les soins de propreté nécessaires, à moins de le sortir de l'appareil. Ainsi pourvue de bretelles et articulée au niveau de l'un des membres inférieurs, la gouttière de Bonnet constitue un excellent appareil, capable de fournir dans le traitement du mal de Pott les meilleurs résultats.

Le point difficile, c'est de préciser le temps pendant lequel l'enfant devra être soumis à l'immobilisation dans la position horizontale. Il est nécessaire pour cela de tenir compte d'un grand nombre de facteurs. Tout d'abord la durée de la maladie : Ce n'est pas avant un an ou dix-huit mois qu'il peut être question de guérison du mal de Pott. Encore, après ce temps, n'a-t-on pas le droit de compter sur une consolidation solide, et, pendant très longtemps encore, il sera nécessaire de soutenir les petits malades au moyen d'appareils portatifs, si l'on veut éviter la production de déformations considérables. L'état général du sujet est également à prendre en considération ; si l'enfant présente un état de santé générale florissant, nous pouvons en conclure que les lésions tuberculeuses des vertèbres sont en bonne voie de guérison. Dans les circonstances inverses, si l'enfant est pâle et amaigri, si ses traits tirés revêtent une expression de souffrance, c'est une raison de croire que le mal de Pott est encore en pleine activité. L'examen de la colonne vertébrale elle-même peut nous renseigner, en nous révélant la présence ou l'absence de douleurs, en nous montrant si la difformité reste stationnaire, ou si elle est encore en voie de progrès. La palpation profonde de l'abdomen nous renseigne sur l'existence ou l'absence d'abcès par congestion ; enfin, la notion de douleurs, de faiblesse ou de contracture du côté des membres inférieurs, peut encore nous guider. Mais, il faut bien le dire, quelque soin que nous apportions à l'examen des malades, il y a des cas où nous restons hésitants. Aussi devons-nous accueillir comme un très grand progrès l'application de la radiographie à l'étude clinique du mal de Pott. C'est surtout au niveau de la région dorsale que son intervention a pour nous un très grand intérêt. A la région lombaire en effet, la palpation profonde de l'abdomen, chez l'enfant dont la paroi abdominale est peu épaisse, suffit dans la plupart des cas pour nous renseigner sur l'existence d'abcès, ou, tout au moins, de masses caséeuses développées au-devant de la colonne vertébrale. A la région dorsale, au contraire, il nous est le plus souvent impossible, par le seul examen clinique, de préjuger l'état exact des lésions. L'emploi de la radiographie nous permet de constater, par les ombres qu'elles développent, l'existence et le volume de masses caséeuses plus ou moins considérables, engainant la colonne vertébrale au niveau du point malade. C'est donc là un nouveau moyen de diagnostic que nous ne devrons pas négliger.

Quand, par un examen aussi circonstancié que possible, nous sommes arrivés à cette conclusion que les lésions sont en bonne voie de guérison, et que l'on peut sans imprudence, commencer à permettre au malade de se tenir debout, il y a encore de nombreuses précautions à prendre. Tout d'abord il convient de limiter soigneusement le nombre d'heures pendant lesquelles le malade aura la permission de marcher ; la marche ne sera permise qu'à l'aide de béquilles. Enfin, et c'est là la question essentielle qui nous reste à résoudre, le malade sera pourvu d'un appareil prothétique soutenant efficacement la colonne vertébrale.

Ces appareils ont été construits avec les matières les plus différentes ; pour ma part, je donne la préférence, toutes les fois que la chose est possible, au cuir moulé. Chez les malades pauvres, le feutre plastique peut également rendre de bons services. Mais, quelle que soit la matière dont le corset est composé, sa construction est astreinte à un certain nombre de règles qui varient suivant le siège et l'étendue du mal vertébral. Si le mal de Pott occupe la région lombaire, un corset ordinaire, c'est-à-dire remontant jusqu'à la région axillaire, suffira. Mais, ce qui importe avant tout, c'est de faire descendre ce corset le plus bas possible, de façon à prendre largement point d'appui sur le bassin. Le bassin est, en effet, le seul point d'appui solide que nous ayons pour agir sur la colonne vertébrale, et tout appareil qui ne possède pas un large point d'appui pelvien est nécessairement sans valeur.

S'agit-il d'un mal dorsal inférieur, siégeant par exemple au niveau de la 10ᵉ vertèbre dorsale, l'appareil pourra être construit d'après les mêmes principes, c'est-à-dire ne pas dépasser par en haut la région axillaire. Mais quand déjà le mal occupe la région dorsale moyenne, au niveau de la 7ᵉ ou de la 8ᵉ vertèbre dorsale, il devient nécessaire de faire remonter plus haut l'appareil, en embrassant complètement les épaules, et allant jusqu'à la base du cou. Enfin, dans le mal dorsal supérieur, celui qui siège au niveau des cinq premières vertèbres dorsales, il faut remonter plus haut encore, et se comporter comme si l'on avait affaire à un mal de Pott cervical, c'est-à-dire surajouter au corset un collier prenant point d'appui sur la nuque et sur le menton, et soutenant exactement l'extrémité céphalique.

Grâce à l'application de ces principes, on peut n'avoir, même dans les variétés dorsales supérieures du mal de Pott, si désavantageuses au point de vue orthopédique, que des difformités insignifiantes. Et c'est précisément parce que, dans la pratique, ces principes sont le plus souvent méconnus, que nous rencontrons si souvent des déformations énormes. Il nous arrive à chaque instant de voir des enfants présentant des gibbosités considérables, consécutives au mal de Pott dorsal supérieur et qui n'ont jamais porté d'autre appareil qu'un corset ordinaire, s'arrêtant au sommet de l'aisselle. Quelle action peut avoir un semblable appareil? Aucune, évidemment ; il représente seulement une véritable cupule dans laquelle repose la gibbosité; mais,

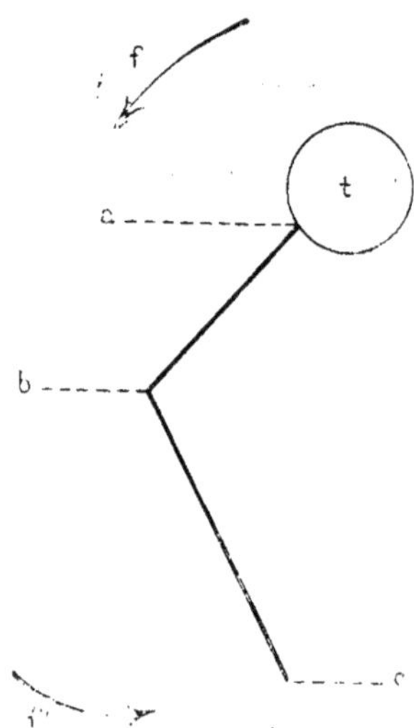

des deux côtés qui, par leur inclinaison réciproque, constituent la déformation angulaire, l'inférieur seul est soutenu, le supérieur est laissé libre. Or, dans ces conditions, non seulement toute espèce de redressement est impossible, mais l'on voit, sous l'influence du poids de la tête et des membres supérieurs, se produire incessamment l'aggravation de la difformité.

Envisageons uniquement pour le moment le côté mécanique de la question : supposons qu'il s'agit de redresser une ligne coudée a, b, c. Nous pourrons y réussir de deux manières, soit en agissant par pression directe sur le sommet de l'angle au point b, soit en agissant sur les deux bras de levier a b, b c, jusqu'à ce qu'ils soient dans la continuité l'un de l'autre, et que toute trace de déviation angulaire ait disparu. Dans le cas particulier du mal de Pott, il est bien évident que toute pression directe exercée sur le sommet de l'angle au point b, est impossible ; car, si elle était suffisante, elle ne tarderait pas à déterminer des escarres. Force est donc d'agir, non pas sur le sommet de l'angle, mais sur ses deux côtés, a b, b c. Et c'est là le point sur lequel nous désirons surtout insister ici. Qui ne voit, en effet, que, si la force est appliquée uniquement sur le bras de levier inférieur b c, le supérieur a b, n'étant pas soutenu, continuera à s'incliner en avant, et cela surtout si, à l'extrémité supérieure de ce bras de levier est appendue une sphère pesante t, représentant le poids de la tête et des membres supérieurs? Si, au contraire, on embrasse dans l'appareil les deux bras de levier, y compris la sphère t, appendue au bras de levier supérieur, on obtiendra le redressement, en agissant suivant la direction des flèches f et f', c'est-à-dire repoussant de bas en haut et d'arrière en avant le bras de levier inférieur, et, au contraire, de haut en bas et d'avant en arrière le bras de levier supérieur. Il suffit d'énoncer de pareils principes pour les rendre évidents à tous les yeux, et l'on s'étonne que, dans la pratique, ils soient si souvent méconnus.

Comme conclusions de cette discussion, nous dirons que dans le mal de Pott, les appareils doivent être en général beaucoup plus étendus que ceux qui sont journellement employés. Vouloir appliquer indistinctement à tous les cas de mal vertébral un modèle unique, c'est faire une thérapeutique irrationnelle, et contraire aux principes les plus élémentaires de mécanique que nous venons de rappeler.

En adoptant ces principes, on arrivera, je ne dis pas à éviter toujours complètement la déformation, mais du moins à n'avoir que des gibbosités extrêmement modérées. Et cela est possible, grâce à deux circonstances qu'il est nécessaire de rappeler ici. La première, c'est que pendant très longtemps, beaucoup plus longtemps qu'on ne le croit généralement, il reste dans le foyer morbide de la mobilité. L'anatomie pathologique et les tentatives de redressement forcé s'accordent à le démontrer. La seconde circonstance qui permet le redressement, c'est que, dans la difformité du mal de Pott, il y a une part importante à faire à la contracture musculaire. Sous l'influence du repos qui supprime les douleurs, sous l'influence de la guérison des abcès, on voit la contracture disparaître, et de ce fait, l'attitude des malades s'améliorer considérablement.

MAL DE POTT

COMMUNICATION

de M. CALOT.

de Berck-sur-Mer.

A l'encontre de la plupart des chirurgiens je n'admets ici, comme dans toutes les manifestations de la tuberculose, d'autre intervention active que celle qui a pour but la correction de la difformité.

S'attaquer directement comme on l'a fait par une intervention sanglante au foyer tuberculeux du mal de Pott, ou à la paralysie, ou à l'abcès par congestion, c'est transformer le mal de Pott fermé en un mal de Pott ouvert.

Si le premier a plus de 95 chances pour 100 de se terminer par la guérison, le deuxième a plus de 95 chances sur 100 de se terminer par la mort.

Je ne puis assez m'étonner que les chirurgiens qui ont tout osé en fait d'opérations sanglantes pour attaquer la paralysie et le foyer ou l'abcès du mal de Pott pour lesquels l'abstention est infiniment préférable, n'aient jamais songé à lutter contre la gibbosité pour laquelle cependant leur intervention aurait été incomparablement plus inoffensive et plus indiquée.

Plus inoffensive si tout ce qu'on fait contre elle se passe en dehors du foyer tuberculeux qui restera fermé.

Plus indiquée, puisque les autres manifestations de la maladie guérissent bien mieux si l'on s'abstient de tout traitement chirurgical, tandis que la gibbosité, si l'on ne s'y oppose, s'installe et s'accroît fatalement.

Or, la gibbosité est ici la manifestation symptomatique particulièrement grave.

Supprimez la gibbosité avec ses conséquences immédiates ou éloignées, et le mal de Pott n'est plus la maladie redoutable que chacun sait. Ne rien faire, cela veut dire s'en tenir aux traitements anciens, car ni les gouttières, ni les corsets ne peuvent en effet empêcher la gibbosité de se produire et de s'aggraver: tous les chirurgiens le savent: et l'on en trouve même l'aveu chez les auteurs qui ont écrit sur la question.

Ces moyens ne peuvent suffire que dans les cas extrêmement bénins et par conséquent exceptionnels.

Pour l'immense majorité des cas, il faut donc un traitement plus sévère, plus précis, plus parfait.

Premier cas. — Le malade arrive sans gibbosité, sans paralysie, sans abcès (ce mal de Pott répond à la coxalgie venue sans déviation).

Notre objectif c'est de faire un traitement qui empêche sûrement la gibbosité de se produire.

Le repos dans la position couchée ne suffit pas, même sur la planche, ou dans la gouttière de Bonnet ou la gouttière plâtrée.

Le seul moyen qui nous permette d'atteindre le but c'est de mettre l'enfant dans un grand appareil plâtré qui maintienne exactement la totalité du tronc, comme le grand appareil de la coxalgie est le seul moyen assuré d'empêcher la déviation de la hanche.

Mais ici, le grand appareil plâtré est encore plus difficile à faire qu'à la hanche. Il faut qu'il maintienne la totalité du tronc, la base du crâne et le bassin, sans cependant gêner le fonctionnement des organes thoraciques ni abdominaux et sans blesser l'enfant.

La difficulté de sa construction, voilà l'écueil. S'il est mal fait il ne remplira pas le but, il peut même être malfaisant ; mais il en est de même pour tous les appareils à des degrés différents. L'orthopédie demande une grande habileté et une grande expérience.

Un appareil bien fait maintient le dos mathématiquement et sauve-garde l'état général de l'enfant.

On le construit dans la suspension avec légère lordose, ce qui nous permet de réaliser ces deux indications du traitement des tuberculoses ostéo-articulaires à savoir la décompression des surfaces malades dans l'immobilisation absolue du rachis et le repos dans le décubitus horizontal.

Cet appareil sera changé le plus rarement possible pour éviter tout traumatisme inutile à l'enfant.

DEUXIÈME CAS. — *Mal de Pott avec abcès.* — Tout se réduit à ceci : n'ouvrir jamais les abcès, les empêcher de s'ouvrir. Donc, les traiter par les ponctions et les injections modificatrices lorsqu'ils menacent la peau.

TROISIÈME CAS. — *Mal de Pott avec paralysie.* — Les opérations sanglantes proposées autrefois pour combattre la paralysie doivent être proscrites : parce qu'elles ont une gravité immédiate très réelle, parce qu'elles ont une gravité éloignée très redoutable, puisqu'elles ont ouvert le foyer tuberculeux et que la fistule qu'elles laissent ne guérira plus, et enfin parce qu'elles n'ont que très peu d'action durable sur la paralysie.

Au contraire, le redressement par la simple suspension et l'appli-cation immédiate d'un grand appareil plâtré, n'a pas de gravité ni immédiate ni éloignée, et guérit toutes les paralysies (peut-être 95 ou 98 sur 100). Si la simple suspension n'a pas suffi, on fait à une séance ultérieure une légère traction et une pression directe sur la gibbosité pour dégager la moelle et on réussit cette fois.

QUATRIÈME CAS. — *Mal de Pott avec gibbosité.* — Si la gibbosité est récente et petite, la suspension avec ou sans chloroforme, avec ou sans légère pression sur la gibbosité, la corrige ; ce redressement dure moins d'une minute et est d'une bénignité absolue.

Appliquer immédiatement un grand appareil plâtré en légère lordose et laisser le malade environ un an dans la position couchée, en ne changeant l'appareil que tous les 6 ou 7 mois si c'est possible.

Si la gibbosité est un peu plus ancienne et plus marquée, faire dans la suspension une pression directe plus énergique, une traction un peu plus forte, mais sans traumatisme inutile. La correction dure encore ici une ou deux minutes, et le traumatisme est, entre des mains exercées, moindre que celui du redressement du genou et de la hanche.

L'appareil plâtré ne doit pas blesser l'enfant, sinon le but n'est pas complètement atteint ; parce que dès lors, l'immobilisation n'est plus absolue. Nous dirons les moyens d'empêcher ces petites blessures.

L'opération sanglante consistant dans l'ablation des extrémités saillantes des apophyses épineuses et l'avivement du périoste des lames, est une intervention qui dure cinq minutes et est d'une bénignité éprouvée.

Elle a de grands avantages :

1° De faciliter le redressement ;

2° D'empêcher que l'appareil ne blesse l'enfant ;

3° De favoriser la consolidation par les néoformations scléreuses et osseuses qu'elle amène.

Si la gibbosité est ancienne et volumineuse, si elle est soudée, c'est-à-dire ne bougeant plus, il ne faut pas y toucher.

Si elle n'est pas soudée, si elle augmente encore, il faut la traiter pour arrêter sa progression ; et le meilleur moyen d'y arriver, c'est de la redresser un peu.

Les enfants doivent rester couchés, si ce n'est lorsque leur état général commande de les faire marcher.

La guérison locale est beaucoup mieux sauvegardée par le décubitus horizontal.

Généralement les enfants garderont ce repos environ un an.

Puis ils se lèvent avec le même grand appareil plâtré emboîtant le crâne (n° 1), ou bien avec un grand appareil s'arrêtant par un col officier à l'union du crâne et de la nuque (n° 2), plus tard avec un petit corset sans col, mais avec « épaulières » (n° 3), qu'on leur laissera longtemps ; on le remplacera plus tard par un corset amovible en celluloïde.

En faisant ainsi on n'aura pas toujours des résultats parfaits, mais on aura des résultats infiniment supérieurs à ceux des anciens traitements, parce qu'on aura lutté avec infiniment plus de vigueur et de persévérance contre la gibbosité tenace et rebelle.

Ce qu'il faut dire surtout c'est que pour les enfants venus à nous pas trop tard, nous avons un moyen sûr d'empêcher la gibbosité d'apparaître ou si elle existe le moyen de la corriger ou de l'atténuer très souvent. Les résultats sont d'autant plus beaux que le traitement nouveau sera mieux connu et mieux appliqué.

DISCUSSION.

M. Villemin. — M. Calot vient de nous dire que la gibbosité se redresse *sous l'ombre d'un danger* par la suspension simple et, sous une autre forme, par des moyens d'une bénignité absolue, que ces manœuvres ne sont pas plus graves que celles que comporte le redressement du genou ou de la hanche. Autant, dans la séance de ce matin, ici même, j'ai été partisan des manœuvres de violence dans le traitement de la scoliose, autant, en ce qui concerne les déviations rachidiennes dues à la tuberculose, je pense, d'accord avec MM. Bradfort, Mouchet et Phocas, qu'on ne saurait jamais être trop prudent.

J'ai toujours eu une crainte instinctive pour le redressement forcé ; je redoute même la suspension simple depuis que le fait suivant a été porté à ma connaissance :

Un enfant d'une dizaine d'années, porteur d'une gibbosité dorsale de dimensions moyennes, fut suspendu selon la technique habituelle pour l'application d'un corset plâtré. Bien que soutenu par le menton et la nuque, sous les bras par deux étriers et la pointe des pieds reposant sur le sol de toute la surface du talon antérieur, le petit patient succomba à des phénomènes asphyxiques au moment de l'application des premiers tours de bande. Aucun agent anesthésique n'avait été employé, aucune violence n'avait été faite. Un abcès froid occupant le médiasin postérieur avait fait irruption dans les plèvres. C'est l'exemple de ce cas malheureux qui me fait dire, contrairement aux assertions de tout à l'heure, que la suspension simple n'est pas absolument innocente, *a fortiori* quand les pieds ne portent pas sur le sol, quand toute la moitié inférieure du corps agit par son poids sur un segment rachidien que la contracture supprimée par le chloroforme n'immobilise plus. Avant d'appliquer un corset plâtré, il est bon d'avertir la famille de tout ce qui peut arriver.

M. le Dr Chipault. — La plupart des orateurs qui sont intervenus dans la discussion en cours sur la réduction des gibbosités pottiques ont eu des résultats médiocres. Je crois qu'à beaucoup ont manqué la conviction et la patience nécessaires et qu'aussi leur technique a été défectueuse ou incomplète. Pour ma part, dans le mal de Pott, au début, j'applique un corset plâtré, toujours très long, dans la position tête en bas. Dans la gibbosité constituée, si elle se réduit par cette position et quelques pressions, sous chloroforme, je fais des ligatures apophysaires ou laminaires et j'applique un corset plâtré ; si elle ne se réduit pas je fais des ligatures apophysaires pour m'opposer au tassement du cal vertébral, atteint d'ostéite raréfiante, et aux déformations progressives des organes. La paraplégie, quoique n'étant pour ainsi dire jamais due à la compression nécessite parfois une laminectomie. J'insiste sur les deux caractéristiques de ma technique : suspension tête en bas, merveilleuse de simplicité, que le malade soit endormi ou non ; ligatures apophysaires. Elle assure à mon avis mieux que toute autre l'immobilisation en bonne position sur la nécessité de laquelle nous sommes tous d'accord ; elle est sans dangers ; elle m'a donné trop de bons résultats pour que je n'insiste pas sur la nécessité de l'appliquer exactement. Mais suivez les indications; faites des ligatures solides, appliquez de très longs appareils plâtrés, n'oubliez pas que le traitement de la tuberculose vertébrale demande des années, et ne soyez pas découragés par les insuccès inévitables dans une affection aussi grave et aussi complexe dans ses manifestations qu'est le mal de Pott. Vous arriverez vite à la conviction que le traitement que je préconise, déprécié par des généralisations intempestives, est, dans les limites que je lui ai assignées dès le début, si on le suit rigoureusement, le meilleur traitement actuel de la tuberculose vertébrale, en tout cas un traitement bien supérieur à toutes les mécaniques orthopédiques qui doivent disparaître absolument de la thérapeutique et à la méthode du redressement forcé sans ligatures que je juge dangereuse et insuffisante.

M. Froelich, fait remarquer que dans la discussion du traitement de la gibbosité on n'a pas encore prononcé le mot de *lordosisation*. C'est cependant à elle que l'on doit les redressements les plus durables. La technique en est très simple. M. F. l'a décrite au Congrès français de chirurgie en 1897.

L'enfant est couché sur le ventre, la tête et les avant-bras croisés sur un petit tabouret, la racine des cuisses sur un autre tabouret. Sur le sommet de la gibbosité on fait passer une anse de bande en toile qui porte, sous le ventre de l'enfant et sous la table, un poids de 1 à 2 kilogrammes; au bout de quelques minutes la contracture musculaire est vaincue, la gibbosité cède un peu, mais surtout il se forme une lordose sus et sous-gibbaire. C'est dans cette position que l'on met l'appareil plâtré qui fixe, comme une virole dont l'axe aurait une convexité antérieure, la colonne dans une attitude corrigée.

La technique est très simple, et le plus souvent ne demande aucun aide, avec un peu de patience, les enfants les plus récalcitrants se prêtent à cette position très peu douloureuse.

Cette lordosisation horizontale lui paraît bien supérieure aux suspensions verticales ou obliques par la tête ou par les poids. Elle est aussi beaucoup plus simple et moins dangereuse.

M. T. Piéchaud, professeur de clinique chirurgicale infantile (de Bordeaux).

Messieurs.

Les communications que nous venons d'entendre et la discussion qui les ont suivies me semblent avoir porté le dernier coup au redressement brusque, à la *cure radicale* de la gibbosité pottique et pour ma part j'en éprouve une réelle satisfaction.

Je n'ai en effet jamais compris comment pouvait s'accommoder de manœuvres violentes une colonne vertébrale entourée d'organes, tels que gros vaisseaux et nerfs importants déplacés ou fléchis, pour la plupart enlizés dans des exsudats en rapport direct avec des tuberculomes qui menacent si souvent les cavités pleurales, les poumons et la moelle elle-même. A juste titre, M. Phocas a dit qu'il y aurait, quoi qu'on fasse, toujours des bossus et je me demande s'il ne vaut pas mieux supporter une déformation, dans bien des cas, que de s'exposer à des accidents mortels.

J'ai toujours résisté à l'enthousiasme de la première heure. Une seule fois, sollicité par les supplications pressantes d'une famille, qui me demandait, quelles qu'en fussent les conséquences, de pratiquer le redressement forcé, j'ai pratiqué cette opération. Il s'agissait d'une fillette de 7 ans atteinte du mal de Pott dorsal inférieur avec gibbosité *moyenne*. Je ne cédai pas sans avoir représenté quelles pouvaient être les complications du redressement brusque et vraiment je ne fus pas encourageant dans cette énumération. L'opération n'exigea que des manœuvres bien simples : la courbure se redressa facilement. Le soir même ma petite opérée était paraplégiée. De tiède que j'étais, je restai complètement refroidi et jamais plus je n'ai fait le redressement forcé.

On nous propose maintenant d'agir par une autre méthode qui est le redressement progressif. Je n'ai pas d'expérience suffisante pour juger cette manière et cependant je vois par les dessins qu'il vient de faire passer sous nos yeux, que M. Calot a obtenu de très beaux résultats. L'avenir jugera, mais je reste toujours en garde contre les complications à craindre en présence d'une lésion très grave qui demande plus à être respectée que violemment traitée.

Pourquoi les orateurs que nous avons entendus ne nous ont-ils pas parlé de l'abcès pottique? Il constitue cependant une des plus graves complications et, durant tout le traitement de la tuberculose vertébrale, guide en quelque sorte le pronostic. Un mal de Pott sans abcès laisse beaucoup d'espoir ; si la suppuration apparaît tout est à redouter parce que l'ouverture du foyer peut entraîner la septicémie. Il serait bien intéressant de savoir si le redressement forcé et mieux le redressement progressif n'ont pas donné trop souvent un coup de fouet à la marche des abcès ossifluents et je veux, en passant, faire constater que les grands appareils réclamés par le redressement ne sont peut-être pas tout ce qu'il y a de mieux pour l'hygiène des pottiques. M. Gourdon, ici présent, doit se rappeler que plusieurs de ses malades ont eu des eschares malgré toutes les précautions qu'il avait prises. Enfermés dans des plâtres depuis la tête jusqu'aux cuisses, même jusqu'aux jambes, ces malades se trouvent à peu près dans les mêmes conditions que si nous les placions dans la gouttière de Bonnet qui est bien pour ces cas le plus mauvais des appareils. Avec cette dernière, la déchéance organique est sûre : comme elle l'est pour la coxalgie traitée de la même manière. La gouttière de Bonnet m'a donné tant de suppurations, j'ai vu tant d'enfants tués par elle que je l'ai depuis longtemps proscrite. Et c'est pour souligner encore ce qu'ont dit les orateurs qui m'ont précédé, que j'insiste sur les précautions d'hygiène indispensables dans la cure du mal de Pott. C'est pour bien affirmer ma conviction que je déclare ne pas admettre qu'il n'existe guère de moyen d'empêcher les complications du mal de Pott.

A mon avis, Messieurs, il existe au contraire deux moyens pour l'éviter: l'immobilisation absolue, radicale et l'application d'un appareil qui la réalise sans offenser les règles les plus élémentaires de l'hygiène.

Comment se fait-il que depuis bientôt douze ans je n'aie pas été obligé d'inciser ou de ponctionner aucun de mes pottiques immobilisés d'après la méthode que j'ai proposée, et dont j'ai plusieurs fois publié la technique? Bien plus, j'ai toujours vu se résorber les abcès existants déjà quand les malades m'ont été conduits, ou apparus peu de temps après le début du traitement parce qu'ils étaient déjà en route vers la fosse iliaque. Au surplus, des exemples pris sur plus de 25 cas demandent à être cités. C'est un jeune homme de 23 ans, porteur d'une gibbosité vertébrale à peine sensible mais atteint d'un abcès de la fosse iliaque considérable contenant au moins un litre de pus, qui après une immobilité de deux ans, a vu sa collection disparaître. C'est une fillette de 6 ans, fort intelligente et docile qui, après dix-huit mois, est restée guérie alors qu'elle présentait un abcès de volume invraisemblable : la paroi abdominale tout entière était soulevée comme dans une ascite ; le pus franchissant l'arcade crurale avait envahi la partie supérieure de la cuisse droite, l'espace de J.-L. Petit avait été forcée en arrière et de la région lombaire on renvoyait jusqu'à la cuisse un mouvement de flot. Tout le monde autour de moi estimait que je devais ponctionner ou inciser : je résistai voyant bien qu'au bout de mon intervention j'avais la septicémie bien menaçante. Ma malade a résorbé son abcès. Agée aujourd'hui de 20 ans, elle est très gibbeuse sans doute, mais elle vit heureuse de son sort et reste un témoignage probant de ce que peut et doit obtenir la prudence dans le traitement du mal de Pott.

Pour que l'immobilité de mes malades soit complète je repousse, si ce n'est pour la convalescence, les appareils autorisant l'attitude assise, à plus forte raison la station verticale et la marche. Le décubitus dorsal est indispensable.

J'ai fait exécuter un appareil qui se réclame des mêmes principes que celui du professeur Lannelongue. C'est un corset en toile, bouclé en avant et muni en haut et en bas, de chaque côté d'un lien fixateur qui le retient à une claie d'osier. Sur les membres inférieurs sont fixés, avec des bandes de flanelle, des liens en caoutchouc qui assurent une extension constante.

La claie qui n'est autre que celle du Dr Courtin ici présent est pourvue d'un matelas peu épais, dur, assurant à la colonne vertébrale un soutien constant. On peut du reste le modifier suivant les cas et la saillie vertébrale.

Ainsi se trouvent réalisées les meilleures conditions d'hygiène. Les enfants dégagés de toute pression possible vivent en contact avec l'air, ne sont souillés ni par l'urine, ni par la sueur, ni par les déjections ; ils peuvent être nettoyés chaque jour et baignés de temps en temps.

Il va sans dire que pour les grandes déformations et le mal de Pott supérieur, d'autres conditions doivent souvent être réalisées.

Contre des cas exceptionnels de nouvelles règles sont à suivre. C'est affaire des appareils dits minerves, c'est peut-être celle du redressement progressif. Je ne parle aujourd'hui que des cas communs pour lesquels nous avons à agir tous les jours. Non seulement nous les guérissons par le procédé que j'indique, mais nous empêchons la gibbosité de se développer et même nous la réduisons souvent.

Je ne peux admettre l'objection qui m'a été faite d'interrompre l'immobilisation par les soins de propreté et les bains. Ma conviction est bien arrêtée à ce sujet. Autrefois, j'admettais comme tout le monde cette loi sacro-sainte de ne jamais, sous aucun prétexte, interrompre même pour quelques instants, l'immobilisation dans le traitement de certaines affections, surtout dans celui de la coxalgie ; mais depuis longtemps, je pense que si l'immobilité est nécessaire, elle l'est peut-être moins que l'hygiène sans laquelle rien ne pourra réussir. Mais entrerait-il dans un esprit judicieux qu'en nettoyant un enfant, en le plaçant avec précaution dans une baignoire d'un modèle spécial, on interrompt le *charme* de l'immobilisation ?

MARDI 7 AOUT

Séance du soir.

SUR LES INDICATIONS THÉRAPEUTIQUES DANS L'APPENDICITE

RAPPORT

par **M.** le docteur **ROUX**,
de Lauzanne.

Il est peu de questions qui aient passionné le monde médical et le grand public autant que l'appendicite : il n'en est pas qui mérite plus que celle-ci de fixer l'attention des chirurgiens.

Cantonnée en apparence dans certaines contrées, cette affection éclatait surtout dans les pays où l'on savait la reconnaître, et, plus encore, dans la clientèle des médecins qui savaient la découvrir : maladie saisonnière au point qu'on a pu, avec quelque raison, la regarder comme épidémique; elle est aussi, au premier chef, une affection familiale où l'hérédité, dans son acception la plus large, joue un rôle de plus en plus important.

L'appendicite a été étudiée partout, dans ces derniers quinze ans, et seules les indications thérapeutiques qu'elle comporte manquent d'unité. Nous félicitons notre Président d'avoir mis à l'ordre du jour du Congrès une discussion si importante.

L'esprit de critique qui honore le corps médical a donné dans l'histoire du siècle le spectacle habituel de batailles scientifiques mémorables, dans lesquelles le dernier mot et la victoire restaient souvent au plus éloquent ou à celui qui savait mettre les rieurs de son côté, malgré une pauvreté d'arguments qui provoquent notre surprise, lorsqu'on pense aux malades.

C'est ce qui m'engage à vous dire dès l'abord que c'est au nom d'un millier d'appendicites — avec plus de six cents opérations à froid — que j'ai accepté la tâche peut-être ingrate de vous présenter un rapport personnel ou, comme nous l'avons entendu définir, « un travail destiné à être attaqué vivement et démoli sans pitié ».

Ce que nous pouvons le plus consciencieusement démolir dans cette assemblée, c'est l'appendicite elle-même. Et nous lui porterons le coup fatal en décidant l'excision « à froid » de tout appendice vermiforme qui a fait parler de lui : nous entendons par là tous ceux qui ont été atteints, ne fût-ce qu'une fois, avec exsudat palpé par un bon médecin, sans se préoccuper si ce diverticule est encore malade et, surtout, sans attendre qu'il s'agisse d'une appendicite à rechute.

Quel que soit l'état dans lequel il se présente à l'examen du malade, c'est un appendice taré, un ennemi dans la place. Nous l'avons vu à l'œuvre et l'examen antomo-microscopique nous montre pourquoi c'est un ennemi irréconciliable : persistance d'un ulcère, d'un calcul, d'une fistule, d'un abcès fongueux; amputation avec formation d'une poche enkystée, vase clos; cicatrice avec microbisme latent : voilà sa tare. Refroidissement, traumatisme, entérite, indigestion, menses, simple hypérémie locale : voilà ses prétextes.

Il est inutile de compliquer le tableau en faisant une classe à part pour l'appendicite chronique, qui n'est souvent qu'un reste, et à laquelle nous n'avons aucune raison de laisser prendre ce qualificatif, même si l'actinomycose ou la tuberculose est en jeu.

Quant à la colique appendiculaire, nous ne croyons pas que ce soit une appellation pratique, tout au moins pas dans l'acception habituelle : il s'agit presque toujours de formes légères de l'appendicite. Nous n'en voulons de meilleure preuve que la lecture attentive du travail dans lequel M. Talamon lui a donné le baptême : une tuméfaction grosse comme un œuf, fût-il de pigeon, n'est plus une colique appendiculaire. Il nous suffit que ce diagnostic ait été posé par un médecin instruit, exact et consciencieux pour nous croire autorisé à intervenir « à froid ».

Lorsque nous aurons excisé tous les appendices notoirement coupables, nous aurons porté, avons-nous dit, un coup mortel à l'appendicite, car nous sommes certain de ne pas exagérer en disant qu'on aura supprimé les trois quarts des appendicites aiguës.

En effet, si l'on questionne attentivement les malades, on se trouve rarement en face d'une première crise : c'est la quatrième, la cinquième, la dix-septième qu'on enregistre. Toutes ces récidives supprimées par l'opération à froid, l'appendicite redeviendra ce qu'elle est encore dans certains pays : une maladie plutôt rare.

Si nous osons recommander dans une aussi large mesure l'intervention à froid, c'est qu'elle est, dans la règle, tout à fait sans danger, puisque l'on peut la pratiquer par centaines sans échec : même en comptant les cas les plus compliqués, ceux dans lesquels il nous est arrivé, par exemple, de réséquer jusqu'à cinquante-huit centimètres d'intestin grêle et gros, de faire des anastomoses ou des résections multiples et de passer à cette besogne deux heures trois quarts, alors que l'opération ordinaire prend huit à quatorze minutes en moyenne, nous n'avons eu que deux échecs sur plus de six cents opérations.

C'est cette bénignité de l'opération à froid qui risque, à notre sens, de compliquer la discussion, puisqu'on va nous la servir au lit du malade, en pleine crise péritonéale aiguë. On a, en effet, depuis quelques années, déplacé la question, et l'on ne discute plus, avec les archéoptéryx de la médecine interne, si l'appendicite est ou non une maladie dans laquelle le chirurgien a son mot à dire : il s'agit, maintenant, de savoir si oui ou non le chirurgien doit se précipiter tête baissée dans le péritoine dès qu'on a prononcé le mot d'appendicite.

À ce point de vue encore, on ne saurait trop louer M. le Président d'avoir rappelé qu'il existe dans l'appendicite aiguë, comme dans toutes les autres maladies, des *indications thérapeutiques*.

La plus urgente des indications est de savoir ce qu'il faut *ne pas faire*, car on a à lutter avec les préjugés du public et ceux plus dangereux — parce qu'ils ont souvent pour base une fausse expérience scientifique — de quelques médecins.

Oubliant qu'une péristaltique normale exige comme premier excitant un certain contenu intestinal et un travail musculaire général, notre génération, hantée par l'idée des résorptions de toxines si chères aux cliniciens actuels, recourt journellement aux laxatifs plutôt qu'à l'ingestion habituelle de fruits et légumes ou autres aliments à résidu abondant.

De là cette manie désastreuse dans le public, qui consiste à donner des purgatifs dès qu'il se présente quelque malaise ressemblant à une indigestion : nous n'avons pas souvenance d'un seul cas d'appendicite dans lequel on n'ait pas commencé les soins et assuré la gravité du mal par un purgatif.

Du côté des médecins, et des meilleurs, on ne parvient pas à se libérer de la détestable habitude de recourir aussi aux purgatifs et, en particulier, au calomel à dose fractionnée avec la morphine.

Pourquoi la morphine? Parce que le malade souffre et surtout parce que le praticien a vaguement le scrupule de faire une bêtise en brassant un ventre si douloureux. Et le calomel? Parce que le médecin se souvient surtout des soupirs de soulagement poussés par lui-même et ses malades au moment d'une débâcle intestinale suivie comme par enchantement de l'euphorie et de la guérison : parce qu'il se laisse effrayer par les signes de pseudo-iléus inflammatoire si souvent observés au début de l'appendicite.

Il oublie, le praticien, que la fameuse débâcle, avec ou sans pus, n'est pas la cause de la guérison, mais qu'elle en est la conséquence, la signature d'un intestin qui recommence à se mouvoir, lorsque l'abcès est franchement enkysté ou vidé, et le reste du ventre rendu à ses préoccupations habituelles.

D'une manière absolue, on proscrira donc les purgatifs dans tout le cours de l'appendicite : même dans la convalescence, on saura les remplacer par des lavements qui eux-mêmes ne seront destinés, en aucun cas, à remonter au-dessus de l'ampoule rectale. S'il est défendu de brasser les intestins avec l'huile de ricin par en haut, il n'est pas permis de les brasser par en bas.

Le repos absolu, sous toutes ses formes, est de rigueur. On interdira tous mouvements, même pour les besoins naturels, et on aura soin, par exemple, de glisser un traversin sous les genoux. On évitera par conséquent de transporter le malade où que ce soit. On forcera l'immobilisation de l'intestin par l'opium administré de préférence par la voie rectale, à plus forte raison s'il y a des vomissements. Pour agir plus vite contre les douleurs quelquefois très vives du début et, peut-être, pour paralyser un peu moins intestins et vessie, on pourra recourir à la morphine en injection.

Ce qu'il ne faut pas faire non plus, c'est de provoquer ou d'encourager les vomissements par l'ingestion intempestive d'aliments quelconques, de remèdes ou de moyens domestiques tels que le café noir, le kirsch, l'alcool de menthe, etc., la diète sera donc absolue pour les premières heures et aussi longtemps qu'il y aura la moindre tendance aux vomissements ou au hoquet.

On se rappellera les expériences de Succi et les typhoïdes et on laissera les malades dans un repos complet anatomique et physiologique. Rien ne sera plus facile que de tromper la soif par quelques gouttes de liquide sur la langue tout au plus, ou de la calmer par de microscopiques lavements, quitte à recourir très exceptionnellement et en cas de détresse, aux injections sous-cutanées d'eau salée, jusqu'au moment où la localisation évidente du foyer permettra d'utiliser plus largement la voie stomacale.

Dès qu'il n'y a plus de vomissements ou de hoquet, il nous paraît ridicule de faire boire les malades par l'hypoderme ou le rectum : les quelques gouttes confiées à l'estomac arrivent à leur adresse avant de réveiller le cœcum et son voisinage.

Si nous ajoutons que la poche de glace aura sa place marquée dans les premiers jours, soit pour calmer la douleur et la phlegmasie, soit pour diminuer le météorisme, jusqu'à ce que les compresses à la Priessnitz la remplacent pour aider à la résorption de l'exsudat, sans nous attarder aux sangsues dont les avantages sont compensés par des inconvénients multiples, nous aurons passé en revue toutes les indications essentiellement négatives qui suffisent dans les cas bénins, de beaucoup les plus nombreux et qui conservent toute leur valeur, à côté de l'opération, dans les cas le plus graves.

Quant à l'intervention sanglante, nous avons dit qu'elle supprimerait à froid les 75 pour 100 des appendicites, en faisant courir fort peu de dangers, et il va sans dire qu'on ferait théoriquement une opération presque à froid, c'est-à-dire inoffensive, dans les premières heures de la crise aiguë. Il n'y a donc rien qui s'oppose à une intervention immédiate dans un très petit nombre de cas, où des circonstances toutes particulières permettent un diagnostic à peu près certain, si les conditions de milieu et d'opérateur sont idéales.

Cependant, même dans ces conditions, nous avons connaissance déjà d'un certain nombre d'opérations inutiles, entreprises pour des appendicites qui n'en étaient pas, où il n'y avait même pas de prétexte analogue, et dont plusieurs ont été suivies de mort.

En attendant que tous les candidats à l'appendicite à rechute se soient mis en règle avec leur cœcum, il arrivera aussi assez fréquemment que des malades auxquels on avait conseillé en vain l'excision à froid, alarmés par les premiers symptômes d'une rechute, accourront au chirurgien : là encore, une intervention immédiate aura bien des chances d'être une sorte d'opération à froid avec tous ses avantages et, plusieurs fois, il nous est arrivé de surprendre une appendicite de ce genre après onze, quatorze ou quinze heures et de trouver le processus vermiforme encore en parfaite liberté.

Par contre, il ne s'ensuit pas que nous osions recommander comme anodine cette excision à froid : c'est une opération souvent délicate, quelquefois très difficile et qui toujours doit être entreprise dans des conditions exceptionnelles de sécurité. Elle ne sera jamais une opération à la portée de tout le monde, à moins d'admettre que des échecs injustifiés sont compensés par quelques succès plus ou moins réels en cas facile.

Il ne faut surtout pas décréter que l'intervention est indiquée dès que le diagnostic est posé, car les cas auxquels nous avons fait allusion constitueront de plus en plus une infime minorité. Le gros contingent sera longtemps encore fourni par des appendicites diagnostiquées ou confiées au médecin après un, deux ou plusieurs jours, alors que dans l'entourage du malade on a tout fait pour assurer la gravité de la crise.

Au moment où l'on appelle le médecin, du moins dans mon pays, il n'est ordinairement plus question d'une sorte d'opération à froid, mais bien d'un vrai remue-ménage, en plein foyer infectieux et en plein ventre, dans un mauvais milieu et quelquefois sur un sujet momentanément en mauvaises conditions de résistance : l'opération devient grave en elle-même. Elle fait courir au malade plus de risques que son mal et, enfin, elle doit fatalement conduire à la formation d'une hernie dans la cicatrice d'une plaie qu'on aura dû laisser ouverte.

Il n'est pas permis de faire croire aux malades ou à leur famille que toute appendicite constitue un danger tel qu'une opération grave soit nécessaire ou justifiée : on ne peut surtout plus parler d'une sorte d'opération « à froid », facile, rapide, anodine : on s'en garderait bien !

Lorsqu'on voit aujourd'hui un chirurgien hésiter à opérer une appendicite aiguë, on croit volontiers qu'il fait machine en arrière : il convient simplement de rappeler qu'au début de son intervention dans cette maladie, celui-ci ne voyait que les cas graves. Maintenant, nous voyons aussi les cas légers, ce ne sont pas les opérations dans la crise qui ont diminué ; ce sont les cas où la temporisation réussit et où l'opération « à froid » seule est nécessaire qui ont augmenté dans une très forte proportion.

Personne n'aura l'idée d'opérer d'emblée l'appendicite la plus sûrement diagnostiquée, lorsque le médecin la découvre par hasard chez un sujet qui vient à la consultation sans douleur, sans fièvre, sans risque, lorsque la plus petite dose de bon sens permet de prévoir une résorption facile et prochaine, pourvu qu'on s'en tienne aux précautions générales que nous avons indiquées.

Dans la règle, on appelle le médecin lorsque la pérityphlite est déclarée et l'appendicite déjà impossible à supprimer par une opération « à froid », ou lorsque en présence d'une certaine irritation péritonéale, le diagnostic n'est pas encore posé : dans aucun de ces cas il ne s'agit d'une opération aussi anodine que la laparotomie exploratrice et les surprises sont trop nombreuses pour qu'il faille citer tous les faits dans lesquels une intervention serait inutile ou plus dangereuse que l'appendicite ordinaire.

Si donc l'état général du malade (faciès souffrant mais non grippé ; bonne qualité d'un pouls accéléré en proportion de la fièvre ; absence de cyanose et de teinte subictérique) n'inquiète pas outre mesure le chirurgien, celui-ci *doit* savoir attendre, car M. Talamon l'a montré depuis longtemps, soit en s'appuyant sur ses observations personnelles, soit surtout en faisant parler nos statistiques, c'est après le quatrième et cinquième jour que les proportions de succès sont le plus grandes.

Et bon nombre d'appendicites localisées, qui nécessiteront quand même une intervention, seront opérées avec plus de succès après quelques jours.

Ordinairement, après les symptômes alarmants du début, les vomissements s'arrêtent, la fièvre baisse, le pouls redevient meilleur, les douleurs cessent et l'observateur attentif assiste à l'évolution d'une péritonite localisée dont l'exsudat, nous le répétons, sera abandonné à la résorption spontanée si tous les symptômes continuent à s'amender ensemble et régulièrement.

On a voulu tirer de l'analyse des urines des renseignements précieux : le seul qui soit utilisable, c'est que l'abondante sécrétion est d'un augure plutôt favorable, la septicémie rapide présentant le phénomène inverse.

L'examen du sang et de la leucocytose en particulier ne paraît pas fournir encore des renseignements utilisables.

Il n'y a réellement pas de formule simpliste, mais il y a pourtant des occasions d'intervenir : lorsque la fièvre persiste avec douleur, augmentation de l'exsudat, pouls rapide et faciès inquiétant, on n'attendra pas une perforation secondaire dans le péritoine.

De même, on recourt à l'incision dès qu'il y aura une dissociation quelconque dans les signes qui marquent la résolution prochaine et assez rapide : un pouls rapide, malgré une température en baisse, est un symptôme qui met le bistouri en main, lorsqu'il n'est pas d'origine banale et passagère. Et si la fièvre prend le caractère hectique, par exemple, avec apathie du sujet, ou bien si l'on observe sa recrudescence ou sa réapparition, l'intervention sera justifiée.

La dissociation d'un pouls rapide et de la température basse sera toujours un avertissement sérieux : la dissociation en sens inverse n'a pas grande importance.

Le réveil de quelques symptômes, en pleine convalescence apparente, devra faire chercher et peut-être ouvrir çà et là une collection purulente.

Il arrive enfin, lorsqu'on a vu beaucoup d'appendicites, qu'on intervient une fois ou l'autre et qu'on incise un abcès localisé, parce que le malade fait *mauvaise impression*, tout court : cette indication, lorsqu'elle se présente, est aussi précise qu'elle est indéfinissable.

L'état paraît-il d'emblée plus grave : le pouls est-il filiforme, les extrémités froides, le malade couvert de sueurs, la respiration haletante et entrecoupée de soupirs et d'accès d'angoisse qui contrastent avec une certaine loquacité ou même certaine jactitation dans une euphorie étonnante; y a-t-il enfin, à côté de la cyanose des pommettes, la teinte subictérique des septicémies, l'opération immédiate, dans les meilleures conditions, offre trop peu de chances pour être tentée. Ces malades-là sont perdus, avec ou sans opération, et il vaut mieux les laisser mourir que de s'habituer à voir mourir aussi en les opérant tous à ce moment, ceux qui rentrent dans la catégorie que nous avons appelée la péritonite réactionnelle du début.

Celle-ci est autre chose que le péritonisme qui accompagne la plupart des appendicites franches : nous en avons parlé à Moscou et l'an dernier au Congrès de Paris. Elle comporte un exsudat plus ou moins louche, souvent très abondant, que nous avons eu l'occasion de percuter, de démontrer, soit à la ponction, soit à l'incision : c'est une vraie péritonite générale.

Et cependant, l'expectation va nous montrer bientôt une appendicite parfaitement localisée, une appendicite vulgaire, tandis que l'exsudat, séreux, séro-fibrineux ou même purulent, sera résorbé ou toléré par le péritoine jusqu'à ce qu'on lui donne issue, si cela devient nécessaire, dans le moment d'accalmie qui va suivre presque toujours.

Il va sans dire que si on opère à ce moment, dans cette période intermédiaire, nous disons en pleine réaction péritonéale, avec les signes les plus inquiétants et sûr du consentement unanime des médecins et de la famille — on aura quelques chances de ne pas tuer tous les malades. Ceux qui partent avaient de quoi, puisqu'on a ajouté, il faut bien le dire, le shock d'une opération grave à une maladie grave, dans un moment critique. Ceux qui guérissent sont enregistrés par les opérateurs comme de merveilleux succès. Et c'est ce qui va rendre notre discussion bien difficile : il est peu d'opérateurs qui consentent à reconnaître que telle brillante laparotomie n'a pas été entreprise pour une péritonite sûrement mortelle. On croirait se diminuer!

Eh bien! Messieurs, nous avons fait souvent la toilette péritonéale et nous ne sommes pas convaincu d'avoir eu une seule fois un vrai succès; nous avons sûrement, par l'opération, hâté la fin de beaucoup de nos malades et nous ne sommes pas assuré que l'un ou l'autre de nos échecs ne fût pas la conséquence plus ou moins immédiate de l'opération; par contre, nous n'avons jamais lu d'observation forçant notre conviction qu'un autre opérateur eût été plus heureux et eût vraiment sauvé un malade par une intervention en pleine péritonite diffuse dans le vrai sens du mot. Il y a toujours quelque réticence sur l'existence de poches ou sur la qualité de l'exsudat, qui nous ont fait penser qu'on s'était plutôt trouvé en face de cette péritonite que nous avons appelée réactionnelle et que, nous le rappelons, l'on avait opérée dans de mauvaises conditions pour le sujet.

Ce qui rend la discussion plus urgente sur ce point, c'est que ce moment de sidération péritonéale remplit naturellement d'inquiétude la famille et le médecin. Et l'opération, si le chirurgien ne sait pas s'y opposer, sera acceptée d'enthousiasme et beaucoup de malades occis le cœur léger.

Presque toujours, jusqu'au quatrième ou cinquième jour, arrive la période d'accalmie plus ou moins complète, avec localisation du ou des exsudats qu'une observation attentive fera toujours découvrir (pourvu qu'on n'oublie pas de les chercher : fosse iliaque, rectum, vagin, synchodrose, sous le diaphragme) et qu'on abandonnera ici encore à la résorption spontanée, si tous les symptômes s'amendent ensemble et régulièrement.

En un mot, malgré un début gravissime en apparence, on voit presque toujours le foyer se localiser et cette appendicite évoluer ensuite comme les cas plus bénins : sinon, c'est-à-dire si les phénomènes de péritonisme persistent avec exsudat, fièvre, etc., on pourra intervenir, après trois ou quatre jours, et souvent dans ces cas une ou plusieurs incisions discrètes, comme nous avons eu l'occasion de le faire en même temps *per vaginam*, dans la fosse iliaque droite et dans l'hypochondre gauche, donneront un meilleur résultat que la grande toilette du péritoine. Le retard apporté à celle-ci, lorsqu'on la tente, sera en tout cas compensé amplement par le relèvement du pouls et le malade sera mieux en état de supporter le shock opératoire que dans la période de sidération initiale.

La simple évacuation du pus est le but immédiat, bien plus que la résection de l'appendice : celui-ci n'est enlevé que s'il se présente complaisamment : — sinon, il sera excisé « à froid » par une incision qui circonscrit la cicatrice et permet la restauration des parois abdominales — qu'il se soit formé ou non une hernie.

Tous nos malades opérés pendant une crise se soumettent volontiers à l'excision ultérieure de l'appendice, qui guérit en même temps la hernie.

L'opération en deux temps de Sonnenbourg nous paraît un accident, un accroc : elle ne saurait être érigée en méthode.

En résumé : faire la résection prophylactique de tout appendice coupable et surprendre, par l'opération improvisée, les cas très exceptionnels qui se prêtent véritablement à l'opération de M. Dieulafoy.

Quant aux cas ordinaires, tels qu'ils se présentent dans la règle...

laisser passer l'orage du début, en *laissant mourir* quelques malades désespérés *pour n'en pas tuer* un plus grand nombre et pour intervenir à un meilleur moment, si c'est utile ou nécessaire, en se rappelant que la médecine ne se laisse pas encore réduire en formules, aussi simples que dangereuses.

Conduit de cette façon, le traitement de l'appendicite ne guérit assurément pas tous les malades qui ne sont pas perdus d'emblée ; mais certains accidents qu'on va dresser devant nous comme fantômes, tels que la pleurésie purulente et l'abcès sous-diaphragmatique, ne sont pas au-dessus de nos ressources : le plus grave de tous et le plus fréquent — celui contre lequel nous luttons personnellement depuis douze ans — la *perforation secondaire dans le péritoine*, aura bien des chances d'être prévenu.

Quant aux autres surprises fatales, comme la pyléphlébite, elles sont décidément trop rares pour qu'on leur offre en sacrifice le péritoine d'un trop grand nombre de victimes.

SUR LES INDICATIONS THÉRAPEUTIQUES DANS L'APPENDICITE

RAPPORT

par M. JALAGUIER.

Une indication générale, n'admettant à mon avis que peu d'exceptions, domine l'histoire thérapeutique de l'appendicite : c'est que tout appendice iléo-cœcal qui a été, ne fût-ce qu'une seule fois, atteint d'appendicite bien caractérisée, doit être considéré comme dangereux et justiciable de l'intervention chirurgicale.

A quelle époque et dans quelles conditions faut-il intervenir ? Aussitôt que le diagnostic d'appendicite est posé, disent les uns. Très rarement pendant la crise aiguë, et seulement « à froid », soutiennent les autres.

Les arguments des interventionnistes hâtifs sont les suivants : lorsqu'une appendicite éclate, il n'est pas possible d'en prévoir l'évolution ; telle appendicite qui donne lieu à des manifestations de début presque insignifiantes peut se compliquer tout à coup des accidents les plus redoutables contre lesquels l'intervention chirurgicale se trouvera souvent impuissante : péritonite suraiguë, intoxication générale de l'économie. L'intervention hâtive supprime tout danger de perforation et d'infection locale ou générale, et, si la perforation s'est déjà produite, l'opération a d'autant plus de chance de sauver le malade qu'elle est plus rapprochée du début des accidents

Le traitement non opératoire est incapable de prévenir ou d'enrayer ces accidents et fait perdre un temps précieux.

En somme, pour les médecins et les chirurgiens de cette école, les indications thérapeutiques dans l'appendicite sont très simples, puisque tout se réduit à une question de diagnostic. Le diagnostic d'appendicite implique l'opération immédiate, quelle que soit la forme et la période de la maladie.

Certes, c'est là une doctrine séduisante, commode et qui supprime pour ses adeptes les préoccupations, je dirai même les angoisses de ceux qui pensent comme moi que l'intervention n'est que rarement indiquée pendant la crise aiguë et qu'il faut tout mettre en œuvre pour conduire le malade jusqu'au moment où l'opération à froid sera praticable avec sécurité.

Je vous demande la permission de rappeler que j'ai été l'un des premiers en France, à défendre cette manière de procéder (¹). Plus mon expérience s'étend et plus ma conviction s'affermit dans ce sens. J'ai observé à l'heure actuelle 560 malades atteints d'appendicite de toutes variétés, et les observations m'ont démontré que, lorsqu'une appendicite est correctement traitée dès son début, l'opération est bien rarement nécessaire pendant l'évolution des accidents aigus ; ce traitement consiste dans l'immobilité, la diète absolue, la glace largement appliquée sur tout l'abdomen, l'opium, et, dans les cas graves, les injections massives de sérum artificiel. On doit s'abstenir rigoureusement, quels que soient les phénomènes d'occlusion, de l'administration des purgatifs et des lavements.

Grâce à cette thérapeutique, les phénomènes inflammatoires et infectieux se localisent et s'atténuent presque toujours et la crise d'appendicite se termine par la résorption spontanée des exsudats. L'examen attentif du malade permet de se rendre compte de l'évolution de la maladie et la localisation des accidents se traduit par des signes cliniques suffisamment précis pour qu'on puisse espérer ne pas se laisser surprendre par des complications irrémédiables.

Il est parfaitement exact que lorsqu'une appendicite débute, on ne peut prévoir dans quel sens elle évoluera, mais le traitement que

<hr>

1. *Bulletin de la Société de chirurgie.* 9 mars 1892, p. 185. — Appendicite, *Traité de chirurgie,* 2ᵉ édition. 1898. t. VI. — *Bulletin de la Société de chirurgie.* 1ᵉʳ février 1899, p. 115.

je viens d'indiquer peut être considéré comme un traitement d'épreuve. Si la localisation doit se faire, on voit, dans l'immense majorité des cas, les accidents s'amender rapidement : la douleur, d'abord diffuse, tend à se limiter à la région de l'appendice, la paroi abdominale recouvre sa souplesse, excepté dans la fosse iliaque droite, les vomissements cessent ou diminuent de fréquence, les caractères du pouls s'améliorent, le visage perd son aspect grippé. Ordinairement on est fixé au bout de 12 ou 24 heures.

Dans bien des cas l'amélioration est si franche au bout de 36 à 48 heures que toute incertitude relativement à la localisation de la péritonite disparaît. Dans les cas graves, après l'atténuation des phénomènes plus ou moins intenses de péritonisme ou de péritonite généralisée, on voit persister pendant quelques jours des symptômes de péritonite circonscrite et d'infection générale. La température est élevée, le pouls vif et rapide, la langue est sale, parfois un peu sèche, les douleurs abdominales restent assez vives avec prédominance vers la fosse iliaque droite ; il y a presque toujours un certain degré de ballonnement avec contracture des muscles du côté droit et hyperesthésie cutanée. La constipation est absolue et l'émission des gaz est supprimée. Il n'est pas rare d'observer, en même temps, de la rétention d'urine ou de la dysurie. D'ordinaire l'expression de la physionomie n'est que peu altérée.

Les choses peuvent rester en cet état pendant 3, 4, 5 jours et même davantage, sans qu'il y ait lieu de désespérer de la terminaison favorable, pourvu que le pouls et la température soient concordants, s'il n'y a pas d'agitation, et, surtout, si l'on peut assister à la formation d'une induration, véritable plastron, qui indique le travail de défense de la séreuse péritonéale. On sera tout à fait rassuré, si, en même temps, reparaît l'émission des gaz.

Le plastron est en général appréciable à partir du 2e, 3e ou 4e jour ; c'est le signe palpable de la localisation de la péritonite. Loin d'être une indication à intervenir, cette induration, cet empâtement, ce plastron, quel que soit le nom qu'on lui donne, est un signe favorable et doit engager à persévérer dans le traitement médical. Cette notion de la valeur pronostique du plastron n'est pas universellement admise. Pour beaucoup de médecins et de chirurgiens, la constatation d'un empâtement commande au contraire l'intervention immédiate. Il m'est arrivé maintes fois d'être appelé pour opérer d'urgence dans ces conditions, du 4e au 10e jour ; j'ai toujours refusé sans avoir eu à m'en repentir, mais j'avoue que souvent la responsabilité m'a semblé lourde

Le plastron ne se trouve pas toujours dans la fosse iliaque droite ; il faut alors chercher si l'on ne découvre pas une induration circonscrite dans un autre point de l'abdomen ou même dans l'excavation pelvienne. Quel que soit le siège de l'induration, sa valeur pronostique reste la même, en admettant, bien entendu, que l'état général demeure satisfaisant et que le pouls soit d'accord avec la température.

La discordance du pouls et de la température se manifeste de deux façons différentes qui n'ont pas la même signification : tantôt, la température s'abaisse pendant que le pouls devient rapide, c'est l'indice presque certain de l'extension de la péritonite. Il n'y a plus à temporiser. Tantôt, au contraire, la température restant élevée, c'est le nombre des pulsations qui diminue pour tomber à 60 et même 50. J'ai observé ce fait sur 5 malades après 4 ou 5 jours de diète absolue et d'administration de l'opium. Je crois que c'est un effet de l'inanition et peut-être aussi de la stercorémie : ces 5 malades ont guéri après des injections très abondantes de sérum artificiel.

J'ai déjà parlé de l'émission des gaz par l'anus ; ce symptôme, dans les cas favorables, est sensiblement contemporain de l'apparition du plastron : il indique que la fin de la crise est proche. Il n'en reste pas moins indispensable de maintenir dans toute leur rigueur l'immobilité et la diète. Si la langue est sèche et la soif vive, on peut permettre l'absorption d'une certaine quantité d'eau (eau bouillie, eau de Vichy, thé, café très léger, etc.) ; on continuera ce régime jusqu'au jour où la défervescence sera complète, défervescence qui se produit le 3e ou le 4e jour dans les cas légers, qui se montre d'ordinaire du 5e au 7e jour et que j'ai vue se faire attendre jusqu'au 10e jour sans modification de l'état local et général : dans les cas de cette catégorie, il est indispensable de soutenir les forces du malade et de favoriser les phénomènes d'élimination par des injections quotidiennes de sérum.

On ne donnera la première tasse de lait que le lendemain du jour où la température sera revenue à la normale. Souvent le thermomètre remonte quelque peu à cette occasion ; il n'y a pas lieu de s'en inquiéter si la douleur locale, qui avait presque complètement disparu, ne présente pas de recrudescence.

On peut considérer, dès lors, la crise aiguë comme terminée, mais il reste encore à provoquer les garde-robes si elles ne se sont pas montrées spontanément après que l'administration de l'opium a été suspendue, opium que je conseille de supprimer aussitôt que les douleurs vives des premiers jours se sont calmées. On administrera, 24 ou 36 heures après la fin de la crise, d'abord un lavement ou des suppositoires, puis une faible dose d'huile de ricin.

Je n'insiste pas sur les précautions que l'on doit prendre jusqu'à la disparition de tout phénomène local. c'est-à-dire jusqu'à la fin de la 3e ou 4e semaine pour les cas d'intensité moyenne, temps qui doit être beaucoup plus long pour les cas graves et lorsque la résorption des exsudats est lente à se faire.

J'ai supposé que l'évolution de l'appendicite, soumise ainsi dès son début au traitement rationnel, se faisait régulièrement vers la guérison spontanée par résolution ou résorption des exsudats. mais je suis bien loin de penser et de dire que les choses se passent toujours ainsi et qu'il faille se renfermer dans une abstention systématique, quels que soient les incidents qui puissent se produire pendant la crise aiguë.

Divers incidents, en effet. peuvent survenir et commander l'intervention chirurgicale.

L'indication d'opérer se présente lorsque, après 24 ou 36 heures du traitement, on ne constate aucune amélioration, lorsqu'il y a de l'agitation, des douleurs vives et lorsque le nombre des pulsations augmente tandis que la température tend à s'abaisser.

L'indication n'est pas moins nette si après une amélioration de courte durée on constate une recrudescence des symptômes qui avaient paru un instant s'amender : réapparition ou augmentation de fréquence des vomissements, élévation ou abaissement anormal de la température, altération des traits, persistance ou augmentation des douleurs.

A partir du 5e ou du 6e jour, la fin de la crise doit s'approcher : si, au lieu de s'abaisser, la température s'élève, s'il y a de grandes oscillations du thermomètre, ou bien si la température, s'abaissant progressivement, n'est pas suivie par un abaissement proportionnel du chiffre des pulsations. s'il y a un ou plusieurs frissons, si les douleurs locales augmentent d'acuité et surtout si elles reviennent par crises, et si l'empâtement s'accroît et devient le siège d'une sensibilité douloureuse intense à sa partie centrale ou bien en dedans de l'épine iliaque et au-dessus de l'arcade crurale. dans toutes ces conditions, l'expectation devient dangereuse ; il convient d'opérer.

Il arrive encore. parfois, qu'après la défervescence et une période de bien-être ayant duré quelques jours. on assiste à une nouvelle poussée imputable presque toujours, soit à la cessation de l'immobilité. soit à un excès d'alimentation. Si cette poussée résiste plus de 24 ou 36 heures à la reprise rigoureuse de la diète et de la glace. il ne faut pas hésiter à intervenir.

Il faut encore opérer, sans attendre le refroidissement complet, lorsque, l'appendicite s'arrêtant dans son évolution favorable, on assiste à une succession de petites crises aiguës ou subaiguës d'une durée variable et plus ou moins rapprochées. Dans l'intervalle de ces crises, on voit persister dans la fosse iliaque ou dans l'excavation un empâtement ou une induration de volume variable. C'est l'appendicite à recrudescences.

Telles sont, très résumées, les indications de l'opération pendant l'évolution d'une appendicite surveillée et dirigée depuis les premières heures par le chirurgien, qui seul, à mon avis, est responsable du moment de l'intervention. Malheureusement, en pratique, il en est rarement ainsi, et bien souvent nous ne sommes appelés à juger de l'opportunité d'une action chirurgicale qu'après un certain nombre de jours pendant lesquels la thérapeutique la plus irrationnelle et la plus néfaste a été mise en œuvre : purgatifs à outrance, lavements forcés, etc. Dans ces conditions, les indications sont quelquefois très difficiles à apprécier.

Je crois qu'en pareille circonstance, il faut s'attacher à établir d'abord le diagnostic exact de la forme de l'appendicite, ou mieux, du stade auquel elle est arrivée. On peut y arriver dans la très grande majorité des cas par l'analyse minutieuse des phénomènes locaux et généraux et par la recherche attentive de ce qui s'est passé depuis le début de la maladie.

On instituera le traitement médical si l'on a quelque raison de penser que la péritonite est plastique et circonscrite. Mais l'on se tiendra prêt à intervenir au premier symptôme alarmant.

L'indication d'opérer sans s'attarder, au traitement médical se présente si l'on constate les symptômes suivants : fièvre vive durant plus de cinq à six jours avec ou sans frissons, diarrhée fétide, état typhoïde, douleur vive, spontanée, revenant par crises, douleur excessive à la pression au niveau de l'empâtement, discordance entre la température et le pouls, etc.

Il faut opérer encore, lorsque la généralisation de la péritonite est un fait accompli : le traitement médical, à cette période n'a plus guère de chance de réussir; mais il ne faut opérer que si la péritonite est caractérisée par une réaction inflammatoire franche, et si l'organisme paraît en état de supporter le traumatisme opératoire. Si le pouls a disparu, ou bien s'il présente des intermittences, je crois qu'il vaut mieux s'abstenir. Dans la forme purulente, inflammatoire de la péritonite généralisée, on a jusqu'au 4ᵉ ou 5ᵉ jour quelques chances de sauver le malade. Dans la forme septique diffuse, au contraire, l'intoxication est tellement rapide que la situation est désespérée après

36 ou 48 heures et, pour ma part, je n'opère plus dans ces conditions.

En effet, j'ai opéré 25 fois pour des péritonites généralisées, et ces opérations ont été pratiquées d'emblée sans que je me sois attardé au traitement médical. J'ai eu 20 morts et 5 guérisons. Dans 13 cas, il s'agissait de péritonites inflammatoires franches à grands enkystements : c'est dans cette série que je compte mes 5 guérisons. 12 fois, j'ai eu affaire à des péritonites septiques diffuses et mes 12 opérés ont succombé. Il faut dire que cette triste série a été observée il y a déjà plusieurs années, à une époque où les péritonites d'origine appendiculaire étaient généralement mal connues et où le chirurgien n'était appelé à intervenir que lorsque les malades se trouvaient dans un état presque désespéré. Depuis le 4 juillet 1897, je n'ai pas eu l'occasion d'opérer un seul cas de péritonite généralisée ; cela ne veut pas dire qu'il ne s'en présente pas encore quelques cas, mais ils sont certainement beaucoup plus rares qu'autrefois parce que l'on sait mieux reconnaître et traiter l'appendicite. En ce qui me concerne, la raison de la diminution du nombre des cas de péritonite dans ma pratique hospitalière tient à ce que, depuis la fin de 1897, je suis chargé d'un service à l'hôpital des Enfants-Assistés, où ne sont pas admis les cas d'urgence. D'autre part, je suis devenu de plus en plus abstentionniste et grâce aux injections massives de sérum, *employées dès le début*, j'ai pu amener à la guérison des malades présentant des appendicites sévères et que j'aurais certainement opérés autrefois. Ces malades, observés depuis trois ans dans la clientèle de la ville, sont au nombre de 11 ; ils étaient tous très gravement atteints : j'ai cru pouvoir porter le diagnostic de péritonite généralisée ou tout au moins en voie de généralisation et 10 ont guéri sans intervention. C'est évidemment une série heureuse, et je n'espère pas toujours de pareils résultats ; on pourra me dire aussi que je n'ai pas la preuve de l'exactitude de mon diagnostic : j'en conviens ; mais ce que je puis affirmer, c'est que j'aurais opéré immédiatement ces 11 malades il y a cinq ou six ans.

Il serait injuste d'opposer sans réserves ces résultats à ceux que j'ai obtenus autrefois par l'intervention. En effet, les malades opérés étaient depuis plusieurs jours en pleine péritonite ; ils étaient pour la plupart profondément infectés et épuisés. Au contraire, ceux qui ont guéri sans intervention ont pu être soumis au traitement médical et aux injections de sérum, quelques-uns tout à fait au début, les autres peu après le début des accidents. Il est bien probable que, si je les avais opérés, la proportion des guérisons aurait été supérieure à *un* pour *cinq*. Il n'en est pas moins vrai que les résultats obtenus par la non-intervention sont des plus favorables et qu'ils m'autorisent.

ce me semble, à persévérer dans mes tendances abstentionnistes.

Voici maintenant la statistique intégrale des malades observés par moi en crise aiguë d'appendicite et non opérés pendant cette crise :

J'ai pu observer pendant la période aiguë 156 cas d'appendicite qui m'ont paru justiciables du traitement médical et de l'expectation. Sur ces 156 cas, la guérison avec résolution a été obtenue 121 fois. (Les 11 cas que je viens de citer sont compris dans cette statistique.)

10 malades ont dû être opérés à chaud, 7 par moi-même et 3 par des collègues. Ils ont guéri. 2 malades ont guéri spontanément après évacuation d'un abcès par le rectum ou la vessie ; 3 malades ont succombé.

Ces 3 cas malheureux réclament quelques commentaires : dans un cas il s'agissait d'une jeune fille de treize ans et demi, auprès de laquelle je fus appelé le 5ᵉ jour d'une appendicite méconnue; l'état était si grave que l'intervention ne me parut pas praticable. Je conseillai des injections massives de sérum. Au bout de douze heures, une amélioration notable s'était produite et j'entrevoyais la possibilité d'opérer. Les accidents reprirent avec une nouvelle intensité et la mort survint en quelques heures.

Dans un autre cas, il s'agissait d'un jeune homme de vingt-deux ans, pour lequel deux de mes meilleurs amis et collègues m'avaient demandé conseil. Nous avions affaire à une appendicite pelvienne nettement circonscrite; le traitement par la glace et l'opium fut institué et tout marcha à souhait : le 20ᵉ jour, le jeune homme paraissait guéri quand il fut emporté en 24 heures par une péritonite foudroyante consécutive, sans doute à la rupture d'un foyer pelvien. Il est bien probable que si nous n'avions pas négligé de pratiquer régulièrement le toucher rectal, l'abcès eût pu être reconnu et évacué.

Enfin, dans un dernier cas, il s'agissait d'un jeune homme de dix-sept ans, observé par moi au 5ᵉ jour d'une péritonite circonscrite pelvienne pour laquelle le traitement médical et les injections de sérum semblèrent d'abord donner un plein succès. Au 15ᵉ jour, tout danger paraissait écarté : le 16ᵉ jour il fut pris d'accidents singuliers : vomissements, diarrhée sanguinolente avec ténesme, frissons, langue et gencives rouges et desséchées : l'aspect du visage était atroce. Je n'avais pas vu le malade depuis plusieurs jours et, comme on me racontait qu'il avait pris la veille et l'avant-veille, sans aucun effet évacuateur, deux doses de 50 centigrammes de calomel, je crus pouvoir mettre ces accidents sur le compte d'un empoisonnement. Le lendemain, l'état était désespéré; aucune intervention n'était possible. Je me demande encore si je me suis trompé et si je n'aurais pas dû attribuer ces accidents à une infection soudaine partie d'un foyer péri-appendiculaire.

Tel est mon bilan. J'ai perdu, il est vrai, 5 malades sur 156, mais il n'en reste pas moins ce fait incontestable que 121 malades atteints d'appendicite aiguë parmi lesquels 52 étaient particulièrement graves, sont arrivés à la résolution sans intervention : 10 ont guéri après intervention ; 2 après évacuation spontanée.

Aurait-on obtenu de meilleurs résultats en opérant d'emblée ces 156 malades ? Je ne puis le croire. Si je le croyais, je deviendrais sans hésiter le plus hâtif des interventionnistes, car je trouve singulièrement enviables le repos d'esprit et la paix intérieure des chirurgiens pour qui tout se borne à poser le diagnostic d'appendicite et à prendre le bistouri. Si l'opéré guérit, et je me plais à reconnaître qu'il guérit le plus souvent, on se félicite d'avoir opéré : on a trouvé l'appendice rouge, turgescent, poisseux, avec des fausses membranes tapissant les anses intestinales voisines : la péritonite était évidemment en voie de généralisation. D'autres fois, l'appendice gangrené était prêt à se perforer ou même perforé, il baignait dans un foyer purulent plus ou moins fétide ; autour du cæcum on trouvait déjà un liquide louche et des fausses membranes, toutes lésions qui semblaient incompatibles avec une guérison spontanée. Si l'opéré succombe, ce qui arrive malheureusement quelquefois, on se persuade que c'est parce que l'on a opéré trop tard, ou bien, avec la plus parfaite bonne foi, on range ce cas malheureux dans la catégorie des opérations pour péritonites généralisées, et l'on se console sans trop de peine de cet insuccès.

Pour moi, le fait qu'on découvre, en opérant un cas aigu, l'appendice gangrené ou perforé, un abcès circonscrit au centre d'un volumineux empâtement, le fait même qu'il y a du liquide plus ou moins louche dans une partie de la cavité abdominale, ne prouve pas du tout que le malade n'aurait pu guérir sans intervention ; la phagocytose péritonéale est d'une activité extrème et les moyens de défense de l'organisme sont puissants quand on ne les contrarie pas. Sur les 156 malades que j'ai suivis pendant leur crise aiguë et parmi lesquels 121 sont arrivés à la résolution, beaucoup avaient présenté des accidents graves avec des indurations et des empâtements parfois énormes. A n'en pas douter, le simple examen clinique permettait d'affirmer que beaucoup d'entre eux avaient des abcès : quelques-uns même avaient présenté dans leur cavité péritonéale des exsudations de liquide donnant lieu à de la matité dans toute la région sous-ombilicale. J'ai opéré à froid 62 de ces malades et, sur 25 d'entre eux, j'ai trouvé des traces d'abcès uniques ou multiples, soit au voisinage de l'appendice, soit entre les anses intestinales, soit dans l'épiploon ; et parmi eux, 9 avaient eu manifestement des destructions de l'appendice par gangrène. Je parle ici seulement de celles de **mes** opérations à froid que j'ai pratiquées sur des malades observés et suivis pendant la crise aiguë. Dans la série de mes autres opérés, j'ai trouvé nombre de fois des lésions semblables.

La constatation de ces faits positifs m'a conduit à devenir de plus en plus abstentionniste pendant la période aiguë.

Des considérations d'un autre ordre viennent encore plaider en faveur de cette manière d'agir : les interventionnistes hâtifs proclament que la résection de l'appendice pratiquée dès les premiers instants est d'exécution aussi facile que la plus simple des résections à froid : je n'en disconviens pas, mais il ne faut pas oublier que l'appendicite n'étant bien souvent que l'expression d'une infection générale et pouvant coïncider avec d'autres manifestations infectieuses gastro-intestinales ou hépatiques, il n'est pas sans danger de troubler par un traumatisme opératoire les efforts que fait l'organisme pour se débarrasser des agents infectieux.

C'est ainsi que l'on a vu parfois succomber à des phénomènes d'ictère grave ou d'urémie des malades opérés au début d'une crise et chez lesquels on ne découvrait que des lésions appendiculaires insignifiantes.

D'autre part on ne saurait nier qu'une opération pratiquée le 2e, le 3e ou le 4e jour, au moment où les phénomènes d'infection générale s'amendent, en même temps que l'infection péritonéale se localise, coure le risque de faire échec à cette tendance favorable et présente certains dangers. N'ayant jamais opéré d'emblée, pendant la période aiguë, excepté dans les cas de péritonites généralisées ou de péritonites circonscrites franchement suppurées, je ne puis prouver cette assertion par des faits personnels, mais une statistique de Broca est très démonstrative à ce point de vue. Broca (l'*Appendicite ; formes et traitement*, Paris, 1900, p. 55) au début de sa pratique chirurgicale, de 1892 à 1895 inclus, a opéré d'emblée à l'hôpital Trousseau 87 appendicites de toutes variétés avec 22 décès. De 1896 à 1898 inclus, influencé, comme il veut bien le dire très amicalement, par ma manière de procéder, il s'est attaché à discerner les cas où la temporisation était admise. Il a opéré 100 malades avec 10 décès seulement. Ces chiffres prouvent jusqu'à l'évidence, comme le dit Broca, que l'opération immédiate est plus grave que l'expectation armée.

L'intervention hâtive expose encore à un autre danger : on sait que certaines affections gastro-intestinales, la gastro-entérite, la fièvre typhoïde, et même la grippe, se manifestent assez souvent à leur début par des symptômes analogues à ceux de l'appendicite. Aussi n'est-il pas très rare que des partisans de l'intervention hâtive aient conseillé et pratiqué, en pareil cas, des opérations parfois nuisibles, toujours inutiles. J'en connais plusieurs exemples dont quelques-uns ont été publiés. Pour ma part, si j'avais été un interventionniste pressé, j'aurais opéré ainsi deux fièvres typhoïdes, deux entéro-colites grippales, une colique néphrétique, et même une pneumonie droite. On m'accordera que c'est là un motif secondaire, il est vrai, mais non sans valeur, de ne pas intervenir en toute hâte et sans avoir le temps d'assurer un diagnostic précis.

Pour résumer cet exposé déjà trop long, je dirai que l'intervention pendant la période aiguë se trouve indiquée seulement dans certains cas rares de péritonites généralisées et dans tous les cas de péritonites enkystées suppurées, incapables de se résorber spontanément.

L'intervention, dans la péritonite généralisée, consiste dans l'évacuation des produits septiques, la résection de l'appendice toutes les fois qu'elle est possible, et l'établissement d'un large drainage. On ne saurait trop insister sur la nécessité d'assurer le libre écoulement des liquides après l'opération et protester assez haut contre les tendances des chirurgiens qui referment le ventre après avoir placé une simple mèche qui bouche et ne draine pas. Le lavage du péritoine n'est indiqué que si la collection purulente est limitée dans une région de la cavité abdominale par une solide barrière d'adhérences.

Pour les péritonites enkystées suppurées, le mode d'intervention varie quelque peu suivant le siège de la collection et je ne saurais m'étendre sur les indications diverses applicables à ces cas. Toutefois, quoi qu'on en ait dit, une indication me paraît capitale, c'est de chercher à pénétrer dans la cavité purulente sans passer par le péritoine libre. Dans ce but, on s'efforcera de ne pas dépasser le champ des adhérences péritonéales ou bien l'on cherchera à aborder l'abcès par un chemin détourné, par exemple, en décollant le péritoine pariétal. Dans quelques cas particuliers, tels que les collections de l'appendicite pelvienne, on pourra être conduit à inciser par le rectum, par le vagin et même par le périnée. S'il faut absolument, pour atteindre l'abcès, traverser le péritoine libre, il est indispensable d'isoler avec le plus grand soin le foyer septique avant de l'ouvrir et de l'évacuer.

Un point de pratique encore discuté est relatif à la recherche de l'appendice dans ces opérations pour collections enkystées. A mon avis, cette recherche ne doit être faite qu'autant qu'elle est compatible avec le respect des adhérences qui protègent la grande cavité péritonéale. Aussi bien la simple ouverture d'un abcès et le drainage suffisent-ils, dans la majorité des cas, pour assurer la guérison. S'il persiste une fistule intarissable, on sera conduit à pratiquer plus tard la résection secondaire de l'appendice, opération toujours délicate et souvent difficile, il est vrai, mais moins dangereuse, à coup sûr, que la recherche acharnée d'un appendice dans les parois d'un foyer septique.

J'ai opéré « à chaud », en suivant cette règle de conduite, dans 24 cas d'appendicites circonscrites suppurées : j'ai eu 22 guérisons et 2 morts. Ces deux insuccès opératoires sont survenus, une fois au 14e jour par hépatite infectieuse suraiguë non suppurée, et une fois en 56 heures par septicémie foudroyante; dans ces deux cas l'opération avait été des plus faciles et des plus rapides: j'avais simplement ouvert un abcès sans chercher l'appendice.

Dans les 22 opérations suivies de guérison, deux fois seulement j'ai enlevé l'appendice gangrené: ces 22 cas ont guéri plus ou moins vite, mais, sauf un, ils n'ont pas de fistule. Ce dernier a été opéré au mois de juin 1899: j'ai trouvé dans l'abcès un gros corps étranger et ce que je croyais être la totalité de l'appendice gangrené. A la fin du mois d'août, la guérison était complète ; mais au mois de janvier 1900, à l'occasion d'une grippe, une nouvelle poussée s'est faite dans ce qui restait d'appendice, un abcès s'est ouvert spontanément, et une fistulette donnant issue à quelques gouttes de pus persiste encore à l'heure actuelle; si elle ne se tarit pas, j'opérerai ce malade dans quelques mois.

On peut rapprocher des cas de cette catégorie, au point de vue des indications ultérieures, les appendicites suppurées évacuées spontanément par l'intestin, la vessie, etc. La guérison définitive, en effet, est assez fréquente, et la résection secondaire de l'appendice n'est indiquée que s'il survient une rechute, rechute qui, en général, ne présente pas beaucoup de gravité.

Après avoir ainsi exposé les indications thérapeutiques pendant la crise aiguë, il me reste à examiner les indications de l'opération « à froid » et à préciser les conditions dans lesquelles elle est applicable.

Une première question se pose, question délicate et qui prête à la discussion : doit-on pratiquer la résection à froid après une crise aiguë unique terminée par une résolution complète? Jusqu'à ces dernières années, étant donné le nombre relativement considérable de malades observés par moi et restés indemnes depuis plusieurs années, j'avais cru pouvoir adopter, comme règle d'attendre, la deuxième attaque avant de proposer l'opération. Mais ayant eu connaissance de trois cas de mort presque foudroyante survenue à l'occasion de la deuxième crise, d'autre part ayant observé chez trois de mes malades que je n'avais pas opérés après la première crise aiguë, une deuxième crise qui a failli les enlever, j'en suis arrivé à considérer l'ablation de l'appendice après une seule crise comme une mesure de prudence pleinement justifiée.

L'opération est quelquefois difficile à faire accepter lorsque la crise est passée et la santé parfaite : les malades ou leurs parents ne comprennent pas qu'il soit nécessaire d'ouvrir le ventre sans une indication palpable. J'ai pour principe, en pareil cas, d'exposer la situation aux intéressés, de leur montrer, d'un côté la possibilité, sinon la probabilité d'une rechute et d'une rechute grave, de l'autre la sécurité absolue au prix d'une opération, somme toute, bénigne. Et après les avoir ainsi dûment avertis, je leur laisse une part de responsabilité dans le parti à prendre. D'ailleurs les indications de l'opération ne sont pas également pressantes pour tous les cas : si la crise aiguë a évolué sans exsudat notable, il est permis de supposer que l'appendice est resté libre et flottant dans le péritoine, et que, par suite, la seconde attaque, si elle se produit, pourra donner lieu aux accidents les plus graves. On devra alors proposer l'opération avec beaucoup plus d'insistance que dans les conditions opposées, c'est-à-dire lorsque l'appendicite s'est accompagnée d'exsudats considérables ayant laissé sans doute autour de l'appendice une barrière d'adhérences. L'âge des sujets et les conditions sociales ont aussi leur importance. Il est en effet reconnu que les attaques d'appendicite sont beaucoup plus graves et les rechutes beaucoup plus fréquentes chez les enfants que chez les sujets âgés. On insistera donc beaucoup plus pour l'opération après une seule crise, chez les enfants, que chez les adultes, et aussi chez les sujets auxquels leur position sociale ne permet pas de se soumettre à des précautions et à un régime destiné à prévenir le retour des accidents.

La perspective de grossesses possibles dans un avenir plus ou moins éloigné, doit, à mon avis, faire conseiller l'opération chez toutes les jeunes femmes qui ont eu une crise bien nette d'appendicite. La grossesse est, en effet, une cause occasionnelle assez fréquente de poussées aiguës sur un appendice préalablement altéré. Pratiquée à froid, l'opération n'affaiblit pas la paroi abdominale et n'expose pas à l'éventration.

L'indication de l'opération à froid étant admise dans ces conditions, il faut bien s'entendre sur la signification de ce terme « à froid ». Il ne suffit pas que les accidents aigus soient calmés depuis quelques jours : il est indispensable que toute inflammation ait disparu, que les exsudats soient résorbés ou du moins aient perdu leur virulence.

Pour les cas légers ayant évolué sans exsudat notable et sans perforation, l'opération peut être faite à froid 15 ou 20 jours après la fin de la crise : mais pour les cas plus sérieux qui ont donné lieu à un empâtement considérable, l'opération doit être retardée pendant six semaines, deux mois et même davantage. Il n'y a pas de limite fixe à la durée de l'expectation, mais on peut dire qu'il faut faire le possible pour n'intervenir que lorsque toute trace palpable de l'induration a disparu depuis au moins 10 ou 15 jours. Il faut savoir résister aux sollicitations et aux instances des malades, car l'opération avant le refroidissement complet expose à certains dangers. La virulence des produits renfermés dans l'appendice et autour de lui dans les adhérences, dans les ganglions lymphatiques, peut se réveiller sous l'influence du traumatisme opératoire et donner lieu à des accidents plus ou moins graves d'infection générale. Au début de ma pratique, je croyais intervenir à froid 15 jours ou trois semaines après la fin d'une crise aiguë de moyenne intensité : il m'est arrivé souvent à cette époque d'observer des accidents post-opératoires sans gravité, je le veux bien, mais qui n'en ont pas moins une certaine importance : élévation de la température entre 38 et 39° pendant deux ou trois jours, aspect subictérique du visage, phlébite dans un cas, pleurésie séreuse dans deux cas. Depuis que, mieux instruit, je retarde beaucoup plus l'intervention, je n'ai plus rien observé de semblable et il me paraît évident que plus l'opération à froid est retardée, moins elle entraîne de dangers. Un autre avantage de ce retard est de simplifier les manœuvres opératoires. L'appendice souvent altéré, déformé, enfoui dans des adhérences, est plus facile à découvrir, le champ des recherches se trouvant plus limité ; on n'a pour ainsi dire plus à compter avec les adhérences et les agglomérations péri-appendiculaires et la résection d'un segment plus ou moins étendu d'intestin devient inutile. Sur 128 opérations à froid, j'ai toujours pu trouver l'appendice, souvent avec difficulté je dois le reconnaître : j'ai dû parfois suturer des perforations ou des déchirures cæcales, mais, jamais je n'ai été forcé de réséquer l'angle iléo-cæcal ce qui me fût certainement arrivé dans quelques cas, si je n'avais pas eu la patience d'attendre la résorption des exsudats péri-appendiculaires. Mes 128 opérés ont guéri [1].

1. Jusqu'à ces derniers jours, je pouvais donner une statistique d'opérations

Telles sont les considérations générales que j'avais à exposer au point de vue des indications thérapeutiques pendant la crise aiguë d'appendicite et après celle-ci. Je ne me berce pas de l'illusion d'être arrivé à la solution définitive de ce problème si difficile, ni d'avoir prévu tous les cas qui peuvent se présenter. Il n'y a pas d'absolu en chirurgie, chaque cas particulier pouvant comporter des indications spéciales.

L'indication de l'intervention dans l'appendicite à rechutes est aujourd'hui universellement admise ; je n'ai donc pas à insister.

A côté de l'appendicite à rechutes, caractérisée par des poussées successives après des intervalles d'accalmie complète, il importe d'étudier les indications opératoires dans l'*appendicite chronique* proprement dite.

L'appendicite chronique s'observe dans deux conditions différentes : le plus souvent il s'agit d'accidents douloureux plus ou moins vagues, dans la fosse iliaque droite, de symptômes dyspeptiques souvent mal caractérisés, d'infection subaiguë avec amaigrissement, troubles que l'on peut assez aisément rattacher à une origine appendiculaire grâce au commémoratif qui vous est fourni parfois d'une crise franche d'appendicite aiguë observée à une époque antérieure, quelquefois plusieurs années avant le moment où l'on examine le malade. Dans d'autres circonstances, plus rares, on ne trouve, dans les antécédents, aucune crise aiguë : on a alors affaire à l'appendicite *chronique d'emblée*, forme connue depuis peu, et sur laquelle Brun et Walther ont eu le mérite d'appeler l'attention.

Cette forme existe d'ordinaire chez des sujets atteints de troubles gastro-intestinaux chroniques parmi lesquels la colite muco-membraneuse occupe la première place. Son évolution est lente, elle ne se complique que rarement d'épisodes aigus et aboutit fréquemment à la sclérose et à l'oblitération plus ou moins complète de l'appendice. Ces altérations chroniques se manifestent quelquefois par le syndrome improprement appelé colique appendiculaire. Dans certaines circons-

à froid exempte de mortalité. Depuis l'achèvement de mon rapport, j'ai opéré 5 malades, ce qui porte à 151 le nombre de mes opérations. J'ai eu le malheur de perdre ma dernière opérée, jeune fille de vingt ans qui avait présenté un grand nombre de crises de gravité progressivement croissante. L'opération fut des plus difficiles : cæcum sous le foie ; appendice enfoui dans des adhérences épaisses et solides, et communiquant largement avec une partie de l'intestin grêle que l'autopsie a montré être la *deuxième portion du duodénum*. Je ne connais pas d'autre exemple de communication appendiculo-duodénale. Ne pouvant amener au dehors l'anse perforée, je dus faire la suture dans la profondeur. L'opération dura plus de deux heures. La mort survint au bout de trente-six heures dans le collapsus. A l'autopsie, on n'a pas trouvé de péritonite. La suture avait bien tenu.

lances elles ne se révèlent que par des troubles dyspeptiques et des douleurs abdominales plus ou moins vagues mais présentant une certaine prédominance vers la fosse iliaque droite. On passe facilement à côté du diagnostic, car les symptômes appendiculaires, souvent mal définis et fugaces, doivent être recherchés avec beaucoup d'attention. La constatation, à une ou plusieurs reprises, du point de Mac Burney à côté d'un cæcum contracté et dur suffit pour permettre d'affirmer l'existence de cette appendicite chronique. J'en dirai autant de la perception par le palper abdominal ou par le toucher rectal d'un appendice induré ou douloureux. Lorsqu'on opère dans ces conditions, il n'est pas rare de constater que l'inflammation chronique de l'appendice s'est propagée aux ganglions lymphatiques du méso-appendice, du mésentère et de méso-côlon. On trouve fréquemment des néoformations séreuses à une assez grande distance sur le côlon ascendant, ou bien encore des adhérences épiploïques et une épiploïte chronique parfois très étendue. L'intégrité apparente de l'appendice contraste souvent avec la gravité de ces lésions à distance ; il n'en est pas moins vrai que la suppression de l'appendice suffit en général pour amener la régression et la guérison de ces lésions secondaires. Dans quelques cas exceptionnels, cependant, lorsque l'épiploïte chronique, très ancienne et très étendue, s'est accompagnée de déviations, de coudures du gros intestin, de l'intestin grêle et même de l'estomac, on peut être conduit à des manœuvres de libération plus ou moins compliquées, parfois même à la résection d'une grande partie de l'épiploon.

Les résultats de l'intervention sont des plus satisfaisants dans cette forme de l'appendicite. On voit disparaître, ou tout au moins s'améliorer, la plupart des troubles fonctionnels ; la colite muco-membraneuse elle même s'en trouve le plus souvent modifiée d'une façon très favorable. L'opération, en pareil cas, paraît donc tout à fait justifiée ; la seule contre-indication se trouve dans l'âge avancé des malades ou dans une altération de l'état général indépendante de l'appendicite chronique, l'obésité, le diabète, par exemple. Comme cette appendicite chronique n'expose, somme toute, que rarement à des accidents aigus graves, l'opération ne doit être entreprise que lorsqu'il s'agit de rendre à un malade l'intégrité de ses fonctions sans mettre sa vie en danger. J'ai, pour ma part, pratiqué 10 résections de l'appendice pour appendicite chronique d'emblée et mes malades s'en sont très bien trouvés.

Je désirerais, en terminant, dire un mot des indications opératoires dans l'appendicite compliquant la grossesse. Malgré tout ce qui a été dit et écrit sur ce sujet dans ces derniers temps, il est évident pour moi, d'après les quelques faits dont j'ai été témoin, que l'état de grossesse ne change rien aux indications thérapeutiques. Je crois qu'il faut toujours chercher à obtenir, par le traitement non opératoire, le refroidissement de la poussée aiguë et n'intervenir à chaud que contraint et forcé, soit par une péritonite généralisée, soit par une péritonite circonscrite suppurée dont il n'est plus permis d'espérer la résorption.

J'ai observé des crises aiguës d'appendicite sur six femmes enceintes. Chez toutes, la résolution a été obtenue par les moyens ordinaires. Deux, qui ont été opérées à froid, ont guéri sans incident, et accouché à terme d'enfants vivants. (L'une a été opérée par Walther, l'autre par moi.) Quatre n'ont pas été opérées; trois ont accouché à terme, une a été perdue de vue. Je n'ai jamais eu l'occasion de voir les cas graves qui ont eu récemment tant de retentissement dans les sociétés savantes et dans la presse et qui ont poussé plusieurs de nos collègues accoucheurs au premier rang des interventionnistes hâtifs. Je ne puis dire quelle eût été ma conduite en présence de ces cas, mais je répète que, d'après ce que j'ai vu, je pense à l'heure actuelle comme en 1898 (*Traité de chirurgie*, 2ᵉ édition, tome VI, p. 682) que l'état de grossesse ne doit pas modifier les indications thérapeutiques dans l'appendicite.

On trouvera peut-être insolite la forme de ce rapport. J'aurais peut-être dû passer en revue, d'une façon complète, les opinions diverses qui ont été émises et les discussions importantes auxquelles elles ont donné lieu. Mais, ne voulant pas sortir des limites restreintes qui m'étaient imposées, il m'a semblé qu'il m'était permis, en raison de mon expérience déjà assez longue, d'exposer cette question d'après mes vues personnelles, et en tenant compte surtout des cas que j'ai moi-même observés. Je l'ai fait en toute sincérité, et si mon rapport n'a pas l'ampleur désirable, je vous demande de m'en excuser.

PRÉSENTATION DE PIÈCE

par **M. RYDYGIER**

Messieurs,

Permettez-moi de vous montrer une préparation très rare et intéressante. Je n'ai trouvé dans la littérature qu'un cas semblable.

Vous voyez ici que l'appendice n'a pas seulement perforé la paroi de l'ileum, il est même entré dans sa lumière et forme un quasi-polype.

TRAITEMENT DE L'APPENDICITE

COMMUNICATION

de M. PAUL REYNIER.

Chirurgien de Lariboisière.

MESSIEURS,

Je ne peux vous dire avec quel plaisir je viens d'entendre le rapport si intéressant de M. Roux, et surtout celui si étudié, si consciencieux, si lucide de mon ami le docteur Jalaguier. Ces rapports viennent en effet à l'appui des idées que j'ai toujours défendues, en même temps que M. Jalaguier, à savoir que l'expectative armée donne plus de succès que l'intervention hâtive, systématique, non raisonnée. Ce sont ces idées que j'ai défendues à la Société de médecine et de chirurgie pratiques en 1896, ce sont celles que j'ai toujours défendues à la Société de chirurgie ; et dans la dernière discussion qui a eu lieu à cette Société, je restais le seul luttant à la fin de cette discussion, pour soutenir cette expectative armée, contre les partisans de l'intervention hâtive. Mais tout ce qu'on m'a objecté n'a pas ébranlé ma conviction. Plus mon expérience personnelle s'accroît, plus j'étudie les faits, plus je crois que les opinions défendues par MM. Jalaguier et Roux sont celles qui sont les vraies. Quand vous êtes appelé dès les premières heures d'une appendicite, le seul traitement doit être la glace, l'immobilité au lit, la diète absolue, l'absence de tout purgatif, et l'opium à l'intérieur.

Mais quand je dis la glace, ce n'est pas la glace comme je la vois mettre trop souvent, par des personnes qui croient faire le traitement par la glace, en faisant toucher le ventre par le fond d'une vessie de glace suspendue à un cerceau. Ainsi à peine 10 centimètres carrés de la peau du ventre se trouvent refroidis. Le traitement par la glace consiste dans l'application de une, deux, ou trois grandes vessies de glace plates, suivant la largeur du ventre, reposant sur celui-ci directement et le couvrant dans son entier, sans qu'on craigne leur poids. Séparez-les simplement de la peau par une épaisseur de flanelle, et surveillez seulement pour que la peau ne devienne pas rouge, de peur des escharres. Que cette glace enfin soit renouvelée scrupuleusement toutes les 2 ou 3 heures, pendant tout le temps qu'il y a quelque chose dans le ventre qui vous préoccupe, par suite, 5, 10, 15 jours au besoin.

Avec ce traitement, toutes les fois que j'ai pu l'appliquer scrupuleusement dès les premières heures, j'ai toujours vu en 24 heures, 48 heures au plus tous les accidents disparaître. Malheureusement nous sommes appelés rarement dès les premiers accidents, et mon expérience personnelle se résume à 12 malades, mais j'ai celle de mes élèves le docteur Marieux, le docteur Deroche qui ont une grosse clientèle, qui souvent voient des appendicites au début, et qui dernièrement encore me disaient que, depuis qu'ils appliquaient ce traitement, ils n'avaient plus d'accidents.

Le plus souvent c'est au bout de 24 heures, de 48, de 62 heures que nous sommes appelés. Alors deux cas se présentent. Ou les accidents sont limités à la fosse iliaque, sans retentissement péritonéal exagéré, ou nous sommes en présence de phénomènes de péritonisme généralisé, ballonnement du ventre, sans localisation appréciable.

Dans le premier cas, instituez le traitement par la glace, et comme vous le dit M. Jalaguier, vous verrez ou tout s'amender ou se limiter de plus en plus, un abcès que vous ouvrirez vers le huitième jour ou le neuvième jour, quand les adhérences se seront faites. J'ai opéré ainsi 50 malades, sans avoir eu de morts à déplorer et j'ai pu chez 51 malades faire retarder l'opération et les opérer à froid, avec une mort, que j'ai due à ma précipitation à l'opérer trop tôt, n'ayant pas laissé complètement refroidir.

Mais renvoyant au rapport de M. Jalaguier, je passe rapidement sur ces faits et j'arrive au cas où nous sommes appelés lorsque le malade est en pleine réaction péritonéale, que nous le trouvons avec le ventre ballonné, les traits tirés, le faciès péritonéal, avec température élevée, ou abaissée, pouls rapide atteignant 120 ou le dépassant, vomissements incessants, voire même fécaloïdes.

Eh bien, là encore, je vais plus loin que mon ami M. Jalaguier. Devant les malades qui ont l'aspect de la péritonite, et quelques-uns de la péritonite septique, quand vous êtes appelé dans les 5 ou 4 premiers jours des accidents, non le sixième, septième, ou huitième jour, car dans ce cas je parlerais autrement, sachant qu'à ce moment je me trouve sûrement en présence de péritonite confirmée, ne pouvant plus rétrocéder, devant ces malades n'intervenez pas. Il faut un certain courage pour venir vous le dire, car un chirurgien peut être accusé dans ce cas-là d'être un timoré, il faut surtout bien plus de courage pour prendre devant le malade cette détermination, car à l'heure actuelle, l'entourage, le médecin, tout le monde vous pousse à l'opération, et comme vous l'a dit M. Jalaguier, l'opération sans discussion, systématique, donne plus de quiétude à l'esprit du chirurgien.

Mais malgré tout, je vous le répète avec encore plus de force que je l'ai dit à la Société de chirurgie, ne vous pressez pas dans ces cas d'intervenir. Faites le traitement par la glace, l'immobilisation et la diète absolue, l'opium, et joignez-y la caféine, les injections de sérum, soit sous-cutanées, soit s'il le faut intraveineuses, et vous aurez plus de succès que par l'intervention. Vous aurez des succès comme je les ai eus, même dans les cas qui vous paraissaient désespérés.

Et pour vous convaincre je ne peux mieux faire que de venir vous apporter ma statistique sur laquelle je base ma conviction, et qui j'espère entraînera la vôtre. J'ai vu 21 de ces cas à réaction périto-néale généralisée, sans localisation appréciable. Dans 9 cas je ne suis pas intervenu, j'ai institué le traitement par la glace, et les injections de caféine et de sérum, et 8 malades sont guéris, un seul est mort, me faisant regretter de n'être pas intervenu.

Or, ces 9 malades, si je ne les ai pas opérés, ce n'est pas par théorie, mais parce que je les trouvais trop bas, pour oser tenter une opération, j'en appelle au témoignage des médecins qui m'avaient demandé, et qui les soignaient avec moi. J'ai donné par ailleurs leurs observations détaillées. Je les rappelle ici brièvement.

Le premier était un malade qui avait été la veille pris de tous les symptômes d'une perforation intestinale. Je le vois 48 heures après le début des accidents avec le docteur Deroche. Il avait un ballonnement généralisé, le pouls rapide, filiforme, la température à 36. On lui fait de la caféine, on applique la glace, et une localisation se produisait, qui, le huitième jour des accidents, me permettait d'ouvrir un abcès contenant des matières fécales, par une incision le long du muscle droit.

J'ai encore à vous citer la malade du docteur Desmons, que nous voyons avec le docteur Beurnier un mardi matin, 3 jours après le début des accidents. Le docteur Beurnier la trouve si mal, avec une température tellement basse, un pouls tellement rapide, que lui, interventionniste de la première heure, me dit de ne pas opérer, et de ne pas faire l'opération, que si les choses continuent à aller de plus en mal, la famille tient absolument à ce qu'on tente quelque chose.

Or, je reviens à 4 heures et je trouve la malade si bas, que je me refuse même à donner cette consolation à la famille. La malade avait des vomissements fécaloïdes, un pouls presque incomptable. Et cependant sous l'influence du sérum, de la caféine, de la glace, le lendemain matin le docteur Desmons me téléphonait qu'elle était sau-vée, et en effet, une localisation se faisait, la température remontait, et le huitième jour j'ouvrais un abcès rétrocœcal, dont l'ouverture était suivie d'une fistule stercorale qui guérissait.

Je vous cite encore ces deux malades que je soigne avec le docteur Paulesco. L'une est vue par moi 4 jours après le début d'accidents d'occlusion liée à une appendicite. Je la trouve, après une purgation avec huile de ricin et gouttes de croton, ayant des vomissements fécaloïdes, le faciès tiré, toutefois le pouls encore bon, à 120, mais bien frappé. — Température 56, 8. — Avec la glace, la caféine, la malade a guéri.

Et ce jeune garçon de 16 ans, que je trouve le 27 mai dans le service du docteur Lancereaux, et que me montre le docteur Paulesco? Il entrait le 25 mai, deux jours après le début d'une appendicite, dans le service. Son médecin lui ordonne de la glace, mais il l'applique pendant une heure, la laisse fondre. Il entre le 25 mai; ventre ballonné, douloureux à la palpation partout, surtout dans la fosse iliaque; faciès tiré, vomissements verts répétés, voix faible, pouls 100. On lui donne un petit lavement purgatif.

26 mai. A la suite de ce lavement, selles abondantes, le ballonnement du ventre persiste, vomissements bilieux incessants, liquide contenant des grumeaux foncés brunâtres.

28 mai. Je le vois le 27 mai au soir, je le trouve me parlant la voix cassée, ayant le faciès tiré, la température à 56, 8, le pouls à 150 avec des vomissements toujours incessants et le ventre toujours ballonné.

Une vessie de glace était bien mise sur le ventre, mais les infirmières l'avaient suspendue à un cerceau, et elle touchait à peine le ventre. Avec le docteur Paulesco, nous le faisons couvrir de glace, on continue l'opium, la caféine.

Sous l'influence de ce traitement, au bout de 48 heures, un mieux s'établissait, et le malade guérissait et était opéré un mois après.

J'ai 9 observations pareilles, dans lesquelles je ne croyais pas en voyant mes malades au début à la possibilité de la guérison et cependant ces malades ont guéri, sauf un que j'ai trouvé le quatrième jour au soir du début des accidents, avec un ballonnement généralisé, le pouls petit, le faciès mauvais avec vomissements bilieux, puis fécaloïdes. Sous l'influence de la glace, des injections de sérum intraveineuses, j'arrivais à voir se localiser une collection que j'ouvrais le huitième jour, mais le malade restait faible, mourait le lendemain de cette intervention, me laissant l'impression à moi comme au docteur Gartner qui le soignait, que nous avions échoué au port.

Opposez à cette statistique celle de mes interventions, ou de celles qui ont été faites dans mon service, par mes assistants: treize fois on es intervenu, toujours parce qu'on trouvait encore le pouls bon et résistant, et le malade paraissant être dans les conditions à supporter une intervention.

Or, sur 15 malades ainsi opérés, j'ai 4 guérisons, 9 morts et cependant j'en ai un qu'avec le docteur Marieux j'ai opéré 24 heures après le début des accidents; je relève 5 opérés le troisième jour, 1 le quatrième, 1 le cinquième, 1 le sixième, 2 passés le huitième jour, 4 malades seulement dans cette série noire ont guéri, 2 opérés par moi, 1 par mon ami Legueu dans mon service, 1 autre par mon interne, à l'heure actuelle le docteur Plœisheim.

Mais je n'ai pas relevé toutes les opérations faites par les chirurgiens de garde dans mon service. Toutes les fois qu'ils ont opéré en pleine poussée péritonéale généralisée avec ce ballonnement du ventre, ces vomissements, ce pouls précipité, je n'ai pas souvenance d'avoir vu guérir un de ces opérés, sauf le malade de M. Legueu, dont je viens de vous parler.

Devant ces faits, comment voulez-vous donc que je puisse conclure autrement qu'en vous disant ce que je vous disais au début. Lorsque vous vous trouverez en présence dans les trois, quatre jours qui suivent le début des accidents, de ces réactions péritonéales généralisées, sans localisation nette, votre malade bénéficiera plus du traitement par la glace, le repos, la diète absolue et l'opium, que de votre intervention.

SUR L'APPENDICITE

DISCUSSION

par M. DURET,

de Lille.

D'après les remarquables rapports de MM. Roux et Jalaguier, qui viennent de nous être lus, et dont la compétence sur ce point de pathologie est hors pair, il semble bien que tous les chirurgiens sont d'accord pour faire, autant que possible, *l'opération à froid*. Comme mon ami Reynier, ils insistent pour qu'on laisse passer l'orage, toutes les fois que cela est possible; et, bien que les accidents soient menaçants, ils trouvent que, dans la grande majorité des cas, les choses finissent par s'arranger, et que l'on opère sûrement plus tard.

Il y a cependant des cas, où il faut intervenir hâtivement, dans la période aiguë; en particulier, lorsqu'il y a dissociation du pouls et de la température; lorsque le pouls est très fréquent, petit, parfois intermittent, la température restant basse et l'état général mauvais. Il n'y a aucune tendance vers la résolution — et, si on ne veut pas intervenir, les malades succombent.

J'ai, pour ma part, depuis dix ans, opéré un grand nombre d'appendicites soit à chaud, soit à froid — et j'ai eu assez constamment des succès. Mais, si j'en juge d'après les cas que j'ai observés dans ces derniers temps, la *gravité de l'appendicite* s'accentue; sa malignité, sa *virulence* s'aggravent.

Récemment, j'opérais, au troisième jour, un jeune garçon de 12 ans, présentant des symptômes de septicémie grave : pouls à 150, température à 58°.5, douleurs intestinales très violentes, faciès mauvais. Après bien des hésitations, j'interviens, parce qu'il est évident qu'il va succomber, si je m'abstiens. Opération des plus simples, des plus méthodiques : quelques gouttes de pus ; je tombe sur l'appendice, recroquevillé dans l'angle iléo-cæcal. Sa moitié libre est dilatée comme le pouce et perforée : calcul fécal du volume d'un grain de café. Suture hermétique de l'intestin. Je ne fais aucune recherche : toute l'intervention s'est passée strictement dans le foyer pathologique, isolé par des adhérences molles. Malgré cette opération idéale, l'enfant succombe en 12 heures. Dans la nuit, 40° : pouls filiforme, agitation ; la septicémie a continué ; les injections répétées de sérum ou de caféine ne l'arrêtent ou ne l'atténuent un seul instant.

Chez une jeune fille de 20 ans, crise aiguë très grave d'appendicite avec température élevée, agitation, pouls très rapide et fréquent. Après 56 heures, l'accalmie semble se faire complète... mais, huit jours après le début, voyant que définitivement le retour à l'état normal ne se fait pas, mon confrère m'appelle.

A l'examen, je trouve un abcès du volume des deux poings, faisant bomber l'abdomen ; en apparence, l'état général n'est pas mauvais, le pouls est à 90, et la température normale. Je me borne à une simple incision du volumineux abcès, avec contr'ouverture lombaire. Tout paraît d'abord devoir se passer simplement ; mais la septicémie continue, s'aggrave même et, quatre jours après, malgré les sérums, malgré des soins répétés, la malade meurt.

Je tire de ces faits — et d'autres semblables que je pourrais citer encore — cette conclusion : qu'il y a des appendicites aiguës, *hypertoxiques, très virulentes*.

Je laisse de côté, bien entendu, les péritonites généralisées, les inondations péritonéales : rien de cela n'existait chez nos malades.

Et bien, dis-je, dans les formes *hypertoxiques*, qu'on intervienne ou qu'on s'abstienne, la septicémie emporte souvent les malades, *quoi qu'on fasse*.

Il ne faut pas cependant s'abstenir, à notre avis, dans ces cas exceptionnellement graves : il faut faire son devoir.

Faire des réserves tant qu'on le voudra, mais agir : car il y a quelques cas où on réussit. Winivarter citait dernièrement un certain nombre de faits de ce genre, où il a pu sauver ses malades, par la simple incision et le drainage, même le péritoine n'étant pas protégé par des adhérences.

Au dernier congrès de chirurgie, j'ai rapporté un cas bien étonnant : chez un homme de 40 ans, ventre distendu au maximum, vomissements fécaloïdes incessants. Les médecins hésitent entre une obstruction et une appendicite. J'interviens au deuxième jour : paroi abdominale infiltrée, verdâtre, pénétrée par les gaz, péritoine noir, lambeaux sphacélés ; par une petite ponction au péritoine, les gaz s'échappent en sifflant, en même temps qu'un jet stercoral. L'ouverture agrandie, il s'écoule un verre à bière de matières stercorales ; pas d'adhérences protectrices. J'annonce l'issue fatale ; et cependant, le lendemain, la fièvre tombe ; le malade guérit avec rapidité.

Il est encore une autre remarque importante à faire : l'expectation, dans le but d'opérer à froid, n'est pas sans inconvénients. Il faut songer à la possibilité, à la fréquence relative des infections secondaires, des lésions à distance, qui ont alors tout le temps de s'établir dans le péritoine, dans le foie, dans les poumons, dans le cerveau. J'ai pu sauver, à grand'peine, un jeune garçon de 10 ans, opéré le huitième jour, d'un gros abcès rétro-péritonéal : il eut de la gangrène pulmonaire et un abcès intra-hépatique, que j'ouvris cinq jours après la première intervention.

J'ai perdu une jeune fille après une intervention très satisfaisante, ayant évacué un verre de pus : la température était tombée, le pouls et le facies bons. Quatre jours après l'opération, je remarquai une inégalité des pupilles, un peu d'agitation ; et, j'annonçai une méningite, qui éclatait dans la nuit et emportait la malade.

Ces faits, que je cite de mémoire, et d'autres qu'on pourrait recueillir, montrent bien que, dans nombre de cas, l'expectation est entourée de grands périls.

A mon avis, c'est aux médecins et chirurgiens à apprécier chaque cas en particulier : souvent la décision à prendre sera très difficile. L'appendicite est une maladie à allures si variées, si protéiformes, parfois si graves, qu'il faut se garder de règles trop absolues, et n'être ni interventionniste ni expectateur à outrance.

On aura bien souvent à résoudre un problème chirurgical très délicat.

M. KIRMISSON. — L'importance de la discussion actuelle n'a pu échapper à personne, et je crois être l'interprète de chacun de vous en adressant nos plus sincères félicitations aux deux rapporteurs. MM. Roux et Jalaguier. Ainsi donc, il est acquis que deux hommes chez lesquels la conscience est à la hauteur du talent chirurgical se prononcent nettement en faveur de l'expectation dans l'appendicite aiguë. Cette constatation est importante à un moment où d'autres voix se font entendre en faveur de l'intervention toujours et quand même dans tous les cas d'appendicite.

Pour moi, pendant très longtemps, je n'ai pas eu l'occasion de prendre position dans le débat, l'appendicite étant très rare aux Enfants-Assistés, comme le rappelait à l'instant, notre collègue M. Jalaguier, mais depuis que je suis arrivé à l'hôpital Trousseau, à la fin de 1897, je me suis trouvé constamment aux prises avec cette terrible maladie. Tout d'abord j'ai été éclectique par tempérament : plus tard, influencé par les opinions qui se faisaient entendre autour de moi, je suis devenu de parti pris interventionniste. Mais cette période a été de très courte durée ; j'ai en effet la conviction intime d'avoir ainsi, dans un ou deux cas, causé la mort de malades qui auraient eu plus de chances de guérison, si on les avait abandonnés à eux-mêmes. En effet, on a beau s'entourer des précautions antiseptiques les plus rigoureuses, il faut aller sculpter l'appendice au milieu d'un foyer septique, et l'on court ainsi les plus grandes chances d'infecter son malade. Je suis bien vite revenu à la doctrine éclectique, et aujourd'hui je n'interviens plus que contraint et forcé dans le cours de l'appendicite aiguë, réservant toutes mes préférences pour l'excision à froid de l'appendice.

Il est un point qui a été touché par notre collègue, M. Jalaguier, dans son rapport et dont je désire dire un mot. Il nous a parlé d'une jeune fille opérée par lui et chez laquelle il a observé des épistaxis, des hémorragies utérines, et des hématémèses. Plusieurs fois j'ai vu des hémorragies au cours de l'appendicite, et j'ai même publié le cas d'une jeune fille qui a succombé à une hématémèse foudroyante à la suite de l'ouverture d'un abcès d'origine appendiculaire. Déjà notre collègue, M. Piéchaud (de Bordeaux) avait publié un cas semblable.

Il y a donc lieu de décrire une septicémie à forme hémorragique dans le cours de l'appendicite, et cette complication redoutable mérite d'être sérieusement étudiée.

MERCREDI 8 AOUT

Séance du soir.

TRAITEMENT DES SUPPURATIONS PAR LES PULVÉRISATIONS ANTISEPTIQUES
A L'AIDE DE L'IPSILEUSE DE M. GUILMETH

COMMUNICATION

de M. PAUL COUDRAY,
de Paris.

Les publications et démonstrations que j'ai déjà faites sur ce sujet ainsi que la thèse récente de mon élève Paul Sempé représentent l'analyse de la question : je me contenterai, dans ce court travail, de présenter la synthèse des faits que j'ai étudiés.

Il y a un peu plus *de deux ans*, un chimiste ingénieux, M. Guilmeth, qui déjà avait introduit dans la pratique un bon agent anesthésique local, le coryl (mélange de chlorure d'éthyle et de méthyle), vint me demander d'expérimenter un procédé d'antisepsie qui consistait à réaliser, dans les plaies infectées de tout ordre, un dépôt instantané d'un antiseptique quelconque, iodoforme, salol, traumatol, etc., etc. : il suffisait pour obtenir ce résultat, de mélanger ces agents antiseptiques à du *chlorure d'éthyle pur* à l'aide d'un dispositif particulier. M. Guilmeth appelait son mélange d'éthyle, *ipsilos* ; le réservoir où se fait ce mélange *ipsileuse*, le tube creux de communication avec l'extérieur *ipsileur*: enfin les mélanges des antiseptiques avec le chlorure d'éthyle sont des *ipsilènes*. Voilà pour la terminologie.

On sait que le chlorure d'éthyle bout à 10°. Or quand on élève la température de ce liquide à 25 ou 50°, ce corps s'échappe de l'appareil en gaz, doué d'une certaine pression, entraînant avec lui les particules finement divisées de l'antiseptique choisi, puis au contact des tissus, il se volatise presque instantanément ; de là, une imprégnation très bonne des surfaces infectées.

Il y a donc : 1° Un effet mécanique, résultat de la pression, par lequel les corps liquides ou solides, adhérents plus ou moins aux drains ou aux parois des parties infectées, sont chassés des plaies ; or ces corps étrangers, caillots sanguins, débris solides résultant des produits de déchéance des tissus, sont souvent rebelles aux lavages ordinaires ; c'est un fait qui se vérifie, pour ainsi dire, à chaque pansement.

2° Outre cet effet mécanique, on obtient un dépôt réel d'antiseptique qui s'opère dans les coins les plus reculés des trajets parfois multiples et compliqués. Vous pouvez vous rendre compte de l'instantanéité de ce dépôt sur le drain que je fais passer devant vos yeux, dépôt obtenu avec l'ipsiléne au menthol. Comme vous le voyez, pour mettre l'appareil en marche, je tourne, de gauche à droite, la tige d'émission ou ipsileur et la communication est établie : je ferme l'appareil en tournant en sens contraire.

Au point de vue de la technique, je dois *insister particulièrement* sur deux remarques concernant le drainage et la pression.

a) Le *drainage* me paraît indispensable d'une manière générale pour deux raisons : d'abord parce que c'est le moyen le plus sûr de guérir les suppurations ; en second lieu, parce que les pulvérisations faites dans des trajets surtout longs et complexes et qui ne sont pas drainés amèneraient des douleurs dues à un excès de pression, les trajets en question tendant à s'oblitérer en quelque point par un accolement de bourgeons ; je me sers de drains ordinaires en caoutchouc rigide et à trous rapprochés. On a pu dire que les drains constituaient une cause d'infection, mais traités par l'imprégnation antiseptique d'iodoforme, ils doivent échapper à ce reproche ; l'expérience que j'ai à cet égard, me permettra d'émettre cette opinion.

b) La *pression* qu'il convient de donner à l'ipsilos est un détail très important. Cette pression est réglée par la température et il suffit de porter cette température à 25 ou 30°. Par les temps *chauds*, l'appareil fonctionne de lui-même ; quand la température est au-dessous de 20°, on met dans la petite caisse qui couronne l'ipsileuse un peu d'eau tiède (à 50 ou 55°). Les pressions plus fortes sont susceptibles d'amener une sensation douloureuse ; au niveau de la mastoïde ou dans le conduit auditif, des phénomènes d'étourdissement et de vertige. En second lieu, en employant les hautes pressions, on amène aussi dans les plaies une dose plus élevée des agents antiseptiques ; ce qui peut avoir des inconvénients. Il est donc préférable d'employer les pressions faibles et de faire deux ou trois petites pulvérisations successives si l'on juge que la première n'a amené qu'une imprégnation insuffisante. Lorsqu'on fait une pulvérisation dans un drain perforant ou à deux issues, drain en anse, on peut faire une première petite pulvérisation qui sert à chasser les corps étrangers, puis une seconde en pinçant le drain à l'un des orifices de sortie ; de la sorte, on a une bonne imprégnation et du drain et des surfaces infectées par les trous rapprochés du drain.

Je ne dirai qu'un mot sur l'antiseptique à choisir. M. Guilmeth a fait des préparations variées : ipsilénes iodé, au traumatol, au salol, au gaïacol, au menthol, à l'eucalyptol ; il pense aussi pouvoir réaliser de la même manière des préparations au permanganate de potasse, à l'aldéhyde formique, à l'oxygène, suivant les préférences de tel ou tel chirurgien. Quant à moi, j'ai expérimenté presque exclusivement l'iodoforme, parce que c'est l'agent qui, d'une manière générale, a fait ses preuves les plus évidentes et les plus constantes et parce qu'il exerce une action un peu spéciale vis-à-vis des lésions tuberculeuses. Dissous dans divers véhicules, l'alcool et l'éther en particulier (le chlorure d'éthyle est un éther) l'iodoforme est rapidement absorbé et par là s'explique l'énergie de son action, comme l'a indiqué de Ruyter. Mais l'action antiseptique ou bactéricide n'est pas seule à considérer ici : il est bien possible que l'iodoforme agisse beaucoup par les actions cellulaires phagocytiques qu'il détermine. Nous avons montré récemment avec M. le professeur Cornil que l'iodoforme employé à doses faibles provoque dans les tissus normaux une néoformation extrêmement riche de leucocytes généralement polynucléaires et de cellules plasmatiques et endothéliales à noyaux multiples et volumineux, éléments qui sont bien armés pour la lutte contre les agents microbiens. Ultérieurement une partie des éléments s'organisent en tissu fibreux.

Quant aux résultats obtenus à l'aide de ce mode d'antisepsie, ils ont été publiés dans la thèse de M. Paul Sempé.

Sur les 50 observations que renferme ce travail ;

5 sont relatives à des plaies *infectées* des parties molles dans lesquelles la guérison nous a semblé rapide.

19 ont trait à des plaies d'origine tuberculeuse.

2 adénites suppurées du cou avec altération ; guérison prompte après incision simple sans grattage, suivie de pulvérisations iodoformées.

6 coxalgies anciennes infectées ou fistuleuses ; 4 guérisons ; 1 cas en voie de guérison ; 1 malade parti très amélioré.

5 maux de Pott avec abcès infectés ou fistuleux ; 1 guéri ; 2 sur le point d'être guéris.

6 ostéites du tarse antérieur ou postérieur.

1 ostéite des os de la face.

1 ostéite du maxillaire inférieur.

6 sont relatives à des ostéites ou ostéo-myélites non tuberculeuses, dont trois mastoïdites, une due à M. Regnier.

A ce sujet, je dois dire, sans vouloir entrer dans le détail, que d'une manière générale le traitement, dans ce dernier groupe de lésions, doit être, en général, précédé d'une opération d'exérèse osseuse pour mettre à nu un foyer profond osseux ou un séquestre, tandis que dans la *tuberculose des os*, du moins chez l'enfant, l'exérèse est restreinte et se borne à une opération de drainage.

La portée de *ce procédé* d'antisepsie me semble très réelle. Ainsi dans les abcès de la coxalgie, comme a bien voulu le dire M. Kirmisson, dans sa communication à la Société de chirurgie, le 29 novembre 1899, ce procédé fournit à la méthode conservatrice un appoint nouveau et intéressant. Dans ces cas graves, de même que dans des cas analogues du mal de Pott que M. Kirmisson m'a confiés, la suppuration très abondante créant un état de septicémie, diminue assez vite ; l'état général de ce fait devient meilleur et dès lors il est tout à fait inutile de penser à pratiquer des opérations d'exérèse ou de résection, car l'indication suppuration *épuisante n'existe plus*.

A fortiori, dans les suppurations de moindre importance, le procédé donne de très bons et rapides résultats.

C'est un vif plaisir pour moi d'avoir eu non seulement les encouragements de M. Kirmisson, mais de M. Reynier qui est devenu un partisan très convaincu de ce procédé d'antisepsie. MM. Ménière et d'Argent l'ont aussi expérimenté, le premier pour les affections suppurées de l'oreille, le second dans quelques affections de la bouche.

TUBERCULOSE EXTERNE AU BORD DE LA MER

COMMUNICATION

de M. le docteur V. MÉNARD,

de Berck-sur-mer.

Le traitement maritime de la tuberculose externe est une des questions les plus importantes de ce temps. Il est d'un grand intérêt pour le monde médical d'être renseigné sur tout ce qui le concerne.

C'est à ce titre que je désire attirer l'attention sur les conditions dans lesquelles se trouvent les malades affectés de tuberculose externe, ganglionnaire, osseuse ou articulaire, sur les côtes de l'Océan et plus particulièrement à Berck.

L'Hôpital maritime reçoit toutes les formes de la tuberculose chirurgicale, mais la tuberculose osseuse et articulaire y occupe la plus large place, plus spécialement dans ses localisations les plus graves.

Sur les 650 à 700 malades de l'hôpital, la coxalgie compte pour plus de 150 : le mal de Pott pour un chiffre un peu plus élevé. Actuellement le mal de Pott et la coxalgie, pris ensemble, occupent 550 lits.

La tuberculose du genou, du coude et du poignet est beaucoup moins fréquente. Le spina-ventosa lui-même, qui affecte si souvent les jeunes enfants, ne se rencontre que chez un assez petit nombre de mes malades et, dans la plupart des cas, il est associé avec d'autres localisations tuberculeuses de plus grande importance.

La prédominance de la coxalgie et du mal de Pott s'explique à la fois par la fréquence relative de ces deux manifestations bacillaires chez l'enfant et par la difficulté du traitement à domicile.

En ville, sur la plage, la proportion entre les différentes localisations tuberculeuses est sensiblement la même. C'est encore la tuberculose de la hanche et du rachis qui occupe le premier rang. Sur 100 malades qui viennent chercher le bénéfice de l'influence maritime, 75 sont des coxalgiques ou des pottiques. Tout comme pour les enfants de l'hôpital, l'extrême difficulté d'instituer un traitement convenable en ville et même un peu partout à domicile engage à recourir au traitement marin.

La tuberculose ganglionnaire vient loin après la tuberculose osseuse et articulaire. L'Hôpital maritime possède au plus une soixantaine d'adénites bacillaires.

La tuberculose articulaire et osseuse tient donc sans contredit le premier rang à Berck par le nombre, aussi bien que par la gravité.

Elle se présente surtout sous ses formes les plus rebelles au traitement : coxalgie et mal de Pott.

Autrefois il avait été décidé par les règlements qu'on enverrait surtout, sinon exclusivement, des convalescents à Berck. Cet article de règlement était même passé dans la légende, si bien que j'ai vu des visiteurs surpris de trouver à l'Hôpital maritime un si grand nombre de malades qui n'étaient nullement à la période de convalescence de leur tuberculose.

Ce qui nous surprend plutôt, nous, c'est qu'un règlement aussi inconséquent ait pu voir le jour.

Si l'on a quelque notion de la marche de la tuberculose, de sa durée longue et accidentée, on pensera que le milieu qui a été favorable à l'évolution heureuse d'une coxalgie ou d'un mal de Pott jusqu'à une période voisine de la guérison est pleinement suffisant pour terminer la cure. Il est vraiment tard d'envoyer à la mer un coxalgique après les deux ou trois ans qu'il lui a fallu pour parvenir à la convalescence.

Si le traitement marin ne devait servir qu'à la convalescence de la tuberculose, il serait entièrement superflu.

En réalité nous voyons un très petit nombre d'enfants au début de leur tuberculose ostéo-articulaire, un nombre assez restreint aussi de cas anciens, pouvant être mis au compte de la convalescence. La grande majorité des malades arrivent avec leur affection en pleine activité. Les altérations sont déjà assez développées : il y a ou il n'y a pas de complications graves ; la réparation n'est pas faite.

Comme il s'agit, à l'Hôpital maritime, d'enfants de la classe pauvre, le traitement a été le plus souvent suivi jusque-là d'une manière irrégulière, intermittente, d'où la gravité des déformations articulaires et la fréquence de la suppuration fermée ou bien ouverte.

Les malades de la ville sont en général moins atteints, ils ont été traités plus tôt et avec plus de suite. Encore y a-t-il nombre d'exceptions à cette règle générale.

Avant d'examiner quel usage il convient de faire de l'influence marine chez les différentes catégories de malades, il faudrait définir cette influence. Peut-être est-il moins facile qu'on ne le pense généralement de répondre à cette question : comment agit la mer sur l'organisme des malades ?

Sans chercher à définir le rôle spécial et direct qui a été dévolu à l'iode, en quantité infinitésimale dans l'air marin, à l'ozone, aux parcelles de chlorure de sodium enlevées par les vents, qu'il nous suffise de constater un fait évident : l'énergie de l'action oxydante de l'air au bord de la mer.

La preuve en est donnée sous les formes les plus vulgaires.

Le fer rouille avec une rapidité extrême à la mer, s'il n'est protégé par un enduit imperméable, vernis ou peinture. Pour entretenir les objets en fer nu, comme le fusil, certaines parties de la bicyclette, il faut des soins très attentifs et très assidus. On sait que le fer est d'un médiocre usage dans les parties extérieures des constructions en vue de la mer.

Les couleurs s'altèrent très vite. Par exemple, les baigneurs sont frappés de ce que les teintes des étoffes sont pâlies, fanées en quelques jours. Les cheveux n'échappent pas entièrement à cette influence décolorante. Spécialement les cheveux blonds ou châtains. Lorsqu'ils sont longs, on voit que leur extrémité libre, plus directement exposée à l'air, est d'une couleur plus claire que la partie plus voisine de la peau et par suite plus cachée. Cette particularité est frappante chez les jeunes enfants dans la population berckoise. Ces enfants sont toute la journée dehors, la tête nue en général. Leurs cheveux sont la plupart du temps très pâles, décolorés, jaune clair, presque blancs à leur extrémité. Si l'on vient à examiner la partie profonde de la chevelure, on lui trouve une coloration plus foncée, et plus pure.

Dans le même ordre d'idées, un autre détail frappe encore davantage les personnes de la ville ou même de la campagne qui arrivent à Berck. Le coup de soleil sur le nez, sur les joues, sur les oreilles, sur le cou, sur les parties découvertes de la peau est très fréquent dans les premiers jours, alors même que le soleil est peu ardent. La brûlure semble produite dans beaucoup de cas presque autant par le vent que par les rayons solaires.

En dehors de cet accident léger, l'épiderme des parties exposées brunit aussi rapidement au bord de la Manche, à Berck, que sous le soleil d'Afrique. La peau des bruns noircit, celle des blonds rougit. La transformation est faite aux bout de trois ou quatre jours.

J'ai attiré l'attention, il y a plusieurs années sur une petite particularité qu'un de mes internes, M. Delmont, avait observée chez nos malades de Berck. Lorsque l'un des membres supérieurs ou inférieurs est le siège d'un foyer tuberculeux, de quelque importance, son épiderme se laisse plus vite et plus profondément brûler au grand air que l'épiderme du membre correspondant du côté sain. C'est ainsi que chez les coxalgiques qui se promènent les jambes et les pieds nus, la peau prend une teinte plus bistrée du côté malade. A ce seul signe, on peut distinguer quel est le côté atteint. Cela veut dire que les tissus, l'épiderme spécialement, offrent une résistance moindre sur le membre malade que sur le membre sain.

Je pourrais multiplier davantage les observations que chacun fait communément et qui toutes démontrent la puissance d'oxydation spéciale à l'air marin.

Faut-il attribuer cette qualité spéciale uniquement à la présence du chlorure de sodium dans l'atmosphère? Ce n'est pas le lieu de soulever cette question qui comporterait sans doute une réponse plus complexe. Quoi qu'il en soit, les propriétés marines ne tardent pas à disparaître dès qu'on s'éloigne du rivage. Elles sont fort atténuées au delà de quelques centaines de mètres en arrière de nos dunes de Berck.

Sans essayer de définir avec plus de précision le mode d'action de l'air marin sur l'organisme, on peut au moins rappeler que la respiration est activée d'une manière évidente. Les habitants de la ville éprouvent en arrivant à la mer une sensation spéciale de bien-être, liée à la respiration de l'air pur. S'ils restent quelques heures à la plage, au début de leur séjour, ils en ressentent une certaine fatigue, une lourdeur des membres que le repos à la campagne ne produit pas. Dans la suite, l'habitude efface cette sensation.

Avec la suractivité respiratoire, vient d'habitude le développement de l'appétit. Il convient d'user de modération ; nombre d'enfants mangent trop les premières semaines : il peut en résulter une fatigue de l'estomac et même un embarras gastrique momentané.

L'excitation des principales fonctions organiques a pour effet un changement rapide dans l'aspect physique. En même temps que l'épiderme du visage se brûle, que le visage se colore, l'embonpoint se prononce, s'exagère même souvent. Dans la suite, l'équilibre s'établit. Les enfants prennent les attributs d'une belle santé, sans engraisser notablement.

Tous ces faits sont évidents. Je ne les ai énoncés que pour exposer brièvement comment je comprends leurs rapports avec la guérison de la tuberculose externe.

Je pense qu'on a trop dit, trop fait entendre, du moins, que l'air marin exerçait une véritable action spécifique sur la tuberculose chirurgicale. Il ne se produit rien de pareil à un traitement spécifique. On ne voit pas la culture bacillaire s'éteindre et les lésions tuberculeuses s'effacer sous l'influence de la mer, comme la syphilis recule devant l'iodure de potassium. Une semblable comparaison ne saurait être faite à aucun degré.

Le progrès et la régression de la culture bacillaire dépendent de la lutte entre deux êtres vivants : le parasite et son porteur.

Deux éléments sont en balance : la résistance de l'organisme humain et la virulence tuberculeuse.

Si le traitement marin avait une action spécifique, il aurait pour effet direct d'éteindre ou d'atténuer la virulence du bacille. On verrait la marche du foyer tuberculeux enrayée. Une arthrite tuberculeuse, par exemple, prise au début, traitée au bord de la mer, dès la période des premiers signes, devrait s'arrêter et se résoudre.

Ce n'est pas là ce que nous voyons. Le foyer tuberculeux, au bord de la mer comme ailleurs, suit son évolution entière, avec des désordres plus ou moins graves sans doute : mais en somme, la guérison, si elle est beaucoup plus fréquente, se fait attendre presque aussi longtemps.

Je serais fort embarrassé, s'il me fallait montrer des cas dans lesquels l'évolution d'une arthrite tuberculeuse s'est arrêtée brusquement à l'une de ses phases. On ne voit pas plus au bord de la mer qu'ailleurs des transformations rapides de la maladie, des guérisons frappantes qui puissent être mises sur le compte d'un arrêt brusque dans l'évolution habituelle de la tuberculose. La culture parcourt toutes ses phases avant de s'atténuer ou de s'éteindre, comme partout ailleurs.

Il semble, au contraire, évident, que l'influence de la mer favorise la guérison en augmentant la résistance du terrain de culture, c'est-à-dire du malade. C'est avec cet esprit qu'il convient de suivre et de traiter les malades et que l'on doit, à mon avis, résoudre un certain nombre de questions de pratique relatives à la direction des tuberculeux au bord de la mer.

D'abord les tuberculeux, porteurs d'un ou de plusieurs foyers cutanés, ganglionnaires, osseux ou articulaires, doivent-ils être exposés sans réserve à l'action de l'air maritime, dès leur arrivée de la ville ou de la campagne au bord de la mer? Pour ma part, je crois que des ménagements sont nécessaires, plus spécialement chez les enfants dont la tuberculose est récente ou a subi une poussée récente. L'excitation vive de nos plages de l'Océan peut occasionner un certain danger en pareil cas. Ce n'est pas là une vue de l'esprit. Un certain nombre de faits, observés par moi-même, viennent à l'appui de ma proposition. J'ai observé plusieurs exemples de méningite tuberculeuse pendant les premières semaines de séjour à Berck et, circonstance intéressante, les enfants dont il s'agit appartenaient pour la plupart à la clientèle de la ville.

Nos malades de l'hôpital ne sont conduits à la mer qu'avec beaucoup de précaution durant le premier mois. Sur le nombre considérable de tuberculeux qui nous arrivent, plus de 500 par an, c'est à peine si j'ai vu trois ou quatre méningites tuberculeuses dans les deux premiers mois de séjour, depuis dix ans.

En ville, les enfants fréquentent la mer plusieurs heures dès le premier ou le deuxième jour. Les parents y mettent un zèle exempt de toute appréhension.

J'ajoute que presque tous les cas de méningite tuberculeuse qui se sont produits dans la clientèle de la ville, à Berck, sont apparus dans les premiers temps du séjour au bord de la mer.

Cette année, une petite fille de 6 ans arrive avec plusieurs manifestations cutanées et deux petits foyers osseux des extrémités, main et pied. Les parents se logent au bord de la mer et vont de suite à la plage. Ils y mettent ensuite quelque retenue sur mon conseil et vont habiter en seconde ligne, à 200 mètres du rivage. Une méningite est survenue.

Une fillette atteinte d'adénopathie bronchique et amenée, il y a quelques mois à Berck fut conduite, dès l'abord, toute la journée au bord de la mer malgré sa fièvre, d'après des conseils inconsidérés. Elle a succombé à une méningite.

La même complication mortelle est survenue dans quelques autres cas, chez des enfants affaiblis, pour lesquels les familles croyaient agir sagement en se précipitant à la plage toute la journée.

Il me semble, au contraire, que la brusquerie même de l'excitation maritime peut tout aussi bien donner un coup de fouet à la culture tuberculeuse et même en occasionner la diffusion en créant des foyers nouveaux, parmi lesquels la méningite. Il est prudent d'observer une certaine réserve pendant les premières semaines. Le malade doit être acclimaté doucement.

On a dit que les foyers tuberculeux subissaient eux-mêmes une poussée au moment où les malades arrivent à la mer. Ce n'est vrai qu'en partie. Je n'ai pas remarqué que la tuberculose osseuse ou articulaire fût jamais modifiée sensiblement pendant les premières semaines du séjour à Berck, que les articulations malades devinssent plus gonflées, plus douloureuses. Si le fait se produit, il doit être fort rare. Je n'ai pu l'observer, malgré que mon attention fût éveillée en ce sens.

Il arrive au contraire assez souvent que les adénopathies bacillaires et plus spécialement celles du cou offrent d'abord à la mer des signes d'excitation. Un ganglion, ou une grappe ganglionnaire, augmente fréquemment de volume d'abord, surtout si l'engorgement est peu ancien. J'ai eu un grand nombre ' fois la preuve de cette proposition. L'explication du fait peut en être donnée, semble-t-il, sans difficulté.

Chez beaucoup d'enfants, affectés d'adénite cervicale bacillaire, la peau et les muqueuses de la tête sont le siège d'altérations superficielles : érosions, ulcérations de la peau de la face et du cuir chevelu, fissures des orifices des cavités principales, hypertrophie des amygdales et de l'appareil glanduleux, du pharynx, etc. Toutes ces surfaces sont irritées, cautérisées légèrement par l'air oxydant de la plage. Il n'en faut pas plus pour que le réseau lymphatique transporte aux ganglions, déjà anciennement altérés, des produits capables de faire naître de nouvelles cultures ou de réveiller des cultures anciennes.

La poussée ganglionnaire est du reste éphémère : elle ne tarde pas à se calmer et s'il n'y a pas d'abcès, on voit ensuite la masse ganglionnaire diminuer peu à peu de volume, avec une lenteur plus ou moins grande, suivant les cas. L'accalmie s'explique aussi facilement que la surexcitation des premiers jours. Les surfaces ulcéreuses de la peau ou des muqueuses se cicatrisent souvent avec rapidité : l'hypertrophie des amygdales et de la muqueuse pharyngée diminue. Les portes d'entrée de l'infection des lymphatiques se trouvent closes ou du moins rétrécies ; la suractivité des grandes fonctions respiratoire et digestive fait le reste.

Lorsque, au bout de quelques semaines, les enfants ont pris l'habitude de vivre à la mer, ils se trouvent bien de passer plusieurs heures à la plage chaque jour. On doit veiller à ce qu'ils soient suffisamment protégés contre le froid, surtout s'il s'agit de sujets jeunes et soumis au repos. Cette précaution observée, je vois de jeunes malades passer une partie de leur journée au bord de la mer, en toute saison, à Berck, et même braver le mauvais temps sans éprouver aucune des complications habituellement mises sur le compte du froid.

Les affections de la gorge, du larynx et des bronches sont exceptionnelles, ce que je suis porté encore à attribuer aux qualités propres de l'air marin.

Cazin avait l'habitude de dire que le séjour à la mer, à Berck, était aussi favorable en hiver qu'en été. On lui attribue ce dicton un peu paradoxal qu'un hiver vaut deux étés. Je pense qu'il y a là une large part d'exagération. Il n'est pas douteux, au contraire, que les longues et belles journées de la belle saison, qui permettent aux malades de vivre en grande partie dehors sur la plage, sont d'un secours beaucoup plus efficace que les journées d'hiver, durant lesquelles les sorties sont nécessairement courtes.

J'ai à la fois sous les yeux, d'un côté, une catégorie de malades qui sortent et sont promenés sur la plage ou à quelque distance derrière les dunes durant toute l'année : ce sont les malades de la ville et aussi les malades de l'hôpital qui peuvent marcher ; et d'un autre côté, le groupe malheureusement nombreux des enfants de l'Hôpital maritime pour lesquels le repos au lit est indispensable. Ceux-ci restent dans leurs dortoirs durant la mauvaise saison.

Il m'est ainsi facile d'apprécier le bénéfice que les malades retirent de leur séjour à la mer dans ces conditions différentes. L'opposition est frappante. Les malades que l'on sort toute l'année ou qui peuvent marcher eux-mêmes ont un état général beaucoup meilleur et ils guérissent mieux.

Il faut donc que les enfants non seulement séjournent à la mer, mais encore qu'ils y vivent au grand air et autant que possible sur la plage même ou dans son voisinage immédiat.

La puissance curative du milieu maritime a été tantôt exagérée avec lyrisme, tantôt diminuée. A côté de ceux qui soutiennent encore que la tuberculose externe guérit aussi bien n'importe où qu'à la mer, il y a une autre catégorie d'enthousiastes pour lesquels la mer suffit à tout, guérit tout à elle seule. Le médecin et le chirurgien s'effacent ;

ils n'ont qu'à suivre les progrès de la cure, sans penser même à aucun traitement complémentaire.

La vérité se place entre ces deux opinions extrêmes. L'influence de la mer a pour effet, avons-nous dit, d'améliorer la santé générale en augmentant l'activité de l'assimilation et de la désassimilation, et par suite d'augmenter la résistance aux infections et le pouvoir réparateur. On a sous les yeux des malades mieux disposés à guérir.

Par suite de je ne sais quel préjugé, quelques-uns ont vu dans ces conditions favorables aux patients un motif d'abstention médicale et chirurgicale. La mer se trouvant être un adjuvant de la cure, la direction du médecin ou du chirurgien deviendrait une vaine parade.

Une pareille déduction est irrationnelle. Les règles de thérapeutique sont les mêmes à Berck que dans les autres milieux. L'intervention par le traitement médicamenteux, et par les opérations petites ou grandes reste soumise d'une manière générale aux mêmes lois.

La seule différence consiste en ce que les conditions sont meilleures pour le tuberculeux dans le milieu marin, que les résultats devront être plus heureux et que les tentatives du médecin et du chirurgien seront plus souvent couronnées de succès.

D'accord avec l'opinion généralement admise à l'heure actuelle, je pense qu'on doit être très économe d'actes thérapeutiques chez les enfants tuberculeux. Le grand acteur de la réparation est l'organisme lui-même. Nous ne guérissons pas les malades. Ils guérissent eux-mêmes, placés dans un milieu favorable. La formule célèbre de A. Paré trouverait ici sa place.

Cependant je ne puis parvenir à comprendre les chirurgiens qui rejettent toute opération à propos d'une arthrite tuberculeuse ou d'une adénopathie du cou, pas plus au reste que les chirurgiens de disposition opposée, qui proposent d'opérer presque tous les cas, de traiter un foyer tuberculeux, quelle que soit sa variété, par une opération correspondante.

Nous avons entendu récemment exprimer ces deux opinions contradictoires relativement à la coxalgie. Les uns se refusent toujours à la résection ; les autres la pratiquent presque constamment. Un collègue plus extraordinaire a, par une conversion qu'il confesse, passé de l'un de ces excès à l'autre. Après avoir opéré toutes les coxalgies, il en est venu ensuite à n'en opérer aucune.

Ce défaut peu commun de pondération doit être lié à la fausse idée que plusieurs se font du rôle exact des opérations chez les tuberculeux.

La plupart des opérations que nous pratiquons dans les foyers tuberculeux ne méritent pas d'être appelées radicales. Car elles n'amènent pas elles-mêmes sûrement la guérison. Je ne fais pas allusion aux amputations qui sont en quelque sorte un renoncement à la cure. Supprimer un segment du membre malade, amputer une jambe pour une tuberculose du cou-de-pied, une cuisse pour une tuberculose du genou, c'est reconnaître notre impuissance de guérir la région malade, genou ou cou-de-pied. Je ne parle ici que des opérations curatives, comme la résection typique ou atypique d'une articulation, l'évidement d'un os tuberculeux, l'ablation d'une masse de ganglions tuberculeux. Ces interventions ne sont pas à proprement parler radicales. On n'est jamais certain d'enlever tout le mal, de mettre le malade à l'abri de la rechute. Mais est-ce là un motif qui justifie l'abandon des opérations plus larges que l'aveugle drainage? Je suis loin de le penser.

De ce qu'une arthrotomie, ou une arthrectomie ne supprime pas tout le foyer tuberculeux, il ne s'ensuit nullement que l'une ou l'autre de ces opérations ne contribue à la guérison. Seule l'expérience résout la question.

Je comprendrais même que les indications pussent être différentes non pas selon les chirurgiens, ce qui étonne, mais selon les milieux. Il me paraît évident que les opérations larges, pratiquées sur les grandes articulations, affectées de tuberculose, fournissent des résultats différents selon qu'elles sont pratiquées à la ville, à la campagne ou à la mer.

S'il est admis que les enfants, qui jouissent du bienfait de la mer, relèvent le pouvoir réparateur de leurs tissus, on est porté à en conclure qu'ils auront plus de chance de guérir à la suite de l'acte opératoire.

Le rôle des interventions dans la tuberculose externe ne va pas jusqu'à guérir radicalement les foyers de culture. Elles ne peuvent avoir cette prétention, parce que si larges qu'elles soient, si complètes qu'elles paraissent, elles ne suppriment probablement presque jamais l'ensemencement d'une manière rigoureuse : il reste toujours assez de bacilles, pour que la culture renaisse, si le terrain s'y prête.

A mon avis, en opérant un foyer tuberculeux, on se propose de supprimer le mieux que l'on peut, un obstacle reconnu d'avance à la guérison, et c'est justement cet obstacle matériel, dont l'existence nous est démontrée dans nombre de cas, qui constitue l'indication opératoire.

Je pourrais citer un grand nombre de circonstances dans lesquelles une altération anatomique déterminée s'oppose à la guérison souvent d'une manière indéfinie sinon absolue. Il suffit d'en rappeler quelques-unes.

Un séquestre invaginé au centre d'une épiphyse empêche la cicatrisation d'une fistule, expose en outre à des désordres graves tels que la multiplication des fistules, la pénétration consécutive d'une articulation voisine. Tout le monde est d'accord sur la nécessité d'enlever le séquestre en drainant largement sa loge.

Un abcès par congestion, qui menace de s'élargir et de s'ouvrir à l'extérieur, et par suite expose le malade au danger grave de l'infection suppurative secondaire, doit être supprimé au même titre. Les ponctions et les injections modificatrices sont les opérations qui viennent le mieux confirmer la définition que j'ai voulu donner. En enlevant incomplètement le contour de l'abcès, en irritant la poche, on enlève l'obstacle à la guérison, on apporte une aide à l'organisme qui fait le reste. Le succès est obtenu dans de telles proportions que la méthode des injections modificatrices dans le traitement de la tuberculose vertébrale ou coxale, compliquée d'abcès, doit être considérée comme le traitement exclusif.

J'ai lu récemment, dans une Revue d'ailleurs excellente sur le traitement de la coxalgie, que les injections modificatrices relèvent de la petite chirurgie. C'est vrai, si l'on veut envisager la bénignité de l'acte opératoire. Mais l'importance et le grand nombre des succès obtenus mettent les injections modificatrices infiniment au-dessus des interventions graves et difficiles pratiquées pour des lésions viscérales peu ou pas réparables, comme les cancers.

Il arrive que les injections modificatrices ne sont pas suivies de la guérison de l'abcès par congestion : un séquestre est au fond du trajet, ou bien la disposition anatomique du foyer tuberculeux est défavorable. En tout cas, l'abcès se reproduit, il tend à s'ouvrir. L'obstacle à la guérison persiste et s'aggrave. C'est dans ces conditions nettement déterminées, que j'ai pratiqué avec des succès très encourageants, puis conseillé la résection aseptique de la hanche.

Loin de moi la prétention d'enlever complètement le foyer tuberculeux de la hanche, malgré le nom de curettage intégral que j'ai donné à l'opération, mais, en opérant largement, avec un soin minutieux, j'ai vu les opérés, plus de 20 enfants et jeunes adultes guérir presque tous par première intention. L'acte opératoire n'a fait encore ici qu'enlever l'obstacle à la réparation.

Le même raisonnement circonscrit les indications opératoires relativement aux adénopathies du cou. L'observation me montre que les ganglions tuberculeux de petit volume, solitaires, en chaîne ou en grappe, diminuent lentement de volume à la mer, durcissent, deviennent mobiles dans la région et, à la longue, s'atrophient spontanément. Au contraire, lorsqu'un ou plusieurs ganglions volumineux sont remplis de caséum, et voués à la fistulisation et à la suppuration, longue et complexe, qui en est la suite, on doit le plus souvent recourir à l'ablation de tout le groupe des gros ganglions.

On laisse sans aucun doute au fond de la plaie des ganglions plus petits et déjà infectés, susceptibles d'augmenter de volume dans la suite. L'expérience me montre qu'au bord de la mer, les interventions pratiquées dans les cas ainsi précisés procurent une très large proportion de succès rapides, alors que l'abstention aurait laissé persister la masse ganglionnaire durant une longue suite d'années.

Dans les cas que je viens de citer, et que je pourrais présenter sous de nombreuses variétés de forme, la guérison est obtenue après la suppression de l'obstacle matériel à la réparation.

Le séquestre, le pus, le caséum ne pouvaient disparaître que par résorption ou élimination. La résorption est très longue, lorsqu'elle est possible: le plus souvent elle ne peut être espérée.

L'élimination expose aux dangers de la suppuration ouverte, toujours très longue, souvent dangereuse pour la vie.

Il me paraît inadmissible que l'on refuse aux malades les bénéfices d'opérations presque exemptes de danger et qui donnent une énorme proportion de succès.

Une sorte de malentendu dans les discussions sur les opérations à pratiquer chez les tuberculeux est né en partie de ce fait que les chirurgiens se trouvaient dans des conditions différentes. Les uns visaient les enfants, d'autres les adultes; ceux-ci des enfants anémiés par le séjour à la ville, ceux-là des enfants transportés à la campagne ou à la mer.

Il est naturel que les mêmes interventions donnent des résultats différents, si les conditions d'âge et de milieu ne sont pas les mêmes.

En ce qui regarde les tuberculeux externes, qui bénéficient du séjour à la mer, au lieu de soutenir que tout secours opératoire leur est interdit, je pense fermement au contraire que les indications sans être plus nombreuses peuvent comprendre des cas plus graves. Les opérations larges sur les grandes articulations et spécialement la résection de la hanche qui, dans la pratique urbaine, donnent des résultats assez médiocres, me fournissent au contraire une proportion très encourageante de succès, bien que je n'opère que dans les atteintes graves, compliquées de suppuration et le plus souvent de suppuration ouverte.

TRAITEMENT DES ARTHRITES TUBERCULEUSES ET PURULENTES
PAR LE DRAINAGE AVEC DES TUBES DE VERRE ET PAR L'ACIDE PHÉNIQUE
PUR, AVEC UN RAPPORT SUR 70 CAS

COMMUNICATION

de M. le docteur PHELPS

de New-York.

L'année passée et l'année d'avant j'ai eu l'honneur de présenter à l'Association américaine d'orthopédie une méthode thérapeutique spéciale des arthritres suppurées. J'ai présenté à cette même séance un travail sur plusieurs cas d'érysipèle traités par l'acide phénique pur dans l'hôpital de la Cité et guéris radicalement par ce moyen.

Depuis la lecture de ce rapport j'ai opéré toutes les arthrites tuberculeuses suppurées par cette méthode. Tous nos cas d'érysipèle ont été traités par les applications d'acide phénique pur et, durant l'année passée, tous les cas traités dans les pavillons et les services chirurgicaux ont avorté ou, du moins, ont été rapidement enrayés et il n'y eu aucun décès signalé à ma connaissance.

En ce qui concerne l'usage de l'acide phénique pur dans les arthrites fongueuses suppurées et sa méthode d'application, j'en recommande l'importance parce que je suis convaincu de sa supériorité sur tous les autres moyens usuels que je connais. Il existe parmi les chirurgiens orthopédiques de grandes divergences d'opinion sur l'opportunité d'opérer les abcès articulaires. Il y a un camp extrême qui préconise de ne rien faire, et Ridlon affirme dans un de ses travaux qu'il n'a pas eu à intervenir une seule fois sur 100 cas. Nous avons un camp qui pense que les abcès qui causent des troubles constitutionnels ou locaux doivent être opérés. Enfin, un dernier parti auquel j'appartiens pense que chaque arthrite suppurée ou tuberculeuse doit être opérée aussitôt que le diagnostic en est fait, et cela pour les raisons suivantes :

Les abcès ne sont jamais l'expression de l'état pathologique d'une articulation. Les abcès les plus vastes, ceux qui causent les troubles constitutionnels les plus graves, sont souvent accompagnés de lésions osseuses insignifiantes ou nulles, tandis qu'au contraire les ostéites les plus sérieuses ne sont souvent compliquées que de tout petits abcès qui ne causent aucun trouble, mais qui détruisent insidieusement toute l'articulation, nécessitant ultérieurement une résection complète et entraînant la mort si l'on n'est pas intervenu hâtivement.

Connaissant ces faits pour les avoir observés des centaines de fois cliniquement, je recommande avec insistance une opération précoce aussi rapidement que le diagnostic est porté pour une arthrite tuberculeuse ou suppurée. L'opération est pratiquée dans un double but :

Le premier, et le plus important, est celui d'explorer la jointure pour se rendre compte des endroits envahis et de l'étendue des lésions.

Le second est celui d'un drainage complet. Une maison vide vaut mieux qu'une maison mal habitée, et sûrement le contact de tissus sains avec des produits tuberculeux et septiques produira de l'infection avec la destruction de l'os et des parties molles, et une infection en rapport avec la durée de la macération et l'étendue de l'infection.

Par exemple un abcès de la hanche, dans bien des cas, ulcère la capsule, envahit le muscle iliaque interne au voisinage du bord antérieur de la capsule; puis, poursuivant sa voie en longeant le bassin, pénètre dans la fosse iliaque. De pareilles lésions résultent presque toujours de la destruction étendue de l'intérieur de l'ilion par suite du drainage insuffisant, à cause de la pression des tissus recouvrant le bassin. Après des mois et des années, vu l'état du malade, lorsqu'une opération est jugée indispensable, le chirurgien trouvera fréquemment qu'il lui faut enlever la crête de l'ilion et supprimer, avec la curette et le ciseau, presque tout le contenu de la fosse iliaque. Cet accident pourrait facilement être évité par une intervention exploratrice précoce, sitôt que la fluctuation est découverte au niveau de l'articulation.

D'autres fois, si l'abcès ne trouve pas sa voie dans la fosse iliaque, le triangle de Scarpa se remplit de pus, des fusées purulentes se produisent à la partie postérieure de la cuisse ou minent la face intérieure des aponévroses de la partie antérieure de la cuisse, détruisant des groupes musculaires tout entiers.

Je ne puis trouver de raison qui permette de laisser un abcès produire de tels dégâts. Très souvent — et je possède toute une liste de ces cas — l'acétabulum se perfore. Le pus se fraie une voie sur la face interne du pelvis, sous le fascia iliaque, aborde le rectum, le perfore, détruit souvent le sphincter ou établit une communication entre l'articulation et le rectum, d'où s'échappent constamment les matières fécales et les gaz.

J'ai opéré des cas semblables, ils sont très graves et difficiles à guérir. Une opération précoce aurait sûrement prévenu cette calamité. Le pus n'envahit jamais la cavité rétro-péritonéale par l'acétabulum, de sorte qu'on peut le découvrir par la palpation.

Du moins on l'a pensé, mais c'est une erreur et les médecins qui l'ont écrit et ceux qui l'ont recopié ensuite n'avaient pas d'observation clinique sur le sujet, et cette erreur ne se serait pas infiltrée dans notre littérature. La seule voie que le pus puisse trouver pour envahir la fosse iliaque est celle que je viens de décrire, due à une rupture de la partie antérieure de la capsule.

Revenons maintenant en arrière et examinons brièvement l'étiologie et la pathologie de ces abcès. Mes remarques concernent seulement la hanche.

L'arthrite de la hanche, soit tuberculeuse, soit purulente, est toujours précédée d'une lésion des os ou des parties molles. Il doit nécessairement, suivant les lois de la bactériologie, y avoir un terrain prédisposé à la réception et au développement des bacilles. Ce terrain se constitue surtout dans le tissu de néoformation d'origine inflammatoire. Lorsqu'un organe est lésé par un traumatisme ou un embolisme, la nature s'efforce de le réparer. S'il ne se produit pas d'inoculation au niveau de cette zone inflammatoire physiologique, l'enfant guérira dans l'espace d'un mois ou deux, après avoir présenté les symptômes de la coxalgie. Cette action inflammatoire normale évolue dans les conditions suivantes :

Après l'accident il se produit une hémorrhagie, puis une émigration de cellules ou plutôt une prolifération cellulaire rapide sur le point lésé.

Le caillot sanguin s'organise. Les cellules se mettent d'elles-mêmes en ligne pour réparer les tissus malades. Des capillaires et des filaments nerveux traversent ce nouveau tissu inflammatoire pour assurer sa nutrition. Peu à peu chaque cellule se transforme suivant la nature du tissu traumatisé, les cellules osseuses produisant de l'os, les autres les parties molles. Au bout d'un certain temps, l'organisation s'achève et le tissu inflammatoire se rétracte. Les capillaires et les filets nerveux disparaissent sous l'influence de la rétractation et la cicatrice apparaît.

Si des bactéries pathogènes flottent dans le torrent circulatoire de l'enfant et qu'elles arrivent au contact du tissu néo-inflammatoire en voie de réparation normale, il se fait une inoculation in situ, les cellules se détruisent les unes après les autres, les bactéries déposent et sécrètent leurs toxines et tout le foyer de réparation physiologique se transforme en cavité purulente ou fongueuse. Cette cavité purulente, remplie de bactéries, est un réservoir d'où rayonne l'infection sur les tissus avoisinants.

Si le foyer malade siège dans la tête ou le col du fémur, il augmente jusqu'à ce que perforation s'ensuive et l'articulation s'infecte secondairement.

Si l'infection se trouve au niveau du cartilage épiphysaire de l'acétabulum, l'articulation s'infecte secondairement, mais presque en même temps que l'acétabulum.

La tête de l'os et l'acétabulum peuvent être infectés secondairement par un abcès de l'intérieur de la capsule, lorsque les parties molles sont primitivement envahies. En d'autres termes, la macération de l'os dans un milieu infecté chargé de bactéries et de toxines virulentes amène la destruction secondaire de tout le tissu osseux. Ces propositions sont acceptées dans le monde chirurgical : la bactériologie, la pathologie et la clinique les ont d'ailleurs démontrées. Je ne puis donc comprendre comment il est possible d'admettre comme règle de conduite la non-intervention dans le traitement d'un processus aussi actif de destruction.

C'est un fait que peut-être un abcès sur dix, soit pour les articulations, soit pour les autres tissus du corps se termine par la résorption. C'est aussi un fait que plus de 50 pour 100 des abcès articulaires se font jour à la surface, de façon à établir un bon drainage et à amener la guérison par un simple moyen mécanique.

Mais que devons-nous faire des autres 50 pour 100 qui produisent des troubles si graves? Comment distinguer les formes bénignes des formes malignes? Nous ne le pouvons pas sans opération exploratrice. La règle suivie dans l'appendicite doit l'être aussi dans les abcès des articulations : précisément il faut adopter, pour les abcès articulaires, les mêmes principes que pour les abcès de n'importe quelle partie du corps, et spécialement ceux de la diaphyse des os longs. Aucun chirurgien de réputation ne songerait à abandonner à la nature un cas d'ostéomyélite ou d'abcès tuberculeux des os.

Ces cas sont toujours opérés, et l'on conserve ainsi la vie et le membre que l'on sacrifierait sans cela.

De nos jours, aucun chirurgien n'abandonnerait à la nature bien des cas d'appendicite. 75 pour 100 des abcès de l'appendice s'ouvrent du côté du péritoine, occasionnant une mortalité de plus de 55 pour 100, tandis que la mort est réduite à moins de 1 pour 100, lorsqu'on opère de bonne heure. Les mêmes arguments peuvent être appliqués aux abcès des articulations. Si l'on opérait à temps toute arthrite suppurée ou fongueuse, la mortalité et la destruction des articulations tomberait à un pourcentage minime, tandis que la mortalité atteint 8 à 12 pour 100 pour les cas non opérés. Quant aux cas où il fallut recourir aux résections et ceux où l'on observe des fistules intarissables pendant des années, je n'en puis fixer le pourcentage, qui doit être très élevé. Je sais que dans ma clinique d'hôpital, qui est largement pourvue de patients provenant de cliniques ou d'autres hôpitaux, plus de 75 pour 100 des malades ont des arthrites chroniques et souvent des lésions du bassin qui durent depuis des années. Et pourtant, si ces cas avaient été examinés à temps et si les abcès avaient été évacués, on aurait pu éviter les résections que je suis obligé de pratiquer. La mortalité pour résection de la hanche atteint probablement 3 ou 4 pour 100.

Certainement, si ces malades avaient été opérés à temps ils n'auraient pas succombé. En outre l'excision de la hanche produit un raccourcissement du membre de deux à trois pouces et demi.

D'après mon opinion, si tous les abcès articulaires étaient opérés de bonne heure, sitôt le diagnostic établi, l'excision ne serait pas nécessaire dans des centaines de cas; tandis que, dans les cas de non-intervention, la résection devient nécessaire dans plus de 25 pour 100 des cas.

Les statistiques de l'Institution de la rue n° 59, de New-York, montrent que les abcès surviennent dans plus de 6 pour 100 des cas traités. Il en est de même à l'hôpital de la rue n° 42. A l'hôpital des Enfants, de Boston, c'est 55 pour 100. Étant donnés 100 de ces abcès, la nature permettra l'ouverture de l'abcès au dehors dans 50 pour 100 des cas, et la guérison s'obtiendra par un simple moyen mécanique. Pour les autres 50 pour 100, grâce à l'ouverture favorable de l'abcès permettant le drainage, grâce aussi à un traitement mécanique soigné, la guérison s'obtient avec un raccourcissement de un à deux pouces avec une atrophie musculaire extrême et définitive. Ces résultats s'obtiennent après des années de traitement orthopédique : 25 pour 100 de ces malades trouvent le chemin de divers hôpitaux et dispensaires de la Cité où l'on soigne pour des complications hépatiques ou rénales, avec destructions osseuses étendues, luxations de la hanche, avec des membres atrophiés et recroquevillés, avec une difformité si grande qu'il faut pratiquer la résection dans la plupart des cas. Voilà ce que j'ai observé pendant quinze ans de pratique dans les dispensaires de New-York; nous pouvons donc examiner la question aussi bien maintenant qu'à toute autre époque.

Les 50 malades qui guérissent ne peuvent éprouver un dommage quelconque d'une incision et d'un drainage soignés, car des mains et des instruments antiseptiques ne peuvent infecter une articulation qui l'est déjà. Aucun médecin expérimenté ne peut déterminer à l'avance quel abcès évoluera favorablement et lequel occasionnera la mort. La seule source de complication possible est l'infection du trajet parcouru par le bistouri : si donc le chirurgien veut protéger complètement la surface de section par les moyens que je vais énumérer, cet accident ne pourra se produire.

La crainte de produire une infection générale quand on intervient sur un foyer tuberculeux n'est pas née de l'observation clinique. Je ne l'ai jamais vue et je ne crois pas qu'elle existe.

Les 50 pour 100 des cas graves mentionnés plus haut peuvent être traités scientifiquement au moment de l'incision par une exploration intelligente de l'articulation. Nous avons vu que la mortalité diminue ou disparaît par ce moyen et que l'on peut éviter les résections pour lésions étendues des os. C'est pourquoi je prétends, et sans crainte de contradiction sérieuse, que dans tous les cas les articulations peuvent être explorées avec intelligence à un moment donné. Et je me base pour le dire sur une observation clinique de quinze ans, portant sur des centaines, je dirai presque sur des milliers de cas d'arthrites suppurées que j'ai observés moi-même. Une hirondelle ne fait pas le printemps, et 55 cas d'abcès de la hanche, choisis et rapportés par le docteur Schaffer à l'Académie de médecine, n'ont pas de poids contre le traitement rationnel de ces abcès basé sur l'étiologie, la pathologie, la bactériologie et l'observation clinique. Nous en dirons autant des succès remportés avec l'aspiration recommandée par Gibney, cas que j'ai suivis longtemps et qui sont devenus très peu satisfaisants. L'aspiration est un leurre pour le chirurgien ; il ne sait jamais s'il ponctionne un abcès dû à un synovite ou à un séquestre étendu, ou à un décollement de la tête du fémur nécessitant une excision immédiate.

Il y a deux ans encore, il était très difficile d'opérer une coxalgie suppurée et de prévenir la suppuration secondaire. Mais depuis l'avènement de l'usage de l'acide phénique pur, comme je l'ai rapporté au dernier congrès, je n'ai plus rencontré de difficultés sur ce point. La médecine est redevable au docteur Senèque Powell, de New-York, d'une des plus importantes découvertes qui aient été faites en chirurgie. Je veux parler des propriétés antidotiques de l'alcool sur l'acide phénique pur. Powell emploie l'acide phénique pur depuis des années pour le traitement des maladies osseuses dans les différentes parties du corps, et il le recommande pour l'érysipèle et les abcès. Je l'ai essayé dans le traitement de l'érysipèle et je le considère comme un spécifique de cette maladie au même titre que la quinine pour la malaria. Ayant remarqué ses bons résultats dans les abcès osseux ou autres, je l'ai appliqué aux arthrites suppurées. Il n'y a aucune différence dans le traitement des abcès articulaires et celui des abcès des os ou des parties molles. Mes observations durant les deux dernières années démontrent la justesse de cette affirmation.

Tout le monde sait que l'acide phénique pur ne peut être absorbé. Comment peut-il donc agir au-delà de la surface malade? Par exemple, dans l'érysipèle cutané les lymphatiques les plus profonds sont envahis. Dans la coxalgie les bactéries se trouvent jusque dans les lymphatiques éloignés de l'articulation : avant que je ne fasse usage de l'acide phénique pur, j'ai souvent vu des abcès apparaître à plus d'un pouce du champ opératoire. Je ne puis l'expliquer que par une théorie : l'acide phénique s'unit à l'albumine des tissus pour former un albuminate éminemment antiseptique. Ce nouveau composé est absorbé par les lymphatiques et détruit les bacilles. Cela doit se passer ainsi, car dans l'érysipèle nous voyons la température tomber, redevenir normale, souvent six heures après la première application. Dans la coxalgie nous observons qu'après son application la température tombe de 105° F. à 100° au bout de douze heures, pour ne plus remonter, à moins qu'il ne se développe de nouveaux foyers.

La méthode d'application consiste simplement en ceci : la cavité de l'abcès est ouverte, l'orifice de la capsule est recherché et élargi, afin de permettre l'exploration de l'articulation. S'il y a ostéite étendue, l'incision est prolongée, la capsule est ouverte sur la moitié ou les deux tiers de sa circonférence, la tête du fémur est luxée du côté du cotyle : on fait largement usage de la curette, puis la cavité est bien nettoyée au sublimé au millième.

On remplit alors l'articulation d'acide phénique pur. Au bout d'une minute, la cavité est entièrement lavée avec de l'alcool pur, puis l'alcool lui-même est remplacé par une solution phéniquée à 2 pour 100.

Au lieu de tamponner la plaie, ou de la suturer, ou de la drainer avec un tube de caoutchouc mou, je me sers de tubes en verre aussi larges que la cavité le permet, que je place dans les parties déclives et que je fais aboutir à la peau. Ces tubes ne permettent pas seulement un drainage parfait, mais, grâce à eux, le chirurgien peut voir au jour le jour ce qui se passe dans l'articulation. Si la suppuration ou la maladie augmentent, on peut faire le curettage au travers du large tube et poser à nouveau de l'acide phénique et de l'alcool. Les tampons peuvent être introduits par le tube pour assurer un parfait drainage de l'articulation. Ces tubes varient de diamètre, d'un demi-pouce à deux pouces et demi, ils sont de longueur variable. Un tube à drainage pour un petit enfant doit être de un demi-pouce d'épaisseur. En d'autres termes, le tube est adapté à la plaie de façon à être aussi large que possible. L'on peut voir déjà les avantages immenses que le chirurgien retire d'inspecter la plaie jour par jour, jusqu'au fond.

Lorsqu'il n'est pas nécessaire d'enlever à la curette des séquestres ou des foyers osseux, la plaie peut être drainée par des tubes étroits. On applique ensuite, pendant la durée du séjour au lit, une extension de neuf à douze livres, après quoi le malade est renvoyé chez lui avec mon appareil et des béquilles. J'ai également observé que lorsqu'il existe une lésion de l'acétabulum et surtout de la tête du fémur, il vaut mieux enlever le trochanter parce que sa proéminence entrave le drainage de la jointure. Son ablation ne diminue en rien l'utilité du membre. Si le grand trochanter est très malade, je l'enlève toujours avec le col et la tête du fémur, parce que j'ai observé qu'on ne

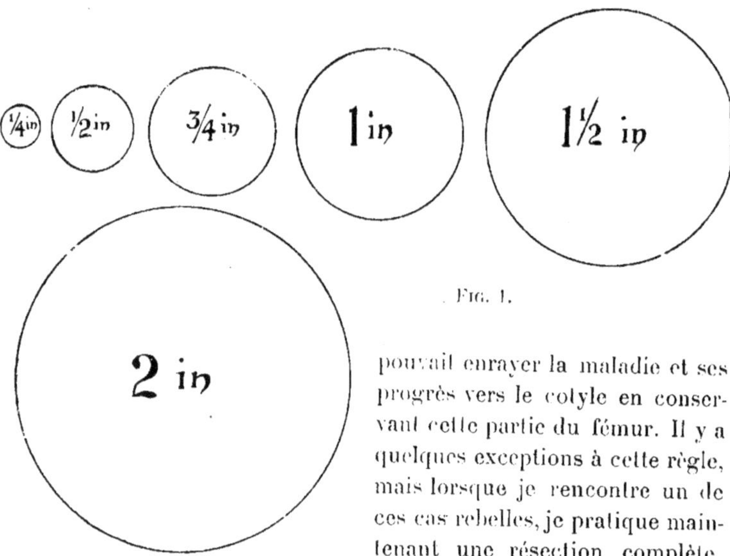

Fig. 1.

pourrait enrayer la maladie et ses progrès vers le cotyle en conservant cette partie du fémur. Il y a quelques exceptions à cette règle, mais lorsque je rencontre un de ces cas rebelles, je pratique maintenant une résection complète.

Lorsque l'abcès a envahi la fosse iliaque, je détache immédiatement le ligament de Poupart, l'épine iliaque supérieure et antérieure, ainsi que les insertions des muscles abdominaux à la crête de l'os iliaque, afin de pouvoir inspecter librement la fosse iliaque, Si le mal s'étend et que l'abcès gagne l'articulation sacro-iliaque, un tube à drainage est placé par derrière dans cette direction.

La figure 1 montre les dimensions exactes des tubes de verre et leurs longueurs allant de un à cinq pouces. Le tube le plus large, long de cinq pouces, est fait pour une résection de hanche chez un adulte. Les autres numéros sont employés pour les arthrotomies simples. Le choix du tube dépend des indications. On les stérilise par

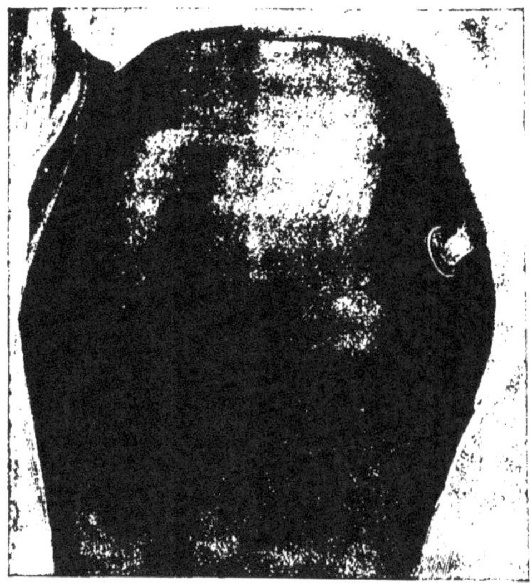

Fig. 2.

l'acide phénique pur au moment de s'en servir. Les figures 2 et 3
montrent les tubes en place et bourrés de gaze pour le drainage. Ce mode de pansement évite bien des souffrances, parce qu'il est facile à enlever tout en assurant un drainage parfait. On peut se servir de ces tubes dans toutes les opérations sur les os. On peut en placer deux ou trois côte à côte si la cavité osseuse est profonde. Le caoutchouc s'affaisse, ce que ne fait pas le verre. En outre, il est sale. Pour traiter convenablement une cavité osseuse, il faut que les parties molles s'adaptent exactement autour du tube.

Voyons maintenant le résultat des 70 opérations que j'ai faites.

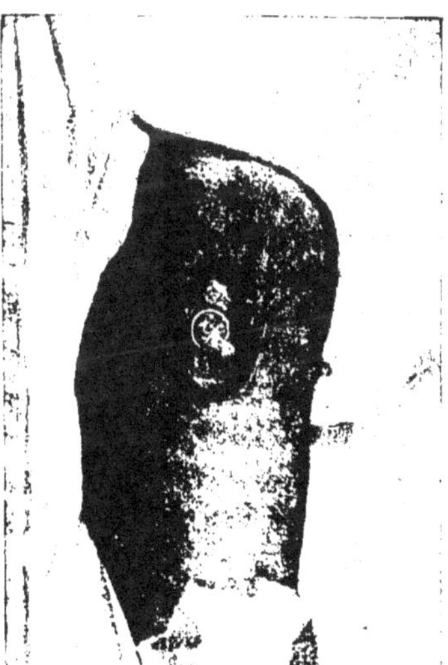

Fig. 3.

Sur ces 70, j'aurais pratiqué, dans ces dernières années, au moins 50 résections. En réalité, sur ces 70 opérations, je n'ai pratiqué que 20 résections. Dans tous les autres cas, l'articulation a été largement ouverte et l'on a enlevé presque dans chaque cas les portions d'os ou de cartilage qui avaient été trouvées cariées. 15 fois la tête du fémur était séparée du col et gisait comme un séquestre au milieu de l'articulation. 12 fois les abcès avaient gagné la fosse iliaque, nécessitant une opération dans cet endroit. Deux fois l'abcès avait franchi le triangle de Scarpa pour apparaître en arrière dans le pli fessier, comme le montre la figure 2. 15 malades soumis à la résection de la hanche ont quitté l'hôpital avec leur appareil un mois après l'opération ; trois sont partis au bout de deux mois ; deux ont dû subir des opérations secondaires : l'un de ces deux a quitté l'hôpital au bout de quatre mois, l'autre qui avait des lésions étendues du bassin, est resté cinq mois dans le service, qu'il quittera dans une semaine ou deux. Enfin, trois autres cas ont été opérés la semaine dernière. Dans tous les cas où l'étendue des lésions nécessitait la résection, les malades ont pu quitter l'hôpital en moyenne trois semaines après l'opération, avec un appareil et des béquilles. Les plaies étaient toutes bien fermées et sont restées telles, excepté les cas mentionnés plus haut.

Lorsque je compare ces résultats avec ceux que j'obtenais avant le traitement des arthrites suppurées par l'acide phénique pur, je suis grandement réjoui. Dans certains hôpitaux, suivant une information, les salles sont encombrées de coxalgies suppurées, dont plusieurs cas sont là depuis des années. Tous ces malades pourraient s'en aller au bout de quelques semaines avec un appareil et des béquilles.

Messieurs, je puis vous parler ainsi à cause des brillants résultats obtenus et à cause du désir que j'ai d'adopter pour l'orthopédie les principes qui sont acceptés par tout le monde chirurgical. Je pense que nous, orthopédistes, nous n'avons pas le droit de violer les lois de la chirurgie. Je tiens à vous dire aussi que l'acide phénique n'est pas un spécifique de la coxalgie, qu'il n'est qu'un simple agent thérapeutique. Cependant, mon opinion est que le traitement chirurgical, aidé de l'acide phénique pur, est plus efficace que tous les autres moyens qui me sont familiers pour la coxalgie.

ABSENCE CONGÉNITALE DOUBLE DU TIBIA

COMMUNICATION

de M. P. E. LAUNOIS

Professeur agrégé, médecin des hôpitaux.

et M. G. E. KUSS

Externe des hôpitaux.

Les auteurs définissent l'absence congénitale du tibia, en tant qu'entité pathologique possédant un tableau symptomatologique caractéristique, « l'absence, à la naissance, du tibia, absence totale ou partielle, alors que le membre inférieur possède ses différents segments, plus ou moins atrophiés, il est vrai, mais relativement bien constitués et possédant (à part le tibia) tous leurs organes essentiels. »

Ils éliminent ainsi de leur description nosologique et de leur statistique les cas d'absence du tibia par amputation congénitale spontanée, par phocomélie, hémimélie, ectromélie.

Leur statistique porte sur 40 cas bien contrôlés et dont ils résument l'histoire en un tableau synoptique accompagné d'un index bibliographique très complet et fort précis.

A propos d'un garçonnet de trois ans qu'ils présentent au Congrès et que l'on peut considérer comme offrant le type parfait d'absence congénitale totale et bilatérale du tibia, les auteurs s'aidant, pour la première fois, en ce cas, de la radiographie, décrivent les caractères de cette malformation hémitérique : hyper-flexion-adduction de la jambe, pied en varus équin extrême, atrophie du membre inférieur, saillies et luxation paradoxale des extrémités épaissies du péroné.

La rotule appliquée et comme incrustée sous les condyles fémoraux, doit à cette position profonde et cachée, d'avoir été, souvent à tort, considérée comme absente.

Ce vice de conformation serait dû à des troubles trophiques locaux, dépendant de la gêne qu'apporterait à la circulation sanguine la compression *médiate*, contre les parois abdominales, des membres inférieurs par l'amnios arrêté en son développement. MM. Launois et Küss établissent une homologie complète entre l'absence du tibia et ses diverses variétés et l'absence du radius, au membre supérieur.

DISCUSSION.

M. le professeur LANNELONGUE. — Les cas analogues à celui-ci sont très rares. Ce qui domine chez ces sujets c'est l'impossibilité de se mouvoir et cette impotence ira en augmentant ; l'enfant finira par marcher à quatre pattes dans la rue ou dans une boîte comme les culs-de-jatte : l'attitude mauvaise des membres inférieurs arrivera à déterminer des modifications graves du côté des hanches. Or la condition première de l'existence de l'homme dans la vie, c'est la marche, et, ici, la chirurgie a le devoir de réaliser pour cet enfant les conditions qui lui permettent de marcher. Il ne peut être question de transplantations osseuses ou de greffes quelconques. Une intervention radicale et prompte est nécessaire.

M. KIRMISSON. — Je n'ai vu qu'une seule fois une absence congénitale du tibia. Dans ces cas on trouve les orteils en nombre normal ou exagéré, tandis que lors d'absence congénitale du péroné un ou plusieurs orteils font défaut. Chez le malade que j'ai vu, la jambe était enroulée autour de la cuisse : l'ostéotomie du péroné a redressé la jambe, mais il reste une grande mobilité qui oblige l'enfant à marcher avec un appareil prothétique. Dans le cas de M. Launois, j'estime qu'il n'y a que la désarticulation du genou à faire.

M. le Dr PRÉCHAUD. — Notre collègue M. Launois, vient de nous poser une question à propos de l'examen qu'il vient de faire devant nous d'un petit malade frappé d'absence congénitale double des deux tibias. Doit-il opérer et quelle est ici l'intervention de choix?

Les observations de MM. Lannelongue et Kirmisson tranchent la question. Il faut intervenir. Je suis du même avis et je crois qu'il faut s'adresser à la désarticulation. Les observations sont rares : je suis heureux de vous apporter un cas des plus intéressants.

Il s'agit d'un enfant de 8 ans, qui me fut présenté à la Clinique de Bordeaux. Ses malformations étaient beaucoup plus accusées que chez le petit sujet que vient de nous présenter M. Launois ; les deux jambes relevées en dedans et en haut heurtaient le ventre et les parties génitales. Malgré cela l'enfant avait appris peu à peu à marcher sur les deux angles formés par la jonction à angle aigu des jambes atrophiées et des cuisses.

Il me parut qu'aucune autre intervention que la désarticulation ne devait être acceptée : je la pratiquai à droite et à gauche à dix jours d'intervalle avec plein succès. Qu'est-il arrivé au point de vue fonctionnel ?

Mon petit opéré était à peine guéri qu'il marchait sur ses deux moignons très réguliers et bien étoffés. Je l'ai revu depuis, il n'est dans son village aucun enfant plus agile, plus habile dans les exercices du corps. Il court, monte aux arbres et sur les échelles.

Mon observation démontre donc que les suites de pareilles interventions chez les sujets affligés d'aussi graves malformations peuvent être bonnes, qu'il vaudra mieux recourir à la suppression du membre qu'à l'ostéotomie qui s'adressant à un os grêle, souvent déformé, ne paraît pas devoir promettre un résultat suffisant.

CURE MARINE DES TUBERCULOSES ARTICULAIRES ET OSSEUSES
RÉSULTATS IMMÉDIATS. RÉSULTATS ÉLOIGNÉS

COMMUNICATION

de M. le docteur CHARLES LEROUX,
de Paris.

L'efficacité du traitement marin n'est plus aujourd'hui discutable : je viens simplement vous exposer les résultats obtenus après dix ans d'exercice dans les établissements que dirige l'œuvre des Hôpitaux marins : Banyuls-sur-Mer et Saint-Trojan.

Ma communication portera uniquement sur les tuberculoses articulaires ou osseuses, dites chirurgicales. Je vous en indiquerai tout d'abord les résultats immédiats, constatés à la sortie des malades, et, ce qui présente plus d'intérêt, les résultats éloignés après 4, 6 et 10 ans.

A. Résultats immédiats.

1° Résultats généraux.

En dix années, 452 enfants atteints de tuberculose articulaire ou osseuse sont sortis de nos deux établissements. Sur ce nombre, on a obtenu :

61 pour 100 de guérisons.

19 pour 100 d'améliorations.

15,5 pour 100 d'état stationnaire.

6,5 pour 100 de décès pendant le séjour.

Je tiens à faire remarquer de suite que, parmi les enfants dont l'état à la sortie était amélioré ou stationnaire, la plupart n'ont fait dans nos établissements qu'un court séjour de quelques semaines ou de quelques mois : or à la mer, comme partout ailleurs, on ne guérit point une coxalgie ou un mal de Pott en un si court espace de temps.

2° Résultats particuliers. Ces chiffres pris en bloc ne donnent qu'une idée fort incomplète des cas traités et des résultats obtenus. Je vous demande la permission d'entrer dans quelques détails et de vous présenter chaque groupe en particulier.

J'ai rangé les tuberculoses articulaires et osseuses dans quatre groupes : 1° mal de Pott; 2° coxalgie; 3° tumeurs blanches des grosses jointures (genou, pied, coude); 4° ostéites, osté-périostites, tumeurs blanches des petites jointures, ordinairement sous forme de manifestations multiples chez le même sujet.

a) Mal de Pott. Beaucoup de ces enfants étaient atteints de la forme grave du mal de Pott, avec abcès ossifluent, trajet fistuleux, etc.; quelques-uns même ont été apportés dans un état de cachexie extrême. Les résultats ont été les suivants : sur 55 malades sortis, on a obtenu 21 guérisons, soit 59 pour 100.

10 améliorations, soit 18 pour 100.

14 états stationnaires, soit 26 pour 100.

8 décès, soit 17 pour 100.

Quelques exemples expliqueront ces résultats :

En 1887, 4 malades sortent, dont deux avaient suppuré; sur ce nombre : 3 guérisons, 1 amélioration. Les deux arthrites vertébrales non suppurées ont guéri, mais avec déviation persistante; le troisième cas a trait à un enfant de 2 ans, Raoul B..., qui présentait un mal de Pott dorso-lombaire avec un énorme abcès par congestion; cet abcès, vidé et largement lavé, a persisté longtemps. La guérison complète a été obtenue en trois ans et sept mois. Le quatrième enfant a été repris quelques mois, amélioré, mais non guéri.

En 1898, 6 maux de Pott sont sortis du sanatorium de Banyuls-sur-Mer: 2 seulement étaient guéris. Cette faible proportion s'explique par les raisons suivantes : deux enfants ont été retirés par leur famille après un séjour de quelques semaines: deux sont arrivés au sanatorium dans un état désespéré et sont morts quelques jours après leur entrée.

Pour les deux cas de guérison, il s'agissait, dans le premier, d'un mal de Pott sans suppuration, mais avec paraplégie. La malade est sortie complètement guérie et marchant bien, après 1856 jours de traitement. Dans le second cas, le mal de Pott s'accompagnait d'un énorme abcès par congestion avec trajet fistuleux au pli de l'aine et d'une profonde cachexie. La guérison a été obtenue après 1540 jours.

Si j'insiste sur ces faits, c'est pour montrer la gravité des affections qui nous sont envoyées. Ce sont des malheureux qui ont épuisé, dans les hôpitaux et les hospices, toutes les ressources médicales et chirurgicales, et qu'en désespoir de cause on expédie à la mer. Cette méthode est déplorable; mais ces faits ne rendent que plus saisissante l'efficacité de la cure marine.

b) Coxalgie. Sur 50 cas on a obtenu :

25 guérisons, soit 50 pour 100.

11 améliorations, soit 22 pour 180.

8 états stationnaires, soit 16 pour 100.

6 décès, soit 12 pour 100.

c) Tumeurs blanches des grosses jointures.

Ce groupe comprend 96 malades : sur le nombre, nous avons

64 guérisons, soit 67 pour 100.

22 améliorations, soit 22 pour 100.

9 états stationnaires, soit 9 pour 100.

2 décès, soit 2 pour 100.

B. RÉSULTATS ÉLOIGNÉS.

Cette analyse des résultats rapprochés ou immédiats de la cure marine est intéressante ; mais cette étude serait incomplète si je ne vous disais maintenant ce que deviennent nos enfants après plusieurs années.

En fait de tuberculose, il faut se méfier des guérisons apparentes. Tous ceux qui, médecins ou chirurgiens, ont étudié cette affection chez l'enfant, savent combien les pseudo-guérisons, les trêves, sont fréquentes ; ils savent aussi que les retours offensifs, même à longue échéance, ne sont pas rares. Ces trêves, nous en avons tous vu, aboutissent souvent à une rechute ; les enfants meurent d'accidents septicémiques, de tuberculose pulmonaire ou de méningite.

Plus d'une fois les partisans et, à plus forte raison, les incrédules de l'action efficace du traitement marin ont dit : « Oui, vous guérissez beaucoup de ces enfants ; mais cette guérison est-elle définitive, et ces enfants, de retour dans un milieu souvent néfaste, restent-ils guéris ? Qui nous dit qu'ils ne succombent point au bout de quelques années ? »

L'objection était grave, et j'ai voulu savoir si les hôpitaux marins faisaient œuvre utile : j'ai dès lors commencé une enquête. J'ai pris tous les dossiers des enfants sortis depuis dix ans avec l'étiquette : *guéris* ; mais pour rendre l'enquête plus précise, je n'ai choisi que les enfants atteints des diverses formes de tuberculose osseuse ou articulaire dont je vous ai parlé. J'ai envoyé des circulaires à Paris, en province, dans tous les coins de la France, aux parents, aux préfets, aux inspecteurs des enfants assistés, etc. Je dois dire que partout j'ai trouvé la plus grande complaisance pour me faciliter la recherche de ces enfants.

Sur 120 lettres expédiées, j'ai reçu 95 réponses très nettes, très précises, qui me permettront de vous indiquer ce que deviennent nos malades, 6, 8 et même 10 ans après leur sortie de nos hôpitaux. Je vous parlerai tout d'abord des résultats d'ensemble, puis des résultats relatifs à chacun des groupes.

Résultats d'ensemble. Sur 98 malades retrouvés en l'espace de dix ans :

> 70 sont restés guéris.   soit 75. 6 pour 100.
> 14 ont rechuté.   soit 14. 8 pour 100.
> 11 sont morts.   soit 11. 6 pour 100.

Le tableau suivant en fournit le détail :

MALADES SORTIS	TOTAL	GUÉRIS EN 1900	RECHUTES	MORTS
En 1890	8	6	2	
— 1891	15	10		5
— 1892	22	16	5	5
— 1893	10	6	4	
— 1894	9	5	1	5
— 1895	7	6	1	
— 1896	10	8	1	1
— 1897	7	6		1
— 1898	8	6	2	1
— 1899	1	1		
Total.	95	70	14	11

On voit donc que, *parmi les guéris*, 6 le sont depuis 10 ans; 10 depuis 9 ans ; 16 depuis 8 ans; 6 depuis 7 ans ; depuis 6 ans au total 45 enfants sont restés guéris après 8 ans et 10 ans, et 27 après 1 à 5 ans.

Ces guérisons sont souvent parfaites: beaucoup de ces anciens malades travaillent, gagnent leur vie. Quelques fillettes, aujourd'hui femmes, sont mariées et l'une d'elles a plusieurs enfants sains. Quelques-uns (dans une proportion difficile à établir) sont restés infirmes ou trop faibles de santé pour travailler.

Parmi les 14 rechutes, 8 ont guéri ultérieurement, quelques-uns après un séjour nouveau dans un sanatorium. Les autres sont encore malades ou ne disent point si la guérison ultérieure a été obtenue. Les rechutes sont ordinairement précoces, souvent dans la première année. Une rechute a eu lieu 5 ans après; dans un autre cas, une fillette atteinte de tumeur blanche du genou a été réséquée; elle est aujourd'hui guérie, mariée et bien portante.

Parmi les 11 décès, 4 ont été constatés dans la première année de leur sortie, 1 dans la deuxième, 1 dans la troisième, 2 dans la cinquième et 3 à une date inconnue. Les causes en ont été : la cachexie tuberculeuse ou septicémique (6 fois), la méningite tuberculeuse (2 fois), la phtisie pulmonaire (2 fois), un amputé est mort quelques mois après sa sortie d'hémorragie, sans indication plus précise.

Résultats particuliers suivant nos 4 groupes.

1° Mal de Pott. Sur 12 malades retrouvés, on constate : 9 guérisons datant de 10 ans: 1 cas, de 8 ans: 1 cas, de 7 ans : 2 cas, de 8 ans : 1 cas, le dernier date d'un an: 1 rechute, avec guérison ultérieure; 2 morts, un et deux ans après la sortie.

2° *Coxalgie*. Sur 26 malades retrouvés, on a :

19 guérisons complètes.

5 rechutes avec survie.

2 décès, 5 ans après la sortie.

Parmi ces coxalgies : 11 étaient suppurées et ont fourni :

6 guérisons.

4 rechutes,

1 décès.

15 étaient sans suppuration et ont fourni :

15 guérisons.

1 rechute.

1 décès.

Les coxalgies suppurées ont donné plus de rechutes que les coxalgies non suppurées, presque un tiers; alors que les coxalgies non suppurées n'ont eu qu'une rechute sur 15 cas.

3° *Tumeurs blanches des grosses jointures*. Sur 24 malades on a constaté :

17 guérisons.

2 rechutes, dont une guérie ultérieurement,

5 décès.

4° *Manifestations multiples* : sur 55 malades retrouvés on a : 25 guérisons complètes :

6 rechutes avec 5 guérisons ultérieures et 5 guérisons incomplètes;

2 décès.

Je m'excuse de tous ces chiffres; mais il en est ainsi dans toute statistique détaillée. Je me résume en disant : la cure marine des tuberculoses chirurgicales donne, dans son ensemble :

61 pour 100 de guérisons.

19 pour 100 d'améliorations.

6.5 pour 100 de décès.

13.5 pour 100 d'états stationnaires.

Les résultats éloignés sont meilleurs qu'on pourrait le supposer, puisque, sur une statistique qui porte sur 95 malades retrouvés en 10 ans, on peut affirmer qu'il y a :

75,6 pour 100 de guérisons maintenues,

14,8 pour 100 de rechutes, avec guérison ultérieure pour quelques cas,

11,6 pour 100 de décès.

Ces résultats seraient meilleurs si les médecins et les administrations hospitalières voulaient bien se conformer aux règles suivantes qui me serviront de conclusions et que je vous demanderai de vouloir bien appuyer de votre autorité :

Conclusions. Le traitement des tuberculoses chirurgicales dans les sanatoriums marins donne d'excellents résultats, mais à deux conditions : 1° y envoyer les enfants dès le début de leur affection, sans attendre la période de suppuration et de cachexie: à agir vite, il y aurait pour les enfants économie de souffrance et, pour les administrations, économie de frais de séjour;

2° Prévoir toujours un séjour prolongé, ordinairement plusieurs années.

A ces conditions seules, on obtiendra des guérisons définitives, les rechutes seront rares et les décès ultérieurs exceptionnels.

TRAITEMENT AMBULATOIRE DES TUBERCULOSES DU MEMBRE INFERIEUR, DE LA COXALGIE ET DE LA TUMEUR BLANCHE DU GENOU EN PARTICULIER

COMMUNICATION

de M. le docteur DUCROQUET.

Il faut dans le traitement de toute tuberculose articulaire réaliser trois conditions fondamentales pour arriver à la guérison :

1° La décompression des surfaces osseuses cariées;

2° L'immobilisation des parties malades ;

3° S'occuper de l'état général de l'enfant.

Dans les villes populeuses où les ouvriers sont miséreux, l'alitement pour ces petits malades condamnés à rester dans le coin d'un taudis sale, mal aéré et mal éclairé, est synonyme de mort, et la marche, la vie extérieure, est pour ces petits êtres une sauvegarde. Nous sommes un peu trop hypnotisés par la localisation osseuse,

Il y a certainement un rapport très grand entre la lésion et l'état
général. Si l'enfant mange et respire à son aise, si sa diététique est
l'objet de beaucoup de soins, sa guérison sera plus prompte. La suralimentation, bref toutes les conditions susceptibles de remettre à flot
l'organisme seront mises en œuvre. La vie au grand air, l'exercice rendent d'immenses services, il ne faut pas nous en priver. D'ailleurs on
peut très bien concilier la décompression des surfaces osseuses et leur
immobilisation avec la marche si l'on sait appliquer un bon appareil.

Le séjour au lit, malgré tout ce qu'on en a dit, est très préjudiciable
aux petits malades, surtout dans la classe pauvre où les conditions
hygiéniques sont tout ce qu'il y a de plus défectueuses. Notre existence n'est pas faite pour le repos au lit. Il est hors de doute que
la vie extérieure est le principal facteur apte à procurer un état physiologique normal.

Au lit l'enfant ne se meut pas, et surtout s'il est soumis à l'extension
continue. Les échanges nutritifs varient. Beaucoup d'enfants sont
gros et gras ; si on leur palpe les membres, on leur trouve un panni-
cule adipeux très épais, et sous ce panicule adipeux, des muscles
d'un volume bien minime. Ils ne présentent que l'apparence de la
santé. Ce sont des malades à nutrition déviée, des obèses qui rentrent
dans la classe des ralentis de la nutrition du professeur Bouchard.
J'ai présent à l'esprit maints exemples d'enfants qui, au bout de quelques années de séjour au lit, étaient, de maigres qu'ils y avaient été
placés, absolument bouffis. Est-ce à dire que ces enfants se portaient
bien ? assurément non. A l'appui de ce fait, je me souviens d'une
jeune enfant de 10 ans, bien proportionnée pour son âge, et sans embonpoint. Atteinte d'un mal de Pott des régions supérieures du rachis,
elle fut immobilisée au lit pendant 5 années, elle arriva à devenir
énorme ; cela ne l'empêcha pas, au bout de ces 5 ans, de faire un mal
de Pott de la partie inférieure du rachis. C'était l'enfant de parents
fort aisés, elle habitait la mer, et je suis bien convaincu qu'étant données
ces conditions hygiéniques, elle eût guéri bien plus promptement si
elle avait été traitée ambulatoirement.

J'ai dit que si l'on palpait les membres de ces enfants maintenus
longtemps au lit, on s'apercevait que les muscles étaient à peu près
disparus, remplacés qu'ils étaient par un énorme panicule adipeux.
Or, il est, je crois, incontestable que la nutrition de l'os lui-même est
en rapport avec celle des parties qui l'avoisinent. Ont-elles une
nutrition languissante, il en est de même de l'os lui-même. Et ne
sait-on pas avec quelle facilité on fracture le fémur dans la coxalgie
lorsque l'on fait le redressement, si l'on ne s'astreint pas à prendre

certaines précautions. L'os est malade, c'est vrai, mais l'immobilité le rend plus friable encore en en diminuant les échanges nutritifs. Je veux dans cet ordre d'idées citer un fait qui m'a toujours frappé. Lorsque l'on a réduit la hanche d'un enfant atteint de luxation congénitale, qu'on a immobilisé cet enfant pendant 5 à 5 mois, lorsque l'on ramène la jambe à la rectitude, il arrive parfois, si l'on n'y prend garde, de fracturer le fémur et cela avec une facilité extrême, ce qui, assurément, eût été plus difficile avant le commencement du traitement. Durant l'immobilisation le fémur, bien que sain, était devenu très peu résistant par trouble nutritif.

Comment le traitement ambulatoire doit-il être envisagé? Traitement ambulatoire ne veut pas dire marche forcée. Il est évident qu'un enfant en pleine période floride ne doit pas marcher. Un genou volumineux, chaud, et dont le moindre mouvement, la moindre percussion occasionne de la douleur doit être immobilisé complètement jusqu'à totale disparition de ces symptômes. La marche n'est permise que lorsque les douleurs sont disparues. Un coxalgique dont la nuit se passe en cauchemars sera, il est évident, condamné au lit jusqu'à leur disparition. Avec une immobilisation bien entendue, 1 mois, 2 au maximum dans les cas ordinaires suffisent à amener la disparition de ces phénomènes douloureux.

La marche est permise : 1° avec un appareil immobilisant simplement l'article ou bien 2° avec un appareil de décharge, c'est-à-dire construit de telle façon que lorsque l'enfant appuie le pied à terre, la pression se fait directement de l'appareil à l'ischion, au lieu de passer par le genou et la hanche avant de se transmettre au bassin. Le malade est en somme dans les mêmes conditions que s'il marchait avec un membre artificiel. Son membre malade est pour ainsi dire inutile.

Dans quelle condition doit-on appliquer un appareil simplement immobilisateur ou un appareil à décharge?

Il faut que la lésion ne prête pas à l'ulcération compressive. Prenons le genou pour exemple. Si la lésion est en *a* sur la surface même du plateau tibial, il y a toute chance pour que le point opposé du fémur se prenne, et chaque fois que le malade posera le pied, la pression du corps pèsera sur la lésion elle-même. Si la lésion se trouve au contraire au-dessus du condyle interne, en *b* par exemple, on n'a pas à craindre d'ulcération compressive du plateau tibial. Vous voyez sur ces deux radiographies des exemples fort nets de ce que je viens d'avancer.

Lorsqu'il s'agit de la hanche, il en est de même, la lésion peut siéger à la partie inférieure du col près de la tête et par suite ne peut se prêter à l'ulcération compressive, elle peut au contraire siéger à la partie supérieure de la tête et par suite est des plus propices à l'ulcération compressive.

La lésion ne prête pas à l'ulcération compressive, immobilisation simple de l'articulation.

La lésion y prête-t-elle, immobilisation de l'articulation réalisant en même temps la décharge. D'ailleurs fort souvent dans ce dernier cas, on est amené à faire un appareil de décharge, la marche sans douleur devenant impossible avec un appareil d'immobilisation simple. Du reste, si le malade souffre par la marche, il faut appliquer un appareil à décharge, quel que soit le point malade. Ordinairement cela se passe ainsi que je l'ai indiqué plus haut.

Trait de la lésion elle-même. — Les indications en sont en général fort nettes. La lésion est-elle nettement intra-articulaire, il est rationnel alors d'essayer d'agir sur elle par les injections dans l'articulation elle-même. Est-elle tout à fait en dehors de l'article, à quoi bon user de ce moyen qui la plupart du temps sera tout à fait inefficace? Il est vrai que dans beaucoup de cas une lésion assez éloignée des surfaces articulaires coïncide souvent avec des lésions des culs-de-sac synoviaux de l'articulation du genou. Il est évident alors que nous avons prise sur ces lésions.

Supposons donc d'abord que nous ayons affaire à des lésions intra-articulaires.

A. *Lésions intra-articulaires.* — Un liquide susceptible d'agir sur les lésions tuberculeuses injecté dans l'articulation pourra avoir quelque action. A quel liquide modificateur devons-nous nous arrêter?

Le choix en est assez grand, l'éther iodoformé, la glycérine iodoformée, le naphtol, le chlorure de zinc, etc. Le naphtol est un des modificateurs les plus puissants des fongosités tuberculeuses. Il en accélère la dégénérescence, mais c'est une arme bien dangereuse, il m'a donné bien des ennuis. Je sais qu'en d'autres mains il y a eu des morts. Il arrive fréquemment lorsque l'on ponctionne une articulation atteinte de tuberculose du genou, par exemple, qu'il s'écoule tout d'abord un peu de synovie, puis de la synovie teintée d'un peu de sang. Cela est dû aux fongosités fermes néoformées dont la trame vasculaire est comme on le sait si friable. Injecte-t-on du naphtol, il est immédiatement absorbé par les vaisseaux sanguins, et de là, consécutivement des symptômes d'intoxication. J'ai eu trois ou quatre alertes des plus sérieuses et j'avoue pour ma part, que je n'injecte du naphtol que lorsque j'ai retiré tout d'abord par la ponction, non de la synovie sanguinolente, mais du pus véritable. Dans cette dernière circonstance on n'a jamais d'ennui. Dans les autres cas, je ne fais aucune injection le plus souvent. L'immobilisation de l'article amène peu à peu d'ailleurs la résorption de ces fongosités. Je me suis servi dans ces derniers temps du liquide de Truneck, qui est formé par les sels du sérum du sang mais en solution plus concentrée. C'est un liquide inoffensif qui m'a paru digne d'attention ; j'en ai trop peu d'expérience encore pour pouvoir en parler. Tant que le malade est en période d'injection, ce qui dure un mois à six semaines ordinairement, je le condamne au repos. La marche ne lui est permise que lorsque son articulation est bien nettoyée.

B. *Lésions extra-articulaires.* — Dans ce cas, comme on le voit sur la radiographie suivante où la lésion siège au-dessus de l'épiphyse en un point extra-articulaire. Il est évident que l'injection d'un liquide dans l'article n'aura aucun retentissement sur la lésion elle-même. Dans ce cas, je me contente souvent de l'immobilisation du membre et quand cela se peut je pratique des injections sclérosantes de chlorure de zinc, ou je fais de la cautérisation profonde intra-osseuse.

Les conditions varient absolument suivant que l'enfant est pris au début ou en cours de traitement.

Pris au début, les conditions sont infiniment meilleures, et lorsqu'il s'agit du genou en particulier on peut espérer arriver à la guérison à peu près complète. J'ai obtenu dans une série peut-être heureuse une suite de résultats vraiment remarquables.

Le point capital est de savoir bien faire l'immobilisation de l'articulation malade. Si l'on sait la réaliser on acquierra des résultats très satisfaisants.

J'envisagerai seulement deux cas, suivant qu'il s'agit de la hanche ou du genou.

Si nous cherchons à nous rendre compte des conditions que doit réaliser un appareil pour obtenir la complète immobilisation de l'articulation de la hanche, nous devons tout d'abord naturellement envisager quels sont les mouvements normaux qui se passent dans cette articulation. Il existe deux grandes variétés de mouvements :

1° Ceux qui changent la direction du membre comme la flexion, l'adduction, l'abduction et l'extension ;

2° Ceux qui se font sans qu'il se produise de changement dans la direction du membre, c'est-à-dire les mouvements de rotation.

Envisager un seul de ces mouvements c'est faire erreur et ne regarder que l'un des côtés de la question.

Examinons d'abord quelle condition doit réaliser l'appareil pour obvier à ces deux catégories de mouvements :

1° Appareils empêchant la déviation de la cuisse sur le bassin.

Nous avons deux os s'articulant ensemble, le fémur et le bassin, nous devons les immobiliser l'un par rapport à l'autre. Nous devons pour cela prendre des points d'appui invariables. Je ne veux parler présentement que de l'immobilisation à l'aide du plâtre.

Si nous entourons le bassin d'une ceinture plâtrée circulaire allant du pubis à l'ombilic, les bandes étant appliquées presque directement sur le corps, nous possédons une ceinture circulaire qui, grâce à un moulage si exactement fait que l'on voit très nettement les épines iliaques représentées à la surface intérieure de l'appareil, ne peut être déplacée ni tournée la partie inférieure du corps se trouvant dans son moulage. Continuons notre appareil jusqu'au-dessous du genou et lorsqu'il est terminé, coupons-le comme le fait Dollinger, juste **au-dessus** de la rotule, en avant et sur les côtés à la partie inférieure des condyles fémoraux, à la partie postérieure du genou échancrons-le de façon à dégager toute cette partie postérieure et partant à permettre à la jambe de se fléchir. Vu d'arrière on voit que l'appareil présente deux petites oreilles latérales qui descendent de chaque côté des condyles.

Cette union du cuissard plâtré à la ceinture pelvienne forme un tout **rigide**, la cuisse ne peut dévier ni en avant, l'appareil s'arrêtant à la partie antérieure du genou, ni sur les côtés, les oreilles latérales de l'appareil prenant point d'appui sur les condyles fémoraux, en arrière la partie postérieure du genou est dégagée, le bord inférieur de l'appareil correspond aux parties molles de la partie postérieure de la cuisse, le point d'appui manque donc mais cela n'a aucune espèce d'importance car nous savons que dans la coxalgie on n'a jamais à combattre l'hyperextension.

Mais cet appareil à ailerons latéraux, quelle que soit l'habileté avec laquelle il ait été construit, est impuissant à empêcher les mouvements de rotation du membre inférieur.

Si l'appareil ne présente pas à sa partie inférieure, les deux ailerons que j'ai signalés pour la prise des condyles et qu'il s'arrête au-dessus de ces derniers que va-t-il se produire? Entre le bord inférieur de l'appareil et le fémur se trouvent les muscles qui le recouvrent, la cuisse va pouvoir entrer en adduction, ce qu'il faut à tout prix éviter: cette adduction est possible, la partie inférieure de la cuisse, pressant sur la partie interne de l'orifice inférieur de l'appareil, les parties molles sont comprimées, muscles et peau, jusqu'au moment où le corps du

fémur sera arrêté par le bord inférieur de l'appareil. Cet accident
m'est arrivé plusieurs fois au début de ma pratique et j'ai été obligé
dans 4 ou 5 cas d'endormir les malades pour leur faire subir un
redressement léger, c'est-à-dire porter la jambe en légère abduction.
L'appareil que l'on a continué de faire dans la coxalgie à la période
de guérison, appareil embrassant le bassin et s'arrêtant souvent à la
partie moyenne ou inférieure de la cuisse, au-dessus des condyles par
exemple est tout à fait défectueux, il est responsable de bien des attitudes vicieuses. Avec l'appareil à ailerons latéraux au contraire on
ne risque absolument rien. Il en serait de même évidemment si l'appareil descendait à mi-jambe, mais à cela il y aurait un grand inconvénient, le genou serait gardé immobile, alors qu'avec l'appareil précédent il peut facilement se fléchir.

2° *Appareil empêchant la rotation du fémur.* — L'appareil précédent
empêche la déviation du membre, sans en empêcher la rotation, or ce
dernier mouvement réveille très souvent la douleur dans la coxalgie.

Pour empêcher la rotation il est absolument nécessaire d'immobiliser le pied lui-même et par suite l'appareil doit descendre jusqu'à la
moitié postérieure du pied, avec un tel appareil il est totalement
impossible d'imprimer des mouvements au genou, on pourrait arriver
au même résultat en pliant le genou sur la cuisse. Un appareil descendant à mi-jambe diminue en grande partie les mouvements de
rotation du fémur, le genou n'ayant pas une forme sphérique, le moulage de cette partie empêche en grande partie les mouvements de
rotation du membre.

Lorsqu'il s'agit d'une immobilisation simple cet appareil suffit
ordinairement.

Mais lorsqu'il s'agit d'un appareil de décharge il est tout à fait
insuffisant.

Dans ce dernier cas j'ai coutume de faire l'appareil dans la position horizontale de façon à pouvoir bien mouler jusque l'ischion. Le
pied est pris dans l'appareil et je place durant la construction de
l'appareil une attelle en fer malléable en forme d'étrier que je place
sous le talon et dont les branches remontent de chaque côté de la
jambe, cette partie incorporée à l'appareil contribue à le consolider.
Dans la pratique de la ville un appareil en celluloïd lui est infiniment
supérieur. Avec cet appareil, chaque fois que l'enfant pose le pied
sur le sol le poids du corps est transmis directement à l'ischion, la
hanche ne supporte aucune pression.

L'appareil s'arrêtant au genou est réservé presque exclusivement
aux coxalgies arrivées à la guérison.

L'appareil descendant à mi-jambe, aux coxalgies dont la lésion ne se prête pas à l'ulcération compressive.

Le grand appareil dans tous les autres cas.

Immobilisation du genou. — Les mouvements du genou sont beaucoup moins complexes que ceux qui se passent dans la hanche.

Il possède cependant lui aussi deux espèces de mouvements :

1° Des mouvements qui changent la direction du membre ;

2° Des mouvements qui se passent dans la direction du membre, la rotation.

1. Des mouvements qui changent la direction du membre, il n'y en a qu'un seul, la flexion.

Pour obvier à ce mouvement il faut immobiliser les deux segments du membre, l'un par rapport à l'autre. Pour immobiliser le fémur nous avons bien un point d'appui aux condyles à sa partie inférieure, mais nous n'avons aucune prise sur sa partie supérieure, pour y arriver nous avons bien un moyen détourné, c'est l'immobilisation de la hanche elle-même, un appareil prenant la hanche et descendant au condyle.

Pour immobiliser la jambe, l'appareil allant des plateaux du tibia au talon suffit à cela, ces deux segments d'appareil unis l'un à l'autre et nous aurons l'immobilisation du genou, du moins pour les mouvements de flexion. Pour empêcher la rotation, il est on le conçoit nécessaire de prendre le pied lui-même dans l'appareil. Pratiquement, dans les formes les plus douloureuses, l'appareil remontant jusqu'à la partie supérieure de la cuisse suffit à calmer les douleurs dans les cas les plus aigus.

Mais lorsqu'il y a une grande tendance à la flexion cet appareil est insuffisant, le fémur tend à venir en contact avec le bord postérieur et supérieur de l'appareil en pressant sur les parties molles.

Pratiquement, l'appareil embrassant les condyles fémoraux suffit à empêcher les mouvements de rotation du fémur, parce que la partie inférieure de la cuisse n'est pas cylindrique, le moulage bien fait empêche les mouvements de rotation de se passer dans cette partie du membre.

Pratiquement, dans les articulations dont la lésion ne se prête pas à l'ulcération compressive, l'appareil allant de la partie supérieure de la cuisse à la partie inférieure de la jambe suffit.

Dans les autres cas on le conçoit, l'appareil doit prendre le pied pour obvier aux mouvements de rotation qui sont douloureux et si cela est nécessaire remonter jusque l'ischion sur lequel le malade prendra point d'appui pendant la marche.

Traitement de la convalescence. — Le traitement ambulatoire prédispose beaucoup moins à l'ankylose que le traitement au lit.

Lorsque la hanche et le genou possèdent des mouvements après la guérison. il ne faut pas quitter les appareils du jour au lendemain. Pour le genou en particulier j'ai coutume de faire un appareil qui permet d'augmenter graduellement l'amplitude des mouvements. On évite ainsi des petites entorses qui sont une amorce à la récidive. Le genou traité dès le début par cette méthode guérit rarement avec ankylose. Pour la hanche les conditions sont moins favorables et les résultats souvent moins heureux, mais ils m'ont paru toujours beaucoup plus favorables que ceux qui étaient obtenus par l'immobilisation seule. La durée du traitement paraît aussi de bien moins longue durée.

GREFFES TENDINEUSES ET MUSCULO-TENDINEUSES
DANS LA PARALYSIE INFANTILE

COMMUNICATION

de M. MAURICE PÉRAIRE,
de Paris.

En 1898. il avait opéré sept enfants atteints de pieds bots acquis avec le concours du docteur Mally. actuellement professeur de médecine à l'école de Clermont-Ferrand. Depuis cette époque il a eu l'occasion d'intervenir cinq fois: dans deux cas. il s'agissait de jeunes filles de quinze à dix-sept ans. Toujours il a obtenu une disparition complète des déformations. une amélioration notable de la marche, et une disparition complète de la fatigue produite par cette marche.

Dans un cas de paralysie spasmodique, le succès a consisté non seulement dans la correction de l'attitude, mais aussi dans la disparition du spasme. C'est d'ailleurs le seul cas de paralysie spasmodique pour lequel il a eu à intervenir.

La technique opératoire n'est nullement difficile. Il a toujours employé les procédés les plus simples d'asepsie. Jamais il ne s'est servi du masque ni des gants de fil comme le fait Vulpius d'Heidelberg. en pareil cas. Pour unir le muscle paralysé au muscle sain, il n'en sacrifie aucun. Il met en connexion le bout périphérique du tendon du muscle malade dédoublé avec le tendon du muscle sain. Il applique de la même façon le muscle sain contre le muscle malade au moyen d'un surjet, après les avoir avivés tous les deux. Il est très facile de voir que les muscles paralysés sont jaunâtres, ont une teinte cireuse tandis que les muscles vivants se différencient par leur coloration rougeâtre.

L'auteur croit que cette opération de greffe musculaire, de transplantation tendineuse, est appelée, non seulement à donner des résultats momentanément brillants, mais aussi des résultats durables sous tous les rapports. Il formule les indications et les contre-indications de la greffe musculaire et sa valeur physiologique.

Indications de l'opération. — Il faut d'abord avoir recours, dit-il, à l'exploration électrique, c'est-à-dire à la méthode de Duchenne (de Boulogne), de Erb, de Remak et des neurologistes allemands actuels, pour déterminer non seulement les muscles paralysés, mais encore leur degré d'altération histologique. Les différentes formes de réaction de dégénérescence, les différents degrés de l'excitabilité électrique permettent de savoir si tel muscle atrophié a subi la dégénérescence totale ou simplement l'atrophie numérique, si on peut espérer lui voir reprendre spontanément sa vitalité, ou s'il est perdu pour toujours.

La *première indication* est donc celle-ci : ne tenter la suppléance que des muscles totalement dégénérés.

Deuxième indication : ne recourir à l'anastomose que s'il reste un certain nombre de muscles sains.

L'opération n'est donc bonne que dans les paralysies à la fois *incurables* et *incomplètes*.

Il résulte des recherches qu'il a faites avec son collaborateur que, dans les paralysies du groupe antéro-externe de la jambe, on peut faire suppléer le jambier antérieur et les péroniers par le triceps, et réciproquement, faire suppléer le triceps par les muscles profonds de la jambe et par les péroniers.

La paralysie isolée du jambier antérieur paraît facilement corrigée par l'anastomose tendon à tendon du jambier et de l'extenseur propre du gros orteil. La paralysie isolée des péroniers peut être corrigée par l'anastomose de leurs tendons avec celui du triceps.

On peut ainsi améliorer dans une large mesure l'état fonctionnel de certains pieds bots paralytiques. L'opération de Phelps, plus ou moins modifiée par les chirurgiens actuels, doit être réservée aux pieds bots ballants, dont la jambe ne contient plus de muscles, ou aux pieds bots négligés qui ont acquis des attitudes vicieuses irréductibles. Il reste donc un certain champ d'action pour cette opération, qu'ils ont pratiquée sur leurs malades avec des suites bénignes et des résultats fort encourageants. Ces malades[1] peuvent accomplir sans fatigue tel trajet familier qui leur demandait jadis un temps beaucoup plus long et de pénibles efforts.

Il y a là un fait chirurgical nouveau et intéressant qui leur paraît digne de fixer l'attention :

En troisième lieu, autres indications d'ordre purement clinique :

Dans le cas de *talus*, il faut greffer les péroniers ou le fléchisseur commun des orteils contractiles sur le tendon d'Achille paralysé.

Dans le cas de *pied bot valgus*, anastomoser le jambier antérieur paralysé adducteur et fléchisseur avec l'extenseur propre du gros orteil contractile, ou avec le long péronier latéral extenseur et abducteur.

Dans le cas de *talus valgus*, réunir le court péronier latéral au long fléchisseur commun des orteils, après avoir passé le premier sous le tendon d'Achille et suturer le long péronier latéral au tendon d'Achille.

Dans le cas de *pied bot varus équin*, on réunit l'extenseur commun des orteils paralysés à l'extenseur propre du gros orteil non paralysé.

Si l'extenseur propre du gros orteil est aussi paralysé, réunir un segment du jambier antérieur à l'extenseur commun des orteils, ou encore ce dernier aux péroniers.

Dans le cas de *pied bot paralytique ballant*, faire la transplantation du muscle extenseur propre du gros orteil sur l'extenseur commun des orteils. Si les muscles élévateurs du bord interne ont prédominance sur les élévateurs du bord externe, emprunter une portion du jambier antérieur et réunir ce segment avec les faisceaux tendineux correspondants du long du péronier latéral.

Pour maintenir parfaite la suture tendineuse, il faut aviver une portion du muscle paralysé. Il faut agir de même sur le muscle suivant, susceptible de bonnes contractions, et les suturer par deux ou trois fils de soie les réunissant bout à bout.

Un appareil plâtré maintient l'immobilité du membre pendant une quinzaine de jours.

Les contre-indications de l'opération leur paraissent être les paralysies totales des muscles de tout un membre, et les attitudes vicieuses irréductibles. Mais l'examen répété des malades et l'expérience qu'ils ont acquise sur ce sujet leur a fait reconnaître que la paralysie totale est plus rare qu'on ne le croit généralement. La paralysie infantile est

1. Voir *Médecine moderne*, Paris, 9ᵉ année, 5 octobre, 12 octobre, 19 et 25 novembre 1898, nᵒˢ 69, 70, 81 et 82. MM. Péraire et F. Mally. *Traitement chirurgical de certains pieds-bots par la greffe musculaire ou tendineuse.*

en effet dès le début limitée à un certain nombre de muscles. Le siège
le plus favorable pour l'opération est la jambe; la cuisse l'est moins.
Les muscles de l'avant-bras se prêtent moins bien à l'intervention:
cependant Vulpius a enregistré un certain nombre de cas très satisfaisants.

Physiologiquement, comment agit la greffe musculo-tendineuse?

En faisant travailler un muscle sain, au lieu d'un muscle malade.
C'est en quelque sorte une prothèse naturelle justifiée par les bons
résultats produits dans les cas de section accidentelle des tendons et
par leur suture à des extrémités tendineuses différentes. Peut-être
peut-on expliquer aussi l'amélioration produite par un changement
dans l'activité réflexe des muscles qui se produit dans les centres
nerveux, grâce à la transmission de la fonction d'un muscle sain sur
un muscle paralysé.

Mais ceci n'est qu'une hypothèse.

En résumé, on peut conclure en disant que la chirurgie orthopédique doit tendre surtout à aider la nature et être éminemment conservatrice.

La greffe musculaire ou tendineuse, appliquée à la cure de pieds
bots résultant de la paralysie infantile, répond à ces desiderata.

Ce que les auteurs ont voulu obtenir, ce n'est pas une régénération
musculaire, à proprement parler, c'est une suppléance fonctionnelle.

Dire que les muscles récupèrent tout ou une partie de leur intégrité,
ce serait beaucoup trop risquer.

Comme suite immédiate, cette opération n'offre aucune espèce de
danger, si elle a été pratiquée bien aseptiquement.

Un ou deux pansements consécutifs et un appareil plâtré pour
maintenir la greffe en bonne position et empêcher les fils de se
casser par les mouvements du malade suffisent amplement.

Quant au procédé opératoire, ils préfèrent la greffe anastomotique
par dédoublement, greffe tendineuse ou musculaire faite en anastomo-
sant une partie du muscle sain avec une partie du muscle paralysé
sans qu'il soit besoin de couper complètement le muscle sain ou le
muscle paralysé pour les réunir l'un à l'autre. L'essentiel est de régler
cette intervention d'une façon logique et de ne point en faire une
panacée universelle.

Ainsi cette opération n'est pas applicable dans les paralysies étendues où l'on ne peut utiliser les muscles voisins. Dans ces cas, il vaut
mieux faire d'emblée l'arthrodèse, l'opération de Phelps, ou la résection des os du tarse.

Enfin, on sera amené à respecter et à favoriser un certain degré d'équinisme, lorsque cette attitude servira à suppléer à un raccourcissement du membre : dans ce cas, on se bornera à corriger l'attitude en valgus ou en varus qui est seule gênante pour le malade.

Sous forme de conclusion, M. Péraire résume son opinion et celle de son collaborateur de la façon suivante :

Lorsqu'il s'agit d'un pied bot paralytique, chez un enfant ou un adolescent, avec lésions nerveuses définitives, l'anastomose musculo-tendineuse est l'opération de choix. Elle leur paraît préférable à la ténotomie. Elle permet d'éviter, dans la grande majorité des cas, les résections étendues du squelette du pied.

La greffe musculaire doit aussi être tentée au membre supérieur comme au membre inférieur dans les cas de paralysie infantile; car c'est le seul procédé qui paraît devoir jusqu'à présent réaliser la correction de la fonction du membre et des attitudes vicieuses par celui-ci.

DE LA LITHOTRITIE ET DE LA TAILLE SUS-PUBIENNE CHEZ L'ENFANT

COMMUNICATION

de M. le docteur DESCHAMPS,

Chirurgien de l'hôpital des Anglais de Liège.

Peut-on faire la lithotritie chez l'enfant? Quand est-elle possible?

Jusqu'en 1894, j'ai toujours pratiqué la taille périnéale ou hypogastrique, la première, tout au début de ma pratique, alors qu'elle était encore généralement admise.

Lors d'un voyage que je fis à Paris, à l'époque du Congrès de chirurgie, j'eus l'occasion de voir pratiquer la lithotritie par Guyon avec un art que je dirai — divin. Il m'en est resté une impression si favorable que je ne pus que m'écrier : « Combien c'est facile. » Aussi je repris mon service hospitalier, bien disposé à profiter de la première occasion. Celle-ci se présenta immédiatement. En mon absence, mon remplaçant avait pratiqué une taille périnéale (quel plaisir de pouvoir, loin de l'œil du maître, montrer son petit talent!), mais, comme j'ai pu m'en convaincre, bien que la vessie eût été largement ouverte, notre jeune opérateur n'avait point trouvé le calcul. Force lui fut d'avouer son mécompte, ajoutant, pour son excuse, que le calcul était enchatonné. Je laissai fermer la plaie, et, après avoir reconnu et fait

reconnaître un tout petit calcul, je fis la lithotritie. Je la fis si bien,
sans incident, que les parents ignorèrent cette nouvelle intervention,
et que je me promis bien de recommencer.

Peu après, je fis une deuxième lithotritie chez un enfant de 9 ans.
La pierre fut aisément saisie, ressaisie, et tout allait si à souhait que
pour peu j'eusse écrit sur mon chapeau : « C'est moi qui suis Guyon,
le grand lithotriteur. » Mais voilà bien triste aventure : impossible de
fermer complètement l'instrument. J'essayai de l'enlever. J'y parvins
par des manœuvres pénibles, non sans avoir lésé le canal de l'urètre.
Le calcul avait été non brisé, mais écrasé, et des particules encrassaient
l'appareil. Il me fallut cependant bien continuer l'opération, obligé toutefois de retirer l'instrument pour le nettoyer, après chaque manœuvre.

Néanmoins, le résultat fut aussi favorable que la première fois. Je
fis alors confectionner un lithotriteur dont la branche femelle était
plus largement fenêtrée en arrière.

Pour une troisième fois, avec cet instrument nouveau, je fis la lithotritie chez un enfant de 11 ans. Le calcul était dur (en voici les fragments), volumineux, et l'instrument dérapa. J'eus des peines infinies
pour l'enlever et force me fut de remettre l'opération à quelques jours.
C'était un samedi, le dimanche je n'allai pas à l'hôpital, le médecin de
service ne me prévint pas, de sorte que le lundi je trouvai l'enfant au
début d'une infiltration urineuse. Je fis la dilatation du col par la
méthode de Dolbeau et je pus ainsi entraîner tous les fragments.

L'incident n'eut pas de suite plus grave.

C'est de ces trois observations que j'ai cru pouvoir poser les règles
de la lithotritie chez l'enfant :

1° Canal suffisamment large pour permettre l'introduction facile de
l'instrument ;

2° Calcul assez dur, non friable, non phosphatique dur :

3° Enfin, peu volumineux.

Ces trois conditions se rencontrent rarement réunies : aussi ce n'est
guère que pour l'instruction de nos internes que nous pratiquons
parfois encore cette opération, leur disant comme Loyola : « *Facite
quod dicunt, secundum autem opera eorum nolite facere* : faites ce
qu'ils disent, ne faites pas ce qu'ils font. »

Un autre motif, mais très secondaire, pour abandonner la lithotritie,
c'est qu'on s'expose parfois à détruire des calculs d'une forme excessivement rare. Voici, en effet, un calcul pesant 25 grammes, arrondi,
et présentant des arborescences telles qu'il en impose pour un polype.
J'ai enlevé ce calcul à un enfant de 7 ans en juillet 1898

Je ne fais donc plus que la taille. Je la fais comme tous. Permettez-moi cependant de dire un mot de la suture et du pansement.

On peut, certes, siphonner comme chez l'adulte ; mais l'indocilité, d'une part, et le défaut de surveillance, d'autre part, tant à l'hôpital qu'en ville, peuvent exposer aux plus grands dangers. De plus, le drain, pour être suffisamment épais, doit être d'assez grand diamètre et, par suite, difficile à placer. S'il est trop mince, il se plie dans la courbe qui se fait de la vessie au récipient.

Cependant, pour pouvoir fermer hermétiquement la vessie, ce que je fais par une suture en étages, il faut être sûr de l'écoulement de l'urine.

La sonde, même fixée au prépuce, est souvent, pendant la nuit, propulsée d'arrière en avant en décrivant une courbe.

La sonde de Pezzer est difficile à placer.

Le cathétérisme rétrograde demande des virtuoses, surtout s'il faut le faire pour le bout antérieur de la sonde.

Je réclame la priorité d'un petit procédé fort ingénieux et qui, bien facile, rend des services immenses.

J'introduis par le canal un numéro relativement gros d'une sonde de Nélaton, puis, lui ayant fait traverser l'ouverture vésicale, je la fends dans l'étendue d'un centimètre environ dans le sens de la longueur. Les deux ailerons ainsi formés sont suturés à la soie, un peu plus haut, sur la sonde, assez étroitement pour la maintenir perpendiculaire à l'axe, assez lâchement pour céder sous une traction un peu énergique. J'ai ainsi un Pezzer extemporané qui m'a toujours parfaitement servi.

Encore un mot. J'ai pu remarquer que les calculs se rencontraient presque toujours dans la même région à Liège, dans le quartier de l'est ; cependant, c'est partout la même eau. J'ai eu l'occasion de réopérer deux enfants dont l'un pour un calcul d'oxalate, il y a quatre ans, et pour deux calculs phosphatiques, que voici, cette année ; et l'autre pour un calcul uratique et un phosphatique, une deuxième fois.

D'où vient cette différence de composition ?

J'ai pratiqué un nombre considérable de tailles ; le plus gros calcul que j'ai extrait chez un enfant et que voici, gros comme un œuf de pigeon, pesait 57 grammes : par contre, j'en ai vu à peine gros comme un pois. En voici un spécimen.

DU MAL DE POTT

DEUXIÈME COMMUNICATION

J'eusse voulu, dans l'avant-dernière réunion, prendre part à la discussion si intéressante qu'a soulevée le traitement des gibbosités pottiques.

Je ne le pouvais sans apporter, à l'appui de mon dire, l'un ou l'autre spécimen des résultats de ma pratique. Je viens de les recevoir.

Nous sommes, je crois, actuellement bien d'accord (*mirabile dictu*) une fois par hasard, pour reconnaître que l'enthousiasme qui a suivi la communication du Dr Calot est bien atténué, si déjà il n'a entièrement disparu. Tous, nous admettons que le redressement des gibbosités n'a pas tenu ses promesses; Calot seul, peut-être, prétendra le contraire. Combien pénible, en effet, de renier son œuvre! Si nous avons, naguère, un des premiers, conjugué au passé le verbe « redresser les bossus », lui prétend d'autant le conjuguer encore au présent et au futur. Que grand bien lui fasse. Bien plus : qu'il a raison, bien que nous n'ayons pas tort! car il fait, lui, ce que tous nous ne pouvons faire : *il désinfecte les bossus.*

Mot étrange, qui demande explication. Toute la thérapeutique actuelle, en effet, tant médicale que chirurgicale, se résume en ce seul mot : désinfection. Elle se fait par des moyens divers, soit, comme dans la diphtérie, par l'injection d'antitoxine, soit, quand c'est possible, pour l'élimination des produits morbides par voie intestinale, soit par les reins, lorsqu'on use du bienfaisant liquide physiologique, on nous l'a dit tantôt pour l'appendicite, soit enfin par la destruction du micro-organisme lui-même, producteur des toxines.

C'est par cette désinfection qu'il faut agir sur les pottiques. Quelle autre action, en effet, attribuer à l'air pur des hauts plateaux qui couronnent le sommet de vos montagnes et des nôtres, ou de nos belles plages du Nord dont une est le théâtre du bienheureux Calot, quand nous, pauvres déshérités, nous avons redressé, nous avons supprimé un symptôme, non sans avoir parfois donné un vigoureux coup de fouet au processus tuberculeux de ces êtres chétifs dont l'étiolement va se continuer dans les lits de nos hôpitaux urbains; tandis que cet air vif et réparateur dont je parlais tantôt, en stimulant l'organisme, eût pu augmenter le nombre et la puissance de leurs globules blancs polynucléaires, et ces phagocytes, ainsi fortifiés, sortir victorieux de la lutte à mort contre le bacille de Koch. Ne cherchez pas ailleurs l'action de l'air salin ni ses heureuses conséquences pour le chirurgien favorisé. Et voilà pourquoi, en ville, nos insuccès sont si grands, et voilà pourquoi, bien qu'il y a trois ans nous ayons obtenu des redressements parfaits (en voici deux spécimens), nous ne redressons plus que bien rarement. Mais à la mer!!! Heureux Calot!!!

Permettez-moi de dire deux mots d'un procédé de cure radicale de la hernie que j'emploie depuis deux ans et qui m'a donné d'excellents résultats.

Les premiers temps sont les mêmes jusque et y compris l'incision de la paroi antérieure du canal inguinal. Cela fait, le sac est saisi par une pince à forcipressure lâche et dont les mords sont encore protégés par une garniture de gutta-percha. Au-dessous de la pince, le sac est ouvert par une incision parallèle à son axe. Les deux bords sont saisis par des pinces de Péan, étalés, et, sous eux, on introduit l'aiguille de Dechamp armée d'un fil de soie ou de gros catgut. On fait la ligature, le sac est laissé. La suture se fait alors comme dans le bassin; seulement, les sutures profondes sont insinuées entre les fils de la réunion cutanée, et liées sur un cylindre de gaze aseptisée. Les sutures profondes peuvent ainsi être retirées plus tard.

Le sac forme bouchon, le cylindre, par sa compression, rapproche la paroi du canal.

J'ai revu assez régulièrement mes opérés et je n'ai constaté ni accident ni récidive. (J'ai eu cependant des récidives par d'autres procédés).

M. Kirmisson. — Messieurs, il ne m'appartient pas de juger les travaux qui vous ont été soumis dans cette session. Je puis cependant affirmer qu'elle a été féconde, et cela grâce à la création d'une section spéciale pour la chirurgie infantile. Déjà, en 1890, à Berlin, j'avais pu juger de l'avantage de cette spécialisation. A Rome, au contraire, en 1894, la chirurgie infantile noyée dans la chirurgie générale a été sacrifiée. Je vous demande donc de formuler le vœu que dorénavant la chirurgie infantile ait une place à part dans le Congrès.

TABLE DES AUTEURS

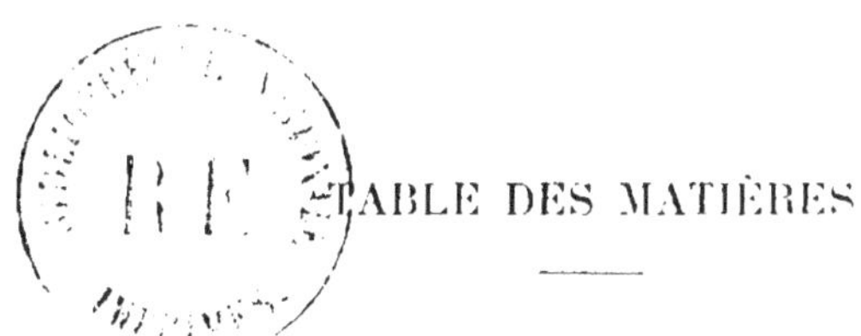

Masson et Cie, Éditeurs

Libraires de l'Académie de Médecine

120, Boulevard Saint-Germain, Paris (VIe)

EXTRAIT

DU

CATALOGUE MÉDICAL

Décembre 1900

La librairie Masson et C⁰ envoie gratuitement et franco de port les catalogues suivants à toutes les personnes qui lui en font la demande.

— **Catalogue général** *contenant, classés par subdivisions, tous les ouvrages publiés à la librairie ainsi que la liste de ses différents journaux et revues.*

— **Catalogues de l'Encyclopédie scientifique des Aide-Mémoire**

    I. *Section de l'ingénieur.*

    II. *Section du biologiste.*

— **Catalogue des ouvrages d'enseignement.**

Des prospectus spéciaux des différents grands Traités publiés par la librairie sont également adressés sur demande.

Traité
de
Pathologie générale

PUBLIÉ PAR

CH. BOUCHARD

MEMBRE DE L'INSTITUT
PROFESSEUR DE PATHOLOGIE GÉNÉRALE A LA FACULTÉ DE MÉDECINE DE PARIS

SECRÉTAIRE DE LA RÉDACTION

G.-H. ROGER

Professeur agrégé à la Faculté de médecine de Paris. Médecin des hôpitaux.

COLLABORATEURS :

MM. ARNOZAN — D'ARSONVAL — BENNI — R. BLANCHARD — BOULAY — BOURCY — BRUN — CADIOT — CHABRIÉ — CHANTEMESSE — CHARRIN — CHAUFFARD — COURMONT — DEJERINE — PIERRE DELBET — DEVIC — DUCAMP — MATHIAS DUVAL — FÉRÉ — FRÉMY — GAUCHER — GILBERT — GLEY — GUIGNARD — LOUIS GUINON — J.-F. GUYON — HALLÉ — HÉNOCQUE — HUGOUNENQ — LAMBLING — LANDOUZY — LAVERAN — LEBRETON — LE GENDRE — LEJARS — LE NOIR — LERMOYEZ — LETULLE — LUBET-BARBON — MARFAN — MAYOR — MENETRIER — NETTER — PIERRET — G.-H. ROGER — GABRIEL ROUX — RUFFER — RAYMOND TRIPIER — VUILLEMIN — FERNAND WIDAL.

6 vol. grand in-8°. avec figures dans le texte.

Sous la puissante impulsion du professeur Bouchard. la pathologie générale a pris une place prépondérante dans les études du monde médical. C'est qu'elle fournit des enseignements indispensables à toutes les branches de la médecine : elle fixe les idées sur les grands problèmes que soulève l'étude de l'homme ; elle éloigne le médecin des changeantes données de l'empirisme et lui apprend à réfléchir sur les phénomènes qu'il observe, à discuter et à comprendre les interventions qu'il doit faire.

Pour être véritablement utile, la pathologie expérimentale doit constamment s'efforcer de réunir et de synthétiser les données de la clinique et de l'expérimentation. C'est dans cet esprit qu'est conçu l'enseignement du professeur Bouchard: c'est dans cet esprit qu'a été écrit le livre dont il dirige la publication. Si tous les collaborateurs ont conservé leur indépendance. tous cependant ont suivi la même idée directrice qui assure à l'œuvre son unité.

Le plan adopté est d'ailleurs fort simple. Il consiste à rechercher par quel mécanisme agissent les causes pathogènes. par quels procédés l'organisme répond à l'attaque, par quels moyens le médecin peut apprécier à leur juste valeur les troubles morbides, les rattacher à leur cause et modifier leur évolution.

C'est la première fois, croyons-nous, qu'une pléiade de savants s'est groupée autour d'un maître illustre. pour élever un pareil monument à l'étude de la pathologie générale. L'intérêt qu'a soulevé cet ouvrage dans le monde scientifique étranger montre que nulle part n'existait l'équivalent d'une telle œuvre, et dès à présent, deux traductions. l'une en italien. l'autre en espagnol. ont été publiées.

Tome V. Fig. 65. Facies myopathique.

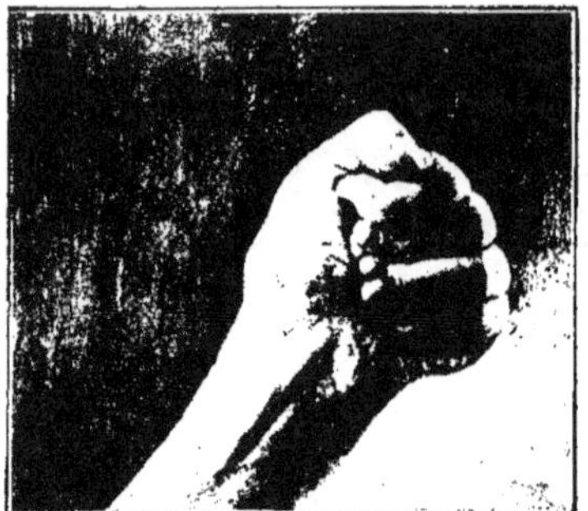

Tome V. Fig. 170. — Déformation de la main par contraction excessive dans un cas de maladie de Parkinson.

DIVISION DE L'OUVRAGE

TOME Iᵉʳ. — 1 vol. grand in-8° de 1008 pages avec figures dans le texte : **18** fr.

Introduction à l'étude de la pathologie générale, par G.-H. ROGER, professeur agrégé à la Faculté de médecine, médecin de l'Hôpital de la porte d'Aubervilliers. — Pathologie comparée de l'homme et des animaux, par G.-H. ROGER et P.-J. CADIOT. — Considérations générales sur les maladies des végétaux, par P. VUILLEMIN, chargé de cours à la Faculté de médecine de Nancy. — Pathogénie générale de l'embryon. Tératogénie, par MATHIAS DUVAL, professeur à la Faculté de médecine de Paris. — L'hérédité et la pathologie générale, par LE GENDRE, médecin des hôpitaux. — Prédisposition et immunité, par BOURCY, médecin des hôpitaux. — La fatigue et le surmenage, par MARFAN, professeur agrégé à la Faculté de médecine de Paris, médecin des hôpitaux. — Les Agents mécaniques, par LEJARS, professeur agrégé à la Faculté de médecine de Paris, chirurgien des hôpitaux. — Les Agents physiques. Chaleur. Froid. Lumière. Pression atmosphérique. Son, par LE NOIR. — Les Agents physiques. L'énergie électrique et la matière vivante, par d'ARSONVAL, membre de l'Institut, professeur au Collège de France. — Les Agents chimiques. Les caustiques, par LE NOIR. — Les intoxications, par G.-H. ROGER.

TOME II. — 1 vol. grand in-8° de 940 pages avec figures dans le texte : **18** fr.

L'Infection, par CHARRIN, professeur agrégé à la Faculté de médecine de Paris, médecin des hôpitaux. — Notions générales de morphologie bactériologique, par GUIGNARD, membre de l'Institut, professeur à l'Ecole de pharmacie. — Notions de chimie bactériologique, par HUGOUNENQ, professeur à la Faculté de médecine de Lyon. — Les microbes pathogènes, par ROUX, professeur agrégé à la Faculté de médecine de Lyon. — Le sol, l'eau et l'air agents des maladies infectieuses, par CHANTEMESSE, professeur à la Faculté de médecine de Paris, médecin des hôpitaux. — Des maladies épidémiques, par LAVERAN, membre de l'Académie de médecine. — Sur les parasites des tumeurs épithéliales malignes, par RUFFER. — Les parasites, par L. BLANCHARD, professeur à la Faculté de médecine de Paris, membre de l'Académie de médecine.

TOME III. — 1 vol. in-8° de plus de 1400 pages avec fig. dans le texte, publié en deux fascicules : **28** fr.

Fasc. I. — Notions générales sur la nutrition à l'état normal, par E. LAMBLING, professeur à l'Université de Lille. — Les troubles préalables de la nutrition, par CH. BOUCHARD, professeur à la Faculté de médecine, membre de l'Institut. — Les réactions nerveuses, par CH. BOUCHARD et G.-H. ROGER, professeur agrégé à la Faculté de médecine de Paris, médecin de l'Hôpital de la porte d'Aubervilliers. — Les processus pathogéniques de deuxième ordre, par G.-H. ROGER.

Fasc. II. — Considérations préliminaires sur la physiologie et l'anatomie pathologiques, par G.-H. ROGER. — De la fièvre, par LOUIS GUINON, médecin des hôpitaux de Paris. — L'hypothermie, par J.-F. GUYON. — Mécanisme physiologique des troubles vasculaires, par E. GLEY, professeur agrégé à la Faculté de médecine de Paris. — Les désordres de la circulation dans les maladies, par A. CHARRIN, professeur agrégé à la Faculté de médecine de Paris, professeur remplaçant au Collège de France, médecin des hôpitaux. — Thrombose et embolie, par A. MAYOR, professeur à la Faculté de médecine de Genève. — De l'inflammation, par J. COURMONT, professeur agrégé à la Faculté de médecine de Lyon, médecin des hôpitaux. — Anatomie pathologique générale des lésions inflammatoires, par M. LETULLE, pro-

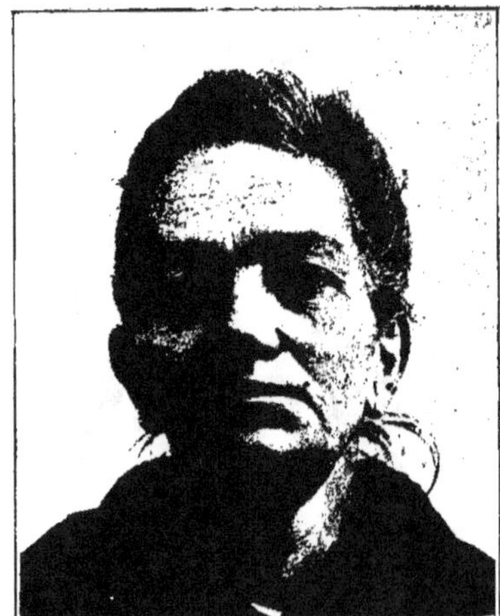

Tome V. Fig. 17. Paralysie bulbaire par névrite périphérique, avec participation du facial supérieur.

fesseur agrégé à la Faculté de medecine de Paris, médecin de l'hopital Boucicaut. —
Les altérations anatomiques non inflammatoires, par P. Le Noir, médecin des hopitaux.
— Les tumeurs, par P. Menetrier, professeur agrégé, médecin de l'hôpital Tenon.

TOME IV. — 1 vol. in-8° de 719 pages avec figures dans le texte : **16** fr.

Évolution des maladies, par Ducamp, professeur à la Faculté de medecine de Montpellier. — Semiologie du sang, par A. Gilbert, professeur agrégé, medecin de l'hôpital
Broussais. — Spectroscopie du sang. Semiologie, par A. Hénocque, directeur-adjoint
du Laboratoire de physique biologique du College de France. — Semiologie du cœur
et des vaisseaux, par R. Tripier, professeur à la Faculté de médecine de Lyon et
Devic, agrégé à la Faculté de Lyon, medecin des hopitaux. — Semiologie du nez et
du pharynx nasal, par M. Lermoyez, medecin de l'hopital Saint-Antoine, et M. Boulay,
ancien interne des hopitaux. — Semiologie du larynx, par M. Lermoyez et M. Boulay.
— Semiologie des voies respiratoires, par M. Lebreton, médecin des hopitaux. —
Semiologie générale du tube digestif, par P. Le Gendre, medecin de l'hôpital Tenon.

TOME V. — 1 vol. in-8° de 1180 pages avec nombreuses figures dans le texte : **28** fr.

A. Chauffard, professeur agrégé à la Faculté de médecine de Paris, medecin des hopitaux : Pathologie générale et Semiologie du foie. — X. Arnozan, professeur à la
Faculté de medecine de Bordeaux : Pancréas. — C. Chabrié, sous-directeur du

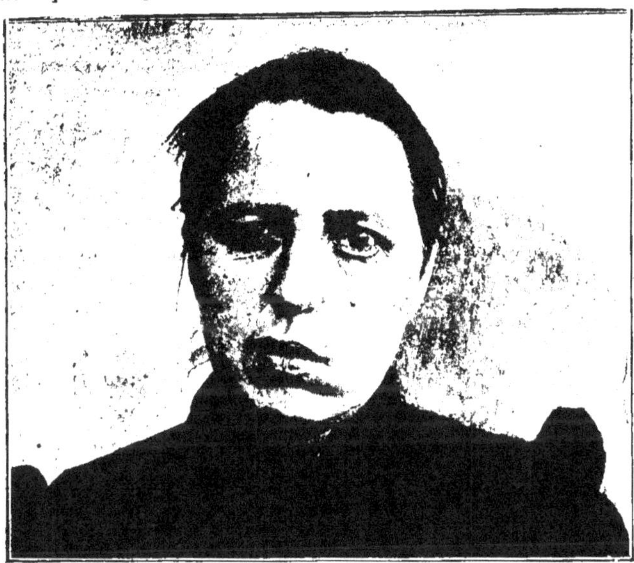

Tome V. Fig. 148. — Paralysie faciale gauche par lésion du rocher.

Laboratoire de Chimie appliquée à la Faculté des Sciences de Paris : Analyse chimique
des urines. — Noel Hallé : Analyse microscopique des urines (histo-bacteriologique). —
A. Charrin, professeur remplaçant au College de France : Le rein, l'urine et l'organisme.
— Pierre Delbet, professeur agrégé à la Faculté de médecine de Paris, chirurgien des
hopitaux : Semiologie des organes genitaux. — J. Dejerine, professeur agrégé à la
Faculté de médecine de Paris, médecin des hopitaux : Semiologie du systeme nerveux.
Cet article comprend plus de 800 pages et est illustré de très nombreuses photogra-
phies, schémas et dessins.)

CONDITIONS DE LA PUBLICATION (Décembre 1900)

Le **Traité de Pathologie générale** est publié en six volumes. Chaque volume est
vendu séparément, et le prix en est fixé suivant l'étendue des matieres.
Les tomes I et II sont vendus chacun. **18** fr. | Le tome IV est vendu . . . . **16** fr.
Le tome III forme 2 part. et est vendu. **28** fr. | Le tome V est vendu . . . . **28** fr.
Il est accepté des **souscriptions** au Traité de Pathologie générale à un *prix à forfait*, quels que soient l'étendue et le prix de l'ouvrage complet.
Ce prix à partir de ce jour a été élevé de **112** francs à **120** francs, *et restera tel,
dans tous les cas, jusqu'à la publication du tome VI.*

CHARCOT — BOUCHARD — BRISSAUD

BABINSKI — BALLET — P. BLOCQ — BOIX — BRAULT — CHANTEMESSE — CHARRIN
CHAUFFARD — COURTOIS-SUFFIT — DUTIL — GILBERT — GUIGNARD — L. GUINON
GEORGES GUINON — HALLION — LAMY — LE GENDRE — MARFAN
MARIE — MATHIEU — NETTER — ŒTTINGER — ANDRÉ PETIT
RICHARDIÈRE — ROGER — RUAULT — SOUQUES — THOINOT
THIBIERGE — FERNAND WIDAL

TRAITÉ DE MÉDECINE

DEUXIÈME ÉDITION
(Entièrement refondue.)

PUBLIÉE SOUS LA DIRECTION DE MM.

BOUCHARD
Professeur à la Faculté de médecine de Paris.
Membre de l'Institut.

BRISSAUD
Professeur à la Faculté de médecine de Paris,
Médecin de l'hôpital St-Antoine.

10 volumes grand in-8°, avec figures dans le texte

En Souscription.. . . . . **150** francs

La deuxième édition du TRAITÉ DE MÉDECINE a été entièrement revisée et augmentée dans de notables proportions. En outre, et pour la commodité des lecteurs, les matières sont réparties en dix volumes qui paraissent successivement.

Chaque volume est vendu séparément.

Jusqu'à ce jour le prix de l'ouvrage reste fixé pour les souscripteurs à 150 francs.

DÉCEMBRE 1900.

Le succès de la première édition du **Traité de Médecine** de MM. Charcot, Bouchard et Brissaud, a rendu nécessaire une seconde édition, et loin de se borner à une réimpression les auteurs ont voulu présenter au public un ouvrage nouveau, gardant le plan et les idées qui avaient assuré le succès sans précédent du traité, lors de son apparition, mais complétant et remaniant la plupart de ses parties et corrigeant les quelques imperfections qui s'étaient glissées dans la première édition. Comprenant désormais 10 volumes, dont 6 déjà ont été publiés, le **Traité de Médecine** reste le plus complet, le plus documenté des livres de ce genre et l'autorité croissante qui s'attache aux noms de ceux qui y collaborent en confirme et en assure le succès persistant.

TOME Iᵉʳ

I vol. grand in-8° de 845 pages, avec figures dans le texte : **16** fr.

Les bactéries, par L. GUIGNARD, membre de l'Institut et de l'Académie de médecine, professeur à l'École de Pharmacie de Paris. — *Pathologie générale infectieuse*, par A. CHARRIN, professeur remplaçant au Collège de France, directeur du Laboratoire de médecine expérimentale (Hautes-Études), médecin des hôpitaux. — *Troubles et maladies de la nutrition*, par PAUL LEGENDRE, médecin de l'hôpital Tenon. — *Maladies infectieuses communes à l'homme et aux animaux*, par G.-H. ROGER, professeur agrégé, médecin de l'hôpital de la Porte d'Aubervilliers.

TOME II

1 vol. grand in-8° de 890 pages, avec figures dans le texte : **16 fr.**

Fièvre typhoïde, par A. CHANTEMESSE, professeur à la Faculté de médecine, médecin des hôpitaux de Paris. — *Maladies infectieuses*, par F. WIDAL, professeur agrégé, médecin des hôpitaux de Paris. — *Typhus exanthématique*, par L.-H. THOINOT, professeur agrégé, médecin des hôpitaux de Paris. — *Fièvres éruptives*, par L. GUINON, médecin des hôpitaux de Paris. — *Erysipèle*, par E. BOIX, chef de laboratoire à la Faculté. — *Diphtérie*, par A. RUAULT. — *Rhumatisme articulaire aigu*, par ŒTTINGER, médecin des hôpitaux de Paris. — *Scorbut*, par TOLLEMER, chef de laboratoire à la Faculté.

TOME III

1 vol. grand in-8° de 702 pages, avec figures dans le texte : **16 fr.**

Maladies cutanées, par G. THIBIERGE, médecin de l'hôpital de la Pitié. — *Maladies vénériennes*, par G. THIBIERGE, médecin de l'hôpital de la Pitié. — *Maladies du sang*, par A. GILBERT, professeur agrégé, médecin des hôpitaux de Paris. — *Intoxications*, par H. RICHARDIÈRE, médecin des hôpitaux de Paris.

TOME IV

1 vol. grand in-8° de 680 pages, avec figures dans le texte : **16 fr.**

Maladies de l'estomac, par A. MATHIEU, médecin de l'hôpital Andral. — *Maladies du pancréas*, par A. MATHIEU, médecin de l'hôpital Andral. — *Maladies de l'intestin*, par COURTOIS-SUFFIT, médecin des hôpitaux de Paris. — *Maladies du péritoine*, par COURTOIS-SUFFIT, médecin des hôpitaux de Paris. — *Maladies de la bouche et du pharynx*, par A. RUAULT, médecin honoraire de la Clinique laryngologique de l'institution nationale des Sourds-Muets.

TOME VI

1 vol. grand in-8° de 612 pages, avec figures dans le texte : **14 fr.**

Maladies du nez et du larynx, par A. RUAULT, médecin honoraire de la Clinique laryngologique de l'Institution nationale des Sourds-Muets. — *Asthme*, par E. BRISSAUD, professeur à la Faculté de médecine de Paris, médecin de l'hôpital Saint-Antoine. — *Coqueluche*, par P. LE GENDRE, médecin des hôpitaux. — *Maladies des bronches*, par A.-B. MARFAN, professeur agrégé à la Faculté de médecine de Paris, médecin des hôpitaux. — *Troubles de la circulation pulmonaire*, par A.-B. MARFAN, professeur agrégé à la Faculté de médecine de Paris, médecin des hôpitaux. — *Maladies aiguës du poumon*, par NETTER, professeur agrégé à la Faculté de médecine de Paris, médecin des hôpitaux.

TOME VII

1 vol. grand in-8° de 550 pages, avec figures dans le texte : **14 fr.**

Maladies chroniques du poumon par A.-B. MARFAN, professeur agrégé à la Faculté de médecine de Paris, médecin des hôpitaux. — *Phtisie pulmonaire*, par A.-B. MARFAN, professeur agrégé à la Faculté de médecine de Paris, médecin des hôpitaux. — *Maladies de la plèvre*, par NETTER, professeur agrégé à la Faculté de médecine de Paris, médecin des hôpitaux. — *Maladies du médiastin*, par A.-B. MARFAN, professeur agrégé à la Faculté de médecine de Paris, médecin des hôpitaux.

Le TOME V sera publié ultérieurement

Traité
de Chirurgie

Publié sous la direction

DE MM.

Simon DUPLAY

Professeur de clinique chirurgicale à la Faculté
de médecine de Paris
Chirurgien de l'Hôtel-Dieu
Membre de l'Académie de médecine

Paul RECLUS

Professeur agrégé à la Faculté de médecine de Paris
Secrétaire général de la Société de chirurgie
Chirurgien des hôpitaux
Membre de l'Académie de médecine

PAR MM.

**BERGER. — BROCA. — Pierre DELBET. — DELENS. — DEMOULIN
J.-L. FAURE. — FORGUE. — GÉRARD-MARCHANT
HARTMANN. — HEYDENREICH. — JALAGUIER. — KIRMISSON. — LAGRANGE
LEJARS. — MICHAUX. — NÉLATON
PEYROT. — PONCET. — QUÉNU. — RICARD. — RIEFFEL. — SEGOND
TUFFIER. — WALTHER**

DEUXIÈME ÉDITION, ENTIÈREMENT REFONDUE

8 forts volumes grand in-8° avec nombreuses figures dans le texte. . .   **150 fr.**

Plus de neuf ans se sont écoulés depuis le jour où fut arrêté le programme du *Traité de Chirurgie*, et, des vingt-quatre collaborateurs du début, aucun, par un rare bonheur, ne manque encore à l'entreprise. Les portes de l'Hôpital et de l'Agrégation se sont ouvertes devant les plus jeunes, le Professorat et l'Académie de médecine en ont élu de plus âgés; tous ont vu s'étendre leur sphère d'activité professionnelle. Aussi pouvons-nous affirmer que ce nouvel ouvrage porte la marque d'une expérience plus mûre et d'une plus grande autorité.

TOME PREMIER. 1 fort vol. de 912 pages avec 218 figures. . .   **18 fr.**

Reclus. Inflammations. — Traumatismes. — Maladies virulentes.	Broca. Peau et tissu cellulaire sous-cutané.
Quénu. Des Tumeurs.	Lejars. Lymphatiques, muscles, synoviales tendineuses et bourses séreuses.

TOME II. 1 fort vol. de 996 pages avec 361 figures. . . . . .   **18 fr.**

Lejars. Nerfs.	Ricard et Demoulin. Lésions traumatiques des os.
Michaux. Artères.	
Quénu. Maladies des veines.	Poncet. Affections non traumatiques des os.

TOME III. 1 fort vol. de 940 pages avec 285 figures . . . . .   **18 fr.**

Nélaton. Traumatismes, entorses, luxations. plaies articulaires.	Quénu. Arthropathies. Arthrites sèches. Corps étrangers articulaires.
	Gérard Marchant. Maladies du crâne.
Lagrange. Arthrites infectieuses et inflammatoires.	Kirmisson. Maladies du rachis.
	Simon Duplay. Oreilles et Annexes.

TOME IV. 1 fort vol. de 896 pages avec 354 figures. . . . . .   **18 fr.**

Delens. Œil et annexes.	Heydenreich. Mâchoires.
Gérard-Marchant. Nez, fosses nasales, pharynx nasal et sinus.	

TOME V. 1 fort vol. de 948 pages avec 187 figures. . . . . . . **20** fr.

Broca. Vices de développement de la face et du cou. Face, lèvres, cavité buccale, gencives, langue, palais et pharynx.
Hartmann. Plancher buccal, glandes salivaires, œsophage et larynx.

Broca. Corps thyroïde.
Walther. Maladies du cou.
Peyrot. Poitrine.
Delbet. Mamelle.

TOME VI. 1 fort vol. de 1127 pages avec 218 figures. . . . . . **20** fr.

Michaux. Parois de l'abdomen.
Berger. Hernies.
Jalaguier. Contusions et plaies de l'abdomen. Lésions traumatiques et corps étrangers de l'estomac et de l'intestin.
Hartmann. Estomac.

Jalaguier. Occlusion intestinale. Péritonites. Appendicite.
Faure et Rieffel. Rectum et Anus.
Quénu. Mésentère. Rate. Pancréas.
Segond. Foie.

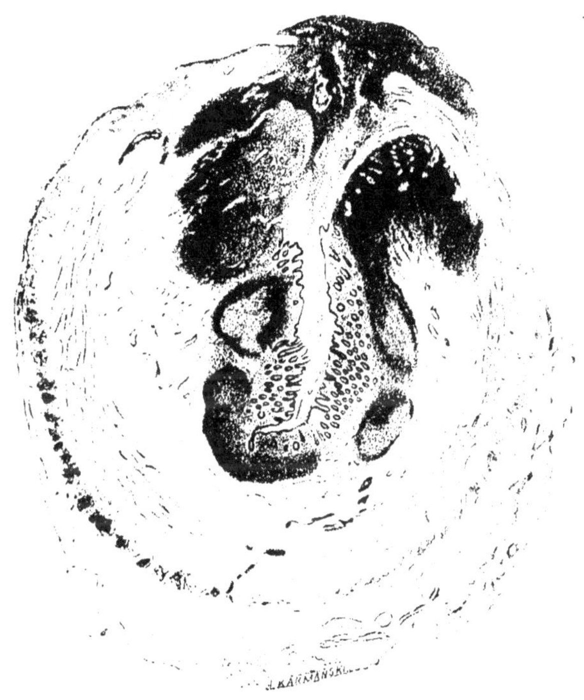

Tome VI. Fig. 116. — Appendicite folliculaire perforante.

TOME VII. 1 fort vol. de 1272 pages avec 297 figures dans le texte. **25** fr.

Walther. Bassin.
Rieffel. Affections congénitales de la région sacro-coccygienne.

Tuffier. Rein. Vessie. Uretères. Capsules surrénales.
Forgue. Urèthre et prostate.
Reclus. Organes génitaux de l'homme.

TOME VIII. 1 fort vol. de 971 pages avec 163 figures dans le texte. **20** fr.

Michaux. Vulve et Vagin.
Pierre Delbet. Maladies de l'utérus.

Segond. Annexes de l'utérus, ovaires, trompes, ligaments larges, péritoine pelvien.
Kirmisson. Maladies des membres.

TABLE ALPHABÉTIQUE des 8 volumes du *Traité de Chirurgie*.

La Pratique
Dermatologique

Traité de Dermatologie appliquée

PUBLIÉ SOUS LA DIRECTION DE MM.

ERNEST BESNIER, L. BROCQ, L. JACQUET

PAR MM.

AUDRY, BALZER, BARBE, BAROZZI, BARTHÉLEMY, BÉNARD, ERNEST BES-
NIER, BODIN, BROCQ, DE BRUN, DU CASTEL, J. DARIER, DEHU, DOMINICI,
W. DUBREUILH, HUDELO, L. JACQUET, J.-B. LAFFITTE, LENGLET, LE-
REDDE, MERKLEN, PERRIN, RAYNAUD, RIST, SABOURAUD, MARCEL SÉE,
GEORGES THIBIERGE, VEYRIÈRES.

*4 volumes richement cartonnés toile formant ensemble environ 3600 pages, très
largement illustrés de figures en noir et de planches en couleurs. En souscription
jusqu'à la publication du Tome II.* . . . . **140** *fr.*
Chaque volume sera vendu séparément.

EXTRAIT DE LA PRÉFACE

..... A tous les titres, il y a intérêt majeur à résumer l'état présent de
la dermatologie à la fin de ce siècle scientifique si fécond et si brillant, et
à l'aube de celui qui le suit, quelque grand qu'il doive être !

Notre but le plus essentiel est, avant tout, de faire œuvre de clinique et de thérapeutique.

Nous voulons fixer les types morbides par des descriptions sobres et précises, appuyées sur des représentations graphiques aussi nombreuses et aussi parfaites que possible, et réaliser ainsi une œuvre de toute utilité, destinée à la grande masse des praticiens.

La thérapeutique des maladies de la peau sera exposée avec une ampleur au moins égale : nous nous sommes attachés à donner place, dans la *Pratique dermatologique*, à tout ce qui peut être utile au médecin praticien pour le traitement de chaque maladie en particulier.

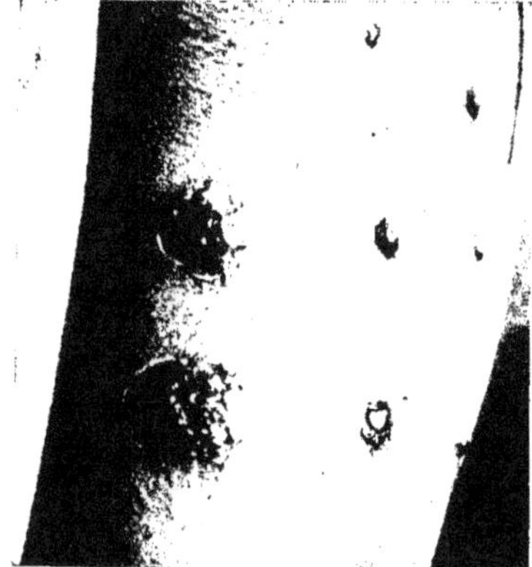

Fig. 225. — Ecthyma.

Que l'on ne se méprenne pas cependant. La *Pratique dermatologique*
ne sera pas un simple manuel illustré renfermant seulement, à propos de
chaque dermatose, un abrégé symptomatologique suivi de formules banales et non contrôlées ; notre but est beaucoup plus élevé. A l'exposé de
chaque question, le médecin dermatologiste trouvera toujours les indications scientifiques principales sur la matière. L'histologie, la bactério-

logie, l'histochimie et l'hématologie seront traitées dans la mesure indiquée par l'état actuel de ces connaissances et par leur importance relative aux dermatoses en particulier. Les plus grands développements seront réservés à la description clinique basée sur l'observation précise et minutieuse des faits, assurés que nous serons, en cela, de faire œuvre durable.

Afin de mieux fixer les types dermatologiques, et pour permettre aux

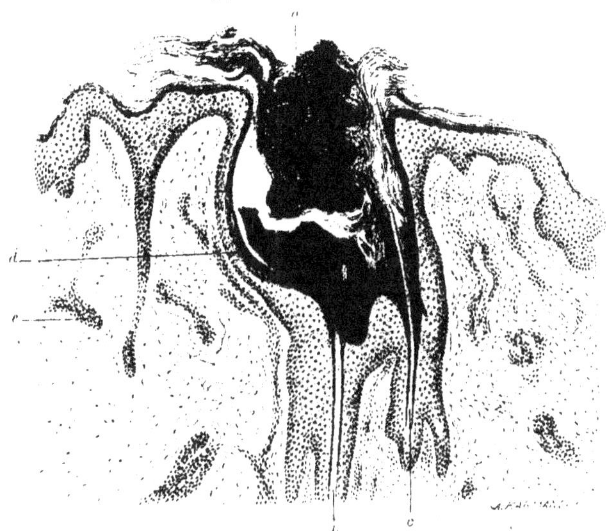

Fig. 23. — Coupe d'acné pustuleuse passant par le comédon.

praticiens de médecine générale de les connaître à coup sûr, nous annexerons au texte, en grand nombre, des planches coloriées et des dessins en noir, aussi exacts que l'on peut actuellement les réaliser.

Et, à titre complémentaire, nous indiquerons, toutes les fois où cela pourra être utile, les numéros correspondants des magnifiques reproductions *ad naturam* accumulées dans le merveilleux musée de l'hôpital Saint-Louis, et dues au talent de Baretta.

TOME PREMIER

1 fort vol. in-8° avec 250 figures en noir et 24 planches en couleurs.
Richement cartonné toile. **36** fr.

Anatomie et Physiologie de la Peau. — **Pathologie générale de la Peau.** — **Symptomatologie générale des Dermatoses.** — **Acanthosis nigricans.** — **Acnés.** — **Actinomycose.** — **Adénomes.** — **Alopécies.** — **Anesthésie locale.** — **Balanites.** — **Bouton d'Orient.** — **Brûlures.** — **Charbon.** — **Classifications dermatologiques.** — **Dermatites polymorphes douloureuses.** — **Dermatophytes.** — **Dermatozoaires.** — **Dermites infantiles simples.** — **Ecthyma.**

SOUS PRESSE : Tome II contenant les articles : *Eczéma*, par ERNEST BESNIER. — *Électricité*, par BROCQ. — *Électrolyse*, par BROCQ. — *Éléphantiasis*, par DOMINICI. *Éosinophilie*, par LEREDDE. — *Épithelioma*, par DARIER. — *Éruptions artificielles*, par THIBIERGE. — *Érythème*, par BODIN. — *Érythrodermie*, par BROCQ. — *Favus*, par BODIN. — *Folliculites*, par HUDELO. — *Furonculose*, par BAROZZI. — *Gale*, par DUBREUILH. — *Greffe*, par BAROZZI. — *Herpès*, par DU CASTEL. — *Icthyose*, par THIBIERGE. — *Impétigo*, par SABOURAUD. — *Kératodermie*, par DUBREUILH. — *Kératose piliaire*, par VEYRIÈRES. — *Langue*, par BÉNARD. — *Lèpre*, par MARCEL SÉE. — *Leucokératose*, par BÉNARD. — *Lichens*, par BROCQ.

Traité d'Anatomie Humaine

PUBLIÉ SOUS LA DIRECTION DE

P. POIRIER   et   A. CHARPY

Professeur agrégé à la Faculté
de médecine de Paris
Chirurgien des hôpitaux

Professeur d'anatomie
à la Faculté de médecine
de Toulouse

AVEC LA COLLABORATION DE

O. AMOEDO — A. BRANCA — B. CUNÉO — P. FREDET
P. JACQUES — TH. JONNESCO — E. LAGUESSE — L. MANOUVRIER
A. NICOLAS — M. PICOU
A. PRENANT — H. RIEFFEL — CH. SIMON — A. SOULIÉ

5 vol. grand in-8° avec figures noires et en couleurs

ÉTAT DE LA PUBLICATION (Décembre 1900)

TOME I. — (*Deuxième édition, revue et augmentée.*) — **Embryologie**. Notions d'embryologie. **Ostéologie**. Considérations générales. Des membres. Squelette du tronc. Squelette de la tête. **Arthrologie**. Développement des articulations. Structure. Articulations des membres. Articulations du tronc. Articulations de la tête. *Un volume grand in-8°, avec 807 figures.* . . . . . **20 fr.**

TOME II. — 1ᵉʳ Fascicule : **Myologie**. Embryologie. Histologie. Peauciers et aponévroses. *Deuxième édition revue et augmentée. Un volume grand in-8°, avec 331 figures* . . . . **12 fr.**

2ᵉ Fascicule : **Angéiologie** (Cœur et Artères). Histologie. *Un volume grand in-8°, avec 145 figures*. . . . . **8 fr.**

3ᵉ Fascicule : **Angéiologie** (Capillaires. Veines). *Un volume grand in-8°, avec 75 figures*. . . . . **6 fr.**

TOME III. — 1ᵉʳ Fascicule : **Système nerveux**. Méninges. Moelle. Encéphale. Embryologie. Histologie. *Un volume grand in-8°, avec 201 figures*. . **10 fr.**

2ᵉ Fascicule : **Système nerveux**. Encéphale. *Un volume grand in-8°, avec 206 figures*. . . . . **12 fr.**

3ᵉ Fascicule : **Système nerveux**. Les Nerfs. Nerfs crâniens. Nerfs rachidiens. *Un volume grand in-8°, avec 205 figures*. . . . . **12 fr.**

TOME IV. — 1ᵉʳ Fascicule : **Tube digestif**. Développement. Bouche. Pharynx. Œsophage. Estomac. Intestins. *Deuxième édition, revue et augmentée. Un volume grand in-8°, avec 201 figures*. . . . . **12 fr.**

2ᵉ Fascicule : **Appareil respiratoire**. Larynx. Trachée. Poumons. Plèvre. Thyroïde. Thymus. *Un volume grand in-8°, avec 121 figures*. . . . . **6 fr.**

3ᵉ Fascicule : **Annexes du tube digestif**. Dents. Glandes salivaires. Foie. Voies biliaires. Pancréas. Rate. **Péritoine**. *Un volume grand in-8°, avec 361 figures*. . . . . **16 fr.**

IL RESTE A PUBLIER

Les Lymphatiques qui termineront le tome II.

Les organes génitaux-urinaires et les **organes des sens** qui formeront le tome V.

Le prolongement caudé du lobule de Spigel dans le lobe droit du foie adulte (*colliculus caudatus* de Haller) obture en partie la fente de Winslow.

Récemment Klaatsch a donné une interprétation tout à fait spéciale de l'hiatus de Winslow. (Voy. *Bibliographie*, p. 1005; ou le premier travail de Brachet (cf. p. 945) et le *Traité d'em-*

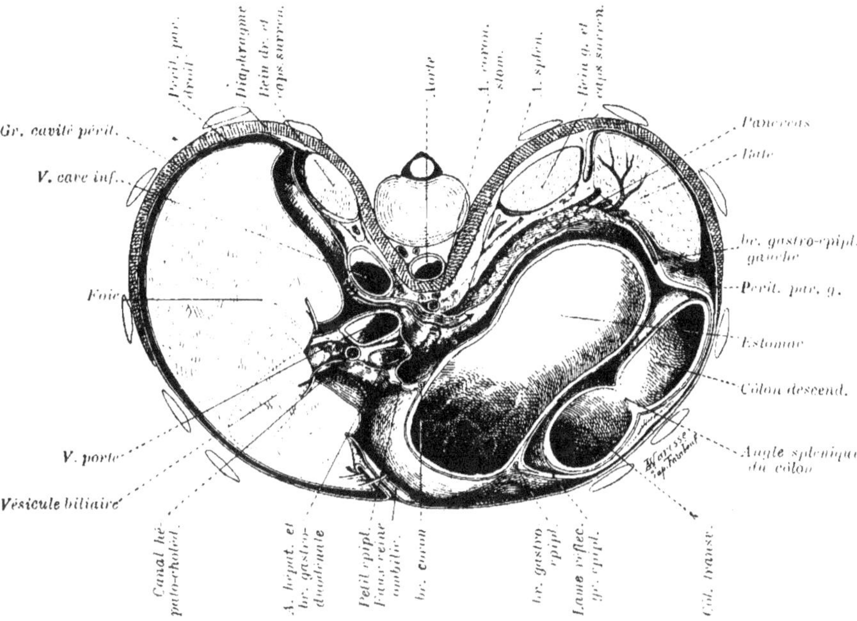

Fig. 577. — Coupe transversale de l'abdomen, au-dessus du seuil de l'hiatus de Winslow, et vue perspective des organes sous-jacents. Reproduction d'un dessin inédit, d'après nature, du Prof. L.-H. Farabeuf. La disposition de l'estomac relativement au côlon est expliquée par le schéma 577 *bis*.

La flèche qui traverse l'hiatus de Winslow, entre la veine cave et la veine porte, franchit l'arc de l'hépatique. Elle peut pénétrer, en arrière de l'estomac, à gauche de la faux de la coronaire (poche rétro-stomacale) ou descendre dans le sac épiploïque.

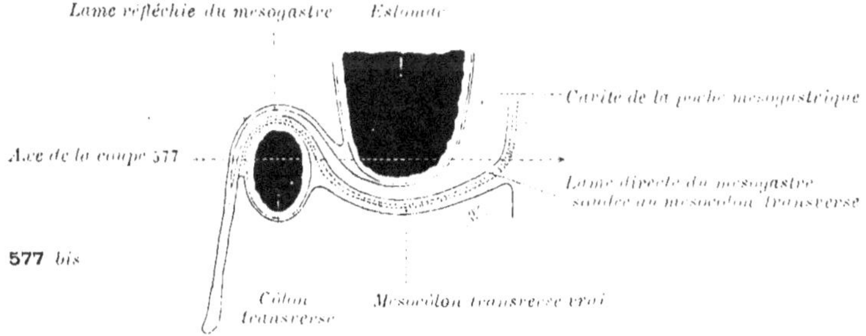

bryologie de Prenant (liv. II, p. 780-781 et 784-785). — Ses théories ont été réfutées par Toldt (*l. c.*, 1893, p. 63), et par Brachet et Swaen.

Pour pénétrer dans l'hiatus de Winslow, il suffit de reconnaître la vésicule biliaire et de suivre son bord droit. On est conduit au niveau du plafond de l'hiatus et on y pénètre aisément, en arrière du ligament hépato-duodénal. On

FREDET.

Traité

DES

Maladies de l'Enfance

PUBLIÉ SOUS LA DIRECTION DE MM.

J. GRANCHER

PROFESSEUR A LA FACULTÉ DE MÉDECINE DE PARIS
MEMBRE DE L'ACADÉMIE DE MÉDECINE, MÉDECIN DE L'HOPITAL DES ENFANTS-MALADES

J. COMBY
MÉDECIN DE L'HOPITAL DES ENFANTS-MALADES

A.-B. MARFAN
AGRÉGÉ, MÉDECIN DES HOPITAUX

5 forts volumes grand in-8°, avec figures dans le texte. . . . . . . **90** francs

Ce *Traité des Maladies de l'Enfance* comble une lacune, et les médecins attendaient avec impatience l'apparition de cet ouvrage. Il existait déjà en effet, traitant des maladies de l'Enfance, plusieurs manuels dont quelques-uns sont fort appréciés, mais nous n'avions pas de traité complet dans lequel les questions de pédiatrie fussent étudiées d'une façon complète. Cet ouvrage paraît en cinq beaux volumes, et la notoriété qui s'attache aux noms des directeurs de cette publication et à ceux des collaborateurs suffit pour lui assurer un plein succès. Les maladies qui y sont traitées ont été confiées, en effet, aux pédiatres qui les ont étudiées d'une façon spéciale. Cette œuvre est pour ainsi dire une œuvre internationale, et parmi les noms des collaborateurs nous trouvons ceux des pédiatres les plus renommés de tous les pays, qui nous font ainsi profiter de l'expérience qu'ils peuvent avoir d'affections qu'ils rencontrent plus que d'autres dans leur champ d'observation. Bien plus, la Médecine et la Chirurgie, ces deux sœurs jumelles qu'on tend bien à tort à séparer sans cesse, ont trouvé le moyen de se retrouver côte à côte au grand profit des lecteurs.

Les 5 volumes se vendent séparément :
Tome I, **18** fr.   Tome II, **18** fr.   Tome III, **20** fr.   Tome IV, **18** fr.   Tome V, **18** fr.

Traité élémentaire

DE

Clinique Thérapeutique

Par le Dr Gaston LYON
Ancien chef de clinique médicale à la Faculté de médecine de Paris.

TROISIÈME ÉDITION REVUE ET AUGMENTÉE

1 *volume grand in-8 de* VIII-1332 *pages. Relié peau.. . . . . .* **20** *fr.*

La seconde édition de ce livre a reçu du public médical le même accueil favorable que la première. Nous trouvant par suite dans l'obligation agréable de préparer une troisième édition, nous avons considéré comme un devoir strict d'y apporter tous nos soins et de justifier ainsi la faveur soutenue dont notre ouvrage a été l'objet.

Un certain nombre de chapitres nouveaux ont été ajoutés avec tous les développements que comporte leur importance ; citons notamment ceux consacrés aux cardiopathies infantiles, aux sténoses du pylore, aux angiocholites infectieuses, aux péritonites aiguës, aux méningo-myélites aiguës, aux polio-myélites, à la peste, etc.

Le chapitre consacré aux dyspepsies a été récrit en entier. Tous les autres chapitres de notre ouvrage ont été l'objet de modifications de détails, quelques-uns même ont été presque entièrement refondus (blennorragie, syphilis, neurasthénie, infections gastro-intestinales infantiles, etc.)

Sur la demande d'un grand nombre de nos lecteurs, une table alphabétique a été ajoutée, qui facilitera les recherches.

Le rôle du médecin change en même temps que se modifient les médications. La mise en œuvre des soins antiseptiques, l'emploi des injections de sérum, tout cela fait que le rôle actif du médecin grandit sans cesse. Nous avons tenu, dans cette édition, à insister sur les détails de direction des traitements, en un mot à justifier, mieux encore que par le passé, notre titre de *Traité de clinique thérapeutique*.

Traité
de Physiologie

PAR

J.-P. MORAT
PROFESSEUR A L'UNIVERSITÉ DE LYON

ET

Maurice DOYON
PROFESSEUR AGRÉGÉ A LA FACULTÉ DE MÉDECINE DE LYON

Ce Traité de Physiologie formera 5 volumes dont voici le détail :

I. — **Fonctions élémentaires.** — Prolégomènes. — Nutrition en général. — Physiologie des tissus en particulier (moins le système nerveux).

II. — **Fonctions d'innervation et du milieu intérieur.** — Système nerveux. — Sang; lymphe; liquides interstitiels.

III. — **Fonctions de nutrition.** — Circulation; calorification.

IV. — **Fonctions de nutrition** (suite). — Digestion; respiration; excrétion.

V. — **Fonctions de relation.** — Sens. — Langage; expression; locomotion. **Fonctions de reproduction**, à l'exception du développement embryologique.

Ces volumes ne seront pas publiés dans l'ordre ci-dessus, mais le seront dans celui de leur achèvement.

Chaque volume sera, pendant tout le cours de la publication, vendu séparément à des prix qui varieront selon l'étendue de chacun.

Toutefois, les éditeurs acceptent, dès à présent, **au prix à forfait de 50 francs,** des souscriptions à l'ouvrage **complet.**

Les souscripteurs payeront en retirant chaque volume le prix marqué; mais le tome V et dernier leur sera fourni gratuitement ou à un prix tel qu'ils n'aient, en aucun cas, payé plus de 50 francs pour le total de l'ouvrage.

Volumes publiés :

III. — **Fonctions de nutrition.** — Circulation, par M. DOYON ; calorification par J.-P. MORAT. 1 volume grand in-8 avec 173 figures noires et en couleurs **12** fr.

IV. — **Fonctions de nutrition** (suite et fin). — Respiration; excrétion, par J.-P. MORAT; Digestion; absorption, par M. DOYON. 1 volume grand in-8 avec 167 figures en noir et en couleurs. . . . . **12** fr.

C'est un grand traité de physiologie, tel qu'il n'en était pas paru depuis la troisième édition (1888) de l'ouvrage classique de Beaunis, que les auteurs ont eu le courage d'entreprendre et qu'ils mèneront certainement à bien, si l'on en juge par le remarquable spécimen qui forme le premier volume.

E. GLEY (*Archives de physiologie*).

... En résumé, à en juger par le spécimen que nous avons sous les yeux, MM. MORAT et DOYON sont en train de doter nos bibliothèques d'un ouvrage précieux et très bien fait en ce sens qu'ils savent le rendre complet sans le grossir démesurément. Leur *Traité de physiologie* conviendra au débutant, à l'étudiant avancé et à toutes les personnes qui ont besoin de prendre une idée générale ou de remonter à l'origine des faits qui ont permis de la dogmatiser.

Dr ARLOING (*Lyon médical*).

TRAITÉ

DE

Physique Biologique

PUBLIÉ SOUS LA DIRECTION DE MM.

D'ARSONVAL	**CHAUVEAU**
Professeur au Collège de France	Professeur au Muséum d'histoire naturelle
Membre de l'Institut et de l'Académie des sciences	Membre de l'Institut et de l'Académie de médecine
GARIEL	**MAREY**
Professeur à la Faculté de médecine de Paris	Professeur au Collège de France
Membre de l'Académie de médecine	Membre de l'Institut et de l'Académie des sciences

SECRÉTAIRE DE LA RÉDACTION

M. WEISS

Professeur agrégé à la Faculté de médecine de Paris

Le **Traité de Physique Biologique** sera publié en trois volumes :

Tome   I. *Mécanique. Actions moléculaires. Chaleur.*
Tome II. *Radiations. Optique.*
Tome III. *Électricité. Acoustique.*

Chaque volume sera vendu séparément.

Le tome I est vendu **25** fr. On souscrit dès maintenant à l'ouvrage complet au prix de **60** fr. — Ce prix restera tel jusqu'à la publication du tome II.

EXTRAIT DE LA PRÉFACE

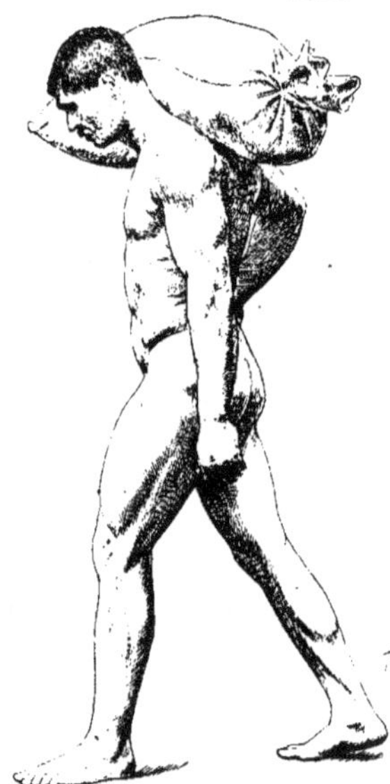

Tome I. Fig. 130. — Marche avec un fardeau sur l'épaule. Moment du double appui.

Au moment où dans les facultés de médecine il s'est produit un changement considérable dans l'enseignemeut de la physique, il a semblé utile de réunir en un ouvrage tous les matériaux qui pouvaient faire le fond de cet enseignement.

Déjà les maîtres qui ont pour ainsi dire fondé la Physique biologique, les Weber, Helmholtz, du Bois-Reymond, Chauveau, Marey, Paul Bert, d'autres encore, ont écrit sur certains points spéciaux des traités importants. — Mais si l'on en excepte les manuels et les traités élémentaires à l'usage des étudiants, il n'a encore paru aucun ouvrage d'ensemble sur la physique biologique. — Il y avait là, semble-t-il, une lacune à combler. . . . .

La Physique pure ne tient dans cet ouvrage qu'une place excessivement réduite. — Sa lecture exige la connaissance des notions générales, toutefois il a paru nécessaire de faire précéder chaque partie d'une sorte d'aide-mémoire rappelant brièvement les principaux faits sur lesquels il pouvait être nécessaire de s'appuyer dans la suite. . . .

L'ouvrage complet comprendra trois volumes.

Nous avons cru devoir placer en tête du premier un court article sur les diverses espèces d'erreur que l'on est exposé à commettre dans les sciences expérimentales, car nous avons remarqué trop souvent que beaucoup de physiologistes ne faisaient pas la distinction convenable entre elles.

Contrairement à notre principe de passer rapidement sur les questions de physique pure, nous avons aussi donné quelque développement à la mécanique et aux actions moléculaires. Il est, en effet, souvent difficile pour le physiologiste de lire des traités de mécanique générale, et nous avons cherché à en exposer les notions les plus indispensables.

Dans ce même volume, se trouve tout ce qui a rapport à la mécanique animale, à la chaleur et aux actions moléculaires, cependant une grande partie des phénomènes de la contraction musculaire a été renvoyée au troisième volume qui contient l'électrophysiologie.

Ce premier volume sera suivi prochainement, nous l'espérons, par un deuxième volume contenant toutes les applications de l'optique géométrique et des radiations.

Enfin le troisième volume est réservé à l'Électricité et à l'Acoustique.

Nous avons fait tous nos efforts pour mener cet ouvrage à bonne fin; il nous semble avoir réuni pour cela les meilleures conditions, il suffit pour s'en convaincre de lire la table de noms de nos collaborateurs et de se rappeler celui de notre éditeur dont l'éloge n'est plus à faire; puissions-nous avoir fait œuvre utile.

TOME PREMIER

1 fort volume in-8° avec 591 figures dans le texte : **25 fr.**

Ce volume contient : Des erreurs dans les mesures. Principes généraux de mécanique, par M. G. WEISS. — Propriétés des solides. Résistance des matériaux. Architecture des os, par M. GARIEL. — Architecture des muscles. Principes généraux de méthode graphique. La contraction musculaire, par M. G. WEISS. — Locomotion humaine, par M. PAUL RICHER. — La locomotion animale, par M. MAREY. — Principes généraux d'hydrostatique et d'hydrodynamique, par M. WEISS. — Cœur. Cardiographie, par M. WERTHEIMER. — Circulation du sang dans les vaisseaux. Pression et vitesse, pouls et sphygmographie, par M. E. MEYER. — Pléthysmographie, par M. HALLION. — Capillarité et tension superficielle. Solubilité des solides. Imbibition, par M. A. IMBERT. — Filtration, par M. GARIEL. — Osmose, par M. A. DASTRE. — Propriétés des gaz. Analyse des gaz. Gaz du sang. Phénomènes physiques de la respiration, par M. J. TISSOT. — Principes généraux de la chaleur, par M. WEISS. — Thermométrie, par M. GARIEL. — Température, par M. J.-P. LANGLOIS. — Calorimétrie. Étuves et régulateurs de température, par M. C. SIGALAS. — Chaleur animale, par M. LAULANIÉ. — Travail fourni par les animaux. Rendement des moteurs animés. Propagation de la chaleur. Protection des animaux, par M. GARIEL. — Influence de la pression sur la vie, par MM. P. REGNARD et P. PORTIER. — Influence des

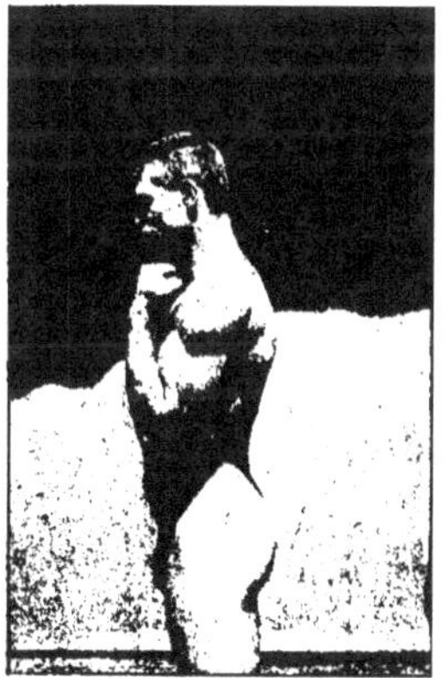

Tome I. Fig. 143. III. — Mouvement rapide. Flexion.

agents atmosphériques sur les éléments cellulaires, par M. A. CHARRIN. — Actions hygrométriques sur les végétaux. Influence de la chaleur sur les végétaux. Actions mécaniques sur les végétaux, par M. MANGIN.

Précis d'Obstétrique

PAR MM.

A. RIBEMONT-DESSAIGNES
Agrégé de la Faculté de médecine.
Accoucheur de l'hôpital Beaujon,
Membre de l'Académie de médecine

G. LEPAGE
Professeur agrégé à la Faculté de médecine
de Paris,
Accoucheur de l'hôpital de la Pitié

CINQUIÈME ÉDITION

AVEC 590 FIGURES DANS LE TEXTE DONT 437 DESSINÉES PAR M. **RIBEMONT-DESSAIGNES**
1 vol. grand in-8" de XXIV-1405 pages, relié toile. . . . . **30 fr.**

Le Précis d'Obstétrique est un bel et bon ouvrage, appelé à rendre de grands services aux praticiens par son plan et son exécution qui sont parfaits. Tenant le milieu entre les Manuels qui tentent les étudiants, mais ne leur apprennent pas grand' chose, et les traités magistraux qu'ils n'ont guère le temps ni les moyens d'aborder, cet ouvrage nous paraît réaliser parfaitement le but des auteurs d'être un livre d'enseignement proprement dit. Et cet enseignement, c'est, dans ses grandes lignes, celui de M. Tarnier et de M. Pinard.

(Revue scientifique.)

Cet ouvrage est appelé à rendre de grands services, non seulement à l'étudiant qui prépare ses examens, mais aussi au praticien, abandonné qu'il est, la plupart du temps, au milieu des multiples difficultés de la clinique et avec une instruction pratique souvent insuffisante....

.... Nous devons aussi parler de la partie iconographique de l'ouvrage; tous les dessins qui sont l'œuvre personnelle de M. Ribemont-Dessaignes joignent à une exactitude photographique un caractère artistique qui donne au livre un aspect particulier.—

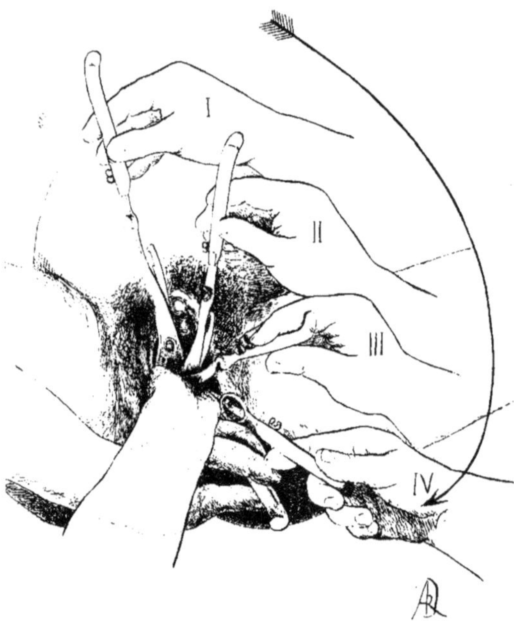

Fig. 440. — Introduction et placement de la cuiller droite sur le sommet en position gauche (variété antérieure).

Ce précis est donc le résumé très complet et très clair de l'art des accouchements; il est pratique pour le clinicien et l'étudiant, en même temps qu'intéressant pour le savant, et les auteurs seront récompensés de leur travail considérable par le succès qu les attend.

(Revue de chirurgie.)

Traité
de Gynécologie

CLINIQUE ET OPÉRATOIRE

Par le Dr Samuel POZZI

Professeur agrégé à la Faculté de médecine, Chirurgien de l'hôpital Broca,
Membre de l'Académie de médecine

TROISIÈME ÉDITION, REVUE ET AUGMENTÉE

1 vol. in-8° de XXII-1270 pages, avec 628 fig. dans le texte. Relié toile. **30 fr.**

..... L'ordonnance générale du traité n'est pas changée, mais de nombreuses additions et des figures multiples sont venues l'enrichir. La thérapeutique chirurgicale des opérations pelviennes, en particulier, a été complètement revisée, et M. Pozzi, tout en restant laparotomiste convaincu, reconnaît à l'hystérectomie vaginale la large place qui lui est due.... Au point de vue thérapeutique, je mentionnerai, comme nouvelles, les pages relatives aux différents procédés d'hystéropexie vaginale recommandés ces derniers temps, celles qu sont consacrées au traitement chirurgical du prolapsus, enfin, et surtout, un petit chapitre relatif à la chirurgie conservatrice des ovaires. — L'anatomie pathologique et la bactériologie tiennent une grande place ; de nombreuses figures originales inédites viennent très heureusement compléter des descriptions qui seraient un peu ardues à la simple lecture.

Partout l'auteur a cherché à être aussi complet que possible, de là une abondance d'indications bibliographiques et de courtes analyses bien fondues ensemble, dont le chercheur tirera grand profit. Mais M. Pozzi a eu soin également de donner toujours son opinion personnelle, permettant ainsi aux jeunes de bénéficier de sa longue expérience. Nous retrouvons ainsi dans cette troisième édition toutes les qualités des deux premières : il est facile d'en prédire le grand succès.

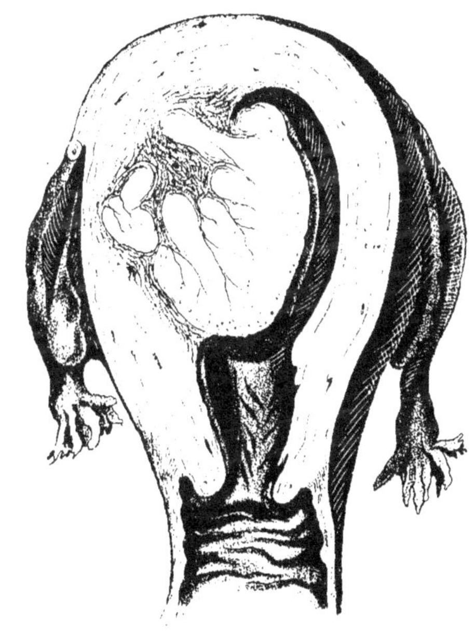

Fig. 251. — Sarcome de la muqueuse utérine.

E. BONNAIRE (*Presse médicale*).

Traité de Chirurgie d'urgence

PAR

FÉLIX LEJARS

Professeur agrégé à la Faculté de médecine
de Paris,
Chirurgien de l'hôpital Tenon
Membre de la Société de chirurgie

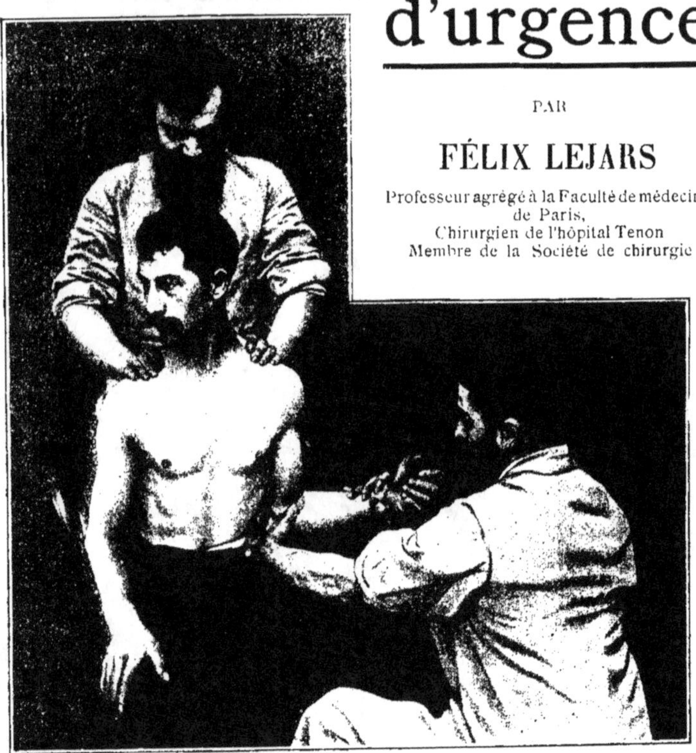

Fig. 131. — Luxation intra-coracoïdienne — Essai de réduction par le procédé de Kocher.
1ʳᵉ manœuvre complémentaire : Le coude est reporté le plus loin possible en arrière.

TROISIÈME ÉDITION, REVUE ET AUGMENTÉE

Plus de **670** figures dont la plupart dessinées d'après nature par le **Dʳ E. DALEINE** et environ **170** photographies originales.

1 volume grand in-8ᵒ, d'environ 950 pages. Relié toile. **25 francs**

Le succès de deux éditions enlevées en quelques mois prouve mieux que tout éloge la valeur et l'utilité du *Traité de Chirurgie d'urgence* du Dʳ F. Lejars.

Fidèle à la méthode qui lui a assuré le succès, le Dʳ Lejars s'est contenté de rendre cette nouvelle édition à la fois plus complète et plus pratique.

Des additions considérables, des remaniements importants ont été faits au texte et des dessins inédits et des photographies originales ont enrichi encore l'illustration déjà hors de pair et universellement appréciée qui fait de cet ouvrage un véritable album.

Ainsi amélioré, le *Traité de Chirurgie d'urgence* se présente pour la troisième fois au public. Il trouvera auprès de lui l'accueil élogieux et empressé qu'il a déjà rencontré et dont les extraits suivants de la presse scientifique ne donnent qu'une incomplète expression.

... Par cette courte analyse, j'aurai voulu engager praticiens et étudiants à lire cet excellent traité. Tous y puiseront avec avantage des notions d'une utilité éminemment pratique et la multiplicité des figures leur facilitera merveilleusement à chaque pas la compréhension du texte....

(Presse médicale.)

... L'auteur a voulu offrir au public un traité essentiellement simple et pratique, permettant à tout médecin, en présence d'un cas de chirurgie d'urgence, de poser une médication thérapeutique et d'être à même de la remplir; c'est à dire l'immense service que cet ouvrage est appelé à rendre partout où le chirurgien de profession fait défaut....

(Revue de Chirurgie.)

... Non e inopportuno aggiungere che alla bontà del libro corrisponde la bellezza dell' edizione, nella quale disegni originali e fotografie sono ritratti con esattezza e finezza non comuni.

(La Clinica Chirurgica.)

Ohne theoretische Auseinandersetzung und ohne viel Gelehrsamkeit führt uns Lejars unmittelbar aus Krankenbett und schildert uns den — vielfach selbsterlebten — Krankheitsfall mitt einer Anschaulichkeit und Klarheit, dass wir glauben, die Gefahr vor unseren Augen zu sehen....

(Klinisch-therapeutische Wochenschrift.)

Der Werth des Buches ruht nicht allein in dem reichem Inhalt, sondern ganz besonders in den vortrefflichen Darstellung, welche vollendet klar, obendrein durch ein Fülle instructivster neuer Zeichnungen ergänzt wird, dann durch den modernen, fortgeschrittenen Standpunkt, welche der Verfasser in allen klinischen und technischen Fragen einnimmt. Die neuesten Erfahrungen und Vorschläge sind berücksichtigt : die Serumtherapie wie die Gelatineinjection, die moderne Hirnchirurgie wie die Fortschritte der Bauchchirurgie und die Naht der Herzwunden; die deutsche Litteratur ist fleissig mit verwerthet.

HELFERICH.

(*Zeitschrift für Chirurgie*.)

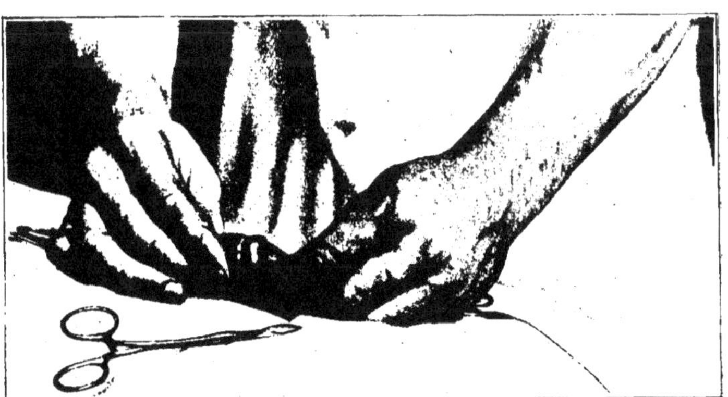

Fig. 250. — Réunion intestinale par le bouton de Murphy (1er temps). Emboîtement à fond les 2 moitiés.

ARTHUS. — *Éléments de Chimie physiologique*, par MAURICE ARTHUS, professeur de physiologie et de chimie physiologique, à l'Université de Fribourg (Suisse). *Troisième édition*, revue et corrigée. 1 vol. in-16 diamant, avec figures dans le texte, cartonné toile. **4 fr.**

BARD. — *Précis d'anatomie pathologique*, par M. L. BARD, professeur à la Faculté de Médecine de Lyon, médecin de l'Hôtel-Dieu. *Deuxième édition, revue et augmentée*. 1 volume in-16 diamant, avec 125 figures, cart. à l'anglaise, tranches rouges. **7 fr. 50**

BAZY. — *Maladies des Voies urinaires, Urètre, Vessie*, par le Dʳ BAZY, chirurgien des hôpitaux, membre de la Société de chirurgie. 2 vol. petit in-8° de l'*Encyclopédie des Aide-Mémoire*.
    I. *Moyens d'exploration et traitement.* 2ᵉ édition.
    II. *Séméiologie.*
    III. *Thérapeutique générale. Médecine opératoire.*
    IV. *Thérapeutique spéciale.*
Chaque volume séparément. **2 fr. 50**

BERLIOZ. — *Manuel de Thérapeutique*, par le Dʳ BERLIOZ, professeur à la Faculté de médecine de Grenoble, avec une préface par M. BOUCHARD, professeur à la Faculté de médecine de Paris. 4ᵉ édition revue et augmentée. 1 vol, in-18 diamant, cartonné toile anglaise, tranches rouges. . . . . **6 fr.**

BLOCQ ET LONDE. — *Anatomie pathologique de la moelle épinière*. 45 *planches en héliogravure*, avec texte explicatif, par PAUL BLOCQ, ancien interne des hôpitaux, chef des travaux anatomo-pathologiques à la Salpêtrière et ALBERT LONDE, directeur du service photographique à la Salpêtrière. Ouvrage précédé d'une préface de M. le professeur CHARCOT. 1 vol. in-4° relié toile. . . . **48 fr.**

BONNIER. — *L'Oreille*, par PIERRE BONNIER. 5 vol. petit in-8° de l'*Encyclopédie des Aide-Mémoire*.
    I. *Anatomie de l'oreille.*
    II. *Pathogénie et mécanisme.*
    III. *Physiologie : Les Fonctions.*
    IV. *Symptomatologie de l'oreille.*
    V. *Pathologie de l'oreille.*
Chaque volume séparément. **2 fr. 50**

BOTTEY. — *Traité théorique et pratique d'hydrothérapie médicale*, par le Dʳ F. BOTTEY, médecin de l'Établissement hydrothérapique de Divonne. 1 volume grand in-8°. **10 fr.**

BOUCHARD (CH.) — *Leçons sur la thérapeutique des maladies infectieuses.* — (*Antisepsie*), professées à la Faculté de médecine de Paris, par M. Ch. BOUCHARD, membre de l'Institut. 1 vol. grand in-8°. **9 fr.**

BRAULT. — *Les Artérites*, par A. BRAULT, médecin de l'hôpital Tenon, chef des travaux pratiques d'anatomie pathologique à la Faculté de médecine. 2 vol. petit in-8° de l'*Encyclopédie des Aide-Mémoire*.
    I. *Les Artérites, leur rôle en pathologie.* 1 vol.
    II. *Les Artérites et les Scléroses.* 1 vol.
Chaque volume séparément. **2 fr. 50**

BRISSAUD. — *Anatomie du cerveau de l'homme.* — *Morphologie des hémisphères cérébraux ou cerveau proprement dit.* Texte et figures par le Dʳ E. BRISSAUD, professeur agrégé à la Faculté de médecine. 1 atlas grand in-4°, de 43 planches gravées sur cuivre, représentant 270 préparations, grandeur naturelle, avec explication en regard de chacune; et 1 volume in-8° de 580 pages, avec plus de 200 figures schématiques dans le texte. 2 vol. reliés toile anglaise. . . . **80 fr.**

— *Leçons sur les maladies nerveuses* (Salpêtrière, 1893-1894), recueillies et publiées par HENRY MEIGE. 1 vol. gr. in-8° avec 240 fig. (schémas et photographies). **18 fr.**

— *Leçons sur les maladies nerveuses* (*Deuxième série* : hôpital Saint-Antoine), recueillies et publiées par HENRY MEIGE. 1 vol. grand in-8° avec 165 figures dans le texte . . . . **15** fr.

BROCA (A.). — *Traitement des tumeurs blanches*. Ostéo-arthrites tuberculeuses des membres chez l'enfant, par A. BROCA, chirurgien de l'hôpital Trousseau, professeur agrégé à la Faculté de médecine. 1 vol. in-8° de l'*Encyclopédie des Aide-Mémoire* . . . . **2** fr. **50**

BROUSSES. — *Manuel technique de massage*, par le Dr J. BROUSSES, médecin-major de 2e classe. 2e édition. 1 vol. in-16, avec nombreuses figures, cartonné toile, tranches rouges . . . . **4** fr.

Centenaire de la Faculté de médecine de Paris (1794-1894), par le Dr A. CORLIEU. 1 vol. in-4°, imprimé par l'Imprimerie Nationale et accompagné d'un album in-4° de 130 portraits des professeurs de la Faculté reproduits d'après des documents authentiques. Les 2 volumes . . . . **100** fr.

CHARRIN. — *Leçons de pathogénie appliquée. Clinique médicale. Hôtel-Dieu* (1895-1896), par A. CHARRIN, professeur agrégé, médecin des hôpitaux, directeur adjoint au laboratoire de Pathologie générale, assistant au Collège de France, Vice-président de la Société de Biologie. 1 vol. in-8° . . . . **6** fr.
— *Poisons de l'organisme*, par le Dr A. CHARRIN. 3 vol. petit in-8° de l'*Encyclopédie des Aide-Mémoire*.
    I. *Poisons de l'urine*. Paris, 1893.
    II. *Poisons du tube digestif*. Paris, 1895.
    III. *Poisons des tissus*. Paris, 1897.
Chaque volume séparément . . . . **2** fr. **50**
— *Les Défenses naturelles de l'organisme* : *Leçons professées au Collège de France*, par A. CHARRIN. 1 vol. in-8° . . . . **6** fr.

CHAUVEL ET NIMIER. — *Traité pratique de Chirurgie d'armée*, par J. CHAUVEL, médecin-principal de 1re classe, professeur à l'École du Val-de-Grâce, et H. NIMIER, médecin-major de 2e classe, professeur agrégé à l'École du Val-de-Grâce. 1 vol. in-8° avec 126 figures dessinées par le Dr J.-E. PESMES, médecin aide-major de 1re classe . . . . **12** fr.

DASTRE. — *Les Anesthésiques. Physiologie et applications chirurgicales*, par M. DASTRE, professeur de physiologie à la Sorbonne. 1 vol. in-8° . . . . . . **5** fr.

DIEULAFOY. — *Manuel de Pathologie interne*, par G. DIEULAFOY, professeur de clinique médicale de la Faculté de médecine de Paris, médecin de l'Hôtel-Dieu, membre de l'Académie de médecine. *Treizième édition entièrement refondue et considérablement augmentée*. 4 vol. in-16 diamant avec figures en noir et en coul., cart. à l'anglaise, tranches rouges **28** fr.
— *Clinique médicale de l'Hôtel-Dieu de Paris*, par le professeur G. DIEULAFOY. 3 vol. gr. in-8°, avec figures dans le texte.
    I. 1896-1897. 1 vol. in-8° . . . . . **10** fr.
    II. 1897-1898. 1 vol. in-8° . . . . . **10** fr.
    III. 1898-1899. 1 vol. in-8° . . . . . **10** fr.

Figure extraite du *Manuel de Pathologie interne*, de M. G. Dieulafoy.

DUCLAUX. — *Pasteur. Histoire d'un esprit*, par E. DUCLAUX, membre de l'Institut, directeur de l'Institut Pasteur, professeur à la Sorbonne et à l'Institut Agronomique. 1 vol. gr. in-8° avec 22 figures dans le texte . . . . **5** fr.
Traité de microbiologie, par E. DUCLAUX.
    Tome I. *Microbiologie générale*. 1 vol. gr. in-8° avec figures . . . . **15** fr.
    Tome II. *Diastases, toxines et venins*. 1 vol. gr. in-8° avec figures . . . **15** fr.
    Tome III. *Fermentation alcoolique*. 1 vol. gr. in-8° avec figures . . . **15** fr.
L'ouvrage formera 7 volumes qui paraîtront successivement.

DUFLOCQ. — *Leçons sur les bactéries pathogènes. faites à l'Hôtel-Dieu annexe*, par P. DUFLOCQ. 1 vol. in-8". . . . . **10** fr.

DUPLAY. — *Cliniques chirurgicales de l'Hôtel-Dieu*, par SIMON DUPLAY, professeur de clinique chirurgicale à la Faculté de médecine de Paris, membre de l'Académie de médecine, chirurgien de l'Hôtel-Dieu. Recueillies et publiées par les Drs M. CAZIN, chef de clinique chirurgicale à l'Hôtel-Dieu, et L. CLADO, chef des travaux gynécologiques à l'Hôtel-Dieu.

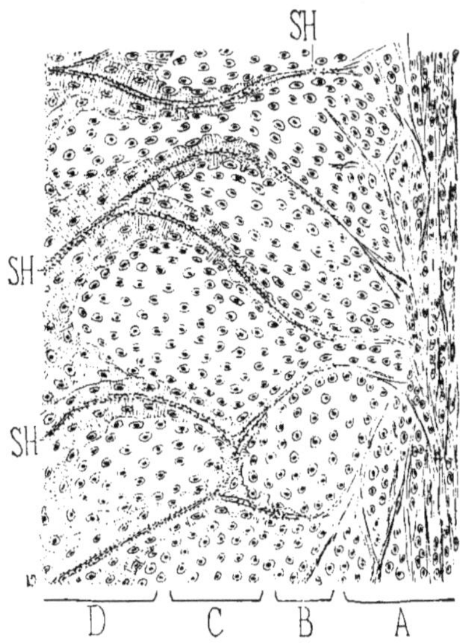

Figure extraite du *Précis d'Histologie*, de M. MATHIAS DUVAL. — Schéma de l'ossification périostique.

1ʳᵉ SÉRIE. 1 vol. in-8" avec figures dans le texte. **7** fr.

2ᵉ SÉRIE. 1 vol. in-8" avec figures dans le texte. **8** fr.

3ᵉ SÉRIE. 1 vol. in-8° avec figures dans le texte. **8** fr.

DUVAL. — *Atlas d'embryologie*, par M. MATHIAS DUVAL, professeur d'histologie à la Faculté de médecine de Paris, membre de l'Académie de médecine. 1 vol. in-4", avec 40 planches en noir et en couleurs, comprenant ensemble 652 figures. Cartonné toile . . . . . **48** fr.

— *Précis d'histologie*, par M. MATHIAS DUVAL, professeur à la Faculté de médecine de Paris, membre de l'Académie de médecine. *Deuxième édition, revue et augmentée.* 1 vol. gr. in-8° avec 427 figures dans le texte. **18** fr.

FAISANS. — *Maladies des organes respiratoires. Méthodes d'exploration, signes physiques*, par LÉON FAISANS, médecin de la Pitié. *Deuxième édition.* 1 vol. petit in-8", de l'*Encyclopédie des Aide-Mémoire*. . . . . **2** fr. **50**

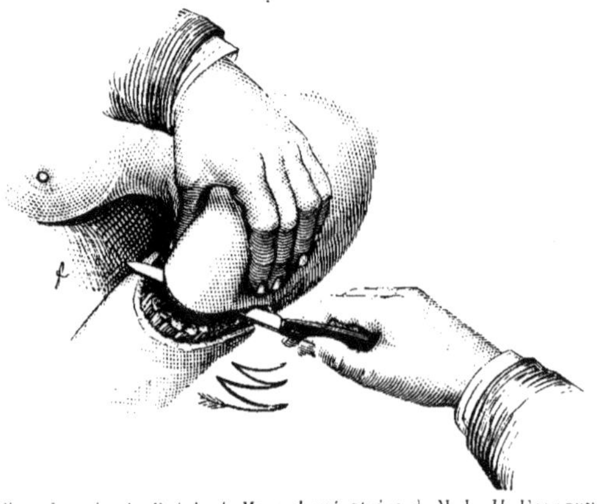

Figure extraite du *Précis de Manuel opératoire*, de M. L.-H. FARABEUF.

FARABEUF. — *Précis de manuel opératoire. Ligatures, Amputations, Résections, Appendice*, par M. L.-H. FARABEUF, professeur à la Faculté de médecine de Paris, membre de l'Académie de médecine. *Quatrième édition entièrement revue.* 1 vol. petit in-8", avec 799 figures. **16** fr.

FÉLIZET. — *Les Hernies inguinales de l'Enfance*, par le Dr G. FÉLIZET, chirurgien de l'hôpital Tenon (Enfants-Malades). 1 vol. grand in-8", avec 73 figures dans le texte. . . . . . **10** fr.

GAUTIER (A.). — *Cours de Chimie minérale et organique*, par M. ARM. GAUTIER, membre de l'Institut, professeur de chimie à la Faculté de médecine de

Paris. *Deuxième édition*, revue et mise au courant des travaux les plus récents.
2 vol. grand in-8°, avec figures dans le texte.
    I. *Chimie minérale*. 1 vol. grand in-8°, avec 244 figures dans le texte. **16 fr.**
    II. *Chimie organique*. 1 vol. grand in-8°, avec 72 figures. . . . . **16 fr.**
— **Leçons de Chimie biologique normale et pathologique.** *Deuxième édition*, publiée avec la collaboration de M. ARTHUS, professeur de physiologie à l'Université de Fribourg. 1 vol. in-8°, avec 110 figures. . . . . **18 fr.**
— **La Chimie de la cellule vivante**, par M. ARM. GAUTIER. *Deuxième édition*. 1 vol. petit in-8° de l'*Encyclopédie des Aide-Mémoire*. . . . . **2 fr. 50**

GILIS. — **Précis d'Embryologie** adapté aux sciences médicales, par PAUL GILIS, professeur agrégé à la Faculté de médecine de Montpellier, avec préface par M. le professeur DUVAL. 1 vol. in-18 diamant, avec 175 figures. Cartonné toile, tranches rouges. . . . . **6 fr.**

GLEY. — **Essais de philosophie et d'histoire de la Biologie**, par E. GLEY, professeur agrégé à la Faculté de médecine de Paris, assistant près la chaire de Physiologie générale au Muséum d'Histoire naturelle. 1 vol. in-16. . . **3 fr. 50**

GOUGUENHEIM et GLOVER. — **Atlas de laryngologie et de rhinologie**, par A. GOUGUENHEIM, médecin de l'hôpital Lariboisière, et J. GLOVER, ancien interne de la clinique laryngologique de l'hôpital Lariboisière. 1 vol. in-4°, avec 37 planches en noir et en couleurs, comprenant ensemble 246 figures, et 47 figures dans le texte. Légendes en langue anglaise et en langue française, relié toile. . . . . **50 fr.**

GRASSET. — **Consultations médicales sur quelques maladies fréquentes.** par le Dr GRASSET, professeur de clinique médicale à l'Université de Montpellier, correspondant de l'Académie de médecine. *Quatrième édition, revue et considérablement augmentée*. 1 vol. in-16, reliure souple, peau pleine. **4 fr. 50**
— **Leçons de Clinique médicale**, faites à l'hôpital Saint-Éloi de Montpellier par le Dr J. GRASSET, professeur de clinique médicale à l'Université de Montpellier, correspondant de l'Académie de médecine, lauréat de l'Institut.
    1re SÉRIE (1886-1890). 1 vol. in-8°, avec 10 planches. . . . . **12 fr.**
    2e SÉRIE (novembre 1890-juillet 1895). 1 fort vol. in-8°, avec une figure dans le texte et 10 planches lithographiées. . . . . **12 fr.**
    3e SÉRIE (novembre 1895-mars 1898). 1 vol. in-8° de VII-826 pages, avec 20 planches hors texte, dont 10 en couleurs et 6 en phototypie.. . . **15 fr.**
— **Traité pratique des maladies du système nerveux**, par le professeur GRASSET, en collaboration avec le Dr RAUZIER. *Quatrième édition*. 2 vol. grand in-8°, avec 33 planches hors texte et 122 figures dans le texte (*Ouvrage couronné par l'Institut : Prix Lallemand*). . . . . **45 fr.**

HAYEM. — **Du Sang et de ses altérations anatomiques**, par G. HAYEM, professeur à la Faculté de médecine de Paris, médecin des hôpitaux, membre de l'Académie de médecine. 1 vol. in-8°, avec nombreuses figures noires et en couleurs dans le texte, relié toile à biseaux. . . . . **32 fr.**
— **Leçons sur les maladies du sang** (*Clinique de l'hôpital Saint-Antoine*). par Georges HAYEM, recueillies par MM. E. PARMENTIER, médecin des hôpitaux, et R. BENSAUDE, chef du laboratoire d'anatomie pathologique à l'hôpital Saint-Antoine. 1 vol. in-8°, avec 4 planches en couleurs. . . . . **15 fr.**

HÉNOCQUE. — **Spectroscopie biologique**, par le Dr ALBERT HÉNOCQUE, directeur adjoint du laboratoire de physique biologique du Collège de France. 3 vol. petit in-8° de l'*Encyclopédie des Aide-Mémoire*.
    I. *Spectroscopie du sang*. Avec figures dans le texte.
    II. *Spectroscopie des organes, des tissus et des humeurs*. Avec figures dans le texte.
    III. *Spectroscopie de l'urine et des pigments*.
    Chaque volume est vendu séparément . . . . **2 fr 50**

KIRMISSON. — **Leçons cliniques sur les maladies de l'appareil locomoteur** (os, *articulations, muscles*), par le Dr KIRMISSON, professeur agrégé à la Faculté de médecine, chirurgien des hôpitaux, membre de la Société de chirurgie. 1 vol. in-8°, avec figures dans le texte . . . . **10 fr.**

Traité des maladies chirurgicales d'origine congénitale, par le Dr E. Kirmisson. 1 vol. in-8°, avec 311 figures dans le texte et 2 planches en couleurs. . . . . **15 fr.**

LACASSAGNE. — *Précis de médecine judiciaire*, par M. A. Lacassagne, professeur à la Faculté de médecine de Lyon. 2ᵉ édition. 1 volume in-18 diamant, avec 47 figures dans le texte et 4 planches en couleur, cartonné à l'anglaise, tranches rouges . . . . **7 fr. 50**

— *Précis d'hygiène privée et sociale*, par M. A. Lacassagne. 4ᵉ édition revue et augmentée. 1 vol. in-16 diamant, cartonné à l'anglaise, tranches rouges. . . . . **7 fr.**

LALESQUE. — *Cure marine de la phtisie pulmonaire*, par le Dr F. Lalesque, ancien interne des hôpitaux de Paris. 1 vol. in-8° avec planches, dessins, tableaux et graphiques. . . . . **6 fr.**

LAMY. — *La syphilis des centres nerveux*, par le Dr Henri Lamy, ancien interne des hôpitaux de Paris. 1 vol. petit in-8° de l'*Encyclopédie des Aide-Mémoire*. . . . . **2 fr. 50**

LANGLOIS. — *Le Lait* par P. Langlois, chef du Laboratoire de physiologie à la Faculté de médecine. 1 vol. p. in-8° de l'*Encyclopédie des Aide-Mémoire*. **2 fr. 50**

LANNELONGUE. — *La Tuberculose chirurgicale*, par O. Lannelongue, professeur à la Faculté de médecine de Paris. 1 vol. petit in-8° de l'*Encyclopédie des Aide-Mémoire* . . . . **2 fr. 50**

LAULANIÉ. — *Énergétique musculaire*, par F. Laulanié, professeur de physiologie à l'École vétérinaire de Toulouse; avec une préface de M. Chauveau, de l'Institut. 1 vol. petit in-8° de l'*Encyclopédie des Aide-Mémoire*. . . . **2 fr. 50**

LAUNOIS. — *Manuel d'Anatomie microscopique et d'Histologie*, par MM. P.-E. Launois, professeur agrégé à la Faculté de Paris, médecin des hôpitaux. Préface de M. Mathias Duval, professeur d'histologie à la Faculté, membre de l'Académie de médecine. *Deuxième édition entièrement refondue*. 1 vol. in-16 diamant, cartonné toile. . . . . **8 fr.**

LAVERAN. — *Du Paludisme* et de son hématozoaire, par A. Laveran, membre de l'Académie de médecine, membre correspondant de l'Institut de France. 1 vol. grand in-8°, avec 4 planches en couleur et 2 planches photographiques . **10 fr.**

— *Traité du Paludisme*, par A. Laveran. 1 vol. grand in-8° avec 27 figures dans le texte et une planche en couleurs . . . . **10 fr.**

· *Traité d'hygiène militaire* par le Dr Laveran. 1 vol. in-8°, avec 270 figures. . . . . **16 fr.**

LEJARS. — *Leçons de chirurgie* (La Pitié 1893-1894), par le Dr Félix Lejars, professeur agrégé à la Faculté de médecine de Paris, chirurgien des hôpitaux. 1 vol. grand in-8°, avec 128 figures. . . . . **16 fr.**

LELOIR ET VIDAL. — *Symptomatologie et anatomie pathologique des maladies de la peau*, par MM. Leloir, professeur à la Faculté de médecine de Lille, et E. Vidal, médecin de l'hôpital St-Louis. Un atlas de 54 planches grand in-8°, tirées en couleur, et accompagnées d'un texte explicatif, relié toile. **70 fr.**

LETULLE. — *L'Inflammation* (Études anatomo-pathologiques), par le Dr Maurice Letulle, professeur agrégé à la Faculté de médecine de Paris. 1 vol. avec 21 figures et 12 planches en chromolithographie hors texte, relié toile. . **20 fr.**

Manuel de pathologie externe, par MM. Reclus, Kirmisson, Peyrot, Bouilly, professeurs agrégés à la Faculté de médecine de Paris, chirurgiens des hôpitaux. Nouvelle édition, illustrée de 720 figures. 4 vol. in-8° avec figures dans le texte. . . . . **40 fr.**

I. *Maladies des tissus et des organes*, par le Dr P. RECLUS, avec figures dans le texte.

II. *Maladies des régions : Tête et Rachis*, par le Dr KIRMISSON, entièrement refondue et augmentée, avec figures dans le texte.

III. *Maladies des régions : Poitrine et abdomen*, par le Dr PEYROT, entièrement refondue et augmentée, avec figures dans le texte.

IV. *Maladies des régions : Organes génito-urinaires*, membres, par le Dr BOUILLY, avec figures dans le texte.

Chaque volume est vendu séparément. . . . . **10 fr.**

MARIE. — *Leçons sur les maladies de la moelle*, par le Dr PierreMARIE, professeur agrégé de la Faculté de médecine de Paris, médecin des hôpitaux. 1 vol. in-8", avec 244 figures dans le texte. . . . . **15 fr.**

— *Leçons de clinique médicale* (Hôtel-Dieu 1894-1895), par le Dr PIERRE MARIE. 1 vol. in-8", avec 57 figures dans le texte. . . . . **6 fr.**

MAURIAC. — *Traitement de la syphilis*, par M. CHARLES MAURIAC, médecin de l'hôpital Ricord (Hôpital du Midi). 1 vol. in-8" . . . . **15 fr.**

MÉGNIN. — *La Faune des cadavres*, *application de l'entomologie à la médecine légale*, par M. P. MÉGNIN, membre de l'Académie de médecine. 1 vol. petit in-8" de l'*Encyclopédie des Aide-Mémoire*. . . . . **2 fr. 50**

MERKLEN. — *Examen et séméiotique du cœur*, *signes physiques*, par le Dr PIERRE MERKLEN, médecin de l'hôpital Laënnec. *Deuxième édition*. 1 vol. petit in-8" de l'*Encyclopédie des Aide-Mémoire*. . . . . **2 fr. 50**

METCHNIKOFF. — *Leçons sur la pathologie comparée de l'inflammation*, faites à l'Institut Pasteur en avril et mai 1891, par ÉLIE METCHNIKOFF, chef de service à l'Institut Pasteur. 1 vol. in-8" avec 65 fig. et 3 pl. en coul. . . . **9 fr.**

MONOD ET TERRILLON. — *Traité des maladies du testicule et de ses annexes*, par MM. Ch. MONOD et O. TERRILLON, professeurs agrégés à la Faculté de médecine de Paris, chirurgiens des hôpitaux. 1 vol. in-8° avec 92 figures dans le texte. . . . . **16 fr.**

MONOD ET VANVERTS. — *L'Appendicite*, par le Dr Ch. MONOD, professeur agrégé à la Faculté de médecine de Paris, chirurgien de l'hôpital Saint-Antoine, membre de l'Académie de médecine, et J. VANVERTS, interne des hôpitaux de Paris. 1 vol. petit in-8" de l'*Encyclopédie des Aide-Mémoire*. . . . . . **2 fr. 50**

OLLIER. — *Traité expérimental et clinique de la régénération des os* et de la production artificielle du tissu osseux, par le Dr OLLIER, chirurgien en chef de l'Hôtel-Dieu de Lyon. Ouvrage qui a obtenu le grand prix de chirurgie. 2 vol. in-8°, avec figures dans le texte et planches en taille-douce. . . . . . . **30 fr.**

— ***Traité des Résections*** et des opérations conservatrices que l'on peut pratiquer sur le système osseux, par le Dr L. OLLIER, professeur de clinique chirurgicale à la Faculté de médecine de Lyon. 3 volumes grand in-8" avec figures. . . . . **50 fr.**

Tome I. *Introduction. — Résections en général*. 1 vol. in-8" avec 127 figures dans le texte . . . . **16 fr.**

Tome II. *Résections en particulier. Membre supérieur*. 1 vol. in-8" avec 156 figures . . . . **16 fr.**

Tome III. *Résections en particulier. Résections du membre inférieur, tête et tronc*. 1 vol. in-8" avec 224 figures. . . . . **22 fr.**

— ***La Régénération des os et les résections sous-périostées***, par le Dr L. OLLIER. 1 vol. petit in-8" de l'*Encyclopédie des Aide-Mémoire*. . **2 fr. 50**

PANAS. — *Traité des maladies des yeux*, par Ph. PANAS, professeur de clinique ophtalmologique à la Faculté de médecine, chirurgien de l'Hôtel-Dieu, membre de l'Académie de médecine, membre honoraire et ancien président de la Société de chirurgie. 2 vol. grand in-8" avec 453 figures et 7 planches en couleurs. Reliés toile. . . . . **40 fr.**

PANAS. — *Leçons de clinique ophtalmologique. professées à l'Hôtel-Dieu*, par Ph. Panas, recueillies et publiées par le Dʳ A. Castan (de Béziers). 1 vol. in-8°, avec figures dans le texte. . . . . **5 fr.**

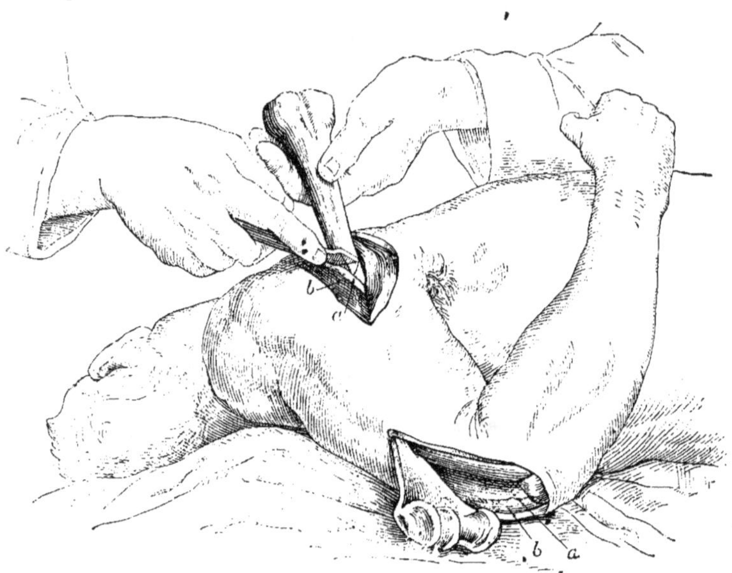

Figure extraite du *Traité des Résections* de M. L. Ollier.

PANAS ET ROCHON-DUVIGNEAUD. — *Recherches anatomiques et cliniques sur le glaucome et les néoplasmes intra-oculaires.* par le professeur Panas et le Dʳ Rochon-Duvigneaud, ancien chef de clinique de la Faculté. 1 vol. in-8°, avec 41 figures dans le texte. . . . . **7 fr.**

POLIN ET LABIT. — *Examen des aliments suspects*, par MM. H. Polin et H. Labit, médecins-majors de l'armée. 1 vol. petit in-8° de l'*Encyclopédie des Aide-Mémoire*. . . . . **2 fr. 50**

PONCET ET BÉRARD. — *Traité clinique de l'actinomycose humaine. Pseudo-actinomycoses et botryomycose.* par Antonin Poncet, professeur de clinique chirurgicale à l'Université de Lyon, ex-chirurgien en chef de l'Hôtel-Dieu, membre correspondant de l'Académie de médecine et Léon Bérard, ex-prosecteur, chef de clinique chirurgicale à l'Université de Lyon, lauréat de l'Académie de médecine. *Ouvrage couronné par l'Académie de médecine et par l'Institut.* 1 vol in-8°, avec 45 fig. dans le texte et 4 planches hors texte en coul. . . **12 fr.**

PONCET ET DELORE. — *Traité de la cystostomie sus-pubienne chez les prostatiques. Création d'un urèthre hypogastrique. Application de cette nouvelle méthode aux diverses affections des voies urinaires.* par Antonin Poncet et Xavier Delore, ex-prosecteur, ancien chef de clinique chirurgicale à l'Université de Lyon. 1 vol. in-8° avec 42 figures dans le texte. . . . . **8 fr.**

— *Traité de l'uréthrostomie périnéale dans les rétrécissements incurables de l'urèthre : création au périnée d'un méat contre nature.* par Antonin Poncet et Xavier Delore. 1 vol. in-8° avec 11 figures dans le texte . . . . **4 fr.**

PROUST. — *La Défense de l'Europe contre le choléra*, par M. le professeur Proust. inspecteur général des services sanitaires. 1 vol. in-8° . . . . . **9 fr.**

— *Douze conférences d'hygiène rédigées conformément aux programmes du*

12 *août* 1890, par A. Proust, professeur à la Faculté de médecine. Nouvelle
édition. 1 vol. in-18. Cartonné toile. . . . . **2 fr. 50**

— **L'Orientation nouvelle de la politique sanitaire,** par A. Proust. 1 vol. in-8°,
avec nombreuses figures et plans dans le texte et une carte en couleurs. **10 fr.**

— **La Défense de l'Europe contre la Peste et la Conférence de Venise
de 1897,** par le professeur Proust. 1 volume in-8° avec figures et 1 carte
en couleurs . . . . **9 fr.**

PRUNIER. — **Les Médicaments chimiques,** par Léon Prunier, membre de
l'Académie de médecine, pharmacien en chef des hôpitaux de Paris, professeur à
l'École supérieure de pharmacie.

I. *Composés minéraux.* 1 vol. grand in-8° avec 137 figures dans le texte. **15 fr.**

II. *Composés organiques.* 1 volume grand in-8° avec 47 figures, dans le
texte. . . . . **15 fr.**

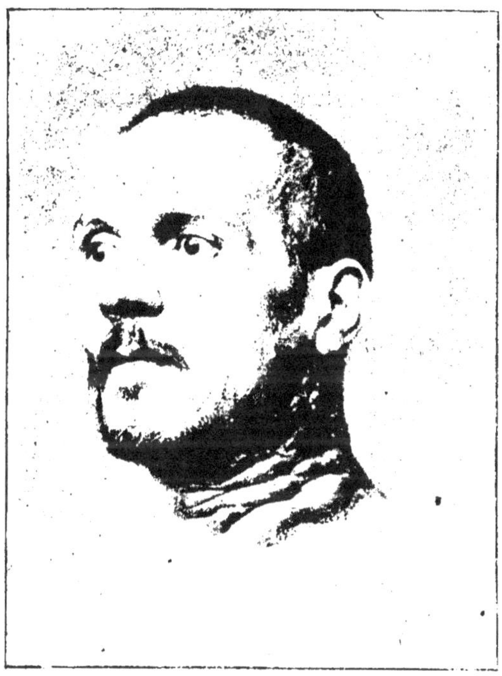

Figure extraite du *Traité clinique de l'actinomycose humaine.*
de MM. A. Poncet et L. Bérard.

RANVIER. — **École pratique des Hautes Études. Laboratoire d'histologie du
Collège de France**. Travaux publiés sous la direction de L. Ranvier, professeur
d'anatomie générale, Membre de l'Institut, avec la collaboration de M. L. Malassez,
directeur adjoint, et des répétiteurs et préparateurs du cours.

Tomes I à XVII (1784-1899). Chaque vol. in-8° avec pl. hors-texte. . . **20 fr.**
Les tomes V et VIII ne se vendent plus séparément.

— **Traité technique d'histologie.** 2° édition entièrement refondue et corrigée,
par M. L. Ranvier. 1 vol. gr. in-8° de 880 pages, avec 414 gravures dans le texte
et 1 planche en chromo. . . . . **12 fr.**

REDARD. — **Traité pratique des déviations de la colonne vertébrale,** par
P. Redard, ancien chef de clinique chirurgicale de la Faculté de médecine de

Paris, chirurgien en chef du dispensaire Furtado-Heine, membre correspondant de l'American Ortopédie Association. 1 vol. grand in-8°, avec 231 figures dans le texte . . . . **12 fr.**

REDARD et **LARAN**. — *Atlas de Radiographie : Chirurgie infantile et orthopédique*, par P. REDARD et F. LARAN. 1 vol. in-4°, contenant 48 planches en photo-collographie, avec leur explication, relié toile. . . . . **25 fr.**

REGNARD. — *La Cure d'altitude*, par le Dʳ PAUL REGNARD, membre de l'Académie de médecine, professeur de physiologie générale à l'Institut national agronomique, directeur-adjoint du laboratoire de physiologie de la Sorbonne. *Deuxième édition*. 1 fort vol. grand in-8°, avec 29 planches hors texte et 110 figures dans le texte, relié toile pleine. . . . . **15 fr.**

RÉNON. — *Étude sur l'Aspergillose chez les animaux et chez l'homme*, par M. RÉNON, ancien interne des hôpitaux de Paris. 1 vol. in-8°, avec figures dans le texte. . . . . **5 fr.**

SOLLIER. — *Guide pratique des maladies mentales* (Séméiologie. — Pronostic. — Indications), par le Dʳ PAUL SOLLIER, chef de clinique adjoint des maladies mentales à la Faculté. 1 vol. in-18 diamant, cartonné toile, tranches rouges. **5 fr.**

SOULIER (H.). — *Traité de thérapeutique et de pharmacologie*, par M. H. SOULIER, professeur à la Faculté de médecine de Lyon, membre correspondant de l'Académie de médecine. *Additionné d'un memento formulaire des médicaments nouveaux* (1901). *Ouvrage couronné par l'Académie des sciences et par l'Académie de médecine*. 2 vol. grand in-8°. . . . . **25 fr.**

TRABUT. — *Précis de Botanique médicale*, par L. TRABUT, professeur d'histoire naturelle médicale à l'École de médecine d'Alger. *Deuxième édition, entièrement refondue*. 1 vol. in-8°, avec 954 figures. . . . . **8 fr.**

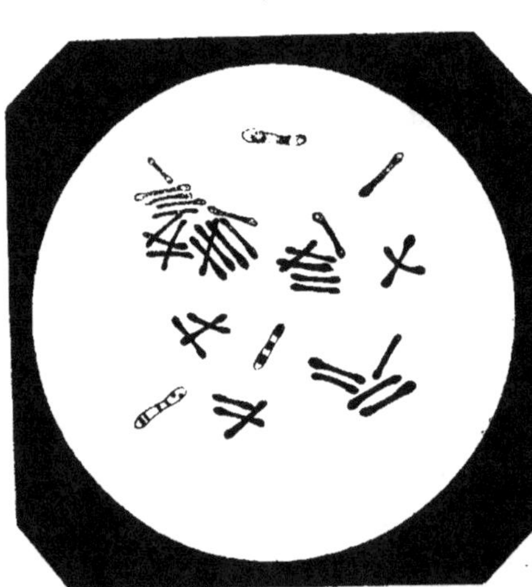

Figure extraite de la *Bactériologie Clinique*, de M. R. WURTZ.
Bacille de la Diphtérie.

TUFFIER. — *Chirurgie du poumon*, par le Dʳ TUFFIER, professeur agrégé à la Faculté de médecine de Paris, chirurgien de l'hôpital de la Pitié. 1 vol. in-8°. . . . . **6 fr.**

WURTZ (R.). — *Technique bactériologique*, par R. WURTZ, professeur agrégé à la Faculté de médecine de Paris, médecin des hôpitaux. *Deuxième édition*. 1 vol. petit in-8° de l'*Encyclopédie des Aide-Mémoire*. . . **2 fr. 50**

— *Précis de bactériologie clinique*, par le Dʳ R. WURTZ. *Deuxième édition*, avec tableaux synoptiques et figures dans le texte. 1 vol. in-16 diamant, cartonné à l'anglaise, tranches rouges. . . . **6 fr.**

ZAMBACO. — *Voyages chez les lépreux*, par le Dʳ ZAMBACO-PACHA, membre correspondant de l'Académie de médecine de Paris, ex-chef de clinique à la Faculté de médecine. 1 vol. in-8°, avec une carte indiquant les localités lépreuses. . . . . **8 fr.**

Les Lépreux ambulants de Constantinople, par le Dʳ ZAMBACO-PACHA, membre associé national de l'Académie de médecine de Paris, membre correspondant de l'Académie de Saint-Pétersbourg, etc. 1 fort vol. in-4°, avec 48 planches hors texte en noir et en couleurs, relié toile . . . . **90 fr.**

L'ŒUVRE MÉDICO-CHIRURGICAL

D' CRITZMAN, directeur

SUITE DE MONOGRAPHIES CLINIQUES

SUR LES QUESTIONS NOUVELLES

En Médecine, en Chirurgie et en Biologie

La science médicale réalise journellement des progrès incessants. Les traités de médecine et de chirurgie auront toujours grand'peine à se tenir au courant. C'est pour obvier à ce grave inconvénient que nous avons fondé ce recueil de Monographies, avec le concours des savants et des praticiens les plus autorisés.

Chaque monographie est vendue séparément. . . . . **1** fr. **25**

Il est accepté des abonnements pour une série de 10 Monographies consécutives au prix à forfait et payable d'avance de **10** francs pour la France et **12** francs pour l'étranger (port compris).

MONOGRAPHIES PUBLIÉES (Octobre 1900).

N° 1. **L'Appendicite,** par le D' FÉLIX LEGUEU, chir. des hôp. de Paris (épuisé).

N° 2. **Le Traitement du mal de Pott,** par le D' A. CHIPAULT, de Paris.

N° 3. **Le Lavage du sang,** par le D' LEJARS, prof. agr., chir. des hôp., membre de la Société de chirurgie.

N° 4. **L'Hérédité normale et pathologique,** par le D' CH. DEBIERRE, prof. d'anatomie à l'Université de Lille.

N° 5. **L'Alcoolisme,** par le D' JAQUET, privat-docent à l'Université de Bâle.

N° 6. **Physiologie et pathologie des sécrétions gastriques,** par le D' A. VERHAEGEN, assistant à la Clinique médicale de Louvain.

N° 7. **L'Eczéma,** *maladie parasitaire,* par le D' LEREDDE, chef de laboratoire, assistant de consultation à l'hôpital Saint-Louis.

N° 8. **La Fièvre jaune,** par le D' SANARELLI, Directeur de l'Institut d'Hygiène expérimentale de Montévidéo.

N° 9. **La Tuberculose du rein,** par le D' TUFFIER, prof. agr., chir. de l'hôp. de la Pitié.

N° 10. **L'Opothérapie.** *Traitement de certaines maladies par des extraits d'organes animaux,* par A. GILBERT, prof. agr., chef du laboratoire de thérapeutique à la Faculté de médecine de Paris, et L. CARNOT, docteur ès sciences, ancien interne des hôpitaux de Paris.

N° 11. **Les Paralysies générales progressives,** par le D' M. KLIPPEL, méd. des hôp. de Paris.

N° 12. **Le Myxœdème,** par le D' THIBIERGE, méd. de l'hôp. de la Pitié.

N° 13. **La Néphrite des saturnins,** par le D' H. LAVRAND, prof. chargé de cours à la Faculté catholique de Lille, lauréat de l'Académie de Paris.

N° 14. **Traitement de la syphilis,** par E. GAUCHER, prof. agr. à la Faculté de méd. de Paris, médecin de l'hôpital Saint-Antoine.

N° 15. **Le Pronostic des tumeurs,** *basé sur la recherche du glycogène,* par le D' A. BRAULT, méd. de l'hôp. Tenon, chef des travaux pratiques d'anatomie pathologique à la Faculté.

N° 16. **La Kinésithérapie gynécologique.** *Traitement des maladies des femmes par le massage et la gymnastique (système de Brandt),* par H. STAPFER, ancien chef de clinique obstétricale et gynécologique de la Faculté de Paris.

N° 17. **De la Gastro-entérite aiguë des nourrissons** (*Pathogénie et étiologie*), par A. LESAGE, méd. des hôp. de Paris.

N° 18. **Traitement de l'Appendicite,** par FÉLIX LEGUEU, prof. agr., chir. des hôp.

N° 19. **Les lois de l'énergétique dans le régime du diabète sucré,** par le D' E. DUFOURT, ancien chef de clinique médicale à la Faculté de Lyon, méd. de l'hôp. thermal de Vichy.

N° 20. **La Peste** (*Épidémiologie, Bactériologie, Prophylaxie, Traitement*), par le D' H. BOURGES, chef du laboratoire d'hygiène à la Faculté de médecine de Paris, Auditeur au Comité consultatif d'hygiène publique de France.

N° 21. **La Moelle osseuse à l'état normal et dans les infections,** par MM. G.-H. ROGER, prof. agr. à la Faculté de méd. de Paris, méd. des hôp., et O. JOSUÉ, ancien interne, lauréat des hôp. de Paris.

N° 22. **L'Entéro-colite muco-membraneuse,** par le D' GASTON LYON, ancien chef de clinique médicale de la Faculté de Paris.

N° 23. **L'Exploration clinique des fonctions rénales par l'élimination provoquée,** par le D' CH. ACHARD, prof. agr. à la Faculté de méd., méd. de l'hôp. Tenon et J. CASTAIGNE, interne lauréat (médaille d'or) des hôp.

N° 24. **L'Analgésie chirurgicale,** par voie rachidienne (injections sous-arachnoïdiennes de cocaïne), par le D' TUFFIER, prof. agr. à la Faculté de médecine de Paris, chir. des hôp.

BIBLIOTHÈQUE
d'Hygiène thérapeutique

DIRIGÉE PAR

Le Professeur PROUST

Membre de l'Académie de médecine, Médecin de l'Hôtel-Dieu.
Inspecteur général des Services sanitaires.

Chaque ouvrage forme un volume in-16, cartonné toile, tranches rouges,
et est vendu séparément : **4 fr.**

Chacun des volumes de cette collection n'est consacré qu'à une seule maladie ou à un
seul groupe de maladie. Grâce à leur format, ils sont d'un maniement commode. D'un
autre côté, en accordant un volume spécial à chacun des grands sujets d'hygiène thérapeutique, il a été facile de leur donner tout le développement nécessaire.

VOLUMES PARUS :

L'Hygiène du Goutteux, par le Professeur PROUST et A. MATHIEU, médecin
de l'hôpital Andral.

L'Hygiène de l'Obèse. par le Professeur PROUST et A. MATHIEU.

L'Hygiène des Asthmatiques. par E. BRISSAUD, professeur à la Faculté de
Paris, médecin de l'hôpital Saint-Antoine.

L'Hygiène du Syphilitique. par H. BOURGES, préparateur au laboratoire
d'hygiène de la Faculté de médecine.

Hygiène et thérapeutique thermales. par G. DELFAU, ancien interne des
hôpitaux de Paris.

Les Cures thermales. par G. DELFAU. ancien interne des hôpitaux de Paris.

L'Hygiène du Neurasthénique (*Deuxième édition*), par le Professeur PROUST
et G. BALLET, professeur agrégé, médecin des hôpitaux de Paris.

L'Hygiène des Albuminuriques, par le Dʳ SPRINGER, chef du laboratoire
de la Faculté de médecine à l'hôpital de la Charité.

L'Hygiène des Tuberculeux, par le Dʳ CHUQUET, ancien interne des hôpitaux de Paris, médecin consultant à Cannes, avec une préface du Dʳ DAREM-
BERG, correspondant de l'Académie de médecine.

Hygiène et thérapeutique des maladies de la bouche, par le Dʳ CRUET,
dentiste des hôpitaux de Paris, avec une préface du Professeur LANNELONGUE,
membre de l'Institut.

L'Hygiène des Diabétiques. par le Professeur PROUST et A. MATHIEU, médecin de l'hôpital Andral.

L'Hygiène des maladies du cœur, par le Dʳ VAQUEZ, professeur agrégé à
la Faculté de médecine de Paris, médecin des hôpitaux, avec une préface du
Professeur POTAIN, membre de l'Institut.

L'Hygiène du Dyspeptique. par le Dʳ LINOSSIER, professeur agrégé à la Faculté de médecine de Lyon. membre correspondant de l'Académie de médecine,
médecin à Vichy.

VOLUME EN PRÉPARATION :

L'Hygiène des maladies de la peau. par le Dʳ G. THIBIERGE, médecin des
hôpitaux de Paris.